Grieve's Modern Manual Therapy

In memory of Barbara Grieve 1916–1991

The Editors have kindly suggested that this edition be dedicated to Barbara Grieve, whose secretarial expertise and administrative skills contributed so much to the successful production of the first edition.

In total and loving commitment she energetically devoted herself to achieving the very best presentation of the final manuscript — everything passing through her hands being thoroughly organized and impeccably turned out on her faithful portable typewriter.

Having taken a lively interest in my training as a physiotherapist, she had the wit to perceive the great potential of neuro–musculo–skeletal medicine. Her enthusiastic efforts to further the welfare of the Manipulation Association of Chartered Physiotherapists also embraced the aims of the International Federation of Orthopaedic Manipulative Therapists. Like the CSP Manipulation courses in the early days to 1975, the MACP and the IFOMT have handsomely acknowledged how much they owe to her.

While she deprecated her talents as a 'self-taught amateur', her considerable achievements truly were a labour of love, as well as of genuine interest in the work. She was the other half of the team, and she warmed whoever was associated with her. She has left a little of herself in so many hearts, worldwide.

For Churchill Livingstone

Commissioning Editor: Mary C. Law
Project Editor: Dinah Thom
Project Manager: Neil A. Dickson
Project Controller: Nicola S. Haig
Indexer: Nina Boyd
Design: Design Resources Unit
Sales Promotion Executive: Maria O'Connor

Grieve's Modern Manual Therapy
The Vertebral Column

Edited by

Jeffrey D. Boyling MSc(Lond) BPhty(Hons)(Qld)
GradDipAdvManipTher(SAIT) MAPA MCSP MErgS MMPAA
Chartered Physiotherapist and Ergonomist, Hammersmith, London; Formerly Senior Teacher,
St Thomas' Hospital School of Physiotherapy, London, UK

Nigel Palastanga MA BA MCSP DMS DipTP
Principal, Cardiff School of Physiotherapy, University Hospital of Wales, Cardiff, UK

Australian Editorial Advisor
Gwendolen A. Jull MPhty GradDipManipTher FACP
Senior Lecturer, Department of Physiotherapy, University of Queensland; Specialist Manipulative Physiotherapist,
Private Practice, Chapel Hill, Queensland, Australia

Canadian Editorial Advisor
Diane G. Lee BSR COMP
Instructor and Examiner, Orthopaedic Division, Canadian Physiotherapy Association; Instructor and Examiner,
North American Institute of Orthopaedic Manual Therapy, British Columbia, Canada

Foreword by
Gregory P. Grieve FCSP DipTP
Formerly Clinical Tutor, Royal National Orthopaedic Hospital, London,
and Norfolk and Norwich Hospital, Norwich, UK

SECOND EDITION

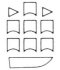

CHURCHILL LIVINGSTONE
EDINBURGH LONDON MADRID MELBOURNE NEW YORK AND TOKYO 1994

CHURCHILL LIVINGSTONE
Medical Division of Longman Group Limited

Distributed in the United States of America by Churchill
Livingstone Inc., 650 Avenue of the Americas, New York,
N.Y. 10011, and by associated companies, branches and
representatives throughout the world.

First edition 1986
Second edition 1994

ISBN 0-443-04348-5

British Library Cataloguing in Publication Data
A catalogue record for this book is available from the British
Library.

Library of Congress Cataloging in Publication Data
A catalog record for this book is available from the Library
Congress.

The
publisher's
policy is to use
**paper manufactured
from sustainable forests**

Produced by Longman Singapore Publishers Pte Ltd
Printed in Singapore

Contents

Contributors

Michael A. Adams BSc PhD
Research Fellow, Department of Anatomy, University of Bristol, Bristol, UK

Wendy Aspinall DipPhysio GradDipManTher MHSC
Instructor and National Examiner for the Orthopaedic Division of CPA; Private Clinical Consultant, Toronto, Ontario, Canada

Nikolai Bogduk BSc(Med) MB BS MD PhD DipAnat HonMMTAA HonFACRM
Professor of Anatomy, Faculty of Medicine, University of Newcastle, Callaghan, New South Wales; Visiting Medical Officer and Director, Cervical Spine Research Unit, Mater Misericordiae Hospital, Newcastle, New South Wales, Australia

David Bowsher MD PhD MRCPEd FRCPath
Director of Research, Pain Research Institute, Walton Hospital; Honorary Consultant, Centre of Pain Relief, Walton Hospital, Liverpool, UK

Jeffrey D. Boyling MSc(Lond) BPhty(Hons)(Qld) GradDipAdvManipTher(SAIT) MAPA MCSP MErgS MMPAA
Chartered Physiotherapist and Ergonomist, Hammersmith, London; Formerly Senior Teacher, St Thomas' Hospital School of Physiotherapy, London, UK

David S. Butler BPhty GradDipAdvManipTher
Private Practitioner, Adelaide; Part-time Lecturer, University of South Australia, Adelaide, Australia

Robert A. Charman FCSP DipTP
Senior Lecturer, School of Physiotherapy, Institute of Health Care Studies, University Hospital of Wales, Cardiff, UK

Alan Coutts BAppSci(Phty) GradDipAdvManipTher
Private Practice, Christies Beach, South Australia

Megan Dalton BPhty(Hons) GradDipAdvManipTher MAPA MMPAA
Lecturer, Department of Physiotherapy, University of Queensland, St Lucia, Brisbane, Australia

G. F. Dommisse OMSS HonMD MB ChB ChM(UCT) MD(Pret) FRCS(Eng) FRCS(Ed)
Associate Professor, Department of Orthopaedics, University of Pretoria, Republic of South Africa

Brian C. Edwards BSc BAppSci MMPAA FACP OAM
Specialist Manipulative Physiotherapist; Honorary Fellow, Curtin University of Technology, Perth, Western Australia

Robert L. Elvey BAppsci(Physio) GradDipManTher
Senior Lecturer in Manipulative Therapy, Curtin University of Technology, Perth, Western Australia

David H. Evans DipPhysio BPT GradDipAdvManipTher
Tutor, Postgraduate Manipulative Therapy Program, University of South Australia; Honorary Consultant in Manipulative Physiotherapy, Royal Adelaide Hospital, South Australia

Clifford Fowler MCSP MCPA COMP
National Examiner, Canadian Manipulative Therapists, Fraser Valley Orthopaedic and Sports Medicine Clinic, Abbotsford, British Columbia, Canada

Louis S. Gifford BSc MCSP SRP
Chartered Physiotherapist, Falmouth, Cornwall, UK

Ruth Grant BPT MAppSc MMPAA
Professor of Physiotherapy; Dean, Faculty of Health and Biomedical Sciences, University of South Australia, Adelaide, Australia

Gregory P. Grieve FCSP DipTP
Formerly Clinical Tutor, Royal National Orthopaedic Hospital, London, and Norfolk and Norwich Hospital, Norwich, UK

Helen M. Jones BAppSci(Physio) Grad DipAdvManipTher
Private Practice, Adelaide, South Australia

Mark A. Jones BS(Psych) PT GradDipAdvManipTher MAppSci(ManipTher)
Co-ordinator and Lecturer, Postgraduate Programmes in Manipulative Therapy, School of Physiotherapy, Faculty

of Health and Biomedical Sciences, University of South Australia, Adelaide, Australia

Gwendolen A. Jull MPhty GradDipManipTher FACP
Senior Lecturer, Department of Physiotherapy, University of Queensland; Specialist Manipulative Physiotherapist, Private Practice, Chapel Hill, Queensland, Australia

David W. Lamb BSc MCSP DipTP COMP
Director, Parkland Physical Therapy, Red Deer, Alberta, Canada; Membership Committee, IFOMT; Examiner, Orthopaedic Division, CPA

Agneta Lando GradDipPhys MCSP SRP MACP
Private Practitioner; Formerly Superintendent Physiotherapist, St Stephen's Hospital, Fulham, London, UK

Diane G. Lee BSR COMP
Instructor and Examiner, Orthopaedic Division, Canadian Physiotherapy Association; Instructor and Examiner, North American Institute of Orthopaedic Manual Therapy, British Columbia, Canada

Janet E. Macintosh BSc(Hons) PhD
Faculty of Medicine, University of Newcastle, Callaghan, New South Wales, Australia

David J. Magee BA DipPT BPT MSc PhD
Professor and Chair, Department of Physical Therapy, Faculty of Rehabilitation Medicine, University of Alberta, Edmonton, Canada

Jill Mantle BA MCSP DipPT
Senior Lecturer, Department of Rehabilitation Sciences, Institute of Health and Rehabilitation, University of East London, London, UK

James T. S. Meadows BSc PT MCPA COMP
Registered Instructor and Examiner, Orthopaedic Division, CPA and North American Institute of Orthopaedic Manipulative Therapy, Edmonton, Canada

Susan Mercer BPhty MSc
Instructor, Department of Physical Therapy, Duquesne University, Pittsburgh, Philadelphia, USA

Juliet M. Moss MCSP DipManTher DipMDT
Private Practice, London, UK

Brian R. Mulligan MNZSP DipMT
Manipulative Therapist and Lecturer in Manual Therapy, Wellington, New Zealand

Christine E. O'Donoghue JP MPhil MCSP
Physiotherapy Practice, St Albans; Formerly Research Physiotherapist, Royal Free Hospital School of Medicine, London, UK

Nigel Palastanga MA BA MCSP DMS DipTP
Principal, Cardiff School of Physiotherapy, University Hospital of Wales, Cardiff, UK

Erl Pettman MCPA COMP
Private Practice, Abbotsford BC; Chief Examiner, Orthopaedic Division, Canadian Physiotherapy Association, Canada

Carolyn A. Richardson BPhty(Hons) PhD
Senior Lecturer, Department of Physiotherapy, University of Queensland, Brisbane, Australia

Sally Roberts PhD
Clinical Scientist, Centre for Spinal Studies, Robert Jones and Agnes Hunt Orthopaedic Hospital, Oswestry, Shropshire, UK

Malcolm G. Robinson GradDipPhys MCSP DipMDT
Chartered Physiotherapist; Member of International Training Faculty, McKenzie Institute (International); Private Practitioner, Sutton Coldfield, West Midlands, UK

Sally A. Ruston BScR(Pt) GradDipManipTher GradDipBiomech PhD
Senior Lecturer, School of Physiotherapy, University of South Australia, Adelaide, South Australia

Greg Schneider MAPA MMPAA FACP
Specialist Manipulative Therapist; Clinical Practice, Sydney; Sessional Lecturer, Cumberland College, University of Sydney, Sydney, New South Wales, Australia

Michael O. Shacklock DipPhysio(Auckland) GradDipAdvManipTher
Private Practitioner, Slater, Butler and Shacklock Pty Ltd, Adelaide, South Australia

Joyce Sherriff MCSP
Superintendent Physiotherapist, King Edward VII Hospital, Windsor, Berkshire, UK

Kevin P. Singer PT MSc PhD
Senior Lecturer, School of Physiotherapy, Curtin University of Technology, Perth, Western Australia

Alison T. Skinner BA MCSP HT DipTP
Senior Lecturer, Middlesex Hospital School of Physiotherapy and University College London, London, UK

Helen Slater BAppSc(Phty) GradDipAdvManipTher
Part-time Lecturer (Postgraduate), University of South Australia; Private Practitioner, Adelaide; Freelance Lecturer, Adelaide, South Australia

Gary L. Smidt PhD PT FAPTA
Professor, Physical Therapy Graduate Program, University of Iowa, Iowa, USA

James R. Taylor MB ChB DTM PhD
Associate Professor, Department of Anatomy, University of Western Australia; Research Fellow, Department of Neuropathology, Royal Perth Hospital, Western Australia

Ann M. Thomson MSc BA MCSP DipTP
Acting Head of School, Middlesex Hospital School of Physiotherapy and University College London, London, UK

Lance T. Twomey DipPhysio BAppSc(WAIT) BSc(Hons)(UWA) PhD(UWA)
Deputy Vice-Chancellor and Professor of Physiotherapy, Curtin University of Technology, Perth, Western Australia

Jocelyn P. Urban PhD DIC
Senior Arthritis and Rheumatism Research Fellow, Physiology Laboratory, Oxford University, Oxford, UK

Fernando Valencia BSc(NSW) MSc(Syd) MCom(NSW) GradDipPhty MAPA MESANZ
Director, Randwick Physiotherapy Centre, Randwick, New South Wales, Australia

Paula M. Van Wijmen DipPhty(Neth) DipMT DipMDT
Manipulative Physiotherapist, Te Aro Physiotherapy, Wellington, New Zealand; Senior Lecturer, McKenzie Institute International

Martin J. Warren BSc MB BS MRCP FRCR
Consultant Radiologist, Luton and Dunstable NHS Trust Hospital, Luton; Formerly Senior Registrar, Radiology, Nuffield Orthopaedic Centre NHS Trust, Headington, Oxford, UK

Dean H. Watson MAppSc MAPA MMPAA
Manipulative Physiotherapist, The Headache Clinic, North Adelaide, South Australia

David R. Worth BAppSc(Physio) MAppSc PhD
Senior Consultant, Rankin Occupational Safety and Health, Adelaide, South Australia

Max Zusman DipPT BAppSc GradDipHthSc MAppSc
Lecturer, School of Physiotherapy, Curtin University of Technology, Perth, Western Australia

Foreword

It is gratifying to write the Foreword to a second edition of this text. An established success after three printings, it was conceived in trepidation and flimsy hope well over 10 years ago. Barbara Grieve would have savoured the occasion, having whole-heartedly shared the prolonged toil and the manifold concerns of producing the first edition.

Because thrust manipulations of the vertebrae have potential for harm as well as good, the manipulative therapist is comprehensively trained in the careful use of localized thrust techniques, with their indications and contraindications, and also in the use of the increasing variety of more moderate means of encouraging regional or localized vertebral movement. A number of these useful additional techniques have been developed by *physiotherapist* manipulators, among them Brian Edwards, Bob Elvey, Olaf Evjenth, Cliff Fowler, Freddy Kaltenborn, David Lamb, Diane Lee, Geoff Maitland and Brian Mulligan. David Butler, Louis Gifford and others have further developed the method of treating abnormal tension in the central and peripheral nervous systems by manual methods, and it is not surprising that an international roll-call of physiotherapists who have made original and significant research contributions, particularly in the Antipodes, would easily fill this page.

The Editors, both experienced physiotherapy teachers, have gathered together a wealth of information and sound instruction. Redundant chapters have been deleted and each of the five main sections has undergone comprehensive updating together with important additions. Of the total of 63 chapters, 46 are new and 17 have been revised and updated. Subjects covered in new chapters include biomechanics of the CNS, diagnostic ultrasound, anatomy of the zygapophyseal joints, kinematics of the pelvic joints, effects of ageing on intervertebral discs, assessment of chronic pain, dizziness, pelvic girdle dysfunction, spinal osteoporosis, clinical reasoning processes, the influence of circadian variations on spinal examination, the significance of temperature testing, CNS tension tests, modern imaging techniques, modified mobilization methods, management of recurrent pain, back pain and pregnancy, manual therapy in water, ergonomics and, finally, conditions (some of them serious) which may masquerade as benign musculo–skeletal problems.

The Editors have cast a wide net to present the best of modern scientific manual treatment for benign neuro–musculo–skeletal conditions of the vertebral column. The baton has been taken up by manifestly capable hands and the success of this second edition is thereby assured.

Halesworth, Suffolk 1994   G. P. G.

Preface to the second edition

The retirement of Gregory Grieve left Churchill Livingstone with a superb text to be continued as well as with the task of finding a replacement editor. The fact that the second edition has been a joint effort is a reflection on the immense contribution to physiotherapy, and manual therapy in particular, that Gregory Grieve has made.

The first edition reflected the leading edge of practice in the early 1980s, and it is to be hoped that this edition reflects the views of manual therapists in the early 1990s. This text is by no means meant to be exhaustive or representative of the full spectrum of work being undertaken. That task represents a dream of past and present editors.

The challenge to validate work has been taken up and it is reflected in the research work included in this text, as well as in the change of emphasis on examination as shown by the appropriate chapters. It is also pleasing to see new material developed by physiotherapists being added to the knowledge base.

It is fitting that this new edition of *Modern Manual Therapy* is being published in the centenary year of the oldest physiotherapy association, the Chartered Society of Physiotherapy. The very roots of the profession are steeped in manual therapy, and it is pleasing that one of the core skills is still at the heart of physiotherapy practice.

It is almost 10 years since the first edition, which is still regarded as a standard text in the subject area, was published. Consequently, the second edition is completely new, with the inclusion of representatives of a new generation of manual therapists keen to display their philosophies and techniques. In addition, long-standing and established practitioners have been able to completely review their contributions as the result of continuing practice and research. The practical application and scientific basis of manual therapy marches on.

Clinical problem-solving has become a part of every therapist's repertoire and this, linked to the need for rigorous quality assurance measures, has increased the need for research to support the use of manual therapy in a cost conscious world.

The authors of the chapters have all produced outstanding work which allows this book to remain at the forefront of physiotherapy practice. No doubt, by the time the next edition is produced yet another group of aspiring manual therapists will be ready to share their professional expertise. The progress of manual therapy moves ever onward.

In conclusion, it is to be hoped that this text will be useful to undergraduates, to practising manual therapists and to the ever increasing number of therapists completing higher degrees.

London and Cardiff, 1994

J. D. B.
N. P.

Preface to the first edition

Churchill Livingstone's invitation to compile and edit a text on Modern Manual Therapy prompted my first concept of a rich and comprehensive totality. Constraints of the possible soon whittled down that vision, yet the chapters are, I hope, a fair representation of what physiotherapists were thinking and doing in the mid-1980s, together with authoritative accounts of some contexts of that work.

I have enjoyed the privilege of being associated with the sixty authors, whose views I may not necessarily share, of course.

Together with excellent contributions from British colleagues, the manifest overseas presence reflects my abiding links with those energetic and restless countries whose citizens have contributed much sound, realistic advancement.

This is not an exhaustive text on technique, nor even a representative vocabulary. Technique is not of prime importance, since technique springs most naturally from the fullest grasp of the nature of the musculo–skeletal problem. More arduous than learning the various ways to push this or tweak and pull that is the task of educating oneself in understanding the problem. This is infinitely worthwhile and rewarding, because it also teaches when not to handle the patient.

Improvement of clinical competence is a demanding business. Ultimately, clinical effectiveness is directly related to the strength of the individual's desire to *be* clinically effective, and it is pointless beseeching deaf heaven, 'Will somebody please tell me what to think', since always there are those only too happy to do this. Workers who seek to improve their clinical efficacy need discrimination and a lively ability to distinguish fact from fancy.

We derive from each other, as the painter Sickert (1860–1942) has expressed it: '. . . the language of paint, like any other language, is kneaded and shaped by all the competent workmen labouring at any given moment; it is, with all its individual variations, a common language and not one of us would have been exactly what he is but for the influence and experience of all the other competent workmen of the period.' Many recent advances in basic knowledge, and alternative ways of thinking about old problems, have already made our yesterdays seem centuries ago, yet we need to recognise sterile propaganda and plain advertisement. Novelty is not progress.

By its nature, manipulative medicine does not enjoy the same scientific basis as anatomy, physiology, molecular biology, pathology or pharmacology, for example. We cannot take the bits apart to see what we are doing, or why we need to do it. Much of what we do is simply what has *been proven on the clinical shop floor* to be effective in getting our patients better — we do not always know precisely why.

We continue to sound as though we know so much, when we know comparatively little. It might be a good thing to admit this. We make much of clinical science, enthusiastically referring to this or that part of the massive mountain of literature which best serves our particular interest, yet Oliver Sacks (1982), who researched the effects of L-dopa on Parkinson's disease, puts the matter clearly: 'We rationalise, we dissimilate, we pretend; we pretend that modern medicine is a rational science, all facts, no nonsense and just what it seems. But we have only to rap its glossy veneer for it to split wide open and reveal to us its roots and foundations, the old dark heart of metaphysics, mysticism, magic and myth.'

As astrology is to the science of astronomy, pure science tends to fall by the wayside as wishful thinking, therapeutic likes, dislikes and old loyalties push to the fore. While it is ordinary commonsense to work in the way in which one feels most comfortable, and most effective, we cannot thereby make a scientific virtue out of expediency.

Professor Lewis Thomas, of the State University of New York at Stony Brook, recently mentions (in *Late Night Thoughts* 1984 OUP) 'Medicine, the newest and youngest of all the sciences, bobs along in the wake of biology, indeed not yet sure that it *is* all that much of a science, but certain that if there is to be a scientific future for medicine it can come only from basic biomedical research.'

Manual therapists may have a long road to travel before we talk an agreed common language, founded on scientific fact, but we can enjoy some solid progress towards that end and are now travelling with confidence.

Halesworth, Suffolk, 1986   G.P.G.

Acknowledgements

Thanks are due to many individuals, without whose interest in and professional approach to manual therapy of the spine this edition would not have been published.

In particular, colleagues in Australia, Canada and the United Kingdom willingly gave constructive criticism which helped to shape the contributor and chapter lists. Special thanks are extended to Gwen Jull and Diane Lee, the corresponding editors in Australia and Canada. Both helped to control the quality and delivery of manuscripts from their respective countries. They also found the time to contribute their own chapters, and their efforts are appreciated.

The staff of Jeffrey Boyling Associates are thanked for their assistance in reading and checking the chapters, as well as for providing useful critical comments on the content.

Like our predecessor, we have enjoyed a cordial and fruitful relationship with the staff of Churchill Livingstone, both in Edinburgh and in overseas countries. In particular, thanks are extended to Mary Law, Dinah Thom and Nicky Haig for the assistance they have given in bringing this new edition to print.

Finally, the patience of our respective families has to be acknowledged. Their tolerance of the evenings and weekends spent reading and re-reading manuscripts has been greatly appreciated.

J. D. B.
N. P.

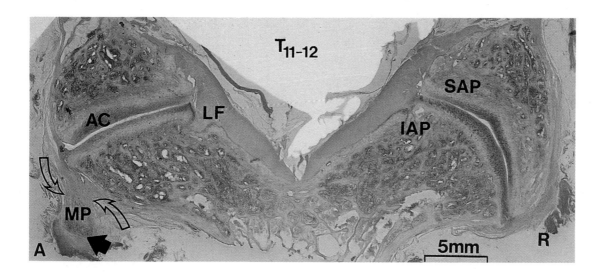

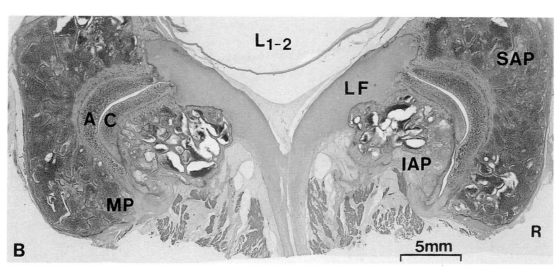

Plate 7.1 **A**. Photomicrograph of a 200 μm-thick transverse section cut in the plane of the superior vertebral end-plate at T11–12 to illustrate a type II unilateral mortice joint on the left formed by the mammillary process MP (arrow) located posteriorly to the inferior articular process IAP. The zygapophysis on the right conforms to a typical sagittally orientated joint. Curved arrows indicate the attachment of the lateral and posterior articular capsular ligaments which are reinforced by the mammillary process. Despite the marked articular tropism, both joint surfaces have a normal histological appearance in this subject. **B**. An example of a bilateral type I mortice joint at L1–2. This section from the lower half of the joint illustrates the extent to which inferior articular processes IAP are embraced by the superior articular process SAP which show a medial tendency in the posterior aspect of the joint. The articular cartilage AC appears normal despite some thinning on the right IAP in the more sagittal component of the joint. LF = ligamentum flavum.

Structure and function

1. The blood supply of the spinal cord and the consequences of failure

G. F. Dommisse

'For the life of all flesh is the blood thereof' Leviticus XVII

'I would have everie man write what he knows, and no more . . .' Montaigne

'It is the function of science to measure what is mensurable and to render mensurable what is not . . .' Galileo

INTRODUCTION

It is a little known yet fundamental fact that the brain and spinal cord, with a combined mass of about 1.5 kg (about 2% of body mass), together consume about 20% of available oxygen in the circulating blood. This is a measure of the metabolic demands of the central nervous system, man's most highly developed organ. When blood flow in the spinal cord is occluded for three minutes, an infarct develops in the grey matter (Fig. 1.1). The posterior spinal ganglion, an integral part of the central nervous system, is equally endowed with blood supply (Fig. 1.2), and equally sensitive to the effects of ischaemia. The

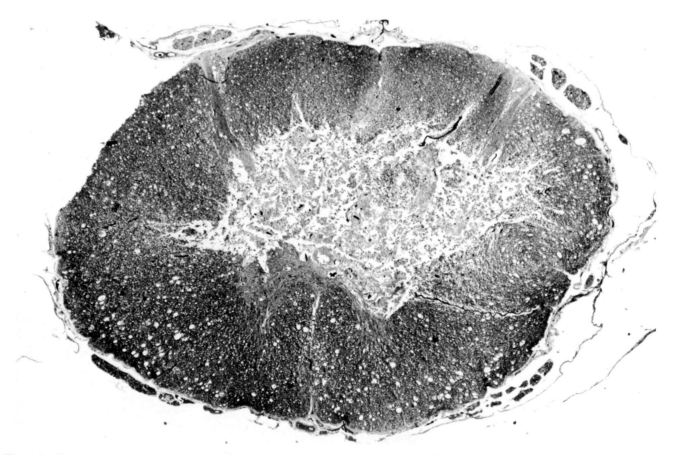

Fig. 1.1 Cross-section of the infarcted spinal cord of a baboon. A central infarct resulted from experimentally induced ischaemia for a period of three minutes. (Reproduced from Dommisse 1980a by courtesy of Professor I. W. Simpson, Department of Pathological Anatomy, Pretoria, and the editor.)

3

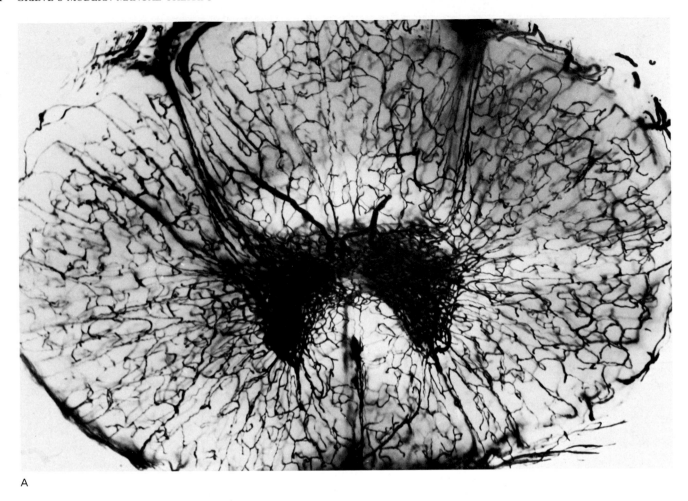

A

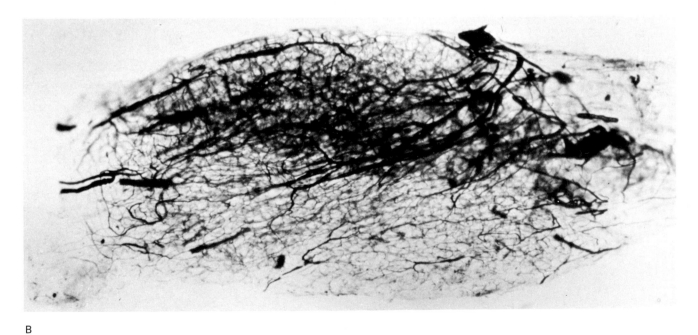

B

Fig. 1.2   A. Cross-section of the spinal cord in the thoracic region. The perforating arteries, and the density of the capillary plexus in the grey matter and the white matter, the well demonstrated (India ink injection, in the specimen cleared by the Spalteholz technique).
B. Section of a posterior spinal ganglion, prepared as in (A). The capillary density compares with that of the grey matter of the cord.

'battered root syndrome' (Bertrand 1975) is due to 'strangulation' consequent upon traumatic, iatrogenically-induced ischaemic fibrosis of the emerging spinal nerve. In this study, a number of parameters were measured and an effort was made to establish norms as well as normal limits. There were more than fifty human cadavers in the series. Six were used for angiograms, and the others were used for a detailed, personally-conducted micro-dissection of the cord 'in situ'. The baboon 'papio ursinus' was used for 'in vivo' studies.

THE PHYSICAL DIMENSIONS OF THE HUMAN SPINAL CORD (DOMMISSE 1973)

Table 1.1 The human spinal cord: physical dimensions

	Adult	Neonate
Average length of spinal cord	40–50 cm	10–12.5 cm
Average length of cervical section	10 cm	–
Average length of thoracic section	20 cm	–
Average length of lumbo-sacral section	15 cm	–
Average mass (cord plus membranes)	91 g	7 g
Average volume (cord plus membranes)	79.2 ml	

THE LUMEN OF THE SPINAL CANAL (Fig. 1.3)

The shape and dimensions vary. In the cervical and thoraco-lumbar zones the canal is relatively capacious. In the thoracic zone proper, from T3/4 to T8/9 vertebral levels, the lumen is narrow, and is narrowest at the T6 vertebra where a cross-section reveals a circular form. In the lumbar and lumbosacral regions it is flattened in the anteroposterior dimension, with a wide lateral diameter, adapted perfectly to accommodate the cauda equina (Dommisse 1975a, 1980a, Eisenstein 1976).

The narrow zone of the spinal canal extends from approximately T4 to T9 vertebral levels, hence a *critical vascular zone* is recognized in this region. Minimal reduction of space, from whatever cause, results in maximal compromise, with a threat of compression and ischaemia of the cord (Dommisse 1974).

THE SPINAL NERVES

The anterior and posterior nerve rootlets join to form the spinal nerves. The posterior spinal ganglion is placed immediately cephalic to the junction of the sensory and motor nerve roots. It occupies a sheltered position in the lateral recess of the canal, beneath the pedicle of the vertebra above (Fig. 1.4).

The nerve roots (Fig. 1.5) take off from the spinal cord at angles which vary according to segmental level, the upper cervical nearly transversely and the thoracolumbar nearly vertically. The elements of the cauda equina pursue a vertical course.

THE NEURAL CANALS (Dommisse 1973, Dommisse & Grobler 1976)

The lateral recess marks the inner entrance, and the intervertebral foramen marks the exit of the spinal nerve in its passage through the neural canal. The length and the incline of the canal vary in the three principal vertebral zones. In the cervical zone, the neural canal is 10–15 mm in length, and it forms a take-off angle of 60–70° with the spine. In the thoracic zone the canal is little more than a window opening (a foramen), through which the nerves pass 'en route' to the trailing edges of the ribs. In the lumbar zone the neural canal is an impressive 'tunnel', about 20–35 mm in length, with a take-off angle of about 45° (Fig. 1.6). The spinal nerve, after passing through the neural canal and after exit from the intervertebral foramen, pursues a laterally and caudally directed course to the periphery. The angle the spinal nerve follows after exit from the neural canal differs in different regions, being nearly 90° in the thoracic region, and less in the cervical and lumbar regions.

The concept of 'an acute upward angulation of the dural sleeve' in the cervical region cannot be supported (Nathan & Feuerstein 1974). The dimensions and boundaries of the neural canals deserve special attention. In the cervical zone they are tightly bounded by the unco-vertebral and para-vertebral joints at front and back, by the pedicles of the adjacent vertebrae above and below, and by the vertebral artery which has a directly anterior relationship to the nerve from C6 to C2 level. The spinal nerve and the vertebral artery are vulnerable in this confined canal, more especially in the elderly, spondylotic individual. Accidental trauma as well as the trauma of forcible manipulation of the neck, whether 'skilled' (sic), or not, are a hazard.

The lumbar neural canals (Fig. 1.6) accommodate an abundance of arteries and veins as well as the posterior spinal ganglion and the spinal nerve. A prolapsed portion of a lumbar disc may be displaced into the neural canal where it compresses the contents of the canal. There is impaction of the ganglion and the nerve, with ischaemic pain. Permanent fibrotic changes ('the battered nerve') develop unless the situation is relieved. Surgical measures which include de-roofing and decompression of the neural canal are indicated for unremitting, intractable pain.

THE BLOOD SUPPLY OF THE SPINAL CORD, THE POSTERIOR SPINAL GANGLIA AND THE SPINAL NERVES

Seven orders of blood vessels are recognized. The capillaries are the vessels of the seventh order, the precapillaries the sixth, the arterioles the fifth, the small arteries the fourth and the aorta the principal or first. All are involved in cord supply, but the most significant are the aorta, the

THE LUMEN OF THE SPINAL CANAL

Mean Diameters			A–P. Diameter Lat. Diameter ×100	
Antero—Posterior	Lateral		MEAN.	RANGE
17 mm	26 mm	C.2	65	62–71
14 mm	25 mm	C.5	56	50–61
15 mm	21 mm	T.I	71	64–80
14 mm	15 mm	T.6	95	81–105
15 mm	16 mm	T.9	92	70–100
16.5 mm	19.3 mm	T.I2	85	81–95
15.6 mm	21.3 mm	L.I	73	69–83
15.6 mm	22 mm	L.3	70	72–75
12 m 18 mm	24 mm 28 mm	L.5 L.5	65	50–81
10 mm 16 mm 16 mm	32 mm 37 mm 33 mm	S.I S.I S.I	41	31–58

Fig. 1.3 The canal is narrowest at the sixth thoracic vertebra. The narrow zone extends from T4–T9 vertebral levels. (Reproduced from Dommisse 1980a by courtesy of the editor.)

medullary feeder arteries (third order), the longitudinal arterial trunks of the cord (fourth order), and those of the smaller orders down to the seventh.

It is fundamental fact that the cord is an *organ*, a solitary integrated organ which extends throughout nearly the full length of the spine. The general concept of a segmented structure is rejected, for there is no evidence of interruption of fibres or cell columns at intersegmental levels.

The study of the blood vessels of the cord is at first bedevilled by the physical fact of its length, but a simplicity and matchless design are seen to emerge, and a number of constant factors (the principles) are observed.

The principles of arterial supply

The capillaries (Fig. 1.2A)

A capillary plexus extends *uninterruptedly* from medulla oblongata to conus medullaris. There is no evidence of a 'glomerular structure' of capillaries, or of end-vessels within the plexus.

Capillary density (Fig. 1.7) is greatest in the grey matter, the site of the neuronal cells. This is because the metabolic demands of the neuronal cells are greater than those the white fibre tracts. For the same reason, the grey matter is more vulnerable, and central lesions of the cord are frequently observed as complicating traumatic lesions of the cervical vertebrae.

The posterior spinal ganglia (Fig. 1.2B) are the site of the primary neuronal cells of the sensory system, and they receive an abundant blood supply, commensurate with the grey matter of the cord.

The spinal nerve rootlets (Fig. 1.5) and the spinal nerves are less generously but nevertheless abundantly supplied. The rootlets, the posterior spinal ganglia and the

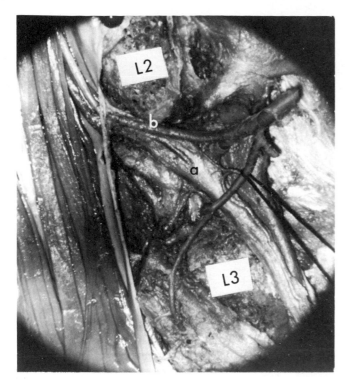

Fig. 1.4 Ventral view of the neural canal. The pedicles of L2 and L3 vertebrae are marked, and the posterior spinal ganglion with radicular artery (a) are sheltered under L2 pedicle. The artery of Adamkiewicz (b) arises at the intervertebral foramen. (Reproduced from Dommisse 1975a by courtesy of the editor.)

proximal portion of the spinal nerves are vulnerable to ischaemia, in the same manner but to a lesser degree than the cord.

The perforating arteries

Three sets of 'perforators' serve the cord. The anterior perforators (Fig. 1.8) supply the major portion of cord substance. They arise from the anterior longitudinal arterial trunk and penetrate the median sulcus. They are largest and most numerous in the cervical and lumbar segments where the ganglionic cells of the brachial and the lumbosacral plexuses are placed. Together with the anterior longitudinal trunk, they are sacrosanct. When occluded, the 'anterior spinal artery syndrome' inevitably follows with motor paralysis, impairment of thermal and pain sensations, and preservation of tactile and pressure sense.

The posterior perforating arteries (Fig. 1.2A) are small, they enter the substance of the cord in the company of the posterior rootlets, and they are distributed in the posterior one-third of the cord. They anastomose with and contribute towards the unbroken plexus of capillaries.

The third or pial set of perforators are small (Fig. 1.2A); they arise from the surface communications between the anterior and posterior longitudinal trunks, and they, too, contribute to the capillary plexus.

Blood flow in the spinal cord

Flow in small vessels is calculated by Poiseuilles' formula:

$$\text{Flow} = \frac{\pi(P_1 - P_2)r^4}{8\,L\eta}$$

in which
P = pressure across the field
r = radius of vessel
L = length of vessel
η = viscosity of the fluid

The blood flow in grey matter is 15.4 times greater than that in white matter. The corollary to this deduction is that the grey matter is 15.4 times more sensitive to ischaemia than the white (Dommisse 1980b).

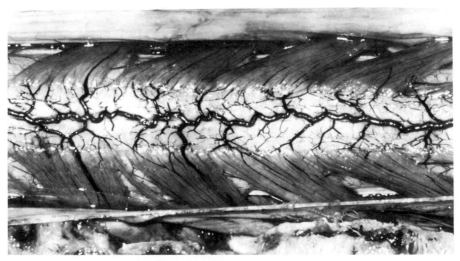

Fig. 1.5 The posterior surface of the spinal cord, with the posterior nerve rootlets. The veins, arteries and capillaries are filled with India ink. Abundant capillary vessels accompany the nerves.

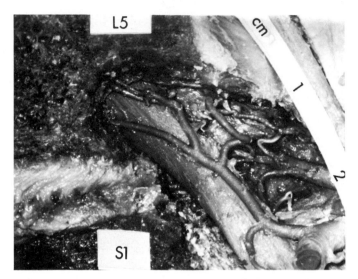

Fig. 1.6 The fifth lumbar spinal nerve on the left. The posterior spinal ganglion nestles under the pedicle of L5. Intraspinal branches of the segmental arteries are seen in the neural canal. The veins have been removed. (Reproduced from Dommisse 1975a by courtesy of the editor.)

The longitudinal arterial trunks

The entire arterial supply of the cord is derived from three great longitudinal arterial trunks, one anterior and two posterolateral. The anterior trunk overlies the anterior median sulcus. Proximally it communicates with the small

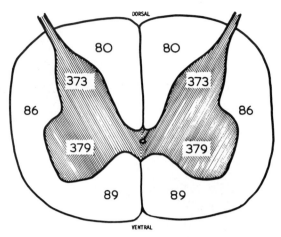

Fig. 1.7 Capillary density of the spinal cord of a baboon. The average number of capillaries/mm² is indicated in figures.

anterior spinal arteries, branches of the left and right vertebral arteries (Fig. 1.9). The direction of flow in these small arteries is either proximodistal *or* the reverse, depending on factors such as unequal intra-arterial pressures, siphon action of one stream upon another, and metabolic supply and demand. It is reasonable to assume a reversibility of flow under varying conditions, as in the circle of Willis at the base of the brain. Both physical and chemical factors are presumed to determine flow.

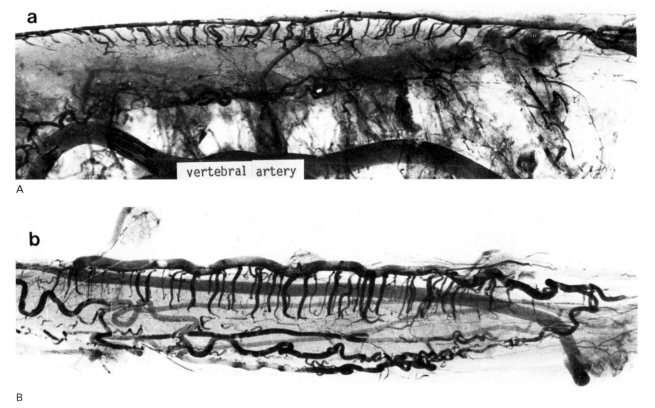

Fig. 1.8 Angiogram of a human spinal cord showing the anterior perforating arteries in the cervical zone (**A**), and lumbar zone (**B**), where they are most prominent.

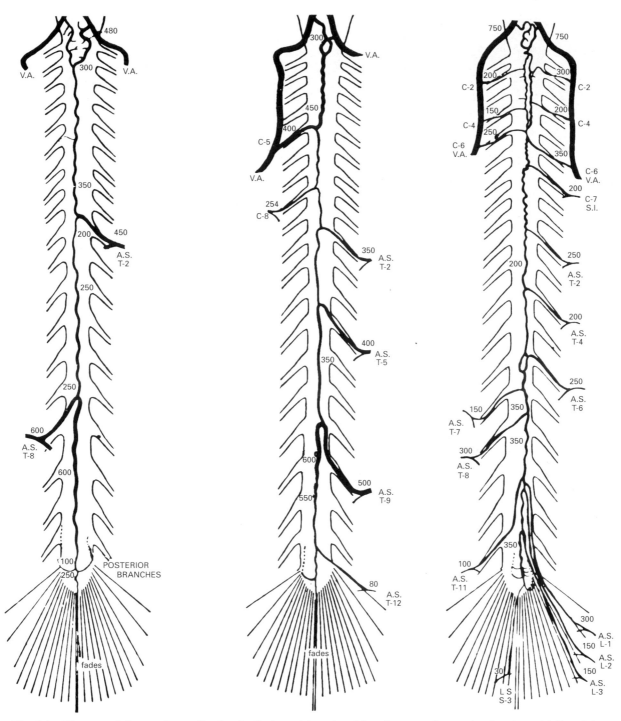

Fig. 1.9 Diagrams of the anterior median longitudinal arterial trunks of three human cadavers, showing the variability of size, number and site of incidence of the medullary feeder arteries. The approximate diameter of the vessels is indicated in micrometres.

The posterior longitudinal trunks are paired vessels extending the length of the cord, smaller than their anterior counterpart, and pursuing a 'weaving' course around and between the posterior nerve rootlets. Proximally, they communicate with the posterior inferior cerebellar branches of the left and right vertebral arteries by means of two posterior spinal arteries. The latter are presumed to permit a flow in both directions. Distally, the anterior and posterior longitudinal trunks communicate freely through a cruciate anastomosis situated over the conus medullaris (Fig. 1.10). The communications at this distal level are probably explained on the same basis as elsewhere, where they constitute alternative routes of supply (Dommisse 1972).

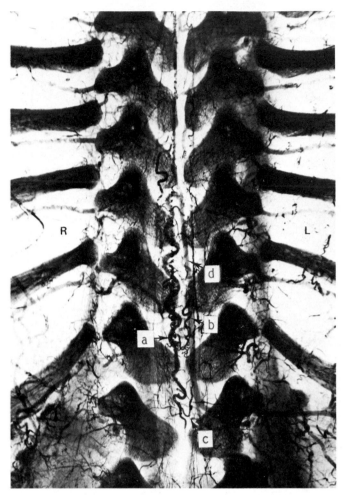

Fig. 1.10 Angiogram of a neonatal human cadaver, showing the anteromedian and the posterolateral longitudinal arterial trunks, and the cruciate anastomosis at the distal end. (a) The anterior median trunk; (b) the posterolateral trunk; (c) the cruciate anastomosis; (d) the artery of Adamkiewicz at the T10/11 level on the left side. (Reprinted from Dommisse 1975b with permission.)

The medullary feeder arteries

Anterior and posterior medullary feeders supply and maintain the longitudinal arterial trunks (Fig. 1.9). They are mainly from the vertebral arteries in the cervical region of the cord, the costocervical trunk at C7–T1–T2 segmental levels, the thoracic aortic segmental arteries (intercostals), in the thorax, and the lumbar aortic segmental arteries (lumbar arteries), at L1–L4/5 levels. More distally, there are occasional contributions from the iliolumbar and lateral sacral arteries.

The site, number and source of origin of the medullary feeders vary from one individual to another, and in no two individuals are they the same. The average number of anterior feeders is 7.5 per cadaver, varying normally from 2 to 17. The corresponding average and variation in posterior feeders are 12.5 average, 6–25 range.

An appreciation of the variability of the medullary feeders is essential knowledge for medical and para-

medical practitioners. There is no way to determine the number or pattern in the individual patient. Obviously, the person endowed with only two anterior feeders is at risk and at a disadvantage for, in such circumstances, both feeder vessels are vital to the maintenance of function. There is no comfort to be had from the 'arteria magna radicularis', the artery of Adamkiewicz, which is reputedly located at the T10–T11 vertebral level on the left side. In this series, the location varied from the T7 and L4 vertebral levels, and in 20% of cadavers it was on the *right* side. In a few, it was replaced by two or more feeder vessels of equal but less impressive size (Adamkiewicz 1881, Kadyi 1889).

Manipulation of the cervical spine is common practice in the spheres of physical medicine and chiropractic. The details of the blood supply of this area are therefore significant.

The cervical zone. The cervical zone extends from C1 to T1 segmental levels, and includes the ganglionic enlargement of the brachial plexus. It enjoys a rich blood supply which has been recorded in 35 cadavers for the anterior vessels, and in 18 cadavers for the posterior vessels in this study. In the adult cadaver, the length of the cervical cord was found to be approximately 10 cm, as compared with 45 cm for the entire cord (Dommisse 1973). A summary of the findings is given below; the reader will appreciate the fact that the figures reflect the diameters of the vessels in the cadaver, not 'in vivo'.

The average number of anterior cervical feeders in 35 cadavers is 3.4 only.

The average diameter of anterior cervical feeders in 35 cadavers is 312 μm.

The average number of posterior cervical feeders in 18 cadavers is 2.8 only.

The average diameter of posterior cervical feeders in 18 cadavers is 170 μm.

The numbers of the anterior and the posterior feeders vary from one to eight per cadaver. There is a concentration of vessels in the lower five neurological segments (C4–T1), conforming with the location of the brachial plexus neurones.

The vertebral arteries supply 77% of the anterior and 51% of the posterior cervical medullary feeder arteries.

The costocervical trunk and its two principal divisions supply 20% only of the anterior, and 37% of the posterior medullary feeders.

Significantly, the costocervical trunk and the proximal thoracic segmental arteries supply 86% (12 out of 14 in this series) of posterior feeders at the level of the thoracic outlet where vascular and neoplastic lesions are known to be common. A selective involvement of the posterior columns of the cord, with degenerative myelopathy, could be attributable to this factor.

The thoracic zone. The thoracic zone is least abundantly supplied. It is also the narrowest zone of the lumen of the spinal canal, and for these reasons it is a critical vascular zone. Traumatic paraplegia consequent upon mid-thoracic lesions (T4–T9) is frequently permanent and complete.

The average number of anterior feeders is 2.3 only.
The average diameter of anterior feeders is 315 μm.
The average number of posterior feeders is 5.3 only.
The average diameter of posterior feeders is 153 μm.

There is a four-to-one preponderance of anterior thoracic feeders on the left side, but there is no concentration at any single level.

When the thoracic blood supply is compared with the cervical, it will be seen that the latter enjoys a 3:2 advantage in numbers, and that the size of the feeders in the two respective areas is strictly comparable. These figures assume greater significance when viewed in perspective, for the thoracic cord (measured from T2 to T9 vertebrae) is approximately 20 cm in length as compared with 10 cm for the cervical cord. The principle of a richer blood supply for a zone of increased ganglionic density is thus seen to be upheld (Dommisse 1973).

The lumbar and sacral zones. The study was continued from the cervical and the thoracic zones to the most caudal aspect of the spine and to the distal extremities of the fifth sacral nerves. This is the zone of the lumbosacral plexus, with an abundant blood supply like the cervical cord.

The average number of anterior feeders is 2.3 only.
The average diameter of anterior feeders is 300 μm.
The average number of posterior feeders is 4.0 only.
The average diameter of posterior feeders is 150 μm.

The 'artery of Adamkiewicz' is a significant medullary feeder, but of no greater functional value than a feeder of similar magnitude situated elsewhere. The common concept that special care exercised at T10 and T11 vertebral levels during invasive procedures is sufficient to ensure the integrity of cord supply, cannot be upheld. Adherence to the concept constitutes a positive risk to cord supply.

The segmental vertebral arteries

There is a pair of segmental vertebral arteries at every intervertebral level. In the neck they are unnamed. In the thorax and abdomen they are well known. They are termed the intercostal and the lumbar arteries. Properly named, they are the thoracic and the lumbar segmental vertebral arteries of the appropriate intervertebral level.

The segmental arteries on left and right sides proceed to the intervertebral foramina of corresponding levels and divide into terminal branches. Accordingly, the intervertebral foramen is an important *arterial distribution point* (Fig. 1.11). Intraspinal branches include the medullary

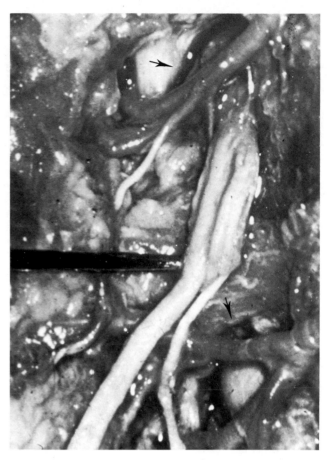

Fig. 1.11 The arterial distribution point of the segmental arteries, at the intervertebral foramen. Intraspinal branches enter the neural canal. A posterior spinal ganglion is at the distal foramen.

feeder arteries at varying levels, radicular arteries for the spinal nerves (radicles) and the posterior spinal ganglia at every level, and arteries which ascend in the canal, which cross the canal to communicate with contralateral vessels forming arterial anastomoses, and which descend. The plexus of arteries supply bony and soft tissue structures, including the dura mater.

Extradural branches supply, among others, the structures of the body wall, the spinal nerves and the sympathetic trunks and ganglia (Dommisse 1972).

Collateral anastomoses or arterial circles

Arterio-arterial anastomoses are common about the vertebral column and are found also in many other regions. The cruciate anastomosis at the knee joint and the circle of Willis at the base of the brain are examples.

Lazorthes et al (1971) report on 'anastomotic substitution pathways' but are cautious about their function: '. . . the anastomotic substitution pathways . . . are potentially valuable but their function is problematical'.

Anastomoses in the thoracic and lumbar regions occur commonly between contralateral and ipsilateral segmental

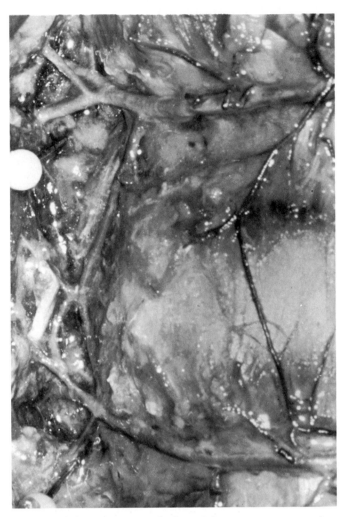

Fig. 1.12   Collateral anastomotic channels between two segmental arteries at the thoracolumbar level. Other anastomotic circles are found within the lumen of the spinal canal.

arteries (Fig. 1.12). The transverse arterial link within the spinal canal referred to earlier is constant and is a source of nutrient vessels for the vertebral body.

The importance of preserving intersegmental arterial circles during surgical approaches to the spine has been stressed by Dwyer and Schafer (1974) and by the author. Thoracic and lumbar segmental arteries should be ligated close to the aorta in order to preserve the collaterals. In the neck, arterio-arterial communications are common between the vertebral, the deep cervical and the ascending cervical arteries. In summary, arterial circles offer alternative routes of supply for the critical structures of the central nervous system, and can be used to the advantage of the patient, during surgical and other invasive procedures.

The direction of blood flow in the longitudinal arterial trunks

The three longitudinal trunks, of cardinal importance, are not arteries in the accepted sense of the word. They are arterial channels or chambers. The direction of flow of blood is not uniformly proximo-distal. Fried et al (1970) injected the subclavian artery of rhesus monkeys with coloured material via a retrograde catheter. Motion photography studies of the 'anterior spinal artery' in the cervical region showed that the flow of dye was directed both cranially and caudally, and accordingly it is suggested that the concept of flow in the length of the vessel be replaced by the concept of an arterial chamber in which the hydrodynamic pressure is maintained by contributions from all the medullary feeder arteries, and the outflow is *across* the chamber, through the perforating arteries, directly to the cord. This is no more than an extension of the principle of an arterial circle, such as the circle of Willis at the base of the brain. It implies a ready reversibility of flow and allows for an increased flow in whatever direction, according to regional demands and threats.

Threats to the arterial chamber may occur at local level, due to injury, disease, or invasive or ill-advised manipulative procedures. Other unfavourable conditions are atheromatous changes common in the aortae of the elderly, surgical procedures involving the heart, the aorta, or the segmental arteries at multiple levels, and following acute hypotension. General factors affecting flow, expressed in Poiseuilles' formula above, are equally important.

The vertebral venous system

The classical Harveian concept of the flow of blood in the form of a one-way stream is inadequate to describe the vertebral venous system, commonly known as Batson's plexus (Batson 1940, 1942, 1957).

Herlihy (1947), in a masterly contribution, laments: 'The vertebral veins receive scant attention, and although anastomoses are mentioned between the azygos system (and groups of other veins), . . . the significance is not stressed . . .'. He continues: 'I shall focus attention upon a great plexus of veins, the vertebral venous plexus (which) . . . lies within the spinal canal, over the bodies and laminae of the vertebrae, and partly in the vertebrae themselves'. Herlihy's contribution is required-reading for the serious student. Only the essence of the article is extracted here.

Reference to the disproportionately large share of cardiac output directed to the brain and spinal cord has been made. It follows that inflow must be matched by outflow if an effective circulation is to be maintained. In order that an even venous outflow from the CNS may be maintained under all physiological conditions, a 'place for the storage of blood' must be available so that an ebb and flow may take place. This storage is in the vertebral venous plexus. Herlihy adds: 'It is a pool for receiving backflow from adjacent veins, hence its many anastomoses . . . Any unequal pressure in the adjacent veins is quickly equalized . . . It has no pressure and hence is more suitable to act as a pressure absorber . . . It has no direction of flow, and this makes possible a quick adjustment and accommodation to a sudden inrush of blood . . .'. Were it not so, the alterations of venous pressure under normal conditions of breathing, coughing, sneezing and parturition among others would interrupt cerebral flow. Even straining at stool would be impossible without a 'blackout'.

The facts quoted above are not new, but they need repetition. In 1817 Bock described the rich plexuses of veins, and in 1819 Breschet — and since then many other researchers — published detailed reports, but it was not until 1942, when Batson described 'the Vertebral Vein System as a Mechanism for the Spread of Metastases' from pelvis and lungs to the brain, that the attention of readers was held. Herlihy more than any other worker drew attention to the normal physiological role. The author has added pictorial records and a diagrammatic representation of the venous system of the brain, the spine and the trunk (Figs 1.13, 1.14).

The practical implications are perhaps greater for the operating surgeon, whose skill and endurance are often taxed by a copious flow of vertebral venous blood, obscuring the operative field and at times endangering the patient's life.

In the field of physical medicine, the prevention of venous thrombosis by means of active and passive movements is a primary objective. Equally important is the supervision of and instruction in deep breathing, in order to promote negative pressure within the thorax and in so doing, to promote venous return. 'Ipso facto', cardiac output is improved.

COMMON SPINAL SYNDROMES

Cervical spondylosis (Long 1983)

Degenerative osteoarthrosis of the cervical spine is common, affecting more than 80% of the population over the age of 55 years. Comparable figures may be inferred for the lower lumbar spine. The presenting symptoms or syndromes of cervical spondylosis are protean. Brain (1963) reported 100 cases with single or combined complaints:

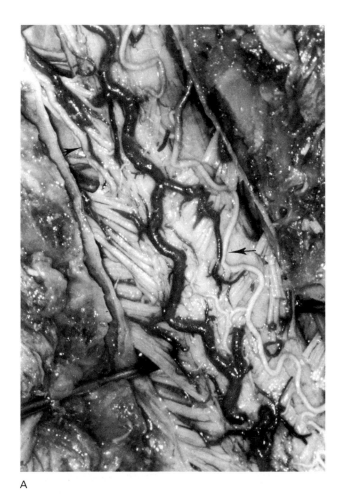

A

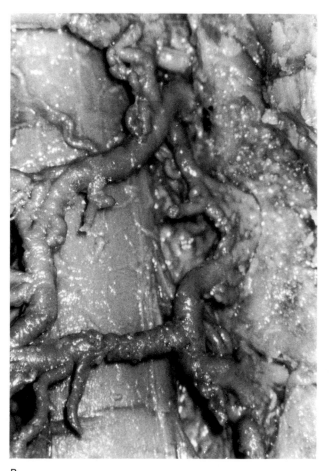

B

Fig. 1.13 **A**. The posterior aspect of the cervical cord of a human cadaver. The large longitudinal venous channel occupies a median position, and the paired longitudinal arterial channels (arrows) are posterolateral. **B**. Dorsal view of the spinal canal in the thoracic region, showing the dural sac and the extradural component of Batson's plexus of veins.

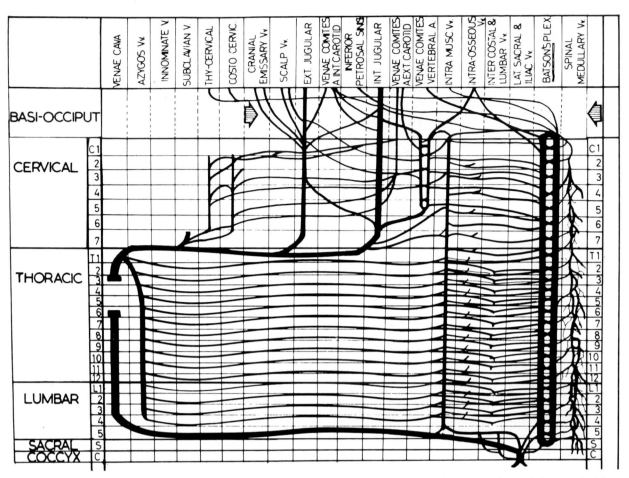

Fig. 1.14 Diagrammatic representation of the venous system, showing the systemic veins, the azygos veins and the complexities of Batson's plexus which communicates with the other venous systems at every level. The veins of the spinal cord drain into the plexus. (Reproduced from Zorab 1974 by courtesy of the editor and publishers.)

Brachial radiculitis	32 cases
Vertigo	17 cases
Pain in neck	13 cases
Attacks of unconsciousness	4 cases
Acute lesions of spinal cord	3 cases
Headache	28 cases
Myelopathy	13 cases
Vertebrobasilar ischaemia	5 cases
Drop attacks	3 cases

Among the acute lesions of the cord were vascular accidents involving the vertebral, the posterior inferior cerebellar and the basilar arteries. The same author comments on precipitating factors leading to these syndromes: 'To accidental trauma to the neck we must now therefore add therapeutic manipulation as a cause of damage to nerve roots, spinal cord or, by way of circulation, the brain . . . it may also occur when the neck has been manipulated by the surgeon or the anaesthetist in . . . surgical procedures in elderly patients . . . known to have cervical spondylosis'.

The warning words are well taken. The spinal column exhibits a range of motion in the sagittal, the coronal and the horizontal planes — flexion and extension, lateral flexion and rotation. *Coupling of motions* is an essential component when movements are forced. Movements on the Y-axis for increasing the physical length of the spine are minimal. White and Panjabi (1978) developed a *stretch test* and reported: 'Based on a study of eight normal subjects, an abnormal stretch test (on the cervical spine) is indicated by an interspace separation of greater than 1.7 mm. Similarly, any excessive relative axial displacement at the interspace in question should make one suspicious of structural damage'.

The vertebral arteries, the medullary feeder arteries and the radicular arteries are at risk within the foramen transversarium and the intervertebral foramina (neural canals). They are relatively or absolutely held by osteophytic spurs or bars, with the amplitude of normal movement reduced.

The diagnosis of radiculitis and radiculopathy is readily overlooked. Jackson (1953), in a classical contribution,

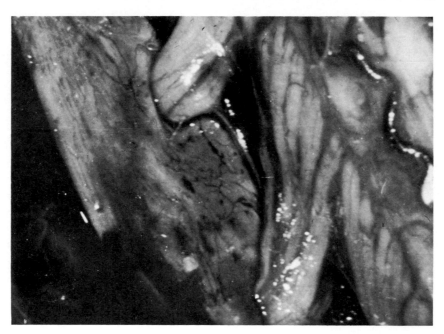

Fig. 1.15 Ischaemic radiculopathy of a cervical spinal nerve, photographed at surgery. Note the plump, healthy appearance of the proximal nerve (Courtesy of Professor R. Lipchitz and Mrs A. Rossouw, Department of Neurosurgery, University of the Witwatersrand.)

warns: 'The importance of cervical investigation in any patient with head, neck, chest, shoulder and arm pain cannot be over-emphasized. The usual diagnosis of arthritis, bursitis, neuritis, muscular rheumatism, fibrositis, fasciitis, tendinitis, pseudo-angina, migraine etc., should not be made until cervical nerve root irritation has been ruled out entirely. Usually these conditions are only secondary manifestations . . .'

Cervical radiculitis and radiculopathy are explained on the basis of temporary or permanent occlusion of the radicular arteries. Irreversible changes of intraneural fibrosis and radiculopathy are the end result (Fig. 1.15).

Myelopathy of the cervical cord

Brain (1963) reported myelopathy in 13 of a series of 100 patients. This is the most sinister and most serious result of chronic 'strangulation' of the cord. The symptoms are vague, sometimes bizarre, and inexorably progressive over the years. The lumen of the canal is narrowed at one or more intervertebral levels by a ridge (an osteophytic bar) across the width of the central spinal canal. When numerous levels are involved, the cord assumes a rosary form. There is patchy necrosis of grey and white matter, graphically illustrated by Ono et al (1977) and by Ogino et al (1983), and demonstrated also in the laboratory animal, the baboon (Fig. 1.16).

The initial symptoms are clumsiness of the hands with wasting of intrinsic muscles, difficulty in walking, and variable sensory loss. The sphincters are sometimes involved at a later stage.

The surgical relief of degenerative myelopathy offers promise when the condition is limited in degree, and in the number of levels involved. Manipulation of the neck is contraindicated. The neurological complications include cerebellar syndromes, tetraplegia and death.

Degenerative arthritis of lumbar spine, with retrolisthesis (Dommisse & Gräbe 1978)

Degeneration of the lower lumbar intervertebral discs (Fig. 1.17) is followed by atrophic changes at the corresponding paravertebral joints, the 'three-joint complex' described by Farfan (1973) and Kirkaldy-Willis and Hill (1979). A state of spinal instability exists, with abnormal mobility in the flexed and extended positions. There is dynamic irritation of the posterior spinal ganglia and the spinal nerves, and the effect is of stenosis of the lateral, neural canals. Direct trauma to the ganglion and nerve, and impairment of blood supply contribute to irreversible intraneural scars.

Chronic arachnoiditis (Fig. 1.18)

The dura mater is a richly vascularized and sensitive structure. In health it presents as a smoothly-rounded sac with lateral extensions ensheathing the spinal nerves. In disease, and following surgical and other invasive procedures (including infiltrations of various types), an inflammatory reaction takes place with permanent fibrotic changes the result. The spinal nerve sheaths are no longer

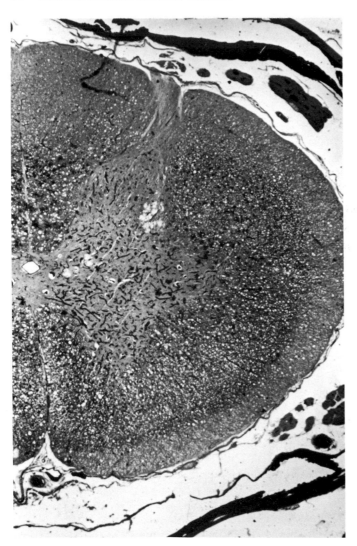

Fig. 1.16 Myelopathy, with a peripheral rim of necrosis, from the spinal cord of a baboon 'papio ursinus', following the experimental induction of ischaemia. The changes resemble those of degenerative myelopathy of the cervical cord of the elderly.

patent (Fig. 1.18B) and the dural sac assumes a 'rat's tail' form (De Villiers 1978). The fibrotic changes are irreversible, and the sensitive nerve structures are permanently embalmed (Symposium 1978).

Vertebrobasilar ischaemia

Syndromes resulting from obstructed bloodflow in the vertebral arteries and the basilar artery, into which the contents of the vertebral arteries flow, embrace an almost unlimited range. Not only are the primary areas of vertebrobasilar supply involved, but also those areas which normally derive their supply from the internal carotid arteries. The primary areas of vertebrobasilar supply are the occipital lobes of the cerebrum, the basal ganglia, the midbrain, the hindbrain (cerebellum, pons, medulla oblongata), the nuclei of the third to twelfth cranial nerves and the long fibre tracts of the spinal cord.

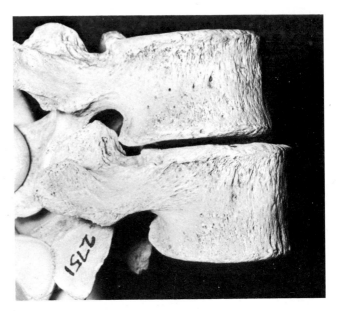

Fig. 1.17 Macerated lumbar vertebrae, demonstrating degenerative narrowing of the disc, local instability, and retrolisthesis. The neural canal is partially occluded, with compression of blood vessels and the spinal nerve.

The 'secondary' areas are those portions of the cerebrum which are normally supplied by branches of the internal carotid arteries, but which, under conditions of stress or disease, or in the presence of congenital anomalies of the cerebral circulation, depend upon the vertebrobasilar system for a back-up supply. This is accomplished through the medium of the arterial circle of Willis at the base of the brain, a system which allows for a direction of flow which may vary according to metabolic demands. Congenital anomalies would possibly account for some of the childhood cases of vertebrobasilar ischaemia reported elsewhere (Zimmerman et al 1978), and the accidents of spinal manipulative therapy in the 35- to 49-year-old age groups (Haldeman 1980).

The term 'ischaemia' requires definition. It is an absolute term and denotes a total cut-off of blood supply to a part. By the same token, it indicates an infarct of the region involved. A large infarct will result in permanent loss of function, but when only a small section is involved, the neighbouring structures may compensate. This phenomenon explains the degree of recovery which may follow upon a stroke. It is not limited to the brain, or even to the central nervous system. It involves all the vital organs of the human body and is nature's incomparable mechanism for preserving life. Sharrard's studies of motor recovery from acute poliomyelitis showed that when only 20% of motor neurons serving a muscle are spared, normal muscle strength can be regained (Sharrard 1955). A similar phenomenon is observed in other organs e.g., lungs and kidneys, where extensive resections of diseased parts may be safely conducted.

Vertebrobasilar ischaemia may result in death or in any

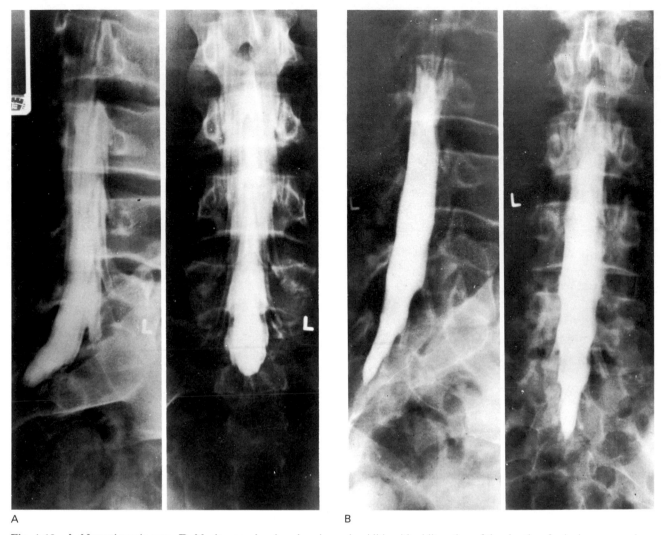

A   B

Fig. 1.18 A. Normal myelogram. **B**. Myelogram showing chronic arachnoiditis with obliteration of the sheaths of spinal nerves, and 'rat's tailing' of the distal extremity of the dural sac.

of a wide variety of syndromes and symptom complexes. They include hemiplegia, quadriplegia, Wallenberg's disease, cranial nerve palsies, vertigo, nausea, vomiting, blurring of vision, speech defects, sensory impairment, motor weakness, Brown–Sequard syndrome, headaches, loss of consciousness, drop attacks and many other neurological deficits (Haldeman 1980).

The circumstances under which vertebrobasilar ischaemia may develop include the following.

Spinal manipulative therapy (SMT)

Haldeman (1980) reviewed the literature and concluded that the complications occurred most commonly in the 35- to 49-year-old age groups and that 'the use of combined rotation and hyperextension during the adjustment is the common etiological factor'. In a series of 25 cases, there were 9 (36%) deaths, one occurring after only three hours, and one after as long as 58 days. Other complica-

tions are enumerated above, all serving to raise the question of whether provocative tests for threatened ischaemia, which are mandatory before SMT, are always dependable (see Ch. 26). They involve hyperextension and rotation of the neck with the patient supine, the shoulders on the couch and the head unsupported. They could be associated with the risk of a vascular accident, more especially in the presence of cervical spondylosis or of a history of a soft-tissue injury of the neck. Unsuspected factors such as congenital abnormalities and variations of the vertebral and internal carotid arteries may also precipitate complications.

The subclavian steal syndrome

First described by Contorni in 1960, subclavian steal involves a reversal of the direction of bloodflow in the vertebral artery, consequent upon occlusion of the first part of the subclavian artery, from atheroma or other factor. The ill effects on cerebral bloodflow may be trivial in the presence of an otherwise healthy arterial tree but are likely to be severe when the internal carotid artery on the ipsilateral side is already compromised, as from atheroma.

Congenital anomalies of the arteries of the central nervous system

Variations in the calibre of the vertebral, the carotid and other major blood vessels occur commonly and remain unsuspected until exposed to stress. Conditions of stress are essentially those imposed by trauma.

Dislocations and subluxations of the cervical spine

Occlusion of the vertebral artery with the symptoms of vertebrobasilar ischaemia has recently been recorded (Louw et al 1990). In their series of 12 cases with facet joint dislocation, either unilateral or bilateral, there were nine cases of vertebral artery occlusion on one or both sides, as demonstrated by intra-arterial, digital subtraction angiography. The average age of the group was 38.8 years, and the range was from 27 to 50 years. The symptoms were typical of vertebrobasilar ischaemia, and the recovery which followed in the entire series was attributable to the youth of the patients and the healthy state of the blood vessels other than those directly involved.

Soft-tissue injuries of the neck

The vertebral artery is exposed to disruptions of the intimal layer, followed by thrombosis which may or may not include the basilar artery. Symptoms persisting longer than three months suggest the need for bloodflow studies by sonar or magnetic resonance angiography, and an endarterectomy procedure to eliminate the obstruction.

Multiple injuries with surgical shock

The hypotension and reduction in cardiac output which are associated with surgical shock lead to a reduction in flow to the brain, which in the presence of a pre-existing vertebrobasilar or carotid shortcoming may have catastrophic effects.

The immediate effects include confusion or loss of consciousness or the ominous state of coma.

Brain damage resulting in an acquired form of cerebral palsy is the all too frequent end result of major trauma.

Hypertension and atheroma

Hypertension is a frequent cause of vertebrobasilar ischaemia, with cerebral symptoms or syndromes as a consequence. Precipitating factors include accidental and iatrogenic trauma.

Idiopathic thrombosis in the vertebrobasilar arterial system in young men (Graham & Adams 1972)

Two cases of the above, and eight cases of idiopathic thrombosis of the internal carotid artery were reported. Albeit rare, it may account for some of the disasters reported elsewhere.

Other pathological conditions associated with vertebrobasilar ischaemia include intrathoracic occlusion of the great vessels (Irvine et al 1963), aneurysm of the vertebral artery within the foramen transversarium (Haldeman 1980), haematoma formation following neck injury in a patient receiving anti-coagulant therapy, and atlanto-axial dislocation in the presence of rheumatoid arthritis of the neck. Congenital malformations of the neck associated with instability on the one hand, or rigidity (as in Klippel–Feil syndrome) on the other, are included in a list of causal or contributory factors of vertebral ischaemia.

The list is not complete, but the reality of a vascular deficiency involving the brain must be kept in mind by all practitioners supplying medical and supplementary medical services. The brain and the spinal cord together constitute a vital organ, and one which, because of its highly specialized construction, is also especially vulnerable.

DISCUSSION

Complaints and syndromes relating to the cervical and lumbar spine affect at least 80% of the general adult population. There is no more serious drain upon the health of the community, and indeed, upon the gross national product, the 'GNP'.

The spinal cord and the brain are the most highly developed structures, and totally dependent upon a superabundant blood supply. A thorough knowledge of the anatomy of cord circulation *is essential knowledge*, before embarking on the management of spinal complaints. Without this knowledge, the would-be healer is embarking upon 'uncharted seas'. Critical zones of vascular supply involve the spinal cord, the posterior spinal ganglia and the spinal nerves under conditions of health. In disease, whether due to congenital, traumatic, inflammatory, neoplastic, metabolic, degenerative or iatrogenic factors, the risk is enhanced. The vertebral arteries and the vertebrobasilar system demand special attention.

Reports of failures and disasters following upon treatment, whether manipulative or surgical, or invasive to a lesser degree, abound in the literature. Catastrophes continue to occur. '. . . the vascular arrangement from patient to patient may underlie not only the presentation of clinical features but also underlie some of the manipulation accidents . . . of which I now have a number of examples in the literature' (Grieve 1983).

The kinematics of the spinal column occupies a position of equal importance. Coupling of motions, a normal phenomenon, imposes limits upon the range to which single-direction motions may be forced. When these limits of motion are exceeded, the normal defence mechanism of the spinal column is undone. When the position is complicated by degenerative, spondylotic changes, the damage is more severe (White & Panjabi 1978).

The spine, the paravertebral joints, the intervertebral discs, the ligaments and muscles, and nervous tissue (including the autonomic nerve fibres and ganglia), fully merit the title 'The Central Axial Organ Spinal Column' of Schmorl and Junghanns (1959). These authors were the first to stress the spinal cord as an *organ* rather than a multisegmented structure. Support for the concept has been built up over the years, and it is realized today that involvement of a part of the spinal cord is involvement of the whole. In traumatic lesions, this phenomenon is clearly observed.

The basic concept of accuracy of diagnosis preceding treatment must be observed. Modern facilities include sonar studies of blood flow and magnetic resonance imaging, with clear resolution of soft tissues as well as bone. Without this facility, diagnosis may be no more than an educated guess. Treatment based upon a guess is empirical and 'taking a chance'. It is common knowledge that in more than 90% of spinal complaints, the diagnosis remains uncertain and the complaint resolves spontaneously within a few days. It follows that treatment is of two main types, firstly of the complaint, e.g. pain. No more than the judicious use of analgesics, combined with rest and selected physiotherapeutic administrations, will generally relieve. Secondly, where a more serious, organic condition exists, in which the vascular supply may be actually or potentially reduced, accuracy of diagnosis is essential as a prelude to active measures. Such active measures include local infiltrations, manipulation, and surgical procedures, all of which are associated with risk.

In this contribution, the complexities and the principles of cord supply are stressed and are related to the intimate anatomy of the part. It is hoped that a closer understanding not only of the physiological anatomy of the spine and the cord will result, but also that there will develop a closer understanding between the medical and the paramedical disciplines involved. In such an important, complicated and common cause of threatened health, an esoteric rather than a general therapeutic approach is desired. Continued research in the non-invasive and invasive techniques of management is necessary at both clinical and laboratory levels.

REFERENCES

Adamkiewicz A A 1881 (a) Über die mikroskopischen Gefässe des Menschlichen Rückenmarkes. Transactions of the 7th Session, International Medical Congress, vol I, pp 155–157
(b) Die Blutgefässe des Menslichen Rückenmarkes: I. Die Gefässe der Rückenmarkssubstanz, Situngsb.d.k. Akad.d.Wissensch., Math.-naturw. Cl.84: 469
(c) Die Blutgefässe des Menschlichen Rückenmarkes: II. Die Gefässe der Rückenmarksoberfläche, Situngsb. d.k.Akad.d.Wissensch., Math.-naturw. Cl.85: 101–130

Bailey R W, Sherk H H, Dunn E J, Fielding J W, Long D M, Ono K, Penning L, Stauffer E S 1983 The cervical spine. The Cervical Spine Research Society. Lippincott, Philadelphia

Batson O V 1940 The function of the vertebral veins and their role in the spread of metastases. Annals of Surgery 112: 138–149

Batson O V 1942 The vertebral vein system as a mechanism for the spread of metastases. American Journal of Roëntgenology and Radium Therapy 48: 715–718

Batson O V 1957 The vertebral vein system. Caldwell Lecture, 1956. American Journal of Roëntgenology Radium Therapy and Nuclear Medicine 78: 195–212

Bertrand G 1975 The 'battered root' problem. Orthopedic Clinics of North America. 6: 305

Brain Lord 1963 Some unsolved problems of cervical spondylosis. British Medical Journal 1: 771–777

Cauthen J C 1983 Lumbar spine surgery: indications, techniques, failures and alternatives. Williams & Wilkins, Baltimore

Contorni L 1960 Il circolo collaterale vertebro-vertebrale nella obliterazione dell' arteria subclavia alla sua origene. Minerva chir 15: 268

De Bakey M E, Crawford E S, Morris G G Jnr, Cooley D A 1961 Surgical considerations of occlusive disease of the innominate, carotid, subclavian and vertebral arteries. Annals of Surgery 154: 698–725

De Villiers P D 1978 The radiology of backache. In: Helfet A J, Greubell Lee D M (eds) Disorders of the lumbar spine. Lippincott, Philadelphia, pp 184–201

Dommisse G F 1972 The blood supply of the human spinal cord from birth. Thesis submitted to the University of Cape Town for the degree of Master of Surgery, Ch M

Dommisse G F 1973 The vascular system of the human spinal cord. Thesis submitted to the University of Pretoria for the doctoral degree M D, p 12

Dommisse G F 1974 The blood supply of the spinal cord. A critical vascular zone in spinal surgery. Journal of Bone and Joint Surgery 56B: 225–235

Dommisse G F 1975a Morphological aspects of the lumbar spine and lumbosacral region. Orthopedic Clinics of North America 6: 163–175

Dommisse G F 1975b Arteries and veins of the human spinal cord from birth. Churchill Livingstone, Edinburgh, p 2

Dommisse G F 1980a The arteries, arterioles, and capillaries of the spinal cord. Annals of the Royal College of Surgeons of England 62: 369–376

Dommisse G F 1980b The blood supply of the spinal cord. In: Owen R, Goodfellow J, Bullough P (eds) Scientific foundations of orthopaedics and traumatology. William Heinemann Medical Books, London, p 109

Dommisse G F, Gräbe R P 1978 The failures of surgery for lumbar disc disorders. In: Helfet A J, Gruebell Lee D M (eds) Disorders of the lumbar spine. Lippincott, Philadelphia, pp 202–216

Dommisse G F, Grobler L J 1976 Arteries and veins of the lumbar nerve roots and cauda equina. Clinical Orthopaedics and Related Research 115: 22–29

Dumanian A V, Frahm C J, Pascale L R, Teplinsky L L, Santschi D R 1965 The surgical treatment of the subclavian steal syndrome. Journal of Thoracic and Cardiovascular Surgery 50: 22–25

Dwyer A F, Schafer M F 1974 Anterior approach to scoliosis. Journal of Bone and Joint Surgery 56-B: 218–224

Editorial 1962 A new vascular syndrome — 'The subclavian steal'. New England Journal of medicine 265: 912

Eisenstein S M 1976 Measurements of the lumbar spinal canal in two racial groups. Clinical Orthopaedics and Related Research 115: 42–46

Farfan H S 1973 Mechanical disorders of the low back. Lee & Febiger, Philadelphia

Fried L C, Doppman J L, Di Chiro G 1970 Direction of blood flow in the primate cervical spinal cord. Journal of Neurosurgery 33: 325–330

Graham D I, Adams H 1972 'Idiopathic' thrombosis in the vertebrobasilar arterial system in young men. British Medical Journal 1: 26–28

Grieve G P 1983 Personal communication

Haldeman S 1980 Modern development in the principles and practice of chiropractic. Appleton-Century-Crofts, New York, pp 360–363

Herlihy W F 1947 Revision of the venous system: the role of the vertebral veins. Medical Journal of Australia 22: 661–672

Irvine W T, Luck R J, Sutton D, Walpita P R 1963 Intrathoracic occlusion of great vessels causing cerebrovascular insufficiency. Lancet i: 1177–1182

Jackson R 1953 The cervical syndrome. American Academy of Orthopaedic Surgeons. Instructional course lectures vol X, pp 65–90

Kadyi H 1889 Über die Blutgefässe des menschlichen Rückenmarkes; nach einer im XV. Bande der Denkschriften der Math.-naturw. Classe der Akademie der Wissenschaften in Kraksau erschienenen Monographie, aus dem polnischen Übersetzt vom Verfasser. Gubrynowicz & Schmidt, Lemberg, Poland

Kirkaldy-Willis W H, Hill R J 1979 A more precise diagnosis for low-back pain. Spine 4: 102–109

Lazorthes G, Gouaze A, Zadeh J O, Santini J J, Lazorthes Y, Burdin P 1971 Arterial vascularization of the spinal cord. Recent studies of the anastomotic substitution pathways. Journal of Neurosurgery 35: 253–262

Long D M 1983 Chronic cervical pain syndromes. In: Bailey R W, Sherk H H, Dunn E J, Fielding J W, Long D M, Ono K, Penning L, Stauffer E S (eds) The cervical spine. The Cervical Spine Society. Lippincott, Philadelphia, pp 424–429

Louw J A, Mafoyane N A, Small B, Neser C P 1990 Occlusion of the vertebral artery in cervical spine dislocations. Journal of Bone and Joint Surgery (Br) 72-B: 679–681

Nathan H, Feuerstein M 1974 Angulated course of spinal nerve roots. Journal of Neurosurgery 32: 349. Quoted in: Gregory P Grieve 1981 Common Vertebral Joint Problems. Churchill Livingstone, Edinburgh, p 56

Ogino H, Tada K, Okada K, Yonenobu K, Yamamoto T, Ono K, Namiki H 1983 Canal diameter, antero-posterior compression ratio, and spondylotic myelopathy of the cervical spine. Spine 8: 1–15

Ono K, Ota H, Tada K, Yamamoto T 1977 Cervical myelopathy secondary to multiple spondylotic protrusions. A clinicopathologic study. Spine 2: 109–125

Santchi D R, Frahm C J, Pascale L R, Dumanion A V 1966 Subclavian steal syndrome: clinical and angiographic considerations in 74 cases in adults. Journal of Thoracic and Cardio-vascular Surgery 51: 103–112

Schmorl G, Junghanns H 1959 The human spine in health and disease. Grune & Stratton, New York

Sharrard W J W 1955 The distribution of the permanent paralysis in lower limbs in poliomyelitis. Journal of Bone and Joint Surgery 37–B: 540–558

Smith R A, Estridge M N 1962 Neurologic complications of head and neck manipulations. Journal of the American Medical Association 182: 5: 528–531

Symposium 1978 Arachnoiditis — nomenclature, etiology and pathology. Spine 3: 21–92

White A A III, Panjabi M M 1978 The basic kinematics of the human spine: a review of past and current knowledge. Spine 3: 12–20

Zimmerman A W, Kumar A J, Gadoth N, Hodges F J III 1978 Traumatic vertebrobasilar occlusive disease in childhood. Neurology 28: 185–188

Zorab P A 1974 Scoliosis and muscle. SIMP research monograph number 4. Lippincott, Philadelphia

2. The dynamic central nervous system: structure and clinical neurobiomechanics

M. O. Shacklock   D. S. Butler   H. Slater

INTRODUCTION

'. . . . . I have found that many neurological disorders in which no mechanical component has ever been suspected do in fact have their origin in tension in the nervous tissue; we are at present, only just beginning to recognise the histological and neurophysiological sequelae of this tension' (Breig 1978)

The central nervous system (CNS) is a dynamic organ like muscle, joint or any other involved in movement. This view and the known pathophysiological consequences of altered nervous system mechanics are not well appreciated. The CNS possesses plastic and elastic properties and, as a consequence, it plays a major role in terms of dynamic responses to forces, as well as its familiar function of impulse transmission. We believe that the mechanical, electrical and physiological components of CNS function are often inseparable; thus, altered mechanics may affect changes in the CNS and ultimately the target tissues which the CNS innervates.

The nervous system as a whole is a mechanically and physiologically continuous structure from the brain to the end terminals in the periphery. This means that mechanical or physiological changes anywhere in the CNS can implicate the whole nervous system. This concept of mechanical and physiological continuity is applicable between the CNS and peripheral nervous system (PNS) and cannot be overemphasized. Assessment and treatment of patients with pain syndromes must take this into account.

The CNS consists of the brain and spinal cord and it is contained within the cranium and spinal canal. The canal bends, twists, lengthens and shortens with movement and, because the CNS is fixed to it at many sites, transmission of even minimal forces to, from and throughout the CNS is inevitable. The CNS responds dynamically to limb movement due to its mechanical continuity with the PNS.

In this chapter, the word 'neuraxis' is used synonymously with the CNS. This is a biomechanically descriptive term (Bowsher 1988) which highlights the fact that, despite many convolutions, the brain and spinal cord possess a longitudinal axis, like an axon, bone, or even the body as a whole. The neuraxis is surrounded by the meninges which are crucial in CNS mechanics, although their structure and functions are quite distinct from the former. The neuraxis, meninges and spinal canal are in fact individual partners forming a 'mechanical triad'. On that account, the aim of this chapter is to present the structure and mechanical behaviour of the neuraxis, with emphasis on clinical neurobiomechanics. We also hope that this chapter will facilitate an understanding of the neuraxis as a dynamic organ and its potential role in symptomatology.

STRUCTURE OF THE NEURAXIS, MENINGES AND SPINAL CANAL

The neuraxis

Microscopic structure

The neuraxis is composed of three basic elements: neurones, interstitial cells (including neuroglia) and connective tissue elements (including blood vessels).

The neurone is the cornerstone of the neuraxis. There are many types of neurone but they all have common features which are essential to normal neural function: reaction to stimuli, impulse transmission and stimulation of other target neurones or tissues. A neurone consists of a cell body and its projections. The projections include dendrites and an axon or nerve fibre, all of which extend from the cell body. Dendrites are generally shorter than the axon—which ranges from a fraction of an inch to several feet long. Axoplasmic fluid is transported bidirectionally inside the axon. This transport enables the movement of cytoskeletal elements, neurotransmitters and neuropeptides along the axon between the cell body and target tissues. In doing so, the neurone exerts influences on its target tissue (neurotrophism) and can respond to demands made by that tissue (neurotropism). When the spinal cord is cut, axoplasm tends to flow from the site of transection. Axoplasm also possesses thixotropic properties, that is, the tendency of fluid to flow increases with repeated movement (Baker et al 1977).

The neurone is surrounded by the plasma membrane of the neuroglial ('nerve glue') cell named the oligodendrocyte which is the equivalent of the Schwann cell in the myelinated peripheral nerve fibre. In forming the myelin sheath, the oligodendrocyte wraps its extended tongue-like membrane around the neurone. The neuroglial cell provides a metabolically balanced environment for the neurone and is situated between vasa nervora and the neurone itself.

Connective tissues provide the neuraxis with the necessary structural support, protecting the neurones from excessive stress. These tissues consist of the meninges and fine connective tissue fibres inside the neuraxis. Blood vessels accompany, and exchange metabolic products with, the neurones via the neuroglia.

On a microscopic level, body movement must affect the relationships between all the above components of the neuraxis. This conceivably results in physiological responses. Even minor trauma or mechanical changes may alter any of the functional or supportive components, resulting in physiological changes.

Brain

Possessing little connective tissue, the brain is a delicate gelatinous organ. It is contained and protected by the skull and meninges which are, from the brain outward, the pia, arachnoid and dura maters. The pia and arachnoid maters are separated by the subarachnoid space which is filled with cerebrospinal fluid (CSF). The brain effectively floats in the CSF and is protected by the shock-absorbing effects of the fluid. The ventricles of the brain are spaces in which CSF is held and they ultimately connect with the subarachnoid space, enabling CSF flow in and around the neuraxis.

The brain is divisible into three main parts, the forebrain, midbrain and hindbrain. These parts are joined and they form a mechanical continuum from the forebrain to the spinal cord, providing the mechanism for the brain tissue to respond to stresses exerted from the cord.

Spinal cord

The spinal cord is the caudal extension of the medulla oblongata and is that part of the neuraxis which is surrounded and protected by the spinal canal. The cord is shaped like a cylinder and is slightly flattened antero-posteriorly. It occupies the upper two-thirds of the spinal canal and terminates caudally as the conus medullaris between the first and second lumbar vertebrae. From here the nerve roots of the cauda equina pass caudolaterally to their intervertebral foramina. The conus, and therefore the neuraxis, is fixed caudally by the filum terminale to the coccyx, providing a mechanism for force transmission between the spine and lower end of the neuraxis.

Like the brain, the cord is surrounded by the meninges and is submerged in CSF. The cord is however uniquely suspended by a series of denticulate ligaments which are described later.

The neurones in the cord are arranged in tracts according to the area of the cord which they occupy, the posterior, lateral and anterior columns. The centrode of the spinal motion segment is about the middle of the intervertebral disc (Gertzbein et al 1985, 1986) which places the neuraxis behind this axis. This dorsal columns are situated further from the axis than the ventral columns; this causes differential loading of the columns during spinal movement (Breig 1978).

Meninges and blood vessels

Leptomeninges

The leptomeninges consist of the pia and arachnoid maters. The pia and arachnoid are continuous with each other and they line the outer surface of the neuraxis and the inner surface of the dura respectively. This configuration is similar to that of the pleura or the peritoneum. The pia is analagous to the visceral part, and the arachnoid to the parietal portion. The leptomeninges are effectively invaginated by the nerve rootlets, nerve roots and blood vessels. The neural structures, blood vessels and connective tissues in the subarachnoid space are thus covered by leptomeningeal cells.

The pia mater is closely associated with the neuraxis, following its contours as a mesh-like covering. It is separated from the neuraxis by the subpial collagen and, more deeply, the subpial space (Millen & Woollam 1961, Parke & Watanabe 1987, Nicholas & Weller 1988). The pia forms a septum on the lateral aspects of the spinal cord and continues laterally to contribute to the denticulate ligaments.

The arachnoid is a thin, loose and transparent membrane and its cerebral and spinal parts are continuous with each other. The arachnoid follows the nerve roots as far laterally as the intervertebral foramen (IVF). Here it is intimately associated with the roots and dura and commences its contribution to the connective tissue of the spinal nerve (McCabe & Low 1969, Sunderland 1974).

Dura mater

The dura mater is a layered tube which encloses the neuraxis, leptomeninges and CSF. It consists of collagen and elastic fibres and plays a major role in the protection of the neuraxis from mechanical and chemical insult.

The cerebral dura attaches to the cranium at the sutures and foramen magnum where it is continuous with the spinal dura.

The spinal dura is a cylindrical sac which attaches to the foramen magnum and posterior aspect of the bodies of C2 and C3. It extends caudally to the S1–2 level and provides laterally directed pouches which, more laterally, serve as protective sleeves for the nerve roots (Gardner et al 1975). The spinal dura is stronger longitudinally than transversely. It also possesses regional differences. The dorsal dura in the cervical region is thicker and stronger than other areas (Haupt & Stofpt 1978), whereas the ventral dura is stronger in the thoracic region. These characteristics may match the mechanical demands made on each region.

Blood vessels

The blood vessels cross the subarachnoid space where they are invested by the leptomeninges. The vessels then pass under a fan-like covering of pia in the subpial space for a short distance before they enter the neuraxis. The subpial space reflects into the neuraxis around the blood vessels, forming perivascular spaces (Hutchings & Weller 1986, Alcolado et al 1988, Nicholas & Weller 1988). In the spinal cord, the blood vessels are surrounded by a protective rhomboid network of fibres which is thought to be continuous with the subpial collagen. The fibres attach to the wall of the perivascular space by sling-like cords called perivascular retinaculae. The elasticity of such a sling is demonstrated by its retraction when it is cut.

The blood vessels are coiled and tortuous at rest but straighten out during elongation of the neuraxis. This feature helps maintain adequate circulation to the neural tissue during extremes of spinal posture (Fig. 2.1).

Innervation of the meninges

In the head, the sinuvertebral nerve (SVN) of the upper three cervical segments supplies the dura and blood

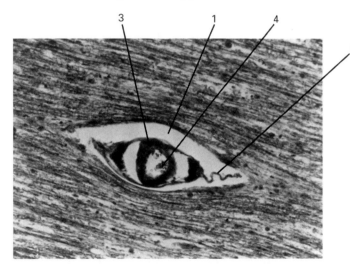

Fig. 2.1 The perivascular connective tissue arrangement: (1) perivascular space; (2) perivascular retinaculum; (3) blood vessel wall; (4) erythrocytes in the blood vessel. Note the bending and approximation of the nerve and glia cells around the blood vessel. (Reproduced from Breig 1978, with kind permission.)

vessels of the posterior cranial fossa, and the remaining dura and blood vessels are supplied by the trigeminal nerve. The SVN passes up through the foramen magnum to supply the dura of the posterior cranial fossa (Gardner et al 1975). The dura and blood vessels have been found to be pain-sensitive by Feindel et al (1960) who electrically and mechanically stimulated these structures in conscious patients. Manual pressure caused pain in the head and eyes and, notably, an occasional contralateral headache in the absence of ipsilateral pain. This is not surprising considering that, in some cases, the trigeminal nerve crosses the midline to anastomose with branches of its contralateral counterpart (Kimmel 1961). This supports the clinical observation that some head pain can respond to treatment of physical signs on the contralateral side.

The spinal dura also produces pain when noxiously stimulated (Falconer et al 1948, Smythe & Wright 1958, El Madhi et al 1981). It is innervated by the SVN after its main branch divides from the ventral ramus of the spinal nerve, returning into the spinal canal through the IVF. The SVN also receives a sympathetic contribution via the grey ramus communicans. The SVN turns around the base of the pedicle, supplying the periosteum, the nerve root sheath and epidural contents. Connective tissues of the dorsal roots and ganglia are supplied by fibres which originate in the dorsal root ganglia (Pedersen et al 1956, Hromada 1963, Edgar & Nundy 1966, Parke & Watanabe 1990).

The intrinsic dural nerve supply extends for as many as four levels rostral and caudal, eight levels in total. This gives the dura the potential to refer pain extrasegmentally to a wide variety of regions as described by Cyriax (1978). Nerve fibres cover the dorsal dura but do not quite reach the midline (Groen et al 1988). The nerve fibres in the dura are coiled and would straighten when the dura is elongated. This is probably a mechanical adaptation designed to protect the nerves from injury. Dural nerve fibres are more abundant in the cervical and lumbar regions—which may be in part why pain occurs more commonly in these regions than in the thoracic region (Cuatico et al 1988, Groen et al 1988) (Fig. 2.2).

Meningeal attachments

Leptomeningeal attachments

Filum terminale. The filum terminale protects the neuraxis from longitudinal stress by elongating and shortening appropriately. It provides limited caudal fixation of the neuraxis and it is a prolongation of the pia mater. Intrathecally, the thin, cord-like filum passes caudally from the base of the neuraxis to pierce and fuse with the dura at the apex of the dural sac. From here it continues to insert extrathecally into the posterior aspect of the coccyx as the filum of the dura (Williams et al 1989). In

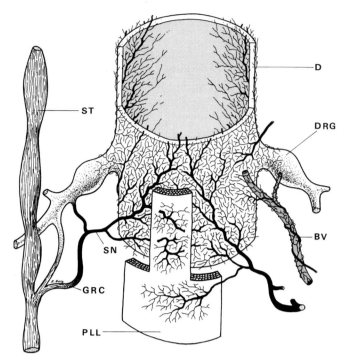

Fig. 2.2 Ventral aspect of the dural sac. Innervation of the dura by the sinuvertebral nerve. (BV) blood vessel; (D) dura; (DRG) dorsal root ganglion; (GRC) gray ramus communicantes; (PLL) posterior longitudinal ligament; (SN) sinuvertebral nerve; (ST) sympathetic trunk. (Reproduced from Butler 1991, with kind permission.)

cases where the filum terminale is too short or thickened, the cord can become tethered, causing increased tension and decreased mobility in the neuraxis (Pang & Wilberger 1982).

Denticulate ligaments. There are 20 to 22 pairs of denticulate ligaments. The tooth-like ligaments are derived from the septum of pia which runs in a continuous line along the entire lateral edge of the cord between the ventral and dorsal rootlets. Each ligament consists of a collagenous core of subpial collagen and a covering layer of leptomeningeal cells. The free lateral edges of these ligaments are concave and run as lateral projections to fuse with the dura and arachnoid between the sites of nerve root emergence from the dura. The uppermost ligament attaches to the rim of the foramen magnum and the lowest blends with the filum terminale (Stoltmann & Blackwood 1966, Noback & Demarest 1975). Because of the relative softness of the nerve rootlets, if they were to rub pathologically against the stronger denticulate ligaments, the nerve rootlets would logically be compromised (Fig. 2.3).

Intermediate leptomeningeal layer and subarachnoid trabeculae. In the thoracic and lumbar regions, a distinct intermediate leptomeningeal (ILL) is loosely attached to the inside of the arachnoid. It is more substantial dorsally than ventrally and, dorsally, it is reflected forward as a trabeculated septum. It crosses the

subarachnoid space to the posterior aspect of the cord where it spreads along the surface of the cord to engulf nerve rootlets and blood vessels. Thin isolated trabeculae also extend from the ILL across the subarachnoid space to the cord (Nicholas & Weller 1988). The ILL allows intermeningeal sliding, and consequently any tethering has the potential to alter movement of the neuraxis and meninges (NAM) and blood vessels. This could have clinical consequences.

Epidural attachments

Ventral attachments. In the cervical region, the dura is attached to the spinal canal wall and IVF by epidural and periradicular connective tissue (Sunderland 1974, Tencer et al 1985). In nine lumbar spines, Spencer et al (1983) found that these fibrous structures could be classified into three types. Although the anatomy of these structures was somewhat variable, generally, the midline attachments connected the dura to the posterior longitudinal ligament centrally. The intermediate attachments connected the anterolateral dura to the lateral part of the posterior longitudinal ligament. The foraminal and most lateral type attached the proximal portion of the nerve root sleeve to the posterior longitudinal ligament and periosteum of the inferior pedicle. The thickest of these tissues occurs at the L4–5 level (Blikra 1969, Parke & Watanabe 1990). Normally these structures limit neural movement, presumably as a protective function. However, in the presence of a space-occupying lesion, they may contribute to tension by preventing compensatory displacement of the neural tissues. If they were to become scarred, they may also cause excessive limitation of neural movement. These attachments are innervated and consequently have the potential to be a direct source of symptoms (Parke & Watanabe 1990).

Dorsal attachments. It has been documented that a dorsal connective tissue band connects the dorsal dura to the internal surface of the vertebral laminae and ligamenta flava in the midline (Blomberg 1986, Savolaine et al 1988). It is not as substantial as the ventral epidural attachments (Parkin & Harrison 1985) but would theoretically limit anterior displacement of the dura (Fig. 2.4).

Nerve rootlets

As collections of nerve fibres, ventral and dorsal nerve rootlets emerge from the spinal cord at the anterolateral and posterolateral aspects respectively. In their distal course they merge to form corresponding ventral and dorsal roots. In the cervical and lumbar regions, some rootlet fibres anastomose with nerve roots of other segments, providing significant normal variation in innervation (Pallie

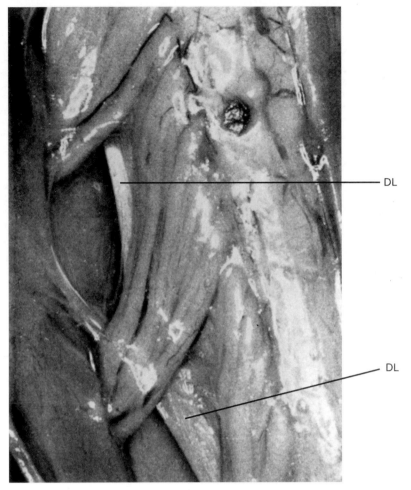

Fig. 2.3 Dorsal view of the spinal cord. A denticulate ligament (DL) emerges from underneath a dorsal nerve root in its lateral course to the arachnoid and dura. The nerve root contacts, and is bent around, the ligament. (Reproduced from Breig 1960, with kind permission.)

1959, Parke & Watanabe 1987, Marzo et al 1989), a point which is clinically important. In the lumbar region, the incidence of these anastomoses ranges from 11 to 30% (d'Avella & Mingrino 1979).

Nerve root complex

Nerve roots

The dorsal nerve root is sensory and the ventral is predominantly motor. Generally, the roots pass caudolaterally, crossing the subarachnoid space to the dural root sleeve. In the subarachnoid space they are covered by pia mater and bathed in CSF (Millen & Woollan 1961). Here the roots receive nutrition from both the CSF and intraneural blood vessels (Parke et al 1981, Rydevik et al 1984b, Parke & Watanabe 1985, Yoshizawa et al 1989). In the cervical region, the nerve roots are angled more horizontally whereas in the lumbosacral region they align more caudally. At the lateral end of their dural sleeve they

pierce the dura before merging into the spinal nerve at the IVF.

The ganglion of the dorsal root is a swelling created by the cell bodies of the dorsal root neurones and it is situated in the IVF (Sunderland 1974). In the irritated state, the ganglion becomes more mechanosensitive than usual (Howe et al 1976). After experimentally induced mechanical insult, the pressure in the ganglion rises and inflammatory changes occur, possibly resulting in a miniature compartment syndrome (Rydevik et al 1988). In this situation, appropriate movement of the nerve roots may pump away excess fluid and improve nutrition. This provides a rationale for passive movement of the DRG in some instances.

Nerve root–meningeal relationships

The nerve root complex (NRC) is a region where forces are transmitted between the neuraxis and spinal nerve.

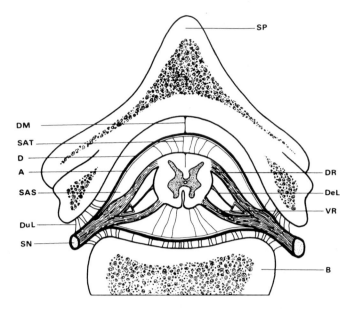

Fig. 2.4 Diagrammatic transverse section of the spinal canal, neuraxis, meninges and attachments. (B) vertebral body; (SP) spinous process; (D) dura; (A) arachnoid; (DR) dorsal root; (VR) ventral root; (DuL) dural ligament; (DeL) denticulate ligament; (DM) dorsomedian septum; (SAS) subarachnoid space; (SAT) subarachnoid trabeculae; (SN) spinal nerve. (Reproduced from Butler 1991, with kind permission.)

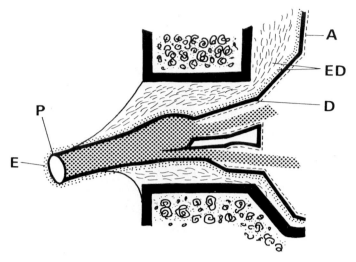

Fig. 2.5 Nerve root complex. (D) dura; (A) arachnoid; (ED) epidural tissue; (NR) nerve root; (E) epineurium; (P) perineurium. (Reproduced from Sunderland 1978, with kind permission.)

The lateral end of the complex is also an area of transition between nerve root and spinal nerve. Here, tension induced by limb and spinal movements passes along the peripheral and spinal nerves and NRC to the dura. The dura distributes the tension along its surface and to the denticulate ligaments (Luttges et al 1986). This mechanism prevents the concentration of neural tension with body movement. Compromise of this protection may lead to neural consequences.

The NRC consists of the two nerve roots, DRG, spinal nerve and connective tissue coverings, (Sunderland 1974). The nerve roots exit the dural theca through openings in the root pouch, one for each root. Here, the dura and arachnoid form a 'bitubular sleeve' which surrounds the roots. In the lumbar region, intrathecally, the lumbosacral nerve roots are freely mobile but, extrathecally, they are attached to the dura and arachnoid by fine strands of connective tissue (Spencer et al 1983). As the neural structures pass through the IVF, the epidural tissue, dura and arachnoid of the nerve root become continuous with the connective tissues of the spinal nerve (McCabe & Low 1969, Haller et al 1972, Sunderland 1974, Spencer et al 1983) (Fig. 2.5).

The NRC is attached to the boundaries of the IVF by connective tissue which permits limited movement (Sunderland 1974, Spencer et al 1983). This is an area of relative fixation around which the NRCs pivot during rostrocaudal sliding of the dura. Altered stresses in this region could compromise the NRC.

Nerve root angulation

Variations in the course of some roots and their sleeves are common, particularly between the levels of C3 and T9 where the roots are angled upward in 76% of cases. Here, intradurally the nerve roots are directed caudolaterally but, because the entrance of the dural sleeve is situated below the level of the IVF, the sleeve and nerve root must bend upward to enter the IVF. This bend can create as much as a 30° angle. The incidence of such angulation increases from C3 to T3 and decreases to T9, usually reaching its maximum at the T2 and T3 levels. As it passes to the IVF, the NRC hooks downward and around the inferior pedicle (Reid 1960a, Nathan & Feuerstein 1970).

Nerve root anomalies

In the lumbosacral region, nerve root anomalies provide variation of innervation and may at times mechanically disadvantage the NRC. Intrathecally, this occurs when a nerve root of one segment joins one of a neighbouring segment before reaching the dural sleeve. Extrathecally, three types of anomalies have been found at operation and in cadavers. In the first type, two nerve roots are housed in one nerve root sheath (conjoined), which then divides just in time to provide a sheath for each root in its correct IVF. Alternatively, the nerve root sheath of one level emerges from the dural sac very close to one of a level below. This results in the sleeve and root coursing too horizontally to the IVF. The second type occurs when two nerve roots exit through a single IVF, leaving one IVF empty. The third type occurs when a nerve root and sleeve anastomose with those of another level. Anomalies may occur in combinations and their incidence has been reported to be between 8.5 and 14% (Keon-Cohen 1968, Hasue et al

1983, Neidre & Macnab 1983, Kadish & Simmons 1984, Kikuchi et al 1986).

Spinal and radicular canals

Spinal canal

The spinal canal is formed by the series of all the vertebral foramina together with the intervening soft-tissue structures. It contains the neuraxis, meninges and epidural structures. The canal is made up of three main surfaces. The anterior surface, or floor, is formed by the posterior surfaces of the vertebral bodies, intervertebral discs and overlying posterior longitudinal ligament. In the lumbar region, the posterior surface of the vertebral bodies is curved anteriorly in the sagittal plane, forming indentations to which the dural sac apposes (Larsen 1985). The lateral surface of the canal is formed by the medial surface of the pedicles whilst the posterior wall, or roof, is provided by the vertebral laminae and ligamenta flava.

The spinal canal possesses regional differences. In the cervical region, the canal is shaped like a rounded triangle, the narrowest point being at C6. In the thoracic region, the canal is more circular and is the least capacious at T6. This means that there is less room to accommodate its contents in the presence of a space-occupying lesion. The lumbar spinal canal provides a progressive transition from an ovoid shape in the upper lumbar region to a triangular shape of the sacral region (Eisenstein 1980).

The epidural region is between the dura and the canal wall and contains fat, the epidural attachments and blood vessels (Dommisse 1975, Parkin & Harrison 1985). Movement of the neuraxis would logically cause sliding of, and changes in pressure and tension in, these blood vessels and attachments.

Radicular canal

The radicular or nerve root canal is a region where the nervous system is particularly susceptible to compromise. It contains the NRC, SVN, blood vessels and fat (Parkin & Harrison, 1985). The canal is formed by the lateral part of the spinal canal and the IVF. The parapedicular part of the canal consists of the gutter on the medial surface of the vertebral pedicle (Fig. 2.6). This bony gutter faces postero-inferomedially and forms an interface against which the NRC runs in contact (Crock 1981, Vital et al 1983, Bose & Balasubramaniam 1984, Lassale et al 1984). Here, and at the IVF, the neural structures can be compromised by conditions, such as thickening of the ligamentum flavum, swelling of the posterior intervertebral joint, osteophytes, disc protrusion, lateral canal stenosis and fibrosis (Frykholm 1951a,b, Epstein et al 1962, Macnab 1971, Epstein et al 1973, Edgar & Park 1974). Like the spinal canal, the radicular canal is relatively unyielding and forms an important interface to the nervous system.

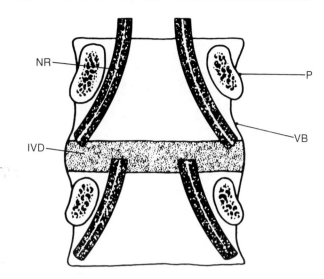

Fig. 2.6 Ventral view of the radicular canal. (N) nerve root; (P) pedicle; (IVD) intervertebral disc; (VB) vertebral body. (Reproduced from Bogduk & Twomey 1987, with kind permission.)

THE NEURAXIS, MENINGES AND SPINAL MOVEMENT

Definitions

Stress: a force or load.

Strain: a change in dimensions of a body produced by a stress, expressed as a percentage of the change in relation to the original unloaded dimension, e.g. a nerve 10 cm long stretched to 11 cm has strained 10%.

Elastic: capable of returning to the original unloaded dimensions.

Response of the neuraxis and meninges to loading

Nerve fibres

When the spinal cord is elongated, the neuroglia, neurones and pial fibres straighten and the distance between the nerve fibres decreases (Fig. 2.7). During longitudinal compression, as in spinal extension, they fold, causing the space between the nerve fibres to expand again (Breig 1978, p 15, Figs 31–36). Stretching the myelinated nerve fibre causes a reduction in the cross-section of its axoplasm and myelin sheath. Transient stretching of peripheral nerves, while not damaging axonal continuity, temporarily decreases conduction (Denny-Brown & Doherty 1945, Gray & Ritchie 1954); presumably this also occurs in the neurones of the spinal cord. The point of failure of the axon in pathological stretching is surprisingly not at the node of Ranvier; instead, it is in short myelinated sections where the normally varying diameter of the nerve fibre is small. Sectioning causes the fibre ends to retract, demonstrating that the axon possesses elastic properties (Schneider 1952).

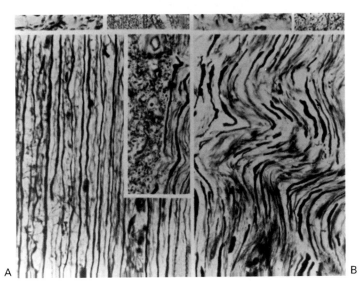

Fig. 2.7 Nerve fibres in the spinal cord. **A**. Flexion. **B**. Extension. (Reproduced from Breig 1978, with kind permission.)

Meninges

The rhomboid nature of the collagen fibres in the pia and arachnoid enables a concertina action by changes in angle between fibres at their intersection. When they are fully tensioned they are more parallel and aligned in the direction of tension, resisting elongation more strongly than in earlier stages of deformation (Fig. 2.8). If compression is added the pial fibres eventually buckle, causing the cord and meninges to wrinkle (Breig 1978, p. 15). The dura possesses plastic and elastic qualities which enable it to resist strongly stresses which could harm the neuraxis (Tunturi 1977).

The filum terminale is the most extensible of the meningeal structures and, when it is pulled caudally, it elon-

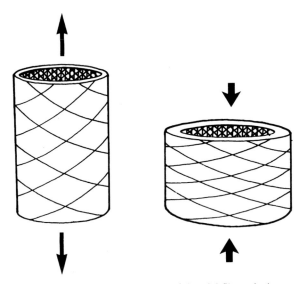

Fig. 2.8 Diagrammatic representation of the pial fibres during neuraxis loading. **A**. Elongation. **B**. Compresion. (Reproduced from Butler 1991, with kind permission.)

gates in a linear fashion (Tani et al 1987). Its main role is to protect the neuraxis from excessive longitudinal stress. It does this by effectively taking up slack in positions of low tension and 'paying-out' to let the neuraxis move in positions of high tension (Tunturi 1977).

When the dura or spinal nerves are pulled during limb or spinal movements most of the force to the neuraxis is transmitted by the denticulate ligaments. This protects the nerve rootlets from excessive stress.

When a space-occupying lesion in the floor of the spinal canal pushes dorsally on the dura, the denticulate ligaments restrict compensatory displacement of the cord and therefore contribute to adverse mechanical tension. Sectioning of the ligaments increases cord movement, relieves tension and can improve neurological changes (Kahn 1947, Cusick et al 1977).

Blood vessels

The blood vessels and nervous tissue of the neuraxis respond simultaneously to stress. The longitudinal vessels, which are normally tortuous and slack at rest, straighten and become narrower with tension. The transverse arteries shorten and wrinkle because the nerve fibres are drawn closer together as the anteroposterior diameter of the cord decreases. This is particularly evident in the posterior columns. Although narrowing of vessels occurs with tension, some resistance to this is provided by the collagen fibres of the perivascular retinaculae (Breig et al 1966, Breig 1978, pp 16, 35).

Spinal position and movement

Spinal movements change the length and shape of the spinal canal and, by virtue of its attachments, the neuraxis is pulled from all directions. This causes the neuraxis to change shape and position in the canal. Gravity also affects the neuraxis (Breig 1978).

Neutral

The neutral position is midway between full flexion and extension and incorporates the spinal curves. In this position, the neuraxis is relaxed in the spinal canal when, in the cervical region, as much as 1 cm lift of the dura from the canal floor is possible (Reid 1960b, Breig et al 1966). The blood vessels and perivascular spaces are quite patent, permitting blood, lymphatic and CSF flow. The axons take up a wavy form in preparation for increased tension with spinal movement (Breig 1978).

Flexion

In full flexion the spinal canal elongates up to 97 mm. The greatest average lengthening in the cervical and lumbar regions (28 mm each) and the least occurs in the thoracic region (3 mm) (Louis 1981). The neuraxis accommodates these dimensional variations by changing its own shape without adverse effects on conduction (Fig. 2.9).

Brain. The increase in distance between the top of the skull and the arch of the atlas with neck flexion causes the brain substance to be pulled taut. The medulla and cord move forward in the canal where the denticulate ligaments and their rostral extensions prevent them from contacting the odontoid process. Flexion also causes the floor of the fourth ventricle of the brain to elongate (Breig & El-Nadi 1966). This suggests that movement of the neuraxis could cause change in CSF flow which may in turn affect the distribution of some neurotransmitters and hormones.

Spinal neuraxis and meninges. The spinal NAM accommodate canal elongation and bending in several ways: ventral displacement, lengthening/strain, axial sliding and angulation of nerve roots.

Ventral displacement. The fact that the neuraxis must take the shortest route between the ends of the canal causes it to bowstring forward. Ventral pressure of the cord on the canal floor causes the cord to take up the shape of the floor and reduce in cross-sectional area. As a result, the dorsal nerve rootlets contact the denticulate ligaments (Breig 1978, p 22) (Fig. 2.3).

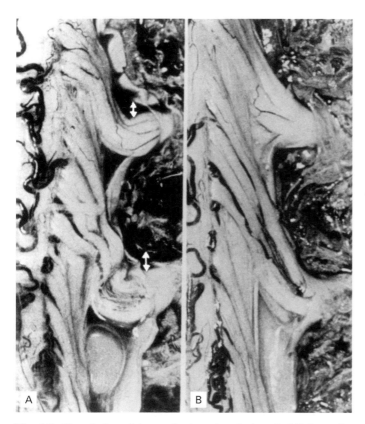

Fig. 2.9 Dorsal view of the cervicothoracic spinal cord while housed on the floor of the spinal canal. **A**. Extension. **B**. Flexion. (Reproduced from Breig 1978, with kind permission.)

Strain/elongation. Strain is considered on two levels: along the entire length of the neural tract and segmentally.

Along the whole length of the neuraxis, axial tension is generated by the neuraxis being pulled from both ends due to the lengthening of the spinal canal with flexion. This occurs by dural fixation at the foramen magnum pulling the pons and medulla rostrally. The filum terminale counters this by pulling caudally from the sacrum. This causes the neuraxis to lengthen, unfolding first, then stretching. Tension generated by the elongation is transmitted as far as the midbrain rostrally and the sciatic nerve caudally (Smith 1956, Breig 1978, Louis 1981). Tightening of the denticulate ligaments is caused rostrocaudally by the elongation of the neuraxis and transversely by the outward pull of the NRCs (Breig & El-Nadi 1966, Adams & Logue 1971).

On a segmental level, strain of neural segments is not uniform. It is higher in areas where the joint sagittal mobility is greater, that is, the low cervical and low lumbar regions. The dural strain at the L5–S1 segment reaches 30%, whereas at L1–2 it is only 15%. In the cervical region, strain peaks at C5–6. The nerve roots also undergo strain during flexion, the greatest of which is 16% in the S1 root (Louis 1981).

Stretching of peripheral nerves decreases intraneural microcirculation (Lundborg & Rydevik 1973). It is likely that the same phenomenon occurs in nerve roots which suggests that nutrition of the nerve roots would fluctuate during normal daily activities. In the case of even a minimally mechanically compromised nervous system, prolonged or repeated spinal flexion, as in gardening or lifting, may cause nerve root circulation to be decreased. This provides a theoretical mechanism of ischaemic neural injury. Symptoms arising from such a primary neural lesion could cause secondary alterations in neuromuscular and joint function. Prolonged neural ischaemia causes inflammatory changes (Denny-Brown & Doherty 1945, Eames & Lange 1967, Hoyland et al 1989), which if in the nerve root, could produce acute symptoms. Frykholm (1951a,b) has found at surgery that such primary changes can occur in the NRC without disc or joint pathology.

Axial sliding. At the L4 spinal level, flexion causes the dura to move up to 3 mm caudally, whereas at L5, there is rostral displacement of 3 mm. The same occurs at C6 where there is caudal sliding at C5 and rostral movement at C6–7. Inevitably there is convergence of the NAM relative to the spinal canal at the low lumbar and low cervical levels, in spite of the NAM simultaneously lengthening. There is also rostral movement above T5 and caudal movement below, causing a relative divergence from the mid thoracic region (Louis 1981) (Fig. 2.10).

The idea of 'relative displacement' is the key point in understanding this paradoxical lengthening and convergence of the neural structures. Lengthening occurs within the nervous system itself whereas movement takes place

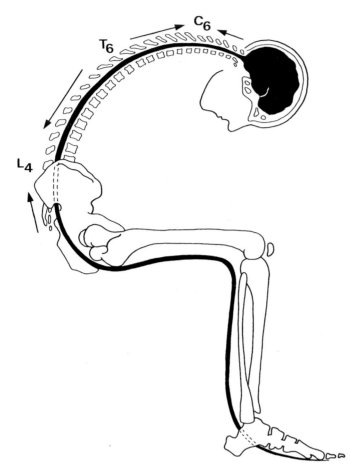

Fig. 2.10 Relative convergence of the neuraxis and meninges toward C5–6 and L4–5, with simultaneous divergence from T7. (Reproduced from Butler 1991, with kind permission.)

between the neural structures and the interface (spinal canal).

When the neuraxis moves, for example rostrally, it moves relative to its interface. Conversely, if the interface moves rostrally around the stationary neuraxis, opposite relative displacement occurs. Alternatively, a component of the interface (e.g. a vertebra) can move with the neural tissues so there is little or no nett displacement at that point, yet both have moved. Each of these phenomena can occur simultaneously at different levels of the spine, so at some segments different movements can occur, while at other levels no relative movement takes place.

In flexion, little relative movement occurs at levels where high segmental mobility enables the vertebral movements to approximate those of the neural structures, namely in the low cervical and low lumbar regions. Greater amounts of relative movement occur where the vertebral movement does not 'keep up' with neural movement, i.e. levels of low segmental mobility. Furthermore, at one level the neural structures can move caudally, yet two levels below they can move rostrally, giving the effect of convergence toward the same point in the canal; never-

theless, the NAM have still lengthened. Above the level of convergence, the posterior vertebral surface moves upward more than the neural structures (as they are fixed caudally by the filum terminale), causing caudal relative displacement. Below the level of convergence, the posterior vertebral surface does not move rostrally as far as the neural structures, causing rostral relative movement (Smith 1956, Reid 1960b, Adams & Logue 1971, Louis 1981).

Nerve root angulation. From extension to flexion, the nerve roots above L3 angle more horizontally whereas those below angle more vertically. This is caused by the dural theca converging toward the L4–5 segment. The nerve roots are forced to pivot about their point of fixation in the IVF. The same occurs in the cervical region, where nerve root angulation follows the dural convergence toward C5–6. The thoracic roots also respond to the axial displacement of the dura away from T6, that is, the T1–6 roots align more vertically and those at T7–12 become more horizontal (Louis 1981).

Extension

From neutral to hyperextension, the spinal canal shortens by as much as 38 mm, causing the neuraxis to slacken and increase in cross-sectional area. Transverse folds also form on its posterior aspect. These folds are most pronounced in the cervical region, where the variations in canal length between flexion and extension are the greatest. In extension, the NAM are loose and can be easily moved passively in all directions. Due to the lack of tension the nerve roots droop away from their neighbouring pedicles (Breig & Marions 1963). Normally, intraneural microcirculation is better in extension than in flexion.

In the lumbar region, extension causes the spinal canal to narrow at the interspaces. This results from inward bulging of the intervertebral discs and ligamenta flava and crowding of the facets (Penning & Wilmink 1981). The cross-section of the IVF also decreases which, if already compromised, could cause a clamping action on the NRC (Panjabi et al 1983). All these effects ultimately cause an increase in the lumbar CSF pressure (Hanai et al 1985).

Lateral flexion

Lateral flexion of the lumbar spine causes the neural structures on the concave side to loosen and those on the convex side to tighten (Fig. 2.11). Tension, causing NRCs on the convex side to be drawn into contact with their adjacent pedicles, is transmitted to the ipsilateral sciatic nerve (Breig 1978, p 161). This corresponds well with the findings of Lew & Puentedura (1985) who, in young asymptomatic subjects, found that contralateral lateral flexion sensitized the response to the straight-leg-raise (SLR) test.

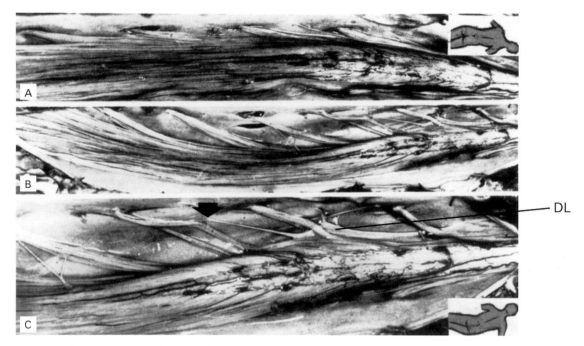

Fig. 2.11 Dorsal view of the lower cord and cauda equina with the dura and arachnoid opened. (DL) denticulate ligament. **A**. Right side lying, positioned in right lateral flexion. The cord, nerve roots and denticulate ligaments become taut on the convex (left) side. **B, C**. Positioned in left lateral flexion, releasing tension in the left neural structures, permitting them to droop with gravity to the downward (right) side. (Reproduced from Breig 1978, with kind permission.)

The cross-sectional area of the IVF is reduced in ipsilateral lateral flexion, thus reducing space for the NRC (Panjabi et al 1983).

Clinically, acute antalgic trunk listing may be caused by a neural lesion. Increased neural tension is likely to cause an anti-tension posture of ipsilateral lateral flexion. This can be distinguished from a disorder of pincer action on the NRC at the IVF which might produce a contralateral lateral flexion posture.

Gravity

The neural structures displace toward the downward side of the spinal canal with gravity, as in right-side lying, when they droop to the right side of the canal (Fig. 2.11). Extension relaxes them and increases the displacement. Flexion tightens them, pulling them back into the centre of the canal (Jirout 1959, 1963, Breig & El-Nadi 1966, Breig 1978).

The total amount of dorsoventral excursion of the neuraxis from prone to supine varies with spinal level, the most occurring at C1 (up to 8.5 mm) (Jirout 1959).

To sensitize an examination or treatment technique, positioning the patient relative to gravity is sometimes useful. An example of this is when a patient describes hip pain when lying on the ipsilateral side with downward leg straightened. This could be interpreted as a unilateral SLR with the neural structures drooping to the downward side of the canal. If the desire is to provoke symptoms, it may be necessary to treat the patient in this position.

Limb movement

Straight-leg-raise test

Standard test. The SLR pulls caudally on the sciatic nerve. This force is transmitted to the neuraxis via the low lumbar and sacral NRCs which move caudolaterally at their IVF (Fig. 2.12). The S1 NRC displaces as much as 10 mm (O'Connell 1943, Charnley 1951, Goddard & Reid 1965). Tension is transmitted as far rostrally as the midbrain (Smith 1956). The SLR also pulls the contralateral NRCs toward the moved limb (Louis 1981).

Sensitizing movements. Medial hip rotation sensitizes the SLR by pulling caudolaterally on the lumbosacral nerve roots (Breig & Troup 1979). Also, hip adduction sensitises the response to the SLR (Sutton 1979), suggesting that the neural structures are stressed with this movement. Ankle dorsiflexion pulls distally on the tibial nerve which alters neural tension during the SLR (Smith 1956). This has been confirmed at surgery when this movement produced movement in the lumbosacral nerve roots while the leg was in the SLR position (Macnab 1988 pers comm). Plantar flexion/inversion of the ankle and foot pulls distally on the common peroneal nerve (Kopell & Thompson 1976, p 45). In cases of intrapelvic division of the sciatic nerve into its peroneal and tibial portions,

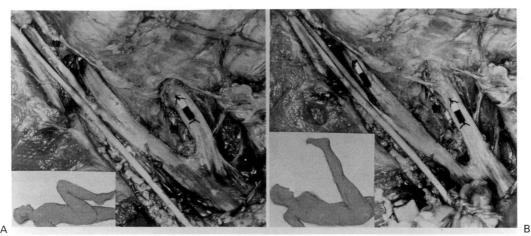

Fig. 2.12   The L4 and 5 spinal nerves as they exit their respective intervertebral foramen and join the lumbosacral trunk. The markers indicate the amount of neural movement at the foramen. **A**. Hip/knee flexion. **B**. Hip flexion/knee extension. (Reproduced from Breig 1978, with kind permission.)

the forces of this movement may concentrate in the L5 nerve root. Positioning the subject in side-lying also affects the response to the SLR and this is thought to be due to the effects of gravity on the neural structures (Miller 1987).

The slump test, which combines the effects of spinal flexion, SLR and dorsiflexion, is used clinically to detect pathomechanics throughout the length of the nervous system (Maitland 1986). Clinically, it is sometimes necessary to sensitize the test by adding combinations of the above movements.

Upper limb tension test

Movements of the upper limb cause movement of the neuraxis in the cervical region (Smith 1956). This occurs via pulling on the peripheral nerves of the upper limb when, due to mechanical continuity, the effects are transmitted to the neuraxis (Sunderland 1974, McLellan & Swash 1976, Elvey 1980). The upper limb tension test (ULTT) combines specific movements which stress the neural structures and is described in Chapter 44 in this volume. The NRCs slide laterally in their IVF, causing the neuraxis and opposite NRC to be pulled toward the test limb. The ULTT therefore mechanically affects the contralateral neural structures. This could be the reason that positioning the opposite upper limb in the ULTT position causes changes in the response to the ULLT of the test side (Rubenach 1985). The SLR can also produce changes in the response to the ULTT (Bell 1987). This may be explained by the caudal movement induced by the SLR being transmitted rostrally to the cervical region.

Prone knee bend

Via the femoral nerve, the prone knee bend (PKB) pulls caudally on the L2, 3 and 4 nerve roots. The femoral nerve passes in front of the hip joint and innervates the muscles of the anterior thigh. Stretching of these muscles with knee flexion stresses the femoral nerve and proximal part of the saphenous nerve (O'Connell 1946). The test is used clinically to detect pathomechanics of the above neural structures. Spinal flexion can be added to the PKB causing further stress in the mid-lumbar nerve roots.

Clinical neurobiomechanics

Link between mechanics and physiology

Dynamic function of the neuraxis is adaptive and protective by preventing the concentration of abnormal stress, allowing normal physiological function. Examples of the failure of the protective mechanisms are demonstrated by tethering or a space-occupying lesion which alters tension, movement and nutrition of the neuraxis, causing conduction and metabolic changes (Cusick et al 1977, Yamada et al 1981). If a tethering structure is sectioned or the neuraxis positioned in low tension, stress, metabolism and conduction can be normalized (Breig 1970, Pang & Wilberger 1982).

Although the concept of normal mechanics preventing the onset of pathophysiological changes is helpful, it is also somewhat inadequate and must be taken further. We hypothesize that regular and appropriate movement of the neuraxis is necessary for optimum physiological function. This is supported by the fact that the vascular supply of the cord is affected by spinal movements (Breig et al 1966). Also, regular stress would theoretically improve nutrition and removal of metabolic waste products. This stress may also help improve or maintain the physical properties of the meninges, since various connective tissues respond beneficially to regular loading (Salter et al 1980).

Axoplasmic flow may also be affected with regular movement in two ways: by the effect of movement on the thixotropic properties of axoplasm and alterations in circulation of the neuraxis with spinal movement. Regular movement 'thins out' axoplasm and improves its flow characteristics. Intraneural microcirculation and axoplasmic flow are decreased in peripheral nerve compression (Rydevik et al 1980, Dahlin & McLean 1986). Therefore even slight mechanical changes in the neuraxis, especially if maintained, might alter impulse traffic to, and trophic effects on, the target tissues. This may further induce functional and structural changes in the target tissues, especially if prolonged. In not considering mechanical treatment of the neuraxis in physiotherapy, treatment of the target tissues alone may in some cases lead to ineffective or temporary results.

The neuraxis and meninges as a mechanical continuum

The neuraxis forms a continuous tract which transmits forces throughout. Loading in one area readily affects local and remote areas in two ways: by transmission of tension and by movement.

Movement of the NAM is a response to tension. It serves to transmit and offset tension and occurs not only in relation to its neighbouring structures, but also between neurones, meninges and blood vessels. If movement is reduced at a point along the tract, for example by an epidural adhesion, tension is no longer offset or dissipated adequately and neural mechanics are altered. Such alterations in mechanics are named pathomechanical changes.

The continuous nature of both the CNS and PNS means that pathomechanics in one area ultimately affect mechanics in other areas. The role of the PNS should not be underestimated. Altered mechanics in a peripheral nerve may lead to changes in the neuraxis. Due to this continuity of the nervous system, for any one tension test to be ideal, all the others must be perfect as well.

The neuraxis in a balanced state

At rest, the neuraxis is in a 'state of readiness for movement'. In this situation, the forces tending to retract and distend it are balanced. The inherent elasticity of the cord and dura is demonstrated by the fact that a gap appears at the site of a transection (Tunturi 1977, Breig 1978, p. 84, Fig. 67). The tendency of the cord and dura to retract is countered in two ways. In the transverse plane it is achieved by the outward pull of the NRCs on the dura via the denticulate ligaments to the cord. Longitudinally, the rostral pull of the brain in the skull and dural fixation at the foramen magnum oppose the caudal pull of the filum terminale. The pull exerted by the filum terminale is relatively small and is exceeded by that of the NRCs and denticulate ligaments. In the dog, by far the greatest retracting effect is via the dura which, when sectioned, causes as much as 20 mm separation of the two ends

(Tunturi 1977). The meningeal attachments and NRCs act as 'guy ropes' which suspend the neuraxis. When spinal movement occurs these 'guy ropes' respond elastically, altering their own dimensions to provide the correct amount and rate of neuraxis movement. This complex protective mechanism is designed to prevent stresses from peaking, allowing optimum neural function.

Mechanical interface

The NAM are surrounded by structures which form a mechanical interface. These structures consist of the cranium and the spinal and radicular canals. The interface is less yielding than the neural tissues which means that when one of its components (e.g. intervertebral disc) fails or alters shape or function, it may ultimately affect neural mechanics and produce symptoms.

Intraneural and extraneural effects

On hypothetical and mechanical bases, some clinical symptom responses to tension tests can be categorized as intraneural or extraneural in origin.

Intraneural effects are more those of tension and cause mechanical effects along the length of the neural structures. An example of this is the opposing rostrocaudal counter-pull caused by simultaneous neck flexion and SLR. Intraneural changes would be indicated by a central lumbar pain which increases when passive neck flexion is added to the SLR which already provoked the pain. In this case, the neural structures are pulled caudally in the spinal canal with the SLR. Then the rostral counterpull induced by neck flexion further increases tension.

The nervous system is relatively mobile, enabling the relationships between its mechanical interface and the nervous system to change. These effects are called extraneural. An example of this is sliding of the neural structures in the spinal canal. A clinical manifestation of extraneural changes would be a lumbar pain which decreases on adding neck flexion to the SLR test. Initially the neural structures are drawn caudally by the SLR, inducing extraneural effects. These effects are reversed by neck flexion which draws the neural structures back up in the canal, reducing the pain.

Structural differentiation

Structural differentiation is used to differentiate between neural and non-neural sources of symptoms. It relies on the principle that the neural structures can be moved in the absence of mechanical effects occurring in the neighbouring non-neural structures. An example of this is when a lumbar pain is altered with head movements when the non-neural structures in the lumbar region are theoretically not moved. The fact that movement of the lumbar neural structures occurs with neck flexion and the non-neural structures remain stationary establishes that the pain is neurogenic. Movement of the local neural structures must always be achieved by movement of a remote part. Another example is when a lumbar pain is altered by dorsiflexion of the foot. Stress is transmitted to the lumbosacral neural structures via the tibial and sciatic nerves, whilst no movement of the non-neural structures occurs. The establishment of the neurogenic nature of symptoms cannot be achieved if the local non-neural structures are moved during the test. An example of a test which fails to be frankly positive would be a lumbar pain which changes with the standard SLR but not with neck flexion or dorsiflexion. Because this movement also moves the lumbar spinal (non-neural) structures (Bohannon et al 1985), the symptoms are not proven to be exclusively neural. Dorsiflexion or neck flexion must be used to confirm the neurogenic nature of the symptoms.

Common sites of compromise

There are sites where the neural structures are particularly susceptible to compromise. The low cervical region has greater mobility than other areas, causing correspondingly greater neural strain locally. In the T5–7 region, the spinal canal leaves little space for adaptive displacement of the neutral tissues, hence we believe that this area is predisposed to developing dysfunction and creating or maintaining disorders of other regions. At the L4–5 level, the neural structures are particularly strongly tethered by dural ligaments which may prevent them adapting to stress (Blikra 1969). This is also an area of relatively high segmental mobility, causing further increased neural strain. Peripherally, the median, ulnar and radial nerves are commonly affected at the elbow and wrist. In the lower limb, the sciatic nerve can be entrapped between the two heads of piriformis. The common peroneal nerve can be compromised at the head of the fibula and the posterior tibial and superficial peroneal nerves are sometimes jeopardized at the ankle (Mackinnon & Dellon 1988). These sites of compromise occur partly because of the anatomy of the interfacing tissue. The most common means of compromise is due to the surrounding non-neural tissues permitting too little space for the nerve, or the interface is too firm and, during repetitive overuse, may cause damage and inflammation in the nerve. These sites are relevant to assessment and treatment of the NAM because pathomechanics or pathophysiology in either the CNS or PNS may affect the other. It is therefore necessary to test the mechanics of the PNS in order to understand the mechanics of the NAM.

Pathomechanics

Tethering. We have classified tethering into two types: longitudinal and adjacent. Although both types ultimately lead to alterations in longitudinal tension, each acts in a different way.

Longitudinal tethering occurs within one component of the nervous system and acts along the neural structure. Examples are an adhesion inside a nerve root or a scarred axon (Denny-Brown & Brenner 1944, Fahrni 1966). In this case, the tethered structure is unable to elongate normally and this causes stress to pass further along the tract than normally (Tani et al 1987), resulting in a 'domino effect'. Normal neural tissues possess such plastic qualities that, if a nerve or nerve root is tightened surgically, within several weeks it adapts by stretching almost to its original length (Dawbin et al 1947, Bora et al 1980). Due to scarring, the neural tissues may not adequately adapt to changes in tension (Millesi 1986).

Adjacent tethering occurs between a nervous system element and its neighbouring structure, limiting sliding between the two. It can occur between neural and non-neural structures, for example the dura and the spinal canal. Tethering can also exist between two neural structures; for example, it may be interneuronal, interfascicular or intermeningeal, reducing movement of the neural structure relative its neighbour. This diminishes the dissipation of tension beyond the point of tethering, causing tension to concentrate between the area of tethering and the site of stress application. An example of this is neck flexion when the dura is experimentally attached to the canal wall in the low cervical region. The upper cervical neural segments undergo greater strain than when the dura is not fixed (Adams & Logue 1971). Conversely, if the subject were to bend from the lumbar region, applying caudal tension, stress would concentrate between the lumbar region and point of tethering in the cervical region. In cases of tethering, mobilization of the neural structures may be warranted.

Abnormal joint mechanics. We believe that the motion segment has an enormous impact on neural mechanics. If a joint which is normally very mobile becomes stiff, neural dynamics will logically change. These changes may be a result of the inability of the motion segment to 'keep up with' neural movement, causing an unaccustomed increase in relative neural movement. The unaccustomed movement could irritate the local neural structures. Local inflammatory changes and fibrosis could follow, further altering neural mechanics (Frykholm 1951a,b, Murphy 1977). These changes could spread rostrally, caudally, or even contralaterally. Excessive or uncontrolled movement of a motion segment may also alter neural dynamics with the potential for symptoms. An aim of treatment would be to optimize intersegmental mobility.

Pincer action. Pincer action occurs when the neural structures are compressed transversely from opposing directions. Examples of this are spinal stenosis or a swollen posterior intervertebral joint pressing against a nerve root in the enclosed IVF (Epstein et al 1962, 1973). In this situation sliding of the NRC would be limited. This pincer action also causes alterations in intraneural microcirculation leading to decreased intraneural venous return, oedema and ultimately fibrosis (Rydevik et al 1984a, Olmarker et al 1988, Hoyland et al 1989, Yoshizawa et al 1989).

Mechanically disadvantaged nervous system. Intrinsically, anatomical variation of a neural structure could theoretically alter its mechanics. The mechanical alteration would depend on the nature of the anomaly. For example, a nerve root which travels in an anomalous fashion around a pedicle would be limited in movement, possibly causing symptoms (Macnab 1971). Two roots in one IVF would be predisposed to compromise by pincer action. The joining of two NRCs by intersegmental cross-bridging may cause tension in one nerve root to transmit more readily to the other.

There may be a range of anomalies from minor to extreme forms of dysraphism which would produce a similar range in mechanical disadvantage. Clinically, this may present as an atypical pattern of symptoms. Anomalies could also produce discrepancies between the degree and chronicity of symptoms and the severity of injury.

Extrinsically, pathology of a mechanical interface structure (disc, joint, canal size or shape) may chronically disadvantage the neural structures.

Detection of anomalous anatomy is performed radiographically and by surgical exploration. Presumably many cases of this type of mechanical disadvantage remain undetected, since many spinal problems are not prolonged, negating the need for detailed investigation.

Hypermobility of the nervous system and redundant nerve roots. If a restraining structure, for example a denticulate ligament or the filum terminale, is overstretched, its ability to resist tension is decreased, causing stress to be transmitted further along the tract than normally. This is confirmed when caudal stress is applied to the filum terminale before and after section of nearby denticulate ligaments. After sectioning, strain of the higher cord segments increases (Tani et al 1987). This type of problem might occur in cases of severe trauma, for example a motor vehicle accident.

Redundant nerve roots of the cauda equina have been reported in the neurosurgery literature whereby some roots are considerably longer than normal. The extra length causes the nerve roots to fold in the dural theca. The folds cause outward pressure on the intact dura and, when the dura is opened and the nerve roots unravelled, can measure up to 12 cm in length. Pathology may result from overbending of the roots as they are accommodated in a relatively fixed space. The roots in this instance can act as a space-occupying lesion which can occlude the subarachnoid space (Cressman & Pawl 1968, Schut & Groff 1968, Fox 1969). This could theoretically cause alterations in nutrition of the nerve roots.

Spread of pathomechanical changes. Pathomechanical changes can spread from a primary source to remote areas, particularly those which are vulnerable due to the local anatomy.

An experimental example of the spreading of pathomechanical changes occurs when the caudal tip of the filum terminale is pulled caudally. The lower segments of the cord elongate less than when the same stress is applied higher at the lower end of the cord (Tani et al 1987). If this tethering were to occur in the lumbar region, neural tension during activities involving flexion would be transmitted further rostrally, altering neural mechanics in the cervical region. Because the remote (cervical) structure is undergoing increased strain, it has the potential to become symptomatic. The remote structures could also remain subclinically compromised due to the original lumbar disorder. The remote disorder could progress to produce symptoms with the possibility of considerable latency between the two problems. In addition to an initial and apparently resolved disorder, a further injury (even minor) may provide the catalyst for symptoms to develop in the remote area (in the cervical region in this case). Remote pathomechanical changes may also induce a previously subclinical condition to become symptomatic. We have noticed that a lumbar disorder which produces positive tension tests frequently precedes the recurrence of an old and, to date, quiescent cervical disorder. Patients sometimes report that familiar neck pains have returned since the onset of an acute low-back problem. Such findings have been reported in the literature as 'brachialgic sciatica' (Torkildsen 1956).

In the PNS, the supinator (posterior interosseous nerve), carpal (median nerve) and cubital tunnels and Guyon's canal (ulnar nerve) are common sites of nerve entrapment. Susceptibility in the lower limb also occurs at the piriformis muscle and peroneal and tarsal tunnels. These neuropathies occur due to the lack of space available to the nerve and the rigid nature of the fibrous or osseous interface. Involvement of a peripheral nerve may lead to a centrally directed spread of symptoms due to altered mechanics and physiology.

The concept of the spread of pathomechanical changes highlights the importance in clinical examination of detailed questioning in relation to past history and spread of symptoms. It also provides a rationale for the treatment of local and remote disorders, supporting the treatment of an old subclinical problem which may maintain or predispose to a more recent one. These disorders may be detectable with detailed examination and, if treated, may be prevented.

SUMMARY

It is inadequate to view the neuraxis as being provided merely with means of protection and adaptation to body movements. It is in fact a dynamic organ which never stops moving. Even when we breath our brain changes its dimensions (Bergland 1985). We believe that not only does the neuraxis depend on optimum mechanical function, but it needs regular, appropriate movement in order to function at a physiological optimum. The link between mechanics and physiology is strong; thus, in physiotherapy, mobilization of the nervous system has enormous potential.

The whole nervous system is mechanically and physiologically continuous throughout and should not be viewed as a segmental structure. This means that mechanical and physiological changes in one area are inevitably linked to, and may cause changes in, other areas. The view that there is no such thing as a discrete lesion of the nervous system provides a rationale to assess and treat areas far remote from the region which would have traditionally been considered to be the source of the symptoms. Due to mechanical continuity, for one tension test to be ideal, so must all the others. We also believe that the PNS plays a role in neuraxis dynamics and it should not be overlooked.

The NAM are encased in a relatively unyielding mechanical interface formed by the cranium and spinal and radicular canals. During normal daily activities forces are transmitted throughout all these structures, and changes in one ultimately affect the others.

The neural structures are vulnerable to insult. Intrinsically, they may be inherently insufficient by anatomical variation and, extrinsically, the more rigid mechanical interface can cause compromise by altering neural dynamics.

Neurogenic symptoms have frequently been considered to be secondary to pathology of an interfacing structure, for example an intervertebral disc, osteophyte or posterior intervertebral joint. Findings at surgery have demonstrated that there need not be such pathology and, based on known pathology and biomechanics, primary neural lesions have the potential to cause clinical presentations similar to those which have been considered to be discogenic (e.g. acute trunk list) or arthrogenic.

Spinal flexion reduces intraneural microcirculation, and neural tissues respond to prolonged or severe ischaemia with inflammation. It is logical that activities involving repetitive and/or sustained flexion have the potential to cause primary inflammatory or ischaemically-based neural lesions. Neurones exert impulse based and trophic influences on their target tissues. Mechanically induced alterations in neuronal function may cause structural and functional changes in these target tissues (muscle, bone, joint, viscera). Thus, many somatic disorders could ultimately be related to neural pathology, and treatment may be ineffective or only temporarily beneficial unless it addresses the neural component.

To facilitate an understanding of some important clinical aspects in relation to the NAM, the relevant structure and clinical neurobiomechanics have been presented. This chapter complements Chapters 44 and 50, which cover assessment and treatment.

REFERENCES

Adams C, Logue V 1971 Studies in cervical spondylotic myelopathy. 1. Movement of the cervical roots, dura and cord, and their relation to the course of the extrathecal roots. Brain 94: 557–568

Alcolado R, Weller R, Parrish E, Garrod D 1988 The cranial arachnoid and pia mater in man: anatomical and ultrastructural observations. Neuropathology and Applied Neurobiology 14: 1–17

Baker P, Ladds M, Rubinson K 1977 Measurement of the flow properties of isolated axoplasm in a defined chemical environment. Journal of Physiology 269: 10p–11p

Bell A 1987 The upper limb tension test—bilateral straight leg raising—a validating manoeuvre for the upper limb tension test. Proceedings of the Fifth Biennial Conference of the Manipulative Therapists Association of Australia, Melbourne

Bergland R 1985 The fabric of mind. Penguin Books, Australia

Blikra G 1969 Intradural herniated lumbar disc. Journal of Neurosurgery 31: 676–679

Blomberg R 1986 The dorsomedian connective tissue band in the lumbar epidural space of humans: an anatomical study using epiduroscopy in autopsy cases. Anesthesia and Analgesia 65: 474–752

Bogduk N, Twomey L 1987 Clinical anatomy of the lumbar spine. Churchill Livingstone, Edinburgh

Bohannon R, Gajdosik R, Le Veau B 1985 Contribution of pelvic and lower limb motion to increases in the angle of passive straight leg raising. Physical Therapy 65: 474–476

Bora F, Richardson S, Black J 1980 The biomechanical responses to tension in peripheral nerve. Journal of Hand Surgery 5: 21–25

Bose K, Balasubramanium P 1984 Nerve root canals of the lumbar spine. Spine 9: 16–18

Bowsher D 1988 Introduction to the anatomy and physiology of the nervous system. Blackwell, Oxford

Breig A 1960 Biomechanics of the central nervous system. Almqvist and Wiksell, Stockholm

Breig A 1970 Overstretching of and circumscribed pathological tension in the spinal cord—a basic cause of symptoms in cord disorders. Journal of Biomechanics 3: 7–9

Breig A 1978 Adverse mechanical tension in the central nervous system. Almqvist and Wiksell, Stockholm

Breig A, El-Nadi A 1966 Biomechanics of the cervical spinal cord. Acta Radiologica Diagnosis 4: 602–624

Breig A, Marions O 1963 Biomechanics of the lumbosacral nerve roots. Acta Radiologica 1 Diagnosis 1141–1160

Breig A, Troup J 1979 Biomechanical considerations in the straight-leg-raising test. Spine 4: 242–250

Breig A, Turnbull I, Hassler O 1966 Effects of mechanical stresses on the spinal cord in cervical spondylosis: a study on fresh cadaver material. Journal of Neurosurgery 25: 45–56

Butler D 1991 Mobilisation of the nervous system. Churchill Livingstone, Edinburgh

Charnley J 1951 Orthopaedic signs in the diagnosis of disc protrusion with special reference to the straight leg raising test. Lancet 1: 186–192

Cressman M, Pawl R 1968 Serpentine myelographic defect caused by a redundant nerve root. Journal of Neurosurgery 28: 391–393

Crock H 1981 Normal and pathological anatomy of the lumbar spinal nerve root canals. Journal of Bone and Joint Surgery 63B: 487–490

Cuatico W, Parker J, Pappert E 1988 An anatomical and clinical investigation of spinal meningeal nerves. Act Neurochirurgica 90: 139–143

Cusick J, Ackmann J, Larson S 1977 Mechanical and physiological effects of dentatotomy. Journal of Neurosurgery 46: 767–775

Cyriax J 1978 Dural pain. Lancet, 2: 919–921

Dahlin L, McLean G 1986 Effects of graded experimental compression on slow and fast axonal transport in rabbit vagus nerve. Journal of the Neurological Sciences 72: 19–30

d'Avella D, Mingrino S 1979 Microsurgical anatomy of lumbosacral spinal roots. Journal of Neurosurgery 51: 819–823

Dawbin W, Cole D, Glasgow G 1947 cited by Falconer et al 1948

Denny-Brown D, Brenner C 1944 The effect of percussion of nerve. Journal of Neurology, Neurosurgery and Psychiatry 7: 76–95

Denny-Brown D, Doherty M 1945 Effects of transient stretching of peripheral nerve. Archives of Neurology and Psychiatry 54: 116–129

Dommisse G 1975 Morphological aspects of the lumbar spine and lumbosacral region. Orthopedic Clinics of North America 6: 163–175

Eames R, Lange L 1967 Clinical and pathological study of ischaemic neuropathy. Journal of Neurology, Neurosurgery and Psychiatry 30: 215–226

Edgar M, Nundy S 1966 Innervation of the spinal dura mater. Journal of Neurology, Neurosurgery and Psychiatry 29: 530–534

Edgar M, Park W 1974 Induced pain patterns on passive straight-leg raising in lower lumbar disc protrusion. Journal of Bone and Joint Surgery 56B: 658–667

Eisenstein S 1980 The trefoil configuration of the lumbar vertebral canal. Journal of Bone and Joint Surgery 62B: 73–77

El Mahdi M, Latif F, Janko M 1981 The spinal nerve root innervation and a new concept of the clinicopathological interrelations in back pain and sciatica. Neurochirurgia 24: 137–141

Elvey R 1980 Brachial plexus tension tests and the pathoanatomical origin of arm pain. In: Idczak R (ed) Aspects of manipulative therapy. Lincoln Institute of Health Sciences, Melbourne

Epstein J, Epstein B, Lavine L 1962 Nerve root compression associated with narrowing of the lumbar spinal canal. Journal of Neurology, Neurosurgery and Psychiatry 25: 165–176

Epstein J, Epstein B, Lavine L et al 1973 Lumbar nerve root compression at the intervertebral foramina caused by arthritis of the posterior facets. Journal of Neurosurgery 39: 362–369

Fahrni W 1966 Observations on straight leg-raising with special reference to nerve root adhesions. Canadian Journal of Surgery 9: 44–48

Falconer M, McGeorge M, Begg A 1948 Observations on the cause and mechanism of symptom-production in sciatica and low-back pain. Journal of Neurology, Neurosurgery and Psychiatry 11: 13–26

Feindel W, Penfield W, McNaughton F 1960 The tentorial nerves and localization of intracranial pain in man. Neurology 10: 555–563

Fox J 1969 Redundant nerve roots in the cauda equina. Journal of Neurosurgery 30: 74–75

Frykholm R 1951a The mechanism of cervical radicular lesions resulting from friction or forceful traction. Acta Chirurgia Scandinavica 102: 93–98

Frykholm R 1951b Cervical nerve root compression resulting from disc degeneration and root-sleeve fibrosis. Acta Chirurgia Scandinavica 160 (suppl): 1–149

Garner E, Gray D, O'Rahilly R 1975 Anatomy, 4th edn. W B Saunders Company, Toronto

Gertzbein S, Seligman J, Holtby R et al 1985 Centrode patterns and segmental instability. Spine 10: 257–261

Gertzbein S, Seligman J, Holtby R et al 1986 Centrode characteristics of the lumbar spine as a function of segmental instability. Clinical Orthopaedics and Related Research 208: 48–51

Goddard M, Reid J 1965 Movements induced by straight leg raising in the lumbo-sacral roots, nerves and plexus, and in the intrapelvic section of the sciatic nerve. Journal of Neurology, Neurosurgery and Psychiatry 28: 12–18

Gray J, Ritchie J 1954 Effects of stretch on single myelinated nerve fibres. Journal of Physiology 124: 84–99

Groen G, Baljet B, Drukker J 1988 The innervation of the spinal dura mater: anatomy and clinical implications. Acta Neurochirurgica 92: 39–46

Haller F, Haller A, Low F 1972 The fine structure of cellular layers and connective tissue space at spinal nerve root attachments in the rat. American Journal of Anatomy 133: 109–124

Hanai K, Kawai K, Itoh Y et al 1985 Simultaneous measurement of intraosseous and cerebrospinal fluid pressures in lumbar region. Spine 10: 64–68

Hasue M, Kikuchi S, Sakuyama Y, Ito T 1983 Anatomic study of the interrelation between lumbosacral nerve roots and their surrounding tissues. Spine 8: 50–58

Haupt W, Stofpt E 1978 Über die Dehnbarkeit und Reibfestigkeit der Dura Mater Spinalis des Menschen. Verhandlungen Anatomische Gesellschaft 72S: 139–144

Howe J, Calvin W, Loesser J 1976 Impulses reflected from dorsal root ganglia and from focal nerve injuries. Brain Research 116: 139–144

Hoyland J, Freemont, Jayson M 1989 Intervertebral foramen venous obstruction, a cause of periradicular fibrosis? Spine 14: 558–568

Hromada J 1963 On the nerve supply of the connective tissue of some peripheral nervous system components. Acta Anatomica 55: 343–351

Hutchings M, Weller R 1986 Anatomical relationships of the pia mater to cerebral blood vessels in man. Journal of Neurosurgery 65: 316–325

Jirout J 1959 The mobility of the cervical spinal cord under normal conditions. British Journal of Radiology 32: 744–751

Jirout J 1963 Mobility of the thoracic spinal cord under normal conditions. Acta Radiologica A Diagnosis 1: 729–735

Kadish L, Simmons E 1984 Anomalies of the lumbosacral nerve roots. Journal of Bone and Joint Surgery 66B: 411–416

Kahn E 1947 The role of the dentate ligaments in spinal cord compression and the syndrome of lateral sclerosis. Journal of Neurosurgery 4: 191–199

Keon-Cohen B 1968 Abnormal arrangement of the lower lumbar canal and first sacral nerves within the spinal canal. Journal of Bone and Joint Surgery 50B(2): 261–265

Kikuchi S, Hasue M, Nishiyama K, Ito T 1986 Anatomic features of the furcal nerve and its clinical significance. Spine 11: 1002–1007

Kimmel D 1961 Innervation of spinal dura mater and dura mater of the posterior cranial fossa. Neurology 11: 800–809

Kopell H, Thompson W 1976 Peripheral entrapment neuropathies. Robert Kreiger Publishing Company, Malabar, Florida

Larsen J 1985 The posterior surface of the lumbar vertebral bodies. Spine 10: 50–58

Lassale B, Morvan G, Gottin M 1984 Anatomy and radiological anatomy of the lumbar radicular canals. Anatomia Clinica 6: 195–201

Lew P, Puentedura E 1985 The straight leg raise test and spinal posture. Proceedings of the Fourth Biennial Conference of the Australian Manipulative Therapists Association, Brisbane

Louis R 1981 Vertebroradicular and vertebromedullar dynamics. Anatomia Clinica 3: 1–11

Lundborg G, Rydevik B 1973 Effects of stretching the tibial nerve of the rabbit. Journal of Bone and Joint Surgery 55B: 390–401

Luttges M, Stodieck L, Beel J 1986 Postinjury changes in the biomechanics of nerves and nerve roots in mice. Journal of Manipulative and Physiological Therapeutics 9: 89–98

McCabe J, Low F 1969 The subarachnoid angle: an area of transition in peripheral nerve. Anatomical Record 164: 15–34

Mackinnon S, Dellon A 1988 Surgery of the Peripheral Nerve. Thieme, New York

McLellan D, Swash M 1976 Longitudinal sliding of the median nerve during movements of the upper limb. Journal of Neurology, Neurosurgery and Psychiatry 39: 566–570

Macnab I 1971 Negative disc exploration. Journal of Bone and Joint Surgery 53A: 891–903

Maitland G D 1986 Vertebral manipulation, 5th edn. Butterworths, London

Marzo J, Simmons E, Kallen F 1989 Intradural connections between adjacent cervical spinal roots. Spine 12: 964–968

Millen J, Woollam D 1961 On the nature of the pia mater. Brain 84: 514–520

Miller A 1987 Neuromeningeal limitation of straight leg raising. Proceedings of the Fifth Biennial Conference of the Manipulative Therapists Association of Australia, Melbourne

Millesi H 1986 The nerve gap. Hand Clinics 2: 651–663

Murphy R 1977 Nerve roots and spinal nerves in degenerative disk disease. Clinical Orthopaedics and Related Research 129: 46–60

Nathan H, Feuerstein M 1970 Angulated course of spinal nerve roots. Journal of Neurosurgery 32: 349–352

Neidre A, Macnab I 1983 Anomalies of the lumbosacral nerve roots. Spine 8: 294–299

Nicholas D, Weller R 1988 The fine anatomy of the human spinal meninges. Journal of Neurosurgery 69: 276–282

Noback C, Demarest R 1975 The human nervous system, 2nd edn. McGraw-Hill, Tokyo

O'Connell J 1943 Sciatica and the mechanism of the production of the clinical syndrome in protrusions of the lumbar intervertebral discs. British Journal of Surgery 30: 315–327

O'Connell J 1946 The clinical signs of meningeal irritation. Brain 69: 9–21

Olmarker K, Rydevik B, Holm S 1988 Intraneural edema formation in spinal nerve roots of the porcine cauda equina induced by experimental, graded compression. Proceedings of the Thirty-Fourth Annual Meeting of the Orthopaedic Research Society, Atlanta, Georgia

Pallie W 1959 The intersegmental anastomoses of the posterior spinal rootlets and their significance. Journal of Neurosurgery 16: 188–196

Pang D, Wilberger J 1982 Tethered cord syndrome in adults. Journal of Neurosurgery 57: 32–47

Panjabi M, Takata K, Goel V 1983 Kinematics of lumbar intervertebral foramen. Spine 8: 348–357

Parke W, Watanabe R 1985 The intrinsic vasculature of the lumbosacral spinal nerve roots. Spine 10: 508–515

Parke W, Watanabe R 1987 Lumbosacral intersegmental epispinal axons and ectopic ventral nerve rootlets. Journal of Neurosurgery 67: 269–277

Parke W, Watanabe R 1990 Adhesions of the ventral lumbar dura: an adjunct source of discogenic pain? Spine 15: 300–303

Parke W, Gammell K, Rothman R 1981 Arterial vascularization of the cauda equina. Journal of Bone and Joint Surgery 63A: 53–62

Parkin I, Harrison G 1985 The topographical anatomy of the lumbar epidural space. Journal of Anatomy 141: 211–217

Pedersen H, Blunck C, Gardner E 1956 The anatomy of lumbosacral posterior rami and meningeal branches of spinal nerves (sinu-vertebral nerves). Journal of Bone and Joint Surgery 38A: 377–391

Penning L, Wilmink J 1981 Biomechanics of lumbosacral dural sac. Spine 6: 398–408

Reid J 1960a Ascending nerve roots. Journal of Neurology, Neurosurgery and Psychiatry 23: 148–155

Reid J 1960b Effects of flexion–extension movements of the head and spine upon the spinal cord and nerve roots. Journal of Neurology, Neurosurgery and Psychiatry 23: 214–221

Rubenach H 1985 The upper limb tension test—the effect of position and movement of the contralateral arm. Proceedings of the Fourth Biennial Conference of the Manipulative Therapists Association of Australia, Brisbane.

Rydevik B, McLean S, Sjöstrand J, Lundborg G 1980 Blockage of axonal transport induced by acute, graded compression of the rabbit vagus nerve. Journal of Neurology, Neurosurgery and Psychiatry 43: 690–698

Rydevik B, Brown M, Lundborg G 1984a Pathoanatomy and pathophysiology of nerve root compression. Spine 9: 7–15

Rydevik B, Holm S, Lundborg G 1984b Nutrition of spinal nerve roots: the role of diffusion from the cerebrospinal. Proceedings of the Annual Meeting of the Orthopaedic Research Society, Atlanta, p 276

Rydevik B, Myers R, Powell H 1988 Tissue fluid pressure in the dorsal root ganglion. Proceedings of the Annual Meeting of the Orthopaedic Research Society, Atlanta, p 135

Salter R, Simmons D, Malcolm B et al 1989 The biological effect of continuous passive motion on the healing of full-thickness defects in articular cartilage. Journal of Bone and Joint Surgery 62A: 1232–1251

Savolaine E, Pandya J, Greenblatt S, Conover S 1988 Anatomy of the human lumbar epidural space: new insights using CT epidurography. Anesthesiology 68: 217–220

Schneider D 1952 Die Dehnbarkeit der markhaltigen nervenfaser des froshces in abhängigkeit von funktion und struktur. Z Naturforsch 7: 38–48 cited by Breig 1978, p 27

Schut L, Groff R 1968 Redundant nerve roots as a cause of complete myelographic block. Journal of Neurosurgery 28: 394–395

Smith C 1956 Changes in length and position of the segments of the spinal cord with changes in posture in the monkey. Radiology 66: 259–265

Smythe M, Wright V 1958 Sciatica and the intervertebral disc. Journal of Bone and Joint Surgery 40A: 1401–1418

Spencer D, Irwin G, Miller J 1983 Anatomy and significance of fixation of the lumbosarcal nerve roots in sciatica. Spine 8: 672–679

Stoltmann H, Blackwood W 1966 An anatomical study of the role of the dentate ligaments in the cervical spinal canal. Journal of Neurosurgery 24: 43–46

Sunderland S 1974 Meningeal–neural relations in the intervertebral foramen. Journal of Neurosurgery 40: 756–776

Sunderland S 1978 Nerves and nerve injuries. Churchill Livingstone, Edinburgh

Sutton J 1979 The straight leg raising test. Unpublished graduate diploma thesis, University of South Australia

Tani S, Yamada S, Knighton R 1987 Extensibility of the lumbar and sacral cord: pathophysiology of the tethered spinal cord in cats. Journal of Neurosurgery 66: 116–123

Tencer A, Allen B, Ferguson R 1985 A biomechanical study of thoracolumbar spine fractures with bone in the canal. Spine 10: 741–747

Torkildsen A 1956 Lesions of the cervical spinal roots as a possible source of pain simulating sciatica. Acta Psychiatrica Scandinavica 31: 333–344

Tunturi A 1977 Elasticity of the spinal cord and dura in the dog. Journal of Neurosurgery 47: 391–396

Vital J, Lavignolle B, Grenier N et al 1983 Anatomy of the lumbar radicular canal. Anatomia Clinica 3: 141–151

Williams P, Warwick R, Dyson M, Bannister L 1989 Gray's anatomy, 37th edn. Churchill Livingstone, Edinburgh

Yamada S, Zinke D, Sanders D 1981 Pathophysiology of 'tethered cord syndrome'. Journal of Neurosurgery 54: 494–503

Yoshizawa H, Kobayashi S, Kubota L 1989 Effects of compression on intraradicular blood flow in dogs. Spine 14: 1220–1225

3. The use of diagnostic ultrasound to observe intersegmental joint motion in the neck

S. A. Ruston

This study was instigated to investigate the possible use of standard diagnostic ultrasound (US) to observe specific anatomical structures in the neck. To ascertain the optimal scanning views, both in vitro and in vivo studies were undertaken. Factors which would inhibit quality images had to be identified. From this basis a pilot study was conducted to evaluate US as a possible in vivo scanning method for the observation and measurement of cervical segmental motion. For this investigation, cervical motion was measured in both cadaveric and in vivo situations using US scanning and a separate digitizing system. Validation of US scanning in the measurement of cervical segmental motion would produce a safe but inexpensive objective measure for future clinical studies.

The wealth of information on the epidemiology and sequelae of low back pain has not been matched with the same enthusiasm for the cervical spine. Information on the anatomy and biomechanics of the cervical spine has often been extrapolated from lumbar spine data. The difficulty in obtaining post-mortem or cadaveric specimens for research work may be a factor in the slower progress. The area of interest for this study was the lower cervical spine from the second (C2) to the seventh (C7) vertebra.

Descriptions of spinal anatomy and biomechanics are made with respect to the functional spinal unit (FSU) or motion segment. This consists of two adjacent vertebrae, the intervening disc and adjoining soft tissues. Anatomical features of interest for US scanning are noted.

ANATOMICAL CONSIDERATIONS OF US SCANNING

To interpret the images produced by US scanning, attention was focussed on the position, complex outline and relationships of the cervical vertebrae, fascia and muscles lying superficially in the posterior and postero-lateral aspects of the neck. The presence of bone, dense fibrous or collagenous tissues was known to reduce or obliterate an ultrasound signal passing through tissue; however, the dense image of the bony structures was required. Figures

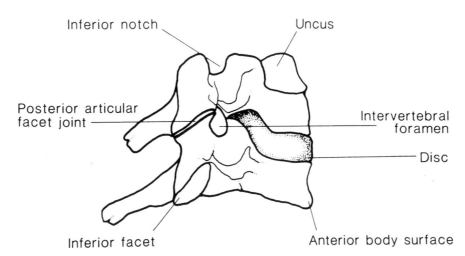

Fig. 3.1 Cervical mobile segment.

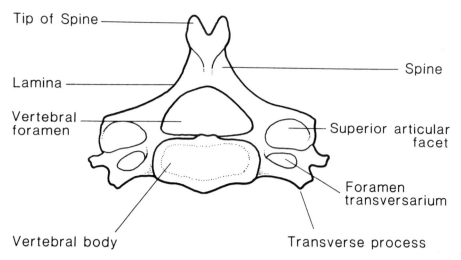

Fig. 3.2   The characteristic bony features of a typical cervical vertebra.

3.1 and 3.2 identify the structures found to be important during US scanning of the cervical spine.

The anterior lordosis of the neck, with its apex between the C4 and C5 levels, is convex in the horizontal plane. Full contact between the skin and the US probe is difficult because most probes vary in length from 12 to 22 cm.

The anterior aspect of the cervical vertebral bodies and the intervening disc spaces were clearly visible from the antero-lateral view. Although this view was not used in the study, it may have value later for observing sagittal rotation or translation. It was not possible to detect the uncinate processes on the lateral and postero-lateral aspects of the vertebral body as they were deep to other shielding bony structures.

Scans in the transverse view showed clearly the variety in size and shape of spinous processes, a factor used for spinal level identification. C2 is usually large and often bifid, whilst those of C3, C4 and C5 are smaller and simple in outline. The lateral articular pillar and pedicles could all be identified using the transverse scanning view, whilst the simple strong shapes of the laminae were very clearly identified in the postero-lateral view. Laminae in the cervical spine are long and narrow, and they overlap with a sharp superior margin adjacent to the ligamentum flavum.

An ultrasound signal will be attenuated as it passes through and across tissue boundaries. The position, structure and density of cervical muscles and fascia in the posterior and postero-lateral aspects was acknowledged. Dissection was undertaken on three embalmed cadavers and one post mortem specimen to note the extent of cervical soft tissue, including the ligamentum nuchae. From the dissections, it was noted that the size, thickness and extent of the fascia and ligamentum nuchae would de-grade any US image obtained in the posterior midline view. It was also noted that the dense posterior muscles of the cervical spine took considerable attachment from the posterior cervical fascia.

CERVICAL MOVEMENT RELEVANT TO US SCANNING

As the cervical spine is a difficult area to image, observe and quantify movement, analysis of cervical spine motion has not been described in detail comparable to that for the lumbar spine. Within the FSU, motion is described as occurring about three axes and within three planes — the Y axis being vertical, the X axis in the direction of progression, and the Z axis directed laterally. The starting position of a movement is usually described from a 'preferred' or the 'natural head posture' position. It is located by gradually reducing a sagittal oscillation of the head and neck to a favoured position for the subject.

It is unlikely that pure movements of translation (glide) or rotation occur within the segment due to the complex articular geometry of the cervical segment and the limiting disc and soft-tissue restraints about the FSU. Motion is said to be combined or coupled when a primary movement about one axis occurs simultaneously with movement about a second axis. In flexion there would be an amount of anterior glide combined with anterior rotation of the cranial vertebra on the caudal vertebra. For the FSU, the instantaneous axis of rotation is complex and is still the subject of research (Amevo et al 1991).

This study considered flexion and extension, lateral flexion and rotation. Interest was focused particularly on the results of lateral flexion and rotation and the combined motion and translation which subsequently occurs.

Flexion

Flexion is a rotation about a transverse axis in a sagittal plane. In the spine, this movement would usually be accompanied by a small degree of anterior translation or glide. The movement may be restricted or guided by the uncovertebral joints on the lateral and posterior lateral aspects of the vertebral body (Penning & Wilmink 1987, Penning 1988). The glide component of flexion is achieved by some translation at the posterior interverte-bral joints and some distortion of the intervertebral discs. Glide between 3.5 and 6 mm has been detected, but White & Panjabi (1978) felt that 3.5 mm is the upper normal limit. Asymmetry or trophism of spinal joints would be a consideration in the type or direction of motion occurring at spinal segments. Degeneration of the uncovertebral joints, affecting the articular facets of the uncovertebral joints, may ultimately cause changes in the range or direction of motion at the FSU. Tension in the posterior muscles and ligaments contribute to a restriction of the range and quality of cervical flexion.

Extension

Spinal extension is essentially the reverse of flexion. The superior articular facets of the FSU glide in a retro or posterior direction on the inferior facet of the FSU. Integrity and flexibility of the joint capsule is required to allow a possible degree of tilt. The intervertebral disc will be in tension anteriorly and its integrity is also necessary for smooth pain-free motion.

Lateral flexion

For the cervical as well as the lumbar spine, it is acknowl-edged (White & Panjabi 1978) that lateral flexion is always combined with a degree of rotation. However, the ratios of the two movements and the directions of the movements are variable and are still being investigated (Mimura et al 1989). The natural mobility of the cervical spine, particularly in the mid-cervical region, may allow unusual patterns of combined or coupled motion. For the lumbar spine the range of motion and the direction of motion have been well described (Pearcy & Whittle 1982).

Rotation

US scanning identified changes in bulk, distribution and tissue texture of the postero-lateral muscle masses; the fascial planes and ligamentum nuchae, as bony structures, were observed during rotation and lateral flexion. Rota-tion will always occur with some lateral flexion, although the ratios of the two movements are still being investi-gated. What is of interest, are the combinations of rotation and translation which produce the final direction of movement.

METHODS OF MEASUREMENT

Direct observation is probably the most used clinical tool, although the accuracy and reliability of this method may be questioned. External devices such as goniometers will allow, at best, an estimation of total motion, although some devices now are better than others (Alund & Larsson 1990) in that they offer a more reliable result. An example is the CROM (cervical range of motion) device.

Measurement by comparing overlaid X-ray films, taken at the extremes of motion, can be used to measure seg-mental motion. This has been described for the cervical spine by Penning (1983). The method requires two sets of films; this may cause concern because of the radiation exposure. This method is technically harder in the cervical spine because the images of the cervical vertebrae are more complex than lumbar vertebrae. Accurate identifica-tion of bony landmarks is difficult. X-rays are excellent for the observation of the skeletal system and are still the clinical tool of choice for many imaging situations. The disadvantages of X-rays are that images are a static repre-sentation of an end-of-range position and that radiation from taking two sets of films is difficult to justify in the non-clinical situation.

By comparing X-ray films from two sources at 90° to each other (stereoradiography), the three-dimensional position of the vertebrae in space can be obtained. Stereoradiography has been used for the lumbar spine for measuring lumbar motion. Analysis of data allows the relative motion of adjacent vertebrae to be described. Exposure to radiation has meant that the technique for in vivo studies is limited. The method has been used in the lumbar spine by Selvik (1977), Stokes et al (1980) and Pearcy and Whittle (1982). With the advent of new tech-nology to describe three-dimensional motion using elec-tromagnetic field sensing, knowledge of the ranges and patterns of movement will improve. At present, specific patterns for normal cervical motion are being investigated (Mimura et al 1989). Data for normal lumbar spine patterns has been achieved (Pearcy & Hindle 1989) and the technology may enable cervical motion to be similarly observed.

Mathematical parameters such as distance and forces can be modelled, but at present they are often very simple models and there is still little information on how the complex musculo-skeletal systems interact. Huelke and Nusholtz (1986) have reviewed the literature of bio-mechanical studies of the cervical spine and their review has illustrated how difficult mathematical modelling can be when applied to the neck. Biplannar photography was used to observe motion between motion segments in cadaver cervical spines, before and after a rotation ma-nipulation (Ruston 1988) for a specific level. The tech-nique was able to demonstrate changes in the segmental motion in cadaver necks, but further extrapolation of results to the in vivo situation would be difficult. In reviewing current imaging methods it was felt that standard diagnostic US might offer the investigator the ability to observe the cervical musculo-skeletal system in both its dynamic and static state. It was felt that the major advantages of US are that US is non-ionizing, non-invasive and has no known long- or short-term side-effects. The equipment is relatively cheap and portable, scanning is comfortable for the patient, and dynamic imaging is possible.

BACKGROUND REVIEW OF DIAGNOSTIC ULTRASOUND (US)

The major technical aspects of US may be found in specific texts on the subject (Powis & Powis 1984, Hussey 1985, Repacholi et al 1987); a review only is given here. Different modes of US are available for different scanning purposes. Simple distance measurements may be taken by an A-scanner, where a pulse-like image is seen. Fluid motion may be scanned using the M-mode, which traces motion against time. These images are created and seen simultaneously, which is in real-time. Static B-scanners are used to form an image by slow, repeated sweeps of the scanner head. An image is produced, line by line, with each sweep of the transducer head. The mode of US used for skeletal scanning is usually the real-time B-scan. The transducer will emit and receive a series of sound pulses, simultaneously creating a two-dimensional image.

Sound is the result of a mechanical disturbance of particles in a source medium, producing within the medium a series of pressure waves of compression and rarefaction. The periodicy or distance between the waves may be measured, and this distance is called the wavelength (λ) or cycle. The number of cycles per second is the frequency of the sound and is measured in Hertz (Hz).

Frequencies commonly used for diagnostic US are usually between 1.5 and 20 MHz. To achieve the optimum images from a real-time B-scanner, a balance has to be sought between the frequency of the signal and the type and depth of tissue to be scanned. The velocity (c) of sound waves is the speed at which sound passes through the medium, and this will depend upon the density (ρ) and compressibility (K) of the medium. The relationship of wavelength to velocity and frequency is usually expressed by the formula:

$$c = 1/\sqrt{K.\rho}$$

Each tissue has its own characteristic impedance (Z) to the passage of sound. This is determined by the ratio of the pressure of the sound waves (p) in the tissue and the velocity of the particles (v) as they are set in motion. Impedance (Z) is also defined as the product of velocity (c) and tissue density (ρ), when the tissue bulk modulus or compressibility is (K).

Table 3.1 Values for the propagation of sound and tissue impedance for some human tissues (adapted from Ziskin & Wells 1980)

Tissue	Coefficient at 1 dB/cm	Speed (m/s)	Acoustic $10^{-6} \times kg/m^2s$
Blood	0.1	1570	1.66
Adipose	0.6	1570	1.39
Muscle	1.0	1590	1.73
Cartilage	5.2	1670	–
Bone	10	3300	5.0

The signal will attenuate or degrade as it passes through tissue and each tissue has its individual attenuation factor. The signal will also decrease as the frequency increases. Therefore, the choice of frequency for a probe requires that the depth and type of tissue be considered. Deep structures usually require a probe with a frequency of 1–5 MHz, and superficial structures, such as eyes, need a probe with a frequency between 5 and 20 MHz. The attenuation of biological tissue is given in u(dB/m). Values for some skeletal tissues are given (Ziskin & Wells 1980) in Table 3.1.

Some of the signal reduction is a result of absorption of energy, but most of the attenuation is from signal reflection or refraction at tissue boundaries. With an ultrasound transducer held perpendicular to the surface, the majority of the signal is transmitted into the medium, with little signal reflection. If the transducer is at an angle to the surface the signal will hit the surface or interface and some of the beam will be reflected, some being transmitted. Because of surface irregularities there is always some scattering of the signal.

Arrays and scanners

Three main designs of probes are used for real-time scanning. The choice would depend upon the equipment and the type of scan to be undertaken. The probes are the mechanical or sector scanner, the multiple element linear array and the multiple element phased array.

Mechanical scanners have either a single or multiple small standard transducer which emits the signal whilst rotating or oscillating at high speed within a casing. Signals are captured each time the transducer faces a 'window' adjacent to the body surface. A cone-shaped image is displayed. Multiple element linear arrays have a strip of small elements, up to 64, giving a probe length up to 180 mm. A disadvantage is that the image may be slow in forming and the final quality may be poor. Multiple-element phased arrays use a line of elements but they are clustered and triggered by cluster. This produces a strong wavefront and faster image production. Focusing of the beam is possible by controlling the firing sequence of the elements. The processing of the images is being improved with each new generation of scanners on the market.

Safety

It should be acknowledged that ultrasound, by its nature, might have some danger for biological tissue. Spatial peaks of energy have been observed. However in real-time B-scanning the peaks of any pulses of energy are reduced. Microstreaming of cellular fluid has been said to occur, and cavitation will also occur only at high intensities (Carstensen 1987).

Experimental ultrasound scanner and probe

Although there are several types of diagnostic scanner available, it was found after testing several scanners that a real-time B-scanner with a phased linear array gave the optimum images. Real-time US images offer both immediate static and dynamic images to the investigator. It should be noted however that, as newer machines become available, the model used in this study will be superseded.

The resolution or ability of a scanner to image an object in both a lateral and axial manner was tested. The resolution of a scanner is determined electronically by manipulation of the signal. In the literature on the use of ultrasound in orthopaedics there is little or no consensus in the choice of scanner. Clarke et al (1985) and Adam et al (1986) used different scanners for imaging the hip joint, and Middleton et al (1986) described a variety of scanners for imaging the shoulder.

The Toshiba Sonolayer, SAL 32 B, with a 5 MHz probe, was found after testing to give the best results. This scanner offered a measurement caliper function, identification characters, direct video output and 16 grey scale levels, which was considered adequate. Lerski (1981) believed that only four grey levels could be detected with any degree of accuracy. The 5 MHz probe had a window of view of 84 mm in length. All images could be seen on the screen and could be recorded directly onto video tape using a small portable video recorder. A freeze-frame facility was useful to capture images for recording.

The images recorded on the VHS video tape were later played back using the Kontron MOP Videoplan Digitising System® and software. This allowed measurements to be taken using a 'pen' and digitizing tablet which could be illuminated from beneath, when measurements from X-ray were required. The accuracy of the digitizing tablet was set at 0.1 mm.

Stand-off medium

Little information was found in the literature on the use of stand-off media for musculo-skeletal scanning. It was anticipated that because of the lordosis in the neck, some form of stand-off medium might be required to maintain good contact between the probe and the neck. A sample of 3M Kitecko® jelly was tested as it had been used in some radiography departments. Above 5 MHz the attenuation of the signal rose rapidly, but below 5 MHz the attenuation was similar to that of soft tissue. The jelly was found to be very friable, and cracks greatly distorted the image signals. Technical data are given below. Lees and McDicken (1984) found that the average velocity of sound in the jelly was less than that for soft tissue (1540 m/s).

A test was undertaken on a two-part silicon gel (Dow Corning® Q7-2218) a polydimethylsiloxane. After many test runs, by altering the proportions of the two-part gel, three blocks were made of varying stiffness. The ability of the blocks to attenuate a 1 MHz A-scan US signal was tested. The scanner used was a Diasonograph NE 4102 machine. The test tank was a large perspex tube 1 m in height and 14 cm in diameter. The tube held distilled water to within 5 cm of the top. Washed sand was placed in the base to reduce the standing waves from the A scan probe which degraded the signal. Two monofilament threads 0.13 mm in diameter were placed diametrically across the tube. The threads were 5 cm apart, and the upper thread was 11 cm below the water surface. The temperature of the water column was left to reach 20°C.

In turn, each of the gel blocks was placed between the threads, and the probe was lowered into the water and the test carried out. The scanner was adjusted to equalize the distal signal of the filament to that of the proximal filament signal. The scanner was adjusted to give equal signal peaks at a frequency of 2 MHz and the time/distance axis was set to the 5 cm distance. The gels, when in place, caused an alteration in the distance reading and amplitude of the distal signal peak. These alterations were noted for each of the three gels in turn. It was found that, for all of the gels, the velocity of sound and the attenuation of signal was less than that given for Kitecko® jelly and body tissue. The final quality of the images was reduced sufficiently for the practice of using a stand-off medium to be discontinued. Only the standard ultrasound contact gel was used.

Resolution of the scanner

Axial and lateral resolution of the scanner was tested using a U-shaped frame with two strands of monofilament (0.13 mm diameter) placed between the frame struts. The frame was lowered into the water-bath so that it could be scanned from the top (axial) and the side (lateral). Using a travelling light microscope to measure the separation of the strands, readings were taken just as the images of the threads merged into one. Results for axial resolution gave a mean distance of 0.4 mm with a range of 0.38 to 0.45 mm. Lateral resolution gave a mean distance of 0.39 mm with a range of 0.37 to 0.44 mm. These results were felt to be well within the range required to detect movement between a spinal motion segment.

COMPARISONS OF MEASUREMENTS MADE WITH THE US SCANNER AND THE DIGITIZING SYSTEM

Test board for horizontal distance measurement

Distances measured by the scanner needed to be tested against another system. Several experiments were carried out using different thicknesses of wire and positions of the probe; an overall summary of results and conclusions is given.

Method

A latex-coated board with several vertical pins attached was constructed. Wires and threads of differing gauges and materials were all tested in the same manner. The material for the test was tied between the vertical pins. Images from this 'calibration' board were recorded, and measurements were taken by standard vernier calipers, the caliper markers on the US scanner screen and the digitizer. The board was submerged in water at room temperature. Measurements were taken with a 5 MHz probe. The US probe was placed normal to the wires, then inclined at 15, 30 and 45°. Two pins were then placed on two adjacent spinous processes of the model spine. With the spine in the water-bath, the probe was applied at very close proximity, again at approximately 4 cm ('normal distance') from the pins, then with the probe just in contact with the water-bath wall (approximately 6 cm).

Result

Results of the effect of probe angulation and the proximity of the probe to the model spine are given in Tables 3.2, 3.3 and 3.4.

Conclusions

Angulation of the probe between 0 and 30° was not found to affect significantly distance measurements between two points. However, above 30° there was a decrease in the quality of the image, or the image was lost from view.

Table 3.2 Changes in measurements with probe in three positions (vertical, 15°, 30°): the mean ($\bar{X}$), standard deviation (SD) and coefficient of variance (CV) for the four groups ($n = 50$ for each group)

	Position of probe			
	Vertical		15°	30°
	Group 1	Group 2		
$\bar{X}$ (mm)	9.80	9.22	8.77	8.41
SD	0.30	0.25	0.33	0.37
CV%	3.06	2.71	3.76	4.39

Table 3.3 Distance between two threads as measured by the digitizer and the scanner with the probe in three positions, comparing the main statistical results

	Position of probe					
	Vertical		15°		45°	
	Digitizer	US	Digitizer	US	Digitizer	US
$\bar{X}$	7.894	8.600	8.169	8.600	8.080	8.600
SD	0.189	0.516	0.225	0.516	0.294	0.516
CV%	2.367	6.000	2.754	6.000	3.637	6.000

Table 3.4 Distance measured between two pins attached to the model spine, with the probe head at different relative distances from the pins

	Position of probe head		
	Near	Distant	Normal
$\bar{X}$ (mm)	9.513	9.190	10.186
SD	0.315	0.168	0.176
CV%	3.316	1.836	1.735

Comparing the same distances measured by the digitizing system and the scanner, there were significant differences between the two systems. From the results, the digitizer was able to measure the distance with greater accuracy than the US scanner. This may well be because the scanner can measure only in increments of 1 mm.

Considering the proximity of the probe to the spine, a significant difference was found between the 'near', 'distant', 'normal' and very close measurements. This may suggest that pressure sufficient to have good contact is correct for the non-distortion of distance measurements.

In vitro cervical scanning

Water-bath

Several designs of water-bath were tried before selecting the best for scanning the in vitro cervical spine. The design used a length of silicon tubing sufficiently wide to enclose the model cervical spine. Silicon allowed good transmission of ultrasound and, being pliable, the spine could be moved within the tube. The tubing was stiff enough to retain a column of water for scanning yet would not buckle with pressure when the probe was applied with a force comparable to the clinical situation.

Model spine

A model cervical spine was made using dried human vertebrae from the first cervical to the first thoracic vertebra. The vertebrae were mounted on a length of stiff silicon tubing placed within the cervical canal. Dense silicon compound was injected carefully into the area normally occupied by the intervertebral disc. The lowest vertebra of the column was embedded in an epoxy resin on the perspex base. This overall arrangement allowed the spine to articulate in a manner similar to the in vivo state.

The model spine within the water-bath offered a realistic phantom for US imaging and the image quality was very acceptable. Recognition of the bony anatomy of the cervical spine was easy, and dynamic motion of the vertebrae could be easily observed. Linear distance between two identified points on the bony skeleton could be measured. Measurements were taken by vernier caliper (dry model), using the calipers of the scanner, and from the digitized image.

In vivo cervical scanning

Views which were useful in vitro were no longer appropriate for in vivo scanning, and considerable time was taken to ascertain the optimum views. These proved to be a postero-lateral view and a transverse view. The postero-lateral view allowed good images of the laminae of the cervical vertebrae (Fig. 3.3). The dense bony masses of the laminae imaged well on US as it was the strong outline of the bony mass that was required. Motion between two or three laminae could be clearly identified. For the transverse view, a good transverse sectional image was easily achieved (Fig. 3.4). However, with this view, motion was noted only in respect to one vertebra.

Overall image clarity was reduced in vivo by the inter-vening body tissue. Signal attenuation within different tissues plus the many tissue boundaries resulted in the degraded US signal. Fascial planes between the para-vertebral muscles were clearly visible in static and dynamic images. It was noted that fascia severely reduced the intensity of the signal, and in midline the ligamentum nuchae reduced the images of vertebrae to faint shadows. In preliminary work it was observed that signal attenuation was very noticeable in subjects with large, fat or very muscular necks. Images were the most difficult to achieve in these subjects.

Postero-lateral view of segmental motion

Method and materials

Twenty female subjects aged between 23 and 37 years (mean age = 29.2 years) with no history of injury, trauma or other musculo-skeletal disorders to the cervical spine, were selected. Information on the procedure was given and consent obtained. For each subject, all the images for the test movements of neutral and lateral flexion were recorded in video tape and the results were later analysed. A null hypothesis was set for this trial: that there would be no significant difference between measurements for the laminae overlap distance as measured by the digitizer for the neutral and lateral flexion positions. Twelve sets of data for each of the two positions and for each of the

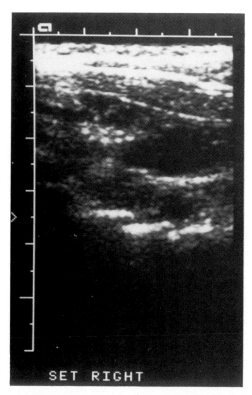

Fig. 3.3 In vivo: postero-lateral view of overlapping laminae below the soft tissue of the neck.

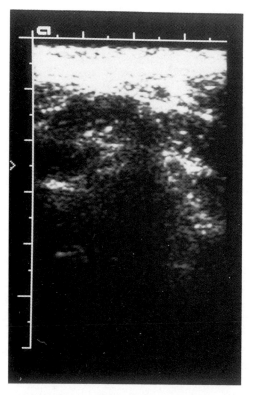

Fig. 3.4 In vivo: transverse scanning view allowing cross-sectional image of the vertebra.

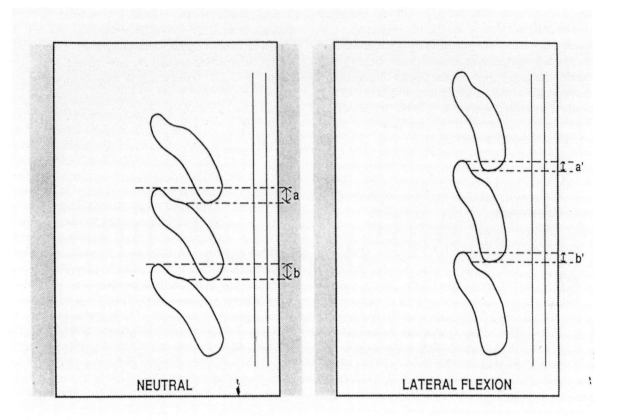

Fig. 3.5 Distance measured by the digitizing system from images of the overlapping laminae.

twenty subjects were obtained and later analysed. The protocol used was as follows.

The subject was seated and the neck area exposed. Standard US gel was applied to the area. The probe was placed longitudinally on the posterior lateral muscle mass of the neck 1.5–2 cm from midline and inclined between the normal and 15° to the normal. From preliminary work, this had been found to give the best images.

With the neck in a preferred neutral position, the subject was asked to laterally flex away slowly from the probe and return the neck to neutral, repeating this twelve times; all images were recorded. Using the digitizing system for neutral and lateral flexion, the overlap distances between two selected laminae were measured (Fig. 3.5).

Results

The combined twelve scores from fifteen of the twenty subjects demonstrated a significant difference ($P = 0.05$ level) in the inter-laminar overlap distance between neutral and lateral flexion, as measured by the digitizing system. Results from four of these subjects chosen at random were subjected to an 'f' test at the $P = 0.05$ level. The significant difference between the results indicated that the digitizing system could detect a difference in the overlap distance when the neck was in the neutral or lateral flexed positions.

Comparison of measurements from X-rays and US scans

X-rays are the standard method of observing spinal structure and position. It was therefore decided to compare distance measured on the US cervical images to the equivalent distances, measured on a plain X-ray film. A null hypothesis was set at the $P = 0.05$ level: that there would be no significant difference between the distance as measured by the two systems. The distance chosen for comparison was the superior, inferior length of an identified lamina.

Method

Two subjects were positioned in the standard manner for a postero-anterior X-ray of the cervical spine. A single X-ray was taken for each subject and the magnification factor of the X-rays was established. US scanning was then undertaken using the postero-lateral view, which allowed the same structures to be visualized. US scans were recorded for each subject. Digitizing of the developed X-ray film was made possible using back illumination of the digitizing tablet.

Results

Calculation of the laminae length was compared between

the two imaging systems. The magnification factors for both X-rays were identical ($P = 0.87$). For each of the two subjects, three set of 10 measurements were taken from both the X-ray and the US scan.

For subject 1, it was found that there was a significant difference in the distance measured for the three data sets, using the two measuring systems (X-ray digitizing and US scanner). For subject 2 there was a significant difference between measurements in two of the three data sets.

Conclusions

These results may reflect the body build of the subjects: subject 1 was more muscular than subject 2. The US images from subject 1 were less defined than those of subject 2, who was of a thin, non-muscular build. The limited ability of the US scanner to measure down to 1 mm separation may also have contributed to these results.

This trial was to ascertain whether it was possible to image the same structures on X-ray and US. This was found to be possible. However, comparing distances taken from the two imaging systems, by digitizer and scanner, was difficult. Recognition should be given to the magnification factors and the probability that increased fibrous tissue will produce a less defined final image.

Effect of manual techniques on range of motion

Previous trials found that it was possible to detect relative segmental motion with US images. An extension of that work was to undertake a pilot study to ascertain whether changes in relative motion could be detected as a result of applying a manual treatment technique to a specific level of dysfunction in an otherwise 'normal' spine.

Clinical examination of the spine usually includes an estimation of the gross range of motion of the region but not always an assessment of segmental motion. The ability of practitioners to determine segmental abnormalities of movement and tissue tension is controversial (Matyas & Bach 1985). For this trial, the clinician was experienced in manual examination and treatment techniques of the spine (Maitland 1986). The transverse scanning view was used in this trial. This would allow the rotation and translation of the vertebra to be observed.

Method

Four female subjects, aged between 22 and 42 years (mean age = 29.5 years) were available for testing. No subject had had any neck injury, other trauma or medical condition to the cervical spine which required medical or physical treatment. All subjects complained of some subjective stiffness at the end of full active rotation and lateral flexion. All subjects were given information on the procedure and their consent was obtained.

The cervical spine motion and motion of the posterior intervertebral joints were examined using central and unilateral pressure techniques (Maitland 1986). A spinal level or segment with demonstrably reduced motion was identified. The US probe was placed transversely across the posterior aspect of the neck at the identified level. The subject was asked slowly to rotate the head to the right and left, then to laterally flex the head away from the probe and return the head to neutral. This sequence was repeated three times and images were recorded on video tape.

The level of abnormal motion was then treated using only unilateral oscillating pressure of the thumbs applied over the previously identified restricted posterior intervertebral joint. To effect a substantial change in the quality of tissue resistance to joint motion, the grade and direction of the mobilization were at the discretion of the therapist. The scanning process was then repeated. Measurements were later taken from the video tape, using the digitizing system.

Consideration had been given to a method of measuring the motion of the vertebra image. In the transverse view a clear cross-sectional image of the vertebra could be obtained; however, only one spinal level was visible. With the equipment available for the trial (and on all US scanners at the time) no fixed reference point from which to take distance readings was available on the machine. A method of measuring relative motion (not actual distances) was achieved by taking a perpendicular distance from the fixed frame of the digitizer image to the posterior border of the vertebral body at the base of the pedicle, for both the left and right sides of the vertebra (Fig. 3.6). These landmarks were clearly visible in all scans.

Results

Dynamic real-time scanning allowed the visualization of translation and rotation of the vertebra in two dimensions. However, the view allowed no comparison of motion between vertebrae.

Mean values for pre- and post-distances for both right and left lateral flexion and rotation (Tables 3.5A and 3.5B) were obtained. Differences in the relative distances were then calculated for the same movements. A negative value was assigned to vertebral rotation to the right.

Conclusions

This test was only one part of work to assess the viability of US to image the cervical spine and observe relative motion. Because of the preliminary nature of the trials, no attempt was made at this stage to increase the sophistication of the test, to include X-ray assessment of subjects, to compare motion between levels, or other sampling factors. Statistically it would be difficult to draw conclusions

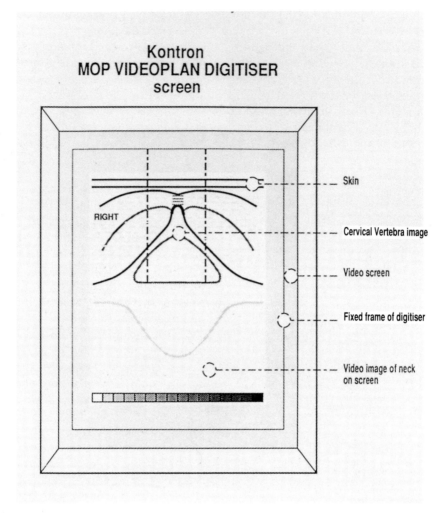

Fig. 3.6   Distances measured by the digitizing system from the fixed frame of the digitizer to the posterior wall of the vertebral body.

Table 3.5A   Means of pedicle distances (left and right), both pre- and post-treatment, producing the final rotation of the vertebra (*n* = 4) during *right rotation*

	Difference in (R) and (L) distances			
Subject	x pre (mm)	x post (mm)	Difference (mm)	Final vertebral rotation
1.	−1.875	−3.283	1.408	Left
2.	−1.760	−0.030	−1.73	Right
3.	2.982	−2.011	4.99	Left
4.	−1.500	−1.413	0.087	Right

Table 3.5B   Means of pedicle distances (left and right), both pre- and post-treatment, producing the final rotation of the vertebra (*n* = 4) during *right lateral flexion*

	Difference in (R) and (L) distances			
Subject	x pre (mm)	x post (mm)	Difference (mm)	Final vertebral rotation
1.	−3.092	−1.941	−1.151	Right
2.	−2.179	−1.337	−0.842	Right
3.	0.568	0.236	0.332	Left
4.	3.338	2.767	0.571	Left

from the four subjects; however, the results of this small sample indicated that this could be an area to develop into a larger pilot project.

The transverse view allowed the visualization of translation motion — which is often mentioned, but has not yet been quantified. It was also noted that, at any level from C2 to C6 which had received mobilization during this test, the movements of lateral flexion and rotation did not have a consistent pattern of movement to the same side (Fig. 3.7). The results for this sample also indicated that no significant difference had been achieved with the manual intervention. This may reflect the lack of severe pathology in the sample as determined by the exclusion criteria, but all subjects reported a subjective feeling of decreased stiffness at the end of range after treatment intervention.

Overall conclusions from the whole study

The realization that observing segmental motion seemed possible only by invasive means, static images or with

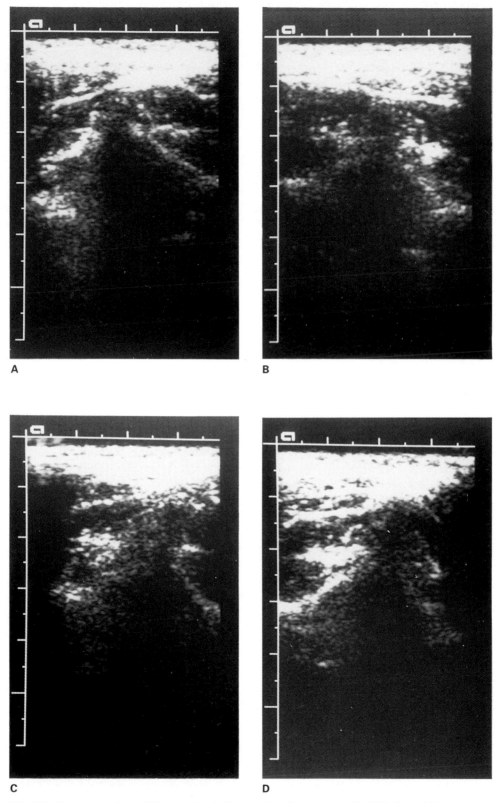

Fig. 3.7   In vivo rotations of the vertebra during a series of movements. **A**. Right lateral flexion.
B. Left lateral flexion. **C**. Right rotation. **D**. Left rotation.

exposure to X-rays, prompted this investigation into the possible use of standard diagnostic US to observe segmental motion in the neck. The ability of the US scanner to display motion in real time was felt to be an advance on traditional static images. The quality of the movements were observed and recorded for the first time. Ultrasound scanning has a successful record in several fields of diagnostic medicine and it is now being used more frequently for musculo-skeletal imaging.

An ultrasound scanner with a phased linear array of 5 MHz was found to be the most suitable for this study. A series of in vitro tests were undertaken to ascertain the practical resolution of the equipment, to test the sensitivity of the equipment for measuring distances at specific angles and to find the optimum scanning planes for cervical vertebrae.

Scanning in vivo was harder than expected, with the lack of resolution due to the dense and fibrous nature of the cervical soft tissue which attenuated the signal. A clear image was difficult to produce when subjects had fat or heavily muscled necks. Two views were established for observing the motion of the cervical vertebrae. Three or four laminae could be visualized with the probe placed longitudinally on the postero-lateral aspect of the neck and a single vertebra was easily imaged with the probe in a transverse position on the posterior aspect of the neck. The advantage of using US scanning was that, for the first time without risk to the subject, in vivo dynamic motion could be observed in the cervical spine. It was clearly seen that the direction of movement of a cervical vertebra was different to that expected from the literature. It was noted that the rotation of the single imaged vertebra could be toward or away from the direction of rotation of the neck and that vertebral translation could also be either away from, or towards, the side of neck lateral flexion. No regular pattern at any segmental level was detected in the small sample tested. This is contrary to the direction of spinal motion usually described for the neck.

Further work

This work has demonstrated that standard diagnostic US can be used to give acceptable, two-dimensional images of structures of the neck and that segmental vertebral motion can be observed. Only one of the optical scanning views allowed relative motion between two vertebrae to be observed. New generations of US equipment will offer superior image quality and variety in shape and size of probes to facilitate scanning on surfaces such as the neck.

Anterior vertebral views should be investigated as the anterior outline of the vertebrae can be easily identified. Rotation and translation in the sagittal plane could then be observed. It is important that further work be undertaken to determine more thoroughly the directions of segmental motion (rotation and translation) with respect to general cervical rotation, lateral flexion and sagittal motion. More information on cervical biomechanics is required and the directions and patterns of movement would be of importance to manual therapists.

A better method of quantifying motion on an ultrasound image, using known reference points, is required. Advances in signal identification technology could be used by manufacturers to produce even better screen images, to provide the ability to 'log' in desired anatomical reference landmarks, to save the data and to bring up the same landmarks on the next image frame so that the relative change in distance could be calculated. At present, X-rays remain the 'gold standard' method in musculo-skeletal imaging for observing and measuring relative motion in the spine. However, the use of diagnostic US technology may well offer a new and safe insight into the dynamic motion of the cervical spine.

REFERENCES

Adam R, Hendry G M A, Moss J, Wild S R, Gillespie I 1986 Arthrosonography of the irritable hip in childhood: a review of 1 year's experience. British Journal of Radiology 59: 205–208

Alund M, Larsson S-E, 1990 Three-dimensional analysis of neck motion: a clinical method. Spine 15: 87–91

Amevo B, Worth D, Bogduk N 1991 Instantaneous axes of rotation of the typical cervical motion segment: a study in normal volunteers. Clinical Biomechanics 6: 111–117

Carstensen E L 1987 Biological effects of acoustic cavitation. In: Repacholi M H, Grandolfo M, Rindi A (eds) Ultrasound medical applications, biological effects, and hazard potential. Plenum Press, New York

Clarke N M P, Harcke H T, McHugh P, Lees M S, Borns P F, MacEwen G D 1985 Real-time ultrasound in the diagnosis of congenital dislocation and dysplasia of the hip. Journal of Bone and Joint Surgery 67B: 406–412

Huelke D F, Nusholtz G S 1986 Cervical spine biomechanics: a review of the literature. Journal of Orthopaedic Research 4: 232–245

Hussey M 1985 Basic physics and technology of medical diagnostic ultrasound. Macmillan, London, ch 2

Lees W R, McDicken W N 1984 Kitecho Jelly Block: end of the waterbath. Proceedings of the British Medical Ultrasound Society, 16th Annual Meeting, Harrogate

Lerski R A 1981 Ultrasound — display and storage. In: Moores B M (ed) Physical aspects of medical imaging. John Wiley, Chichester, p 141

Maitland, G D 1986 Vertebral manipulation. 5th edn. Butterworth, London, pp 43–102

Matyas T A, Bach T M 1985 The reliability of selected techniques in clinical arthrometrics. Australian Journal of Physiotherapy 31: 175–199

Middleton W D, Reinus W R, Totty W G, Melson G L, Murphy W A 1986 Ultrasonographic evaluation of the rotator cuff and biceps tendon. Journal of Bone and Joint Surgery 68: 440–450

Mimura M, Moriya H, Wanatabe T, Takahashi K, Yamagata M, Tamaki T 1989 Three-dimensional motion analysis of the cervical spine with special reference to the axial rotation. Spine 14: 1135–1139

Pearcy M J, Hindle R J 1989 New method for the non-invasive three dimensional measurement of human back movement. Clinical Biomechanics 4: 73–79

Pearcy M J, Whittle M W 1982 Movements of the lumbar spine measured by three dimensional X-ray analysis. Journal of Biomedical Engineering 4: 107–111

Penning L 1983 Roentgenographic evaluation. In: Sherk H H (ed) The cervical spine. JB Lippincott, Philadelphia, ch 3

Penning L 1988 Differences in anatomy, motion, development and ageing of the upper and lower cervical disk segments. Clinical Biomechanics 3: 37–47

Penning L, Wilmink J T 1987 Rotation of the cervical spine: a CT study in normal subjects. Spine 12: 732–738

Powis R L, Powis W J 1984 A thinker's guide to ultrasound imaging Urban & Schwarzenberg, Baltimore

Repacholi M H, Grandolfo M, Rindi A (eds) 1987 Ultrasound medical applications, biological effects and hazard potential. Plenum Press, New York

Ruston S A 1988 Movements of the cervical spine observed by diagnostic ultrasound. PhD thesis, University of Strathclyde, Glasgow

Selvik G 1977 A roentgen stereophotogrammetric method for the study of the kinematics of the skeletal system: principles and application. University of Lund, Sweden

Stokes I A F, Medlicott P A, Wilder D G 1980 Measurement of painful intervertebral joints. Medical and Biological Engineering and Computing 18: 694–700

White A A, Panjabi M M 1978 Clinical biomechanics of the spine. JB Lippincott, Philadelphia, pp 30–42

White A A, Johnson R M, Panjabi M M, Southwick W O 1975 Biomechanical analysis of clinical stability in the cervical spine. Clinical Orthopaedics and Related Research 109: 85–96

Ziskin M C, Wells P N T 1980 Tissue characterization. In: Wells P N T, Ziskin M C (eds) New techniques and instrumentation in ultrasonography. Churchill Livingstone, New York, ch 11

4. Movements of the head and neck

D. R. Worth

INTRODUCTION

The cervical spine should be considered as a universally mobile axial structure capable of a wide range of mobility. It has been customary to describe the movements of the cervical spine as rotational movements of the head and neck in one of the mutually orthogonal planes referred to as sagittal, frontal and horizontal.

Whilst it may be clinically useful to describe these movements as flexion, extension, lateral flexion and rotation respectively, this offers only a description of whether the head alone is moving forward or backwards, sideways to the left or right, or turning to the left or right. This does not describe what is taking place in the cervical vertebral column as a whole or the change in position of a particular vertebra relative to its neighbour as a function of movements of the head and neck.

In kinematic terms, movements of the head and neck will result in altered relationships between the cervical vertebrae in combinations of rotations and translations about or along one or more of the axes of movement.

To appreciate fully the ranges of in vivo cervical spine movements, all of the intervertebral rotation and translation ranges should be considered. The coordinate axes used and positive rotation angles (in a right-hand sense) are shown in Figure 4.1. The X-axis is a transverse axis; translations along it are to the left or right, and rotations about it are flexion–extension. The Y-axis is a frontal (longitudinal) axis with translations superiorly or inferiorly and axial rotations to the left or right. The Z-axis is a sagittal axis with translations anteriorly or posteriorly, and rotations about it are lateral flexion to the left or right.

THE GROSS RANGES OF HEAD AND NECK MOVEMENTS

The range of movement of the cervical spine is examined clinically by observation or measurement of the movement of the head relative to the trunk. However, several factors will not be observed using this technique, possibly resulting in erroneous clinical judgements. The range of head movement bears no relation to the range of neck

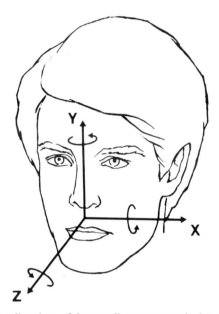

Fig. 4.1 The directions of the coordinate axes used, also showing positive translations and rotations.

movement, and the total range of movement equals the sum of head and neck movement (Adams & Logue 1971). The cervical spine should firstly be thought of as the upper and lower cervical spine with the division occurring both morphologically and physiologically at C2–C3. The cervical spine has two normally occurring curves, the larger lordotic curve in the lower cervical spine and a reversal of this in the upper cervical spine when the head and neck are observed in the neutral position. This observation is consistent with the development of the cervical lordosis as a secondary curve imposed between the primary dorsal and upper cervical curves. The persistence of the primary upper cervical curve is responsible for the maintenance of the horizontal disposition of the line of vision. It is therefore possible to flex and extend the upper cervical spine independently of the lower cervical spine and vice versa. Furthermore, it is possible to extend the upper cervical spine and flex the lower cervical spine at the same time. In fact, bilateral contraction of the sterno-cleido-mastoid muscles results in flexion of the lower and extension of the upper cervical spine.

Careful observation of a lateral X-ray of the cervical spine in full flexion reveals two curves: a slightly lordotic upper cervical spine and a kyphotic lower cervical spine (Fig. 4.2). The curvatures in the upper and lower cervical spine change independently whilst the head and neck move from full flexion to full extension (Dimnet et al 1982). In full extension the whole cervical spine is in a lordotic curvature (Fig. 4.3). The degree of upper and lower curvature as a result of cervical spine flexion will be affected by the order of performing the flexion movement.

If the subject flexes the head and neck as far as possible, starting from the neutral position, a full range of flexion (or maximum kyphotic curve) will occur in the lower cervical spine. Comparing the full flexion X-ray to the full extension X-ray there may appear to be less upper cervical flexion (atlanto-occipital) in the flexed position. If, in an attempt to obtain full upper cervical flexion, the subject is instructed to flex the upper cervical spine first and then the lower, the result is a slight increase in upper cervical flexion still less than neutral, and a decrease in lower cervical flexion.

To obtain lateral X-rays of full range flexion of both the upper and lower cervical spine it is necessary to examine upper cervical flexion with the lower cervical spine in neutral (Fig. 4.4) and then the lower cervical spine in full

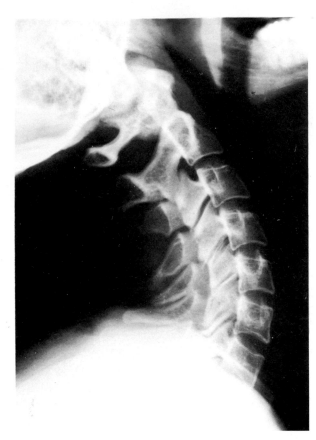

Fig. 4.3 X-ray of the cervical spine in the position of full extension.

flexion with the upper cervical spine slightly extended (Dirheimer 1977, Worth 1988) (Fig. 4.2).

Therefore, in order to examine clinically cervical flexion and extension the same differentiation between upper and lower cervical spine must be applied. Compare (A) and (B) in Figure 4.5.

There are several possible explanations for the differentiation of movement between the upper and lower cervical spine. In some individuals the chin may make contact with the chest in the position of full flexion, resulting in a passive extension of the upper cervical spine (Dirheimer 1977). This simple mechanical explanation does not explain the smaller range of upper cervical flexion in the position of full head and neck flexion compared to neutral in persons whose chin fails to abut the sternum.

The final deflection of the upper cervical spine is more likely to be the result of passive insufficiency of the sterno-cleido-mastoid muscles. Passive insufficiency of a muscle occurs when a full range of motion at any joint or joints which that muscle crosses is limited by that muscle's length (O'Connell & Gardner 1972). When the upper and lower cervical spines are flexed as fully as possible at the same time, the available length of the sterno-cleido-mastoid is insufficient to permit upper cervical flexion to occur. This is despite any synergistic contraction of the anterior suboccipital muscles and the supra and infra hyoid muscles (Kapandji 1974a).

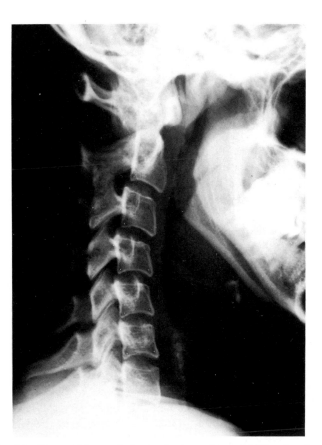

Fig. 4.2 X-ray of the cervical spine in the position of full head and neck flexion.

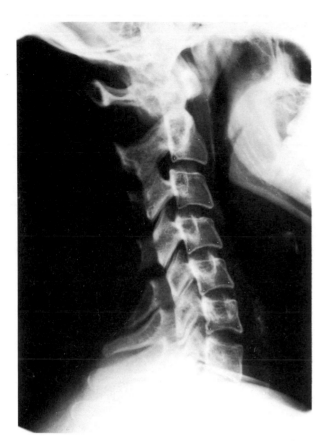

Fig. 4.4 X-ray of the cervical spine with the upper cervical spine in flexion and lower cervical spine in neutral. This position is obtained by instructing the patient to tuck the chin as far as possible without bending the neck forward.

Other structures may also play a similar role. If such a structure is ligamentous, then the mechanism explaining the upper and lower cervical differentiation is passive co-ordination. Joints are passively coordinated when at least one of the participating bones is not acted upon directly by muscles or, more rarely, when there is a physical link across two or more of the joints of the set (Barnett et al 1961a). If the length of the ligamentum nuchae is insufficient to allow the maximum separation of all the spinous processes as well as the occiput from the posterior tubercle of the atlas, then in full flexion the gap between the basi-occiput and posterior atlantal arch will appear to be less than in the neutral position.

The structures within the spinal canal should also be considered. The spinal cord and related structures, having a fixed attachment above and spanning the lower cervical joints, may have insufficient length to permit the full stretch of flexion of both upper and lower cervical spine. The head may extend at the end of the movement to relieve this stretch by virtue of passive coordination.

Thus, whilst it is true that the total range of cervical spine movements equals the sum of the head and neck movement, it is important that these two parts of the movement are measured independently of each other when the full range of cervical flexion is being assessed. This applies especially when the passive range of cervical flexion is being examined using palpation tests of passive intervertebral mobility.

In considering the quantification of gross cervical spine

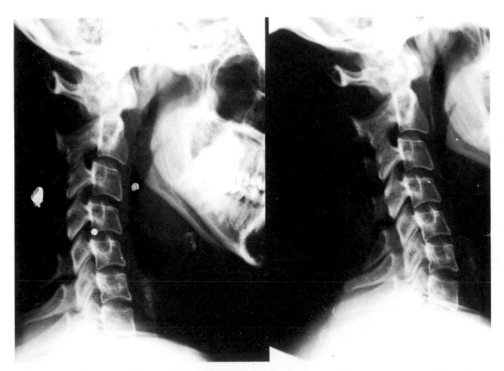

Fig. 4.5 **A**. The same X-ray as shown in Figure 4.2, full flexion. **B**. The same X-ray as shown in Figure 4.4, upper cervical flexion. Note the wider occipito-atlantal distance, the differences in the upper and lower curvatures when compared to (A).

Table 4.1 Average reported gross cervical spine range of movement

	Flexion–extension	Flexion	Extension	Left lateral flexion	Right lateral flexion	Total lateral flexion	Left rotation	Right rotation	Total rotation
Schoening & Hannan (1964)		38.6	43.7	38.0	36.0		58.0	58.8	
Ferlic (1962)	127 SD 19.5					73 SD 15.6			142 SD 17.1
Bennett et al (1963)		54.0	93.2	–	–		75.0	76.0	
Snyder et al (1975)	103.7					71.0			136.5
O'Driscoll & Tomenson (1982)	M: 108.8 ± 8.9 F: 104 ± 2.9					169.8 ± 4.5 186.1 ± 3.9			129.8 ± 3.2 132.5 ± 2.7
Colachis & Strohm (1965) (C2–T1)		24	16						
Alund & Larsson (1990)	140 ± 18					91 ± 12			153 ± 16

mobility, it is important to take into account several factors which will affect the reliability and the validity of measurement. These include measurement of simultaneous head and neck movement, the error of using an artificial zero neutral position within a plane of movement, measuring two-dimensionally a three-dimensional movement, and attributing significance of alleged restricted movement to intrinsic cervical structures.

The need to differentiate between upper and lower cervical mobility, as explained, is reflected in the diverse values recorded for cervical mobility in Table 4.1. Colachis and Strohm (1965) measured a total range of 40° flexion–extension between C2 and T1. They used a radiographic technique measuring total flexion and extension range by superimposing T1 and taking the superior apex of T1 as the pivot point for the line representing the shortest distance between C2 and T1. The angles this line made between neutral, flexion and extension respectively represented the range.

Their results compared to other workers (Table 4.1) illustrate the effect of excluding the range of the upper cervical spine when measuring sagittal plane rotation. This reduces the total range to about one-third of the average total range (112°). All the techniques employed in other studies (Table 4.1) used either pointers or goniometers placed on, or attached to, the subjects' heads. In this way, movement of the head was recorded but with no consideration of how head movement affected the lower cervical spine.

O'Driscoll and Tomenson (1982) used a spirit inclinometer placed vertically and sagitally on the crown of the subject's head, and the range of flexion and extension was read directly. For lateral flexion and rotation, the inclinometer was placed in the frontal and horizontal plane respectively.

Ferlic (1962) used a pointer attached to a football helmet. The pointer cast a shadow on a background grid, and the angles created by the shadows of the pointer were measured on the grid with a protractor.

Another source of error was that some workers measured sagittal plane rotation using an arbitrary neutral position or point representing zero (Table 4.1). This also occurred for left and right rotation and lateral flexion. This is a major source of error since it is impossible to replicate the position of zero for both the head and cervical spine (O'Driscoll & Tomenson 1982). Therefore, only the measurement of the full range of movement in each plane, which is not affected by this error, should be considered.

A sophisticated and precise method of measurement of head and neck movement was described by Snyder et al (1975) who examined 96 normal subjects using photogrammetry. Simultaneous firing of three cameras occurred when the subject reached the extreme range of movement of flexion, extension, left and right rotation for the measurement of full movement in each plane (Table 4.2).

By comparing the findings of Snyder et al (1975) (Table 4.1), Ferlic (1962) and O'Driscoll & Tomenson (1982) it can be seen that there is general agreement in the range of sagittal and horizontal plane rotation, with a dramatic disagreement in the lateral flexion or frontal plane rotation reported by O'Driscoll & Tomenson (1982).

This departure from the finding by Ferlic (1962) and Snyder et al (1975) is most likely due to error brought about by the technique used by O'Driscoll & Tomenson (1982). When lateral flexion is performed there is a coupled range of ipsilateral rotation. A bubble goniometer will register an erroneous amount of lateral flexion unless

Table 4.2 Mean range of rotation (after Snyder et al 1975)

Subjects	Plane of rotation		
	Sagittal	Horizontal	Frontal
Females			
18–24 years	124.1	150.6	86.0
35–44	104.6	143.6	73.9
62–74	84.3	123.6	56.3
Males			
18–24 years	129.0	149.5	86.3
35–44	102.7	137.1	73.0
62–74	76.6	113.9	48.0
All females	104.2	139.3	72.0
All males	103.3	133.7	69.8
All subjects	103.7	136.5	71.0

the coupled rotation is corrected by ensuring that the head is in the frontal plane or that lower cervical rotation is compensated for by de-rotation of the upper cervical spine. This has obvious clinical implications since lateral flexion range of the head therefore bears no relationship to intervertebral lateral flexion ranges.

Many of the problems with reliability and validity were overcome by Alund and Larsson (1990) who measured neck motion during movements of the head relative to the trunk. They used five electrogoniometers with known precision to measure simultaneously the range of motion in three planes. The validity of their procedure was found to be significant by comparing the electrogoniometric measurement with sagittal plane radiographic measurement of flexion–extension. The radiographic procedure inter-observer variability was ±2°. Test–re-test reliability was significant with an interval of one week between examinations. This procedure differentiated qualitatively between upper and lower cervical flexion. Lower cervical flexion showed an initial upper cervical extension. This was interpreted as the chin pushing slightly forward at the start of the movement. When the chin is first pulled in and the neck then flexed there was a forward rotation of the head. Then, when the neck is flexed, the initial forward rotation was reversed. When rotation was recorded, coupled lateral flexion occurred in the ratio of 0.05. When lateral flexion was recorded, coupled rotation occurred in the ratio of 0.53.

Whilst both the three-dimensional techniques (Snyder et al 1975, Alund & Larsson 1990) account for precision and accuracy there are differences in their recorded ranges in all three planes. The results of Alund & Larsson (1990) relate closely to those of Bennett et al (1963) in flexion–extension and rotation and to those of Ferlic (1962) in flexion–extension and lateral flexion.

A three-dimensional bubble goniometer was developed by Kadir et al (1981) for use as a simple clinical tool with high inter- and intra-observer reliability.

Measurement of gross movements of the head and neck are obtainable with precision and accuracy. Differences in reported ranges (Table 4.1) reflect differences in methodology and subjects; however, more significantly, they do not reflect intersegmental cervical movements.

Thus, what appears to be a simple concept — the range of head and neck movements — is extremely complicated.

MOVEMENTS OF THE CRANIOVERTEBRAL JOINTS

Marked variability exists in the reported ranges of mobility at the craniovertebral joints (Tables 4.3 and 4.4). This reflects different measurement techniques, various methods of describing movements, lack of reliability and validity studies, and errors of measurement.

Movement of the atlanto-occipital joints

Flexion–extension

The movement of greatest amplitude at the craniovertebral junction is that of flexion–extension or nodding (Steindler 1955, Jackson 1966, Smith 1968). Some authors describe this as flexion and extension (Hollinshead 1967,

Table 4.3 Ranges of movements of the atlanto-axial joints

Source	Flexion–extension	Lateral flexion	Axial rotation
1. Werne (1957) (1959)	About 10° (2°–21.5°)	0	About 47° (22–50°)
2. Fick in Werne (1957)	Insignificant	0	60°
3. Poirier & Charpey in Werne (1957)	11°	4 mm	30–80°
4. Braakman & Penning (1971)	Up to 35°	5°	35°–40° in each direction
5. Hohl & Baker (1964)	10–15°	0–8 mm causing 15° axis rotation	30° in each direction
6. Fielding (1957)	Flexion 5° Extension 10°	'Some lateral shift of atlas'	Up to 90°
7. White & Panjabi (1975)	Compiled range 2°–21° Representative angle 10°	0	Compiled range 22°–58° Representative angle 47°
8. Dvorak et al (1987a)	No values	No values	64.4°
9. Dvorak et al (1987b)	No values	No values	86.1°
10. Penning & Wilmink (1987)	No values	No values	81°
11. Wackenheim (1974)	(a) Odontoid-basion distance may decrease 1–2 mm or increase 1–5 mm or not alter, in flexion	No values	No values
	(b) Distance between posterior tubercle C1 and spinous process C2 may increase 1–8 mm in flexion; in extension it diminishes by 1–7 mm	No values	No values

Table 4.4 Ranges of movements of the atlanto-occipital joints

Source	Flexion–extension	Lateral flexion	Axial rotation
1. Werne (1957)	About 13°	About 8°	0
(1959)	(3°–32.5°)	(4°–13.5°)	
2. Fick in Werne (1957)	50°	30°–40°	0
3. Poirier & Charpey in Werne (1957)	50°	14°–40°	0
4. Braakman & Penning (1971)	Up to 30°	5°	0
5. Fielding (1957)	Flexion 10° Extension 25°	'Some lateral shift of atlas' 35°	0
6. White & Panjabi (1975)	Compiled Range 4°–33° Representative angle 13°	Compiled Range 4°–14° Representative angle 8°	0
7. Kapandji (1974b)	15°	3°	Linear displacements of occiput 2–3 mm in direction of rotation and contralateral flexion
8. Dvorak et al (1987a)	No values	No values	10–25°
9. Dvorak et al (1987b)	No values	No Values	8°
10. Penning & Wilmink (1987)	No values	No values	2° Linear displacement of atlas 4.4 mm in opposite direction to head rotation
11. Wackenheim (1974) Measurements of linear displacements	Distance between basion and superior aspect of anterior arch of atlas increased 1–3 mm; distance between posterior margin of foramen magnum and superior aspect of posterior arch of atlas decreased 1–3 mm	Overlap of articular margins; no values given	No values given

Warwick & Williams 1989). Steindler (1955) and Barnett et al (1961b) describe the movement as both a rocking or angular movement and a gliding movement of the occiput. The glide of the occiput scans in the opposite direction to the angular movement. The axis of movement resembles that of the knee joint and shifts during the movement, i.e. 'forms an evolute' (Steindler 1955).

Lateral flexion

This movement has a variety of descriptions. Several authors suggest that lateral flexion occurs only in the coronal plane (Werne 1959, Hollinshead 1967, Last 1972, Shapiro et al 1973, Warwick & Williams 1989). Using a model, Werne (1957) reported that this is possible about a sagittal axis centred within the skull; this implies that lateral flexion includes a gliding movement with the rocking component.

Other authors describe lateral flexion as a lateral tilt associated with a simultaneous rotational movement at the atlanto-occipital joint (Steindler 1955, Hall 1965, Basmajian 1971, Kapandji 1974b). Steindler (1955) explains that the lateral tilt is associated with a contralateral rotation within this joint.

Furthermore, Jirout (1973) contends that lateral flexion at the atlanto-occipital joint occurs together with rotation at the atlanto-axial joint, and Smith (1968) concurs with this.

Rotation

Many authors believe that rotation of the atlanto-occipital joint does not occur because of the restricting configuration of the articular surfaces (Werne 1959, Last 1972. Dunkster et al 1978, White & Panjabi 1978). Romanes (1972) comments that the configuration limits the rotation to a small movement. Those anatomists promoting the concept of contralateral rotation with side tilting at the atlanto-occipital joint accept rotation. While Romanes (1972) does not actually state that the two movements are interconnected, he describes a slipping movement of one occipital condyle forwards and the other back as the total excursion of rotation at the joints. The resultant position is described as an oblique tilt (Steindler 1955, Hall 1965, Basmajian 1971, Romanes 1972, Kapandji 1974b). This tilt necessarily involves a lateral movement combined with rotation. Attempts to explain the nature of this movement often describe the atlas as a 'washer', being like an interposed meniscus or sesamoid bone between the occiput and the axis. This concept implies a gliding or linear displacement between the occiput and atlas rather than defining a true rotary movement (Braakman & Penning 1971, Von Torklus & Gehle 1972, Shapiro et al 1973, Penning 1978). The recent use of computerized axial tomography (CT) has made the examination of in vivo cervical spine rotation possible. Tables 4.3 and 4.4 indicate rotation ranges for the atlanto-axial and atlanto-occipital joints measured from CT studies (Dvorak et al 1987a, b, Penning & Wilmink 1987).

Penning and Wilmink (1987) report lateral displacement of the atlas of 4.4 mm relative to the foramen magnum in a direction contralateral to the direction of rotation of the head.

Movement of the atlanto-axial joints

Rotation of the atlanto-axial joints

Rotation of the atlanto-axial joint is said to be accompanied by a screw-like action, accounting for vertical translation of atlas in relation to axis (Werne 1957). Rotation to the right is checked by the tension of those fibres of the right alar ligament which are attached to the dens in front of the axis of movement and those of the left alar ligament which are attached to the process behind the axis of movement (Warwick & Williams 1989).

Flexion and extension of the atlanto-axial joints

Flexion of the atlanto-axial joint is seen by separation of the spinous process of the axis relative to the posterior arch of the atlas, and approximation in extension (Fielding 1957, Werne 1957, Wackenheim 1974). This movement also involves gliding of the atlantal arch superiorly on the odontoid in extension and inferiorly in flexion (Steindler 1955). Generally, the width of the atlanto-odontoid space diminishes during extension and may increase during flexion (Wackenheim 1974).

Lateral flexion of the atlanto-axial joints

The atlas alters its relationship with the axis during lateral flexion of the head and neck. Lateral flexion of up to 15° (without rotation of the head) produces rotation of the axis. Beyond 15° this is accompanied by further atlanto-axial rotation and lateral displacement of the atlas on the axis (Hohl & Baker 1964).

Functional and anatomical descriptions of ranges of movement of the craniovertebral joints

Differences in reported atlanto-occipital flexion–extension range are as wide as 10° and 35° (Werne 1957, Hohl & Baker 1964, White & Panjabi 1975, Penning 1978, Worth & Selvik 1986). Extension from full flexion results in anterior translation of the basiocciput relative to the atlas. This translation for a point in the occiput coincident with the centre of gravity of the atlas is approximately 5.5 mm for an extension–flexion range of approximately 18.5° (Worth & Selvik 1986). During extension from full flexion, a small amount of anterior translation of the atlas relative to the axis is normal. This is limited by the transverse ligament of the atlas.

Axial rotation between atlas and axis results in contralateral lateral flexion between the atlas and occiput (Worth & Selvik 1986, Kapandji 1974b). Lateral flexion is of the order of 8% of the axial rotation (Worth & Selvik 1986). Conversely, Worth and Selvik (1986) found that when lateral flexion of the head was induced, ipsilateral axial rotation between the atlas and axis occurred.

When testing the passive range of rotation, the therapist should note the passive range of the coupled contralateral lateral flexion at the atlanto-occipital joint.

Worth and Selvik (1986) also found that axial rotation to the left resulted in translation of the occiput to the left relative to the atlas and confirmed that this translation was approximately 2–3 mm (Kapandji 1974b) up to 4.4 mm (Penning & Wilmink 1978). There is controversy concerning the vertical translation of the atlas on the axis during axial rotation. Kapandji (1974b) says that this occurs as a spiral or helical movement of the order of 2–3 mm. However, this was not found by Worth and Selvik (1986).

Approximately the same amount of lateral flexion occurs between occiput and atlas, and atlas and axis. This lateral flexion is coupled with ipsilateral axial rotation between the atlas and axis.

Table 4.5 presents the ranges of movement at the atlanto-occipital and atlanto-axial functional spinal units. Tables 4.6, 4.7 and 4.8 give the coupled ranges of movement which occur during flexion–extension, rotation and lateral flexion (Worth & Selvik 1986).

Table 4.5 Table of means ± the confidence limits of the principal manipulated ranges of motion of the craniovertebral joints of the sample of 13 specimens*

	Extension to flexion	Axial rotation (right to left)	Lateral flexion (left to right)
0–C1	18.63 ± 1.51 (0.70)	3.43 ± 1.02 (0.39)	3.97 ± 1.54 (0.59)
C1–C2	13.33 ± 2.35 (0.90)	35.16 ± 7.39 (2.83)	4.07 ± 2.01 (0.77)

* The bracketed number is the standard deviation of the mean.

Table 4.6 Mean rotation effects of X-axis rotation

	Full flexion from full extension		
	X rotation	Y rotation	Z rotation
0–C1	18.63°	0.79° (right rotation)	0.60° (left lateral flexion)
C1–C2	13.33°	2.22° (right rotation)	0.28° (right lateral flexion)

Table 4.7 Mean rotation effects of Y-axis rotation

	Right-to-left axial rotation		Lat. flexion
	X rotation	Y rotation	Z rotation
0–C1	1.54° (extension)	3.43°	2.69° (right)
C1–C2	0.87° (extension)	35.16°	2.91° (left)

Table 4.8   Mean rotation effects of Z-axis rotation

	Left-to-right lateral flexion		
	X rotation	Y rotation	Z rotation
0–C1	0.33° (extension)	0.33° (right rotation)	3.97°
C1–C2	0.70° (flexion)	7.16° (right rotation)	4.07°

MOVEMENTS OF THE CERVICAL SPINE (C2–C7)

Intersegmental movements of the cervical spine have usually been examined by radiographic methods. These methods could be categorized into the following measurement techniques:

1. Direct X-ray measurement
2. Overlay technique
3. Modified overlap technique
4. Angular measurement from lines drawn on X-rays
5. Cineradiography
6. Biplanar X-ray photogrammetry.

Some of these measurement techniques have been used in cadaveric studies and some during in vivo studies. In some studies a combination of measurement techniques has been used.

Cadaver subjects have been chosen in studies of intersegmental mobility of the spine in preference to living subjects by several workers for the following reasons:

1. To prevent errors of measurement in uniplanar radiographs of living subjects
2. To validate measurements either in a cadaver or in an in vivo experiment
3. To allow invasive or destructive techniques to be used.

Table 4.9 indicates a wide disparity of some of the reported ranges of intervertebral mobility. To understand this it is necessary to have some insight into the various techniques used. What follows is a brief summary of how some of the reported ranges in Table 4.9 were obtained, together with comments on other relevant studies.

Direct X-ray measurements

Measurements of the intersegmental ranges in the cervical spine were taken directly from radiographic cadaveric studies (Ball & Meijers 1964, Ten Have & Eulderink 1980, 1981a, b).

Ball and Meijers (1964) examined 21 post mortem specimens (C1 to T2). Twelve were healthy, four had simple disc degenerative changes, two had ankylosing spondylitis, one had gross rheumatoid arthritis, one had polyarthritis and one had Reiter's disease. These pathologies may have affected the measured intersegmental ranges, bringing into question the validity of these results.

Flexion and extension were simulated by a force applied to the specimen through a line from the atlas suspended over a pulley. At the extreme of flexion and extension radiographs were taken. Angles of rotation were created by the images of steel pins inserted into the anterior surface of each vertebral body. They reported the mean ranges in nine normal subjects as shown in Table 4.9.

This experimental technique was put to clinical use in a study of the effects of degenerative changes in the ageing cervical spine upon intervertebral mobility (Ten Have & Eulderink 1981a) and the effect of degenerative changes

Table 4.9   Average reported ranges of cervical intervertebral movement

Authors reporting sagittal plane Rotation ranges	0/1	1/2	2/3	3/4	4/5	5/6	6/7
Dunkster et al (1978)	–	9.0	10.0	13.0	13.0	20.0	11.5
Penning (1978)	30.0	30.0	12.0	18.0	20.0	20.0	15.0
Mestagh (1976)	–	–	11.0	14.5	18.0	19.5	16.0
White & Panjabi (1978)	13.0	10.0	8.0	13.0	12.0	17.0	16.0
Buetti–Bauml (1954)	–	–	10.5	17.0	21.0	22.5	18.0
Bhalla & Simmons (1969)	–	–	9.0	14.0	22.0	18.0	19.0
Werne (1957)	13.0	10.0	–	–	–	–	–
Fielding (1957)	35.0	15.0	–	–	–	–	–
Worth (1980)	18.6	13.3	–	–	–	–	–
Lysell (1969)	–	–	4.9	10.2	13.0	14.5	13.5
Baake (1931)	–	–	12.6	15.4	15.1	20.4	17.0
Kottke & Mundale (1959)	–	11.0	11.0	16.0	18.0	21.0	18.0
Johnson et al (1977)	18.8	13.7	12.0	17.6	20.1	21.9	20.7
Ball & Meijers (1964)	–	–	9.5	15.1	18.1	20.2	17.6
Aho et al (1955)	–	13.6	12.7	16.1	21.8	27.6	15.7
Worth (1988)	–	–	9.9–11.7	13.6–15.7	16.0–18.5	15.5–18.8	12.8–15.3
Dvorak et al (1988)		12	10	15	19	20	19
Frontal plane rotation ranges Lysell (1969)	–	–	7.9	9.8	9.1	9.0	8.4
Dunkster et al (1978)	–	–	–	–	13.0	15.0	12.0
Horizontal plane rotation ranges Lysell (1969)	–	–	6.0	9.8	10.3	8.0	5.7

alone upon cervical intervertebral mobility (Tcn Have & Eulderink 1981b).

Whilst cadaveric experiments may allow high levels of precision, they are not easily generalized to the in vivo situation. Nevertheless, such cadaver X-rays may certainly be used as controls to test in vivo measurement technique for accuracy.

Overlay technique

Several studies used a well known technique which, for simplicity, is referred to here as the 'overlay technique' (Penning 1960, 1978, Dunkster et al 1978, Dvorak et al 1988).

The overlay technique has two main objectives: to locate the instantaneous axis of rotation of the cervical vertebrae and to calculate the angles of intervertebral rotation in the sagittal plane.

For the determination of mobility in various mobile segments a larger lateral film of the fully flexed cervical spine is overlaid by a smaller lateral film of the fully extended cervical spine. The images of the vertebral bodies and spinous processes of C7 in both films are superimposed as precisely as possible. Using the hard edge of the smaller film a line is drawn on the larger film. This process is repeated for C6 — and so on up the cervical spine. The angle between the first and second lines represents the range of movement between C7 and C6, and so on.

Penning (1978) reports 10° of lateral flexion and 70° of axial rotation in the craniovertebral joint, and 70° of lateral flexion and axial rotation for C3–C7 using the overlay technique.

Dunkster et al (1978) used the overlay method to measure sagittal plane rotation range in a subject group similar to that of Penning. They report some lateral flexion ranges but do not report details of the technique used. It is interesting to note the differences between the findings of Dunkster et al and Penning in all levels except for C5/6, which is the same (Table 4.9).

This technique was used to compare active and passive ranges (Dvorak et al 1988). The passive ranges were found to be 2° greater than the active ranges at all levels except C1/2 and C5/6, where the increase was 3°.

The overlay technique had the advantage of superimposing an infinite number of points around the periphery of the lateral image of a vertebra. Inter-observer reliability was reported as significant by Dvorak et al (1988). However they state that further information may be obtained by determining the centre of rotation at each level or by determining the ventral and dorsal gliding movements of each segment.

In using the overlay technique for determination of the instantaneous axes of rotation of the cervical motion segments, Amevo et al (1991a) found high inter- and intra-observer differences in individual subjects.

Qualitative analysis suggested that identification of the two radiographic images of the vertebrae and their tracing was the greatest source of error for this technique.

Prior to Dvorak et al (1988) and Amevo et al (1991a) the reproducibility of the overlay technique was not supported in the literature by tests of precision or accuracy.

Modifications of the overlay technique

Buetti-Bauml (1954) developed a modified overlay technique which was a precursor to the overlay technique reported by Penning (1960).

Buetti-Bauml (1954) used carbon paper to trace the images of two adjacent vertebrae from the flexion to the extension X-ray, superimposing the images of the lower vertebrae; then, lines were drawn along the posterior borders of both upper vertebral bodies — the angle between these lines representing the sagittal rotation ranges (Table 4.9).

Since then a number of workers have used the overlay technique with various modifications (Buetti-Bauml 1954, Parera 1975, Mestagh 1976, Schlicke et at 1979, Worth 1986, Dvorak et al 1988, Amevo et al 1991a–d).

Parera (1975) used a multivariate approach to study symptomatic and asymptomatic subjects. In this study, the measurement of range of intervertebral rotation and the location of the axis of that rotation was achieved with the use of the overlay technique. The major contribution of this work was that some of the errors of measurement in the overlay techniques were overcome by conducting a reliability trial to establish the 'best fit' method of accurately superimposing the image of the vertebra in one X-ray over the image of the same vertebra in the succeeding X-ray.

Mestagh (1976) used 33 healthy young adults, superimposing the images of the lower vertebra of a motion segment in the flexion and extension films and measuring the angles between the lines drawn along the inferior margins of the upper vertebra. The same technique was used for lateral flexion range using two antero-posterior X-rays with the subject in the extremes of left and right lateral flexion. A trigonometric formula was used to measure horizontal rotation.

An innovative approach to the problems of bony landmark identification was adopted by Schlicke et al (1979) using a modified overlay technique. These authors studied five males and three females between the ages of 23 and 37 years under mechanical cervical traction in supine with a load of 1/3 of the subjects body weight. An initial lateral X-ray was taken prior to the load being applied, and a second X-ray was taken 3 minutes after the application of the load. They state that 'two points on a rigid body completely define its position in a plane and with these two points both translation and rotation of a rigid body can be determined. Difficulty arises in being able

Table 4.10 Cervical spine rotation and displacements as a result of vertical loading (Schlicke et al 1979)

Average displacements			
C2–3	0.33	±	0.53
C3–4	0.69	±	0.38
C4–5	0.92	±	0.38
C5–6	0.68	±	0.49
Average	0.70	±	0.5
Average rotation range (flexion)			
C2–3	0.04	±	1.58
C3–4	1.54	±	2.05
C4–5	1.34	±	1.63
C5–6	0.66	±	1.52
Average	0.9	±	2.4

to recognize a specific anatomical point on a patient's X-ray film'.

Superimposition of the same vertebra in successive X-rays was referred to as the 'best fit' method. Having done this, two very small pin holes were made on the film at the upper anterior and posterior corners of the vertebral body. This was repeated for all cervical levels so that the pin holes became repeatable points between successive X-rays. The measurements were made from the pin holes rather than the 11 defined anatomic parts. Results included average anterior and superior separation and average rotation as a function of cervical traction (Table 4.10).

The ranges of cervical spine sagittal plane mobility were examined in a group of normal subjects using the overlay technique with the following modifications designed to enhance precision and accuracy (Worth 1986):

1. The extension X-ray was reversed into a photographic negative.
2. The X-rays were covered with acetate foil and superimposed using a bright light point with a variable control in the light box.
3. Visual parallax was reduced by positioning of the light box.
4. The superimposition of vertebral images was performed according to the technique of Parera (1975).
5. Fine pointed precision centre dividers were used to make puncture holes to be used as markers in the vertebral images as used by Schlicke et al (1979).
6. The subject was kept parallel to the film plane using a three-dimensional goniometer (Kadir et al 1981) and a calibration procedure.

This study reported translation ranges as well as flexion–extension ranges. Table 4.11 gives the 95% confidence interval for the ranges of flexion–extension, ventrodorsal and cephalocaudad translations.

The importance of the changes in the intersegmental relationships between the translations and sagittal plane rotation was demonstrated in a study of motor vehicle accident victims (Worth 1988).

Table 4.11 The 95% confidence interval for ranges of movement of C2–C7 of 55 normal subjects as measured using the functional X-ray and geometric measurement technique

Segment	Degrees of flexion–extension range	Ventrodorsal translation range (mm)	Cephalocaudad translation range (mm)
C2–3	9.87 – 11.71	2.67 – 3.19	–1.17 – –0.89
C3–4	13.58 – 15.74	3.27 – 3.83	–1.60 – –1.28
C4–5	16.00 – 18.48	2.62 – 5.18	–2.00 – –1.56
C5–6	15.48 – 18.76	2.89 – 3.57	–2.14 – –1.66
C6–7	12.80 – 15.32	1.81 – 2.41	–1.78 – –1.38

The average flexion–extension range from C2 to C7 in the group involved in rear-end collisions depended on the displacement in both the ventrodorsal and cephalocaudad translations. However at C1–C2, flexion and extension ranges depended almost exclusively on the cephalocaudad translation and not on the ventrodorsal translation. This difference was observed despite the fact that 'rear-end' victims demonstrated virtually normal average C1–C2 flexion–extension range radiographically (Worth 1986). This implies that neither standard radiography nor conventional functional radiography of the cervical spine is sufficiently sensitive to reveal these subtle translation departures from normal. It is likely, therefore, that false-negative radiological reports increase the tendency to label cervical soft-tissue injury victims as neurotic.

Both 'rear-end' and 'head-on' groups were significantly less mobile than normal subjects in flexion–extension range at the atlanto-occipital segment ($P < 0.05$). This effect was less marked in the 'head-on' groups than in the 'rear-end' groups (Table 4.12).

Thus, notwithstanding the fact that the symptomatic group of subjects had previous post-injury radiographs which predominantly were reported as normal, the experimental technique of functional cervical spine radiographs detected significant differences from the normal group.

Recent work has been directed to the reduction of errors occurring during X-ray studies of cervical spine kinematics using modified overlay techniques. X-ray kinematic studies have been applied to segmental ranges of rotatory and translatory movement, gross cervical spine movement and the behaviour of the instantaneous axis of rotation of the typical cervical motion segment (Worth &

Table 4.12 Difference in range of movement at the atlanto-occipital segment in normal, 'head-on' and 'rear-end' subjects using the upper cervical technique*

	Mean range of C0–1 flexion–extension in 52 motor vehicle accident victims		
	Normal	Rear-end	Head-on
Observed range	11.21°	5.80°	7.77°
Amount of lost range		5.41° (48.3%)	3.44° (30.7%)

* 'Rear-end' subjects lost 48.3% of sagittal plane rotation and 'head-on subjects' lost 30.7% of sagittal plane rotation by comparison with normal subjects ($P < 0.05$).

Selvik 1986, Worth 1988, Van Mameren et al 1990, Amevo et al 1991a).

The overlay concept (Buetti-Bauml 1954, Penning 1960) was enhanced for precision by Parera (1975) and used with a high level of reliability by Worth (1986). This involved calibration in order to reduce radiographic distortion to a minimum, calculation of the magnification factor, and alignment of the subject as close as possible to the central focus. The plane of rotation was monitored to maintain parallelism to the film plane, and reproducibility was demonstrated using the test–re-test reliability approach (Worth 1986).

Van Mameren et al (1990) however failed to demonstrate sufficient intra-examiner reliability using a fast method of determining the outlines of bony structures on cervical spine X-rays and concluded that neither total range of movement nor segmental range of movement was suitable as a parameter of cervical spine mobility using this method. They suggested that plotting the instantaneous centre of rotation might be a suitable parameter to employ with this method of measurement.

Radiological centres of rotation for cervical spine flexion movement were determined by Penning (1960). These centres were defined by Penning (1960) as instantaneous centres of rotation, being centres based on the two end positions of full flexion and full extension. Penning's centre for C2/3 was located in the dorsocaudal part of the body of C3, for C6/7 at the middle of the cranial endplate of C7, and for C3/4 to C5/6 intermediate positions.

Substantial measurement problems were found when using the overlay method of calculating the location of the instantaneous axes of rotation in the cervical vertebrae (Amevo et al 1991a).

Amevo et al (1991b) improved the overlay technique by reducing the error in tracing the vertebral outlines and by the application of specific criteria for fitting a coordinate system on the tracings of vertebral bodies.

This modified overlay technique was used to plot the locations of the instantaneous axes of rotation of the cervical motion segments C2/3 to C6/7 from the flexion–extension X-rays of 40 normal subjects (Amevo et al 1991c). There was little technical error, and the data obtained indicated the locations of the instantaneous axes of rotation of the typical cervical motion segments. Whilst this study confirmed Penning's findings that the instantaneous axes of rotation lie in the bodies of the subjacent vertebrae and appear similarly distributed, Amevo et al (1991c) were able to express the locations in digital terms in both absolute and normalized values.

Amevo et al (1991d) went on to compare the locations of the instantaneous axes of rotation of the cervical motion segments of the normal group to a symptomatic group of 109 patients with uncomplicated neck pain. The locations of the instantaneous axes of rotation were abnormal in 57% of patients and marginally abnormal in a further 26%.

It is important to note that all the patients' conventional plain X-rays had not been diagnostic and had not revealed any radiological abnormality.

The segmental source of pain was determined by provocation discography or zygapophyseal joint blocks.

Whilst there was no correlation between the location of an abnormal instantaneous axis of rotation and the demonstrated segmental source of pain, there was a significant correlation between the presence of pain and an abnormal axis. This may indicate other causes of pain or other associated causes for an abnormal axis such as muscle spasm (Amevo et al 1991d).

Angular measurement from lines drawn on X-rays

Several workers measured the intersegmental cervical spine ranges of movement from angles drawn directly onto X-ray images of cervical vertebrae (Aho et al 1955, Kottke & Mundale 1959, Bhalla & Simmons 1969, Johnson et al 1977, Worth 1986, Penning & Wilmink 1987).

Bhalla & Simmons (1969) measured the range of cervical spine intervertebral sagittal plane rotation in 20 healthy adults between 18 and 23 years. Intersecting lines were drawn along the posterior borders of each cervical vertebra from T1 up to C2. The angulation at each level was calculated relative to the line representing the posterior margin of the vertebra body of T1. Each cervical level was measured in flexion and extension and the sum of these two angles was the range (Table 4.9). This study was reported as reliable and stated 'the same figures can be obtained in consecutive trials on the same patient. This was demonstrated several times during the study when more than one set of radiographs was taken during the course of one evaluation and the development of the technique'. Every fifth frame of cineradiographs of cadaver specimens during flexion and extension was also measured, and the cadaver ranges corresponded consistently to the ranges of the 20 in vivo subjects. The sources of measurement error in the X-ray technique were recognized, and the following steps were taken to control them:

1. To prevent synchronous motion the heads of the subjects were kept parallel to the plane of sagittal rotation by an apparatus which was attached to the film stand.
2. The magnification factor was largely eliminated by keeping the distance from the subject's head to the X-ray plate fixed.

Kottke & Mundale (1959) measured cervical spine intervertebral sagittal plane rotation in 78 males aged 15–30 years from the occiput to C7. A line inferior to the atlas from the base of the tubercle to the base of the neural arch was used as the line of reference. The angles formed by lines through the bases of the bodies of the lower six cervical vertebrae and the line of reference were measured in flexion and extension. A line from the tubercle of the root of the zygoma to the postero-lateral tubercle of the foramen magnum was used as the reference line for the skull. The flexion and extension angles were added to give the range (Table 4.9).

Johnson et al (1977) studied the range of cervical intervertebral sagittal plane rotation, gross frontal plane and horizontal plane rotation of the head and neck in 44 healthy subjects from 20 to 36 years of age. The sagittal plane rotation was measured with the subject's head in neutral, full extension and full flexion. Lines were drawn on the X-rays tangential to the base of the skull at the foramen magnum and the basiocciput, along the inferior margin of the ring of the atlas, and through the tips of the inferior lips of each vertebral body from C2 to T1. The lines were extended until they intersected and the resulting angles were measured. Lines converging anteriorly were recorded as flexion angles and lines converging posteriorly were recorded as extension. The extension and flexion angles were added to give the range (Table 4.9).

Frontal plane rotation was measured as the angle made by a plastic rod with radiopaque beads at each end, held in the teeth and a line drawn tangential to the superior margins of the transverse processes of T1. Horizontal plane rotation was measured using overhead photographs of the head and shoulders with the subject wearing a cap fitted with reference marks.

Aho et al (1955) studied cervical spine sagittal plane rotation in three groups of subjects: 15 outpatients with normal cervical spine; 18 subjects with a radiological diagnosis of chondrosis; 15 subjects with advanced morphological change due to osteochondrosis and spondyloarthrosis deformans. In this technique lines were drawn joining the anterior and posterior tips of the inferior margin of each vertebra from C2 to C7. A second line joined the upper anterior corner and the lower posterior corner of the same vertebrae and was extended to intersect with the first line of the vertebra below forming angles representing the angle of intervertebral rotation. The ranges for the normal group are given in Table 4.9.

Cervical spine intersegmental rotation was measured in 26 healthy subjects using CT scans with the head fixed in full range left and right rotation (Penning & Wilmink 1987). Lines were drawn through symmetrical landmarks, and the films were superimposed to allow measurement between lines depicting relative vertebral rotation. Test–re-test reliability was significant. However, positioning led to C3–C5 tending to be parallel to the CT plane of investigation, whilst above and below there was tilting of the bony images interfering with the symmetry of the landmarks. Reported ranges were: C0/1 — 1°, C1/2 — 40.5°, C2/3 — 3.0°, C3/4 — 6.5°, C4/5 — 6.8°, C5/6 — 6.9°, C6/7 — 5.4°, C7/T1 — 2.1°. Coupled lateral flexion to the side of rotation measured 25.2° between C2 and T1.

The comparative reliability of the lines and angles and the overlay technique was examined by Worth (1986). The lines and angles technique was found to be unreliable at the mid-cervical levels (C2/3, C3/4, C4/5) for measurement of flexion–extension. This is the area of greatest flexion–extension range where there is a likelihood of greater variability and error of measurement.

Cineradiography

Cineradiography has been used to display cervical spine movements (Fielding 1957, 1964, Jones 1960, 1967, Woesner & Mitts 1972, Bleasel et al 1973).

The literature fails to reveal any quantitative measurements using this technique. Woesner and Mitts (1972) compared cineradiography with conventional radiography. They suggested that efficient use of routine plain film X-ray would provide most of the information regarding abnormal motion that could be detected by using either method.

Biplanar X-ray photogrammetry

Hallert (1958, 1970) applied the principles of photogrammetry to the X-ray imaging of the human body. He demonstrated that it was possible to represent the three-dimensional location of a rigid body with the aid of two simultaneous images of the object taken from two different planes.

X-ray photogrammetry has been used to study cervical spine intersegmental mobility in cadavers (Lysell 1969, Worth & Selvik 1986) and in living subjects (Suh 1974, Mimura et al 1989).

Lysell (1969) used biplanar X-ray photogrammetry with 28 cervical spines taken from fresh cadavers. They were X-rayed in both the frontal and sagittal planes whilst the specimen was in a fixed position. He pointed out that the following problems exist when measuring vertebral movement on single plane X-rays:

1. Linear error. Small errors in the measurement of linear distances may result in significant errors in the calculation of angles of rotation when using these measured distances as input data in trigonometric formulae.
2. Synchronous motion. A plain X-ray reduces a three-dimensional object to a two-dimensional image of that object. This may result in movements in planes other than that of the image not being detected.
3. Reproducibility. Reproducible points within the vertebrae may not be easily identified from one X-ray

to the next, either in the same plane or another plane. Reproducibility will be affected by any tendency of the subject not to be parallel to the film plane whilst the X-ray is being taken.

In this experiment these problems were overcome by using the biplanar technique which resulted in measurement of angular rotation ranges in three planes (sagittal, frontal and horizontal) as a function of movement in one of these planes. Implanted metal markers were used instead of bony landmarks to ensure accurate identification of the measuring point in all the X-rays.

The results described a pattern of cervical motion where, in extension, the superior vertebra in a motion segment tilts back and slides back. The reverse occurred in flexion. An index for the amount of intervertebral translation was developed; this was called the top angle (T angle). This index was reduced in the presence of increasing degenerative change. In contrast, the range of movement was not reduced with increasing joint degenerative change.

There was coupling in the frontal and horizontal planes, but during sagittal rotation (flexion, extension) no significant synchronous movement was found. Ranges of intervertebral rotation movement in the sagittal, frontal and horizontal planes measured in this experiment are given in Table 4.9.

Reliability and validity of the modified overlay technique of measurement of flexion–extension and cephalo-caudad and ventro-dorsal translation of cervical segments was studied using cadaveric X-ray photogrammetric results as criteria (Worth 1986).

It is important to note that despite the advantages of cadaver experimentation there are serious disadvantages. The greatest problem is that whilst the techniques used in cadaver experiments overcome some of the technical limitations on precision, most of the techniques are not able to be used on living subjects. It is therefore not readily possible to generalize results of cadaver studies to in vivo situations. Furthermore, cadaver simulation of cervical movements often falls short of the actual movements.

Suh (1974) applied X-ray photogrammetry to the cervical spine. The method was cumbersome and logistically not appropriate for investigation of large numbers of clinical subjects.

In a recent study (Mimura et al 1989), twenty normal males were X-rayed using biplanar radiography to produce three-dimensional analysis of movements. Subjects were X-rayed in a reference frame in neutral, full left and right rotation. Axial rotation and coupled movements were calculated within a vertebral three-dimensional coordinate system using bony landmarks. The occiput was marked with four steel ball markers attached to the skin. The atlas was not measured due to lack of suitable bony landmarks. Accuracy was quoted as 1 mm for translation

— 1.5° for rotation. Lateral flexion–rotation couping was observed ipsilaterally below C3/4 and contralaterally above C2/3. This technique presents the problems of requiring special apparatus and software, does not recognize the atlas and specific occipital landmarks, and measures the cranio-vertebral movements in one segment (C0–C2) only.

X-ray photogrammetry is complicated and relies on biplanar identification of landmarks. The best landmarks in this technique are metal implants. It is generally not an efficient method for in vivo examination of cervical spine intersegmental movements. However, it is an excellent tool for the validation and reliability testing of other less complicated measurement techniques.

CERVICAL SPINE KINEMATICS

This section deals with the patterns of cervical spine movements which provide the head and neck with a large amount of mobility. This mobility helps to orient the sensory organs of the head and neck in response to internal and external stimuli. By a complex integration of changing relationships between the components of the functional spinal units, purposeful movements of the head and neck occur. This forms the raw material of kinematics which is the description of motion in mathematical terms (Selvik 1974).

It is well established that lateral flexion results in a coupled range of ipsilateral rotation at each of the cervical motion segments (Lysell 1969). This is usually compensated for by a de-rotation at the atlanto-axial level (Kapandji 1974a). This explains why it is possible for the face of a subject performing lateral flexion to remain in the frontal plane. However, the coupled range of ipsilateral rotation below the atlanto-axial joint will still be occurring. The amount of coupled rotation when lateral flexion takes place has been studied in cadavers (Lysell 1969). However, it is extraordinarily difficult to replicate such studies in living subjects as such a study requires biplanar X-ray photogrammetry and the use of marker implants to act as reproducible indentifiers. This supports the most common use of flexion–extension functional X-rays, which are uniplanar and reproducible and involve little or no coupled movements (Lysell 1969).

The notion of coupled lateral flexion and rotation suggests that the axis of rotation is likely to be close to the zygapophyseal joint on the side to which the subject is turning. This also suggests that the contralateral articular surface of the cephalad vertebra is sliding up and forward in a flexion-like fashion. If this is the case then a rotation or lateral flexion movement abnormality should predict a flexion–extension abnormality which can be palpated.

Between C2 and C7, flexion and extension take place in the sagittal plane by means of rotation of a vertebra about an axis situated in the body of the vertebra below

(Penning 1978). The location of this axis implies that, during flexion–extension movements, the vertebra slides upward and forward when flexing and downward and backward when extending. This observation, and an important relationship between flexion–extension (sagittal plane rotation) and two translations, has recently been confirmed (Worth 1986). This relationship was found to be a linear one which depends upon the values of two independent variables: cephalocaudad and ventrodorsal translation. Subtle changes in this relationship are not easily detected on routine cervical radiographic examinations, or hitherto in functional radiographic studies. Flexion–extension range increases as the positive value for ventrodorsal translation increases, and the negative value for cephalocaudad translation also increases. In anatomical terms, this means that the range of extension from full flexion will increase by a predictable amount according to the prescribed amounts of ventrodorsal and cephalocaudad translation. In clinical terms, the linear relationship between flexion–extension and translations may allow the therapist to determine which component of the movement of a cervical motion segment is likely to be abnormal in a subject whose flexion–extension range reproduces the relevant symptoms (Worth 1986).

In flexing from a position of extension, a cervical vertebra slides upward and forward over its subjacent neighbour (Lysell 1969) combining the Z and Y axis translation with X axis rotation. This is an important consideration in examining for abnormal patterns using tests of passive intervertebral movements. Postero-anterior pressures with the patient prone may not elicit the same information as palpation of the articular pillars during flexion from full extension. The former test is more likely to reveal which motion segment is most productive of the symptoms of which the patient is complaining, whereas the latter is more likely to reveal which joints present an abnormal pattern of movement, and the two may not coincide. This indicates the reason why both passive physiological intervertebral movements and passive accessory movements are included in a patient examination of the cervical spine which will extend from C0/1 to T4/5 (approxi-

mately). For example, palpation may reveal C2/3 as the motion segment responsible for the patient's symptoms since unilateral vertebral pressures over one of the posterior vertebral joins of that segment reproduce the patient's symptoms, and perhaps some guarding muscle spasm is noted during palpation. Thus, movement of the segment appears to be restricted by pain and spasm when palpated. However, passive motion testing may reveal restricted movement in the C3/4 motion segment or other distal segments. This restriction should also be palpated for both reproduction of symptoms and loss of accessory movements even if it seems asymptomatic. This is necessary because abnormal patterns of movement may be the cause of persistent irritability in the joint above, i.e. in this example of C2/3. The irritability in C2/3 may be temporarily relieved by treatment but is likely to recur unless the neighbouring motion segments are restored to as normal a pattern of movement as possible.

There are clinical implications of the presence of abnormally located instantaneous axes of rotation and disturbances in the linear relationships between sagittal plane rotation and translations which lead to speculation about pain sources.

The presence of these observed kinematic disturbances, particularly despite the almost total absence of reported radiological abnormality, indicates the importance of the more sensitive techniques which identify subtle changes in movement patterns (Worth 1986, Amevo et al 1991b).

These kinematic disturbances must be due to soft-tissue abnormality in any structure which can affect cervical spine mobility. These structures could be muscular, ligamentous, neural or vascular and may be intimately related to, or be remote from, the joints. They may be within or outside the spinal canal.

Now that it is possible to measure the relationship between the presence of symptoms and abnormal kinematics in the cervical spine, a great deal of work is necessary to understand more about the causal relationships. We may then apply our treatment confident that we are treating an abnormal functional spinal unit which is responsible for the patient's symptoms.

REFERENCES

Adams C B T, Logue V 1971 Studies in spondylotic myelopathy 2. The movement and contour of the spine in relation to the neural complications of cervical spondylosis. Brain 94: 569–586

Aho A, Vartainen O, Salo O 1955 Segmentary antero-posterior mobility of the cervical spine. Annales Medicinae Internae Fenniae 44: 287–299

Alund M, Larsson S (1990) Three-dimensional analysis of neck motion. A clinical method. Spine 15: 87–91

Amevo B, Macintosh J E, Worth D R, Bogduk N 1991a Instantaneous axes of rotation of the typical cervical motion segments: 1. An empirical study of technical errors. Clinical Biomechanics 6: 31–37

Amevo B, Worth D, Bogduk N 1991b Instantaneous axes of rotation of the typical cervical motion segments: II. Optimization of technical errors. Clinical Biomechanics 6: 38–46

Amevo B, Worth D, Bogduk N 1991c Instantaneous axes of rotation of the typical cervical motion segments : a study in normal volunteers. Clinical Biomechanics (in press)

Amevo B, Aprill C, Bogduk N 1991d Abnormal instantaneous axes of rotation in patients with neck pain. Spine (submitted for publication)

Baake S N 1931 Rontgenologische Beobachtungen Uber die Bewegungen der Wirbelsaule. Acta Radiologica (Stockholm) (suppl 13)

Ball J, Meijers K A E 1964 On cervical mobility. Annals of Rheumatic Diseases 23: 429–438

Barnett C H, Davies D V, MacConaill M A 1961a Synovial joints — their structure and mechanics. Longman, London, pp 260–268

Barnett C H, Davies D V, MacConaill M A 1961b Synovial joints, their structure and mechanics. Longman, London, pp 170–199

Basmajian J V (ed) 1971 Grant's method of anatomy .Williams & Wilkins, Baltimore

Bennett J G, Bergmanis L E, Carpenter J K, Skowlund H V 1963 Range of motion of the neck. Journal of the American Physical Therapy Association 43: 45–47

Bhalla S K, Simmons E H 1969 Normal ranges of intervertebral joint motion of the cervical spine. Canadian Journal of Surgery 12: 181–187

Bleasel K, Connelley T J, Dan N G 1973 Cervical spondylitic myelopathy: the use of cine-radiography to select certain cases for surgery. Proceedings of the Australian Association of Neurologists 9: 213–218

Braakman R, Penning L 1971 Injuries of the cervical spine. Excerpta Medica, Amsterdam, pp 3–30

Buetti-Bauml C 1954 Funktionelle Roentgendiagnostik der Halswirbelsaule. Thieme Verlag, Stuttgart, pp 20–24

Colachis S C, Strohm B R 1965 Radiographic studies of cervical spine motion in normal subjects. Flexion and hyperextension. Archives of Physical Medicine and Rehabilitation 46: 753–760

Dimnet J, Pasquet A, Krag M H, Panjabi M M 1982 Cervical spine motion in the sagittal plane: kinematic and geometric parameters. Journal of Biomechanics 15: 959–969

Dirheimer Y 1977 The craniovertebral region in chronic inflammatory rheumatic diseases. Springer-Verlag, Berlin, p 23

Dunkster S B, Colley D P, Mayfield F H 1978 Kinematics of the cervical spine. Clinical Neurology 25: 174–183

Dvorak J, Hayek J, Zehnder R 1987a CT — functional diagnosis of the rotatory instability of the upper cervical spine — 2. An evaluation on healthy adults and patients with suspected instability. Spine 12: 726–731

Dvorak J, Panjabi M M, Gerber M, Wichmann W 1987b CT — functional diagnostics of the rotatory instability of upper cervical spine. 1. An experimental study on cadavers. Spine 12: 197–205

Dvorak J, Froehlich D, Penning L, Baumgartner H, Panjabi M M 1988 Functional radiographic diagnosis of the cervical spine: flexion/extension. Spine 13: 748–755

Ferlic D 1962 The range of motion of the 'normal' cervical spine. Bulletin of the Johns Hopkins Hospital 110: 59–65

Fielding J W 1957 Cineroentgenography of the normal cervical spine. Journal of Bone and Joint Surgery 39A: 1280–1288

Fielding J W 1964 Normal and selected abnormal motion of the cervical spine from the second cervical vertebra to the seventh cervical vertebra based on cineroentgenography. Journal of Bone and Joint Surgery 46A: 1779–1781

Hall M C 1965 The locomotor system: functional anatomy. Thomas, Illinois

Hallert B 1958 The basic geometric principles of X-ray photogrammetry. AB Henrik Lindstahls Bokhandel I Distribution, Stockholm

Hallert B 1970 X-ray photogrammetry basic geometry and quality. Elsevier, Amsterdam

Hohl M, Baker H R 1964 The atlanto-axial joint. Journal of Bone and Joint Surgery 46A: 1739–1752

Hollinshead W J 1967 Textbook of anatomy. 2nd edn. Harper & Row, New York

Jackson R 1966 The cervical syndrome. 3rd edn. Thomas, Illinois, pp 5–20

Jirout J 1973 Changes in the atlas-axis relations on lateral flexion of the head and neck. Neuroradiology 6: 215–218

Johnson R M, Hart D L, Simmons E F, Ramsby G R, Southwick W O 1977 Cervical orthoses. Journal of Bone and Joint Surgery 59A: 332–339

Jones M D 1960 Cineradiographic studies of the normal cervical spine. California Medicine 93: 293–296

Jones M D 1967 Cineradiographic studies of abnormalities of the high cervical spine. Archives of Surgery 94: 206–213

Kadir M, Grayson M F, Goldberg A A S, Swain M C 1981 A new neck goniometer. Rheumatology and Rehabilitation 20: 219–226

Kapandji I 1974a The physiology of the joints Vol 3. The trunk and vertebral column. 2nd edn. Longman, New York, pp 218–228

Kapandji I 1974b The physiology of the joints. Vol 3. The trunk and vertebral column. 2nd edn. Longman Group, New York, pp 178, 182, 184

Kottke F J, Mundale M O 1959 Range of mobility of the cervical spine. Archives of Physical Medicine and Rehabilitation 40: 379–382

Last R J 1972 Anatomy: regional and applied. 5th edn. Churchill Livingstone, Edinburgh

Lysell E 1969 Motion in the cervical spine, an experimental study on autopsy specimens. Acta Orthopaedica Scandinavica suppl 123: 4–61

Mestagh H 1976 Morphological and biomechanical properties of the vertebroaxial joint (C2/3). Acta Morphologica Neerlando-Scandinavica 14: 19–30

Mimura M, Moriya H, Watnabe T, Takahashi K, Yamagata M, Tamaki T (1989) Three-dimensional motion analysis of the cervical spine with special reference to the axial rotation. Spine 14: 1135–1139

O'Connell A L, Gardner E B 1972 Understanding the scientific bases of human movement. Williams & Wilkins, Baltimore, p 38

O'Driscoll S L, Tomenson J 1982 The cervical spine. Clinics in Rheumatic Diseases 8: 617–630

Parera C E 1975 Functional cervical studies in vestibular dysfunction. Advances en Radiologia O R l, Marban (ed) Madrid pp 229–317

Penning L 1960 Functioneel rontgenoderzoek bij degenerative en traumatische aandoeningen der laag-cervical bewegingssegmenten. Proefschrift, Groningen, pp 1–11

Penning L 1968 Functional pathology of the cervical spine. Excerpta Medical, Amsterdam, pp 28–33

Penning L 1978 Normal movements of the cervical spine. American Journal of Roentgenology 130: 317–326

Penning L, Wilmink J T 1987 Rotation of the cervical spine. A CT study in normal subjects. Spine 12: 732–738

Romanes G J (ed) 1972 Cunningham's textbook of anatomy. Oxford University Press, Oxford

Schlicke L H, White A A, Panjabi M M, Pratt A, Kier L 1979 A quantitative study of vertebral displacement and angulation in the normal cervical spine under axial load. Clinical Orthopaedics and Related Research 140: 47–49

Schoening H A, Hannan V 1964 Factors related to cervical spine mobility, part 1. Archives of Physical Medicine and Rehabilitation 45: 602–609

Selvik G 1974 A roentgen stereophotogrammetric method for the study of the kinematics of the skeletal system. Thesis, Department of Anatomy and Department of Diagnostic Radiology, University of Lund, Lund, Sweden

Shapiro R, Youngberg A A, Rothman S L G 1973 The differential diagnosis of traumatic lesions of the occipito-atlanto-axial segment. Radiological Clinics of North America XI 3: 505–525

Smith B A 1968 Cervical spondylosis and its neurological complications. Thomas, Illinois

Snyder R G, Chaffin D B, Schneider L W, Foust D R, Bowman B M, Baum J K 1975 Basic biomechanical properties of the human neck related to lateral hyperflexion injury. Highway Safety Research Institute, University of Michigan Final Technical Report UM-HSRI-BI 75-4: 455–485

Steindler A 1955 Kinesiology of the human body. Thomas, Illinois, p 147

Suh C H 1974 The fundamentals of computer aided X-ray analysis of the spine. Journal of Biomechanics 7: 161–169

Ten Have H A M J, Eulderink F 1980 Degenerative changes in the cervical spine and their relationship to mobility. Journal of Pathology 132: 133–159

Ten Have H A M J, Eulderink F 1981a Mobility and degenerative changes of the ageing cervical spine. A macroscopic and statistical study. Gerontology 27: 42–50

Ten Have H A M J, Eulderink F 1981b Degenerative changes in the cervical spine and their relationship to mobility. Journal of Pathology 132: 133–159

Van Mameren H, Drukkers J, Sanches H, Beursgens J 1990 Cervical spine motion in the sagittal plane (1) range of motion of actually performed movements, an X-ray cinematographic study. European Journal of Morphology 28: 47–68

Von Torklus D, Gehle W 1972 The upper cervical spine. Butterworths, London, p 9

Wackenheim A 1974 Roentgen diagnosis of the cranio-vertebral region, Springer-Verlag, Berlin, pp 96–102

Warwick R, Williams P L (eds) 1989 Gray's anatomy. 35th edn. Longman, London, pp 416, 417

Werne S 1957 Studies in spontaneous atlas dislocation. Acta Orthopaedica Scandinavica Supplementum, No. XXIII, p 47

Werne S 1959 The possibilities of movements in the cranio-vertebral joints. Acta Orthopaedica Scandinavica 28: 165–173

White A A, Panjabi M M 1975 Spinal kinematics. In: Research status of spinal manipulative therapy NINCDS. Monograph no 15. US Department of Health, Education and Welfare, p 93

White A A, Panjabi M M 1978 The clinical biomechanics of the occipitoatlantoaxoid complex. Orthopaedic Clinics of North America 9: 867–878

Woesner M E, Mitts M G 1972 The evaluation of cervical spine motion below C2: a comparison of cine roentgenographic and conventional roentgenographic methods. American Journal of Roentgenology, Radium Therapy and Nuclear Medicine 115: 148–152

Worth D R 1980 Kinematics of the cranio-vertebral joints. In: Idczak R (ed) Aspects of manipulative therapy. Lincoln Institute of Health Sciences, Victoria, pp 39–44

Worth D R 1981 Cervical spine kinematics. Unpublished report, Higher Degrees Committee, School of Medicine, Flinders University of South Australia

Worth D R 1986 Cervical spine kinematics. Doctoral thesis, Flinders University of South Australia

Worth D R 1988 Biomechanics of the cervical spine. In: Grant R (ed) Physical therapy of the cervical and thoracic spine. Churchill Livingstone, New York

Worth D R, Selvik G 1986 Movements of the craniovertebral joints. In: Grieve G (ed) Modern manual therapy of the vertebral column. Churchill Livingstone, Edinburgh, p 53

5. The menisci of the cervical synovial joints

S. Mercer

Intra-articular inclusions are said to be typical of synovial joints in general (Williams et al 1989), and the synovial joints of the vertebral column have been shown to contain various types of inclusion. Most descriptions of these intra-articular inclusions are found in the European literature (Santo 1935, Zaccheo & Reale 1956, Dorr 1958, Penning & Tondury 1963, De Marchi 1963, Tager 1965, Emminger 1972, Kos & Wolf 1972, Tondury 1972, Benini 1979). Only a few occur in the English-language journals and then, largely with respect to the lumbar zygapophyseal joints where their form, incidence and disposition has been reported (Hadley 1961, Hadley 1964, Engel & Bogduk 1982, Bogduk & Engel 1984, Jones et al 1989, Singer et al 1990).

Until recently the few studies of menisci in the cervical synovial joints had been largely descriptive and based on histological or whole-mount sections of the joints (Santo & Schminke 1932, Santo 1935, Tondury 1941, Penning & Tondury 1963, Emminger 1972, Yu et al 1987). Three types of intra-articular inclusions are found in the cervical synovial joints: intra-articular fat pads, fibro-adipose meniscoid structures and capsular rims. At least one type of structure is found in each synovial joint (Mercer & Bogduk (in prep)).

INTRA-ARTICULAR INCLUSIONS

Intra-articular fat pads

Articular fat pads occupy the space bounded by the joint capsule and the perimeter of the articular cartilage, and therefore remain outside of the joint space. They have wide bases attached to the joint capsule and rounded free borders. Microscopically, fat pads are composed primarily of adipose tissue with associated loose connective tissue and blood vessels. Connective tissue septa divide the adipose tissue into lobules which are collectively surrounded by layers of connective tissue which also provide support for the blood vessels and attachment of the pad to the joint capsule. The pads are covered by the adipose type of synovial membrane.

Fat pads occur most frequently at the atlanto-occipital joints where they are located either medial or lateral or both to the constriction of the superior articular facet of the atlas. At lower levels of the cervical spine their presence is rare and their disposition irregular (Table 5.1).

Fibro-adipose meniscoids

Fibro-adipose meniscoids are the most commonly found intra-articular inclusion in joints at all levels of the cervical spine except at the atlanto-occipital joint where the fat pads predominate (Table 5.1). Each meniscoid has a thick base attached to the joint capsule but tapers to a thin fibrous end which protrudes into the joint cavity for varying distances ranging from 2 to 5 mm. They are freely mobile over the articular surfaces. The disposition of these structures depends on the shape and orientation of the articular facet.

At the lateral atlanto-axial joints meniscoids are crescentic in shape, being located along the medial, dorsomedial, lateral or ventrolateral margins of the joint. Where the inferior facet is oval the meniscoid stretches across the ventrolateral or across both the ventrolateral and dorsomedial margins of the articular surface. In lateral atlanto-axial joints, where the inferior facet is rounded,

Table 5.1 Prevalence of intra-articular inclusions in the cervical synovial joints by type and segment

| Segment | Number studied | Prevalence | | |
		Fat pads	Fibro-adipose meniscoids	Capsular rims
AO	30	28(93%)	4(14%)	12(40%)
C1–2	30	0(0%)	29(97%)	2(7%)
C2–3	30	2(7%)	25(83%)	7(23%)
C3–4	30	0(0%)	30(100%)	4(13%)
C4–5	30	2(7%)	30(100%)	6(20%)
C5–6	30	1(3%)	28(93%)	3(10%)
C6–7	30	2(7%)	28(93%)	8(27%)
Total	210	35(17%)	174(83%)	42(20%)

AO = atlanto-occipital joint; C1–2 = lateral atlanto-occipital joint; C2–3 etc. zygapophyseal joints.
Taken from a study which examined 210 cervical synovial joints (Mercer & Bogduk, in prep).

the meniscoid occurs along the ventral or along both the ventral and dorsal poles of the joint. The fibro-adipose meniscoids occur at the ventrolateral or dorsomedial poles in zygapophyseal joints which have oval facets and at the ventral or dorsal poles in the joints having circular facets.

On the basis of histological examination the fibro-adipose meniscoids may be divided into three regions: basal, middle and apical. The basal region consists of either a core of adipose tissue interwoven and covered by connective tissue that is continuous from the joint capsule, or is composed only of connective tissue and blood vessels. The middle region is comprised of denser connective tissue. The apical region and its free borders are composed exclusively of collagen which is orientated on the surface but unorientated internally. The fibro-adipose meniscoids are totally covered by synovial membrane which is of the fibrous type in the apical region and over the free borders and either of the adipose or fibrous type in the basal region.

Capsular rims

Capsular rims are stiff, wedge-shaped invaginations of the joint capsule. They occur around the margins of the articular surfaces and do not enter the joint space. Rather, they occupy the space between the joint capsule and the facet margin. The presence of capsular rims at each level was rare, being most likely to occur at the atlanto-occipital level (Table 5.1). They also tend to occur anywhere around the facet margin but with some preponderance towards the dorsal or lateral margins. In the zygapophyseal joints, when capsular rims and fibro-adipose meniscoids are present, they tend to be continuous at the anterior and posterior poles.

Microscopically, capsular rims appear to be internal thickenings of the joint capsule as the connective tissue is a continuation of the fibrous tissue of the capsule. Blood vessels are randomly dispersed throughout the connective tissue. The capsular rims are covered by synovial membrane of the fibrous type.

FUNCTIONAL SIGNIFICANCE

The suggested functions of the fibro-adipose meniscoids or intra-articular foldings have been: compensation for joint incongruency (Santo & Schminke 1932, Putz & Pomaroli 1972), distribution of synovial fluid (Santo & Schminke 1932), preservation of articular facet edges (Santo and Schminke 1932, Tondury 1941), transmission of forces (Putz & Pomaroli 1972), and fillers of cavities or spaces left open during motion (Tondury 1941, Dorr 1958, Putz & Pomaroli 1972). In these studies no attempt was made to relate type, incidence or disposition of the intra-articular inclusions to function.

At the atlanto-occipital joints the predominant structures were articular fat pads which were located in the recesses at the constriction of the superior articular facets of the atlas. Their site suggests that they could be acting as displaceable space fillers. In the neutral position the fat pads would fill the non-articular portions of the joint and, during motion, would move, as occurs with the non-articular fat pads in the knee joint. For this purpose neither synovial fluid nor fibrous tissue would serve as well as fat. Synovial fluid is not designed to fill cavities but rather to act as a lubricant, while fibrous tissue would cause the joint to be stiff. The presence of articular fat pads in the zygapophyseal joints is so rare that they probably have no significant function at these levels.

The fibro-adipose meniscoids predominate at the lateral atlanto-axial joints, and in the zygapophyseal joints they are located along the principal axes of motion. They occur in those joints that translate with the superior facets subluxing within the normal range of motion thus exposing the joint surface. Being located along the articular margins and attached to the joint capsule the fibro-adipose meniscoids would protect the exposed cartilage during joint motion by maintaining a film of synovial fluid between themselves and the cartilage. Otherwise the only protection possible for the exposed cartilage would be synovial fluid, and in a gliding joint its viscosity would hinder freedom of movement.

Capsular rims, being stiff, wedge-shaped invaginations of the joint capsule would fill the space around the rim of the joint where the articular surfaces diverge. Although they are rarely present their highest incidence is at the atlanto-occipital joints which are weight-bearing but have a more restricted range of motion than the weight-bearing atlanto-axial joints. At the atlanto-occipital joint they would fill the space around the rim and so distribute forces.

CLINICAL SIGNIFICANCE

The presence of these intra-articular inclusions in the cervical synovial joints invites consideration of their possible role in movement dysfunction. Because of their size and presence in such small joints, imaging of these structures is difficult so that discussion of their role in joint pathology must be speculative. Two possible roles of intra-articular inclusions in movement dysfunction are in joint stiffness and in acute locked neck.

Histological examination of the intra-articular inclusions revealed the presence of fatty and fibrous connective tissue. In the knee joint it is known that the adipose tissue of the intra-articular fat pads is the first tissue to proliferate following joint immobilization (Enneking & Horowitz 1972, Akeson et al 1980). Similar changes could occur in those cervical synovial joints containing articular fat pads or fibro-adipose meniscoids having an adipose tissue core in their basal region. These structures could act as the nidus for the proliferation of fatty tissue in immobilized cervical joints. The presence of fibro-adipose meniscoids within the joint cavity also provides an ideal site for fibrous tissue proliferation which could develop into adhesions between the articular cartilage. This mechanism for the development of adhesions has been demonstrated in the knee joint (Enneking & Horowitz 1972, Akeson et al 1980). The stiffness of cervical joints evident on manual examination, as reported in the physiotherapy literature (Jull 1986), could be accounted for by fibrous tissue proliferation and such adhesions. These might well be precipitated by intra-articular haemorrhage following injuries to cervical joints, such as capsular tears or subchondral fractures.

Intra-articular inclusions have been implicated in the acute locked neck. The clinical features of this disorder are: sudden onset of unilateral mid-cervical pain and movement restriction which may have developed following a quick, unguarded movement of the head and a tendency for repeated episodes with no history of trauma. The patient presents with a protective deformity of lateral flexion and rotation away from the side of pain with pain increasing on attempted lateral flexion and rotation towards the affected side.

Mechanical dysfunction of a zygapophyseal joint on the involved side has been suggested as the underlying cause (Maitland 1978, Spraque 1983). Dorr (1958) specifically implicated the role of the menisci in this mechanical problem, suggesting that the menisci slide into the joint, become trapped and so apply tension to the joint capsule resulting in pain and motion restriction. Pinching of the menisci was the mechanism that Kos and Wolf (1972) proposed for the development of sudden catching neck pain and blockage of the joint in the neutral position. They stated that squeezing of the menisci between the articular surfaces caused the surrounding muscles to reflexly contract, thus restricting movement. Manipulation would result in separation of the articular surfaces thus releasing the squeezed meniscus.

Of relevance to the discussion of the role of the menisci in the development of acute locked neck is the posture and motion restriction exhibited by the patient. The classical posture is one of lateral flexion and slight rotation away from the painful side with increased pain on attempted movement towards the painful side (McNair 1986), not pain and motion restriction in the neutral position. This condition is also particularly responsive to manipulative therapy, with longitudinal movement cephalad, rotation away from the side of pain, and transverse thrust manipulation being the treatments of choice (Maitland 1978, Spraque 1983, McNair 1986). Longitudinal movement cephalad causes an opening of the zygapophyseal joint space. Rotation and transverse thrust result in further superior and anterior motion of the

contralateral inferior articular facet with gapping of the joint cavity. Following one of these techniques the patient is able to regain a neutral head position or move towards the painful side (Maitland 1978).

A proposed explanation for the pathology of acute locked neck which responds to manipulative therapy is one of extrapment of the fibro-adipose meniscoid. This mechanism of menisci extrapment has been proposed to account for the development and response to manipulative therapy of acute locked back (Bogduk & Jull 1985). In the mid-cervical region, the most common clinical site of pain associated with acute locked neck, fibro-adipose meniscoids are the most prevalent form of intra-articular inclusion. They are also the only structures which are large and protrude into the joint cavity. In the motion of lateral flexion and rotation away from the painful side, the inferior articular facet of the involved joint glides superiorly and anteriorly taking the fibro-adipose meniscoid with it, due to the attachment of the meniscoid to the stretching joint capsule. If, on the return movement the meniscoid becomes deflected on the articular margin it would buckle, causing tension on the innervated joint capsule resulting in pain and muscle spasm. Maintenance of the classic posture associated with acute locked neck would minimize pain while movement towards neutral or the painful side would place increasing tension on the joint capsule and an increase in pain and muscular spasm. Examination of the manipulative therapy techniques stated to be successful in treating acute locked neck reveals that they would open the joint space and allow the menisci to straighten, therefore facilitating its return into the joint cavity.

Lewit's (1987) criticism of the extrapment theory of menisci in the lumbar zygapophyseal joints arises as the result of a semantic misinterpretation. The original European theory of meniscus entrapment refers to the role of menisci in stiff joints locked in a neutral position whereas the meniscus extrapment theory relates to joints locked at extremes of physiological subluxation after flexion in the lumbar spine and lateral flexion and rotation of the cervical spine. The blockage or stiffness in neutral with associated restriction of motion is consistent with the fibro-adipose meniscoids precipitating an intra-articular fibrosus.

CONCLUSION

Although the morphology of the cervical fibro-adipose meniscoids is well known, conjectures as to their physiological function and pathological significance remain only speculative. To date, there have been no imaging techniques whereby these structures can be visualized in vivo. However, it appears that these structures can be resolved with good quality MRI. Future refinements of MRI may well prove to be the tool by which the clinical and pathological significance of cervical meniscoids might be explored in a conclusive manner.

In the meantime, the theory of cervical meniscus extrampment is attractive because it is consistent with the experience of manipulative therapists who treat acute locked neck and the manual techniques found to be effective for this condition.

REFERENCES

Akeson W H, Amiel D, Woo S L Y 1980 Immobility effects on synovial joints. The pathomechanics of joint contracture. Biorheology 17: 95–100

Benini A 1979 Das kleine Gelenk der Lendenwirbelsäule. Zur Kenntnis seiner funktionellen Anatomie unter besonder Berücksichtigung der meniskoiden Einschlusse. Fortschritte der Medizin 97: 2103–2106

Bogduk N, Engel R 1984 The menisci of the lumbar zygapophysial joints. A review of their anatomy and clinical significance. Spine 9: 454–460

Bogduk N, Jull G 1985 The theoretical pathology of acute locked back: a basis for manipulative therapy. Manual Medicine 1: 78–82

De Marchi G F 1963 Le articolazioni intervertebrali. La Clinica Ortopedica 15: 26–32

Dorr W M 1958 Über die Anatomie der Wirbelgelenke. Archiv für Orthopädische und Unfallchirurgie 50: 222–234

Emminger E 1972 Les articulations interapophysaires et leurs structures meniscoides vues sous l'angle de la pathologie. Annales de Medicine Physique 15: 219–238

Engel R, Bogduk N 1982 The menisci of the lumbar zygapophyseal joints. Journal of Anatomy 135: 795–809

Enneking W, Horowitz M 1972 The intra-articular effects of immobilization of the human knee. Journal of Bone and Joint Surgery 54A: 973–985

Hadley L A 1961 Anatomico-roentgenographic studies of the posterior spinal articulations. American Journal of Roentgenography 86: 270–276

Hadley L A 1964 Anatomico-roentgenographic studies of the spine. Thomas, Springfield, p 175

Jones T R, James J E, Adams, J W, Garcia J, Walker S L, Ellis J P 1989 Lumbar zygapophyseal joint meniscoids: evidence of their role in chronic intersegmental hypomobility. Journal of Manipulative and Physiological Therapeutics 12: 374–385

Jull G A 1986 Clinical observations of upper cervical mobility. In: Grieve G P (ed) Modern manual therapy of the vertebral column. Churchill Livingstone, Edinburgh

Kos J, Wolf J 1972 Die 'Menisci' der Zwischenwirbelsäule und ihre mögliche Rolle bei Wirbelblockierung. Manuelle medizine 10: 105–114

Lewit K 1987 'The theoretical pathology of acute locked back: a basis for manipulative therapy' by N. Bogduk and G. Jull. Manual Medicine 3: 69

McNair J F S 1986 Acute locking of the cervical spine. In: Grieve G P (ed) Moden manual therapy of the vertebral column. Churchill Livingstone, Edinburgh

Maitland G D 1978 Acute locking of the cervical spine. Australian Journal of Physiotherapy 24: 103–109

Mercer S, Bogduk N The menisci of the cervical synovial joints (in prep)

Penning L, Tondury G 1963 Entstehung, Bau und Funktion der meniskoiden Strukturen in den Halswirbelgelenken. Zeitschrift für Orthopaedie und ihre Grenzgebiete 98: 1–14

Putz R, Pomaroli A 1972 Form und Funktion der Articulatio Atlanto-axialis Lateralis. Acta Anatomica 83: 333–345

Santo E 1935 Zur Entwicklungsgeschichte und Histologie der Zwischenscheiben in den kleinen Gelenken. Zeitschrift für Anatomie und Entwicklungsgeschichte 104: 623–634

Santo E, Schminke A 1932 Zur normalen und pathologischen Anatomie der Halswirbelsäule. Centralblatt für Allgemeine Pathologie und Pathologische Anatomie 55: 369–372

Singer K P, Giles L G F, Day R E 1990 Intra-articular synovial folds of thoracolumbar junction zygapophyseal joints. Anatomical Record 226: 147–152

Spraque R B 1983 The acute cervical joint lock. Physical Therapy 63: 1439–1444

Tager K H 1965 Wirbelmenniskus oder Synovial Fortsatz. Zeitschrift für Orthopädie und ihre Grenzgebiete 99: 439–447

Töndury G 1941 Beitrag zur Kenntnis der kleinen Wirbelgelenke. Zeitschrift für Anatomie und Entwicklungsgeschichte 110: 568–575

Töndury G 1972 Anatomie fonctionelle des petites articulations du rachis. Annales de Medicine Physique 15: 173–191

Williams P L, Warwick R Dyson M, Bannister L H (eds) 1989 Gray's anatomy. 37th edn. Churchill Livingstone, Edinburgh, pp 470–476

Yu S, Sether L, Haughton V M 1987 Facet joint menisci of the cervical spine. Correlative MR imaging and cryomicrotomy study. Radiology 164: 79–82

Zaccheo D, Reale E 1956 Contributo allo conoscenza delle articolazioni tra i processi articolari delle vertebre dell'oumo. Archivo Italiano di Anatomica e di Embriologia 61: 1–16

6. Clinical anatomy and biomechanics of the thoracic spine

F. Valencia

INTRODUCTION

The intent of this chapter is to review aspects of applied anatomy and biomechanics of the thoracic spine which are relevant to the understanding of thoracic motion disorders. The conclusions drawn are based on experimental and computer-simulation data from the literature, combined with analysis of the anatomical geometry of the joints involved. Details of anatomy are also derived from cadaveric dissections by the author performed in order to confirm and expand knowledge.

The interdependence between anatomical and biomechanical characteristics of the musculoskeletal tissues of the thoracic spine is explored. The role of these characteristics in the functions of the spine, i.e. force transmission, movement and protection of neurological structures, is systematically described. Finally, the anatomical relationship between the neurological and musculoskeletal tissues is outlined based on cadaveric dissections performed by the author.

Biomechanics uses the laws of physics and engineering to analyse the movement of various musculoskeletal components and the forces acting on these body parts during normal daily activities. The dynamic components of the system are external forces and muscular control. The collagenous tissues (i.e. ligaments, intervertebral disc, joint capsules, tendons) contribute to the static mechanics (stability) of the musculoskeletal system. The elastic behaviour of their components prevents excessive movement due to their morphological or intrinsic characteristics.

Pathological changes of trauma to musculoskeletal tissues may result in vertebral movement disorders. They, in turn, may alter the neural space with subsequent neurophysiological and neuropathological effects that may culminate in clinical neuromuscular dysfunction (Reid 1960). Recognition of the relative importance of the various factors involved in motion disorders (pathological, circulatory, congenital, and biomechanical) is a prerequisite to appropriate intervention. The therapeutic problem may then be solved by choosing the modality or modalities that will most safely, effectively, and economically provide results.

Understanding of the clinical anatomy and biomechanics in musculoskeletal clinical intervention is important. This information needs to be interpreted and transformed accurately into therapeutic guidelines.

Anatomical and biomechanical analysis has become a very important element in the development of manual therapy techniques designed to restore normal musculoskeletal function.

FUNCTIONAL ASPECTS OF THE VERTEBRAL COLUMN

The spinal column as a whole has three main functions:

1. Transmission of forces from the head and trunk to the pelvis and lower extremities
2. Movement of the trunk in order to place the head and arms in functional positions
3. Protection of spinal cord, the spinal roots, and their membranes.

In order to fulfil these functions, the whole column and its components show pertinent characteristics which combine to form a mechanical system which is very efficient and effective in transmitting forces while allowing large degrees of mobility without compromising the delicate structures of the nervous system. Weight bearing and force transmission are accomplished by the presence of curves, the structure and strength of the vertebral bodies plus the contribution from the zygapophyseal joints.

The existence of the spinal curves gives the vertebral column a higher resistance to weight bearing. Their shape correlates directly with the interrelation of shapes and sizes of the discs and vertebral bodies.

The thoracic kyphosis is a primary curve which may be considered as a persisting curve of the embryonic axis (Frazer 1965). The apex of this curve is generally accepted to be at the T7 to T8 level. This curve is the result of the lesser anterior vertical height of the thoracic vertebral bodies. On the other hand, the cervical and lumbar lordosis are accounted for mainly by the corresponding differences in the intervertebral disc heights. A slight lateral curve is evident sometimes in the coronal plane in the thoracic region. It has been suggested that this curve may be the result of use of the right hand or the presence of the aorta (Rouviere 1927, Steindler 1955, Davis 1959, Frazer 1965) or developmental asymmetries (Taylor 1983).

Strong vertebral bodies are designed to sustain mainly compressive loads and therefore become larger as the superimposed load increases caudally (Frazer 1965). Cancellous bone forms almost the entire part of the body with strong lamellae running vertically in the direction of force transmission. This porous structure enables cancellous bone to have a high energy storage capacity (Carter & Hayes 1976).

The intervertebral discs, which connect the vertebral bodies, represent more than one-fifth of the total length of the spinal column. Due to this fact a large degree of flexibility is achieved. This effect is the result of superimposition of small amounts of movement available at each level. Therefore, their structure provides both stability, by connecting the vertebral bodies strongly together, and flexibility, by allowing intervertebral movement.

The functional necessities of the vertebral column as a whole are also served by the intrinsic characteristics of the vertebral arches. They protect the spinal cord, spinal roots, and their membranes. They provide anchorage for the muscles controlling the movement of the spine. Finally, they guide the movement of the intervertebral segments as well as contributing to some extent to the load-bearing function of the spinal column (King et al 1975, Louis 1985).

At rest, the geometrical characteristics of the facets contribute to weight bearing. The proportion of weight bearing taken by these joints varies between 0 and 33% depending on the posture adopted (King et al 1975).

FUNCTIONAL ANATOMY OF THE THORACIC VERTEBRAL SEGMENT

The functional unit of the vetebral column is the motion segment which is constituted by two adjacent vertebrae and their intervening soft tissues. Cervical and lumbar segments present two compartments. The thoracic spine presents a third compartment. The study of the functional anatomy and biomechanics of the spine is simplified by considering the details of the various compartments of the vertebral segment.

Anterior compartment

The anterior compartment is formed by the two superimposed vertebral bodies, the intervertebral disc, and the longitudinal ligaments. The anterior longitudinal ligament is a strong band of tissue which is made up of several layers of fibres which vary in length but are closely interlaced with one another. This ligament is narrower but thicker in the thoracic spine relative to the cervical and lumbar areas (Rouviere 1927, Williams et al 1989). The posterior longitudinal ligament also is thicker in the thoracic region. It is wider at the disc level and narrower at the vertebral body (Rouviere 1927) (Fig. 6.1).

Posterior compartment

The corresponding posterior compartment is formed by the vertebral arches, the zygapophyseal joints, the transverse and spinous processes, and the ligaments joining them. The articular capsules of the thoracic joints are attached to the lateral margins of the articular processes of adjacent vertebrae. These capsules are reinforced anteriorly and posteriorly by the ligamentum flavum (capsular fibres) and by a posterior ligament, respectively (Rouviere 1927). The laminae, spinous, and transverse processes are connected by various ligaments. The ligamentum flavum attaches to the anterior surface of the lamina above, along an oblique line directed superolaterally (Tobias & Arnold 1967). The inferior border of the ligament attaches to the superoposterior aspect of the lamina below. It extends laterally into the intervertebral foramen forming its posterior boundary or roof. The ligament is composed of a large number of elastic fibres which have a 2:1 ratio with respect to the collagen fibres (Nachemson & Evans 1968). This elastic property of the ligamentum flavum has been shown to give a considerable amount of static compression to the vertebral segment (Nachemson & Evans 1968). The ligament undergoes fibrosis with increasing age, and this has led to speculative overrating of its role in decreasing the intervertebral foramen (Ramsay 1966).

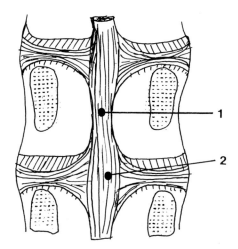

Fig. 6.1 Posterior view of thoracic vertebral segment. The pedicles have been cut to show the arrangement of the posterior longitudinal ligament. The ligament narrows over the vertebral body (1) and widens over the intervertebral disc (2).

The spinous processes are connected by the interspinous and supraspinous ligaments. The interspinous ligaments tend to blend superiorly with the articular capsules and posteriorly with the supraspinous ligament (Fig. 6.2). The latter is a more distinct entity in the thoracic spine compared to its counterpart in the lumbar area where it blends with the fibres of the erector spinae aponeurosis and the posterior layer of the thoracolumbar fascia (Heylings 1978, Bogduk 1984). Cephalically, the supraspinous ligament attaches to the spinous process of the seventh cervical vertebra, blending with the elastic ligamentum nuchae.

The transverse processes are connected firstly to one another by the intertransverse ligaments which, in the case of the thoracic spine, are cord-like. The other ligaments attaching to the transverse processes are those that connect them with the ribs.

Costal compartment

In the case of the thoracic spine, the ribs constitute a third compartment of the vertebral segment. The ribs attach to the transverse processes of the thoracic vertebrae by various ligaments. The superior costotransverse ligament runs from the inferior aspect of the transverse process to the superior aspect of the transverse process to the superior aspect of the rib below, but it is not present on the first rib. At the last rib, the costotransverse ligament becomes the lumbocostal ligament which runs to the L1 transverse process (Frazer 1965). The superior costotransverse ligament may be considered as two bands, an anterior layer whose medial border limits the foramen through which the spinal nerve exits from the intervertebral canal, and a posterior band which passes more laterally to attach to the tuberosity of the rib. The anterior part of the ligament blends with the medial aspect of the intercostal aponeurosis, while the posterior band is continuous with the external intercostal muscle (Rouviere 1927, Williams et al 1989). The costotransverse ligament occupies the space between the anterior aspect of a transverse process and the posterior aspect of the neck of the articulating rib. The lateral costotransverse ligament runs from the tip of a transverse process to the posterior aspect of the tubercle of its articulating rib (Frazer 1965). The lamellocostal ligament connects the inferior aspect of the lamina of the vertebra above to the posterior aspect of the neck of the rib below. Its lateral aspect blends with the posterior band of the superior costotransverse ligament (Rouviere 1927) (Fig. 6.3).

STABILITY OF THE THORACIC SPINE

Various intrinsic characteristics of the thoracic spine allow it to contribute to the overall function of the spine in weight bearing and force transmission.

The intrinsic morphological equilibrium of the spine provided by the ligaments and intervertebral discs makes it a well-balanced mechanical unit. Its integrity depends on the relationship between the anterior and posterior compartments. The normal nucleus pulposus acts hydrostatically, and during loading there is a uniform distribution of pressure (Nachemson 1960). The disc tends to separate the vertebral bodies, subjecting the ligaments and annular fibres to tensional stresses. On the other hand, the ligaments have been shown to prestress the disc and therefore provide intrinsic pressure to the unloaded disc. As long as the integrity of the vertebral unit is maintained, the two forces are in equilibrium. In fact, in vitro removal of the posterior elements results in instability of the vertebral unit in the three planes of motion (White & Hirsch 1971, Markolf 1972, Panjabi et al 1981, Chazal et al 1985).

The vertebral column is constantly subjected to rotational stresses in the coronal and sagittal planes due to gravitational forces. In the thoracic spine the line of gravity tends to increase the kyphotic curve (Asmussen 1960). In order to overcome this force, resistance is provided by the ligaments of the posterior compartment as well as by the muscular activity of the paravertebral muscles.

Stresses in the horizontal plane are overcome by the intervertebral disc and the articular facets. The annular fibres attach to the cartilagenous end plates in the inner zone as well as attaching directly to the periphery of the vertebral body. This arrangement provides powerful resistance to translation and shear deformation in the

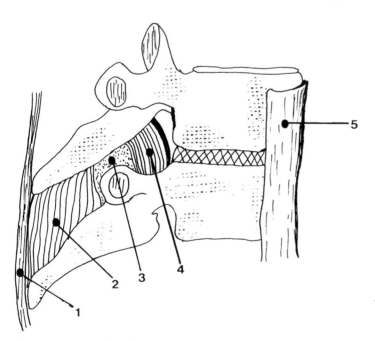

Fig. 6.2 Lateral view of the thoracic vertebral segment. The ligaments shown are: (1) supraspinous; (2) interspinous; (3) ligamentum flavum; (4) capsule of facet joint; (5) anterior longitudinal.

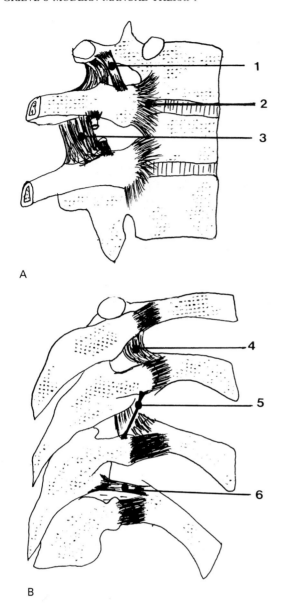

Fig. 6.3 A. Anterolateral view of the thoracic vertebral segment. This figure shows the anterior (1) and posterior (3) layers of the superior costotransverse ligament. The costovertebral joint is represented by (2). **B**. Posterolateral view of the thoracic vertebral segment. This figure shows the posterior aspect of the superior costotransverse ligament (4), the intertransverse ligament (5) and the lamellocostal ligament (6).

horizontal plane (Hirsch & Sonnerup 1968). Contact of the facets prevents anterior displacement of the vertebral unit (White & Hirsch 1971).

Mechanical stability is further enhanced in the thoracic area by the rib cage. The ribs are attached by strong ligaments at the vertebral end, a semi-rigid articulation with the sternum, and a strong intercostal aponeurosis. It has been calculated that the presence of the rib cage provides considerable stability to the thoracic spine due to the characteristics of the costovertebral joints and the presence of the sternum. The relative values of stability have been computed using a mathematical model (Andriacchi et al 1974). A significant two-fold increase in the stiffness

values of the spine due to the presence of the rib cage has been reported with the removal of the sternum resulting in a decrease in stiffness. It has also been demonstrated that the load-bearing capacity of the spine increased by three-fold when the rib cage was intact (Andriacchi et al 1974). More stability is provided by increases in intrathoracic pressure which convert the thorax into a solid unit capable of transmitting large forces (Morris et al 1961).

FLEXIBILITY OF THE THORACIC SPINE

One of the factors affecting the amount and direction of intervertebral movement in any particular segment is the elastic behaviour of the musculoskeletal components. In general terms the most restricting element, in the case of the thoracic spine, is the intervertebral disc. The height of the thoracic discs is small compared to those in the lumbar area (Reuben et al 1979). The ratio of average disc diameter to height is two to three times higher in thoracic than in lumbar segments (Kulak et al 1975). These geometrical differences result in thoracic discs showing elastic properties more like those of a solid material (Horst & Brinckmann 1981). During axial compression, the thoracic discs (T5–T6; T10–T11) behave in a more viscous manner than do the lumbar discs. This has been hypothesized to be due to a different structure of the collagen fibres or their framework (Koeller et al 1984). The collagen fibres composing the annulus fibrosus are arranged, on average, in some six to nine concentric layers. From a lateral view the fibres of the annulus depart from the vertebral margin of the vertebra below at an acute angle of 27 to 30% and insert into the upper vertebra at identical but reversed angles. In adjacent lamellae these fibres are arranged in a helicoid manner (Galante 1967). This criss-cross arrangement of the lamellae, together with the bonding between individual and neighbouring fibres, forms a tight seal against penetration of the nucleus under high pressure as long as degenerative changes have not occurred (Hickey & Hukins 1980). The thoracic nucleus pulposus has a relatively smaller size and a lower capacity to swell in comparison to the cervical and lumbar areas (Beadle 1931), although its water content seems to be similar to that in the lumbar spine (Koeller et al 1984).

The flexibility of the intervertebral disc during flexion, extension, and lateral flexion has been found to be approximately the same for the thoracic as for the lumbar discs (Markolf 1972). It has been proposed that this is due to the neutralizing effect of cross-sectional area and disc height on stiffness. Disc height tends to reduce stiffness whereas cross-sectional area increases it. This ratio of disc diameter to height results in a decrease of the circumferential stresses so dominant in the lumbar region (Kulak et al 1975).

During torsional deformation, the thoracic vertebrae

bearing ribs attaching to the sternum present increased resistance to motion. Since this high resistance to torsional stresses is also characteristic of the lumbar spine, the discs of the intermediate segments (i.e. T10–11; T11–12; T12–L1) may be considered as an elastic component representing a site of structural weakness (Markolf 1972).

MOVEMENT IN THE THORACIC SPINE

The close interaction between articular physiological and accessory movements, which is so important in the understanding of the normal biomechanical integrity of peripheral joints, is also present in the vertebral segment. The physiological movements are those which describe the anatomical patterns of motion, i.e. flexion, extension, lateral flexion and axial rotation. The corresponding accessory movements are represented by intervertebral translation and rotation.

Biomechanical considerations

The movement of one vertebra with respect to the other in a motion segment has six degrees of freedom. They are: translation along the antero-posterior (Z), lateromedial (X), and superoinferior (Y) axes, and rotation around each of these axes (Fig. 6.4).

Intervertebral movement is rarely uniplanar. It is necessary to remember when describing traditional patterns of motion (flexion, extension, lateral flexion, and axial rotation) that they conform to traditional anatomical descriptions rather than representing the true nature of intervertebral motion. In reality, coupling of two or more of the uniplanar motions occurs concurrently or successively (White 1969, Panjabi et al 1976). Simple coupling of movement occurs between translatory or rotational movements about or along one axis, and translation or rotation along or about another axis, e.g. sagittal rotation (Rx) will combine with anteroposterior translation (Tz) during flexion and extension of the spine. This type of coupling is stronger in the sagittal plane than in the coronal and horizontal planes (Panjabi et al 1976).

It has been shown that the relative amounts of movement (flexibility) of the thoracic intervertebral segments in the various planes obey the following trends: there is equal flexibility during translation in the lateromedial (X) and anteroposterior (Z) axes, but less in the superoinferior (Y) axis. Similar degrees of flexibility occur during rotation in the coronal and horizontal plane; however, in the sagittal plane the amount of motion is more restricted (Panjabi et al 1976).

The rotatory and translatory elements of motion are

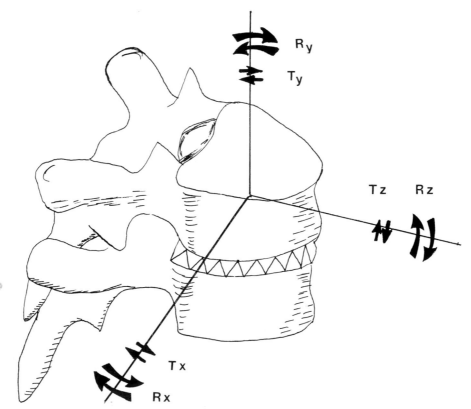

Fig. 6.4 Six degrees of freedom of the thoracic vertebral segment. Translation along the anteroposterior axis (Tz); translation along the lateromedial axis (Tx); translation along the superoinferior axis (Ty); rotation around the Z axis (Rz); rotation along the X axis (Rx); rotation around the Y axis (Ry).

small in the thoracic spine. It has been determined that an average intervertebral horizontal translatory displacement of 1 mm and sagittal plane rotation of 1.4° may be obtained when the intervertebral segment is subjected to forces of 43% of the body weight (Panjabi et 1981). Determining with exactitude the amount of motion in the various components of movement presents technical difficulties.

The representative angles of physiological movement in the various planes have been measured for the various thoracic levels (White 1969). The values are represented in Table 6.1.

More complex coupling results from combining the anatomical patterns of motion. In the upper thoracic spine there is relatively identifiable and consistent coupling of axial rotation and lateral flexion. The direction of coupling is such that the spinous processes move towards the convexity of the lateral curve. In the middle and lower areas of the thoracic spine this pattern still exists; however, it is not as marked (MacConail & Basmajian 1969).

The extent of coupling in the thoracic segments is dependent on the slope of the superior articular facets. The slope of these facets varies according to the level. In the upper thoracic segments this is similar to the cervical spine (45–60° with respect to the horizontal). In the middle segments the slope is closer to 90°, representing true thoracic segments, while the lower vertebral levels approximate the lumbar characteristics (Fig. 6.5).

Role of the articular facets during segmental movement

The alignment of the articular facets determines their mechanical role during movement of the vertebral segment. In the thoracic spine the superior articular facet is almost flat and faces posteriorly, superiorly, and slightly laterally. The inferior articular facet is oriented in a recip-

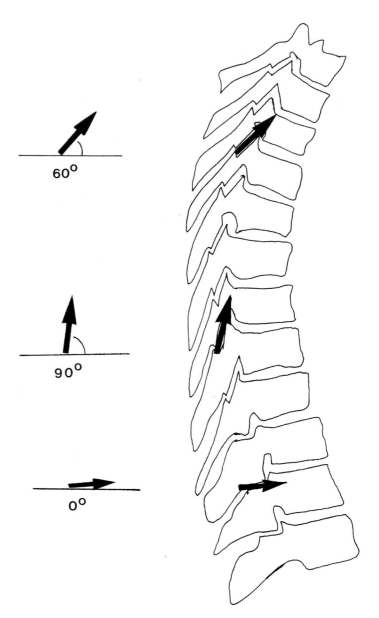

Fig. 6.5 Geometrical orientation of the zygapophyseal joints in the thoracic spine. The obliquity of their planes is shown by the arrows. The angle with respect to the horizontal changes according to the level from close to 60° in the upper levels to close to 0° in the lower levels.

rocal manner. The combined plane of these facets forms the arc of a circle in the horizontal plane (Davis 1959). The location of the centre of this arc varies according to the level in question. In the upper two thoracic vertebrae it lies well in front of the vertebral body. Progressing downwards, the point approaches the anterior border and enters the vertebral body only to leave it again in the lower thoracic region. This reflects the change in medial orientation of the facets at the various levels of the thoracic spine (Davis 1959).

It has been found that the inferior facet has a greater radius than the superior facet (Davis 1959). This has been thought to reflect the intra-articular incongruence and looseness peculiar to synovial joints which permits free-

Table 6.1 Physiological movement in the thoracic spine*

Level	Amount (degrees)
Sagittal plane (flexion–extension)**	
T1–2 to T5–6	4
T6–7 to T9–10	6
T11–12 to T12–L1	9–12
Coronal plane (lateral flexion)	
T1–2 to T9–10	6
T10–11 to T12–L1	7–9
Transverse plane (axial rotation)	
T1–2	9
T2–3 to T7–8	8
T8–9 to T12–L1	2–7

*The ranges of motion for the various thoracic levels in the sagittal, coronal and transverse planes are adapted from White and Panjabi (1978)
**In the sagittal plane flexion makes the major contribution to these figures with only 30–42% attributed to extension.

dom of movement. In any synovial joint the position of full congruence of the articular facets has been named the close-packed position. It has been described as occurring in the vertebral joints when full extension is achieved (MacConail & Basmajian 1969).

Traditionally, the movement between the articular facets has been described as of a gliding type. It has been thought that the articular movement serves 'only as a guide or pilot' to the intervertebral movement (Steindler 1955). However, facet contact or guidance with anterior shear and loss of contact with posterior shear must also be considered when analysing vertebral movement (Panjabi et al 1984).

The zygapophyseal joints are oriented in oblique planes which face backward and upward. At rest, the upward-facing component of the slope contributes to weight bearing (Fig. 6.6). The proportion of weight bearing taken by these joints varies between 0 and 33% depending on the posture adopted (King et al 1975). The backward-facing component of the slope stabilizes the vertebral segment against forward translation. During movement of the vertebral segment, the slope of the articular facets predisposes to the coupling of movements. Anterior translation is limited by the contact of the two facets (Fig. 6.6). Therefore, further translation can only occur due to the forward tilting of the superior vertebra which results in upward gliding of the inferior articular process.

The facets offer little resistance to movement during axial rotation. Their movement approximates lateral gliding. Movement in the coronal plane during lateral flexion results in unilateral facet contact, with some degree of posterior translation due to the slope of the facets.

Anatomical considerations during segmental movement

The distance between the vertebral bodies increases during extension whilst that between the vertebral arches decreases. The reverse occurs during flexion. A tensile stress is placed on the anterior elements, which act as a check on further widening of the intervertebral space. The posterior longitudinal ligament and posterior annulus are subjected to compression. The inferior facets of the superior vertebra descend on the slope of the superior facets of the vertebra below. Contact of either the spinous processes or the inferior aspect of the articular facet of the vertebra above with the soft tissues and superior aspect of the lamina below will prevent further rotation. Further translation in the horizontal plane may then occur due to separation of the articular facets. This motion is limited eventually by the articular capsule and the anterior compartment (Fig. 6.7).

During lateral flexion, in the coronal plane, rotation causes vertical compression of the ipsilateral articular facets. The ipsilateral inferior articular facet rides downward and backward along the slope of the superior articular process. This posterior translation results in axial rotation being coupled with lateral flexion. During axial rotation in the upper and middle regions of the thoracic spine the articular facets provide almost no resistance to the movement. Rotation of the intervertebral disc rather than translation predominates in this movement. Both lateral flexion and axial rotation are considerably limited by the costovertebral joints and the rib cage.

Due to their morphological configuration, the costovertebral joints allow only very small degrees of gliding movement. The heads of the ribs are closely connected to the vertebral bodies by the radiate and interarticular ligaments (Williams et al 1989). Similarly, the costotransverse joint is stabilized by strong ligaments binding the tubercle and neck of the rib with the transverse process. The nature of the gliding motion available at this joint is determined by the shape and direction of the articular surfaces. In the upper six ribs, the articular surfaces on the tubercles are oval in shape and convex from above downwards. The anterior surfaces of the transverse processes are concave. Therefore, the supero-inferior movement at the costotransverse joint results in rotation of the rib on its long axis. The articular surfaces of the tubercles of the lower four true ribs are flat. The corresponding articular surfaces on the transverse process are on its superior aspect. This results in posteromedial gliding of the ribs without any rotation. The costovertebral joints have been found to exhibit high stiffness in lateral movement, especially in the midthoracic region (Schultz et al 1974).

The anterior ends of the ribs are connected to the costal cartilages, which in turn join the sternum by the costosternal joints. With the exception of the first, the costosternal joints are synovial joints. The interchondral articulations between the 6th, 7th, 8th and 9th costal cartilages are also synovial. Sometimes the 5th–6th and the 9th–10th have synovial characteristics; however, the

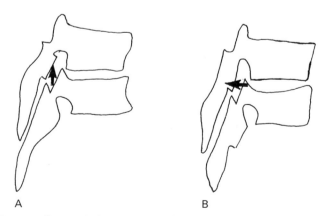

A   B

Fig. 6.6 Geometrical components of the slope of the superior articular process. The upward facing component (**A**) contributes to weight bearing. The backward facing component (**B**) resists posterior translation.

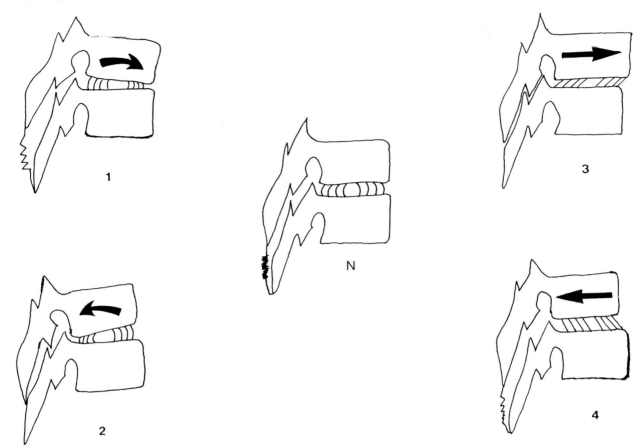

Fig. 6.7   Anatomical changes during thoracic vertebral segment movement from neutral (**N**). During anterior rotation (**1**) the distance between the components of the posterior compartment increases while the anterior compartment decreases. The reverse occurs during posterior rotation (**2**). During anterior translation (**3**) impaction of the facets prevents further anterior movement. Further movement can occur only by superior gliding of the facets. Posterior translation (**4**) is limited mainly by the intervertebral disc.

later is usually fibrous. The individual components of the rib cage are quite flexible and therefore allow movement between ribs during vertebral motion in the various planes. As a whole, the rib cage increases the stiffness of the thoracic vertebral column mainly due to the presence of the sternum (Andriacchi et al 1974).

INNERVATION OF THE THORACIC SPINE

The thoracic dorsal root ganglia are situated partly outside the intervertebral foramina attached by connective tissue to its floor and anterior wall. The thoracic spinal nerve trunks are very short (of the order of 2–5 mm).

Ventral rami

The ventral rami run anterior to the superior costo-vertebral ligament. They follow a lateral and slightly anterior pathway on their way to the intercostal space. Small articular branches are given at this point from their medial and superior aspects to innervate the costovertebral joints of the same level.

Dorsal rami

The thoracic dorsal rami arise from their common trunks just outside the intervertebral foramina. They vary in length, but they are usually between 3 and 5 mm. They curve dorsally around the lateral aspect of the zygapophyseal joint, and here two to four articular branches are given off.

The dorsal ramus then immediately enters an osseoligamentous foramen, formed by the inferior aspect of the transverse process above, the superior aspect of the neck of the rib below, the superior articular facet medially and the medial aspect of the anterior band of the superior costotransverse ligament laterally.

Once the dorsal ramus passes the osseoligamentous foramen it runs posterolaterally on the costotransverse ligament. In this part of its course the dorsal ramus lies between the anterior band of the superior costotransverse ligament and the Y-shaped ligamentous structure formed medially by the lamellocostal ligament and laterally by the posterior band of the superior costotransverse ligament.

The dorsal ramus then appears deep to the longissimus muscle, lateral to the semispinalis muscle and medial to the levator costae muscle. At this level the ramus divides into its terminal branches. Close to this division, a small articular branch is given off to the costotransverse joint of the level below. Sometimes it is adherent to the lateral branch of the dorsal ramus but by careful dissection they can be separated.

Branches of the dorsal rami may be divided into two groups according to the distribution of their terminal branches. In the superior group (T1–7), the lateral branch is muscular while the medial branch is musculocutaneous. In the inferior group (T8–12), the lateral branches are musculocutaneous while the medial branches are only muscular. The T6 to T8 levels are transitional and their branches may be distributed in various ways (Johnston 1908, Piersol 1919).

In the superior group, the medial branch forms an S-shaped curve; this has been described by Johnston (1908) as a mechanism for the protection of these nerves during flexion of the spine. After separation from the dorsal ramus the medial branch divides into three sub-branches (Fig. 6.8) which run medially around the intertransverse ligament and pass between the tendons of multifidus and semispinalis cervicis. The most superior of these sub-branches runs medially on multifidus to reach the midline and eventually it becomes superficial. In the upper two levels, a small branch may reach the interspinalis muscle. The middle sub-branches are distributed to the posterior aspects of multifidus and the rotatores. The most inferior sub-branch gives innervation to the anterior aspect of fascicles of the semispinalis as they run superiorly.

The superficial course of the medial branches of the dorsal rami in the superior group varies according to the description of various authors (Johnston 1908, Hovelacque 1927, Hovelacque et al 1937, Grant 1972, Williams et al 1989, Rohen & Yokochi 1983). In general, it can be said that the cutaneous branches of the dorsal rami in the superior group exit from the muscular mass close to the midline and then run laterally, the T2 being the longest and reaching the acromion after running along the scapular spine.

The lateral branches of this superior group are mainly muscular. They run posterolaterally from their point of separation from the dorsal ramus towards the costotransverse joint. They pass lateral to this joint forming a shallow groove in the periosteum of the rib. Small branches are given off at this level to innervate the

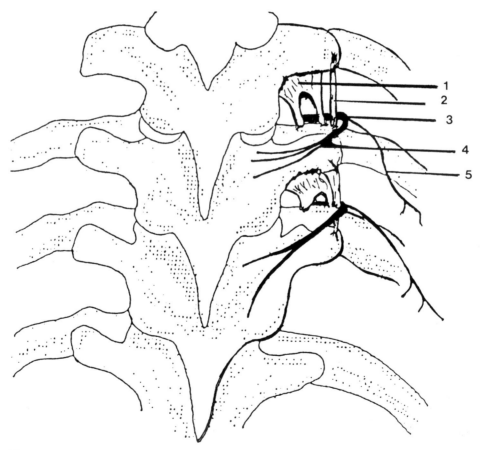

Fig. 6.8 Posterior view of the distribution of the dorsal rami in the thoracic spine. This figure represents the dorsal rami (3) as they pass under the Y ligamentous structure (1) and around the intertransverse ligament (2). The medial (4) and lateral (5) branches of the dorsal rami are also represented.

levatores costae muscles. Past the rib, the lateral branches run laterally deep to longissimus giving branches to those fascicles of this muscle attaching to the first or second level above. They then penetrate the anterior aspect of the iliocostalis and are distributed in that muscular mass.

In the inferior group the medial branches are smaller and usually divide into two sub-branches (Fig. 6.8) which are distributed to the multifidus, rotatores, semispinalis thoracis and spinalis thoracis. The larger lateral branches of this group are musculocutaneous. They follow a similar course to their counterparts in the superior group, as far as the level of the costotransverse joints. Then they proceed on an oblique and posterior pathway deep to erector spinae giving branches to those fascicles attaching one or two levels above.

Some small branches interconnecting adjacent medial branches of the dorsal rami have been observed by the author. Tiny twigs arise from these branches for the innervation of the anterior aspect of the zygapophyseal joints.

However, their incidence and precise distribution need to be studied further in order to determine the true segmental innervation of these articulations.

Sinuvertebral nerves

The sinuvertebral nerve is formed by a spinal and a sympathetic root. The spinal root arises from the lateral end of the spinal nerve. According to Hovelacque 1927 and Hovelacque et al 1937, in 25% of cases this spinal root is made up of two parts which arise, one close to the other, from the superior border of the spinal nerve and very rarely from its posterior aspect.

The origin of the sympathetic root varies. It may arise directly from either the sympathetic ganglion above or below, the ramus communicantes or by combination of any of these three origins.

The spinal and sympathetic roots of the sinuvertebral nerve join outside the intervertebral foramen. The nerve

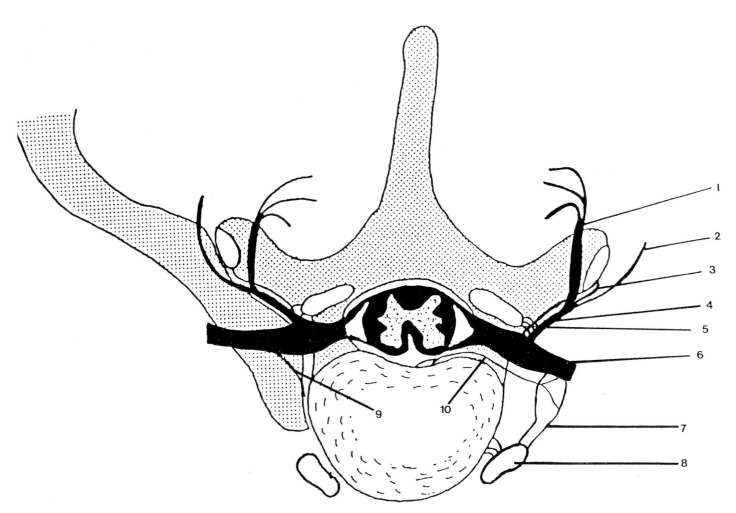

Fig. 6.9 Horizontal view of the distribution of a typical thoracic spinal nerve. Articular branches (9) of the ventral rami (6) are distributed to the costovertebral joint. The articular branches of the dorsal rami (4) are distributed to both the zygapophyseal joint (5) and the costotransverse joint (3). The medial (1) and lateral (2) branches are distributed to the posterior elements of the thoracic spine. The sinuvertebral nerves (10) are formed by a sympathetic root from the ramus communicantes (7) and a spinal root from the ventral ramus (6). The sympathetic ganglion (8) given small branches which penetrate the anterolateral corner of the vertebral body.

then travels in from the spinal nerve among the veins of the area. From its initial part collateral branches are given off to supply the periosteum of the vertebral arch and neck of the rib (Hovelacque 1927, Hovelacque et al 1937).

Once in the spinal canal the nerve divides into its terminal branches. Two types of terminal branches have been described by Hovelacque (1927) and Hovelacque et al (1937). Short ones are distributed to the longitudinal venous plexus, and long ones, which run obliquely in the epidural space, to be distributed to the posterior aspect of the vertebral bodies, the anterior aspect of the laminae, the posterior longitudinal ligament and the dura mater. He reported that he never saw ascending or descending terminal branches of the sinuvertebral nerve interconnections between the branches inside the spinal canal.

More recent studies of the sinuvertebral nerve in the thoracic region have presented different views about certain details of its formation and distribution. Buskirk (1941) studied the distribution of the sinuvertebral nerve in cat and human fetal material. By histological techniques, in sections of vertebral columns from the 8th cervical to the 10th thoracic levels, he observed ascending terminal branches in the upper thoracic levels. These branches extended up to six or more levels. He also described branches which extended outwards into the intervertebral foramen.

Edgar and Nundy (1966) claimed that the spinal root of the sinuvertebral nerve arose from the anterior ramus rather than the spinal nerve as described by Hovelacque (1927). In the thoracic spine they found that this root sometimes had contributions from the dorsal ramus. They also described ascending (in the cervical) and descending (in the cervical and lumbar) terminal branches of the sinuvertebral nerve in the spinal canal. However, they did not mention whether any of these branches were present in the thoracic spine.

A summary of the innervation of a typical thoracic segment is presented in Figure 6.9.

REFERENCES

Andriacchi T, Schultz A, Belytschko T et al 1974 A model for studies of mechanical interactions between the human spine and rib cage. Journal of Biomechanics 7: 497

Asmussen E 1960 The weight carrying function of the human spine. Acta Orthopaedica Scandinavica 29: 276

Beadle O A 1931 The intervertebral discs. His Majesty's Stationery Office, London. In: White A A 1969 Analysis of the mechanics of the thoracic spine in man. Acta Orthopaedica Scandinavica (suppl 127)

Bogduk N 1984 The applied anatomy of the thoracolumbar fascia. Spine 9: 164

Buskirk C Van 1941 Nerves in the vertebral canal. Archives of Surgery 43: 427

Carter D R, Hayes W C 1976 Bone compressive strength. The influence of density and strain rate. Science 194: 1174

Chazal J, Tanguy A, Bourges M et al 1985 Biomechanical properties of spinal ligaments and a histological study of the supraspinal ligament in traction. Journal of Biomechanics 18: 167

Davis P R 1959 The medial inclination of the human thoracic intervertebral articular facets. Journal of Anatomy 93: 68

Edgard M A, Nundy S 1966 Innervation of the spinal dura mater. Journal of Neurology Neurosurgery and Psychiatry 29: 530

Frazer J E 1965 Frazer's anatomy of the human skeleton. Churchill Livingstone, London

Galante G O 1967 Tensile properties of the human lumbar annulus fibrosus. Acta Orthopaedica Scandinavica (suppl 100)

Grant J C B 1972 An atlas of anatomy. 6th edn. Williams & Wilkins, Baltimore

Heylings D J A 1978 Supraspinous and interspinous ligaments of the human lumbar spine. Journal of Anatomy 125: 127

Hickey D S, Hukins D W L 1980 Relations between the structure of the annulus and the function and failure of the disc. Spine 5: 106

Hirsch C, Sonnerup L 1968 Macroscopic rheology in collagen material. Journal of Biomechanics 1: 13

Horst M, Brinckmann P 1981 Measurement of the distribution of axial stress on the end plate of the vertebral body. Spine 6: 217

Hovelacque A 1927 Anatomie des nerfs craniens et radichiens et du sisteme grand sympathique chez l'homme. 1st edn. Gaston Doin et Cie, Paris

Hovelacque A, Monod O, Evrard H 1937 Le thorax anatomie medico-chirurgicale. 1st edn. Librairie Malaine, Paris

Johnston H M 1908 The cutaneous branches of the posterior prymary divisions of the spinal nerves and their distribution in the skin, Journal of Anatomy and Physiology 43: 80

King A I, Prasad P, Ewing C L 1975 Mechanisms of spinal injury due to caudocephalad acceleration. Orthopaedic Clinics of North America 6: 19

Koeller W, Meier W, Hartmenn F 1984 Biomechanical properties of human intervertebral discs subjected to axial dynamic compression. A comparison of lumbar and thoracic discs. Spine 9: 725

Kulak R F, Schultz A B, Belytschko T et al 1975 Biomechanical characteristics of vertebral motion segments and intervertebral discs. Orthopaedic Clinics of North America 6: 121

Louis R 1985 Spinal stability as defined by the three column spine concept. Anat Clin 7: 33

MacConail M A, Basmajian J V 1969 Muscles and movements: a basis for human kinesiology. Williams & Wilkins, Baltimore

Markolf K L 1972 Deformation of the thoracolumbar intervertebral joints in response to external loads. A biomechanical study using autopsy material. Journal of Bone and Joint Surgery 54: 511

Morris J M, Lucas D B, Bresler B 1961 Role of the trunk in stability of the spine. Journal of Bone and Joint Surgery 43: 327

Nachemson A 1960 Lumbar intradiscal pressure. Experimental studies on post mortem material. Acta Orthopaedica Scandinavica (suppl 43)

Nachemson A L, Evans J H 1968 Some mechanical properties of the third human lumbar interlaminar ligament (ligamentum flavum). Journal of Biochemistry 1: 211

Panjabi M M, Brand R A, White A A 1976 Mechanical properties of the human thoracic spine as shown by three dimensional load displacement curves. Journal of Bone and Joint Surgery 58: 642

Panjabi M M, Hausfeld J N, White A A 1981 A biomechanical study of the ligamentous stability of the thoracic spine in man. Acta Orthopaedica Scandinavica 52: 315

Panjabi M M, Krag M H, Dimnet J C et al 1984 Thoracic spine centres of rotation in the sagittal plan. Journal of Orthopaedic Research 1: 387

Piersol G A 1919 Human Anatomy. 7th edn. J B Lippincott, Philadelphia

Ramsay R H 1966 Anatomy of the ligamenta flava. Clinical Orthopaedics 44: 129

Reid J D 1960 Effects of flexion extension movements of the head and spine upon the spinal cord and nerve roots. Journal of Neurology Neurosurgery and Psychiatry 23: 214

Reuben J D, Brown R H, Nash C L et al 1979 In vivo effects of axial loading on healthy adolescent spines. Clinical Orthopaedics 139: 17

Rohen J W, Yokochi C 1983 Color atlas of anatomy. A photographic study of the human body. 1st edn. Igaku-Shoin, New York

Rouviere H 1927 Anatomie humaine. Descriptive et topographique. Masson, Paris

Schultz A B, Benson D R, Hirsch C 1974 Force deformation properties of costosternal and costovertebral articulations. Journal of Biomechanics 7: 311

Steindler A 1955 Kinesiology of the human body. Charles C Thomas, Springfield, IL

Taylor J R 1983 Scoliosis and growth. Patterns of assymmetry in normal vertebral growth. Acta Orthopaedica Scandinavica 54: 596

Tobias P V, Arnold M 1967 Man's anatomy. Witwatersrand University Press, Johannesburg

White A A 1969 Analysis of the mechanics of the thoracic spine in man. Acta Orthopaedica Scandinavica (suppl 127)

White A A, Hirsch C 1971 The significance of the vertebral posterior elements in the mechanics of the thoracic spine. Clinical Orthopaedics 81: 2

White A A, Panjabi M M 1978 The basic kinematics of the human spine. A review of past and current knowledge. Spine 3: 12

Williams P, Warwick R, Dyson M, Bannister L H (eds) 1989 Gray's anatomy. 37th edn. Churchill Livingstone, London

7. Anatomy and biomechanics of the thoracolumbar junction

K. P. Singer

INTRODUCTION

Current stylized descriptions of the vertebral column, which reinforce concepts of symmetry and what is believed to be normal, cloud the true idiosyncratic nature and form of our biology. This is particularly true of the human vertebral column and, in particular, the transitional regions, which have been described as 'ontogenically restless' by Schmorl and Junghanns (1971). These departures from contemporary anatomical teaching are important to the astute clinician yet have largely been ignored due to the considerable research focus on the lumbar and cervical regions.

The thoracolumbar junction (TJ) is typically depicted in anatomical texts as showing an abrupt change in the orientation of the zygapophyseal joints of the last thoracic vertebra (Fig. 7.1). This 'distinguishing feature' (Pick 1890) is represented by inferior articular processes which 'turn to face laterally' (Testut & Latarjet 1948, Sobotta & Uhlenhuth 1957, Hamilton 1976, Williams & Warwick 1980), a concept that is perpetuated in clinical sources (Hoppenfeld 1977, Gehweiler et al 1980, Parke 1982, Malmivaara 1989). To gain any appreciation of the diversity of this transitional region, the interested reader must search the anthropological, anatomical and radiological literature.

A number of early reports described cranial and caudal variations in the segmental location of the thoracolumbar transition (Humphry 1858, Struthers 1875, Hasebe 1913, Schertlein 1928, Kühne 1932, Stewart 1932, Lanier 1939, Terry & Trotter 1953, Allbrook 1955), asymmetry of the TJ zygapophyseal joints (Barclay-Smith 1911, Whitney 1926, Shore 1930), and a mortice-like configuration of the TJ zygapophyseal joints in which the superior articular processes embraced those from the vertebra above (Topinard 1877, Le Double 1912, Davis 1955). These variations in TJ location and morphology were reported to be so common that attempts to provide a systematic framework for differentiating between thoracic and lumbar regions were considered by Todd (1922) to be impractical.

Recently, a comprehensive anatomical study of the T10–11, T11–12, T12–L1 and L1–2 segments was undertaken by Singer (1989a) using CT archives from over 600 patient examinations, complemented with histology performed on 75 cadaveric TJs. From this work, the concept of an abrupt transition representing the normal anatomy of the TJ has been challenged (Singer et al 1989a). A gradual or progressive change from T10–11 to T12–L1 appears to be the most common junctional

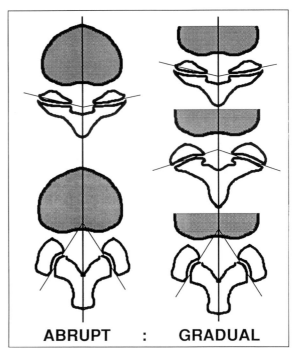

Fig. 7.1 Schematic illustration depicting the common representation of the change in zygapophyseal joint orientation at the thoracolumbar junction. The transition (left) is described as an abrupt change from the coronal plane of the lower thoracic zygapophyseal joints to the predominantly sagittal planes of the first lumbar segment. The classification of an abrupt transition was based on an angulation difference between adjacent paired joints of >120°. In contrast, the gradual pattern depicts an intermediate segment interposed between the more coronally and sagittally orientated levels. Right and left joint angles were calculated by plotting a line of best-fit through the joint margins in relation to the sagittal midline.

85

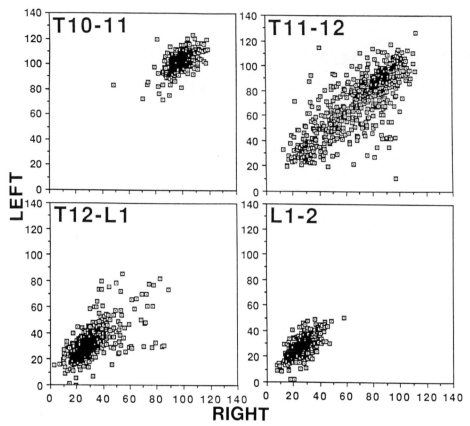

Fig. 7.2 Scattergrams depicting the dispersion of right and left zygapophyseal joint angles for the T10–11, T11–12, T12–L1 and L1–2 segmental levels. The relative consistency of coronal and sagittal joint orientations at T10–11 and L1–2 respectively, is emphasized in the tight cluster of data points. The marked variation evident at T11–12 and T12–L1 is evidenced in the scatter about the diagonal, which indicates both the diversity in level of the transition and also the extent of asymmetry or tropism between joint pairs.

pattern (Fig. 7.2), supporting the anecdotal observation by Struthers (1875) who described a TJ transition pattern in which the zygapophyseal joints of the middle level adopted an intermediate orientation between the sagittal and coronal planes of adjacent segments. In contrast, the text book description of an abrupt transition, as defined in these studies (Fig. 7.1), applied to approximately 30% of the population examined.

Of interest was the apparent sexual dimorphism in transition patterns, which indicated that the more gradual form of transition was largely a female characteristic (Singer et al 1989a). The trend for females to show a two-fold higher incidence of the gradual transition pattern compared to males, may be related to adaptations to different mechanical demands. The female role as child-bearer has resulted in the evolution of a broader pelvis which, in concert with a deeper lumbar lordosis (Williams & Warwick 1980), may produce greater axial rotation of the thoracic and thoracolumbar vertebral column, particularly during gait. Consequently, the progressive form of transition may be an adaptation to minimize stress concentration between these mobile segments of this transitional region.

DEVELOPMENT

An early signal to the stabilizing role of the human TJ appears in the sequence of ossification of the vertebral centra. A number of reports have indicated that the first sites of ossification are consistently located in the lower two thoracic and first lumbar vertebral bodies before a progressive cranial and caudal pattern of ossification commences in the adjacent vertebrae (Noback & Roberston 1951, Bagnall et al 1977, Birkner 1978). Similarly, by about two years of post-natal life the vertebral ring apophyses from T10 to L1 appear to ossify first (Louis 1983). These predictable ossification patterns have prompted Bagnall et al (1977) to suggest that the use of trunk musculature and associated fetal movement in utero acted to facilitate early skeletal development of the TJ elements in response to this early mechanical stress being applied to the vertebral column.

Anatomically, the thoracolumbar transitional zone also marks an increase in the size of the vertebral bodies and intervertebral discs (Fig. 7.3) (Cyriax 1929, Davis 1980, Berry et al 1987), associated with a larger vertebral canal to accommodate the lumbar enlargement of the spinal cord and conus (Gonon et al 1975, Louis 1983).

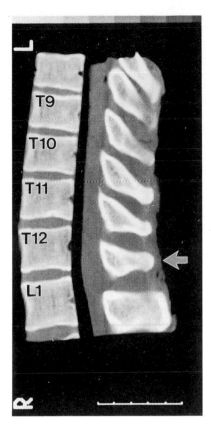

Fig. 7.3 Median sagittal CT slice through the thoracolumbar junction depicting the progressive change in vertebral body and intervertebral disc dimensions from the 'rectangular' thoracic shape to the typical 'square' profile of lumbar vertebrae. The direction of the spinous processes is observed to attain an almost horizontal direction at T12. This transitional 'anticlinal' spinous process (arrow) marks the start of the more substantial lumbar spinous processes.

THORACOLUMBAR CURVATURE

Of the physiological curvatures of the column, the lordotic curves of the cervical and lumbar regions permit greater mobility than do the longer thoracic kyphotic curve (Kapandji 1977). The thoracic region, with its anterior concavity, affords protection to the thoracic and upper abdominal viscera, and tension on the spinal cord is reduced due to the attendant rib cage which impedes thoracic flexion (Humphry 1858).

Changes in the thoracolumbar curvature appear to vary widely in response to different physiological postures (Strasser 1913) and to increasing age (Singer et al 1990c). These curve characteristics are also influenced by spinal fractures and resulting deformity (Willén et al 1990). In the normal orthograde posture, the location of the line of gravity in relation to the vertebral column appears to be consistently located through the transitional regions (Humphry 1858, Braune & Fischer 1889, Åkerblom 1948, Nathan 1962, Anderson 1982). Despite changes in the magnitude of the curves from one region to another, they appear to compensate each other in order to maintain a 'balance' in relation to the line of gravity (Steindler

1955). This reciprocal change in curvature of the thoracic kyphosis and lumbar lordosis produces an inflexion point which is located commonly between T11 and L1 (Stagnara et al 1982, Singer et al 1990c).

The strategy of locating an inflexion point at an area of mechanical and morphological transition may afford protection in the form of reduced localized bending stress, at least for sagittal plane motion. This contrasts with the curve apices which sustain the greatest deflection under static loading and clinically, at least for the mid-thoracic region, an increased risk of vertebral fractures (Kazarian 1978, Lampmann et al 1984). However, if the bending moment is applied suddenly, the thoracic column tends to 'pivot' over the mechanically 'stiffened' thoracolumbar junctional region, usually resulting in fracture (Levine & Edwards 1987).

In considering the functional significance of the TJ inflexion point, the dynamic role of the vertebral column as a whole must be examined. During static axial loading, the TJ shows little 'warping' or rotational deformity in the horizontal plane, compared to adjacent thoracic and lumbar regions (Kazarian 1972). This mechanical characteristic appears to reflect the increased stability of this region during loaded postures. The morphology of the thoracolumbar mortice joint, which may aptly be described as an 'anti-torsion' device, appears to contribute to the resistance against torsional stress of the TJ segments (Markolf 1972, Singer et al 1989b). Any explanation which seeks to account for the localized incidence of vertebral body compression fractures at the TJ (Rehn 1968) must consider not only the anatomical and aetiological factors contributing to the problem, but other factors such as the biomechanical capacities of the mobile segments and the change in curvature at the TJ.

LOAD-BEARING BY THE THORACOLUMBAR JUNCTION MOBILE SEGMENTS

Weight-transmission down the axial skeleton in the erect posture is believed to be primarily through the vertebral bodies and intervertebral discs, which progressively increase in size from C1 to L5 (Pooni et al 1986). However, the zygapophyseal joints also contribute to axial weight-bearing (El-Bohy et al 1989) depending on their relationship to the line of gravity. At the TJ, the upper lumbar vertebral bodies demonstrate a relatively marked increase in cross-sectional dimension compared with the thoracic vertebrae (Gonon et al 1975, Davis 1980, Berry et al 1987). Vertebral trabecular density appears to show greater mean density values for the lower thoracic compared with upper lumbar vertebral levels, while the product of mid-vertebral body cross-sectional area and the associated vertebral trabecular density were similar for each vertebra from T10 to L1 (Singer & Breidahl 1990b). This finding may suggest that, at the TJ, a relatively equal axial weight-bearing load may be accommodated by each verte-bra despite a caudal increase in the physical dimension of the lumbar vertebrae.

The tendency for the anterior aspect of each vertebral body to demonstrate a significantly higher trabecular den-sity measure (Singer & Breidahl 1990b) may be accounted for by the greater flexion loading sustained by the low thoracic and upper lumbar vertebrae. The consistent finding of anterior vertebral osteophytes, demonstrated frequently in the concavity of the thoracic region, has been clearly shown by Shore (1935) and Nathan (1962) to represent an important weight-bearing mechanism for the vertebral column.

AXIAL LOAD-SHARING BETWEEN ANTERIOR AND POSTERIOR ELEMENTS

In an anatomical study attempting to quantify the pro-portion of weight-bearing shared between the vertebral mobile segments, Pal & Routal (1987) suggested that the vertebrae intersecting the line of gravity would undergo the highest axial loading. Nachemson (1960) and Pal & Routal (1987) have, in general, tended to discount the posterior elements as less significant contributors to direct transmission of axial loads. However, the work of Yang & King (1984) has shown that lumbar zygapophyseal joints can contribute up to 47% of axial load bearing. This relationship depends on the distance of each vertebra from the line of gravity.

Similarly, the marked increase in pedicle cross-section area at the TJ (Zindrick et al 1986, Berry et al 1987) appears purposefully designed to facilitate the transmis-sion of load between the anterior and posterior elements relative to changes in posture.

As each synovial joint is designed to sustain load trans-mission across the articular surfaces (Radin 1976), the TJ zygapophyseal joints were studied to consider their poten-tial for axial load transmission. This feature was evident from frontal CT scans of the TJ zygapophyseal joints, which demonstrated the medial taper and enclosure offered by these joints (Singer 1989b). At the level of the mortice joint and above, the inferior articular processes would appear to abut against the lamina in axially loaded postures and in end-range spinal extension (Grieve 1981).

ZYGAPOPHYSEAL JOINT TROPISM AT THE THORACOLUMBAR JUNCTION

Differences in zygapophyseal joint planes (tropism) is another common feature at the TJ (Fig. 7.4). In this instance, tropism >20° between joint planes showed a two-fold higher frequency in males (Singer 1989a). The rationales proposed to account for tropism are many and varied. Debate exists between those who advance either a genetic or functional thesis, or both. For example, per-formance of manipulative tasks using the dominant upper extremity was the reason suggested by Whitney (1926) for TJ zygapophyseal joint asymmetry. Odgers (1933) was of the belief that the multifidus muscle controlled the de-velopment of lumbar zygapophyseal joint sagittalization

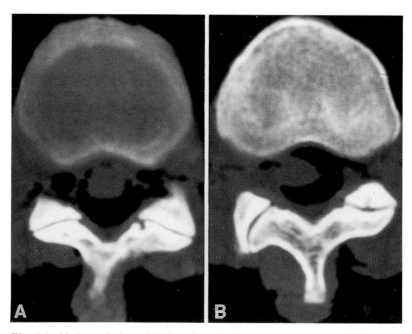

Fig. 7.4   Horizontal plane CT slices through the superior end-plate at T11–12 in two individuals. The gradual transitional pattern depicted in (**A**) accounted for 70% of the series studied. Marked articular tropism between the right and left articular planes is represented in (**B**). These two examples emphasize the diversity of zygapophyseal joint orientation at the thoracolumbar transitional junction.

and would account for the variety of articular plane orientations between joint pairs; a view upheld by Pfeil (1971) and Lutz (1967). In the model proposed by Putz (1976, 1985), lateral mechanical shear stresses on the articular surfaces were considered to be responsible for shaping the zygapophyseal joints. This latter view is sustained when considering the influence of scoliosis, whereby the articular surfaces adapt their orientation as a consequence of the deformity (Giles 1982).

The investigations by Huson (1967), Cihak (1981), Reichmann (1971), Hadley (1976) and Med (1980), who studied zygapophyseal joint orientation in the developing vertebral column, have almost invariably recorded that the orientation of all joints lie close to the coronal plane in utero. However, in utero variation in the development of the zygapophyseal joints has been reported, some individuals showing the eventual adult form and shape of the lumbar zygapophyseal joints (Reichmann 1971).

Zygapophyseal joint tropism occurs most frequently at T11–12 (Malmivaara et al 1987, Singer et al 1989a), which has been described by Veleanu et al (1972) as the 'headquarters' for the TJ. The highly variable orientations in the zygapophyseal joints present at this level may indicate an intermediate stage in the evolution of this transitional region. The gradual form of transition (Fig. 7.4), which was found in the majority of cases, is probably the most developed form for this region (Singer et al 1989a).

MORTICE JOINTS

Early descriptions of interlocking zygapophyseal joints (Hildebrandt 1816, Humphry 1858), and the TJ 'mortaise' joint coined by Topinard (1877) and others (Le Double 1912, Davis 1955), have been extensively reported. Davis (1955, 1961) suggested that the 'mortice' effect could be gauged according to development of the mammillary processes and their projection behind the inferior articular processes. This morphological feature was examined radiographically, with the use of CT, and histologically, to provide a quantitative description of the relationship of the mammillary processes to TJ zygapophyseal joint orientation (Plate 7.1). The most common segmental level demonstrating mortice joints was T11–12, followed by T12–L1 (Davis 1955, Malmivaara et al 1987, Singer 1989b).

Of interest was the presence of unilateral mortice joints, defined previously by Malmivaara et al (1987), and their association with zygapophyseal joint tropism. It was evident from the CT studies performed by Singer et al (1990a) that unilateral mortice joints frequently possessed a mammillary process on the side of the coronally orientated joint, which appeared to form a posterior buttress for the adjacent inferior articular process (Plate 7.1A).

According to the comparative studies reported by Vallois (1920) and Kaplan (1945), the mammillary processes are most evident at the TJ in those primates who achieve an orthograde posture during ambulation. Speculation by both writers suggests that these processes develop in response to the activity of the multifidus muscle which, from electromyographic studies performed by Donisch and Basmajian (1972), appears to function primarily as a stabilizer of adjacent vertebral segments during axial rotation. This finding might suggest that the multifidus acts more as an antagonist to rotation at the TJ, and thereby reinforces the morphological role of the zygapophyseal joints in preventing torsion. The laminar fibres of multifidus, which attach to the mammillary processes immediately below, would tend to act closer to the horizontal plane, whereas the fibres passing superiorly to the spinous process of the cranial segments might function as a 'brake' to flexion coupled with rotation. This may further ensure that the joints remain relatively approximated, as a strategy to reduce segmental mobility.

INTRA-ARTICULAR SYNOVIAL FOLD PROTRUSIONS

Histologically, intra-articular synovial folds have been demonstrated consistently in the TJ zygapophyseal joints (Singer et al 1990b). This finding complements similar observations reported on zygapophyseal joints of the lumbosacral junction (Giles 1987) and the lumbar (Dörr 1958, Töndury 1940, Kirkaldy-Willis 1984), thoracic (Ley 1975) and cervical (Töndury 1940, Bland 1987) regions. According to Töndury (1972), these intra-articular synovial folds act as displaceable space-fillers which deform to accommodate incongruities between the articular surfaces during normal joint excursions. The relative change in orientation of the TJ zygapophyseal joints may also account for differences in the morphology of these inclusions. Fibro-adipose folds, noted more in coronally orientated joints, may be suited to the marked translatory movements performed by these joints. In contrast, fibrous folds predominated in the more sagittally orientated joints (Singer et al 1990b), occasionally showing histological evidence of fibrosis at their tips to suggest that these folds may become tractioned or compressed. The mechanical situations favouring this occurrence may include sudden torsional forces or compression due to joint approximation during flexion or extension postures.

ACCESSORY OSSIFICATION CENTRES AT THE THORACOLUMBAR JUNCTION

The development of the TJ zygapophyseal joints is often associated with the appearance of vertebral process variants (Hayek 1932, Heise 1933). Accessory ossification centres appearing adjacent to the spinous, transverse

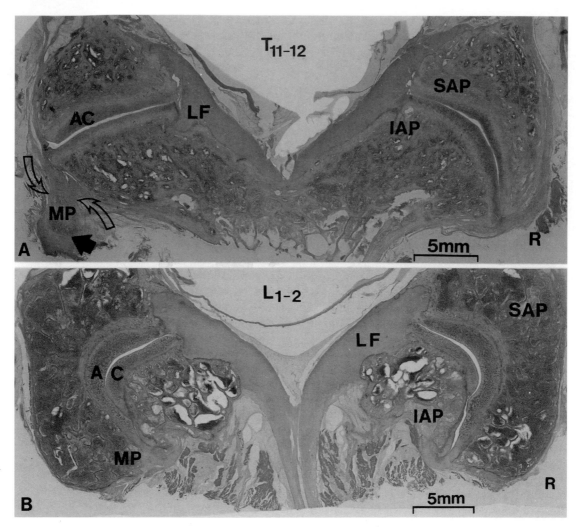

Plate 7.1   A. Photomicrograph of a 200 μm-thick transverse section cut in the plane of the superior vertebral end-plate at T11–12 to illustrate a type II unilateral mortice joint on the left formed by the mammillary process MP (arrow) located posteriorly to the inferior articular process IAP. The zygapophysis on the right conforms to a typical sagittally orientated joint. Curved arrows indicate the attachment of the lateral and posterior articular capsular ligaments which are reinforced by the mammillary process. Despite the marked articular tropism, both joint surfaces have a normal histological appearance in this subject. **B**. An example of a bilateral type I mortice joint at L1–2. This section from the lower half of the joint illustrates the extent to which inferior articular processes IAP are embraced by the superior articular process SAP which show a medial tendency in the posterior aspect of the joint. The articular cartilage AC appears normal despite some thinning on the right IAP in the more sagittal component of the joint. LF = ligamentum flavum. (This plate is reproduced in colour at the front of the volume.)

and mammillary-accessory processes are a relatively rare finding, occurring in approximately 1–2% of the populations studied by Pech and Haughton (1985) and Singer and Breidahl (1990a). Rudimentary costal elements are more frequently observed, and appear to be more common in men than women (Schertlein 1928). The clinical significance of these variations is their possible confusion with fractures at the TJ (Keats 1979, Singer & Breidahl 1990a) and their contribution to miscalculations of vertebral levels.

BIOMECHANICS OF THE THORACOLUMBAR JUNCTION

Limitation to regional spinal and segmental mobility

occurs by virtue of the shape of the vertebral bodies, the thickness of the intervertebral discs, and the relative orientation of the zygapophyseal joints (Fick 1911, Pearcy 1986).

In the thoracic region, the almost vertical alignment of the zygapophyseal joints, together with the costovertebral joints and the splinting effect of the ribs, precludes any marked tendency towards flexion. Similarly, thoracic extension and rotation are limited due to the constraint afforded by the posteriorly projecting lamina and approximation of spinous processes. The stabilizing role of the thoracic cage is lessened in the lower thoracic segments due to the greater mobility afforded by the floating ribs.

Several in vitro investigations have been performed on the thoracolumbar vertebral column to determine the mobility of these segments (White 1969, Kazarian 1972, Markolf 1972). In general, the influence of variation in transition patterns has been largely overlooked. However, the consistent findings from these studies has been the limitation in segmental mobility due to the specialized morphology of the zygapophyseal joints. Kazarian (1972) has drawn attention to the idiosyncratic motion behaviour of the lower thoracic vertebral elements, particularly when loaded axially; similarly, Markolf (1972) has emphasized the torsional resistance afforded by the TJ segments. An in vivo study was performed by Gregersen and Lucas (1967) to examine segmental mobility patterns throughout the thoracolumbar spine but they did not attempt any special study of the TJ region.

AXIAL ROTATION AT THE THORACOLUMBAR JUNCTION

The change of zygapophyseal joint orientation at the TJ has been interpreted by anatomists and clinicians as signifying an abrupt change in the mobility of these joints, particularly in the horizontal plane (Humphry 1858, Levine et al 1988). It is interesting to note that White and Panjabi (1978) base mobility information for T12–L1 on extrapolations from adjacent lower thoracic and upper lumbar segments. The different regional orientations of the TJ zygapophyseal joints permit mainly rotation in the thoracic segments and sagittal range in the lumbar region

(Davis 1959, Gregersen & Lucas 1967, Evans 1982). For example, the upper lumbar joints, through approximation of the articular surfaces, also restrict mobility, particularly extreme extension (Davis 1955), or flexion (Kummer 1981); indeed, the posterior elements of the upper lumbar segments are positioned to afford stability in the plane of the intervertebral disc (Farfan 1983) and appear to minimize excessive torsional forces (Stokes 1988).

Singer et al (1989b) used CT studies of subjects who were positioned in a rotated posture to consider the potential for segmental displacement at the TJ. They were able consistently to demonstrate ipsilateral compression and contralateral separation of the sagittally directed articular surfaces in their volunteers, whereas coronally directed joints tended to show translatory displacement of the articular facets, as depicted in Figure 7.5 (Singer et al 1989b). Similarly, those subjects possessing a mortice type of joint demonstrated little motion relative to adjacent segments.

Other anatomical, developmental and degenerative mechanisms would appear to increase the resistance to torsion, for instance, the ingrowth into the ligamentum flavum by laminar spicules (Davis 1955, Allbrook 1957) which, in some instances, results in ossification of the ligamentum flavum (Kudo et al 1983). The orientation of the laminar fibres of multifidus muscle may also serve to increase the axial 'stiffness' of the TJ (Donisch & Basmajian 1972).

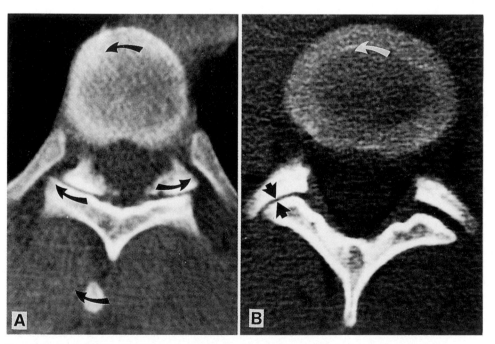

Fig. 7.5 A. CT slice taken through the superior end-plate of T10–11 with the subject in comfortable end-range right trunk rotation to illustrate the extent of axial translation of the zygapophyseal joints. The spinous process of the cranial segment confirms the axial displacement induced through the subject's rotated posture. **B**. The same subject scanned through the superior end-plate at L4–5 showing the relative approximation and separation of zygapophyseal joints produced through a sustained right trunk rotation position.

The notion that rotation is restricted in the upper lumbar region, due to predominantly sagittal orientation of the zygapophyseal joints, is not new. Hildebrandt (1816), and numerous commentators over the ensuing decades, have dismissed lumbar inter-segmental rotation as minimal (Humphry 1858, Lewin et al 1962, Kummer 1981, Farfan 1983, Putz 1985). Actual rotation is said to be produced through displacement of adjacent vertebrae, which induces lateral shear forces within the intervertebral disc (Gregersen & Lucas 1967), flexibility of the neural arch (Farfan 1983, Stokes 1988) and, to a lesser extent, by compliance of the articular surfaces (Lewin et al 1962).

SPINAL EXTENSION AT THE THORACOLUMBAR JUNCTION

At the TJ, a 'close-packed' joint position may be achieved when the thoracolumbar column is extended, as a result of the medial taper of the zygapophyseal joints (Singer 1989b) and the 'mortice-like' disposition of the articular surfaces and the mammillary processes (Topinard 1877). This approximation would, to coin Davis' (1955) description, act to 'lock' the TJ segments.

The tendency for the mortice joint to act as an 'axis', or pivot, has been further demonstrated by loading autopsy vertebral columns into extension and then examining the alteration in spinal curvature in relation to the unloaded position (Singer, unpublished observations). In the loaded posture, a noticeable discontinuity of the thoracolumbar curve at the junctional region was noted. This finding would appear to indicate that a close-packed position is achieved at the TJ when the inferior articular process abuts onto the laminae of the vertebra below (Grieve 1981).

BIOMECHANICS OF SPINAL INJURIES AT THE THORACOLUMBAR JUNCTION

The TJ has been the focus for many clinical and surgical reports due to the high frequency of serious spinal trauma located within the lower thoracic and upper lumbar mobile segments (Rehn 1968, Rostad et al 1969, Schmorl & Junghanns 1971, Denis 1983, Larson 1986). In this context, the transition has been classically regarded as mechanically disposed to trauma, being less capable of withstanding axial and torsional stresses at a point of marked anatomical and mechanical change (Humphry 1858, Macalister 1889). The localization of injury to the TJ has been attributed to the difference in mobility between the thoracic and lumbar regions, given the tendency, during rapid hyperflexion, for the 'stiff' thoracic segments to act as a long 'lever' which pivots over the lumbar spine (Jefferson 1927, Levine et al 1988). The majority of traumatic injuries at the TJ involve the vertebral bodies, usually producing a compression or burst fracture (Rehn 1968, Denis 1983, Lindahl et al 1983, Willén et al 1990). However, descriptions of TJ injuries do not appear to have considered the influence that transitional variations of the zygapophyseal joints might play in the mechanism of injury and the type of trauma sustained. As predicted, an abrupt transition pattern at the TJ tended to localize trauma to these segments, particularly when rotation was a known contributor to the injury mechanism (Singer et al 1989c).

PATHOANATOMICAL RELATIONSHIPS AT THE THORACOLUMBAR JUNCTION

Veleanu et al (1972) indicated that similar patterns of osteoarthritis are demonstrated in the lower thoracic zygapophyseal joints and upper lumbar region, due to these elements sustaining similar stresses as the lumbar spine. This appears to reinforce speculation by Lewin (1964), who suggested that the thoracolumbar mortice joint morphology might predispose to the early development of osteoarthritis.

In a preliminary study into the effects of tropism on osteoarthritic changes of the lumbosacral zygapophyseal joints, Giles (1987) found evidence to suggest that the more sagittally orientated joints showed greater signs of degeneration compared with the more coronally disposed joint. This observation was confirmed for the TJ by Malmivaara et al (1987) in an investigation of macerated vertebrae. However, a careful histological examination of hyaline articular cartilage by Singer et al (1990a) did not reveal any correlation between articular cartilage degeneration and tropism. On the contrary, there appeared to be evidence to suggest that zygapophyseal joint tropism and the presence of a well developed mammillary process ensured the integrity of the articular surfaces (Singer et al 1990a) (Plate 7.1). Mortice joints appeared similarly to act in a protective way (Plate 7.1).

Davis (1955) suggested that the mortice joint morphology might act as an 'axis' for flexion forces, resulting in localized TJ vertebral compression fractures. This theory may also relate to the high frequency of vertebral endplate lesions (Schmorl's nodes) in this region (Resnick & Niwayama 1978, Hilton 1980) (Fig. 7.6). According to Malmivaara et al (1987), this pattern of end-plate injury appears most commonly in the lower thoracic vertebrae. Similarly, there is also a high incidence of osteoarthritis in the zygapophyseal and costovertebral joints of the lower thoracic segments (Shore 1935, Nathan et al 1964). Recent studies by Malmivaara and co-workers have concentrated on the pathologies involving the vertebral bodies and intervertebral discs of the TJ (Malmivaara et al 1987, Malmivaara 1987, 1989). Their studies have been based on cadaveric investigations of 24 thoracolumbar spines and have described the pathoanatomical relationships

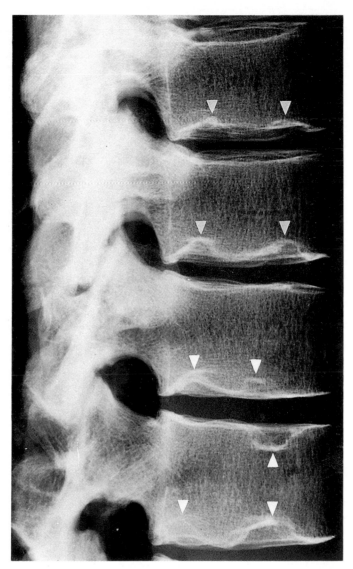

Fig. 7.6 A plain radiograph illustrating multiple end-plate lesions (arrowheads) (Schmorl's nodes) at the thoracolumbar junction in a 36-year-old male. Despite these lesions at every level the intervertebral disc heights do not show any marked reduction. Compare with Figure 7.3.

between Schmorl's nodes, costovertebral joint osteoarthritis, vertebral body osteophytosis, and intervertebral disc degeneration. Their thesis proposes that patterns of TJ degeneration are closely linked to the transitional characteristics of the anterior and posterior elements depending on their respective capabilities for resisting torsional and compressive forces applied to this region.

CLINICAL ANATOMY OF THE THORACOLUMBAR JUNCTION

Transitional variations in zygapophyseal joint orientation appear often at both the thoracolumbar and lumbosacral junctions (Singer 1989a). The observation of multiple anomalies present at several transitional junctions has

been documented previously by Kühne (1932), Schmorl and Junghanns (1971), MacGibbon and Farfan (1979) and Wigh (1980). This tendency has several implications for the clinical assessment and management of patients with spinal pathology. Schwerdtner (1986) found that patients with structural variations at the lumbosacral junction tended to show poor responses to manipulative therapy and recommended conservative management when treating these patients. Similarly, Wigh (1979) noted that surgical patients with thoracolumbar and or lumbosacral transitional variations were more likely to have inappropriate surgery. Wigh (1980) suggested that part of the difficulty in diagnosing the symptomatic level appeared to stem from the incorrect identification of accessory ossification centres and vestigial ribs.

Some clinical features and syndromes appear to be specific to the TJ. For example, investigations reported by McCall et al (1979) and Maigne (1980, 1981) have suggested that irritation to the lateral branches of the dorsal rami from the low thoracic and upper lumbar segments at the TJ may be confused with low back pain syndromes as these nerves become cutaneous over the buttocks and the region of the greater trochanter.

Clinical statements about the mechanical capability and treatment of the TJ mobile segments, as expressed by Lewit (1986) and Maigne (1980), contrast with biomechanical data which indicates that this region acts to resist torsional forces (Singer et al 1989b). Therefore, the appropriateness of manipulative treatments of this transitional region, as advocated by Maigne (1980) (Fig. 7.7), may need to be reappraised.

Markolf (1972) has suggested, on biomechanical grounds, that the first segment above the transitional level with coronally orientated zygapophyseal joints would be more susceptible to torsional stress. This speculation was not confirmed within the context of a preliminary study of TJ spinal injuries reported by Singer et al (1989c); however, thoracic disc herniations appear more frequently in the lower thoracic segments compared with the middle and upper thoracic region (Chin et al 1987, Ryan et al 1988). While the overall incidence of thoracic discal herniation is low, approximately 4% according to Bury & Powell (1989), the relationship between the level of lesion and the TJ transition may be strongly related, as mechanical aetiologies, often involving rotation, are implicated in the production of symptoms (Russell 1989).

Intra-articular synovial fold protrusions have been demonstrated in the superior and inferior joint 'spaces' of the TJ zygapophyseal joints and, less frequently, at the middle third of the joint (Singer et al 1990b). Investigations by Giles and Harvey (1987) have indicated the presence of free nerve endings in the substance of similar synovial folds within lower lumbar zygapophyseal joints. It may be assumed that compression or traction of these structures could produce pain. The specific morphology of the TJ

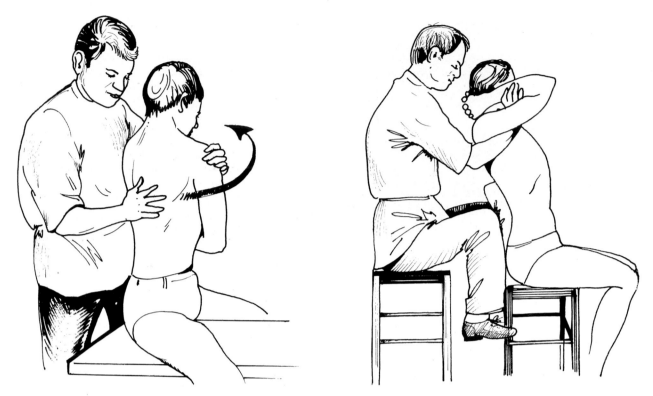

Fig. 7.7   Rotary and extension manipulations have been advocated for the thoracolumbar junction. Both would presumably result in 'locking' of this transitional region, which would, in turn, *increase* the local stress on these segments (redrawn from Maigne 1980 with kind permission of the Archives of Physical Medicine and Rehabilitation).

zygapophyseal joints appears to dictate the type and location of intra-articular synovial inclusions (Singer et al 1990b). Therefore, forceful mobilization techniques which compress or apply torsion to these joints (Maigne 1980) may, in fact, be provocative of symptoms (Fig. 7.7). Similarly, the pain centralization phenomenon described by Donelson et al (1990), following repeated or sustained thoracolumbar extension, may well evoke complaint from the zygapophyseal joints due to the compression of intra-articular structures.

From the foregoing discussion it would appear that conservative treatment of painful disorders arising from the TJ may be more appropriate than some of the recommended mechanical therapies (Grieve 1981, Singer & Giles 1990). The clinical impression advanced by Lewit (1986) that the TJ is designed for rotation appears to contradict the anatomical and biomechanical studies reported on this region (Singer 1989b, Singer et al 1989b). The capacity for regional mobility of the vertebral column according to morphological studies such as these must continue to serve as the basis for rational mechanical therapies.

A review of the anatomy of the TJ (Singer 1989a) re-veals that, in a majority of the individuals studied, the posterior elements of the TJ exhibit anatomical features consistent with reducing stress through an area of considerable morphological and functional variation, principally through a gradual transition in the orientation of the zygapophyseal joints.

This finding challenges the notion that the TJ is necessarily a 'weak point' of the vertebral column. The TJ represents the most variable of the vertebral transitional regions in terms of zygapophyseal joint orientation, tropism, and in the segmental level of transition. The mortice arrangement at the T11–12 and T12–L1 zygapophyseal joints appears to limit rotation and extension. Therefore, examination procedures and any manual therapy interventions should consider these factors for the effective management of patients with mechanical dysfunction at the thoracolumbar transition.

Acknowledgements

The author recognizes with pleasure the contributions to these investigations by Dr Peter Breidahl, Mr Robert Day and Dr Lynton Giles.

REFERENCES

Åkerblom B 1948 Standing and sitting posture: with special reference to the construction of chairs. A-B Nordiska, Bokhandeln

Allbrook D 1955 The East African vertebral column. American Journal of Physical Anthropology 13: 489–511

Allbrook D 1957 Movements of the lumbar spinal column. Journal of Bone and Joint Surgery 39B: 339–345

Anderson J 1982 The thoracolumbar spine. Clinics in the Rheumatic Diseases 8: 631–653

Bagnall K, Harris P, Jones P 1977 A radiographic study of the human fetal spine. [2] The sequence of development of ossification centres in the vertebral column. Journal of Anatomy 124: 791–798

Barclay-Smith E 1911 Multiple anomaly in a vertebral column. Journal of Anatomy 45: 144–171

Berry J, Moran J, Berg W, Steffee A 1987 A morphometric study of human lumbar and selected thoracic vertebrae. Spine 12: 362–367

Birkner R 1978 Normal radiologic patterns and variances of the human skeleton. Urban & Schwarzenberg, Baltimore

Bland J 1987 Disorders of the cervical spine. Saunders, Philadelphia

Braune W, Fischer O 1889 Über den Schwerpunkt des menschlichen Köpers mit Rücksicht auf die Ausrüstung des duetschen Infansteristen. Cited in: Åkerblom 1948

Bury R, Powell T 1989 Prolapsed thoracic intervertebral disc: the importance of CT assisted myelography. Clinical Radiology 40: 416–421

Chin L, Black K, Hoff J 1987 Multiple thoracic disc herniations: case report. Journal of Neurosurgery 66: 290–292

Cihak R 1981 Die Morphologie und Entwicklung der Wirbelbogengelenke. Die Wirbelsäule in Forschung und Praxis 87: 13–28

Cyriax E 1929 On certain absolute and relative measurements of human vertebrae. Journal of Anatomy 54: 305–308

Davis P 1955 The thoraco-lumbar mortice joint. Journal of Anatomy 89: 370–377

Davis P 1959 The medial inclination of the human thoracic intervertebral articular facets. Journal of Anatomy 93: 68–74

Davis P 1961 The thoraco-lumbar mortice joint in West Africans. Journal of Anatomy 95: 589–593

Davis P 1980 Engineering aspects of the spine. Mechanical aspects of the spine. Mechanical Engineering Publications, London, pp 33–36

Denis F 1983 The three column spine and its significance in the classification of acute thoracolumbar spinal injuries. Spine 8: 817–831

Donelson J, Silva G, Murphy K 1990 Centralization phenomenon. Its usefulness in evaluating and treating referred pain. Spine 153: 211–213

Donisch E, Basmajian J 1972 Electromyography of deep muscles in man. American Journal of Anatomy 133: 25–36

Dörr W 1958 Über die Anatomie der Wirbelgelenke. Archiv für Orthopädische und Unfallchirurgie 50: 222–243

El-Bohy A, Yang K-H, King A 1989 Experimental verification of facet load transmission by direct measurement of facet lamina contact. Journal of Biomechanics 22: 931–941

Evans D 1982 Biomechanics of spinal injuries. In: Gonza E, Harrington I (eds) Biomechanics of musculoskeletal injury. Williams & Wilkins, Baltimore, pp 163–224

Farfan H 1983 Biomechanics of the lumbar spine. In: Kirkaldy-Willis W (ed) Managing low back pain. Churchill Livingstone, New York, pp 9–21

Fick R 1911 Spezielle Gelenke und Muskelmechanik. Handbuch der Anatomie und Mechanik der Gelenke. Gustav Verlag Fischer, Jena

Gehweiler J, Osborne R, Becker R 1980 The radiology of vertebral trauma. Saunders, Philadelphia

Giles L 1982 Leg length inequality with postural scoliosis: its effect on lumbar apophyseal joints. MSc thesis, University of Western Australia

Giles L 1987 Lumbo-sacral zygapophyseal joint tropism and its effect on hyaline cartilage. Clinical Biomechanics 2: 2–6

Giles L, Harvey A 1987 Immunohistochemical demonstration of nociceptors in the capsule and synovial folds of human zygapophyseal joints. British Journal of Rheumatology 26: 362–364

Gonon G, Rousson B, Fischer L, Morin A, Bouchet A 1975 Donnes metriques concernant l'arc posterieur au niveau du rachis dorso-lombarire de D8 a L5. Association des Anatomistes Comptes Rendus 58: 867–875

Gregersen G G, Lucas D 1967 An in vivo study of the axial rotation of the human thoracolumbar spine. Journal of Bone and Joint Surgery 49A: 247–262

Grieve G 1981 Common vertebral joint problems. Churchill Livingstone, Edinburgh, p 14

Hadley L 1976 Anatomico-roentgenographic studies of the spine. C C Thomas, Illinois

Hamilton W 1976 Textbook of human anatomy. 2nd edn. Macmillan, London

Hasebe K 1913 Die Wirbelsäule der Japaner. Zeitschrift für Morphologie Jahrbuch 43: 449–476

Hayek H 1932 Über lendenrippen. Fortschritte auf dem Gebiete der Rontgenstrahlen und der Nuklearmedizin. Erganzungsband 45: 582–592

Heise H 1933 Über anomalien der lendenwirbelsäule. Deutsche Zeitschrift für Chirurgie 227: 349–367

Hildebrandt G 1816 Handbuch der anatomie. Cited in Humphry 1858

Hilton R 1980 Systematic studies of spinal mobility and Schmorl's nodes. In: Jayson M (ed) The lumbar spine and back pain. Pitman, Bath, pp 115–134

Hoppenfeld S 1977 Orthopaedic neurology: a diagnostic guide to neurologic levels. Lippincott, Philadelphia

Humphry G 1858 A treatise on the human skeleton. Macmillan, London, pp 169–171

Huson A 1967 Les articulations intervertébrales chez les foetus humain. Comptes Rendus des Association D'Anatomists 138: 676–683

Jefferson G 1927 Discussion on spinal injuries. Proceedings of the Royal Society of Medicine 20: 625–637

Kapandji I 1977 The physiology of the joints, vol 3. The trunk and vertebral column. 2nd edn. Churchill, Edinburgh, pp 16–17

Kaplan E 1945 The surgical and anatomic significance of the mammillary tubercle of the last thoracic vertebra. Surgery 17: 78–92

Kazarian L 1972 Dynamic response characteristics of the human vertebral column. Acta Orthopaedica Scandinavica (suppl 146)

Kazarian L 1978 Identification and classification of vertebral fractures following emergency capsule egress from military aircraft. Aviation Space and Environmental Medicine 49: 150–157

Keats T 1979 An atlas of normal roentgen variants that simulate disease. 2nd edn. Year Book Medical Publishers, Chicago

Kirkaldy-Willis W 1984 The relationship of structural pathology to the nerve root. Spine 9: 49–52

Kudo S, Ono M, Russell W 1983 Ossification of thoracic ligamenta flava. American Journal Roentgenology 141: 117–121

Kühne K 1932 Die Vererbung der Variationen der menschlichen. Wirbelsäule Zeitschrift für Morphologie Anthropologie 30: 1–221

Kummer B 1981 Biomechanik der Wirbelgelenke. Die Wirbelsäule in Forschung und Praxis 87: 29–34

Lampmann L, Duursmar S, Ruys J 1984 CT densimetry in osteoporosis. Martinus Nijhoff, Boston

Lanier R 1939 The presacral vertebrae of American white and Negro males. American Journal of Physical Anthropology 3: 341–420

Larson S 1986 The thoracolumbar junction. In: Dunsker S B, Schmidek H, Frymoyer J, Kahn A (eds) The unstable spine. Grune & Stratton, Orlando, pp 127–152

Le Double A-F 1912 Traite des variations de la colonne vertébrale de l'homme. Vignot-Freres, Paris

Levine A, Edwards C 1987 Lumbar spine trauma. In: Camins E, O'Leary P (eds) The lumbar spine. Raven Press, New York, pp 183–212

Levine A, Bosse M, Edwards C 1988 Bilateral facet dislocations in the thoracolumbar spine. Spine 13: 630–640

Lewin T 1964 Osteoarthritis in lumbar synovial joints. Acta Orthopaedica Scandinavica (suppl 73)

Lewin T, Moffett B, Viidik A 1962 The morphology of the lumbar synovial intervertebral joints. Acta Morphologica Neerlando-Scandinavica 4: 299–319

Lewit K 1986 Muscular pattern in thoraco-lumbar lesions. Manual Medicine 2: 105–107

Ley F 1975 Contribution a l'etude des cavités articulaires interapophysaires vertébrales thoraciques. Archives D'Anatomie D'Histologie et D'Embryologie 57: 61–114

Lindahl S, Willén J, Nordwall A, Irstam L 1983 The 'crush-cleavage' fracture. A 'new' thoracolumbar unstable fracture. Spine 8: 181–186

Louis R 1983 Surgery of the spine. Springer-Verlag, Berlin, p 10

Lutz G 1967 Die Entwicklung der kleinen Wirbelgelenke. Zeitschrift für Orthopädie und ihre Grenzgebiete 104: 19–28

Macalister A 1889 A textbook on human anatomy. Griffin, London, p 129

MacGibbon B, Farfan H 1979 A radiologic survey of various configurations of the lumbar spine. Spine 4: 258–266

McCall I, Park W, O'Brien J 1979 Induced pain referral from posterior lumbar elements in normal subjects. Spine 4: 441–446

Maigne R 1980 Low back pain of thoracolumbar origin. Archives of Physical Medicine and Rehabilitation 61: 389–395

Maigne R 1981 The thoracolumbar junction syndrome. Low back pain, pseudo-visceral pain, pseudo-hip pain and pseudo-pubalgia. Semaine des Hopitaux de Paris 57: 545–554

Malmivaara A 1987 Disc degeneration in the thoracolumbar junctional region. Evaluation by radiography and discography in autopsy. Acta Radiologica 28: 755–760

Malmivaara A 1989 Pathoanatomical changes in the thoracolumbar junctional region of the spine. Annals of Medicine 21: 367–368

Malmivaara A, Videman T, Kuosma E, Troup J 1987 Facet joint orientation facet and costovertebral joint osteoarthrosis, disc degeneration, vertebral body osteophytosis and Schmorl's nodes in the thoracolumbar junctional region of cadaveric spines. Spine 12: 458–463

Markolf K 1972 Deformation of the thoracolumbar intervertebral joints in response to external loads. Journal of Bone and Joint Surgery 54A: 511–533

Med M 1980 Prenatal development of intervertebral articulation in man and its association with ventrodorsal curvature of the spine. Folia Morphologica 28: 264–267

Nachemson A 1960 Lumbar intradiscal pressure. Acta Orthopaedica Scandinavica (suppl 43)

Nathan H 1962 Osteophytes of the vertebral column. An anatomical study of their development according to age, race and sex: with considerations as to their etiology and significance. Journal of Bone and Joint Surgery 44A : 243–268

Nathan H, Weinberg H, Robin G, Aviad I 1964 The costovertebral joints: anatomico-clinical observations in arthritis. Arthritis and Rheumatology 7: 228–240

Noback C, Roberston G 1951 Sequences of appearance of ossification centres in the human skeleton during the first five prenatal months. American Journal of Anatomy 89: 1–28

Odgers P 1933 The lumbar and lumbo-sacral diarthrodial joints. Journal of Anatomy 67: 301–317

Pal G, Routal R 1987 Transmission of weight through the lower thoracic and lumbar regions of the vertebral column in man. Journal of Anatomy 152: 93–105

Parke W 1982 Applied anatomy of the spine. In: Rothman R, Simeone F (eds) The spine. Saunders, Philadelphia

Pearcy M 1986 Measurement of back and spinal mobility. Clinical Biomechanics 1: 44–51

Pech R, Haughton V 1985 CT appearance of unfused ossicles in the lumbar spine. American Journal of Neuroradiology 6: 629–631

Pfeil E 1971 Stellungsvarianten der Gelenkfortsätze am Lendenkreuzbein-Übergang. Zentralblatt für Chirurgie 93: 10–17

Pick T 1890 Gray's anatomy: descriptive and surgical. Longmans, London

Pooni J, Hukins D, Harris P, Hilton R, Davies K 1986 Comparison of the structure of human intervertebral discs in the cervical, thoracic and lumbar regions of the spine. Surgical and Radiologic Anatomy 8: 175–182

Putz R 1976 Beitrag zur Morphologie und Rotationsmechanik der kleinen Gelenke der Lendenwirbelsäule. Zeitschrift für Orthopädie 114: 902–912

Putz R 1985 The functional morphology of the superior articular processes of the lumbar vertebrae. Journal of Anatomy 143: 181–187

Radin E 1976 Aetiology of osteoarthrosis. Clinics in Rheumatic Diseases 2: 509–522

Rehn J 1968 Die knöchernen Verletzungen der Wirbelsäule Bedeutung des Erstbefundes für die spätere Begutachtung. Die Wirbelsäule in Forschung und Praxis 40: 131–138

Reichmann S 1971 The postnatal development of form and orientation of the lumbar intervertebral joint surfaces. Zeitschrift für Anatomie Entwicklungsgeschichte 133: 102–123

Resnick D, Niwayama G 1978 Intravertebral disk herniations: cartilaginous Schmorl's nodes. Radiology 126: 57–65

Rostad H, Solheim K, Siewers P, Lie M 1969 Fracture of the spine. Acta Orthopaedica Scandinavica 40: 664–665

Russell T 1989 Thoracic intervertebral disc protrusion: experience of 76 cases and review of the literature. British Journal of Neurosurgery 3: 153–160

Ryan R, Lally J, Kozic Z 1988 Asymptomatic calcified herniated thoracic disks: CT recognition. American Journal of Neuroradiology 9: 363–366

Schertlein A 1928 Über die haufigsten Anomalien an der Brustlendenwirbelsäulengrenze. Fortschritte auf dem Gebiete der Rontgenstrählen und der Nuklearmedizin. Erganzungsband 38: 478–488

Schmorl G, Junghanns H 1971 The human spine in health and disease. 2nd American edn. Grune & Stratton, New York, pp 55–60

Schwerdtner H 1986 Lumbosakrale Übergangsanomalien als Rezidivursache bei chirotherapeutischen Behandlungstechniken. Manual Medizin 24: 11–15

Shore L 1930 Abnormalities of the vertebral column in a series of skeletons of Bantu natives of South Africa. Journal of Anatomy 64: 206–238

Shore L 1935 On osteo-arthritis in the dorsal intervertebral joints. A study in morbid anatomy. British Journal of Surgery 22: 833–849

Singer K 1989a Variations at the human thoracolumbar transitional junction with reference to the posterior elements. PhD thesis, University of Western Australia

Singer K 1989b The thoracolumbar mortice joint. Radiological and histological observations. Clinical Biomechanics 4: 137–143

Singer K, Breidahl P 1990a Accessory ossification centres at the thoracolumbar junction. Surgical and Radiologic Anatomy 12: 53–58

Singer K, Breidahl P 1990b Vertebral body trabecular density at the thoracolumbar junction using quantitative computed tomography. A post-mortem study. Acta Radiologica 31: 37–40

Singer K, Giles L 1990 Manual therapy considerations at the thoracolumbar junction: an anatomical and functional perspective. Journal of Manipulative and Physiological Therapeutics 13: 83–88

Singer K, Breidahl P, Day R 1988 Variations in zygapophyseal orientation and level of transition at the thoracolumbar junction. A preliminary CT survey. Surgical and Radiologic Anatomy 10: 291–295

Singer K, Breidahl P, Day R 1989a Posterior element variation at the thoracolumbar transition. A morphometric study using computed tomography. Clinical Biomechanics 4: 80–86

Singer K, Day R, Breidahl P 1989b In vivo axial rotation at the thoracolumbar junction: an investigation using low dose CT in healthy male volunteers. Clinical Biomechanics 4: 145–150

Singer K, Willén J, Breidahl P, Day R 1989c A radiologic study of the influence of zygapophyseal joint orientation on spinal injuries at the thoracolumbar junction. Surgical and Radiologic Anatomy 11: 233–239

Singer K, Giles L, Day R 1990a Influence of zygapophyseal joint orientation on hyaline cartilage at the thoracolumbar junction. Journal of Manipulative and Physiological Therapeutics 13: 207–214

Singer K, Giles L, Day R 1990b Intra-articular synovial folds of the thoracolumbar junction zygapophyseal joints. Anatomical Record 226: 147–152

Singer K, Jones T, Breidahl P 1990c A comparison of radiographic and computer-assisted measurements of thoracic and thoracolumbar sagittal curvature. Skeletal Radiology 19: 21–26

Sobotta J, Uhlenhuth E 1957 Atlas of descriptive anatomy. 7th English edn. Hafner, New York, p 24

Stagnara P, Mauroy J, de Dran G, Gonon G, Costanzo G, Dimnet J, Pasquet A 1982 Reciprocal angulation of vertebral bodies in a sagittal plane: approach to references for the evaluation of kyphosis and lordosis. Spine 7: 335–342

Steindler A 1955 Kinesiology of the human body: under normal and pathological conditions. C C Thomas, Illinois

Stewart T 1932 The vertebral column of the Eskimo. American Journal of Physical Anthropology 16: 51–62

Stokes I 1988 Mechanical function of facet joints in the lumbar spine. Clinical Biomechanics 3: 101–105

Strasser H 1913 Die Rumpfhaultungen. Lehrbuch der Muskel und Gelenkmechanik. Springer, Berlin, pp 244–320

Struthers J 1875 On variations of the vertebrae and ribs in man. Journal of Anatomy and Physiology 9: 17–96

Terry R, Trotter M 1953 Osteology. In: Schaeffer J P (ed) Morris' human anatomy. New York, McGraw-Hill, p 102

Testut L, Latarjet A 1948 Traité d'anatomie humaine, vol 1, 9th edn. Dion, Paris, p 69

Todd T 1922 Numerical significance in the thoracolumbar vertebrae of the mammalia. Anatomical Record 24: 261–286

Töndury G 1940 Beitrag zur Kentniss der Kleinen Wirbelgelenke. Zeitschrift für Anatomie Entwicklungsgeschichte 110: 568–575

Töndury G 1972 Anatomie fonctionelle des petites articulations de rachis. Annales de Medecine Physique 15: 173–191

Topinard P 1877 Des anomalies de nombre de la colonne vertebrale chez l'homme. Revue D'Anthropologie 6: 577–649

Vallois H 1920 La signification des apophyses mammillaires et accessories des vertèbres lombaires. Comptes Rendus Societie de Biologie 83: 113–115

Veleanu C, Grün U, Diaconescu M, Cocota E 1972 Structural peculiarities of the thoracic spine. Their functional significance. Acta Anatomica 82: 97–107

White A 1969 Analysis of the mechanics of the thoracic spine in man. Acta Orthopaedica Scandinavica (suppl 127)

White A, Panjabi M 1978 Basic kinematics of the spine. Spine 3: 12–29

Whitney C 1926 Asymmetry of vertebral articular processes and facets. American Journal of Physical Anthropology 9: 451–455

Wigh R 1979 Phylogeny and the herniated disc. Southern Medical Journal 72: 1138–1143

Wigh R 1980 The thoracolumbar and lumbosacral transitional junctions. Spine 5: 215–222

Willén J, Anderson J, Tomooka K, Singer K 1990 The natural history of burst fractures in the thoracolumbar spine T12 & L1. Journal of Spinal Disorders 3: 39–46

Williams P, Warwick R 1980 Gray's anatomy. 36th edn. Churchill Livingstone, London, pp 277, 284

Yang K, King A 1984 Mechanism of facet load transmission as a hypothesis for low back pain. Spine 9: 557–565

Zindrick M, Wiltse L, Doornik A et al 1986 Analysis of the morphometric charateristics of the thoracic and lumbar pedicles. Spine 12: 160–166

8. Structure and function of lumbar zygapophyseal (facet) joints

J. R. Taylor   L. T. Twomey

INTRODUCTION

The zygapophyseal joints are synovial joints between the articular processes which project upwards and downwards from the lateral parts of the laminae. They are often called facet joints and sometimes described as 'interlaminar joints'. An accurate knowledge of their structure and geometry is essential for a clear understanding of their function and an informed appreciation of the malfunctions to which they may be subject as a consequence of injury or ageing. They are traditionally described in major anatomical texts as planar or flat (Warwick & Williams 1973, Romanes 1981), but this is accurate only for the cervical and thoracic facets. More recent editions admit the curved nature of some zygapophyseal articular surfaces (Warwick & Williams 1980). Adult lumbar facets are curved or biplanar in the transverse plane. Two zygapophyseal joints and an intervertebral disc form the articular triad which unites two vertebrae in a stable amphiarthrosis. The disc and its associated zygapophyseal joints both contribute in different ways to movement and to stability. Generally, the disc, which is the stronger structure, by its thickness and compliance controls the ranges of movement possible while the facet orientation determines the type of movements permitted and restrains or opposes movements which might damage the disc. Thus, the lumbar facets provide a most important protection for the disc, shielding it from most of the shearing forces which might tear or disrupt it and preventing that range of axial rotary movements which would overstretch its obliquely oriented annular fibres. Without normal zygapophyseal joints the disc could not sustain the normal loads of weight-bearing and movement and the motion segment would become unstable (Kirkaldy-Willis 1983). This is seen, for example, where instability develops following facet removal in decompression laminectomies (Hopp & Tsou 1988) or when the facet's stabilizing influence no longer operates, as in spondylolisthesis (Farfan 1973, Penning & Blickman 1980).

THE LUMBAR FACETS: THEIR STRUCTURE AND GEOMETRY

Development

The lumbar facets are originally flat in the coronal plane in infants (Lutz 1967, Taylor & Twomey 1987), but in older children and in adults they are usually curved in the transverse plane, due to their manner of growth. Growth of both facets in later infancy and childhood takes place in a posterior direction from the lateral margins of the original coronally oriented parts. This gradually adds the larger sagittally oriented portion as each lumbar facet grows throughout childhood. During this growth, the junction of the coronal and sagittal components is rounded off by remodelling. Zygapophyseal joints remain capable of remodelling throughout life. Facet shape changes are observed, due to altered loading, in joints where there is persistent malposition of the facets in an unstable motion segment (Taylor et al 1989).

Adult anatomy

The lumbar facets are curved or biplanar in transverse section (Figs 8.1, 8.2) or as viewed in computed tomograms of the lumbar spine (CT scans); they are flat in sagittal section and approximately parallel to the posterior surface of the vertebral body (Taylor & Twomey 1986). Like the vertebral bodies, the articular processes contain cancellous bone, but their shell of compact bone is thicker than that of the vertebral bodies, particularly at their medial margins. A lumbar inferior articular process (IAP) projects downwards from the lower lateral part of the lamina on each side. Each IAP presents a convex facet, directed forwards and medially, to engage closely with the slightly larger concave facet on the superior articular process (SAP) of the vertebra below (Fig. 8.2). The concave SAP projects backwards and upwards from the junction of the pedicle and lamina at the root of the transverse

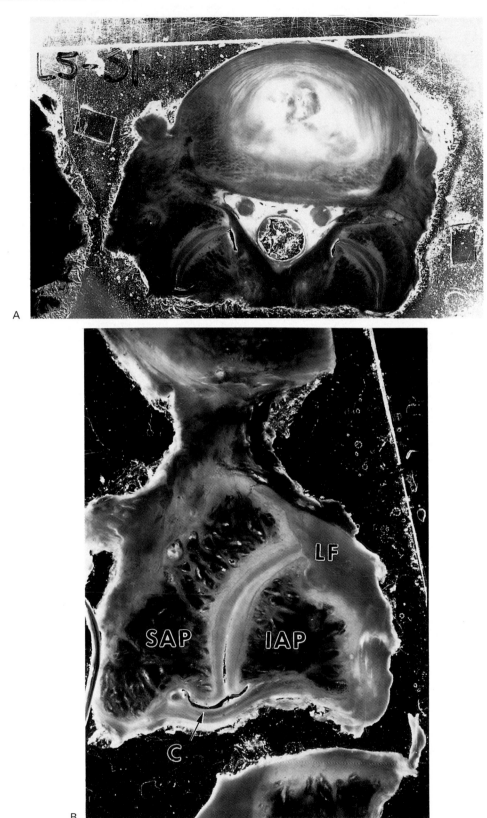

Fig. 8.1   Lumbar facet joints: 2 mm-thick transverse sections. **A.** The lumbo-sacral motion segment, sectioned through the two symmetrical facet joints and the lower margin of the intervertebral disc. The spinal canal contains sacral nerve roots within the circular dural sac, and the S1 nerve roots can be seen in the lateral recesses of the triangular bony spinal canal. **B.** Transverse section of a left facet joint. The concave surface of the superior articular process (SAP) of the lower vertebra is congruous with the convex surface of the inferior articular process (IAP) of the upper vertebra. The surfaces are lined by smooth articular cartilage overlying compact subchondral bone plates which have a whitish appearance. The ligamentum flavum (LF) encloses the joint anteriorly and a fibrous capsule (C) encloses the posterior aspect of the joint.

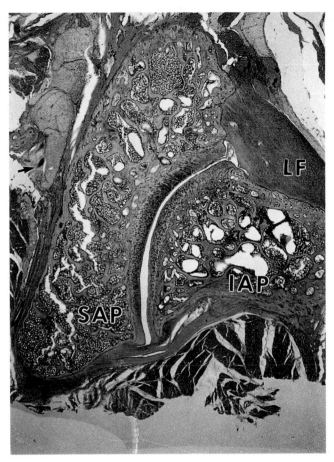

Fig. 8.2 Lumbar L3–4 facet joint: 100 μm stained transverse section at 'mid-joint' level. This facet joint shows normal chondrocytes evenly distributed through the smooth articular cartilage. The anterior part of the joint approximates to the coronal plane, and the posterior part curves round into the sagittal plane. The ligamentum flavum (LF) encloses the joint in front. The posterior fibrous capsule is in two parts separated by a small fat pad behind the inferior articular process (IAP). The long superficial capsular fibres are attached to the back of the IAP at some distance medial to the joint line. Part of the multifidus muscle overlies the capsule. The arrow indicates a branch of the dorsal ramus passing back around the superior articular process.

process on each side. Its articular surface faces backwards and medially. It can be regarded as having an anterior, coronally oriented part (the antero-medial third of the facet) and a sagittally oriented posterior part (the posterior two-thirds of the joint). The facets are slightly larger in their vertical dimension (about 15 mm) than in their transverse dimension (about 12 mm). Just lateral to the posterior margin of each lumbar SAP a mamillary process projects backwards for the lower lateral attachment of the flat tendon of a lumbar multifidus muscle, which descends obliquely across the joint from a spinous process two segments above. Below each SAP there is a small fossa on the back of the lamina (the pars interarticularis) for the fat pad which fills the inferior joint recess. This fossa is largest in the lower lumbar vertebrae. The fat pad of the inferior recess is mostly extracapsular (Fig. 8.3); it communicates with the joint cavity and its extracapsular part

is enclosed by the multifidus muscle as it crosses obliquely to the SAP below (Taylor & McCormick 1991). Between the SAP and IAP, on each side, is that part of the lamina called the pars interarticularis. The narrowest part or isthmus of the pars interarticularis, just below the SAP and the root of the transverse process, is vulnerable to stress fracture. This part is readily recognized on oblique X-rays of the lumbar spine as the 'neck of the Scotty dog', the 'muzzle' being the transverse process and the 'ear' being the SAP. The body and legs of the imaginary dog are formed by the lamina plus spinous process and IAPs, respectively (Fig. 8.7).

As viewed in transverse section or in CT scans, the facets from L1 to L5 progressively change their orientation from a predominantly sagittal orientation at L1 to a more nearly coronal orientation at S1. Measurements of the angle formed by the joint plane (the SAP) with the median plane (Kenesi & Lesur 1985, Taylor & McCormick 1987) show an increase in this angle from L2 down to S1 (Fig. 8.6). The angular change in degrees is greatest between the SAP of L4 and the SAP of L5. This change in angle may relate to the changing posture of the individual lumbar vertebrae with descent towards the lumbo-sacral junction, as the lower vertebrae are increasingly tilted forwards. Davis (1961) has pointed out that the greater the forward tilt the larger the force vector tending to push the upper vertebra forwards off the lower vertebra. The greater width in the coronal plane of lower lumbar facets permits distribution of this anteriorly directed load over a larger area.

Joint tropism

Asymmetry of zygapophyseal joint angles is quite common (Badgeley 1941, Farfan & Sullivan 1967, Cihak 1970, Kenesi & Lesur 1985) and it is regarded by some as a contributory cause of low back pain (Farfan & Sullivan 1967).

In our studies of CT scans of the lower lumbar spine (L3–4 to L5–S1) from 193 patients investigated for low back pain and 68 'controls' with no history of back pain requiring treatment, we found joint angle asymmetry of 10° or more in 22% of controls and 28% of the back-pain patients. Tropism is most frequent at the lowest two levels, where 30% of joints show 10° or more of asymmetry. If a higher threshold of 20° difference between right and left is used, only 3.5% of joints are affected. Comparing numbers of patients affected by this amount of tropism, rather than numbers of joints, 14% of back pain patients and 8.8% of controls show lumbar facets (L3–4 to L5–S1) with tropism >20°. This degree of tropism is more common in younger patients than in older patients, suggesting a developmental origin for the more marked degrees of tropism. This degree of tropism is more common in the back pain group than in controls. How-

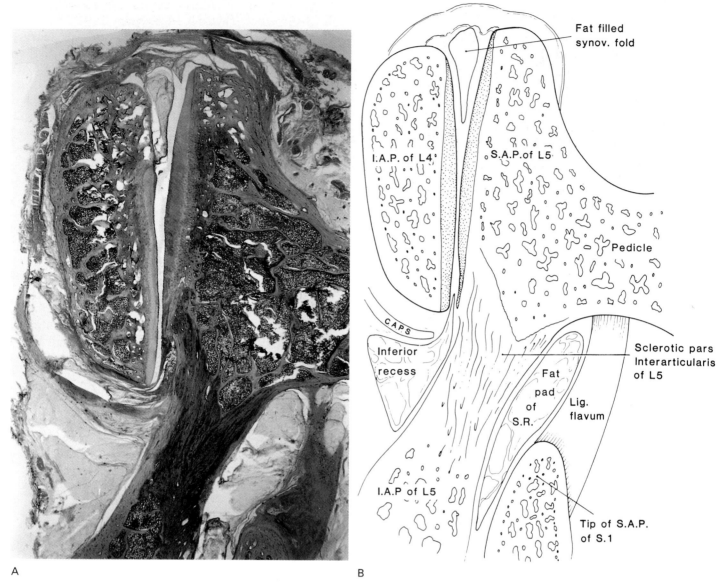

A   B

Fig. 8.3 Lower lumbar facets in sagittal section. **A.** Stained sagittal section. **B.** Diagrammatic representation of section. A 100 μm stained sagittal section through the centre of L4–5 and the medial part of L5–S1 with a diagram illustrating the parts shown in the section. Note the synovial lined fat pad extending 3–4 mm down into the joint from the superior recess (SR) under the ligamentum flavum. Each lower lumbar facet joint has a capsular opening at its lower pole through which the large, cushioning fat pad, which lies outside the joint under the multifidus muscle, communicates freely with the joint. The part projecting into the joint is lined by synovial membrane. That part of the lamina separating the inferior recess of L4–5 from the superior recess of L5–S1 is called the pars interarticularis. This part may be fractured in sporting injuries, connecting the two joint cavities.
SAP = superior articular process: IAP = inferior articular process; CAPS = capsule.

ever, the origin of tropism and its relation to back pain are complex problems. Some zygapophyseal asymmetry is developmental and it may lead to back-ache as a consequence of the asymmetrical mechanical forces acting on the motion segment — but some tropism is also acquired, for example, due to facet remodelling following the development of segmental instability. In this case the tropism could not be held to be the cause of any associated back pain.

Articular cartilage and subchondral bone plate

The articular cartilage is on average 1 mm thick on each facet (Fig. 8.1) with a regular thickness and a smooth surface in young people (Twomey & Taylor 1985). It shows chondrocyte hypertrophy in the coronal component of the SAP, quite frequently in young adults, with multiple splits appearing in this hypertrophic zone, again selectively in the coronal part of the SAP (Fig. 8.4). Complete loss of

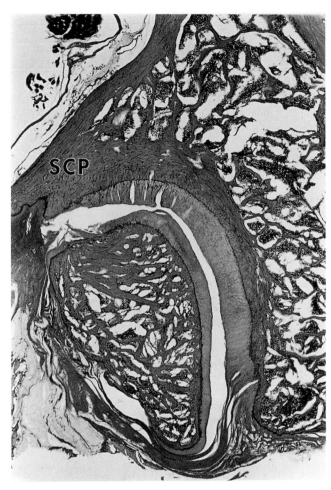

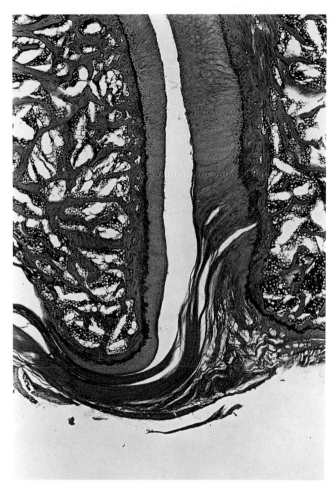

Fig. 8.4 Transverse 100 µm stained section of L3–4 showing chondromalacia (splitting) of the articular cartilage on the coronal part of the concave superior articular process. The subchondral bone plate (SCP) under this cartilage is thickened.

Fig. 8.5 A higher-power view of the posterior part of the joint shown in Fig. 8.4 showing the direct continuity of the capsule and the articular cartilage on the concave facet. This continuity can lead to traction damage at the margin of the cartilage, as shown. The cartilage is split and the dark 'tide mark' where the cartilage attaches to the subchondral bone plate is thickened and irregular. The convex facet shows extension of the articular cartilage beyond its normal confines, around its posterior margin under the capsule, as a response to pressure from the overlying capsule.

cartilage with ageing was rare in our series, but a number of middle-aged and elderly subjects showed selective loss of cartilage from the posterior parts of the facets; others showed metaplastic extension of cartilage around the posterior margins of the IAPs, due to pressure and rubbing of the IAPs against the posterior capsule, giving an appearance like 'wrap-around bumpers' on the back of each IAP (Fig. 8.5). This may be associated with loosening of the joint and stretching of its capsule, with posterior subluxation of the IAP relative to the SAP (Taylor et al 1989).

The subchondral bone plate (SCP), a fairly compact layer of bone which supports the cartilage, varies in thickness, from 0.5 mm to 1.4 mm in different parts of the adult joint. In the SAP, it is thicker in the coronal component than in the sagittal component. This 'wedge-shaped' appearance (Fig. 8.1) becomes increasingly evident with growth of the joint (Taylor & Twomey 1985). The SCP changes in other respects with growth and development. It is thin and ill-defined in the infant when the lumbar

joints are coronally inclined like thoracic facets. It is vascular in the child and younger adolescent, as the sagitally oriented part of the joint grows backwards from the original coronal part. It becomes thicker, especially anteriorly, and less vascular in the adult (Taylor & Twomey 1986). Frequently, sclerotic changes are observed in the thicker coronal component of the joint in adolescent males, young adults of both genders and middle-aged adults. Its relative thickness in the coronal part, compared to the sagittal part, changes from a proportion of 1.5-to-1 in children, to 3-to-1 in adults. The SCP loses thickness in the elderly but maintains its characteristic wedge shape. The SCP of the IAP is not wedge-shaped as a rule, but is little thicker centrally than peripherally. Sclerotic changes are uncommon in the convex IAP compared to the concave SAP.

The joint capsule

Synovial joints have a fibrous capsule enclosing the joint; it is strong and tight enough to give joint stability, but lax enough in certain positions to permit the physiological ranges of movement. This capsule is lined on its inner aspect by synovial membrane. This secretes the synovial fluid which lubricates and nourishes the articular cartilages. Between the fibrous and synovial layers there is a variable vascular, fatty layer, which enables the synovial folds to accommodate their shape to fill any potential space around the articular margins (Giles & Taylor 1987).

The zygapophyseal joint capsule is sometimes described as 'thin and loose' (Warwick & Williams 1980), or 'lax' (Romanes 1981). This is not the impression gained from a study of fresh, intact post mortem lumbar joints, where the posterior capsular fibres and the ligamentum flavum appear quite tight with the facets held in close apposition. It is not usually possible to separate the articular surfaces using a slowly applied twisting manual force in intact unfixed autopsy spines, but where there is segmental instability with an abnormally slack capsule a CT scan of the specimen can demonstrate diastasis of the articular surfaces when axial torque is applied to the specimen (McFadden & Taylor 1990). So the anterior ligamentum flavum and the posterior fibrous capsule appear taut and closely applied to the anterior and posterior margins of normal joints, but the capsule around the polar recesses is loose. This arrangement accommodates vertical sliding of the facets due to the looseness at the polar recesses, by the obliquity of the posterior fibres and the elasticity of the anterior fibres. Unstable motion segments have demonstrable damage to the intervertebral disc and often unilateral damage to a zygapophyseal joint.

Transverse sections of the zygapophyseal joint (Fig. 8.1) show that the anterior capsule is formed by the ligamentum flavum, which is about 3 mm thick at the joint line (Hirsch et al 1963, Taylor & Twomey 1986). The ligamentum flavum has an extensive attachment to the anterior surface of the IAP, and laterally it wraps around the anterior aspect of the SAP, attaching to it and forming the posterior boundary of the lower half of the intervertebral foramen. Superiorly, the ligamentum flavum passes from the tip of the SAP directly upwards to the junction of the lamina and pedicle above, enclosing the fat pad of the superior joint recess between itself and the pars interarticularis of the vertebra above (Fig. 8.3). The direction of the fibres in the ligamentum flavum is almost vertical in the medial interlaminar portion, but the capsular fibres of the ligamentum flavum are oblique, passing downwards and laterally around the anterior margin of the SAP. The posterior fibrous capsule is usually in two parts, collectively 1 mm thick. The deep, short capsular fibres are attached near or into the articular margins, including the posterior margin of the articular carti-

lage; the superficial part forms a long sheet which passes from the mamillary process and posterior margin of the SAP across the joint line and the posterior surface of the IAP to an attachment 7 mm or more medial to the joint line (Fig. 8.2); its long fibres are angled slightly downwards as they pass laterally to allow for the principal movement of flexion (Farfan 1973, Taylor et al 1990). A small fat pad separates the superficial and deep posterior capsular fibres and fat with synovial membrane lines the

AVERAGE JOINT PLANE

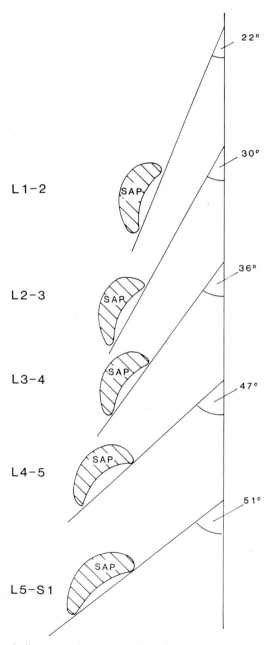

Fig. 8.6 A diagrammatic representation of the change in joint angles from L1–2 to L5–S1, based on measurements in CT scans from over 200 patients (fewer data were available for the upper two joints). Note that the angle increases from above down, and the greatest increase in angle occurs between L3–4 and L 4–5.

deep surface of the capsule. The posterior fibrous capsule is well innervated, but we found relatively few nerve fibres in the ligamentum flavum (Giles & Taylor 1987). It is important to note that direct continuity of the posterior fibrous capsule with the posterior margin of the articular cartilage is common (Fig. 8.5), particularly at the posterior margin of the SAP, and that some fibres of multifidus attach to this part of the capsule as well as to the mamillary process. The lumbar multifidus is usually described as arising from the mamillary processes and inserted into the spinous processes allowing it to rotate the spinous processes. However, the close application of its flat tendons to the back of the joint capsules and its attachment close to the joint line provokes comparison to the rotator cuff of the shoulder. The muscle is probably a stabilizer of the zygapophyseal joint. It should be noted that decalcified, dehydrated transverse sections of the joints gape open in their posterior parts when this muscle is no longer active to maintain congruity of the joint surfaces, whereas the anterior articular surfaces are held together by the elasticity of the ligamentum flavum. The potential influence of the direct capsular attachment to the posterior margin of the articular cartilage, in contributing to detachment of a cartilage flap from the subchondral bone plate, should also be noted. Sprains of the posterior capsule appear quite common in middle life (Twomey & Taylor 1988). Alternatively parts of the articular cartilage may be torn off, leaving the capsule intact. This may be related to the observation of selective loss of cartilage from the posterior parts of the facets in some older subjects (Taylor & Twomey 1986).

The joint recesses, synovium and 'menisci'

The ligamentum flavum encloses an intracapsular superior joint recess containing a fat pad between itself and the roof of the IAP. This fat pad is lined by synovial membrane which projects downwards as a fat-filled synovial fold for about 3 mm between the articular surfaces (Fig. 8.3). The pad becomes fibro-fatty with ageing and is often described as a meniscus, since transverse sections near the upper pole of the joint show it completely traversing the joint from front to back. A meniscus is not normally seen in the middle third of zygapophyseal joints, but examples of enlarged fat pads which extend from the joint recesses right through the joint to mid-joint levels are found in 4% of lumbar spinal joints (Taylor & McCormick 1991). Some of these joints with enlarged fat pads are also unstable, and the extension of the synovial lined fibro-fatty pad appears to be an attempt to fill up the space in a 'loose' joint.

At the inferior recess, the fibrous capsule merges with the ligamentum flavum. A small gap or rounded hole in the capsule is usually found here, through which the large extracapsular fat pad of the inferior joint recess communicates with the fat filled synovial fold which projects upwards between the articular surfaces. Using fresh, unfixed autopsy material, this fat pad can be seen to move freely in and out of the lumbar zygapophyseal joint during passive movements (McFadden & Taylor 1990); this probably acts both as a damping and a lubricating mechanism (Fig. 8.3). The synovial folds of the joint recesses are innervated and may be sources of pain when inflamed (Giles & Taylor 1987). Synovial fold inflammation may be caused by trauma or by irritation from joint debris in an arthritic joint. This would be expected to lead to pain and local muscle spasm. Small synovial fringes also form triangular space-fillers around the posterior and anterior margins of the joint. These are smooth, rounded and glistening, with a vascular content and a villous surface in young fresh joints, where they are capable of adapting freely to the changing shape of the moving joint, acting as lubrication 'space-fillers' around the joint margins and secreting the synovial fluid essential to articular cartilage nutrition (Giles & Taylor 1982). They become stiffer and more triangular in shape in older subjects, with fibrous change at their tips where they project and are nipped or compressed between the joint margins. They become larger and more fibrous with ageing, particularly if the joint capsule becomes slack (Taylor & Twomey 1986).

'Locking' of Z joints

A different, pathological type of joint inclusion or 'meniscus', which has potential significance in relation to 'locked back', is the fibrocartilaginous inclusion created by the tearing off of part of the articular cartilage of a zygapophyseal facet, where the articular cartilage is firmly attached to the posterior joint capsule. A high percentage of normal joints have direct continuity of the posterior fibrous capsule with the posterior articular cartilage margin. Joint movement produces tension on the capsule; this tension is augmented by the partial attachment of the multifidus muscle into the capsule and a part of the articular cartilage may be sheared off the underlying bone, keeping its capsular attachment. This small flap, detached from the articular surface, would move about in the posterior joint as the capsule moves and it may be displaced within the joint, especially in loose joints subjected to torsional strain. Displacement of this fibrocartilaginous inclusion is capable of 'locking' the joint in a manner comparable to a torn knee joint meniscus. Since the posterior capsule itself is well innervated, the abnormal capsular strain would cause acute back pain and muscle spasm (Taylor & Twomey 1986, 1987).

The relation of joint structure of joint function and movement

The zygapophyseal joints are essential to the stability of

the motion segment and control its movements (Adams & Hutton 1983, Taylor & Twomey 1986). Two zygapophyseal joints and one intervertebral disc form an articular triad, which is supported by various ligaments and segmental muscles constituting a spinal motion segment. The thickness and compliance of the intervertebral disc are the principal determinants of the range of movement in each segment while the zygapophyseal joints act as 'guide rails', determining, by their orientation, the planes in which these movements can take place (Gregerson & Lucas 1967). The predominantly sagittal orientation of the lumbar facets prevents true axial rotation of more than one or two degrees per motion segment and appears designed to limit lumbar movements to the sagittal and coronal planes. It can be appreciated that the obliquely oriented fibres of the anulus fibrosus could be overstretched and torn if axial rotation was permitted to accompany flexion. With each physiological movement, the lumbar disc changes shape and a rocking movement of one vertebra upon another occurs in the sagittal or coronal plane around a midline axis or fulcrum, near the posterior margin of the disc. At the same time, upward and downward gliding movements occur between the articular facets of the zygapophyseal joints. In flexion and extension both IAPs slide upwards then downwards on the SAPs. In lateral bending the upward and downward gliding alternates on the two sides.

The lumbar zygapophyseal joints also act as restraints at the end-ranges of movements, e.g. in full extension the tips of the IAPs abut on the lamina below, bringing extension to a halt. Terminal extension is damped by the inferior recess fat pad which occupies a hollow on the lamina, below the tip of the IAP, but in rapid extension the abutment of the sharp tip of the IAP imposes stress on the lamina below, which may be responsible for the sclerotic changes frequently observed there. By a different mechanism, the facets play an important role in limiting flexion and in preventing forward slide of the upper vertebra on the lower vertebra, which would injure the disc. A forward compression of the convex IAP into the concavity of the SAP near the end of flexion builds up loading on the facets, which restrains flexion and forward translation (Taylor & Twomey 1986). The lumbar SAPs, in contrast to cervical and thoracic SAPs, are almost parallel to the long axis of the spine. This is important for stability in a part of the spine which must bear high loads. In full flexion from a standing position, the weight of the upper body (and any load in the hands) would tend to make a lumbar vertebra slide forwards on the next adjacent lower vertebra, but the IAPs, passing down on each side like hooks behind the SAPs of the next vertebra, stabilize the vertebra and prevent forward slide with excessive shear in the disc. The movement of flexion is principally a forward rotation around an axis in the posterior disc, but there is always a small amount of forward translation (up to 3 mm

is regarded as normal). This causes a build-up of pressure between the closely apposed facets, which, together with the increased tension in the joint capsules, ligamenta flava and interspinous ligaments, and lumbodorsal fascia, brings flexion to a halt. Cadaver experiments suggest that the build-up of compression between the apposed facets during flexion is quantitatively the most effective of these restraints. Studies in living subjects show that the erector spinae is not active in full flexion (Kippers & Parker 1985) but that the thoracolumbar fascia, which completely envelops the lumbar post-vertebral muscles, excercises some restraint on flexion.

Forces transmitted through the facets: facet injuries and spondylolysis

The importance of the lumbar articular facets in load bearing may have been underestimated by some authors, since in the axial load bearing of static erect posture, they are said to bear 16% of the axial load (Hutton & Adams 1980), though Yang & King (1984) suggested that they could carry 25% of body weight and perhaps more in arthritic joints. This ignores the frequency with which the spine is loaded in flexion in occupational and sporting activities and the loading in extension which accompanies many sporting activities (Twomey et al 1990). Studies of the articular surfaces of the lumbar facets show that chondromalacia (Fig. 8.4), with splitting of the articular cartilage in the coronally oriented part of the SAP, plus thickening of the subchondral bone plate, is very common in young adults (Eisenstein & Parry 1987, Taylor & Twomey 1987). Our posterior release experiments (Twomey & Taylor 1983) and observations of chondromalacia in the coronal component of the SAP in active young people suggest repetitive high loading of this coronal part of the SAP. The distribution of dense haematoxylin staining in the subchondral bone plates and the pars interarticularis (Fig. 8.3), reflecting sclerotic changes, appears to indicate a pathway of stress from the SAP through the pars interarticularis to the IAP. These observations, together with the frequency of spondylolysis in young athletes (Fig. 8.7), all support the view that high loads are imparted to the facets, particularly in flexion.

The restraining forces in the compressed SAP in full flexion are transmitted down through the pars interarticularis (Fig. 8.3). The sclerotic changes we observed so frequently in the pars interarticulares of the lower lumbar vertebrae of adolescents and young adults indicate the high levels of stress in the pars associated with sporting activities which may cause spondylolysis, a common stress fracture in young athletes. In motor vehicle accidents the loads on the lumbar facets frequently produce small articular fractures, as well as capsular tears or sprains (Twomey et al 1989, Taylor et al 1990). Deceleration forces are borne by the lumbar facets in a similar manner

POSTERIOR OBLIQUE VIEWS

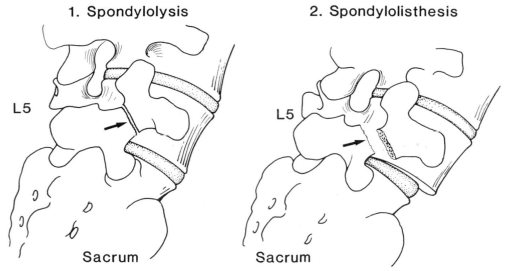

Fig. 8.7 A diagram of postero-lateral oblique views of the lumbo-sacral spine showing spondylolysis — a fracture through the pars interarticularis, and spondylolisthesis — a forward slip of the upper vertebra where there was a bilateral spondylolysis.

to lumbar facet loading at end-range. The biomechanical distribution of forces in flexion loading of the lumbar articular triad contrasts with the situation in the cervical motion segment. Cervical facets, which have a 45° angle with the long axis of the spine and are designed to allow translation with flexion, give less protection to the cervical discs (Taylor & Twomey 1990). A study of cervical autopsy material from motor vehicle accidents shows relatively few facet fractures but more frequent disc injuries with moderately frequent capsular tears with haemarthrosis in cervical zygapophyseal joints (Taylor & Twomey 1991).

NEUROLOGY OF ZYGAPOPHYSEAL JOINTS: NERVE SUPPLY AND ROOT CANAL STENOSIS

Nerve supply

The zygapophyseal joints are closely related to the spinal nerves and to their dorsal rami which supply them. As the spinal nerve issues from the intervertebral foramen it divides into its primary rami. The dorsal ramus divides into medial and lateral branches almost immediately and the medial branch winds backwards around the base of the SAP. It descends between the mamillary and accessory processes under cover of the mamillo-accessory ligament, supplying the posterior capsule and the inferior recess of the corresponding joint and terminating by supplying the superior recess of the joint below.

Nerve root canals

The lumbar nerve roots and spinal nerves normally lie in the wider superior parts of the intervertebral canals, well

SEGMENTAL INSTABILITY AND FORAMINAL STENOSIS

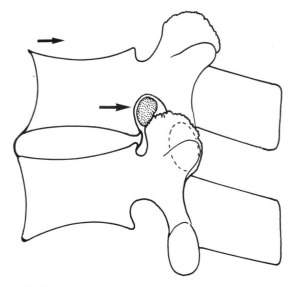

Fig. 8.8 A diagram showing how the superior articular process (SAP) may 'entrap' the spinal nerve (arrowed) in the intervertebral foramen due to a combination of ageing and degeneration including: (a) shortening of the lumbar motion segment, due to end-plate bowing or disc thinning; (b) osteophytic enlargement of the SAP margin; (c) lordotic posture; (d) retrolisthesis of the upper vertebra associated with motion segment instability. Of these, we consider retrolisthesis to be the most important cause of foraminal stenosis with nerve root entrapment by the superior articular facet.

above the tips of the SAPs which are partially covered and 'smoothed out' by the ligamenta flava. A number of factors related to ageing or pathology may alter the relation of the facets to the spinal nerves. These factors include arthritic enlargement of the facets, with osteophytosis of the SAP, anterior displacement of the SAP into the intervertebral foramen, associated with retrolisthesis of the vertebra above the foramen and overriding of the facets, or shortening of the lumbar column due to loss of disc height or osteoporosis, with associated loss of height of the intervertebral foramen. Any one of these or any combination of them may bring the nerve roots within reach of the SAP (Fig. 8.8). In this case, nerve root canal stenosis is present, either with change of the spinal canal to a trefoil shape, giving lateral recess stenosis or with intervertebral canal stenosis (Fig. 8.8). In either case, nerve root entrapment may occur. When an IAP slips backwards in motion segment instability the SAP of the vertebra below moves forwards into the foramen. In instability, nerve root canal stenosis may be a dynamic problem rather than a permanent structural narrowing.

Pain and sciatica may follow weight-bearing on a sloppy unstable motion segment, due to creep in a degenerate disc gradually producing a more stenotic nerve root canal during the later part of the working day. In erect posture, retrolisthesis and creep of the IAPs of a damaged motion segment into an increased lordosis, would also narrow the root canal (Kirkaldy-Willis 1983, Taylor et al 1989).

It can be appreciated from this brief account of the lumbar facet joints that a thorough knowledge of their structure gives a better understanding of their function as guides and restraints of movement and protectors of the intervertebral discs from damage and the spinal nerves from entrapment. Degenerative or traumatic failure of the facets (or surgical removal) can lead to damage to unprotected discs; spinal stenosis may result from facet hypertrophy, with chronic back pain. Trauma to the soft capsular, articular and synovial tissues can cause acute back pain and stiffness or acute locked back.

REFERENCES

Adams M A, Hutton W 1983 The mechanical function of the lumbar joints. Spine 8: 327–330

Badgeley E D 1941 The articular facets in relation to low back pain. Journal of Bone and Joint Surgery 23/2: 481–496

Cihak R 1970 Variations of lumbosacral joints and their morphogenesis. University of Carolina Medicine 16: 145–165

Davis P 1961 The thoraco-lumbar mortice joint in West Africans. Journal of Anatomy 95: 589–593

Eisenstein S M, Parry C R 1987 The lumbar facet arthrosis syndrome. Journal of Bone and Joint Surgery 69B: 3–7

Farfan H F, Sullivan J D 1967 The relation of facet orientation to intervertebral disc failure. Canadian Journal of Surgery 10: 179–185

Farfan H F 1973 Mechanical disorders of the low back. Lea & Febiger, Philadelphia, pp 1–247

Giles L, Taylor J R 1982 Intra-articular protrusions in the lower lumbar apophyseal joints. Bulletin of the Hospital for Joint Diseases XLII: 248–254

Giles L, Taylor J R 1987 Human zygapophyseal joint capsule and synovial fold innervation. British Journal of Rheumatology 26: 93–98

Gregerson G G, Lucas D B 1967 An in vivo study of axial rotation of the human thoracolumbar spine. Journal of Bone and Joint Surgery 49: 247

Hirsch C 1963 The anatomical basis of lower back pain. Acta Orthopaedica Scandinavica 33: 1–17

Hopp E, Tsou P M 1988 Postdecompression lumbar instability. Clinical Orthopaedics and Related Research 227: 143–151

Hutton W, Adams M A 1980 The forces acting on the neural arch and their relevance to low back pain. Engineering aspects of the spine. Mechanical Engineering, London, pp 49–55

Kenesi C, Lesur L 1985 Orientation of the articular processes at the L4, L5 and S1; possible role in pathology of the intervertebral disc. Anatomica Clinica 7: 43–47

Kippers V, Parker A W 1985 Electromyographic studies of erectores spinae: symmetrical postures and sagittal trunk motion. Australian Journal of Physiology 31: 95–105

Kirkaldy-Willis W H 1983 Managing low back pain. Churchill Livingstone, New York, pp 1–174

Lutz G 1967 Die entwicklung der kleinen wirbelgelenke. Z Orth 104: 19–28

McFadden K D, Taylor J R 1990 Axial rotation in the lumbar spine and gaping of the zygapophyseal joints. Spine 15: 295–299

Penning L, Blickman J R 1980 Instability in lumbar spondylolisthesis: a radiologic study of several concepts. American Journal of Roentgenology 134(2): 293–301

Romanes G J R 1981 Cunningham's anatomy. 12th edn. Oxford University Press, Oxford

Taylor J R, McCormick C C 1987 Variation and asymmetry in lower lumbar zygapophyseal joint angles. Proceedings of the Australian Orthopaedic Association, Perth, 1987, p 64

Taylor J R, McCormick C C 1991 Lumbar facet joint fat pads. Neuroradiology 33: 38–42

Taylor J R, Twomey L T 1985 Vertebral column development and its relation to adult pathology. Australian Journal of Physiotherapy 31: 83

Taylor J R, Twomey L T 1986 Age changes in lumbar zygapophyseal joints: observations on structure and function: Spine 11: 739–745

Taylor J R, Twomey L T 1987 The lumbar spine from infancy to old age. In: Twomey L T, Taylor J R (eds) Physical therapy of the low back. Churchill Livingstone, New York, ch1

Taylor J R, Twomey L T 1990 Disc injuries in cervical trauma. Lancet 2: 1318

Taylor J R, Twomey L T 1991 The effects of whiplash trauma on cervical joints. Spine (in press)

Taylor J R, McCormick C C, Willen J 1989 Lumbar zygapophyseal incongruity as a sign of motion segment instability. Journal of Anatomy 165: 299–300

Taylor J R, Twomey L T, Corker M 1990 Bone and soft tissue injuries in post mortem lumbar spines. Paraplegia 28: 119–129

Twomey L T, Taylor J R 1983 Sagittal movements of the human lumbar vertebral column – a quantitative study of the role of the posterior vertebral elements. Archives of Physical Medicine and Rehabilitation 64: 322–325

Twomey L T, Taylor J R 1985 Age changes in the lumbar articular triad. Australian Journal of Physiotherapy 31: 106–112

Twomey L T, Taylor J R 1988 Zygapophyseal joints of the lumbar spine. Proceedings of the 5th Biennial Congress of the Manipulative Therapists Association of Australia, Melbourne 1988, pp 377–398

Twomey L T, Taylor J R, Oliver M 1988 Sustained flexion loading, rapid extension loading of the lumbar spine and physiotherapy of related injuries. Physiotherapy Practice 4: 129–138

Twomey L T, Taylor J R, Taylor M 1989 Acute injuries to lumbar zygapophyseal joints. Australian Medical Journal 151: 210–217

Warwick R, Williams P L 1973 Gray's anatomy. 35th edn. Churchill Livingstone, Edinburgh

Warwick R, Williams P L 1980 Gray's anatomy. 36th edn. Churchill Livingstone, Edinburgh, p 446

Yang K M, King A I 1984 Mechanism of facet load transmission as an hypothesis for low back pain. Spine 9: 557

9. Biomechanics of the lumbar motion segment

M. A. Adams

INTRODUCTION TO THE 'MOTION SEGMENT'

A 'motion segment' consists of two adjacent vertebrae and the intervening disc and ligaments. Being the basic functional unit of the osteoligamentous spine, it is sometimes referred to as a 'functional spinal unit' (FSU). Muscle tissue is not included, so the motion segment is essentially a passive structure which responds to forces applied to it, either by the musculature in vivo or by a materials testing machine in vitro.

Motion segments are used in most experimental investigations of spinal mechanics because they are the smallest repeating units of the spine, and so enable maximum use to be made of cadaveric material. Also, there is a fundamental difficulty associated with experiments on longer spinal segments (see for example, Yamamoto et al 1989) and that is the lack of control over the intermediate 'floating' vertebrae which, in life, are stabilized by numerous muscle attachments. The stabilizing effect of muscle action can be simulated in vitro by embedding the upper and lower surfaces of the motion segment in cups of fixative so that loads can be applied evenly to the surfaces of the vertebrae, and their relative movements carefully controlled.

Nevertheless, motion segment experiments have limitations of their own. The longitudinal ligaments and the supraspinous ligaments span more than one vertebral level and so are weakened in a motion segment. The fixative may prevent the outer vertebral body end-plates from deforming in the same way as the inner end-plates, which are in contact with the intervertebral disc, and this may lead to excessive deformation of the inner end-plates.

Also, of course, there are problems in relating the mechanical properties of dead tissues to those of living spines. Although the water content of intervertebral discs is little affected by death, at least in the rabbit (Galante 1967) there is some slight evidence that death may alter the disc's creep behaviour (in the pig: Keller et al 1990). This latter result should be treated with caution, however, because the authors failed to demonstrate a mechanical

'steady state' before the experimental animals were killed, and so the changes in creep behaviour attributed to death may have been caused by incomplete recovery from the creep test performed before death occurred. Freezing and thawing has little effect on the tensile properties of small samples of disc tissue (Galante 1967) or the compressive properties of whole discs (Smeathers & Joanes 1988). Similarly, prolonged testing in a laboratory does not significantly affect the gross mechanical properties of motion segments (Panjabi et al 1985). Testing at ambient room temperature rather than body temperature slows the rate of disc creep by about 10% (Koeller et al 1986) and affects the elastic properties of ligaments in a way which is consistent with a slight thermal contraction of the tissue (Hasberry & Pearcy 1986). The importance of these changes need not be exaggerated, because they are small compared to the naturally occurring differences found between tissues from different individuals.

MECHANICAL PROPERTIES OF INDIVIDUAL SPINAL STRUCTURES

Annulus fibrosus

The annulus consists of about 15–25 concentric lamellae (Marchand & Ahmed 1990) which contain and prestress the nucleus pulposus (Nachemson 1960). The collagen network of each lamella is orientated at about 30° to the horizontal, and the orientation alternates in successive lamellae as shown in Figure 9.1. Detailed dissections under a binocular microscope have shown that the fibre angle can vary between 20° and 55° over a short distance, so that the fibres take a curved course. Also, the annulus contains many structural irregularities, with lamellae splitting and merging with each other (Marchand & Ahmed 1990).

The primary mechanical function of the annulus is to contain the hydrostatic pressure of the nucleus pulposus, and so it is essentially a tensile structure, designed to withstand high circumferential 'hoop stresses' when the disc is

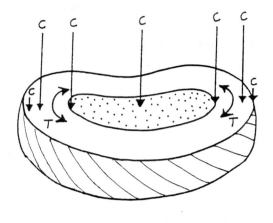

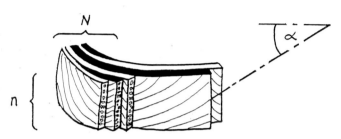

Fig. 9.1 An intervertebral disc. **Upper**: the soft nucleus pulposus (dotted) is surrounded by the concentric lamellae of the annulus fibrosus. Compressive stresses (C) generate a hydrostatic pressure in the nucleus and a tensile 'hoop' stress (T) in the annulus. **Lower**: the number of lamellae (N) varies between 15 and 25, and the number of collagen fibre bundles stacked vertically in a given lamella (n) varies between 20 and 62. The angle α is generally 30° but can vary locally between 0° and 90° (Marchand & Ahmed 1990).

subjected to compressive loading. This is reflected in its tensile properties: small samples of annulus are stiffest and strongest when stretched circumferentially (Galante 1967). Also, the fact that the outer annulus is stiffer and has better elastic recovery than the inner annulus (Galante 1967) is consistent with the 'hoop stress' model because the theory of thick-walled pressure vessels predicts higher circumferential stresses in the outermost part of the wall.

Compressive loading, however, is less important than bending in causing posterior disc prolapse (see Combined Bending and Compression: Disc Prolapse — p. 120). Bending causes the annulus to be stretched vertically (perpendicular to the end-plates) and it is then much less stiff (Galante 1967) but it nevertheless has considerable strength: about 3.7 MN/m² in the outer posterior annulus, and 1.7 MN/m² in the outer anterior annulus (Green & Adams 1992). Vertical tensile failure generally occurs at the annulus–bone junction, but the very outermost fibres, which are the last to fail, pull apart at mid-disc height. Much of the tensile stiffness, and by implication, strength, is attributable to interactions between the collagen fibres and the hydrated proteoglycan gell of the matrix, rather than to the number of intact collagen fibre bundles passing from one vertebra to the next (Adams & Green 1992).

This may be significant because it implies that cells can effect substantial mechanical repair of the annulus by producing proteoglycans, rather than collagen which has a turnover time of many years (Maroudas 1982). Collagen–proteoglycan interactions may also explain the high resistance of the annulus to cyclic ('fatigue') loading: if the applied stress is less than 50% of the ultimate tensile stress, then fatigue failure is unlikely to occur even if 10 000 loading cycles are applied (Green & Adams 1992).

Degenerative changes increase the number of discontinuities in the annulus (Marchand & Ahmed 1990) and reduce its mechanical strength (Galante 1967). This may explain why the anterior annulus is stiffer and stronger than the posterior (Galante 1967).

The compressive properties of small samples of annulus have not been tested in the same way. However, it is known that the annulus as a whole is capable of resisting high compressive forces perpendicular to the end-plates, even when nucleus pulposus material is removed (Markolf & Morris 1974, Brinckmann & Grootenboer 1991). Also, high peaks of *compressive* stress have been demonstrated in the matrix of all regions of the annulus except the most peripheral 2–4 mm (McNally & Adams 1992) so the annulus is obviously more than just a tensile structure. In fact, the annulus is a 'prestressed fibre composite' in which the fibres (collagen) are constantly in tension as they resist the swelling tendency of the hydrophilic matrix (proteoglycan–water gel). External loading of the disc increases both the compressive stresses in the matrix and the tensile forces in the restraining collagen.

Nucleus pulposus

The nucleus is a highly hydrated proteoglycan–water gel which is loosely held together and bound to the hyaline cartilage end-plates by a sparse and random collagen network (Roberts et al 1989). The swelling pressure of the proteoglycans is resisted by tensile stresses in the surrounding annulus, and so the nucleus behaves like a pressurized fluid, and exhibits a considerable hydrostatic pressure even when no external forces are applied to the disc (Nachemson 1960). With normal ageing, the water content of the adult nucleus falls from about 85% to 75% (Adams & Hutton 1983a) and the material appears to coalesce into several discrete fibrous bodies, separated by areas of softer material, which are probably responsible for the typical 'hamburger' shape often seen in discograms (Adams et al 1986). Further degenerative changes cause internal disruption of the lamellar structure of the annulus, but the hydrostatic properties of the nucleus persist even when the discograms are abnormal (Nachemson 1965, McNally & Adams 1992). If released from the confining annulus, nucleus material will absorb water and swell up by 200–300% within a few hours (Dolan et al 1987). This doubtless happens when a disc prolapses and

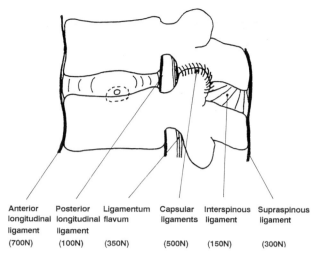

| Anterior longitudinal ligament (700N) | Posterior longitudinal ligament (100N) | Ligamentum flavum (350N) | Capsular ligaments (500N) | Interspinous ligament (150N) | Supraspinous ligament (300N) |

Fig. 9.2 Sagittal view of a lumbar motion segment showing the intervertebral ligaments. Typical values of tensile strength are shown for each ligament; these are based on data from several sources (see text). The centre of rotation for sagittal-plane movements (O) usually lies within the region enclosed by the dotted line. (Posterior on right).

may explain why some patients experience a gradual onset of symptoms.

Intervertebral ligaments

The mechanical properties of individual ligaments have been evaluated by pulling apart their bony vertebral attachments, a technique which avoids damaging the ligaments in the clamps of the testing machine. Typical values of the tensile strengths of the intervertebral ligaments are compared in Figure 9.2. Values of failure stress and strain are not given because there is a lack of accurate data on ligament cross-sectional area and resting length. Approximate values of stress and strain have been reported by Adams et al (1980) and Chazal et al (1985).

The anterior longitudinal ligament has a strength of about 600 N (Myklebust et al 1988) when tested in situ, but only 330 N when stripped from the underlying bone and held in clamps (Tkaczuk 1968). The difficulty in drawing a precise boundary between disc and ligament may account for some of this discrepancy. At low values of strain, the ligament is easily extensible because its collagen network has a wavy or 'crimped' structure which gradually straightens out as the ligament is stretched. The crimps are straight at a strain of about 10% (Hukins et al 1990) and failure occurs at about 50% strain (Chazal et al 1985).

The posterior longitudinal ligament is much weaker than the anterior ligament, with a typical strength of only 53 N (Myklebust et al 1988). Evidently, it does not play a significant mechanical role in protecting the intervertebral disc from flexion injury, but it may serve to deflect any prolapsed disc material away from the spinal cord. The ligament has both capsulated and uncapsulated nerve endings (Hirsch et al 1963, Korkala et al 1985) and its

primary function may be to act as a 'nerve net' to detect abnormal deformation of the underlying disc.

The ligamentum flavum is strong and extremely extensible, being able to recover from strains of up to 80% (Nachemson & Evans 1968). This is attributable to its high elastin content and to a loose alignment of the (uncrimped) collagen network about the long axis of the ligament (Hukins et al 1990). The ligament prestresses the disc in the normal upright posture (Nachemson & Evans 1968) and it may be inferred that its primary mechanical function is to provide a smooth posterior lining to the spinal canal — one that does not become slack, or buckle, in lordotic postures. The ligamentum flavum provides most of the resistance to bending of the motion segment at small angles of flexion, and about 13% of its resistance in full flexion (Adams et al 1980).

The capsular ligaments of the apophyseal joints are short but extremely strong. Their true strength was probably underestimated in the experiments of Cyron & Hutton (1981a) and Myklebust et al (1988) because the vertebrae anchoring the ligaments were pulled apart in the vertical direction. The resulting force–deformation graphs showed two distinct peaks (Cyron & Hutton 1981b), suggesting that the capsular ligaments are grouped into two main bundles of similar strength but different length. The ligaments are probably deployed so that they provide maximum resistance to flexion movements, with the group of shorter fibres located at the anterior margin of the joint where they are closer to the centre of rotation in the discs and therefore are stretched less (Adams 1980). These ligaments provide almost 40% of a motion segment's resistance to forward bending, and in full flexion resist an average tensile force of 591 N (Adams et al 1980). They also resist backwards bending (Yang & King 1984, Adams et al 1988, Hedtmann et al 1989) and may resist lateral flexion also, so their function appears to be to stabilize the spine and protect the disc from excessive bending in any direction.

The interspinous ligament forms a broad membrane between adjacent spinous processes, and the predominant fibre direction is approximately posterior-superior to anterior-inferior (Rissanen 1960, Heylings 1978). During spinal flexion movements of small magnitude, the ligaments provide negligible resistance (Adams et al 1980, Hindle et al 1990) presumably because the fibres are being re-orientated, rather than stretched. However, at larger flexion angles, the tensile force in the ligament can rise to at least 100 N without damage (Hindle et al 1990). If two vertebrae are pulled vertically apart, the interspinous ligament is found to have a tensile strength of about 100 N (Dumas et al 1987, Myklebust et al 1988). For the reason discussed above in connection with the capsular ligaments, this method of testing is likely to under-record the strength of a broad ligament which, in life, would be called upon to resist flexion movements.

The supraspinous ligament is weak or absent in the lower lumbar spine (Rissanen 1960, Hukins et al 1990). Average strength values at the elastic limit are 77 N for the levels L1–3 and 49 N for L3–5 (Dumas et al 1987). It is possible that the high strength values obtained by Myklebust et al (1988) were due to the inclusion of thoracolumbar fascia.

The fibres of the interspinous and supraspinous ligaments are interconnected, so any attempt to separate them by making a cut at their common boundary reduces their combined tensile stiffness by 40% (Dumas et al 1987). This suggests that, mechanically, they should be treated as a single unit. When considered together, the two ligaments have a tensile strength of about 160 N at 39% strain (Adams et al 1980). Because they act on a long lever arm posterior to the centre of rotation in the disc, they provide about 20% of the motion segment's resistance to flexion near the elastic limit, and are the first structures to be damaged in hyperflexion (Adams et al 1980). Ruptures of the interspinous ligament are found in about 20% of adult cadaveric lumbar spines (Rissanen 1960).

Vertebrae

Mechanical tests on cadaveric material have shown that most of the compressive strength of the vertebral body comes from the network of trabeculae, since careful removal of the cortex weakens the structure by between 10% (McBroom et al 1985) and 35–45% (Yoganandan et al 1988). The contribution of the cortex can be as high as 75% in old and osteoporotic specimens (Rockoff et al 1969, Yoganandan et al 1988). It has been suggested that the vertebral body might be hydraulically strengthened at rapid strain rates by the presence of trapped fluid, but this theory is not supported by experiment (Hutton et al 1979).

The mechanics of spondylolysis has been investigated by measuring the resistance of the neural arch to a posteriorly-directed force acting on the inferior articular processes. Strengths between 600 N and 2800 N were recorded, at displacements of up to 1.2 mm (Cyron et al 1976). The large displacement values suggest that spondylolysis, in life, is more likely to occur as a fatigue fracture (Cyron & Hutton 1978).

COMPRESSION

Compression forces acting on the spine in vivo

The lumbar spine is compressed by the weight of the upper body, and by the tensile forces acting in the muscles and fascia of the trunk. In the erect standing posture, superincumbent body weight is about 55% of whole body weight, or about 380 N for an average man. However, in vivo measurements of intradiscal pressure suggest that the overall compressive force on the lumbar spine is about 500 N (Nachemson 1981) so the stabilizing activity of trunk muscles, and of the psoas (Nachemson 1966) must make a relatively small contribution of about 120 N.

During forward bending and lifting activities, the situation is reversed, and the compressive force attributable to tension in the back muscles and fascia greatly exceeds that due to body weight. The reason for this is shown in Figure 9.3. The spine pivots about the centre of the intervertebral discs, and the effective lever arm of the back muscles is 7–8 cm (McGill & Norman 1987a). The lever arm of the weight being lifted can be about 30–45 cm, so in static equilibrium the tensile force in the muscles must be about 5–6 times as great as the weight being lifted. This simple 'moment arm analysis' ignores the antagonistic activity of trunk muscles other than the erector spinae, but the potential errors are not large since the other muscles are relatively small (McGill et al 1988) and show much lower levels of electrical activation during heavy lifting (McGill & Norman 1987b, Potvin et al 1991).

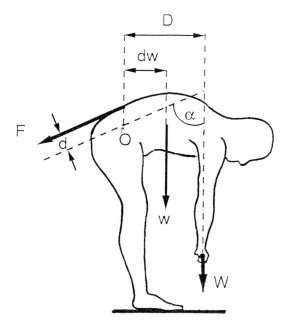

$$F \times d = W \times D + w \times dw - M$$

$$C = F + (W + w) \times \cos \alpha$$

F = tensile force in the back muscles
d = lever arm of back muscles
O = centre of rotation in L5-S1 intervertebral disc
W = weight lifted
D = lever arm of weight lifted
w = weight of upper body
dw = lever arm of weight of upper body
M = bending moment resisted by osteo-ligamentous spine
C = compressive force acting on lumbo-sacral spine
α = inclination of upper body to the vertical

Fig. 9.3 'Moment arm analysis' shows that the compressive force acting on the lumbar spine (C) rises to high levels during heavy lifting.

The possible role of a raised intra-abdominal pressure in reducing spinal compression (Bartelink 1957) is the subject of some debate (McGill & Norman 1987b). However, the combination of a pressurized abdomen and a broad belt can probably reduce the compressive force on the lumbar spine by about 1000 N (McGill et al 1990).

During dynamic lifting movements, the lumbar spine is rapidly extended from an initial position of flexion (Davis et al 1965, Adams & Dolan 1991) and the extra muscle force required to provide the angular acceleration of the upper body can increase the compressive force on the spine by up to 70% during the fastest movements (Dolan & Adams 1993a). Also, the compressive force may be further increased by about 20% as a result of acceleration down the long axis of the spine (McGill & Norman 1985).

The effect of compression on lumbar motion segments

When a motion segment is subjected to pure compression, so that it neither bends nor twists, then most of the compressive force is transmitted through the vertebral bodies and intervertebral discs (Adams & Hutton 1980). However, if the height of the intervertebral disc is reduced by creep loading or simulated disc injury (Dunlop et at 1984) then the apophyseal joints can resist a small fraction of the applied compressive force. If, in addition, the motion segment is wedged in 2 or 4° of extension, in order to simulate a lordotic posture such as erect standing, then the apophyseal joints resist about 16% of the compressive force on average, and up to 70% where pathological disc narrowing is present (Adams & Hutton 1980). Most of this force is transmitted across the articular surfaces, but there is evidence of extra-articular impingement also (Dunlop et al 1984, El-Bohy et al 1989) and a mathematical model has suggested that some compressive force is resisted by the joint ligaments and capsule as they are deformed by the inferior articular processes (Yang & King 1984).

The intervertebral disc resists compression by a special mechanism. The nucleus pulposus acts rather like a pressurized fluid and converts much of the vertical compressive stress into a circumferential ('hoop') tensile stress and a radial compressive stress in the annulus fibrosus (Nachemson 1960). The radial stress causes the annulus to bulge radially outwards, by about 0.2 mm, when the compressive force rises from 300 N to 1000 N, and it bulges a further 0.2 mm when the force rises to 2000 N (Brinckmann & Horst 1985). Deformations of similar magnitude occur in the adjacent vertebrae, where the bony end-plates of the vertebral bodies are forced to bulge into the vertebra by the (virtually) incompressible nucleus pulposus. End-plate deflections can be as great as 0.6 mm when the compressive force reaches 7500 N (Brinckmann et al 1983).

Recent measurements of stresses acting inside intervertebral discs show that the above mechanism is an over-simplification. In young non-degenerated discs, a hydrostatic pressure (where the horizontal and vertical components of stress are equal to each other) can be demonstrated not only in the nucleus, but throughout most of the annulus as well (McNally & Adams 1992: see Fig. 9.4). This confirms earlier measurements (Horst & Brinckmann 1981) which suggested that a young disc behaves like a 'bag of fluid' and so can be modelled as a thin-walled pressure vessel (Brinckmann & Grootenboer 1991). After the age of about 40 years, the hydrostatic behaviour is usually confined to the nucleus, and peaks of (anisotropic) stress are more commonly observed,

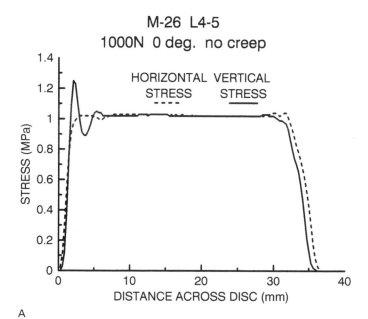

A

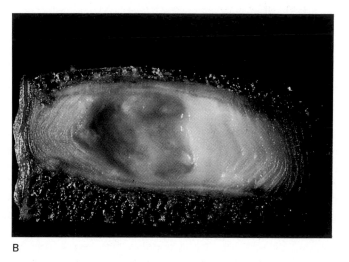

B

Fig. 9.4 A. The distribution of compressive stress acting across the sagittal midline of a young intervertebral disc. Posterior on left. Areas in which the vertical and horizontal stresses are the same can be assumed to be acting like a fluid. This 26-year-old male specimen was subjected to a pure compressive force of 1000 N when the stress distribution was measured. **B.** Sagittal section of a disc of similar age.

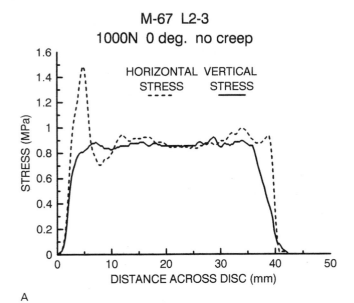

A

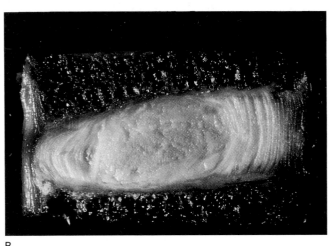

B

Fig. 9.5 A. The distribution of compressive stress acting across the sagittal midline of an elderly intervertebral disc. Note the anisotropic stress peak in the posterior annulus. **B.** Sagittal section of a disc of similar age.

particularly in the posterior annulus (Fig. 9.5). In the outermost 2–4 mm of annulus, little if any compressive stress can be recorded in any disc (McNally & Adams 1992) suggesting that this highly fibrous region has insufficient matrix to couple the tensile stress in the collagen fibres with the pressure-sensitive membrane of the pressure transducer. (The absence of high compressive stresses in the matrix of the peripheral annulus may explain why nerve endings appear to be confined to this region of the disc: Yoshizawa et al 1980, Bogduk & Twomey 1991).

The distribution of stress inside a disc varies considerably with the angle of flexion or extension (see Backwards Bending (Extension) — p. 117, and Forward Bending (Flexion) — p. 118) and stress peaks in the annulus are much greater after a period of creep loading (see Time-dependent Effects — p. 122). This latter result highlights

the importance of nuclear volume in disc mechanics. If this volume is reduced following rupture of the vertebral end-plates or discectomy, then the disc behaves like a flat tyre: it loses height and bulges radially, and the pressure within it falls by as much as 30% (Brinckmann & Horst 1985, Brinckmann & Grootenboer 1991). Also, high peaks of compressive stress can appear in the posterior annulus following end-plate fracture or disc prolapse (Adams et al, unpublished data 1992). These stress peaks imply radial forces acting to pull the lamellae in different directions and they may explain why the inner lamellae tend to bulge internally into the nuclear space after denucleation (Seroussi et al 1989). Conversely, if the volume of the nucleus is increased by injecting fluid into it, then radial bulging decreases (Brinckmann & Horst 1985) disc height increases (Brinckmann & Horst 1985) and nuclear pressure increases (Andersson & Schultz 1979).

Pure compression causes the thin vertebral body end-plates to bulge as much as, or even more than, the annulus (see above) so it is not surprising that compressive overload damages the end-plates rather than the disc. It makes no difference if the loading is applied rapidly or slowly (Perey 1957) or if thousands of loading cycles are applied (Liu et al 1983, Brinckmann et al 1988) or even if the inner posterior annulus is artificially weakened prior to loading (Brinckmann 1986). The hypothesis that compression causes primary disc damage has been thoroughly disproved. Vertebral endplate fracture may itself be a clinical problem, and its effect on disc mechanics (see above) may lead to degenerative changes in the long term. However, more direct links between mechanical overload, disc prolapse, and back and leg pain will be considered later under the heading Combined Bending and Compression: Disc Prolapse — p. 120.

Compressive strength of lumbar motion segments

The compressive strength of lumbar motion segments varies between about 2 kN and 14 kN depending on the size, age, sex and physical strength of the individual from which they were taken, and also on the level in the lumbar spine (Perey 1957, Eie 1966, Hansson et al 1980, Hutton & Adams 1982, Brinckmann et al 1989). The average compressive strength of motion segments from young men of average body mass, tested in slight flexion, is 10 kN (Hutton & Adams 1982). It now appears that the flexion angle has little effect on compressive strength (Granhed et al 1989, Adams et al 1992). In living people, vertebral strength can be predicted to an accuracy of about 1 kN from measurements of quantitative computed tomography (Brinckmann et al 1989) or bone mineral content (Hansson et al 1980). Competitive weight lifters have extremely dense vertebrae, and their spines may be much stronger than any tested so far in vitro (Granhed et al 1987).

Repetitive (fatigue) loading causes motion segments to fail at lower loads than single loading cycles, and the compressive strength falls off rapidly as the number of loading cycles increases (Brinckmann et al 1988, Hansson et al 1987). For example, if 10 000 N were required to crush a motion segment in a single loading cycle, then failure would be expected after about 10 cycles at 7000 N or 5000 cycles at 5000 N. Fatigue damage is unlikely to accumulate unless the compressive force rises above 30% of the ultimate compressive strength.

Can the lumbar spine be crushed in heavy lifting?

It has been suggested that the lumbar spine is in danger of being crushed during heavy lifting, and various relieving mechanisms have been proposed to prevent this from happening (Bartelink 1957, Gracovetsky & Farfan 1986, Aspden 1989). However, a sober appraisal of spinal loading, based on the detailed anatomical studies of Bogduk, suggests that compressive forces do not rise to damaging levels (McGill & Norman 1987a, Potvin et al 1991). Of course, champion weightlifters generate enormous compressive forces on their spines, but there is no reason to suppose that their spines are not well adapted to resist them (see above). In some cases, the 'adaptation' may take drastic forms, since there is a strong link between heavy manual work and vertebral osteophytosis (Videman et al 1990).

An interesting qualification to the general rule of 'horses for courses' is suggested by a small-scale cadaveric study (Porter et at 1989). This showed that the compressive strength of motion segments increased with the level of physical activity of the person before death. However, there was also evidence that the strengthening was more pronounced in the vertebrae than in the discs, so that the discs of active people were more vulnerable to prolapse under high loads, in the manner described later under the heading Combined Bending and Compression: Disc Prolapse — p. 120. This suggests that the very low metabolic rate of intervertebral discs (Maroudas 1982, Bayliss et al 1988) may prevent them from adapting to increased mechanical demands as quickly as the adjacent vertebrae. The discs, then, would be particularly vulnerable to injury several weeks or months after a move to a physically demanding occupation: at this time they would still be attempting to 'catch up' with the increasing strength of the spinal muscles and bones. This may explain why young manual workers are prone to develop symptomatic disc prolapse early in their working lives (Varma 1987).

SHEAR

Shear forces acting on the lumbar spine in vivo

The upper surfaces of the sacrum and the L5 vertebral body are inclined at a considerable angle to the horizontal, and so the lower lumbar vertebrae experience a gravitational shear force acting to move each vertebra forwards over the one below. During forward bending movements, all of the lumbar vertebrae are subject to forward shear. Walking with a back-pack can generate shear forces of about 570 N on the lower lumbar spine (Hutton et al 1977). However, the lumbar musculature has many muscle slips which arise from the transverse and spinous processes and pass posteriorly and inferiorly to insert on the sacrum and ilium (Bogduk & Twomey 1991). These muscles are capable of resisting the intervertebral shear force (Potvin et al 1991) but it is not certain whether or not they do this in practice.

The effect of shear on lumbar motion segments

If a motion segment is loaded in combined compression and shear (in life, the two would rarely be separated) then the neural arch resists about 70% of the shear component, while the disc resists the rest (recalculated from data of Cyron et al 1979). However, if the apophyseal joints are removed, the disc 'creeps' forward in response to repetitive shear forces (Cyron & Hutton 1981b). This suggests that in an intact motion segment, sustained loading will soon cause most or all of the intervertebral shear force to be resisted by the apophyseal joints (or muscles). Although small, the joint surfaces are orientated to resist horizontal forces, and the strength of the neural arch in resisting shear is considerable: when loaded in a direction perpendicular to the pars interarticularis, the inferior articular processes can resist shearing forces of between 600 N and 2800 N before failure occurs in the pars or in the pedicles (Cyron et al 1976).

If the apophyseal joints are orientated assymetrically in the horizontal plane, then cyclic loading in shear and compression causes the upper vertebra to rotate in the horizontal plane towards the side of the apophyseal joint with the more oblique (frontal plane) orientation (Cyron & Hutton 1980).

TORSION

Torque acting on the lumbar spine in vivo

Torsion causes rotation of the spine about its long axis, and it occurs in activities such as discus throwing. Torsion is effected primarily by the muscles of the abdominal wall which act on long levers (the ribs) and which compress the spine as well as twist it. Back muscles such as multifidus, longissimus and iliocostalis attach to much shorter levers (the spinous and transverse processes) and so are poorly placed to twist the spine. Gravity has very little effect on the torque acting on the spine, whereas it can apply high bending stresses to it (see Forward Bending (Flexion) — p. 118). However, a force applied to an outstretched arm may subject the lumbar spine to an impulsive torque.

Centre of axial rotation

The centre of axial rotation is poorly defined and probably moves during a twisting movement. If a lumbar motion segment is subjected to a pure torque, the centre of rotation generally lies in the posterior annulus fibrosus (Cossette et al 1971). This location gives the motion segment its minimum torsional stiffness for torques up to about 20 Nm (Adams & Hutton 1981) and so may be assumed to be the centre of rotation in vivo also. The orientation of the lumbar apophyseal joints might be taken to imply that the centre of rotation lies near the spinous processes (Fig. 9.6) but this pre-supposes that these joints are designed to facilitate axial movement, whereas the experimental evidence indicates that they act to limit it and increase the stability of the vertebral column. At high values of torque, there is bony contact between the apophyseal joint surfaces on the side towards which the spine is being twisted (see below) and it is likely that the centre of rotation then moves close to this joint.

The effect of torsion on lumbar motion segments

When lumbar motion segments are subjected to a combination of compression and torsion, axial rotation is severely limited by the apophyseal joints. In non-

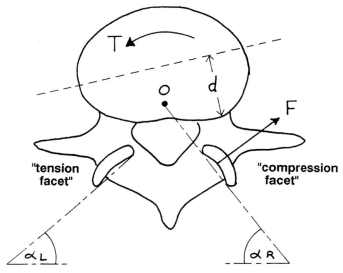

Fig. 9.6 View of a lumbar motion segment in the transverse plane (anterior on top). The centre for axial rotation (O) lies in the posterior annulus, so the 'compression facet' is ideally orientated to resist the applied torque (T). Note that the apophyseal joints are often asymmetrical ($\alpha_L \neq \alpha_R$). This may encourage bending of the motion segment about a slightly oblique axis, and cause the maximum bending stresses to act at the posterolateral corner of the disc which lies furthest (distance d) from the oblique axis.

degenerated spines, only 1 to 2° of movement to each side is permitted before inelastic deformation (damage) occurs in the 'compression' joint (Adams & Hutton 1981). A similar range of lumbar movement has been measured on living people (Gregersen & Lucas 1967, Lumsden & Morris 1968, Pearcy & Tibrewal 1984a). Old motion segments, and those with degenerated discs, can rotate by as much as 8°, presumably because of the extra 'play' caused by the loss of articular cartilage from the articular surfaces (Adams & Hutton 1981). The elastic limit is usually reached with a torque of about 12–30 Nm, most of which is resisted by the compression joint and the disc. The force acting on this joint is then about 250–500 N (Adams & Hutton 1981). Bony resistance to axial rotation explains why motion segments are stiffer in torsion than in bending: typically, a bending moment of 10.6 Nm causes about 5.5° of flexion and 3.0° of extension, but a torque of 10.6 Nm causes only 1.5° of axial rotation (Schultz et al 1979). Bony resistance also explains why the increase in intradiscal pressure caused by torsion is less than 15% of that caused by forward or lateral bending of the motion segment (Schultz et al 1979).

If the apophyseal joints are removed, then the disc can be twisted by about 9° before the first sign of damage (Adams & Hutton 1983b). Axial rotation is resisted by only half of the collagen fibres in the annulus, because every second lamella has a fibre orientation which could offer only token resistance (compare Figs 9.1 and 9.6). This may explain the circumferential disruption and separation of individual lamellae, with tearing of their vertebral attachments, when ultimate failure occurs at angles between 11 and 32° (Farfan et al 1970). Torsional failure does not resemble disc prolapse, which is essentially a radial lesion, and discograms taken after torsional failure show no leaking of contrast medium through the annulus (Farfan et al 1970). Also, the posterior/posterolateral location of most prolapses does not suggest an aetiology based on torsion, because these are the parts of the disc closest to the centre of axial rotation, and therefore subject to the smallest torsional stresses. Fatigue loading in axial rotation likewise causes damage to the apophyseal joints rather than to the disc (Liu et al 1985).

It has been hypothesized that lumbar flexion might increase the range of axial rotation by allowing more 'free play' in the tapered tips of the inferior facets. However, experiments on cadaveric spines and on living people both suggest that forward bending movements actually *decrease* the range of axial movement (Gunzburg et al 1991) because they increase the forward shear force on the lumbar vertebrae and close up any gap appearing between the articular surfaces.

The obliquity of the apophyseal joints in the horizontal plane has little effect on the range of axial rotation (Ahmed et al 1990, Gunzburg et al 1991) even when coupled movements are taken into consideration (Duncan &

Ahmed 1991) so it is unlikely that asymmetrical apophyseal joints could lead to torsional damage to the discs. The association between facet tropism and the side of disc prolapse (Farfan & Sullivan 1967, Noren et al 1991) may be due to the asymmetrical neural arch allowing asymmetrical bending of that motion segment. A combination of lateral and forward bending can lead to postero-lateral disc prolapse, as described later under the heading Combined Bending and Compression: Disc Prolapse — p. 120.

BACKWARDS BENDING (EXTENSION)

Backwards bending of the lumbar spine in vivo

The curvature, or lordosis, of an excised cadaveric lumbar spine is about 41° on average (Farfan et al 1972) whereas the curvature in living people standing erect is about 54–60° (Andersson et al 1979, Frymoyer et al 1984). It follows that considerable backwards bending movements occur whenever a person stands up after sitting down, and

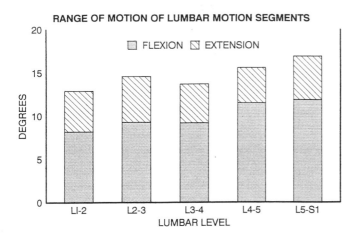

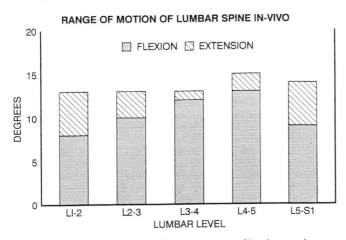

Fig. 9.7 The range of sagittal-plane movement of lumbar motion segments (**top**) is compared with that of living people (**bottom**). The in vivo measurements are relative to erect standing, so the lower figure indicates that standing entails considerable extension of the spine between L2 and L5. The range of flexion at L5–S1 appears to be reduced in vivo, possibly by the iliolumbar ligament.

that little additional backwards bending is possible before the limit of movement is approached (Pearcy et al 1984: see Fig. 9.7). Activities that are likely to increase the standing lordosis are those which involve lifting objects above head height, when it becomes mechanically advantageous to lean backwards in order to 'get under the weight' and keep it close to the axis of the body.

The effect of backwards bending on lumbar motion segments

Motion segments are stiffer in backwards bending than in forwards or lateral bending (Schultz et al 1979) suggesting that there is some bony resistance to movement. Contact stresses on the apophyseal joint surfaces increase rapidly with angle of extension, and tend to become concentrated in the lower margins of the articular surfaces (Dunlop et al 1984, Shirazi-Adl 1991). Extension causes the posterior annulus to bulge outwards and the mid-sagittal diameter of the spinal canal is reduced by about 2 mm (Schonstrom et al 1989). The stress distribution inside the disc is greatly affected by extension. Just 2° of movement is usually sufficient to create high peaks of compressive stress in the posterior annulus (Adams et al 1992, McNally & Adams 1992). Stresses elsewhere in the disc are considerably reduced because, at this angle, the apophyseal joints resist about 16% of the applied compressive force (Adams & Hutton 1980). Exceptionally, extension can actually *reduce* the stresses acting on the posterior annulus, while increasing them on both the anterior annulus and apophyseal joints (Adams, unpublished data 1992). This curious example of 'stress-shielding' has been noted on several motion segments to date and it may possibly explain the success of extension exercises in relieving central back pain in some people (Donelson et al 1991).

The limit of extension movement is marked by inelastic, non-recoverable deformation of the motion segment at some angle between 3 and 8° (mean 5°) and an average bending moment of about 28 Nm (Adams et al 1988). Beyond the elastic limit, damage usually occurs first in the spinous processes or in the interspinous ligament nipped between them. If the spinous processes are particularly widely spaced, then the facet joints can be damaged first in hyperextension. The intervertebral disc resists about 30–40% of the applied bending moment in full extension, but shows no apparent sign of being damaged before the neural arch (Adams et al 1988).

If a motion segment is wedged in hyperextension and then compressed rapidly to failure, the outcome can, in rare cases, be an anterior prolapse of the intervertebral disc (Adams et al 1988). The mechanism is doubtless similar to that described in detail for posterior prolapse (see Combined Bending and Compression: Disc Prolapse — p. 120) and the fact that anterior prolapse is much more difficult to achieve is probably due to the greater strength and thickness of the anterior annulus compared to the posterior annulus.

If the neural arch is removed and the remaining vertebral body–disc–vertebral body unit subjected to fatigue loading in backward bending and compression, then the stress peaks in the posterior annulus cause the outer lamellae to bulge posteriorly, and this deformation persists after cessation of loading (Adams et al 1988). In life, the deformation may be reversed by the diurnal exchange of fluid, but it is conceivable that if the loading were severe enough, the damage might not be reversed, but accumulate until a gross posterior protrusion of the disc occurred. This mechanism could explain the hairpin bending and posterior ruptures which occur in the discs of rats' tails when they were fixed in permanent hyperextension (Lindblom 1952). If a complete rupture exists in the posterior annulus, then repeated extension movements can force injected contrast medium down the fissure and into the spinal canal (Gill et al 1987).

LATERAL BENDING

Lateral bending of the lumbar spine in vivo

The full range of lateral bending, from side to side, is about 10° per lumbar level in the upper lumbar spine, but this falls to 3° at L5–S1 (Pearcy & Tibrewal 1984a) where the iliolumbar ligaments restrict movement (Leong et al 1987, Yamamoto et al 1990). There is a slight tendency for coupling to occur between lateral bending and axial rotation, but the effect is slight and inconsistent, and is probably under muscular control in living people (Pearcy & Tibrewal 1984a). Much of the coupling observed in cadaveric specimens may be attributable to the method of loading, and in particular, to the lack of substantial compressive and shear pre-loads. Pure lateral bending is probably a rare phenomenon in life (aerobics classes excepted) but it is frequently combined with forward bending in awkward asymmetrical lifting tasks, and during digging and shovelling. These activities also involve torsion, but the torsional component must be small, for the reasons discussed under Torsion — p. 115.

The effect of lateral bending on lumbar motion segments

This has not been studied in detail. A bending moment of 10.6 Nm causes about 4.4° of lateral bending, with nearly all of the resistance coming from the disc (Schultz et al 1979). The rise in nuclear pressure associated with this much lateral bending is greater than that observed when the same bending moment is applied to produce forward flexion (Schultz et al 1979). Lateral bending is probably limited by the apophyseal joints and the intertransverse ligaments.

FORWARD BENDING (FLEXION)

Forward bending of the lumbar spine in vivo

The lumbar spine exhibits its greatest range of angular movement in forward bending. When a healthy person bends forwards to touch his toes from the upright standing position, each lumbar motion segment is flexed between about 8°, at L1–2, and 11° at L4–5 and L5–S1 (Adams & Hutton 1982, Pearcy et al 1984). Typical values are shown in Figure 9.7. Not surprisingly, smaller movements are observed in people with back pain (Pearcy et al 1985). Movement at the lumbosacral junction is less, on average, than that at L4–5 and shows greater interindividual variability (Fig. 9.7). In vitro motion segment studies (see below) show that an L5–S1 motion segment is just as mobile as L4–L5, so it is possible that structures such as the iliolumbar ligament prevent some people from fully flexing this joint when trying to touch their toes (Leong et al 1987, Yamamoto et al 1990).

Forward bending of the lumbar spine is a common movement. Sitting unsupported on an upright chair requires about 20–30° of lumbar flexion (Andersson et al 1979, Dolan et al 1988). Sitting on the floor requires about 35° (Dolan et al 1988) while activities such as picking objects up off the floor or putting on a sock tend to flex the lumbar spine right up to its physiological 'toe-touching' limit (Adams & Dolan 1991). Even weightlifters can flex their lumbar spine close to this limit when lifting heavy weights (Cholewicki & McGill 1992). Flexion is initiated by the abdominal muscles, but is usually continued by the gravitational moment of the upper body, acting under the varying restraint of the back muscles. As full flexion is approached, the electromyographic activity of the back muscles falls to very low levels and the upper body then 'rests' on the passively stretched muscles, ligament and fascia of the lower back (Floyd & Silver 1951, Schultz et al 1985).

Centre of rotation

In healthy subjects bending forwards, the centre of rotation of the lumbar motion segments lies in the middle of the intervertebral disc, close to the endplate of the inferior vertebra (Pearcy & Bogduk 1988). It moves slightly during a full flexion movement indicating that flexion involves a component of forward translatory movement as well as rotation. Degenerative changes in a motion segment can result in the instantaneous centre of rotation taking a long and tortuous path during a full flexion movement (Gertzbien et al 1985) but much of this may be attributable to experimental error and to the precise compressive and shear forces acting on the motion segment.

The effect of forward bending on lumbar motion segments

Cadaveric motion segments have been subjected to a physiological combination of bending, shear and compression in order to simulate someone bending down to touch their toes (Adams et al 1980). The motion segment offers little resistance to bending for the first few degrees (the 'neutral zone': Panjabi et al 1982) but the resistance rises rapidly to about 50–60 Nm as the elastic limit is approached (Adams et al 1980, Adams & Dolan 1991). This limit is marked by a decrease in bending stiffness and an increase in hysteresis energy, and it probably represents the threshold of injury to the motion segment (Yoganandan et al 1989). It has been reported that no overt damage occurs at bending moments of 70 Nm and less (Miller et al 1986) but the instrumentation used in this experiment may have lacked the sensitivity to detect the first signs of damage at the elastic limit. Beyond this limit, the motion segment still has reserves of strength, and complete disruption requires a flexion angle of about 20° and a bending moment of 150 Nm (Osvalder et al 1990).

The mobility of cadaveric motion segments varies with lumbar level and age in much the same way as in living people (Fig. 9.7) suggesting that, in life, the range of lumbar flexion is determined largely by the mobility of the osteoligamentous spine, rather than by the extensibility of the back muscles. However, the two are doubtless related, and at the elastic limit, the osteoligamentous lumbar spine resists only half of the forward bending moment of the upper body, or about 50 Nm (Adams et al 1980).

Although the mobility and strength in bending of motion segments vary considerably, the shape of the bending moment–flexion angle curve is remarkably consistent. This becomes evident when values of flexion are expressed as a percentage (F) of the full range of flexion for that specimen and, likewise, bending moment is expressed as a percentage (B) of the bending moment required to bend that specimen to the elastic limit. The two normalization procedures reduce the variability arising from differences in specimen mobility and strength, respectively, and make it possible to express the forward bending properties of motion segments in a single equation relating F and B (Adams & Dolan 1991). The significance of this finding is that it enables bending stresses acting on the lumbar spine in life to be quantified from measurements of lumbar flexion. The procedure is valid only if the bending properties of the cadaveric spines are assessed under physiologically-relevant loading conditions, since the bending properties are dependent on the prevailing compressive force. Increasing the compressive preload from 400 N to 1300 N increases a motion segment's resistance to flexion by about 30% (Adams & Dolan 1991) and further small increases occur when the compressive force rises to 2200 N and 4400 N (Janevic et al 1991).

In full flexion, the bending moment applied to a motion segment is resisted by the capsular ligaments of the apophyseal joints (39% on average) the intervertebral disc (29%) the interspinous and supraspinous ligaments (19%) and the ligamentum flavum (13%) (Adams et al 1980). The interspinous and supraspinous ligaments simply re-align at low angles of flexion, but are the first structures to be damaged when the elastic limit is exceeded. Further hyperflexion can then damage the capsular ligaments and finally the disc–vertebral body junction fails (Adams & Hutton 1982). The articular surfaces of the apophyseal joints probably play a minor role, if any, in resisting flexion (Adams et al 1980). (However, they will appear to offer substantial resistance if the loading regime consists primarily of forward shear rather than bending: Twomey & Taylor 1983).

Intradiscal pressure increases by up to 80% in full flexion (Table 9.1) and this is mostly due to increased tension in the posterior ligaments. This increase becomes less pronounced as the compressive force rises, and is insignificant when the compressive force reaches 2000 N (Adams et al 1992). Flexion increases the radial bulging of the anterior annulus (Lin et al 1978) and, in a minority of discs, generates high vertical compressive stresses in the anterior annulus (McNally & Adams 1992, Adams et al 1992). In most discs, however, flexion removes peaks of compressive stress from the posterior annulus and equalizes stress right across the disc (Fig. 9.8).

If the neural arch is removed, then flexion (and extension) have very little effect on the stresses in the nucleus pulposus, at any load (Table 9.1).

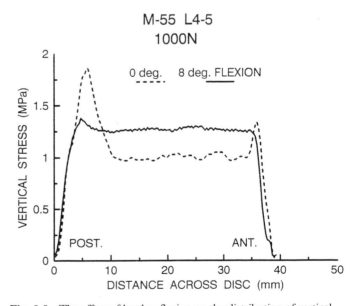

Fig. 9.8 The effect of lumbar flexion on the distribution of vertical compressive stress in a mature intervertebral disc. Flexion removes the stress peak in the posterior annulus and increases, slightly, the pressure in the nucleus pulposus.

Table 9.1   The effect of flexion and extension on the pressure in the nucleus pulposus (IDP). Changes in pressure are expressed as a percentage increase (+) or decrease (–) of the pressure recorded in the neutral position (0°) for the same compressive force. Values are the mean for observations on five motion segments (occasionally, $n = 3$ or 4). Numbers in brackets are the standard error of the mean.

Compressive force (N)	Increase (+) or decrease (–) in IDP (%)					
	4° Extension	2° Extension	0°	50% Flexion	75% Flexion	100% Flexion
Intact motion segment						
500	–35 (8)	–4 (4)	0	+10 (1)	+50 (11)	+130 (42)
1000	–35 (25)	–1 (3)	0	+4 (1)	+25 (8)	+88 (25)
3000	–19 (13)	–2 (2)	0	+1 (1)	+7 (3)	+30 (6)
Disc–vertebral body unit						
500	+7 (13)	+4 (1)	0	+3 (3)	+15 (8)	+44 (20)
1000	+1 (8)	+5 (1)	0	0 (3)	+7 (6)	+13 (22)
3000	–1 (6)	+2 (1)	0	–1 (2)	+2 (4)	+3 (9)

The position of the centre of sagittal rotation implies that the posterior annulus must be stretched by about 50% in the vertical direction, and this has been confirmed by X-ray studies on living people (Adams & Hutton 1982, Pearcy & Tibrewal 1984b). Collagen fibres cannot stretch as much as this without rupturing, so the 50% deformation must involve some re-orientation of the fibres within each lamella (Rolander 1966, Klein & Hukins 1982). Also, the fibres of the posterior annulus gain some 'slack' from the reduction in radial bulging that accompanies flexion. During a movement of short duration, the fluid content and volume of the posterior annulus remain constant, and so the vertical stretching must be accompanied by thinning in the horizontal direction. This has been confirmed experimentally using a radioactive tracer technique (Adams & Hutton 1986b). It may also be inferred from the movement of metal beads implanted in the disc (Seroussi et al 1989).

The forward bending properties of lumbar motion segments vary with the fluid content of the intervertebral discs, and therefore show a marked diurnal variation in life (Time-dependent Effects — p. 122).

COMBINED BENDING AND COMPRESSION: DISC PROLAPSE

The previous section has shown that forward bending increases the hydrostatic pressure in the nucleus pulposus and stretches and thins the posterior annulus fibrosus. Nuclear pressure can be raised further by increasing the overall compressive force applied to the motion segment. Not surprisingly, therefore, a combination of bending and compression has the potential to rupture the intervertebral disc, as shown in Figure 9.9, and this mechanism of disc prolapse has been confirmed in cadaver experiments. Two distinct types of lesion were produced, depending on whether the bending and compression were applied in a single severe loading cycle, or in thousands of less severe cycles (fatigue loading).

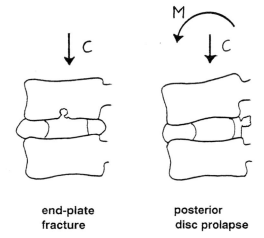

end-plate fracture   posterior disc prolapse

Fig. 9.9   (**Left**) When a motion segment is loaded in pure compression (C), the pressure in the nucleus pulposus rises and fractures the vertebral end-plate. (**Right**) A combination of compression (C) and bending (M) raises the pressure in the nucleus, and also stretches and thins the posterior annulus fibrosus. This can become the 'weak link' of the motion segment, and the outcome is then a posterior prolapse of the disc.

Prolapse as a hyperflexion injury (Adams & Hutton 1982)

The laminae were removed from lumbar motion segments so that the posterior annulus could be clearly seen. The specimens were then flexed about a slightly oblique axis in order to severely stretch one of the posterolateral corners of the disc; while so positioned, the specimens were compressed rapidly to failure.

Of sixty-one motion segments tested, twenty-six failed by posterior disc prolapse, and in eighteen of these, a fragment of nucleus pulposus burst through the posterior annulus to lie outside the disc. The other specimens sustained fractures of the vertebral body. The average compressive force required to cause prolapse was 5488 N (range 2760 N to 12 968 N). The bending moment was not recorded, but the average flexion angle was 15.8° (range 9 to 21°). The flexion angles given in the original

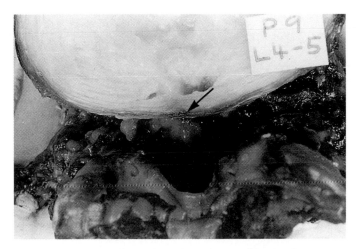

Fig. 9.10 Posterior disc prolapse (arrow) created in vitro by a simulated hyperflexion injury. Note that there is no gross distortion of the posterior lamellae in the vicinity of the prolapse, indicating that the 'door has closed' behind the expelled fragment of nucleus pulposus.

paper (Adams & Hutton 1982) were all 3° too low because of a zero error in the scale used to measure flexion. Prolapse occurred most readily in slightly degenerated L4–L5 and L5–S1 discs from cadavers aged between 40 and 50 years; in fact, all of the discs meeting all of these criteria prolapsed. However, even young discs showing no apparent degenerative changes could prolapse.

In subsequent experiments (including: Dolan et al 1987, Porter et al 1989) this type of prolapse has been produced as a matter of routine, and without removing the neural arch (Fig. 9.10). In all cases though, the interspinous and supraspinous ligaments were stretched beyond their elastic limit.

Some details of these experimental 'prolapses' may be of clinical interest. Prolapse occurred in an instant, sometimes with an audible 'pop', and in one case the displaced nuclear material was projected through the air for a distance of about 50 cm! The displaced material emerged either on the posterolateral margin of the disc opposite to the side of lateral bending, or behind the posterior longitudinal ligament. In the latter case, it might burst through the ligament, or remain covered by it, giving the impression of an incomplete disc protrusion. The material could sometimes be sucked back into the disc by bending the specimen forwards and pulling the vertebrae apart, but it always returned to its original position after the 'manipulation' had ceased. No further nuclear material was extruded if the loading cycle was repeated. (Recent experiments have shown that this is because prolapse reduces the pressure in the nucleus pulposus and generates high stress peaks in the posterior annulus: Adams & McNally, unpublished results 1992). Subsequent sectioning of the disc revealed no gross distortion of the annulus; indeed the exit path of the nuclear material was usually difficult to locate. If fluid was injected into the disc after it had prolapsed, it flowed down the fissure to reach the displaced material (Dolan et al 1987).

Prolapse as a fatigue injury (Adams & Hutton 1985a)

Motion segments were wedged in forward and lateral flexion, as described above, but this time the elastic limit of the posterior ligaments was not exceeded. The specimens were then subjected to 40 compressive loading cycles per minute for up to 6 hours, with a peak compressive force of about 1000 N–3000 N. The fatigue loading decreased disc height and increased the range of flexion (see Time-dependent-Effects — p. 122) so in order to maintain a high bending moment, the flexion angle was increased by 1–3° during the testing period, without damage to the ligaments. Of 29 specimens tested in this manner, six developed a radial fissure in the posterolateral corner of the disc opposite the side of lateral bending, and there was a gradual 'leaking' of soft nuclear material into the intervertebral foramen. Discograms were taken before the loading period in order to demonstrate that the fissures were not present before testing.

The six discs which prolapsed were from the L4–L5 and L5–S1 levels of cadavers aged between 15 and 44 years, and none showed any marked degenerative changes other than the large posterolateral radial fissure created during the test. Many other fatigue-loaded discs showed distortions and disruptions of the lamellae. Often, these were suggestive of incomplete radial fissures whose posterior growth had been checked by the outermost one or two lamellae.

The radial fissures created in these experiments resemble those found in random cadaveric material (Hirsch & Schajowicz 1953) but they are not the same as the discrete peripheral tears or 'rim lesions' described by Osti et al (1990). Radial fissures grow from the inside out, and usually affect the posterior and posterolateral annulus (Lindblom 1952) whereas peripheral tears spread from the outside in, and affect the anterior annulus only.

Radial fissures appear to have been created in discs subjected to cyclic loading in combined bending, compression and torsion (Gordon et al 1991). It is not yet clear just what effect, if any, the torsion had on the outcome.

Prolapse in vivo

The two types of prolapse are compared in Figure 9.11. Their relevance to living people has been considered previously (Adams & Hutton 1988). Briefly, there appears to be no valid reason why living discs should not prolapse if loaded as severely as the cadaveric ones in the hyperflexion experiment, and this could easily happen during some traumatic incident. However, disc prolapse is not usually preceded by trauma, and it is pertinent to compare the severity of loading in the fatigue experiment with normal 'wear and tear' loading in life. The compressive forces used (about 1000 N–2000 N in most cases) could easily occur in life, but the flexion angles and

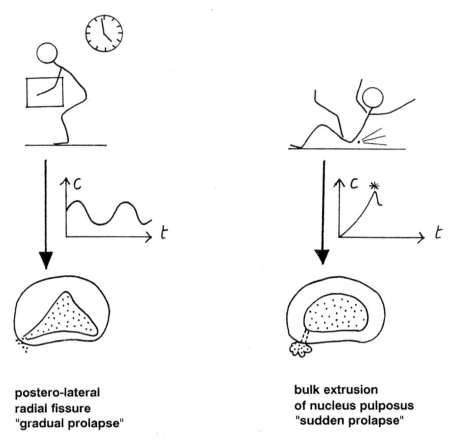

**postero-lateral
radial fissure
"gradual prolapse"**

**bulk extrusion
of nucleus pulposus
"sudden prolapse"**

Fig. 9.11   A comparison of the two types of disc prolapse simulated in vitro. Repetitive 'fatigue' loading can create posterolateral radial fissures and gradual 'leaking' of nuclear material (**left**) whereas a hyperflexion injury can cause sudden bulk extrusion of a fragment of nucleus (**right**).

relentless nature of the loading may not. Recently, it has become possible to measure lumbar flexion continuously during bending and lifting activities and it has been shown that the normal limit of flexion (as defined by the toe-touching posture) is frequently approached or exceeded, even when the knees are bent (Adams & Dolan 1991, Potvin et al 1991, Cholewicki & McGill 1992). However, the back muscles ensure that this physiological limit is about 10° short of the 'elastic limit' referred to in the cadaver experiments (Adams & Hutton 1986a). It remains to be seen just when this margin of safety is reduced or eliminated. Preliminary work in our own laboratory suggests that it is much reduced in the early morning (Time-dependent Effects) and when the back muscles become fatigued.

Despite these difficulties, it is reasonable to accept the mechanical aetiology of disc prolapse, as described above, at least until some other aetiology can be demonstrated. A finite element model has been developed to explain the precise mechanisms involved (Shirazi-Adl 1989) and epidemiological surveys confirm a strong association between acute disc prolapse and the forward bending and lifting activities simulated in the cadaver experiments (Kelsey et al 1984).

The fact that prolapsed disc material removed at sur-

gery appears to be different from normal tissue (Hendry 1958, for example) does not mean that the changes occurred *before* prolapse, since the evidence from animal experiments shows quite clearly that gross changes will appear very quickly *after* prolapse (Lipson & Muir 1981, Osti et al 1990). Even if surgery is performed within hours of prolapse occurring, this is long enough for most of the proteoglycans to leach out of the displaced nuclear material (Dolan et al 1987).

TIME-DEPENDENT EFFECTS

Effect of loading rate on motion segment mechanics

The mechanical properties of intervertebral discs and ligaments depend on the rate of loading. During rapid loading cycles, the fluid trapped in the tissue has no time to move anywhere, and the material is relatively resistant to deformation. It behaves like an elastic solid, and springs back to position as soon as the load is removed. Slow loading cycles, however, gradually squeeze fluid out of the regions of highest stress, and the material's resistance to deformation decreases. When the load is removed, the material is slow to regain its former shape, and its behaviour is termed 'visco-elastic'.

The compressive stiffness of a motion segment increases by about 30% when the loading frequency is increased by a factor of 1000, from 0.01 Hz to 10 Hz (Smeathers & Joanes 1988). Energy dissipation (hysteresis) decreases by 60%. The compressive strength of lumbar vertebrae increases by up to 30% when they are crushed rapidly, and this increase is not simply due to fluid being trapped within the body of the vertebra (Hutton et al 1979). A motion segment's resistance to bending increases by about 15% when the duration of loading decreases from 10 s to 3 s, but little further increase occurs in 1 s loading cycles; conversely, sustained bending for 10 minutes reduces the motion segment's passive resistance to bending by about 40% (Adams et al 1992, unpublished data). The tensile stiffness of the interspinous ligament increases by 15–30% when the duration of loading decreases from about 20 s to 1 s (Hindle et al 1990). These results serve as a warning that mechanical properties measured under slow 'quasi-static' loading conditions are not a reliable guide to mechanical behaviour under dynamic loading conditions.

Intervertebral disc creep

If a load is suddenly applied to an intervertebral disc, the disc deforms immediately. This initial deformation is termed 'elastic' because it is completely reversed as soon as the load is removed. If the load is not removed, then the motion segment shows a slowly increasing deformation which is termed 'creep' (Fig. 9.12). Creep occurs in many materials and is caused by a variety of different mechanisms, but in the disc it is due primarily to the slow expulsion of fluid through the tiny pores of the extracellular matrix. In addition, some disc height loss may be attributable to extra radial bulging of the disc, secondary to a reduction in the volume of the nucleus (The Effect of Compression on Lumbar Motion Segments — p. 113). In life, the high swelling pressure of the proteoglycans in the matrix ensures that the creep process is reversed when the deforming load is removed, and the fluid should be re-absorbed in half the time it took to expel it (Urban & Maroudas 1980). In cadaver experiments, a full recovery of disc height can occur if the disc is in contact with saline, but the disc's mechanical properties are not completely restored (Smeathers & Joanes 1988).

Motion segment creep has been measured in response to sustained compressive loading. A force of 1000 N (which is appropriate to simulate light manual labour: Nachemson 1981) causes a creep height loss of about 1.5 mm over four hours (Adams & Hutton 1983a). Most of this loss occurs in the first hour (Fig. 9.12) but creep continues beyond 4 hours at a greatly reduced rate. During the 4-hour period, the disc loses about 10% of its total water content. Old and degenerated discs lose less water than young discs, but the height loss is about the same (Adams & Hutton 1983a). Axial loading appears to expel a higher proportion of water from the annulus compared to the nucleus (Adams & Hutton 1983a) but this may possibly be due to post-mortem changes in the permeability of the vertebral body end-plate. After 24 hours of loading at 981 N, the water loss from the nucleus and annulus is 8% and 11% respectively (Kraemer et al 1985).

If a motion segment is compressed while wedged in flexion, then the increased intradiscal pressure (Table 9.1) expels more water from the disc, especially from the nucleus (Adams & Hutton 1983a). High intradiscal stress gradients associated with eccentric loading (Horst & Brinckmann 1981, McNally & Adams 1992) also redistribute water within the disc and this can leave the motion segment wedged in slight flexion, even after the load has been removed (Twomey & Taylor 1982, Adams & Hutton 1985a).

The effect of disc creep on motion segment mechanics

Creep has a profound effect on the mechanical properties of the motion segment. These may well be of practical clinical significance because of the diurnal pattern of creep and recovery described in the following section.

Disc height loss is accompanied by increased radial bulging, according to the flat tyre analogy (Compressive Strength of Lumbar Motion Segments — p. 114). This has not been measured directly, but it may be inferred from measurements of increased radial bulge following partial discectomy (Brinckmann & Grootenboer 1991) or end-plate fracture (Brinckmann & Horst 1985). Alternatively, if the volume of the nucleus is increased by means of a fluid injection, then the radial bulge decreases and disc height increases (Brinckmann & Horst 1985).

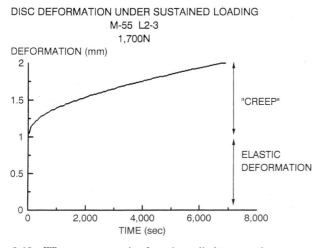

Fig. 9.12 When a compressive force is applied to a motion segment, there is an immediate 'elastic' deformation (height loss). If the load is not removed, there follows a gradual time-dependent deformation called 'creep'.

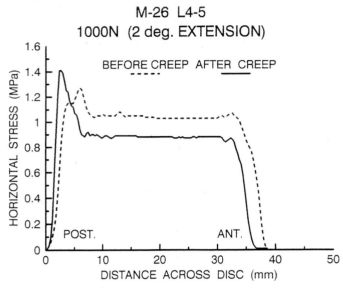

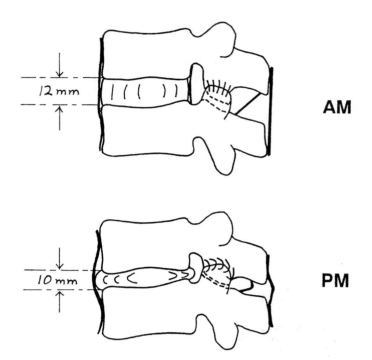

Fig. 9.13 The effect of sustained (creep) loading on the distribution of compressive stress inside an intervertebral disc. Creep reduces the hydrostatic pressure in the nucleus pulposus, and increases any anisotropic stress peaks in the annulus. Much greater effects can be seen in some older discs.

Fig. 9.14 Diagrammatic summary of the effects of creep on motion segment mechanics. (**AM**) Before creep (corresponding to the early morning, in life) the disc is swollen with fluid, and the ligaments are taut. (**PM**) After creep (corresponding to later in the day) the disc has less height and bulges more, the ligaments are slack, and the apophyseal joints come into close contact.

Stress distributions within a disc are affected by creep loading. Creep increases the compressive stress on the annulus and decreases the pressure in the nucleus (McNally & Adams 1992: see Fig. 9.13). A motion segment's resistance to forward bending falls by about 70%, with the disc being particularly affected, and posterior disc prolapse becomes more difficult to simulate (Adams et al 1987). These effects are probably caused by increased slack in the collagen network of the peripheral posterior annulus after water has been expelled from the disc.

After creep, the disc behaves more like an elastic material, and dissipates less 'hysteresis' energy during a loading/unloading cycle (Koeller et al 1986). This actually improves the disc's function as a shock absorber during locomotion because it minimizes the risk of thermal damage to the avascular tissue (see Posture During Dynamic Movement — p. 125).

Adjacent structures are affected by the loss of disc height that accompanies creep loading (Fig. 9.14). The apophyseal joint surfaces come into closer apposition and start to resist a proportion of the compressive force acting on the lumbar spine (Adams & Hutton 1980) and there is a risk of extra-articular impingement of the inferior articular process on the lamina below (Dunlop et al 1984). The intervertebral ligaments gain some slack and so provide less resistance to bending movements (Adams et al 1987, Hedtmann et al 1989) and they pre-stress the disc less in flexed postures.

In vivo diurnal variations in spinal mechanics

The typical diurnal cycle of daily activity and nightly rest

leads to a diurnal cycle in disc water content and height, for the reasons discussed above. During the course of a day, body height is reduced by about 20 mm (De Pukey 1935; Tyrrell et al 1985, Krag et al 1990). This value is compatible with the creep height lost by cadaveric motion segments (see Adams et al 1987) and so the mechanical properties of the osteoligamentous spine in vivo should show a variation between morning and evening similar to that shown by cadaveric specimens before and after creep loading.

The most profound of these changes are the increased loading of the apophyseal joints in the afternoon, and the greatly increased bending stiffness of the osteoligamentous spine, and consequent risk of disc prolapse, in the early morning (Adams et al 1990). It might be expected that in a living person the back muscles would compensate for these changes in the underlying spine. For example, muscle action to decrease the lumbar lordosis would reduce apophyseal joint loading, and a restricted range of flexion movement would reduce stresses due to bending. However, this appears not to happen to any significant extent in practice, and bending stresses on the intervertebral disc probably increase by about 300% in the early morning (Adams et al 1987).

There is plenty of anecdotal evidence suggesting that back injuries are particularly common in the early morning, but there is only a little scientific data to back this up (Evans et al 1980, Baxter 1987). Accidents attrib-

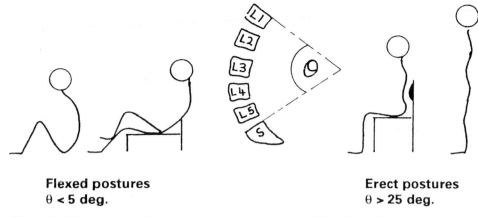

Flexed postures
θ < 5 deg.

Erect postures
θ > 25 deg.

Fig. 9.15 The curvature of an excised cadaveric lumbar spine (θ) is about 40° on average. In life, it is useful to distinguish between 'flexed postures', which greatly reduce the normal lumbar lordosis, and 'erect postures' which largely maintain or increase it.

utable to diurnal variations in spinal mechanics are difficult to distinguish from those caused by reduced alertness, or fatigue at the end of a long working shift.

Since different spinal structures are more heavily loaded at different times of the day, diurnal variations in patients' signs and symptoms may provide valuable clues about the underlying pathology (Adams et al 1990, Porter & Trailescu 1990).

POSTURE

This word is open to a variety of interpretations, but is used here to describe the curvature of the lumbar spine in the sagittal plane, as shown in Figure 9.15.

Posture during dynamic movement

Figure 9.16 shows schematically how the bending moment on a lumbar motion segment varies throughout the full range of sagittal movement. It is apparent that in between full flexion and full extension there is a comparatively safe range of movement where there is only a small risk of the type of bending injuries described under Backwards Bending (Extension) (p. 117), Forward Bending (Flexion) (p. 118) and Combined Bending and Compression: Disc Prolapse (p. 120). Note that the centre of this zone corresponds to slight lumbar flexion. The lordotic stance characteristic of erect standing (about 2° of extension) is at one edge of the zone because it is associated with high stress concentrations acting on the apophyseal joints (Backwards Bending of the Lumbar Spine in vivo — p. 117) and the posterior annulus fibrosus (Fig. 9.13).

The size of the 'safe zone' varies greatly between a particularly stiff spine and a very mobile one. This suggests that good sagittal mobility may protect the lumbar spine by allowing it to stay well within the 'safe zone' during normal daily activities. There is some experimental evi-

dence in support of this: during forward bending and lifting activities, the peak bending stresses acting on the osteoligamentous lumbar spine are increased by up to 100% in people with a particularly low range of lumbar sagittal movement (Dolan & Adams 1993).

Compressive stresses within cadaveric intervertebral discs also show a most favourable distribution when the spine is moderately flexed (Adams et al 1992: see Fig. 9.8). Flexion to 75% of the full range allowed by the ligaments often removes peaks of anisotropic stress from the posterior annulus, but without creating similar peaks in the anterior annulus. Admittedly, this amount of flexion does tend to increase the hydrostatic pressure in the nucleus because it removes forces from the apophyseal joints, and increases tension in the posterior ligaments. However, the pressure increase disappears when the

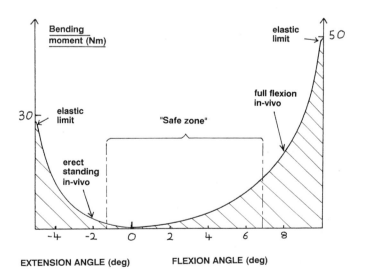

Fig. 9.16 In between flexion and extension there is a range of movement in which the bending stresses on the spine remain low. Within this 'safe zone' the discs and ligaments of the lumbar spine are relatively safe from injury, although there remains some risk of compressive injury to the vertebral bodies.

applied compressive force exceeds 2000 N (Adams et al 1992) because the compressed anterior annulus is able to 'stress-shield' the nucleus at high loads, as was suggested previously (Adams & Hutton 1985b). Full flexion appears less advantageous because it increases nuclear pressure even when the compressive force is high, and it probably generates high *tensile* stresses in the peripheral posterior annulus (Adams et al 1992). Conversely, extension angles appropriate to simulate the lordotic standing posture often create high *compressive*, stress peaks in the posterior annulus, especially after sustained ('creep') loading (Adams et al 1992, McNally & Adams 1992: see Fig. 9.13).

It would appear, therefore, that a position of moderate flexion reduces the risk of bending injuries and optimizes the distribution of stresses in the intervertebral discs. It is also the most favourable configuration for absorbing energy during locomotion, when the curvature of the lumbar spine varies during different phases of the gait cycle. In a slightly flexed spine, the intervertebral discs and ligaments do not absorb much of this energy because they offer little resistance to small angular movements (Fig. 9.16). It is therefore left to the trunk musculature and their tendons to absorb energy by opposing the changes in spinal curvature. Tendons are particularly good at absorbing strain energy and are more able than the avascular intervertebral discs to dissipate any potentially damaging heat (hysteresis energy) generated during the process.

Static postures

In static postures it is comparatively rare for the lumbar curvature, as defined in Figure 9.15, to lie between about −25 and −5° (Dolan et al 1988). Usually the spine slumps either into flexion or lordosis, and it is useful to distinguish between 'flexed postures', which involve a considerable reduction of the lumbar lordosis seen in erect standing, and 'erect postures' which maintain or increase this lordosis.

The experiments on cadaveric lumbar motion segments described in this chapter show that flexed postures have the following advantages: they reduce stress concentrations in the apophyseal joints (The Effect of Backwards Bending on Lumbar Motion Segments — p. 117); they reduce the disc's tendency to bulge posteriorly (p. 119); they remove peaks of compressive stresses from the posterior annulus (p. 119); and they also improve the transport of nutrients into those regions of the disc where the supply is thought to be precarious (Adams & Hutton 1983a, 1986b). On the other hand, erect postures reduce the hydrostatic pressure in the nucleus pulposus (Table 9.1) but this benefit is apparent only at low load levels, where mechanical damage is unlikely to occur.

These results may explain the obvious preference that many people show for sitting with the legs crossed, or raised up, or for standing with one leg on a bar rail, and so on. All of these habits cause the lumbar spine to flex to a greater or lesser extent (Dolan et al 1988). Of course, it is beneficial to support the lumbar spine in the sense of providing a firm surface for it to rest against, but there is no reason why this support should force the lumbar spine into a lordosis. As discussed above, some lumbar lordosis is desirable during locomotion because of its shock-absorbing action, but during static postures it is neither 'natural' nor beneficial. It is interesting to note that lumbar disc degeneration is comparatively rare in certain Third World countries where many people adopt extremely flexed squatting postures (Fahrni & Trueman 1965).

Postural recommendations for healthy backs do not necessarily apply to people suffering with low-back pain. Many patients experience symptom relief from an exaggerated lordosis (Donelson et al 1991, Williams et al 1991) no doubt because it reduces mechanical loading on whatever tissue is causing the pain. However, this does not mean that lordotic posture should be advocated as a means of preventing 'mechanical' back problems in the first place. To take a simple analogy, you might use crutches to relieve the pain from a sprained ankle, but you would probably not consider using them to safeguard a healthy leg!

REFERENCES

Adams M A 1980 The mechanical properties of lumbar intervertebral joints with special reference to the causes of low back pain. PhD thesis, Polytechnic of Central London

Adams M A, Dolan P 1991 A technique for quantifying bending moment acting on the lumbar spine in vivo. Journal of Biomechanics 24: 117–126

Adams M A, Green T P 1992 The contribution of collagen-proteoglycan interactions to the tensile stiffness of the annulus fibrous. International Society for the Study of the Lumbar Spine, Chicago USA, May 1992

Adams M A, Hutton W C 1980 The effect of posture on the role of the apophyseal joints in resisting intervertebral compressive force. Journal of Bone and Joint Surgery 62-B: 358–362

Adams M A, Hutton W C 1981 The relevance of torsion to the mechanical derangement of the lumbar spine. Spine 6: 241–248

Adams M A, Hutton W C (1982) Prolapsed intervertebral disc. A hyperflexion injury. Spine 7: 184–191

Adams M A, Hutton W C 1983a The effect of posture on the fluid content of lumbar intervertebral discs. Spine 8: 665–671

Adams M A, Hutton W C 1983b The mechanical function of the lumbar apophyseal joints. Spine 8: 327–329

Adams M A, Hutton W C 1985a Gradual disc prolapse. Spine 10: 524–531

Adams M A, Hutton W C 1985b The effect of posture on the lumbar spine. Journal of Bone and Joint Surgery 67-B: 625–629

Adams M A, Hutton W C 1986a Has the lumbar spine a margin of safety in forward bending? Clinical Biomechanics 1: 3–6

Adams M A, Hutton W C 1986b The effect of posture on diffusion into lumbar intervertebral discs. Journal of Anatomy 147: 121–134

Adams M A, Hutton W C 1988 Mechanics of the intervertebral disc. In: Ghosh P (ed) The biology of the intervertebral disc. CRC Press, Boco Raton, Florida

Adams M A, Hutton W C, Stott J R R 1980 The resistance to flexion of the lumbar intervertebral joint. Spine 5: 245–253

Adams M A, Dolan P, Hutton W C 1986 The stages of disc degeneration as revealed by discograms. Journal of Bone and Joint Surgery 68-B: 36–41

Adams M A, Dolan P, Hutton W C 1987 Diurnal variations in the stresses on the lumbar spine. Spine 12: 130–137

Adams M A, Dolan P, Hutton W C 1988 The lumbar spine in backward bending. Spine 13: 1019–1026

Adams M A, Dolan P, Hutton W C, Porter R W 1990 Diurnal changes in spinal mechanics and their clinical significance. Journal of Bone and Joint Surgery 72B: 266–270

Adams M A, McNally D S, Chinn H, Dolan P 1992 Posture and the compressive strength of the lumbar spine (submitted for publication)

Ahmed A M, Duncan N A, Burke D L 1990 The effect of facet geometry on the axial torque-rotation response of lumbar motion segments Spinc 15: 391–401

Andersson G B J, Schultz A B 1979 Effects of fluid injection on mechanical properties of intervertebral discs. Journal of Biomechanics 12: 453–458

Andersson G B J, Murphy R W, Ortengren R, Nachemson A L 1979 The influence of backrest inclination and lumbar support on lumbar lordosis. Spine 4: 52–58

Aspden R M 1989 The spine as an arch: a new mathematical model. Spine 14: 266–274

Bartelink D L 1957 The role of abdominal pressure in relieving the pressure on the lumbar intervertebral discs. Journal of Bone and Joint Surgery 39-B: 718–725

Baxter C E 1987 Low back pain and time of day: a study of their effects on psychophysical performance. PhD thesis, University of Liverpool, UK

Bayliss M T, Johnstone B, O'Brien J P 1988 Proteoglycan synthesis in the human intervertebral disc. Variation with age, region and pathology. Spine 13: 972–981

Bogduk N, Twomey L T 1991 Clinical anatomy of the lumbar spine. Churchill Livingstone, Edinburgh

Brinckmann P 1986 Injury of the annulus fibrosus and disc protrusions. An in vitro investigation on human lumbar discs. Spine 11: 149–153

Brinckmann P, Grootenboer H 1991 Change of disc height, radial disc bulge and intradiscal pressure from discectomy: an in vitro investigation on human lumbar discs. Spine 16: 641–646

Brinckmann P, Horst M 1985 The influence of vertebral body fracture, intra-discal injection, and partial discectomy on the radial bulge and height of human lumbar discs. Spine 10: 138–145

Brinckmann P, Frobin W, Hierholzer E, Horst M 1983 Deformation of the vertebral end-plate under axial loading of the spine. Spine 8: 851–856

Brinckmann P, Biggerman M, Hilweg D 1988 Fatigue fracture of human lumbar vertebrae. Clinical Biomechanics 3 (suppl 1)

Brinckmann P, Biggemann M, Hilweg D 1989 Prediction of the compressive strength of human lumbar vertebrae. Clinical Biomechanics 4 (suppl 2)

Chazal J, Tanguy A, Bourges M et al 1985 Biomechanical properties of spinal ligaments and a histological study of the supraspinal ligament in traction. Journal of Biomechanics 18: 167–176

Cholewicki J, McGill S M 1992 Lumbar posterior ligament involvement during extremely heavy lifts estimated from fluoroscopic measurements. Journal of Biomechanics 25: 17–28

Cossette J W, Farfan H F, Robertson G H, Wells R V 1971 The instantaneous centre of rotation of the third lumbar intervertebral joint. Journal of Biomechanics 4: 149–153

Cyron B M, Hutton W C 1978 The fatigue strength of the lumbar neural arch in spondylolysis. Journal of Bone and Joint Surgery 60-B: 234–238

Cyron B M, Hutton W C 1980 Articular tropism and stability of the lumbar spine. Spine 5: 168–172

Cyron B M, Hutton W C 1981a The tensile strength of the capsular ligaments of the apophyseal joints. Journal of Anatomy 132: 145–150

Cyron B M, Hutton W C 1981b The behaviour of the lumbar intervertebral disc under repetitive forces. International Orthopaedics 5: 203–207

Cyron B M, Hutton W C, Troup J D G 1976 Spondylolytic fractures. Journal of Bone and Joint Surgery 58-B: 462–466

Cyron B M, Hutton W C, Stott J R R 1979 Spondylolysis — the shearing stiffness of the lumbar intervertebral joint. Acta Orthopaedica Belgica 45: 459–469

Davis P R, Troup J D G, Burnard J H 1965 Movements of the thoracic and lumbar spine when lifting: a chrono-cyclographic study. Journal of Anatomy 99: 13–26

De Pukey P 1935 The physiological oscillation of the length of the body. Acta Orthopaedica Scandinavica 6: 338

Dolan P, Adams M A 1993 The relationship between EMG activity and extensor moment generation in the erector spinae muscles during forward bending activities. Journal of Biomechanics (in press)

Dolan P, Adams M A 1993 The effect of lumbar and hip mobility on the bending moment acting on the lumbar spine. Clinical Biomechanics (in press)

Dolan P, Adams M A, Hutton W C 1987 The short-term effects of chymopapain on intervertebral discs. Journal of Bone and Joint Surgery 69-B: 422–428

Dolan P, Adams M A, Hutton W C 1988 Commonly adopted postures and their effect on the lumbar spine. Spine 13: 197–201

Donelson R, Grant W, Kamps C, Medcalf R 1991 Pain response to sagittal end-range spinal motion: a prospective randomised multicentered trial. Spine 16: 6 suppl 5206–5212

Dumas G A, Beaudoin L, Drouin G 1987 In situ mechanical behaviour of posterior spinal ligaments in the lumbar region. An in vitro study. Journal of Biomechanics 20: 301–310

Duncan N A, Ahmed A M 1991 The role of axial rotation in the etiology of unilateral disc prolapse: an experimental and finite-element analysis. Spine 16: 1089–1098

Dunlop R B, Adams M A, Hutton W C 1984 Disc space narrowing and the lumbar facet joints. Journal of Bone and Joint Surgery 66-B: 706–710

Eie N 1966 Load capacity of the low back. Journal of Oslo City Hospitals 16: 73–98

El-Bohy A A, Yang K-H, King A I 1989 Experimental verification of facet load transmission by direct measurement of facet lamina contact pressure. Journal of Biomechanics 22: 931–941

Evans J H, Greer W, Pearcy M J, Frampton S, Daniel J 1980 Back problems in a mining/smelting company. In: Engineering aspects of the spine. Institute of Mechanical Engineers Conference Publications 1980–82. c134/80: 79–82. Published by Mechanical Engineering Publications Ltd, London for the Institute of Mechanical Engineers

Fahrni W H, Trueman G E 1965 Comparative radiological study of the spines of a primitive population with North Americans and North Europeans. Journal of Bone and Joint Surgery 47B: 552–555

Farfan H F, Sullivan J D 1967 The relation of facet orientation to intervertebral disc failure. Canadian Journal of Surgery 10: 179–185

Farfan H F, Cossette J W, Robertson G H, Wells R V, Kraus H 1970 The effects of torsion on the lumbar intervertebral joints: the role of torsion in the production of disc degeneration. Journal of Bone and Joint Surgery 52-A: 468–497

Farfan H F, Huberdeau R M, Dubow H I 1972 Lumbar intervertebral disc degeneration. Journal of Bone and Joint Surgery 54-A: 492–510

Floyd W F, Silver P H S 1951 Function of erectores spinae in flexion of the trunk. Lancet 1: 133–134

Frymoyer J W, Newberg A, Pope M H, Wilder D G, Clements J, Macpherson B 1984 Spine radiographs in patients with low back pain. Journal of Bone and Joint Surgery 66-A: 1048–1055

Galante J O 1967 Tensile properties of the human lumbar annulus fibrosus. Acta Orthopaedica Scandinavica (suppl 100)

Gertzbein S D, Seligman J, Holtby R, Chan K H, Kapasouri A, Tile M, Cruickshank B 1985 Centrode patterns and segmental instability in degenerative disc disease. Spine 10: 257–261

Gill K, Videman T, Shimizu T, Mooney V 1987 The effect of repeated extensions on the discographic dye patterns in cadaveric lumbar motion segments. Clinical Biomechanics 2: 205–210

Gordon S J, Yang K H, Mayer P J, Mace A H, Kish V L, Radin E L

1991 Mechanism of disc rupture — a preliminary report. Spine 16: 450–456

Gracovetsky S, Farfan H 1986 The optimum spine. Spine 11: 543–571

Granhed H, Jonson R, Hansson T 1987 The loads on the lumbar spine during extreme weight lifting. Spine 12: 146–149

Granhed H, Jonson R, Hansson T 1989 Mineral content and strength of lumbar vertebrae: a cadaver study. Acta Orthopaedica Scandinavica 60: 105–109

Green T P, Adams M A 1992 Fatigue failure of the annulus fibrosus. British Orthopaedic Research Society, Birmingham, UK, September 1991

Gregersen G G, Lucas D B 1967 An in vivo study of the axial rotation of the human thoracolumbar spine. Journal of Bone and Joint Surgery 49-A: 247–262

Gunzburg R, Hutton W, Fraser R 1991 Axial rotation of the lumbar spine and the effect of flexion. Spine 16: 22–29

Hansson T, Roos B, Nachemson A 1980 The bone mineral content and ultimate compressive strength of lumbar vertebrae. Spine 5: 46–55

Hansson T, Keller T, Spengler D 1987 Mechanical behaviour of the human lumbar spine. II Fatigue strength during dynamic compressive loading. Journal of Orthopaedic Research 5(4): 479–487

Hasberry S, Pearcy M J 1986 Temperature dependence of the tensile properties of interspinous ligaments of sheep. Journal of Biomedical Engineering 8: 62–66

Hedtmann A, Steffen R, Methfessel J, Kolditz D, Kramer J, Thols M 1989 Measurement of human lumbar spine ligaments during loaded and unloaded motion. Spine 14: 175–185

Hendry N G L 1958 Hydration of the nucleus pulposus and its relation to intervertebral disc derangement. Journal of Bone and Joint Surgery 40-B: 132–144

Heylings D J A 1978 Supraspinous and interspinous ligaments of the human lumbar spine. Journal of Anatomy 125: 127–131

Hickey D S, Hukins D W L 1980 Relation between the structure of the annulus fibrosus and the function and failure of the intervertebral disc. Spine 5: 106–116

Hilton R C, Ball J, Benn R T 1979 In vitro mobility of the lumbar spine. Annals of the Rheumatic Diseases 38: 378–383

Hindle R J, Pearcy M J, Cross A 1990 Mechanical function of the human lumbar interspinous and supraspinous ligaments. Journal of Biomedical Engineering 12: 340–344

Hirsch C, Schajowicz F 1953 Studies on structural changes in the lumbar annulus fibrous. Acta Orthopaedica Scandinavica 22: 184–231

Hirsch C, Inglemark B, Miller M (1963). The anatomical basis for low back pain. Acta Orthopaedica Scandinavica 33: 1–17

Horst M, Brinckmann P 1981 Measurement of the distribution of axial stress on the endplate of the vertebral body. Spine 6: 217–232

Hukins D W L, Kirby M C, Sikoryn T A, Aspden R M, Cox A J 1990 Comparison of structure, mechanical properties and functions of lumbar spinal ligaments. Spine 15: 787–795

Hutton W C, Adams M A 1982 Can the lumbar spine be crushed in heavy lifting? Spine 7: 309–313

Hutton W C, Stott J R R, Cyron B M 1977 Is spondylolysis a fatigue fracture? Spine 2: 202–209

Hutton W C, Cyron B M, Stott J R R 1979 The compressive strength of lumbar vertebrae. Journal of Anatomy 129: 753–758

Janevic J, Ashton-Miller J A, Schultz A B 1991 Large compressive preloads decrease lumbar motion segment flexibility. Journal of Orthopaedic Research 9: 228–236

Keller T S, Holm S H, Hansson T H, Spengler D M 1990 The dependence of intervertebral disc mechanical properties on physiologic conditions. Spine 15: 751–761

Kelsey J L, Githens P B, White A A et al 1984 An epidemiologic study of lifting and twisting on the job and risk for acute prolapsed lumbar intervertebral disc. Journal of Orthopaedic Research 2: 61–66

Klein J A, Hukins D W L 1982 Collagen fibres reorientate in the annulus fibrosus of intervertebral discs during bending and torsion, measured by X-ray diffraction. Biochemica Biophysica Acta 719(1) 98–101

Koeller W, Muehlhaus S, Meier W, Hartmann F 1986 Biomechanical properties of human intervertebral discs subjected to axial dynamic compression — influence of age and degeneration. Journal of Biomechanics 19: 807–816

Korkala O, Gronblad M, Liesi P, Karaharju E 1985 Immunohistochemical demonstration of nociceptors in the ligamentous structures of the lumbar spine. Spine 10: 156–165

Kraemer, J Kolditz D, Gowin R 1985 Water and electrolyte content of human intervertebral discs under variable load. Spine 10: 69–71

Krag M H, Cohen M C, Haugh L D, Pope M H 1990 Body height change during upright and recumbent posture. Spine 15: 202–207

Leong J C Y, Luk K D K, Chow D H K, Woo C W 1987 The biomechanical function of the iliolumbar ligament in maintaining stability of the lumbosacral junction. Spine 12: 669–674

Lin H S, Liu Y K, Adams K H 1978 Mechanical response of the lumbar intervertebral joint under physiological (complex) loading. Journal of Bone and Joint Surgery 60-A: 41–55

Lindblom K 1952 Experimental ruptures of intervertebral discs in rats' tails. Journal of Bone and Joint Surgery 34A: 123–128

Lipson S J, Muir H 1981 Proteoglycans in experimental intervertebral disc degeneration. Spine 6: 194–210

Liu Y K, Njus G, Buckwalter J, Wakano K 1983 Fatigue response of lumbar intervertebral joints under axial cyclic loading. Spine 8: 857–865

Liu Y K, Goel V K, Dejong A, Njus G, Nishiyama K, Buckwalter J 1985 Torsional fatigue of the lumbar intervertebral joints. Spine 10: 894–900

Lumsden R M, Morris J M 1968 An in-vivo study of axial rotation and immobilisation at the lumbosacral joint. Journal of Bone and Joint Surgery 50-A: 1591–1602

McBroom R J, Hayes W C, Edwards W T, Goldberg R P, White A A 1985 Prediction of vertebral body compressive fracture using quantitative computed tomography. Journal of Bone and Joint Surgery 67-A: 1206–1213

McGill S M, Norman R W 1985 Dynamically and statically determined low back moments during lifting. Journal of Biomechanics 18: 877–885

McGill S M, Norman R W 1987a Effects of an anatomically detailed erector spinae model on L4/L5 disc compression and shear. Journal of Biomechanics 20: 591–600

McGill S M, Norman R W 1987b Reassessment of the role of intra-abdominal pressure in spinal compression. Ergonomics 30: 1565–1588

McGill S M, Patt N, Norman R W 1988 Measurement of the trunk musculature of active males using CT scan radiography: implications for force and moment generating capacity about the L4/L5 joint. Journal of Biomechanics 21: 329–341

McGill S M, Norman R W, Sharratt M T 1990 The effect of an abdominal belt on trunk muscle activity and intra-abdominal pressure during squat lifts. Ergonomics 33: 147–160

McNally D S, Adams M A 1992 Internal intervertebral disc mechanics as revealed by stress profilometry. Spine 17: 66–73

Marchand F, Ahmed A M 1990 Investigation of the laminate structure of lumbar disc annulus fibrosus. Spine 15: 402–410

Markolf K L, Morris J M 1974 The structural components of the intervertebral disc. Journal of Bone and Joint Surgery 56-A: 675–687

Maroudas A 1982 Nutrition and metabolism of the intervertebral disc. In: White A A, Gordon S L (eds) Symposium on ideopathic low back pain. C V Mosby, St Louis

Miller J A A, Schultz A B, Warwick D N, Spencer D L 1986 Mechanical properties of lumbar spine motion segments under large loads. Journal of Biomechanics 19: 79–84

Myklebust J B, Pintar F, Yoganandan N et al 1988 Tensile strength of spinal ligaments. Spine 13: 526–531

Nachemson A L 1960 Lumbar intradiscal pressure. Acta Orthopaedica Scandinavica (suppl 43): 1–104

Nachemson A 1965 In vivo discometry in lumbar discs with irregular nucleograms. Acta Orthopaedica Scandinavica 36: 418–434

Nachemson A 1966 Electromyographic studies on the vertebral portion of the psoas muscle. Acta Orthopaedica Scandinavica 37: 177–190

Nachemson A 1981 Disc pressure measurements. Spine 6: 93–97

Nachemson A L, Evans J H 1968 Some mechanical properties of the third human lumbar interlaminar ligament (ligamentum flavum). Journal of Biomechanics 1: 211–220

Noren R, Trafimow J, Andersson G B J, Huckman M S 1991 The role of facet joint tropism and facet angle in disc degeneration. Spine 16: 530–532

Osti O L, Vernon-Roberts B, Fraser R D 1990 Annulus tears and intervertebral disc degeneration: an experimental study using an animal model. Spine 15: 762–767

Osvalder A L, Newman P, Lovsund P, Nordwall A 1990 Ultimate strength of the lumbar spine in flexion — an in vitro study. Journal of Biomechanics 23: 453–460

Panjabi M M, Goel V K, Takata K 1982 Physiologic strains in the lumbar spinal ligaments. Spine 7: 192–203

Panjabi M M, Krag M, Summers D, Videman T 1985 Biomechanical time-tolerance of fresh cadaveric human spine specimens. Journal of Orthopaedic Research 3: 292–300

Pearcy M J, Bogduk N 1988 Instantaneous axes of rotation of the lumbar intervertebral joints. Spine 13: 1033–1041

Pearcy M J, Tibrewal S B 1984a Axial rotation and lateral bending in the normal lumbar spine measured by three-dimensional radiography. Spine 9: 582–587

Pearcy M J, Tibrewal S B 1984b Lumbar intervertebral disc and ligament deformations measured in vivo. Clinical Orthopaedics and Related Research 191: 281–286

Pearcy M J, Portek I, Shepherd J 1984 Three-dimensional X-ray analysis of normal movement in the lumbar spine. Spine 9: 294–297

Pearcy M J, Portek I, Shepherd J 1985 The effect of low-back pain on lumbar spinal movements measured by three-dimensional X-ray analysis. Spine 10: 150–153

Perey O 1957 Fracture of the vertebral endplate. A biomechanical investigation. Acta Orthopaedica Scandinavica (suppl 25)

Porter R W, Trailescu I F 1990 Diurnal changes in straight leg raising. Spine 15: 103–106

Porter R W, Adams M A, Hutton W C 1989 Physical activity and the strength of the lumbar spine 14: 201–203

Potvin J R, McGill S M, Norman R W 1991 Trunk muscle and lumbar ligament contributions to dynamic lifts with varying degrees of trunk flexion. Spine 16: 1099–1108

Rissanen P M 1960 The surgical anatomy and pathology of the supraspinous and interspinous ligaments of the lumbar spine with special reference to ligament ruptures. Acta Orthopaedica Scandinavica (suppl 46): 1–100

Roberts S, Menage J, Urban J P G 1989 Biochemical and structural properties of the cartilage end-plate and its relation to the intervertebral disc. Spine 14: 166–174

Rockoff S D, Sweet E, Bleustein J 1969 The relative contribution of trabecular and cortical bone to the strength of human lumbar vertebrae. Calcified Tissue Research 3: 163–175

Rolander S D 1966 Motion of the lumbar spine with special reference to the stabilising effect of posterior fusion. Acta Orthopaedica Scandinavica (suppl 90): 1–144

Schonstrom N, Lindahl S, Willen J, Hansson T 1989 Dynamic changes in the dimensions of the lumbar spinal canal: an experimental study in vitro. Journal of Orthopaedic Research 7: 115–121

Schultz A B, Warwick D N, Berkson M H, Nachemson A L 1979 Mechanical properties of human lumbar spine segments. Part 1. Response in flexion, extension, lateral bending and torsion. Journal of Biomechanical Engineering 101: 46–52

Schultz A B, Haderspek-Grib K, Sinkora G, Warwick D N 1985 Quantitative studies of the flexion-relaxation phenomenon in the back muscles. Journal of Orthopaedic Research 3: 189–197

Seroussi R E, Krag M H, Muller D L, Pope M H 1989 Internal deformations of intact and denucleated human lumbar discs

subjected to compression, flexion and extension loads. Journal of Orthopaedic Research 7: 122–131

Shirazi-Adl A 1989 Strain in fibers of a lumbar disc. Analysis of the role of lifting in producing disc prolapse. Clinical Biomechanics 14: 96–103

Shirazi-Adl A 1991 Finite-element evaluation of contact loads on facets of an L2-L3 lumbar segment in complex loads. Spine 16: 533–541

Shirazi-Adl A, Ahmed A M, Shrivastava S C 1986 Mechanical response of a lumbar motion segment in axial torque alone and combined with compression. Spine 11: 914–927

Smeathers J E, Joanes D N 1988 Dynamic compressive properties of human lumbar intervertebral joints: a comparison between fresh and thawed specimens. Journal of Biomechanics 21: 425–433

Stokes I A F 1988 Mechanical function of facet joints in the lumbar spine. Clinical Biomechanics 3: 101–105

Stokes I A F, Bevins T M, Lunn R A 1987 Back surface curvature and measurement of lumbar spinal motion. Spine 12: 355–361

Thurston A J, Harris J D 1983 Normal kinematics of the lumbar spine and pelvis. Spine 8: 199–205

Tkaczuk H 1968 Tensile properties of human lumbar longitudinal ligaments. Acta Orthopaedica Scandinavica (suppl 115)

Twomey L, Taylor J 1982 Flexion creep deformation and hysteresis in the lumbar vertebral column. Spine 7: 116–122

Twomey L T, Taylor J R 1983 Sagittal movements of the human lumbar vertebral column: a quantitative study of the role of the posterior vertebral elements. Archives of Physical Medicine and Rehabilitation 64: 322–325

Tyrrell A R, Reilly T, Troup J D G 1985 Circadian variation in stature and the effects of spinal loading. Spine 10: 161–164

Urban J P G, Maroudas A 1979 The measurement of fixed charge density in the intervertebral disc. Biochimica et Biophysica Acta 586: 166–178

Urban J P G, Maroudas A 1980 The chemistry of the intervertebral disc in relation to its functional requirements. Clinics in Rheumatic Diseases 6: 51–76

Varma K M K 1987 First episode of low back pain. PhD thesis, University of Liverpool, UK

Videman T, Nurminen M, Troup J D G 1990 Lumbar spinal pathology in cadaveric material in relation to history of back pain, occupation and physical loading. Spine 15: 728–740

Williams M M, Hawley J A, McKenzie R A, van Wijmen P M 1991 A comparison of the effects of two sitting postures on back and referred pain. Spine 16: 1185–1191

Yamamoto I, Panjabi M M, Crisco J J, Oxland T 1989 Three-dimensional movements of the whole lumbar spine and lumbo-sacral joint. Spine 14: 1256–1260

Yamamoto I, Panjabi M M, Oxland T R, Crisco J J 1990 The role of the iliolumbar ligament in the lumbosacral junction. Spine 15: 1138–1141

Yang K H, King A I 1984 Mechanism of facet load transmission as a hypothesis for low back pain. Spine 9: 557–565

Yoganandan N, Myklebust J B, Wilson C R, Cusick J F, Sances A Jr 1988 Functional biomechanics of the thoracolumbar vertebral cortex. Clinical Biomechanics 3: 11–18

Yoganandan N, Ray G, Pintar F A, Myklebust J B, Sances A Jr 1989 Stiffness and strain energy criteria to evaluate the threshold of injury to an intervertebral joint. Journal of Biomechanics 22: 135–142

Yoshizawa H, O'Brien J P, Smith W T, Trumper M 1980 The neuropathology of intervertebral discs removed for low-back pain. Journal of Pathology 132: 95–104

10. Kinematics of the pelvic joints

D. G. Lee

HISTORICAL REVIEW

The obstetricians of Hippocrates' era were apparently the first to have recorded interest in the function of the pelvic girdle (Weisl 1955). At that time, the sacro-iliac joints were thought to be immobile, except during pregnancy. From the 17th century to date, the classification, composition and biomechanics of the pelvic girdle have been debated.

Bernhard Siegfried Albinus (1697–1770) and William Hunter (1718–1783) (Lynch 1920) were the first anatomists to demonstrate that the sacro-iliac joint was a true synovial joint. Von Luschka, in 1854, was the first to classify the joint as diarthrodial. In 1909, Albee's studies confirmed that the joint was lined with a synovial membrane and contained by a well-formed articular capsule. It wasn't until 1938 that the variations in the articular cartilage lining the iliac and sacral surfaces were noted (Schunke 1938).

Mobility of the sacro-iliac joint has been recognized since the 17th century; however, the specific articular biomechanics are still unvalidated (Vleeming 1990). Since the middle of the 19th century, both post-mortem and in vivo studies have been done in an attempt to clarify the movements of the sacro-iliac joints and the pubic symphysis and the axes about which these movements occur (Meyer 1878, Albee 1909, Goldthwait & Osgood 1905, Sashin 1930, Weisl 1954, 1955, Colachis et al 1963, Egund et al 1978, Wilder et al 1980, Lavignolle et al 1983, Walheim & Selvik 1984, Miller et al 1987, Sturesson et al 1989, Dijkstra et al 1989, Vleeming et al 1990b, Vleeming 1990).

Briefly, the investigative methods include manual manipulation of the sacro-iliac joint both at surgery and in a cadaver (Fothergill 1896, Jarcho 1929, Chamberlain 1930, Lavignolle et al 1983), X-ray analysis in various postures of the trunk and lower extremity (Albee 1909, Brooke 1924), roentgen stereophotogrammetric and sterioradiographs after the insertion of tantalum balls into the innominate bone and sacrum (Egund et al 1978,

Walheim & Selvik 1984, Sturesson et al 1989), and inclinometer measurements in various postures of the trunk and lower extremity after the insertion of Kirschner wires into the innominate bone and sacrum (Pitkin & Pheasant 1936, Colachis et al 1963).

The results of these studies have lead to proposals of both function and consequently dysfunction of the pelvic girdle.

ANATOMY

Sacro-iliac joint

The sacro-iliac joint is classified as a synovial joint or diarthrosis (Bowen & Cassidy 1981). The L-shaped articular surface of the sacrum is contained entirely by the costal elements of the first three sacral segments

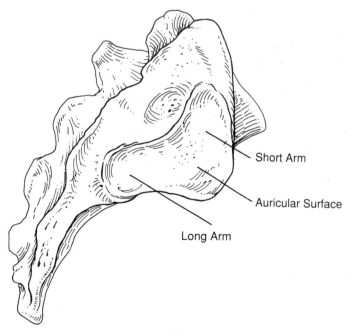

Fig. 10.1 The lateral aspect of the sacrum. (Reproduced with permission from Lee 1989 and the publishers Churchill Livingstone.)

131

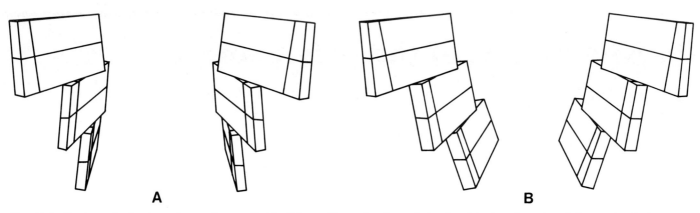

Fig. 10.2 Steriometric drawings of two pelves studied by Solonen illustrating the variation found in the orientation of the sacral articular surface. (Redrawn from Solonen 1957 and reproduced with permission from Lee 1989 and the publishers Churchill Livingstone.)

Table 10.1 Orientation of the articular surface of the sacrum in the coronal and transverse planes*

Coronal plane	
90% narrow inferiorly at S1	A & B in Figure 10.2
85% narrow inferiorly at S2	B in Figure 10.2
80% narrow superiorly at S3	A in Figure 10.2
Transverse plane	
S1 and S2 narrow posteriorly	
S3 narrows anteriorly	

* Solonen 1957.

(Fig. 10.1). The short arm lies in a cephalocaudad plane within the first sacral segment. The long arm lies in an anteroposterior plane within the second and third sacral segments. The contours of the articular surface are highly variable, depending upon the age of the individual (Weisl 1954, Solonen 1957, Kapandji 1974, Bowen & Cassidy 1981, Walker 1984, 1986, Lee 1989, Vleeming et al 1990a, Vleeming 1990). The orientation of the articular surface of the sacrum in both the coronal and the transverse planes has been studied by Solonen (Table 10.1) (Fig. 10.2). Grieve notes that 'Each joint exhibits at least two planes slightly angulated to one another and often three — their disposition and area are not always similar when sides are compared in the same individual' (Grieve 1981). The L-shaped articular surface of the ilium is found on the medial aspect of the bone and its orientation follows that of the sacrum.

Several investigators have noted (Schunke 1938, Bowen & Cassidy 1981, Walker 1986, Vleeming et al 1990a, Vleeming 1990) the macroscopic and microscopic differences between the iliac and sacral articular cartilage. The ilium is lined with a type of fibrocartilage (Bowen & Cassidy 1981) which is bluer, duller and more striated than the hyaline cartilage which lines the sacrum (Fig. 10.3). Paquin et al (1983), in contradiction, concluded from their histological, biochemical research that the iliac cartilage was a special form of hyaline cartilage. The sacral hyaline cartilage is 3–5 times thicker than the iliac fibrocartilage (Fig. 10.4) (Schunke 1938, MacDonald & Hunt 1951, Bowen & Cassidy 1981, Vleeming et al 1990a, Vleeming 1990).

In most specimens, ridges and depressions can be found in both the cartilage and the underlying bone. The sinusoidal nature of these curves increases with advancing age, and they are also noted to be more frequent in males (Fig. 10.5) (Vleeming et al 1990a, Vleeming 1990).

By the third decade the superficial layers of the iliac fibrocartilage are fibrillated, and crevice formation and erosion has begun. In the fourth and fifth decades, in both men and women, the articular surfaces increase in irregularity and coarseness (Fig. 10.6) (Vleeming et al 1990a, Vleeming 1990). Plaque formation and peripheral erosion of cartilage can progress to subchondral sclerosis of bone on the iliac side (Bowen & Cassidy 1981). The articular capsule thickens and para-articular osteophytosis may be present. Even with these anatomical changes, Vleeming et al, in a sacro-iliac joint mobility study of four

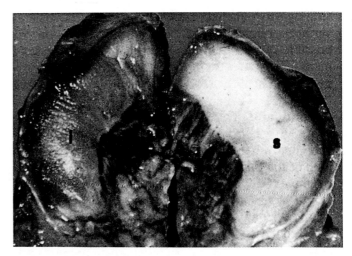

Fig. 10.3 Sacro-iliac joint of a male, 3 years of age (the sacral surface is on the right). Note the dull, striated fibrocartilage which lines the articular surface of the ilium. (Reproduced with permission from Bowen & Cassidy 1981 and the publishers Harper and Row.)

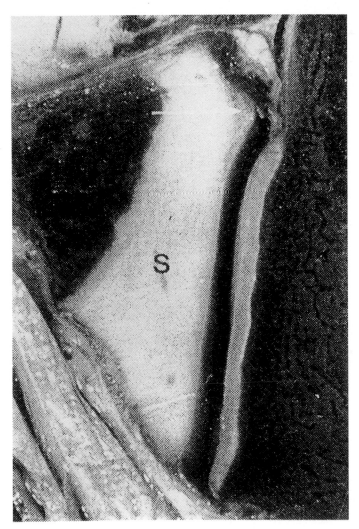

Fig. 10.4 A coronal section through the sacro-iliac joint of a male 12 years of age. Note the planar articular surface as well as the variation in the depth of the articular cartilage. S indicates the sacral side of the joint. (Reproduced with permission from Vleeming et al 1990 and the publishers Harper and Row.)

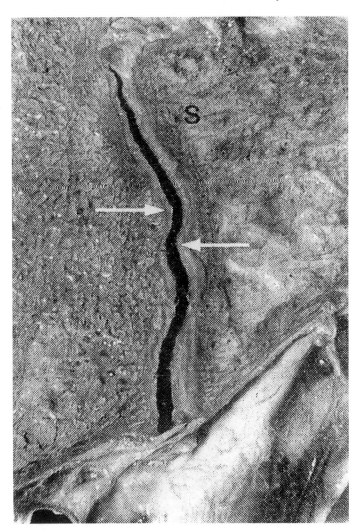

Fig. 10.5 A coronal section through the sacro-iliac joint of a male over 60 years of age. Note the sinusoidal nature of the articular surface as well as the reduction in articular cartilage. (Reproduced with permission from Vleeming et al 1990 and the publishers Harper and Row.)

cadavers aged 65–82 years, noted that 'Most sacroiliac joints were mobile, allowing for the combination of nutation and contranutation — total rotation of up to 4 (degrees). In younger persons larger rotation can be expected' (Vleeming et al 1990c). Since the total range of motion is small, even in youth, any study of articular biomechanics of the sacro-iliac joint should be done on specimens younger than 40 years.

The joint capsule is composed of two layers, an external fibrous layer which contains abundant fibroblasts, blood vessels and collagen fibres, and an inner synovial layer (Bowen & Cassidy 1981). The capsule is supported by overlying ligaments, some of which are the strongest in the body. They include the ventral sacro-iliac ligament, interosseus sacro-iliac ligament, dorsal sacro-iliac ligament, sacrotuberous ligament, sacrospinous ligament and the iliolumbar ligament. Vleeming et al (1989a, b) in two very

interesting studies on the influence of the sacrotuberous ligament on the motion of the sacro-iliac joint, confirms the clinical impression that the sacrotuberous ligament plays a significant role in stabilizing the sacrum against 'nutation' or forward rotation when subjected to vertical loading. He also notes that the gluteus maximus, piriformis and occasionally the biceps femoris muscles have direct attachment into the sacrotuberous ligament, and that contraction of these muscles increases the tension within the ligament and thus provides a dynamic support.

Pubic symphysis

This articulation contains a fibrocartilagenous disc and has no synovial tissue or fluid; it is therefore classified as a symphysis. The fibrocartilagenous disc separates a thin

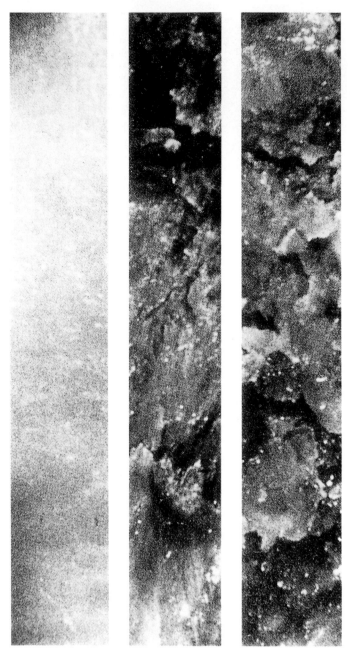

Fig. 10.6   Photomicrographs of the iliac fibrocartilage of (**left**) a male 12 years of age, and (**centre, right**) males over 60 years of age. (Reproduced with permission from Vleeming et al 1990 and the publishers Harper and Row.)

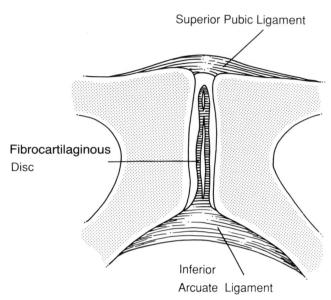

Fig. 10.7   A coronal section through the pubic symphysis. (Redrawn from Kapandji 1974 and reproduced with permission from Lee 1989 and the publishers Churchill Livingstone.)

this stability is vital to both the kinetic and kinematic function of the pelvic girdle.

KINEMATICS OF THE PELVIC GIRDLE

Terminology

'Osteokinematics' refers to the study of motion of bones (Williams et al 1989). 'All bones move at joints, but the kinematics of a bone does not require any inquiry into the kinematics of the joint at which the bones move. The bone is considered simply as an object moving in space, an object that can be studied without opening the joint' (MacConaill & Basmajian 1977). 'Arthrokinematics' refers to the study of motion of joints. 'Intra-articular kinematics or arthrokinematics has to do with the movement of one articular surface upon another ... Articular surfaces can spin and/or slide upon each other' (MacConaill & Basmajian 1977).

Osteokinematics of the pelvic girdle

'Traditionally, motion of the pelvis has been considered one of the primary parameters in any investigation of human locomotion. However, motion of the pelvis is not to be confused with motion in the pelvis' (Reynolds 1980).

Motion *of the pelvis* can occur in all three body planes, i.e. flexion/extension in the sagittal plane during forward and backward bending, lateral flexion in the coronal plane during side-bending, and axial rotation in the transverse plane during twisting of the trunk. During these habitual movements, motion also occurs *within the pelvis*. The quantity of movement available and the specific axes of

layer of hyaline cartilage which covers the adjacent bones (Fig. 10.7). A cavity is commonly found in the posterosuperior aspect of the disc, though rarely before the age of 10 (Williams et al 1989). This is a non-synovial cavity and may represent a chronological degenerative change. The supporting ligaments of this articulation include the superior pubic ligament, inferior arcuate ligament, posterior pubic ligament and the anterior pubic ligament.

The pubic symphysis is a very stable articulation, and

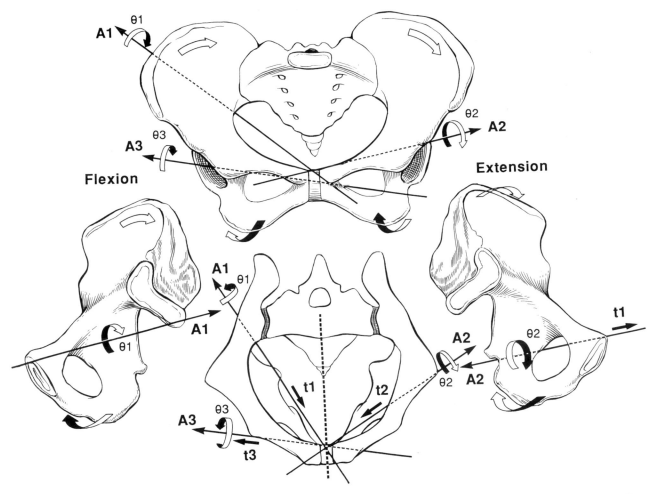

Fig. 10.8 The axes of innominate rotation. **A1.** Posterior rotation of the right innominate bone on the sacrum at the right sacro-iliac joint. **A2.** Anterior rotation of the left innominate bone on the sacrum at the left sacro-iliac joint. **A3.** Posterior rotation of the right innominate bone on the left innominate bone at the pubic symphysis. **t1.** Anterior translation of the right innominate bone at the right sacro-iliac joint which occurs during posterior rotation (A1 motion). **t2.** Anterior translation of the left innominate bone at the left sacro-iliac joint which occurs during anterior rotation (A2 motion). **t3.** Lateral translation of the right innominate bone at the pubic symphysis which occurs during posterior rotation (A3 motion). (Reproduced with permission from Lavignolle et al 1983 and the publishers Springer Verlag.)

innominate and sacral motion are still controversial (Vleeming 1990). Lavignolle's in vivo study (Lavignolle et al 1983) of two women and three men under 25 years of age reported that 10–12° of posterior innominate rotation (flexion) together with 6 mm of anterior translation and 2° of anterior innominate rotation (extension) with 8 mm of anterior translation along the rotary axis is possible. The axis of innominate rotation is not thought to lie in the coronal plane but to run obliquely in a posterolateral direction (Fig. 10.8). The craniocaudal orientation of this axis varies during anteroposterior rotation (Fig. 10.8, A1, A2). This study was conducted in the non-weight-bearing position, and Vleeming (1990) notes that this is probably a significant factor in the quantity of motion reported. Sturesson's in vivo study of 21 women from 19 to 45 years of age, and four men from 18 to 45 years age, was conducted in the weight-bearing position and found that only 2.5° of innominate rotation occurred and that

translation was limited to 0.5–1.6 mm. He felt that the other authors (Weisl 1954, 1955, Colachis et al 1963) had overestimated the mobility within the pelvic girdle.

It appears that while the quantity of motion is still in question, the direction of motion of the innominate bones and the sacrum is agreed.

Forward and backward bending in the sagittal plane

Forward bending of the trunk results in a posterior displacement of the pelvic girdle as a unit which shifts the centre of gravity behind the pedal base (Fig. 10.9). The innominate bones flex bilaterally on the femoral heads and the sacrum initially flexes and then extends between the two innominate bones with no apparent rotation or lateral bend. The axis of innominate rotation is oblique in a posterolateral direction; the iliac crests and the PSISs approximate while the ischial tuberosities and the ASISs

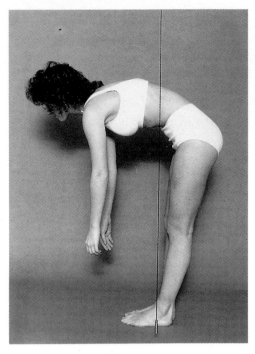

Fig. 10.9 Forward bending of the trunk from the erect standing position. (Reproduced with permission from Lee 1989 and the publishers Churchill Livingstone.)

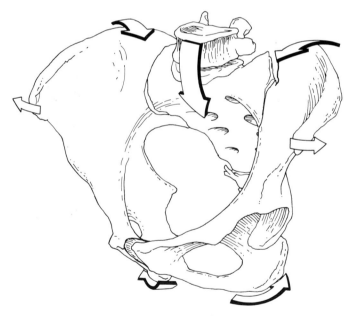

Fig. 10.10 The osteokinematic motion of the pelvic girdle during forward bending of the trunk. (Reproduced with permission from Lee 1989 and the publishers Churchill Livingstone.)

separate (Fig. 10.10) (Weisl 1954, 1955, Colachis et al 1963, Mitchell et al 1979, Lavignolle et al 1983, Dvorak & Dvorak 1984). The opposite rotation of the innominate bones has also been observed (Lee 1989) and is possibly dependent upon the anteroposterior dimension of the sacrum (S1 to S3) in the transverse plane.

Backward bending of the trunk results in an anterior displacement of the pelvic girdle which shifts the centre of gravity anterior to the pedal base. The innominate bones extend bilaterally on the femoral heads and the sacrum relatively flexes between the two innominate bones with no rotation or lateral bend.

Lateral bending in the coronal plane

Side-bending of the trunk on the lower limbs occurs during rapid lateral motion of the body. Left lateral flexion of the pelvic girdle is initiated by displacing the upper legs to the right, thus maintaining the line of gravity central within the pedal base (Fig. 10.11). The pelvic girdle as a unit laterally flexes to the left. Within the pelvic girdle itself, right intrapelvic torsion occurs (Lee 1989). During this motion, the right innominate bone posteriorly rotates relative to the anteriorly rotating left innominate bone and the sacrum rotates to the right (Fig. 10.12). The innominate bones are the driving force behind the sacral rotation during both lateral flexion and rotation (Pitkin & Pheasant 1936). Rotation of the sacrum occurs about an oblique axis. The exact location of this axis has yet to be determined via scientific methods. The rotary axis cannot be vertical since right sacral rotation results in a deepening of the left sacral sulcus, an anterior displacement of the left sacral base, a shallowing of the right sacral sulcus, a posterior displacement of the right sacral base, a posterior displacement of the right inferior lateral angle of the sacrum, and an anterior displacement of the left inferior lateral angle of the sacrum (Lee 1989). These positional

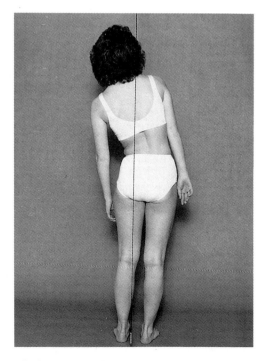

Fig. 10.11 Left lateral bending of the trunk. (Reproduced with permission from Lee 1989 and the publishers Churchill Livingstone.)

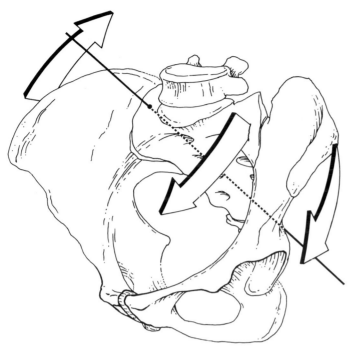

Fig. 10.12 The osteokinematic motion of the pelvic girdle during left lateral bending of the trunk. (Reproduced with permission from Lee 1989 and the publishers Churchill Livingstone.)

relationships of the sacrum to the coronal body plane suggest an oblique axis of sacral rotation.

Axial rotation in the transverse plane

During left axial rotation, the pelvic girdle as a unit rotates to the left on the displaced femoral heads. Within the pelvic girdle itself, left intrapelvic torsion occurs. The right innominate bone anteriorly rotates, the left innominate bone posteriorly rotates, and both bones passively drive the sacrum into left rotation.

Arthrokinematics of the pelvic girdle

The arthrokinematics of the sacro-iliac joint are still hypothetical. The early investigators (Meyer 1878, Pitkin & Pheasant 1936, Pratt 1952) felt that sacral flexion/extension occurred about a stationary transverse axis requiring an inferior glide of the sacrum along the short arm of the articular surface together with a posterior glide along the long arm. In 1954, Weisl refuted this theory of sacral rotation about a fixed transverse axis noting that the arcuate groove and gutter along which the articular

surfaces were proposed to slide appeared only later in life and that overriding of the reciprocal elevations and depressions would lead to a wide separation of the articular surfaces. He felt that separately each sacro-iliac joint could move both supero-inferiorly and postero-anteriorly, but when the two joints were conjoined at the pubic symphysis, only the postero-anterior movement could occur. Anterior translation of the innominate bone (6–8 mm) conjoined with both anterior and posterior rotation of the innominate bone has been confirmed (Lavignolle et al 1983), although the quantity of this translation is disputed (0.5–1.6 mm) (Sturesson et al 1989).

The arthrokinematics which occur during sacral rotation have not been studied, although several theories have been proposed (Pratt 1952, Mitchell et al 1979, Fowler 1986). It has been suggested (Beal 1982, Meadows 1985) that sacro-iliac joint motion may in fact be due to deformation of the thick intra-articular cartilage rather than specific sliding of the articular surfaces.

Both vertical and lateral translation (2 mm) of the pubis bone has been noted (Walheim & Selvik 1984) to occur at the pubic symphysis in active straight-leg raising, standing on alternating legs and unilateral abduction of the hip. As well, sagittal rotation (flexion/extension) about a paracoronal axis and coronal rotations (abduction/adduction) about a sagittal axis of up to 3° have been reported (Fig. 10.8) (Walheim & Selvik 1984).

CONCLUSION

Significant knowledge pertaining to the anatomy and biomechanics of the pelvic girdle has accrued over the last 50 years. Today, the chronological changes in the anatomy of the sacro-iliac joint are well known and this knowledge is reflected in the subjects recruited for kinematic research of the pelvic girdle. The in vivo research appears to be moving towards validating or refuting the biomechanical theories of function upon which clinicians have based the examination and treatment of dysfunction within the pelvic girdle (Lee 1989). As biomechanics of the region are more fully understood, examination and treatment specificity will follow.

Acknowledgements

The author would like to gratefully acknowledge the assistance of Frank Crymble who prepared the original line drawings in this chapter.

REFERENCES

Albee F H 1909 A study of the anatomy and the clinical importance of the sacroiliac joint. Journal of the American Medical Association 53: 1273–1276

Beal M C 1982 The sacroiliac problem: review of anatomy, mechanics, and diagnosis. Journal of the American Osteopathic Association

81: 667–679

Bowen V, Cassidy J D 1981 Macroscopic and microscopic anatomy of the sacroiliac joint from embryonic life until the eighth decade. Spine 6: 620–628

Brooke R 1924 The sacro-iliac joint. Journal of Anatomy 58: 299–305

Chamberlain W E 1930 The symphysis pubis in the roentgen examination of the sacroiliac joint. American Journal of Roentgenology 24: 621–625

Colachis S C, Worden R E, Bechtol C O, Strohm B R 1963 Movement of the sacroiliac joint in the adult male: a preliminary report. Archives of Physical Medicine and Rehabilitation 44 : 490–498

Dijkstra P F, Vleeming A, Stoeckart R 1989 Complex motion tomography of the sacroiliac joint. Fortschritte auf dem Gebiete der Rontgenstrahlen und der Nuklearmedizin 150: 635–642

Dvorak J, Dvorak V 1984 Manual medicine diagnostics. Thieme Stratton, New York

Egund N, Olsson T H, Schmid H 1978 Movements in the sacro-iliac joints demonstrated with roentgen stereophotogammetry. Acta Radiologica 19: 833–846

Fothergill W E 1896 Walcher's position in parturition. British Medical Journal 2 : 1290–1292

Fowler C 1986 Muscle energy techniques for pelvic dysfunction. In: Grieve G P (ed) Modern manual therapy of the vertebral column. Churchill Livingstone, Edinburgh

Goldthwait J E, Osgood R B 1905 A consideration of the pelvic articulations from an anatomical, pathological and clinical standpoint. Boston Medical and Surgical Journal 152: 593–602

Grieve G P 1981 Common vertebral joint problems. Churchill Livingstone, Edinburgh, p 29

Jarcho J 1929 Value of walcher position in contracted pelvis with special reference to its effect on true conjugate diameter. Surgery, Gynecology and Obstetrics 49: 854–858

Kapandji I A 1974 The physiology of joints III: the trunk and vertebral column, 2nd edn. Churchill Livingstone, Edinburgh, pp 58–60

Lavignolle B, Vital J M, Senegas J et al 1983 An approach to the functional anatomy of the sacroilliac joints in vivo. Anatomia Clinica 5: 169–176

Lee D 1989 The pelvic girdle: an approach to the examination and treatment of the lumbo-pelvic-hip region. Churchill Livingstone, Edinburgh

Lynch F W 1920 The pelvic articulations during pregnancy, labor, and the puerperium. Surgery, Gynecology and Obstetrics 30: 575–580

MacConaill M A, Basmajian J V 1977 Muscles and movements; a basis for human kinesiology, 2nd edn. Krieger, New York, chs 2, 3

MacDonald G R, Hunt T E 1951 Sacro-iliac joints observations on the gross and histological changes in the various age groups. Canadian Medical Association Journal 66: 157–163

Meadows J 1984 Pelvic arthro kinetics. In: Gilraine F, Sweeting L (eds) Proceedings of the Fifth International Seminar on Manual Therapy, International Federation of Orthopaedic Manipulative Therapists, Vancouver, p 96–99

Meyer G H 1878 Der mechanismus der symphysis sacroiliaca. Archiv für Anatomie und Physiologie 1: 1–19

Miller J A A, Schultz A B, Andersson G B J 1987 Load–displacement behavior of sacroiliac joints. Journal of Orthopaedic Research 5: 92–101

Mitchell F L, Moran P S, Pruzzo N A 1979 An evaluation and treatment manual of osteopathic muscle energy procedures. Mitchell, Moran and Pruzzo, Missouri

Paquin J D, Van der Rest M, Marie P J, Mort J S, Pidoux I, Poole A R, Roughley P J 1983 Biochemical and morphologic studies of cartilage from the adult human sacroiliac joint. Arthritis and Rheumatism 26: 887–894

Pitkin H C, Pheasant H C 1936 Sacroarthrogenetic telalagia II. A study of sacral mobility. Journal of Bone and Joint Surgery 18: 365–374

Pratt W A 1952 The lumbopelvic torsion syndrome. Journal of the American Osteopathic Association 51: 97–103

Reynolds H M 1980 Three-dimensional kinematics in the pelvic girdle. Journal of the American Osteopathic Association 80: 277–280

Sashin D 1930 A critical analysis of the anatomy and the pathologic changes of the sacro-iliac joints. Journal of Bone and Joint Surgery 12: 891–910

Schunke G B 1938 The anatomy and development of the sacroiliac joint in man. Anatomical Record 72: 313–331

Solonen K A 1957 The sacro-iliac joint in the light of anatomical roentgenological and clinical studies. Acta Orthopaedica Scandinavia Supplement 27 9–127

Sturesson B, Selvik G, Uden A 1989 Movements of the sacroiliac joints. A roentgen stereophotogrammetric analysis. Spine 14: 162–165

Vleeming A 1990 The sacro-iliac joint. A clinical-anatomical, biomechanical and radiological study. Rotterdam

Vleeming A, Stoeckart R, Snijders C J 1989a The sacrotuberous ligament: a conceptual approach to its dynamic role in stabilizing the sacro-iliac joint. Clinical Biomechanics 4: 201–203

Vleeming A, Van Wingerden J P, Snijders C J, Stoeckart R, Stijnen T 1989b Load application to the sacrotuberous ligament: influences on sacro-iliac joint mechanics. Clinical Biomechanics 4: 204–209

Vleeming A, Stoeckart R, Volkers A C W, Snijders C J 1990a Relation between form and function in the sacroiliac joint. Part I: Clinical anatomical aspects. Spine 15: 130–132

Vleeming A, Stoeckart R, Volkers A C W, Snijders C J 1990b Relation between form and function in the sacroiliac joint. Part II: Biomechanical aspects. Spine 15: 133–135

Vleeming A, Van Wingerden J P, Dykstra P F, Stoeckart R, Snijders D J, Stijnen T 1990c Mobility in the SI-joints at high age; a kinematic and roentgenologic study. In: Vleeming A The sacro-iliac joint. A clinical-anatomical, biomechanical and radiological study. Rotterdam

Walheim G G, Selvik G 1984 Mobility of the pubic symphysis. Clinical Orthopaedics and Related Research 191: 129–135

Walker J M 1984 Age changes in the sacroiliac joint and their importance to manual therapy. In: Gilraine F, Sweeting L (eds) Proceedings of the Fifth International Seminar on Manual Therapy, International Federation of Orthopaedic Manipulative Therapists, Vancouver, p 250–257

Walker J M 1986 Age-related differences in the human sacroiliac joint: a histological study; implications for therapy. Journal of Orthopaedic and Sports Physical Therapy 7: 325–334

Weisl H 1954 The articular surfaces of the sacro-iliac joint and their relation to the movements of the sacrum. Acta Anatomica 22: 1–14

Weisl H 1955 The movements of the sacro-iliac joint. Acta Anatomica 23: 80–91

Wilder D G, Pope M H, Frymoyer J W 1980 The functional topography of the sacroiliac joint. Spine 5: 575–579

Williams P L, Warwick R, Dyson M, Bannister L H (eds) 1989 Gray's anatomy, 37th edn. Churchill Livingstone, Edinburgh

11. Factors influencing ranges of movement in the spine

L. T. Twomey   J. R. Taylor

INTRODUCTION

The vertebral column uniquely combines the opposing qualities of mobility and stability by incorporating a large number of mobile segments, each amphiarthrosis allowing only a few degrees of movement. The thickness of each intervertebral disc, the compliance of its fibrocartilage and the dimensions and shape of its adjacent vertebral end-plates are of primary importance in governing the extent of movement possible. The shape and orientation of the vertebral arch articular facets, with the ligaments and muscles of the arch and its processes, guide the types and amount of movements possible and provide restraints against excessive movement.

At each level in the vertebral column there are three interacting joints allowing and controlling movement. This unique combination is known as the articular triad or the mobile segment. However, in the cervical region, the presence of the uncovertebral joints, which develop from about 8 years of age, add further complexity to the cervical segments. While each articular triad allows only a few degrees of movement, spinal movement usually involves a complex interaction of mobile segments at multiple levels. The thickness of each intervertebral disc, the compliance of its fibrocartilage, and the dimensions and shape of its adjacent vertebral end-plates are of primary importance in governing the extent of movement possible.

The anterior elements (vertebrae and discs) of the mobile segments have the potential to allow ranges of movement in different planes depending on disc dimensions (thickness and horizontal dimensions) and disc stiffness.

Disc dimensions

A large range of movement would occur when disc height was relatively great and vertebral end-plate horizontal dimensions relatively short (Fig. 11.1). Adolescent and young adult females have shorter vertebral end-plates (Fig. 11.1, a) than males, while disc height (Fig. 11.1, b1,

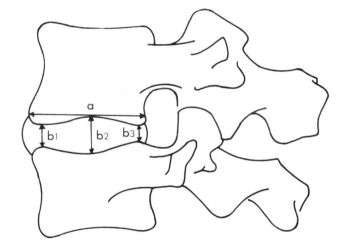

ANTERIOR VERTEBRAL ELEMENTS

a = vertebral end-plate

b = disc thickness

Fig. 11.1 The anterior vertebral elements (mobile segment); a = vertebral end-plate, b = disc thickness.

b2, b3) and disc stiffness are substantially the same. Thus, females possess the necessary combination of dimensions for a larger range of movements than is possible in males (Taylor & Twomey 1984, Twomey & Taylor 1987). In old age, when male and female vertebrae and disc shapes become very similar, and hormonal differences are reduced, the range of movement of the lumbar spine in men and women becomes almost identical (Fig. 11.2).

Disc stiffness

The general reduction in movement ranges in both sexes is attributable to increased disc stiffness. This has been demonstrated by the lumbar posterior release experiment of Twomey and Taylor (1983) which demonstrates a 40% increase in disc stiffness in the elderly.

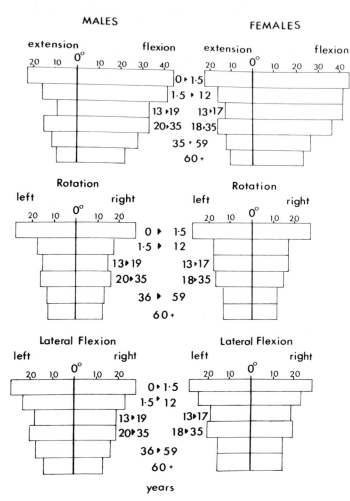

Fig. 11.2 Age changes in the range of lumbar movements in both sexes (Taylor & Twomey 1981a).

tion of facetal joint surfaces (Taylor & Twomey 1986) and by the increasing tension developed in the ligaments and muscles (Vernon-Roberts & Pirie 1977, Adams & Hutton 1983). In the thoracic spine, the presence of the ribs is a major factor in limiting movement and is assisted in this by the forward slope of the facets in the frontal plane (Töndury 1972).

There is considerable individual variation in facetal orientation, both within the three spinal regions and between individuals. Asymmetry of facetal orientation at specific vertebral levels is present in about 30% of all individuals and is known as 'tropism'. Where tropism occurs at a particular level, there is a difference in the motion of that segmental level and a change in the forces imposed on other structures, particularly the intervertebral discs (Hagg & Wallner 1990).

Planes of movement

The movements possible at each spinal motion segment are traditionally described as being in the sagittal (flexion–extension), coronal (lateral flexion), and horizontal (axial rotation) planes. Each movement occurs along one of three coordinate axes: *x*, *y* and *z* (Fig. 11.3). Thus, all mobile segments of the lumbar spine possess 6 degrees of freedom, and each movement consists of an angular or rotary displacement together with translation of a vertebra on its subjacent vertebra. It is rare for movement to occur exclusively in a single plane. Movements are generally 'coupled' in habitual movement (White & Panjabi 1978), and they occur across the standard descriptive planes of motion.

CONTROL OF THE DIRECTIONS OF MOVEMENT

It is the posterior elements of the vertebral column which are responsible for directing and controlling spinal movement. Thus, the articular facets and ligament and muscles of the vertebral column govern the type and extent of movement possible at each spinal level. Facet orientation differs significantly in each of the three functional spinal regions and largely determines the direction and amounts of movement available. Thus, in the cervical spine, the facetal surfaces which are 45° to the horizontal encourage a significant amount of motion in all three planes and provide very little protection for the intervertebral discs. Movement ranges are thus limited by ligament and muscle tension and not by bone apposition. However, in the lumbar spine, the vertical and largely sagittal orientation of the strong biplanar joint facets provides a very effective 'block' to the movements of extension, axial rotation and side flexion. Lumbar flexion is limited by both the apposi-

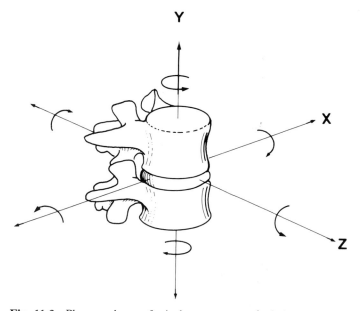

Fig. 11.3 Planes and axes of spinal movement: sagittal plane movements occur about the x axis, coronal plane movements occur about the z axis, and horizontal plane movements around the y axis.

THE LUMBAR SPINE

In recent years, the movements and mechanics of the lumbar spine have received more concentrated research attention than have cervical and thoracic regions. Furthermore, most of the principles of movement and mechanical behaviour originally established for the lumbar spine are applicable to the other regions. For these reasons, the movements of the lumbar spine will be considered first and in greater detail.

Ranges of lumbar movement

Despite the availability of simple, reliable methods for measuring spinal mobility, these have not been applied to studies of normal spine movement until recently. The literature records considerable variation in the values given for the ranges of movements of the lumbar spine. This variation stems largely from the different measurement methods used and the differences in age, sex, race, and numbers of subjects studied. The clinical measurements most frequently used include indirect estimates of spinal mobility from measurement of (i) the distance from the fingertips to the floor when the patient bends forward, and (ii) the use of a tape measure to measure the increase in distance between two skin landmarks, often the S1 and L1 spinous processes. These methods are inaccurate, and they give no direct measure of the range (angular deflection) of spinal movement. The former is dependent on hamstring muscle length and the latter fails to show a reasonable level of consistency between repeated measures. Published studies of lumbar spinal movement have concentrated mostly on sagittal and coronal plane movements and include:

1. Direct measurement in living subjects, utilizing a wide variety of equipment (Dunham 1949, Leighton 1966, Lindahl 1966, Gregersen & Lucas 1967, Moll & Wright 1976, Taylor & Twomey 1981a)
2. Radiographic studies (Wiles 1935, Tanz 1953, Rolander 1966, Froning & Frohman 1968)
3. Cadaveric studies that have mostly involved a single mobile segment in a small number of specimens (Virgin 1951, Hirsch 1955, Rolander 1966, King & Vulcan 1971, Panjabi 1977, Twomey 1981)
4. Photographic techniques (Keegan 1953, Davis et al 1965)
5. Theoretical studies based on mathematical models (Panjabi 1973, Schultz et al 1973, Gracovetsky et al 1977).

Estimates of the range of sagittal motion of the lumbar region vary widely from 121° in a young male acrobat (Wiles 1935), to 21.8° in elderly women (Tanz 1953). However, Begg and Falconer (1949) considered 70° to be the 'normal' average total range of lumbar flexion-extension. Few studies have attempted to measure axial rotation in the lumbar spine, largely because of methodological problems. It has proven difficult to measure lumbar rotation in the living either directly or radiographically with any degree of accuracy, and cadaveric studies have been confined mostly to motion segments rather than to the whole lumbar column. Some authorities maintain that rotary movement does not exist as a separate entity in the lumbar region (Kapandji 1974), or that if rotation does occur, it is in spite of the fact that the facets are designed to prevent it (Lewin et al 1961). Other sources have assessed the total range of rotation as between 5 and 36° of movement (Gregersen & Lucas 1967, Lumsden & Morris 1968, Loebl 1973).

Clinical measurement

In an effort to provide instrumentation that would be relatively easily applied in the clinical situation and provide reasonably accurate objective data, two instruments have been devised to measure lumbar sagittal- and horizontal-plane movement, and have been tested in clinical trials (Farrell & Twomey 1982, Twomey & Taylor 1987). The lumbar spondylometer is non-invasive, has good inter-person and inter-test reliability, and measures lumbar sagittal motion (Fig. 11.4). Since its base rests on the sacrum, the measurement is not confounded and invalidated by the inclusion of hip motion. Tests of its accuracy made by comparing living subjects with fresh, cadaveric specimens suggest that it underestimates the range of movement by an average of 1° (Twomey 1981). Inter- and intra-operator repeatability trials show high correlation (Farrell & Twomey 1982). The lumbar spondylometer is comparable in accuracy and in some respects in principle to an inclinometer, but with a more complex geometry (Dunham 1949); it is also easier to use in a clinical situation where separate readings from two inclinometers would be required. Its use requires a thorough knowledge of the surface anatomy of the lumbar region, with consistently accurate placement of the cushions, and the precise location of the L1 process.

Similarly, the external measurement of lumbar rotation in the clinical situation has been made possible by the development of the lumbar rotameter (Taylor & Twomey 1981a). It is a reliable instrument, the measurements correlate well with those from cadaveric spines, and it shows a maximum variation of 5° in a total range of 56° (Twomey & Taylor 1987). However, the apparatus is cumbersome, and for that reason it is generally preferred as a research tool rather than as a commonly used clinical instrument.

Ranges of lumbar movement for both sexes in six age-group categories using the spondylometer and the rotameter together with the gravity inclinometer (Leighton 1966) for side flexion are listed in Table 11.1.

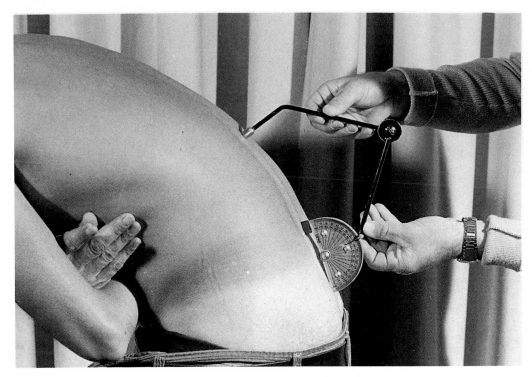

Fig. 11.4   The lumbar spondylometer.

Age changes in ranges of movements

Table 11.1 clearly demonstrates a decline in the ranges of all lumbar movements in the living with increasing age. This decline parallels the reductions observed in cadaveric studies by other authors (Tanz 1953, Allbrook 1957, Hilton et al 1979, Twomey 1981, Nachemson 1985).

In old age the ranges of lumbar movement in men and women become almost identical. It would appear that when hormonal differences are reduced, sexual differentiations in vertebral shape, posture, and spinal-movement ranges disappear.

The general reduction in ranges in both sexes occurs as a result of increased 'stiffening' of the intervertebral disc in association with disc-shape changes involving increases in the antero-posterior length and concavity of the vertebral end-plate (Twomey & Taylor 1983).

A reason often provided for the decline in average ranges of movements in ageing populations (i.e. a general

tendency to thinning of intervertebral discs in old age) has recently been shown to be false (Taylor & Twomey 1981a, Twomey & Taylor 1985a, b). In old age most discs increase in volume, become thicker centrally, and more convex at the disc–vertebra interface. Only about 30% of discs become thinner. The principal reason for decreased range of movement is increased disc stiffness (Twomey & Taylor 1983).

The 40% increase in disc stiffness with age is associated with well-documented histological and biochemical changes. These include an increase in the total number of collagen fibres and in the ratio of type I to type II collagen; a decrease in water content; and a change in the proteoglycan ratios where the proportion of keratin sulphate:chondroitin sulphate increases (Adams et al 1977, Bushell et al 1977). There is also an associated increase in 'fatigue failure' of collagen in older cartilage. It is uncertain whether it is collagen fibres that undergo 'fatigue' or

Table 11.1   The mean and standard deviation for the total ranges of sagittal, horizontal and coronal plane movements in living subjects (population 960 persons)

Age	Sagittal range (flexion–extension)		Horizontal range (rotation to both sides)		Coronal range (side flexion)	
	male	female	male	female	male	female
5–12 years	58° ± 9°	58° ± 9°	34° ± 6°	34° ± 6°	47° ± 6°	47° ± 6°
13–19 Years	45° ± 10°	57° ± 8°	30° ± 4°	34° ± 4°	38° ± 5°	37° ± 4°
19–35 years	42° ± 6°	42° ± 7°	33° ± 6°	33° ± 6°	40° ± 5°	40° ± 5°
35–59 years	38° ± 7°	38° ± 9°	26° ± 6°	27° ± 6°	32° ± 4°	30° ± 3°
60+ years	30° ± 7°	28° ± 9°	22° ± 5°	20° ± 4°	28° ± 4°	30° ± 5°

splitting or whether it is collagen fibres that separate (Stockwell 1979). Collectively, these changes and the associated decrease in compliance render the disc fibrocartilage less capable of acting efficiently as a shock absorber or joint, and of evenly transmitting loads along the vertebral column (Nachemson 1976, Twomey & Taylor 1983).

Control of flexion

Muscular control of flexion

The lumbar back muscles exert considerable control over active ranges of lumbar movement. Erector spinae and multifidis are principally responsible for all movements by active contraction in extension and by exerting an eccentric control (i.e. by paying out) on movements that are gravity-assisted. Thus, trunk flexion in standing or sitting is controlled by an eccentric contraction of these muscle groups. In exerting this control, the muscles tend to restrict the total range of movements that the joints and ligaments would allow, particularly in the sagittal plane (Taylor & Twomey 1981a). This helps to explain why cadaveric studies show a slightly greater range of lumbar sagittal movement than is usually recorded in living subjects (Twomey 1981).

It has been shown that after suitable warm-up exercises the ranges of lumbar flexion increase by a few degrees (Taylor & Twomey 1981a), and that a change in posture from the upright posture to the side-lying position brings about an additional increase, giving a total range which equates with the ranges observed in the cadaveric studies. It would appear that warm-up exercises achieve their effect by relaxation or stretching of the sacrospinalis muscle group and by progressive loading of the ligamentous elements, and it is not unreasonable to assume that the slightly larger increase obtained in side-lying is due to the elimination of antigravity activity in the long back muscles. Kippers and Parker (1983) have shown an 'electrically silent' phase in the back muscles at the limit of lumbar flexion. While they conclude that the spine is supported passively by tension in postvertebral connective tissue structures at this point, it may also be due in part to passive elastic tension of the posterior muscles themselves. Indeed, the opposed zygapophyseal facets play the greater restraining role (Twomey & Taylor 1983).

Each lumbar multifidus muscle attaches strongly to a mamillary process on a superior articular process and also into the capsule of a zygapophyseal joint. It acts as a rotator cuff muscle and maintains the approximation and congruity of the zygapophyseal facets on the posterolateral aspect of the joint (the ligamentum flavum maintains the articular surfaces in close apposition on the anteromedial side of the joint). The close relation of this muscle to the joint capsule and its similar innervation would readily explain how, with other postvertebral muscles, it would

severely limit flexion and rotation in any painful condition of the joints.

Other factors controlling lumbar flexion

Adams et al (1980), in a sequential posterior release experiment, quantified the relative parts played by the supraspinous ligamentum flavum, the facet joint ligamentous capsule and the intervertebral disc in resisting flexion of individual lumbar mobile segments. They concluded that the capsular ligaments and the intervertebral disc play the most important roles, with the ligamentum flavum and the supraspinous interspinous ligaments making lesser contributions. They remark that it is surprising that the relatively unimpressive capsular ligaments should exert such large restraining forces and admit to technical problems in sectioning all capsular fibres — thus making it difficult to distinguish the role of capsular forces from articular facet forces exerted through the bony articular processes.

However, Twomey and Taylor (1983) showed that it is the intact facetal joints which have a greater restraining influence than the ligamentous complex in flexion, as well as in extension (Fig. 11.5). Their associated radiological study demonstrates that in the intact osteo-ligamentous spine there is 2–3 mm of ventral translation of one vertebra on the next which occurs with the forward rotation component of flexion. The lumbar facets guide the forward rotation and resist the ventral slide, and when the pedicles are cut, a greater amount of ventral slide accompanies further rotation. Thus, ventral zygapophyseal joint loading increases to the point where the articular forces act so as to prevent further flexion. The lumbar bony

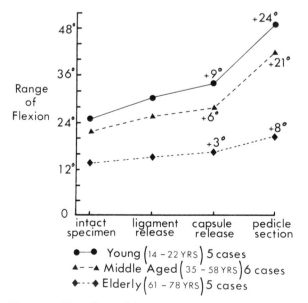

"POSTERIOR RELEASE": EFFECT on RANGE of FLEXION

Fig. 11.5 The effects of the serial release of the posterior vertebral elements on the range of lumbar flexion (Twomey & Taylor 1983).

vertebral arches thus provide an essential restraint, preventing transmission of shearing stresses to the intervertebral discs leading to instability, with danger to the caude equina and nerve roots in the intervertebral canals.

There are interesting age differences in the flexion responses to the sectioning procedure. Following ligamentous release, and also — more dramatically — following pedicle section, the 'available' increase in movement range is much reduced in elderly subjects compared to young subjects. This shows that the compliance of young discs is much greater, and that changes in the stiffness of intervertebral discs which occur with age are mainly responsible for the observed decrease in lumbar range of movement with ageing.

'Creep' in the lumbar spine. Stiffness in intervertebral discs and the progressive loading of the zygapophyseal joints are the factors bringing the normal range of flexion to a halt. However, sustained loading in flexion does produce further flexion of the spine. This movement is due to 'creep', which is the progressive deformation of a structure, in this case the vertebral column, under constant load when the forces are not large enough to cause permanent damage to the vertebral structures.

Axial 'creep'. In the normal erect posture, approximately 12–25% of axial compressive load on the lumbar spine is borne by the zygapophyseal joints, while the rest is carried by the intervertebral discs (Nachemson 1960, Miller et al 1983), which are well suited to this purpose. When axial loads to intervertebral discs are maintained, the discs progressively lose height until the chemical forces developed within them equal those mechanical forces applied externally (Kazarian 1975). Provided that the forces used are below the levels that would cause permanent damage, then the greater the external force the greater the loss of height that occurs (Kazarian 1975).

During the day, a person's body weight acts as an axial compression force through the vertebral column, and the subsequent 'creep' brings about a reduction in stature. When body weight is relieved (e.g. at night in bed) and axial loads are reduced, the intervertebral discs and other soft tissues are able to rehydrate and stature increases (Koreska et al 1977). It has recently been demonstrated that a period of rest in full flexion brings about a more rapid increase in stature than does rest in the fully extended position (Tyrell et al 1985). This presumably occurs because flexion acts as a distracting force on the lumbar region, causing the discs to 'imbibe' water at a greater rate.

'Creep' in flexion. When full range lumbar flexion is maintained under load for a period of time, the articular triad is distorted so that the anterior disc region is 'squeezed' while the posterior region is stretched; the zygapophyseal joint surfaces are compressed tightly together as the coronal part of the articular surfaces bear most of the load, and the soft tissues adjust by 'creep'

(Kazarian 1975, Twomey & Taylor 1982). 'Creep' in flexion is observed as progressive ventral movement into further flexion, so that the end-point of flexion is increased (i.e. range increases). The amount of 'creep' in the elderly is greater than in the young, and both the 'creep' and the recovery from 'creep' take place over a longer period of time. During the process, fluid is extruded from the soft tissues and they become relatively deprived of their nutrition (Adams & Hutton 1983). Repetitive loading causes cartilage degeneration and bone hypertrophy in the various elements of the articular triad (Taylor & Twomey 1986).

If the amount of 'creep' involved after prolonged load bearing in flexion is considerable, then recovery back to the original starting posture (hysteresis) is extremely slow. It takes considerable time for the soft tissues to imbibe fluid after is has been expressed during prolonged flexion loading. Many occupational groups (e.g. stonemasons, bricklayers, roofing carpenters and the like) regularly submit their lumbar spines to this category of insult. They work with their lumbar column fully flexed and under load for considerable periods of time. There is often little movement away from the fully flexed position once it has been reached, and little opportunity for recovery between episodes of work in this position. It is therefore not at all surprising to find so many bricklayers, for instance, with chronic back pain and with occasional episodes of acute pain. These occupational groups need considerable ergonomic advice and require alterations to their working conditions if this situation is to be rectified (Twomey et al 1988).

Control of extension

The control of lumbar extension has not been investigated and analysed to quite the same extent as flexion. In the erect standing or sitting postures, the movement is initiated by contraction of the long back-extensor muscles, and then controlled by the eccentric contraction of the abdominal muscle group once the movement has begun. The range of extension from the neutral erect standing position is much less than the range of flexion, but the muscular control mechanisms are very similar.

The range of extension is not controlled by ligamentous tension, but ceases when the two inferior articular processes at any level are forced against the laminae of the vertebrae below, or perhaps when the spinous processes 'kiss'. This is witnessed by the build-up of compact bone in the lamina beneath the inferior joint recess. Extension occurs around an axis in the posterior part of the intervertebral disc at that level. This position probably does not place the soft tissues under the same constant strain as flexion does except at the limits of lordosis after prolonged standing when zygapophyseal joints probably take a larger amount of the load of body weight. When hyperextension occurs, it is likely that the axis of movement shifts even further posteriorly and is located where the tips of the inferior facets articulate with the laminae. This would cause stretching of the anterior soft tissues, notably the anterior longitudinal ligament and the anterior anulus fibrosus, which are extremely strong and capable of withstanding such forces. It is apparent from our investigations that considerable osteoarthritic change takes place in the articular cartilage and subchondral bone at the inferior polar region of the zygapophyseal joints. These areas correspond to the areas of impact and compression in extension (Twomey & Taylor 1987).

'Creep' in extension. Examples of prolonged maintenance of an extended posture or of loading in extension are rare, and few if any occupational groups have such a working situation. Brunnstrom (1966) describes the position of the line of gravity in erect standing as passing anterior to the thoracic vertebrae and through the lumbar vertebrae. Theoretically, prolonged standing, (i.e. axial loading with body weight) would tend to increase thoracic kyphosis (by 'creep') but not alter lumbar lordosis. However, present evidence indicates that in prolonged standing there is a tendency for the axial load of body weight to increase lumbar lordosis. In this way, the zygapophyseal joints will take an increasing proportion of the load of body weight. Although long, continued loading in lordotic posture is rare, a number of sports activities involve full extension movements of an explosive nature. These may be repetitive movements and may involve high peaks of loading in full extension. Thus, fast bowlers in cricket, gymnasts, and high-jumpers are three groups who place tremendous impact forces through this posterior arch complex. At heel strike during these sports, the chisel-like inferior articular processes are forced down suddenly onto the laminae of the vertebrae below. The forces involved are very considerable, as the load borne by the facets increases dramatically with the amount of extension of the region (Yang & King 1984). Repetition over long periods of time results in soft-tissue inflammation and bone sclerosis that may become obvious on radiographic examination, but which may later result in fracture and perhaps displacement. The bone area that absorbs this force is the isthmus between the zygapophyseal facets, i.e., the pars interarticularis. As is well known, this is the site at which spondylolysis occurs. It is even more likely that the repetitive combination of alternative explosive full extension followed suddenly by full forceful flexion places enormous strain on the pars interarticularis region. This extension/flexion repetition moment at the pars may cause fatigue fracture in a similar way to that of fatigue in metal caused by successive opposite movements (Twomey et al 1988).

Considerable research on the mechanics of this region has taken place in recent years, and the reader is referred to the series of papers on the posterior vertebral elements in the journal *Spine*, Volumes 3 and 4, 1983.

THE CERVICAL SPINE

The general principles of movement as described in the lumbar spine are also applicable to the cervical region. The major differences which modify cervical movement are that cervical discs are proportionally thinner and their horizontal dimensions are smaller than are lumbar discs, and the articular facets provide little stability and protection to the cervical discs. The range of motion available at each segmental level is larger in the cervical spine (in all directions) than in the lumbar spine (White & Panjabi 1978). A large number of instruments have been devised to measure the ranges of cervical movement (Buck et al 1959, Ferlic 1962, De Fibaugh 1964, Newell & Nichols 1965, Leighton 1966, Kadir et al 1981, Tucci et al 1986, Worth 1988). Most clinical and research workers now use Myrin goniometers, usually attached to a helmet (Gooch 1992).

Sagittal motion in the cervical spine involves both the rotation of an upper about a lower vertebra and also considerable ventral translation of the upper vertebra. The ventero-dorsal amount of translation is proportionally greater in the cervical rather than the lumbar spine (White & Panjabi 1978). Both axial creep and creep in flexion are factors which affect the range of motion available in the neck, and little information is currently available on cervical creep under conditions of sustained loading. However, a recent unpublished study of cervical creep in living persons by Gooch (1992), indicates that it is a significant occurrence.

Panjabi et al (1988) published a three-dimensional movement analysis of the upper cervical spine. This comprehensive cadaveric study documented the ranges of all movements available at the atlanto-occipital and atlanto-axial joints. These results are shown in Table 11.2.

They showed that the greatest range of intervertebral movement in the spine was axial rotation at the atlanto-axial level.

In another recent study, Dvorak et al (1988) have provided segmental ranges of sagittal plane movements in 59 living subjects in the cervical spine. Their study clearly showed that the passive range of cervical movement at each level was 2–3° greater than the active range (Table 11.3). This increase in range is almost certainly due to the greater reliance on soft tissues for stability in the neck and on the considerable changes which occur to cervical

Table 11.2 Ranges of movement of the atlanto-occipital (C0–1) and atlanto-axial (C1–2) joints*

	C0–1	C1–2
Flexion	3.5°	11.5°
Extension	21.0°	10.9°
Lateral bending (one side)	10.9°	6.7°
Axial rotation (one side)	6.7°	38.9°

* Adapted from Panjabi et al (1988).

Table 11.3 Ranges of sagittal movement in the cervical spine performed actively and passively*

Level	Active	Passive
C2–3	10	12
C3–4	15	17
C4–5	19	21
C5–6	20	23
C6–7	19	21

* Adapted from Dvorak et al (1988).

Table 11.4 Ranges of sagittal motion (in degrees) in the cervical spine as measured by van Mameren (1988)

C0–1	3.0 →	30.8
C1–2	8.4 →	27.0
C2–3	10.2 →	15.8
C3–4	12.3 →	22.1
C4–5	14.0 →	25.2
C5–6	17.5 →	26.3
C6–7	6.7 →	23.5

intervertebral discs during maturation. Cervical discs progressively show a natural fissuring beginning in the postero-lateral corners of each disc and proceeding across the posterior half of the disc with increasing age (Kraemer 1981, Taylor & Twomey 1991).

In a recent intricate X-ray study of the patterns of motion in the cervical spine, van Mameren et al (1990) from the University of Maastricht in The Netherlands, showed the difficulty in obtaining consistent measurements for cervical sagittal movement. They clearly demonstrated the variability in cervical ranges of sagittal movement in 10 subjects measured in a variety of ways. They were unable to determine whether these problems were time-dependent, due to intra-individual variability as to the direction in which the movement was made (i.e. from full flexion to full extension, or vice-versa) (van Mameren 1988, van Mameren et al 1990). In measuring from full extension to full flexion, van Mameren (1988) found the ranges of segmental sagittal motion from his 10 subjects as given in Table 11.4.

Van Mameren's data on the total range of sagittal movement in the cervical spine averaged 123.8° when measured from full extension to full flexion, and 118.7° when measured from full flexion to full extension. However, he carefully points to the great variability in the data, both within and between individuals, when measured from radiographs of living people.

Horizontal and frontal plane movements in the cervical spine are complex and difficult to measure as the movements of rotation and side-flexion are usually coupled (Worth 1988). Thus, measures of range of either rotation or side-flexion movements are quite variable depending on the amount of coupling involved. For this reason it makes little sense to provide the reader with a chart of ranges of these motions.

The human vertebral column is a complex multi-segmented rod which serves as the axial support of the body, protects the spinal cord, acts as a shock absorber and yet allows for complex movement in all directions. At segmental level, each articular triad of joints adds its own unique contribution to the total pattern of movement which occurs. However, movement can never take place at just one segment, but necessarily involves the interaction over longer spinal lengths, with movement in one region often requiring complementary or compensatory movement in another. Thus, lumbar flexion in forward bending may be associated with cervical extension and/or rotation as the individual maintains the sight of an object. Fundamentally, spinal movement occurs as discs compress and as the orientation and size of the facet joints allow for the extent and direction of movements. When this primary unit is damaged or disturbed, movement disorders (including restriction) will follow.

REFERENCES

Adams M A, Hutton W C 1983 The mechanical function of the lumbar apophyseal joints. Spine 8: 327–330

Adams P, Eyre D R, Muir H 1977 Biochemical aspects of development and ageing of human lumbar intervertebral discs. Rheumatology and Rehabilitation 16: 22–29

Adams M A, Hutton W C, Stott M A 1980 The resistance to flexion of the lumbar intervertebral joint. Spine 5: 245–253

Allbrook D 1957 Movements of the lumbar spinal column. Journal of Bone and Joint Surgery 39B: 339–345

Begg A G, Falconer M A 1949 Plain radiographs in intraspinal protrusion of lumbar intervertebral discs: a correlation with operative findings. British Journal of Surgery 36: 225–239

Brunnstrom S 1966 Clinical kinesiology. 2nd edn. F A Davis, Philadelphia

Buck C A, Dameron F B, Dow M J, Skowlund H V 1959 Study of normal range of motion in the neck utilizing a bubble goniometer. Archives of Physical Medicine and Rehabilitation 60: 390–392

Bushell G R, Gosh P, Taylor F K, Akeson W H 1977 Proteoglycan chemistry of the intervertebral disc. Clinical Orthopaedics and Related Research 129: 115–119

Davis P R, Troup J D G, Burnard J H 1965 Movements of the thoracic and lumbar spine when lifting: a chrono-cyclophotographic study. Journal of Anatomy 199: 13–26

De Fibaugh J J 1964 Measurement of head motion. Pt II. Journal of the American Physical Therapy Association 44: 163–168

Dunham W F 1949 Ankylosing spondylitis: measurement of hip and spine movements. British Journal of Physical Medicine 12: 126–129

Dvorak J, Froehlich D, Penning L, Baumgartner H, Panjabi M M 1988 Functional radiographic diagnosis of the cervical spine. Flexion/extension. Spine 13: 748–755

Farrell J P, Twomey L T 1982 Acute low back pain: comparison of two conservative treatment approaches. Medical Journal of Australia 1(4): 160–164

Ferlic D 1962 The range of motion of the 'Normal' cervical spine. Bulletin of the Johns Hopkins Hospital 110: 59–65

Froning E C, Frohman B 1968 Motion of the lumbosacral spine after laminectomy and spine fusion. Journal of Bone and Joint Surgery 50A: 897–918

Gooch L 1992 In vivo-creep of the cervical spine. Master's degree thesis in preparation. Curtin University, Western Australia

Gracovestky S, Fardan H F, Lamy C 1977 A mathematical model of the lumbar spine using an optimized system to control muscles and ligaments. Orthopedic Clinics of North America 8: 135–153

Gregersen G, Lucas D B 1967 An in-vitro study of the axial rotation of the human thoraco-lumbar spine. Journal of Bone and Joint Surgery 49A: 247–262

Hagg O, Wallner A 1990 Facet joint asymmetry and protrusion of the intervertebral disc. Spine 15: 356

Hilton R C, Ball J, Benn R T 1979 In-vitro mobility of the lumbar spine. Annals of the Rheumatic Diseases 38: 378–383

Hirsch K 1955 The reaction of the intervertebral discs to compression forces. Journal of Bone and Joint Surgery 37A: 1188–1196

Kadir N, Grayson M F, Goldberg A A J, Swain M L 1981 A new neck goniometer. Rheumatology and Rehabilitation 20: 219–226

Kapandji I A 1974 The physiology of the joints. Vol 3, Trunk and vertebral column. 2nd edn. Churchill Livingstone, London

Kazarian L E 1975 Creep characteristics of the human spinal column. Orthopedic Clinics of North America 6: 3–15

Keegan J J 1953 Alterations of the lumbar curve related to posture and seating. Journal of Bone and Joint Surgery 35A: 589–603

King A I, Vulcan A P 1971 Elastic deformation characteristics of the spine. Journal of Biomechanics 4: 413–429

Kippers V, Parker A W 1983 Hand positions at possible critical points in the stoop-lift movement. Ergonomics 26: 895–903

Koreska J, Robertson D, Mills R H, Gibson D A, Albisser A M 1977 Biomechanics of the lumbar spine and its clinical significance. Orthopedic Clinics of North America 8: 121–133

Kraemer J 1981 Intervertebral disc lesions: causes, diagnosis, treatment and prophylaxis. Georg Thieme Verlag, Stuttgart

Leighton J R 1966 The Leighton flexometer and flexibility test. Journal of the Association for Physical and Mental Rehabilitation 20: 86–93

Lewin T, Moffett B, Viidik A 1961 The morphology of lumbar synovial intervertebral joints. Acta Morphologica Neerlando-Scandinavica 4: 229–319

Lindahl O 1966 Determination of the sagittal mobility of the lumbar spine. A clinical method. Acta Orthopaedica Scandinavica 37: 241–254

Loebl W Y 1973 Regional rotation of the spine. Rheumatology and Rehabilitation 12: 223

Lumsden R M, Morris J M 1968 An in-vitro study of axial rotation and immobilisation at the lumbosacral joint. Journal of Bone and Joint Surgery 50A: 1591–1602

Miller J A A, Haderspeck K A, Schultz A B 1983 Posterior element loads in lumbar motion segments. Spine 8: 331–337

Moll J, Wright V 1976 Measurement of spinal movement. In: Jayson M I V (ed) The lumbar spine and back pain. Grune & Stratton, New York, ch 6, pp 93–112

Nachemson A L 1960 Lumbar intradiscal pressure. Acta Orthopaedica Scandinavica (suppl 43)

Nachemson A L 1976 The lumbar spine. An orthopaedic challenge. Spine 1: 59–71

Nachemson A L 1985 Lumbar spine instability: a critical update and symposium summary. Spine 10: 290–291

Newell D J, Nichols J R 1965 The accuracy of estimating neck movements. Annals of Physical Medicine 8: 120–124

Panjabi M M 1973 Three-dimensional mathematical model of the human spine structure. Journal of Biomechanics 6: 671–680

Panjabi M M 1977 Experimental determination of spinal motion segment behaviour. Orthopedic Clinics of North America 8: 169–180

Panjabi M M, Dvorak J, Duranceau J, Yamamoto I, Gerber M, Rauschning W, Buff H U 1988 Three-dimensional movements of the upper cervical spine. Spine 13: 727–730

Rolander S D 1966 Motion of the lumbar spine with special reference to the stabilising effect of posterior fusion. Acta Orthopaedica Scandinavica (suppl 90)

Schultz A B, Belytshko T P, Andriacchi T P, Galante J O 1973 Analog studies of forces in the human spine: mechanical properties and motion segment behaviour. Journal of Biomechanics 6: 373–383

Stockwell R A 1979 Biology of cartilage cells. Cambridge University Press, Cambridge

Tanz S S 1953 Motion of the lumbar spine. A roentgenologic study. American Journal of Roentgenology 69: 399–412

Taylor J R, Twomey L T 1981a Age-related change in the range of movement of the lumbar spine. Journal of Anatomy 133: 473

Taylor J R, Twomey L T 1981b Sagittal and horizontal plane movement of the human vertebral column in cadaveric and in the living. Rheumatology Rehabilitation 19: 223

Taylor J R, Twomey L T 1984 Sexual dimorphism in human vertebral shape: its relation to scoliosis. Journal of Anatomy 138: 218–286

Taylor J R, Twomey L T 1986 Age changes in lumbar zygapophyseal joints. Observations on structure and function. Spine 11: 739–745

Tondury G 1972 Functional anatomy of the small joints of the spine. Annales de Medicine Physique XV: 2

Tucci S M, Hicks J E, Gross E G, Campbell A, Danoff J 1986 Cervical motion assessment: a new simple and accurate method. Archives of Physical Medicine and Rehabilitation 67: 225–230

Twomey L T 1981 Age changes in the human lumbar spine. PhD thesis, University of Western Australia

Twomey L T, Taylor J R 1982 Flexion creep deformation and hysteresis in the lumbar vertebral column. Spine 7: 116–122

Twomey L T, Taylor J R 1983 Sagittal movements of the human lumbar vertebral column: a quantitative study of the role of the posterior vertebral elements. Archives of Physical Medicine and Rehabilitation 64: 322–325

Twomey L T, Taylor J R 1985a Age changes in the lumbar intervertebral discs. Acta Orthopaedica Scandinavica 56: 496–499

Twomey L T, Taylor J R 1985b Age changes in the lumbar articular triad. Australian Journal of Physiotherapy 31: 106–112

Twomey L T, Taylor J R 1987 Physical therapy of the low back. Churchill Livingstone, New York

Twomey L T, Taylor J R, Oliver M 1988 Sustained flexion loading, rapid extension loading of the lumbar spine and the physical therapy of related injuries. Physiotherapy Practice 4: 129–138

Tyrrell A R, Reilly T, Troup J D G 1985 Circadian variation stature and the effects of spinal loading. Spine 10: 161

Van Mameren H 1988 Motion patterns in the cervical spine. PhD thesis, University of Maastricht

Van Mameren H, Drukker J, Sanches H, Beursgens J 1990 Cervical spine motion in the sagittal plane (I). Range of motion of actually performed movements, an X-ray cinematographic study. European Journal of Morphology 28: 47–68

Vernon-Roberts B, Pirie C J 1977 Degenerative changes in the intervertebral discs of the lumbar spine and their sequela. Rheumatology and Rehabilitation 16: 13–21

Virgin W J 1951 Experimental investigations into the physical properties of the intervertebral disc. Journal of Bone and Joint Surgery 33B: 607–611

White A A, Panjabi M M 1978 The clinical biomechanics of the spine. J B Lippincott, Philadelphia

Wiles P 1935 Movements of the lumbar vertebra during flexion and extension. Proceedings of the Royal Society of Medicine 28: 647

Worth D R 1988 Biomechanics of the cervical spine. In: Grant R (ed) Physical therapy of the cervical and thoracic spine. Churchill Livingstone, New York

Yang K H, King A I 1984 Mechanism of facet load transmission as a hypoythesis for low back pain. Spine 9: 557–565

12. The innervation of the intervertebral discs

N. Bogduk

INTRODUCTION

The study of the innervation of intervertebral discs has had a long and chequered history, characterized by negative studies and positive studies, and by reviews that either denied or proclaimed that these structures had a nerve supply. When this topic was addressed in the first edition of this text (Bogduk 1986) it was at a time when the issue was still considered controversial; insufficient numbers of people knew of the results of then contemporary studies, and many still believed that the discs had no innervation. This is no longer the situation. The innervation of the lumbar discs has been established and reconfirmed, and since the first edition of this text the innervation of the cervical discs has been elucidated.

This chapter provides an opportunity to consolidate the history of research into the innervation of the intervertebral discs and constitutes an update of a recent review (Bogduk 1988).

THE LUMBAR DISCS

The study of the innervation of the lumbar intervertebral discs has followed two parallel lines of investigation. One has been the search for nerve endings in the discs; the other has been the determination of the source of these endings.

Jung and Brunschwig (1932) undertook the first search for nerve endings in the lumbar discs. Although they found unmyelinated nerve fibres and nerve endings in both the anterior and the posterior longitudinal ligaments, they found neither nerve fibres nor nerve endings in the discs themselves. In contrast, Tsukada (1938, 1939) reported finding both myelinated and unmyelinated nerve fibres in the annulus fibrosus and nerve endings in the notochord and nucleus pulposus. It is noteworthy, however, that of all the studies that have addressed the innervation of the intervertebral discs, those of Tsukada (1938, 1939) remain the most enigmatic, for no-one since has verified the presence of nerve endings in the nucleus pulposus

and, indeed, some authorities have even challenged the accuracy of Tsukada's findings in the annulus fibrosus (Pedersen et al 1956).

It was Roofe (1940) who published the first unequivocal evidence of nerve fibres in the annulus fibrosus. He reported 'many' unmyelinated fibres in the annulus fibrosus which terminated in 'naked nerve endings' and provided photographic evidence of his observations. Although he emphasized that nerve fibres occurred in the annulus fibrosus, Roofe (1940) commented that 'no nerve tissue was observed within the disc itself'. While seemingly contradictory, this remark was probably meant to imply the absence of nerve fibres in the nucleus pulposus.

Roofe's report (Roofe 1940) was limited to the results of his histological studies, and although suspecting that the nerves he found in the fourth and fifth lumbar discs arose from the third and fourth lumbar spinal nerves, he commented that the origin had still to be determined. However, Spurling and Bradford (1939), Spurling and Grantham (1940), and later, Bradford and Spurling (1945) stipulated that the source of these nerves was the sinuvertebral nerve, which they illustrated as a long, descending branch from the L2 spinal nerve. Roofe was credited with this description (Spurling & Grantham 1940), but it was never formally published or endorsed by him.

Lazorthes et al (1947) seized upon this description of the sinuvertebral nerves, for it contradicted those in the classical German and French literature (von Luschka 1850, Soulie 1905, Hovelacque 1925, 1927). The classical literature maintained that each sinuvertebral nerve arose from two roots: a somatic root from the spinal nerve at each segmental level, and an autonomic root from a grey ramus communicans. The nerve so formed passed through the intervertebral foramen to divide into a major ascending branch and a smaller descending branch, which together supplied the vertebral venous plexuses, the dura mater, the vertebral bodies, and the posterior longitudinal ligament. A distribution to the intervertebral discs, however, was never specifically mentioned.

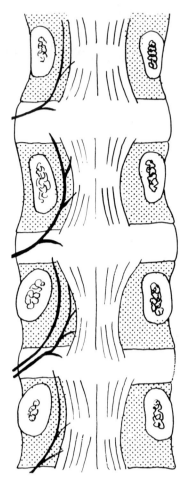

Fig. 12.1 A sketch of the anatomy of the left lumbar sinuvertebral nerves as described by Lazorthes et al (1947) and confirmed by Pedersen et al (1956) and Bogduk et al (1981).

Lazorthes et al (1947) studied 100 nerves in 10 lumbar vertebral columns and found no examples of nerves like those described by Spurling and colleagues (loc cit). Two-thirds of the nerves they dissected were single trunks that ramified at their level of entry and formed an ascending branch to the level above (Fig. 12.1). The nerves were distributed to the dura mater, the posterior longitudinal ligament, the vertebral bodies and the intervertebral discs at and above their level of origin. The remaining one-third of their specimens were multiple filaments rather than single nerve trunks, but nevertheless, with a similar distribution.

Two years later Herlihy (1949) entered the debate on the anatomy of the sinuvertebral nerves, but without contributing any original work. He simply contrasted the descriptions of Lazorthes et al (1947) with those of Buskirk (1941). Quoting Buskirk (1941), Herlihy (1949) claimed that the lumbar sinuvertebral nerves formed a continuous chain of nerve fibres running longitudinally within the vertebral canal. This differed from the interrupted, essentially bisegmental described by Lazorthes et al (1947). Reference to Buskirk's original publication

(Buskirk 1941), however, revealed that what he described was, in fact, the distribution of sympathetic fibres within the vertebral venous plexus, not the somatic branches of the sinuvertebral nerves. Moreover, his studies were performed on cats and at thoracic levels. Thus, his data do not constitute a legitimate challenge to the descriptions of the lumbar sinuvertebral nerves given by Lazorthes et al (1947).

Wiberg (1949) contributed to his debate and illustrated the lumbar sinuvertebral nerves as each ramifying its level of entry and communicating with the nerves of adjacent levels opposite the middle of the interposed vertebral body, a description similar to that of Lazorthes et al (1947). Wiberg's attempts at histological studies, however, failed to demonstrate any nerve fibres in the annulus fibrosus (Wiberg 1949).

In a paper on the embryology of the vertebral column, Ehrenhaft (1943) briefly mentioned the presence of nerve bundles beneath the posterior longitudinal ligament and 'within the annulus fibrosus proper'. Ikari (1954), on the other hand, failed to find any nerve endings in the annulus fibrosus.

In 1956, Stillwell (1956) reported an exhaustive study of the innervation of the vertebral column in the monkey, which, while itself not evidence of what occurs in humans, nonetheless served to foreshadow what the human anatomy might be. He reported branches from the sinuvertebral nerves to the posterior portions of the annulus fibrosus and branches to the lateral portions from the grey rami communicantes. The anterior longitudinal ligament received branches from the sympathetic trunk, and the posterior longitudinal ligament was innervated by the sinuvertebral nerves. Stillwell (1956) remarked that the nerves to the annulus fibrosus were confined to the surface of the disc, for he found none within the annulus itself.

In the same year, Pedersen et al (1956) described the lumbar sinuvertebral nerves in what has become a classical paper in the literature on the lumbar spine. Although apparently unaware of the earlier work of Lazorthes et al (1947) they confirmed exactly the descriptions of the French investigators (Fig. 12.1).

At this stage of history, attention briefly changed from the skeletal distribution of the sinuvertebral nerves to their distribution to the dura mater. Bridge (1959) described the dural innervation in cats, dogs, and in some human specimens, and the dural innervation in humans was later elaborated by Kimmel (1961) and Edgar and Nundy (1966), and more recently by Groen et al (1988).

The story of the intervertebral discs resumed in 1959 when Malinsky (1959) published an exhaustive report on the ontogenetic development of nerve terminations in human lumbar intervertebral discs. He found that the inner part of the annulus fibrosus and the nucleus pulposus were devoid of nerve fibres and nerve endings throughout their whole ontogenetic development. In contrast, he consistently found nerve fibres and nerve endings in the outer zone of the annulus fibrosus and on its surface.

Malinsky's studies demonstrated that, during the prenatal period, nerves are abundant in the annulus fibrosus where they form simple free nerve endings, and they increase in number in older fetuses. During the postnatal period, various types of non-encapsulated receptors occur, and in adult material five types of nerve terminations can be found: simple and complex free nerve endings, 'shrubby' receptors, others that form loops and mesh-like formations, and clusters of parallel free nerve endings. On the surface of the annulus fibrosus, various types of encapsulated and complex unencapsulated receptors occur. They are all relatively simple in structure in neonates, but more elaborate forms occur in older and mature specimens.

Within a given disc, Malinsky (1959) reported that receptors are not uniformly distributed. The greatest number of endings occurs in the lateral region of the disc, and nearly all the encapsulated receptors are located in this region. Following postnatal development, there is a relative decrease in the number of receptors in the anterior region, such that, in adults, the greatest number of endings occurs in the lateral regions of the disc, a smaller number in the posterior region, and the least number anteriorly.

While not approaching the detail provided by Malinsky (1959), Hirsch et al (1963) and later Jackson et al (1966) confirmed the presence of free nerve endings in the annulus fibrosus of lumbar intervertebral discs, although they found them only in the most superficial laminae of the annulus. The latter authors also reported finding encapsulated receptors on the ventrolateral surface of the discs in neonates (Jackson et al 1966).

In 1976, the first review of the innervation of the spine was published, based on the data then available. Edgar & Ghadially (1976) acknowledged the failure of Jung and Brunschwig (1932), Wiberg (1949) and Ikari (1954) to find evidence of nerve fibres in the lumbar intervertebral discs, but they highlighted the detection of nerve fibres in the outer laminae of the annulus fibrosus by Malinsky (1959), Hirsch et al (1963) and Jackson et al (1966). Their review also encompassed the Japanese literature, including the studies of Tsukada (1938, 1939) and a lesser known study by Shinohara (1970), who apparently confirmed the presence of nerve fibres in the outer layers of the annulus fibrosus. He also reported that in degenerative discs, nerve fibres could be found accompanying granulation tissue into the deeper layers of the annulus and even into the nucleus pulposus.

Contrasting reviews were written by Wyke (1976, 1980) who concluded that nerve terminals in the intervertebral discs 'rapidly degenerate and disappear, so that in the mature human spine no nerve endings of any description remain in the nucleus pulposus or annulus fibrosus of the

intervertebral discs in any region of the vertebral column'. This conclusion was made in spite of the observations of Malinsky (1959), Hirsch et al (1963), Jackson et al (1966) and Shinohara (1970). Paradoxically, Malinsky (1959) was even cited by Wyke (1976, 1980) to support his negative conclusions.

It seems that Wyke (1976, 1980) did not consider the possibility that those few studies that failed to demonstrate nerves in the lumbar discs might have been compromised by technical difficulties. Even under the best of conditions, metallic-ion stains for nerves in connective tissue are notoriously capricious. Negative results, therefore, can be false-negative and as an investigative technique, metallic-ion stains are of value only when positive.

Nevertheless, reviews like those by Wyke (1967, 1980)

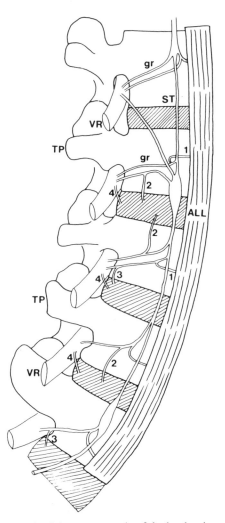

Fig. 12.2 A sketch of the nerve supply of the lumbar intervertebral discs outside the vertebral canal (reproduced from Bogduk 1983). The anterior longitudinal ligament (ALL) receives recurrent branches (1) from the grey rami communicantes (gr) and sympathetic trunk (ST). Laterally the discs receive branches (2) from these same sources. Posterolaterally they receive branches (3,4) from the grey rami and ventral rami (VR). The latter (4) may not be specific disc branches but may represent terminal trunks of microscopic plexuses covering the lateral aspect of the disc and stemming from the grey rami.

apparently were not without influence, for others have stated that the lumbar discs lack an innervation (Lamb 1979, Anderson 1980). However, such conclusions are based more on opinion, dysinformation or lack of information rather than on facts, and are unjustified even given the literature only up to 1976. Fortunately, to dispel such negative conclusions absolutely, additional studies have further elaborated the innervation of the lumbar discs.

Prompted by Stillwell's observations in the monkey (Stillwell 1956), Taylor and Twomey (1979) and then Bogduk et al (1981) investigated the nerve supply to the human lumbar intervertebral discs. The latter group confirmed that, posteriorly, the discs were innervated by the sinuvertebral nerves (Fig. 12.1) and established that the anterior longitudinal ligament was supplied by recurrent branches of the grey rami communicantes. Their additional revelation was that, laterally, the discs were innervated by branches of the grey rami communicantes, and that, posterolaterally, they receive branches from the grey rami communicantes and direct branches from the ventral rami (Fig. 12.2). The latter finding confirmed the brief report by Taylor & Twomey (1979), and the overall pattern of innervation described by Bogduk et al (1981) was reminiscent of that described by Stillwell (1956) in the monkey and has been endorsed by more recent studies (Paris 1983).

Although their study was directed principally to determining the source of innervation of the lumbar disc, Bogduk et al (1981) did report finding nerve fibres within the outer third of the annulus fibrosus, but a contemporary histological study explored this phenomenon in more detail. Yoshizawa et al (1980) studied specimens of intervertebral discs removed at operation for anterior and posterior lumbar interbody fusion and found abundant nerve endings with various morphologies throughout the outer half of the annulus fibrosus. The varieties of nerve endings found included free terminals, often ending in club-like or bulbous expansions or complex sprays, and, less commonly, terminals forming convoluted tangles or glomerular formations that were occasionally demarcated by a 'capsule-like' condensation of adjacent tissue. In contrast to the report of Shinohara (1970), these workers found no evidence of in-growth of nerve fibres into areas of disc degeneration.

More recent studies have employed modern, immunohistochemical techniques to search for nerve fibres in lumbar disc. These techniques stain for specific transmitter substances within nerves. The substances investigated have been substance P, calcitonin gene-related peptide (CGRP) and vaso-active intestinal polypeptide (VIP), all of which are known to be present in nociceptive afferent fibres.

Substance P, CGRP and VIP have been found to be present in the annulus fibrosus of rat discs (Weinstein et al 1988) and of human discs obtained at operation (Konttinen et al 1990), although, in human material, immunoreactivity appears far more frequently in the posterior longitudinal ligament than in the annulus fibrosus (Konttinen et al 1990).

THE CERVICAL DISCS

Compared to the lumbar intervertebral discs, the cervical discs have been less studied. Such descriptions of the innervation of cervical discs as occur in the clinical literature (Cloward 1959, 1960) have been based on conjecture or extrapolations of data on the lumbar discs. Similarly, statements that deny an innervation of the cervical discs (Wyke 1976, 1980) are based on extrapolations of incomplete reviews of lumbar data, and they conspicuously overlooked the available literature on the cervical discs.

Hovelacque (1925, 1927) described the cervical sinuvertebral nerves as arising from the so-called vertebral nerve: the sympathetic plexus accompanying the vertebral artery. However, he offered no further description of their distribution within the vertebral canal. Although not describing them in his texts, Hovelacque (1925, 1927) illustrated branches of the vertebral nerve entering the lateral aspects of the cervical intervertebral discs.

Until recently, apart from these two descriptions, there had been no further studies of the cervical sinuvertebral nerves, and indeed, Cloward (1960) proclaimed that these nerves were so small as to defy normal, anatomical methods.

Again, until recently, the only histological study of cervical discs had been an infrequently quoted report by Ferlic (1963) who examined fetal and adult discs obtained at operation. In the fetal material he found 'many nerve fibres . . . in the anterior and posterior ligaments, and in the superficial or most peripheral layers of the annulus fibrosis (sic)'. In the adult material he identified nerve fibres in two of the eighteen sections studied.

Prompted by this limited, though encouraging literature and by the positive findings of nerves to and within lumbar intervertebral discs, Windsor et al (1985) and Bogduk et al (1985, 1989) undertook studies of the gross and histological innervation of the cervical intervertebral discs.

With respect to the cervical sinuvertebral nerves, these investigators established that these nerves at the C3–C8 levels resembled those of the lumbar region (the C1 and C2 sinuvertebral nerves differed in their anatomy for lack of intervertebral discs at these levels, and their distribution to the atlanto-axial joint complex and the dura mater of the posterior cranial fossa and upper cord has been described elsewhere (Kimmel 1961)).

Each of the C3–C8 sinuvertebral arises from a somatic and an autonomic root. The somatic root stems from the ventral ramus at each segmental level while the autonomic roots are derived from the vertebral nerve. At upper cervical levels, the autonomic roots arise from the terminal branches of the vertebral nerve. At lower levels they are definitive branches of that sympathetic plexus, and can be traced back, at mid-cervical levels, to grey rami communicantes from the sympathetic trunk, and at lower cervical levels, to branches of the stellate ganglion. The somatic and autonomic roots of each sinuvertebral nerve join medial to the vertebral artery, in the intervertebral foramen.

Once formed, each sinuvertebral nerve runs obliquely upwards and medially through the intervertebral foramen, anterior to the spinal nerve, crossing the back of the intervertebral disc and then the back of the vertebral body above (Fig. 12.3). The principal branch of the nerve then continues rostrally circumventing the supradjacent pedicle, running parallel to the edge of the posterior longitudinal ligament. This branch finally ramifies in the posterior longitudinal ligament and the peridiscal connective tissue of the segment next above (Fig. 12.3). En route, it

furnishes minor branches to the periosteum of the pedicle and vertebral body, the epidural veins, and substantial branches directly dorsally to the dura mater. A major branch consistently arises just above the disc at the level of origin of each sinuvertebral nerve. This passes transversely to end in the posterior longitudinal ligament, and supplies small, descending branches to the subadjacent disc (Fig. 12.3).

The C3 sinuvertebral nerve differs somewhat from this typical pattern because of the absence of a disc at the C2 level. As at other levels, this nerve runs obliquely through the intervertebral foramen and forms a transverse branch to the posterior longitudinal ligament and the intervertebral disc at its level of origin; however, rostrally it continues a prolonged course within the vertebral canal to join the C1 and C2 sinuvertebral nerves to supply the

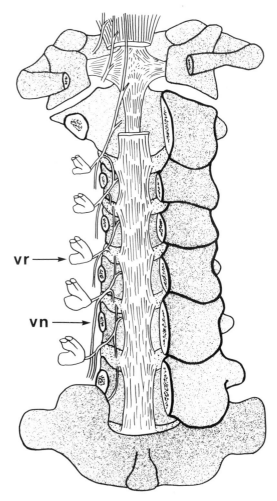

Fig. 12.3 A sketch of the cervical sinuvertebral nerves (reproduced from Bogduk et al 1988). At typical cervical levels each sinuvertebral nerve arises from the vertebral nerve (vn) and the ipsisegmental ventral ramus (vr) and passes upwards in the vertebral canal ramifying in the ipsisegmental disc and the disc above. The C1, C2 and C3 sinuvertebral nerves supply the ligaments of the atlanto-axial joints.

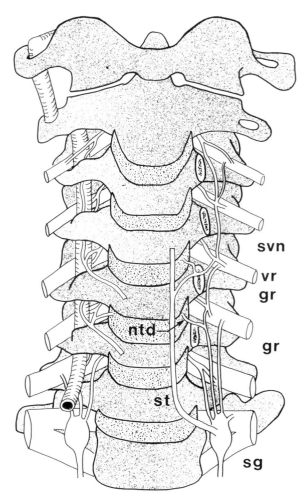

Fig. 12.4 A sketch of the vertebral nerve (reproduced from Bogduk et al 1988). The right vertebral artery is drawn in situ with nerves accompanying it. The left vertebral artery has been removed to reveal the connections of these nerves. Grey rami communicantes (gr) reach the cervical ventral rami (vr) from the stellate ganglion (sg) and sympathetic trunk (st). Communicating loops between the grey rami and ventral rami create the vertebral nerves, from which the sinuvertebral nerves (svn) arise and enter the intervertebral foramina. Branches of the grey rami and vertebral nerve furnish nerves to the lateral aspects of the discs (ntd).

atlanto-axial joints and the craniocervical dura mater (Kimmel 1961) (Fig. 12.3).

In addition to the sinuvertebral nerves, Bogduk et al (1989) found other branches of the vertebral nerves supplying the cervical discs, in essence confirming the illustrations of Hovelacque (1925, 1927). These branches include fine filaments running with, but distinct from, the sinuvertebral nerves, that end in the posterolateral corner of the discs. Other branches include larger definitive nerves passing medially from the vertebral nerve to enter directly, the lateral aspect of the adjacent disc (Fig. 12.4).

Because of the intimate relationship between the prevertebral muscles on the front of the cervical discs, Bogduk et al (1989) included in their study dissections of the prevertebral branches of the cervical ventral rami which supplied prevertebral muscles, expecting to find branches from them to the disc. This exploration, however, failed to demonstrate any such branches, and the authors concluded that, if they existed, they were too small to be resolved by microdissection.

In their histological studies, Bogduk et al (1989) were frustrated by technical problems in their attempts to stain nerve fibres in cadaveric discs. However, they did succeed in demonstrating neural tissue in two operative specimens of C5–6 discs. Using a cholinesterase stain, they revealed nerve fibres and nerve endings within the outer third of the annulus fibrosus. The endings included not only free nerve endings, but also what appeared to be complex unencapsulated endings (Fig. 12.5). The quality of staining achieved, however, precluded any more defini-

tive study or classification of the morphology of these endings.

While derived from only a limited number of specimens, these histological observations were nonetheless clearly positive and corroborated the report of Ferlic (1963). Taken together, these two studies vindicate the notion that, like the lumbar discs, the cervical discs are innervated. From the dissection studies of Bogduk et al (1989) it would appear that the source of this innervation is from the cervical sinuvertebral nerve posteriorly and from the vertebral nerve laterally.

One description of cervical sinuvertebral nerves, not based on any formal anatomical study, maintains that the lower cervical sinuvertebral nerves send long descending branches to thoracic levels (Wyke 1970). No such nerves were identified in the studies of Bogduk et al (1989), and it was suggested that this spurious description was based on an extrapolation of the erroneous description of descending branches of lumbar sinuvertebral nerves made by Spurling and co-authors (loc cit) which has now been dispelled (see above).

The fact that the vertebral nerve is predominantly derived from the sympathetic nervous system (Monteiro & Rodrigues 1931, Lazorthes & Cassand 1939, Laux & Guerrier 1939, 1947, Guerrier 1949, Bogduk et al 1981a) suggests that the branches from this nerve to the cervical discs would be autonomic in nature. This may be so, in part, because such vessels as may occur in the discs would require an efferent innervation, but it is pertinent to note that the vertebral nerve is not exclusively sympathetic. It

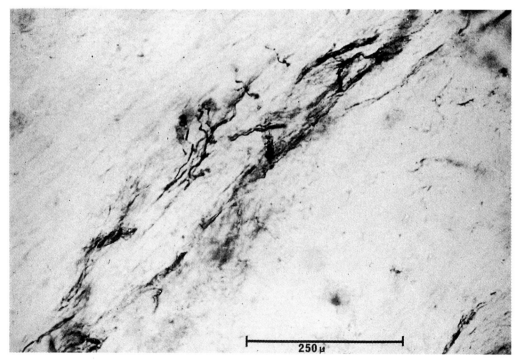

Fig. 12.5 A photomicrograph of nerve endings stained for cholinesterase evident in the outer half of the antero-lateral sector of an intervertebral disc obtained at operation (reproduced from Bogduk et al 1988).

has substantial connections with the cervical ventral rami (Bogduk et al 1981a), which raises the possibility that the vertebral nerve also conveys somatic afferents. Indeed, this has been verified at upper cervical levels where, in studies of human fetuses, Kimmel (1959) traced afferent fibres from the vertebral artery that ran through the vertebral nerve to the C2 spinal nerve and had cell bodies in the dorsal root ganglia. Thus, it is feasible that a similar phenomenon could occur at lower cervical levels with respect to afferents from the discs using the vertebral nerve to reach the somatic nervous system. Consequently, branches from the sinuvertebral nerve to the cervical discs should not be viewed as exclusively autonomic in nature. Similar arguments have been advanced with respect to the branches to the lumbar discs from grey rami communicantes (Bogduk et al 1981b).

Despite the relative paucity of data on the cervical discs, those studies that have been done are positive, demonstrating that macroscopically and histologically the cervical discs do have an innervation. Thus, the data on cervical discs are in accord with those on the lumbar discs.

THE DEFINITIVE WORK

In 1990, knowledge about the innervation of intervertebral discs underwent a quantum leap when Groen et al (1990) reported the results of their studies of human fetuses, elaborating a short earlier study restricted to the cervical intervertebral discs (Groen et al 1979). These investigators revealed that the entire human vertebral column is covered by extensive and dense microscopic nerve plexuses lying anterior and posterior to the vertebral bodies and intervertebral discs. Anteriorly, these plexuses stem from the sympathetic trunks and the grey rami communicantes. Posteriorly, they stem from multiple filaments derived from the grey rami communicantes as they approach the segmental ventral rami in the intervertebral foramina. Transverse sections reveal that elements of both the anterior and posterior vertebral plexuses penetrate both the vertebral bodies and the intervertebral discs. Branches entering the vertebral bodies accompany blood vessels deeply into the bone. Branches to the intervertebral discs are restricted to the outer layers of the annulus fibrosus (Figs 12.6, 12.7).

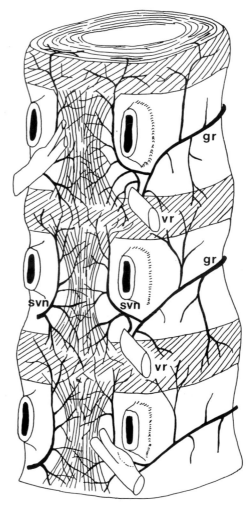

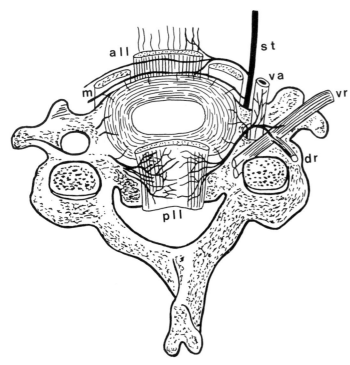

Fig. 12.6 A sketch of the innervation of the plexuses surrounding a cervical intervertebral disc (based on Groen et al 1990). The sinuvertebral nerves form a dense plexus accompanying the posterior longitudinal ligament (pll). Anteriorly, branches of the sympathetic trunk (st) supply the front of the disc and form a plexus accompanying the anterior longitudinal ligament (all). vr = ventral ramus, dr = dorsal ramus, va = vertebral artery, m = prevertebral muscles.

Fig. 12.7 A sketch of the plexuses of the lumbar intervertebral discs (based on Groen et al 1990). The sinuvertebral nerves generate a plexus accompanying the posterior longitudinal ligament from which the intervertebral discs are innervated. Laterally, the grey rami communicantes generate fine plexus over the surfaces of the discs before reaching the ventral rami (vr). Upon dissection, elements of this plexus may appear as direct branches to the disc from the ventral rami (cf. Fig. 12.2).

What these studies revealed was that the sinuvertebral nerves both in the lumbar region and in the neck constitute only a fraction of the nerves that innervate discs. Indeed, the sinuvertebral nerves represent only the larger filaments that are sufficiently large so as to be visible upon microdissection; the majority of filaments innervating the discs are too small to be found reliably by dissection, but are clearly revealed in microscopic studies.

The revision called for by the studies of Groen et al (1990) is that no longer can the intervertebral discs be held to receive specific 'articular' branches but that each is regularly and extensively innervated by multiple, microscopic nerves, amongst which more macroscopic, sinuvertebral nerves occur.

FUNCTION

The function of disc nerves is still open to speculation. Because of the association between disc nerves and the sympathetic nervous system, both in the lumbar and in the cervical regions, previous investigators seem to have been obliged to acknowledge that possibly these nerves have a vasomotor function. However, this acknowledgement seems more of a gesture respectful of the traditional views of the functions of apparent sympathetic nerves than a proper reflection of the function of these nerves. The annulus fibrosus has only a meagre blood supply, incommensurate with the density of its innervation, and moreover, most of the nerve endings in the annulus fibrosus are unassociated with blood vessels.

Disc nerves can be interpreted as analogous to the sensory nerves found in the thoracic and lumbar splanchnic nerves and those found in the vertebral nerve. As discussed above in the context of the nerves to the cervical intervertebral discs, disc nerves are sympathetic only in so far as they follow the course of sympathetic nerves to get to their destination; otherwise, there are no grounds to consider them other than somatic sensory fibres. Moreover, the presence in disc nerves of substance P, CGRP and VIP indicates that they are sensory.

Explicit electrophysiological studies have yet to be conducted on disc nerves. Consequently, one can speculate as to their function only on the basis of circumstantial, anatomical evidence. Their close relationship to the collagen of the annulus fibrosus suggests a mechanoreceptive function. At one extreme, these nerves may well be able to transduce changes in strain in the annulus fibrosus rendering them essentially proprioceptive in nature. Indeed, Malinsky (1959) postulated such a role for the encapsulated receptors located on the surface of lumbar discs, but it seems equally plausible for more deeply located, free nerve endings.

At the other extreme, free nerve endings are classically associated with nociception. However, it is not satisfying to proclaim that the discs receive nociceptive nerves simply in case the disc ever becomes painful. On teleological grounds, nociception is more satisfyingly regarded as a fortuitous extension of the mechanoreceptive function of disc nerves; they are designed to detect stresses within the normal range of movement of the annulus fibrosus, but are capable of signalling impending or actual tissue damage if these stresses become severe. Whatever the teleological arguments, it is in this regard that disc nerves have their greatest clinical relevance: in the context of disc pain.

DISC PAIN

Discography is a radiological technique in which contrast medium is injected into the nucleus pulposus of a disc to depict its internal structure. It was originally devised as a procedure to verify disc herniation (Lindblom 1948, 1950, 1951a, b). However, it was noted that, in some instances, injection of the disc reproduced the patient's customary back pain and referred pain, even when no herniation was present. This prompted the belief that discs could be a source of pain by means other than by herniation and nerve root compression.

Despite vehement resistance and views to the contrary (Meyer 1963, Sneider et al 1963, Holt 1964, 1968, Taveras 1967, Wilson & MacCarty 1969, Klafta & Collis 1969, Clifford 1986, Shapiro 1986a, b, Scullin 1987), many investigators have endorsed the notion that intervertebral discs can be a primary source of pain and that provocation discography is the one means of establishing this diagnosis (Hirsch 1949, Friedman & Goldner 1955, Smith 1959, Cloward 1959, 1960, 1963, Keck 1960, Collis & Gardner 1962, Butt 1963, Feinberg 1964, Wiley et al 1968, Patrick 1973, Collins 1975, Simmons & Segil 1975, Van Niekerk 1979, Brodsky & Binder 1979, Park 1980, Kikuchi et al 1981, Milette & Melanson 1982, 1987, McCutcheon 1986, Perkins 1986, Bernard 1987, 1990, Errico 1987, Colhoun et al 1988, McFadden 1988).

This notion has been challenged on the basis that because the discs lack an innervation, they could not possibly be a source of pain. Given the data covered in this review, however, this challenge cannot be sustained. The intervertebral discs are endowed with the anatomical substrate for nociception and, therefore, must be viewed as potential sources of pain.

Alternative explanations for the pain of discography either have not been offered or have been ambiguous or speculative — like simply 'nerve root irritation' or leakage of contrast medium into the vertebral canal. Neither of these alternative mechanisms has been verified; moreover, neither mechanism explains the pain of discography when normal saline is used or when contrast medium is clearly retained wholly within the disc. It is, therefore, an inescapable conclusion that the pain of discography must arise from within the disc and is mediated by the nerves to the disc.

This controversy has recently come to a head. Opposition to discography has been based largely on the cynical studies of Holt (1968), but a recent review has soundly refuted this work on methodological grounds (Simmons et al 1988). The Executive Committee of the North American Spine Society (1988) came out in support of discography as a valid diagnostic technique, only to be challenged by Nachemson (1989). A cardinal source of contention has been that discography is not valid because reportedly normal discs in asymptomatic individuals can be made to hurt (Holt 1968). However, this issue has now been laid to rest.

In a meticulously stringent study, Walsh et al (1990) compared the responses to discography of patients with and without symptoms of low back pain. Disc injection was performed in all subjects by the one operator who was masked as to the status of the subject; injection pressure was monitored by manometry, and patient responses were recorded on videotape and scored by two independent observers other than the operator. Only patients with back pain reported reproduction of pain upon discography; no asymptomatic individuals reported what could be construed as disc pain. Through this study, lumbar discography was shown to be a highly specific diagnostic test. Provocation discography is not positive in normal individuals; it is positive only in patients with back pain, and implies that the symptomatic disc has undergone some sort of change that renders it symptomatic.

Another reservation about discography has been that the morphology of the disc, as revealed by discography, does not correlate well with whether or not the disc is symptomatic. However, this is so only with respect to the appearance of the disc on plain radiographs. Antero-posterior and lateral radiographs of a discogram are difficult to interpret, for they do not provide a three-dimensional perspective of the distribution of contrast medium within the disc. What may appear on antero-posterior and lateral views to be a degenerated or disrupted disc with chaotic dispersal of contrast medium can be shown to be a more specific, focal disruption if a third, top view is obtained.

Studies on cadaveric lumbar discs have shown that rather than dispersing randomly through a deranged disc, contrast medium spreads through radial fissures and extends circumferentially in the annulus fibrosus (Videman et al 1987). This specific circumferential spread cannot be deduced from antero-posterior and lateral radiographs, but it is clearly evident if CT scans of the injected disc are obtained.

In a multi-centre survey, Vanharanta et al (1987) examined the appearances of discs on CT-discography and correlated these with the reproduction of pain reported by patients during the provocation phase of discography. These investigators used the Dallas discogram scale (Sachs et al 1987) which recognizes four grades of internal anular disruption: grade 0, in which contrast medium was confined to the nucleus pulposus; grade 1, in which contrast medium extended along a radial fissure but no further than the inner third of the annulus fibrosus; grade 2, in which contrast medium extended along a radial fissure into the inner two-thirds of the annulus fibrosus; and grade 3, in which contrast medium extended along a radial fissure as far as the outer third of the annulus fibrosus. They found that grade 0 and grade 1 discs were rarely painful, but over 70% of grade 3 discs were painful and over 70% of patients with pain reproduction upon discography exhibited grade 3 anular disruption. Grade 2 discs exhibited an intermediate correlation with pain reproduction. Consequently, pain reproduction is directly proportional to the radial extent of internal annular disruption.

What is striking about this correlation is that it parallels exactly the density of innervation of the disc. The nucleus pulposus and inner annulus fibrosus are devoid of nerve endings, and so would not be expected ever to be painful. Nerve endings sometimes extend to the middle third of the annulus fibrosus, and so this segment of the annulus could be expected to be symptomatic in some individuals — whereas the outer third of the annulus fibrosus is regularly innervated, so that it becomes highly likely that damage to this segment of the annulus would be symptomatic.

The studies of Vanharanta et al (1987) provide for the first time in the history of back pain research, a clear association between a detectable morphological change and reproduction of pain. Exactly how annular disruption becomes painful has not been proven, but, on theoretical grounds, several mechanisms may pertain.

It should be appreciated that, morphologically and functionally, discs resemble ligaments. Both consist of orientated collagen fibres; both stabilize joints; and both are innervated. In the appendicular skeleton, there is no dispute that straining even a normal ligament to extremes can be painful. Moreover, it is well appreciated that an injured ligament will become painful when subjected to a stress normally tolerated by an uninjured ligament, and this phenomenon is used in various clinical tests to diagnose ligament 'sprain' clinically. The same principle is applicable to intervertebral discs.

When normal saline or contrast medium is injected into a normal, or an asymptomatic intervertebral disc, it should not be painful. The intact inner layers of the annulus fibrosus prevent the stress of injection being transmitted to any appreciable extent to the nerve endings in its outer third.

An injured or diseased disc, on the other hand, is more likely to be painful, or painful at lesser pressures of injection for various possible reasons.

In the presence of a radial fissure, the fissure itself need not be the actual source of pain. Rather, it is the intact, remaining lamella of the annulus fibrosus that are more likely to be the source of pain. In an intact disc, any given sector of the annulus fibrosus is accustomed to withstanding a certain stress during activities of daily living, and each lamella of the annulus fibrosus will share this stress more or less equally. If some of the lamellae are disrupted, as in the case of a radial fissure, fewer lamellae remain intact to sustain the normal tensile loads imparted on the disc. Consequently, the relative stress sustained by these lamellae increases. For example, if a fissure extends through two-thirds of the annulus fibrosus, the remaining one-third must be sustaining three times their accustomed tensile load.

It can be perceived that, at some stage in the development of a radial fissure, the load imparted on the remaining annulus fibrosus exceeds a threshold at which those innervated fibres of the outer third of the annulus fibrosus become painful. The exact criteria that render an annulus fibrosus symptomatic have not been fully defined. The size of the radial fissure is but one factor, the longer the fissure the more likely the remaining fibres are to be subjected to excessive stresses. However, it is possible that even a severely disrupted annulus fibrosus may not become symptomatic if other structures in the affected segment protect the annulus from being subjected to excessive stresses.

Such mechanisms underlie the mechanical basis by which annular disruption could become symptomatic. A second mechanism is chemical nociception.

If it is accepted that disc degradation, or degeneration, involves an inflammatory-like proteolytic process within the nucleus, it is conceivable that this process could extend into the annulus. By progressively eroding deeper layers of the annulus, and by extending radially along fissures, this process could eventually reach innervated portions of the annulus. There, the degradation process would provide an abundant supply of enzymes and inflammatory substances that putatively could excite the nerve endings within the annulus. Under these circumstances the annulus would be rendered symptomatic even in the absence of mechanical stresses.

In some situations both chemical and mechanical processes may be involved. Inflammatory mediators present in the outer third of the annulus fibrosus would sensitize the nociceptive nerve endings located therein. This would provide a basis for continuous low-grade chemical nociception, but would also render the annulus fibrosus more sensitive to mechanical stresses; whereupon, even normal movements of the affected segment would become painful.

Through a combination of any or all of these, albeit theoretical, mechanisms, the production of disc pain can be understood. There is no need to invoke extra-discal explanations for causing the pain when plausible explanations confined to the disc are available — particularly when they are no different from the explanation of pain from ligaments and joints in the appendicular skeleton, about which there is no controversy.

Provocation discography, however, is not without its liabilities, and these, like its rationale, are fundamentally related to the way in which discs are innervated. The rationale of provocation discography is that if a disc is symptomatic, then stressing it should reproduce the patient's pain. However, the primary liability of this rationale stems from how effectively a disc may be stressed by intranuclear injections. If provocation does reproduce the right sort of pain, there is no issue, other than confirming that the patient is not mistaking this pain for pain arising from adjacent segmental levels. This can be done by testing adjacent levels on a single-blind basis and retesting the putatively symptomatic disc.

On the other hand, failure to reproduce pain does not necessarily exclude discs as the source of symptoms, for, along the lines outlined above, the test injection may fail to stress adequately an otherwise symptomatic disc. This pertains particularly in the case of torsion injuries of the annulus fibrosus where the lesion lies in the outer third of the annulus fibrosus but the inner annulus remains intact and the nucleus is unaffected; radial fissures are absent. In these circumstances, the rise in nuclear pressure during discography may be insufficient to strain the outer laminae of the annulus and therefore fail to activate the nerves to the disc. In this way, provocation discography is liable to false-negative results. However, this does not detract from its value as a diagnostic test when results are clearly positive.

To reinforce their diagnosis, some practitioners add a subsequent injection of local anaesthetic — so-called analgesic discography (Roth 1976). This test, however, while valuable when positive, is very liable to be falsely negative. It should be appreciated that the mechanism of analgesic discography differs physically from that of provocation discography. Provocation discography depends simply on the transmission of induced stress from the nucleus to the innervated portion of the annulus, i.e. the propagation of a force. Analgesic discography, in contrast, depends on the actual material dispersion of local anaesthetic from the nucleus to the innervated portions of the annulus. In a disc whose inner annulus is substantially intact, these inner lamellae would form a physical barrier to the dispersion of local anaesthetic, preventing it from reaching the nerves of the disc, or at least substantially slowing its diffusion. Under such circumstances, the inner annulus might not prevent the transmission of the stress in provocation discography, allowing pain to be provoked, but an injection of local anaesthetic might not relieve the pain. Such a paradoxical approach should not be viewed as a contradiction, but merely a function of the structure of the disc, the distribution of nerves within it, and the physical differences between inducing a strain and infiltrating a local anaesthetic.

When analgesic discography provides prompt relief of pain, the implication is that the local anaesthetic has been able to diffuse rapidly from the nucleus pulposus to the innervated outer third of the annulus. In such cases, the local anaesthetic probably reaches the innervated and symptomatic portions of the annulus along radial fissures. Lacking a physical barrier, the anaesthetic rapidly disperses to its desired site of action.

DISCUSSION

At present, the diagnosis of intrinsic disc pain can be made only on the basis of discography, supplemented, for satisfaction, by the morphological appearances of annular disruption on CT-discography. There are no clinical or manual tests whereby primary intrinsic disc derangement can be diagnosed. Farfan (1985) has described a variety of tests which can be used putatively to distinguish torsion injury and compression injury to an intervertebral disc, but the external and internal validity of these tests have not been established. If a clinical method of identifying internal disc derangement is to be established, studies are urgently required in which the results of clinical examination are correlated against the results of provocation discography and CT discography. Until such studies are completed, the diagnosis of primary disc pain will remain the province of radiologists who practise discography and have CT at their disposal.

REFERENCES

Anderson J 1980 Pathogenesis of back pain. In: Grahame R, Anderson J A D (eds) Low back pain. Eden Press, Westmount, Quebec, vol 2, ch 4

Bernard T N 1987 Don't discard diskography. Radiology 162: 285

Bernard T N 1990 Lumbar discography followed by computed tomography: refining the diagnosis of low-back pain. Spine 15: 690–707

Bogduk N 1983 The innervation of the lumbar spine. Spine 8: 286–293

Bogduk N 1986 The innervation of the lumbar intervertebral discs. In: Grieve G P (ed) Modern manual therapy of the vertebral column. Churchill Livingstone, Edinburgh, ch 14

Bogduk N 1988 The innervation of intervertebral discs. In: Ghosh P (ed) The biology of the intervertebral disc. CRC Press, Boca Raton, vol 1, ch 5

Bogduk N, Lambert G A, Duckworth J W 1981a The anatomy and physiology of the vertebral nerve in relation to migraine. Cephalalgia 1: 11–14

Bogduk N, Tynan W, Wilson A S 1981b The nerve supply to the human lumbar intervertebral discs. Journal of Anatomy 132: 39–56

Bogduk N, Windsor M, Inglis A 1985 The innervation of the cervical intervertebral discs. Presented at the XIIth International Anatomy Congress, London, August 17–22

Bogduk N et al 1988

Bogduk N, Windsor M, Inglis A 1989 The innervation of the cervical intervertebral discs. Spine 13: 2–8

Bradford K, Spurling R G 1945 The intervertebral disc. 2nd edn. Charles C Thomas, Springfield, Illinois

Bridge C J 1959 Innervation of spinal meninges and epidural structures. Anatomical Record 133: 553–561

Brodsky A E, Binder W F 1979 Lumbar discography. Its value in diagnosis and treatment of lumbar disc lesions. Spine 4: 110–120

Buskirk C 1941 Nerves in the vertebral canal. Archives of Surgery 43: 427–432

Butt W P 1963 Lumbar discography. Journal of the Canadian Association of Radiologists 14: 172–181

Clifford J R 1986 Lumbar discography: an outdated procedure. Journal of Neurosurgery 64: 686

Cloward R B 1959 Cervical diskography. A contribution to the aetiology and mechanism of neck, shoulder and arm pain. Annals of Surgery 130: 1052–1064

Cloward R B 1960 The clinical significance of the sinu-vertebral nerve of the cervical spine in relation to the cervical disk syndrome. Journal of Neurology Neurosurgery and Psychiatry 23: 321–326

Cloward R B 1963 Cervical discography. Acta Radiologica Diagnosis 1: 675–688

Colhoun E, McCall I W, Williams L, Cassar Pullicino V N 1988 Provocation discography as a guide to planning operations on the spine. Journal of Bone and Joint Surgery 70B: 267–271

Collins H R 1975 An evaluation of cervical and lumbar discography. Clinical Orthopaedics and Related Research 107: 133–138

Collis J S, Gardner W J 1962 Lumbar discography — an analysis of 1000 cases. Journal of Neurosurgery 19: 452–461

Crock H V 1986 Internal disc disruption: a challenge to disc prolapse fifty years on. Spine 11: 650–653

Edgar M A, Ghadially J A 1976 Innervation of the lumbar spine. Clinical Orthopaedics 115: 35–41

Edgar M A, Nundy S 1966 Innervation of the spinal dura mater. Journal of Neurology Neurosurgery and Psychiatry 29: 530–534

Ehrenhaft J L 1943 Development of the vertebral column as related to certain congenital and pathological changes. Surgery, Gynecology and Obstetrics 76: 282–292

Errico T J 1987 The role of diskography in the 1980s. Radiology 162: 285–286

Executive Committee of the North American Spine Society 1988 Position statement on discography 13: 1343

Farfan H F 1985 The use of mechanical etiology to determine the efficacy of active intervention in single joint lumbar intervertebral joint problems. Spine 10: 350–358

Feinberg S B 1945 The place of diskography in radiology as based on 2320 cases. American Journal of Roentgenology 92: 1275–1281

Ferlic D C 1963 The nerve supply of the cervical intervertebral discs in man. Bulletin of the Johns Hopkins Hospital 113: 347–351

Friedman J, Goldner M Z 1955 Discography in evaluation of lumbar disk lesions. Radiology 65: 653–662

Groen G J et al 1979

Groen G J, Baljet B, Drukker J 1988 The innervation of the spinal dura mater: anatomy and clinical implications. Acta Neurochirurgica 92: 39–46

Groen G J, Baljet B, Drukker J 1990 Nerves and nerve plexuses of the human vertebral column. American Journal of Anatomy 188: 282–296

Guerrier Y 1949 Les nerfs vertebraux. Acta Anatomica 8: 62–90

Herlihy W F 1949 The sinu-vertebral nerve. New Zealand Medical Journal 48: 214–216

Hirsch C 1949 An attempt to diagnose the level of a disc lesion clinically by disc puncture. Acta Orthopaedica Scandinavica 18: 132–140

Hirsch C, Ingelmark B E, Miller M 1963 The anatomical basis for low back pain. Acta Orthopaedica Scandinavica 33: 1–17

Holt E P 1964 The fallacy of cervical discography. Journal of the American Medical Association 188: 799–801

Holt E P 1968 The question of lumbar diskography. Journal of Bone and Joint Surgery 50A: 720–725

Hovelacque A 1925 Le nerf sinuvertebral. Annales d'Anatomie Pathologique et Anatomie Normale Medico-Chirurgicale 2: 435–443

Hovelacque A 1927 Anatomie des nerfs craniens et rachidiens et du systeme grande sympathique. Doin, Paris

Ikari C 1954 A study on the mechanisms of low back pain. The neurohistological examination of the disease. Journal of Bone and Joint Surgery 36A: 195

Jackson H C, Winkelmann R K, Bickel W M 1966 Nerve endings in the human lumbar spinal column and related structures. Journal of Bone and Joint Surgery 48A: 1272–1281

Jung A, Brunschwig A 1932 Recherches histologiques des articulations des corps vertebraux. Presse Médicale 40: 316–317

Keck C 1960 Discography: technique and interpretation. AMA Archives of Surgery 80: 580–586

Kikuchi S, MacNab I, Moreau P 1981 Localisation of the level of symptomatic cervical disc degeneration. Journal of Bone and Joint Surgery 63B: 272–277

Kimmel D L 1959 The cervical sympathetic rami and the vertebral nerve plexus in the human foetus. Journal of Comparative Neurology 122: 141–161

Kimmel D L 1961 Innervation of spinal dura mater and dura mater of posterior cranial fossa. Neurology 10: 800–809

Klafta L A, Collis J S 1969 The diagnostic inaccuracy of the pain response in cervical discography. Cleveland Clinic Quarterly 36: 35–39

Konttinen Y T, Gronblad M, Antti-Poika I et al 1990 Neuroimmunohistochemical analysis of peridiscal nociceptive neural elements. Spine 15: 383–386

Korkala O, Gronblad M, Liesi P, Karaharju E 1985 Immunohistochemical demonstration of nociceptors in the ligamentous structures of the lumbar spine. Spine 10: 156–157

Lamb D W 1979 The neurology of spinal pain. Physical Therapy 59: 971–973

Laux G, Guerrier Y 1939 Innervation de l'artère vertebrale. Annales d'Anatomie Pathologique et d'Anatomie Normale Medicochirurgicle 16: 249–255

Laux G, Guerrier Y 1947 Innervations de l'artere vertebrale. Comptes Rendus de l'Association des Anatomistes, 34: 298–300

Lazorthes G, Cassan J 1939 Essai de schematisation des ganglions etoile et intermediare. Comptes Rendus de l'Association des Anatomistes, 28: 193–210

Lazorthes G, Pouhes J, Espagno J 1947 Etude sur les nerfs sinu-vertebraux lombaires. Le nerf de Roofe, existe-t-il? Comptes Rendus de L'Association des Anatomistes 34: 317–320

Lindblom K 1948 Diagnostic disc puncture of intervertebral disks in sciatica. Acta Orthopaedica Scandinavica 17: 231–239

Lindblom K 1950 Technique and results in myelography and disc puncture. Acta Radiologica 34: 321–330

Lindblom K 1951a Technique and results of diagnostic disc puncture and injection (discography) in the lumbar region. Acta Orthopaedica Scandinavica 20: 315–326

Lindblom K 1951b Discography of dissecting transosseous ruptures of intervertebral discs in the lumbar region. Acta Radiologica 36: 13–16

Malinsky J 1959 The ontogenetic development of nerve terminations in the intervertebral discs of man. Acta Anatomica 38: 96–113

McCutcheon M E 1986 CT scanning of lumbar discography: a useful diagnostic adjunct. Spine 11: 257–259

McFadden J W 1988 The stress lumbar discogram. Spine 13: 931–933

Meyer R R 1963 Cervical diskography: a help or hindrance in evaluating neck, shoulder, arm pain. Radiology 90: 1208–1215

Milette P C, Melanson D 1982 A reappraisal of lumbar discography. Journal of the Canadian Association of Radiologists 33: 176–182

Milette P C, Melanson D 1987 Lumbar diskography. Radiology 163: 828–829

Mixter W J, Barr J S 1934 Rupture of the intervertebral disc with involvement of the spinal canal. New England Journal of Medicine 211: 210–215

Monteiro H, Rodrigues A 1931 Sur les variations du nerf vertebral. Comptes Rendus de l'Association des Anatomistes, 21: 406–419

Nachemson A 1989 Editorial comment: lumbar dicography — where are we today? Spine 14: 555–557

Paris S V 1983 Anatomy as related to function and pain. Orthopedic Clinics of North America 14: 475–489

Park W 1980 The place of radiology in the investigation of low back pain. Clinics in the Rheumatic Diseases 6: 93–132

Patrick B C 1973 Lumbar discography: a five year study. Surgical Neurology 1: 267–273

Pedersen H E, Blunck C F J, Gardner E 1956 The anatomy of the lumbosacral posterior rami and meningeal branches of spinal nerves (sinu-vertebral nerves). Journal of Bone and Joint Surgery 38A: 377–391

Perkins P G 1986 Lumbar discography. Journal of Neurosurgery 65: 882–883

Roofe P G 1940 Innervation of annulus fibrosus and posterior longitudinal ligament. Archives of Neurology and Psychiatry 44: 100–103

Roth D A 1976 Cervical analgesic discography. A new test for the definitive diagnosis of the painful-disk syndrome. Journal of the American Medical Association 235: 1713–1714

Sachs B L, Vanharanta H, Spivey M A et al 1987 The relationship of pain provocation to lumbar disc deterioration as seen by CT/discography. Spine 12: 287–294

Scullin D R 1987 Lumbar diskography. Radiology 162: 284

Shapiro R 1986a Lumbar discography: an outdated procedure. Journal of Neurosurgery 64: 686

Shapiro R 1986b Current status of lumbar diskography. Radiology 159: 815

Shinohara H 1970 A study on lumbar disc lesions. Journal of the Japanese Orthopaedic Association 44: 553

Simmons E H, Segil C M 1975 An evaluation of discography in the localisation of symptomatic levels in discogenic disease of the spine. Clinical Orthopaedics 108: 57–69

Simmons J W, Aprill C N, Dwyer A P, Brodsky A E 1988 A reassessment of Holt's data on: 'the question of lumbar discography'. Clinical Orthopaedics and Related Research 237: 120–124

Smith G W 1959 The normal cervical diskogram. Radiology 81: 1006–1010

Sneider S E, Winslow O P, Pryor J H 1963 Cervical diskography: is it relevant? Journal of the American Medical Association 185: 163–165

Soulie A 1905 Nerfs rachidiens. In Poirier P, Charpy A (eds) Traite d'anatomie humaine. 2nd edn. Masson, Paris, vol 3

Spurling R G, Bradford F K 1939 Neurologic aspects of herniated nucleus pulposus. Journal of the American Medical Association 113: 2019–2022

Spurling R G, Grantham E G 1940 Neurologic picture of herniation of the nucleus pulposus in the lower part of the lumbar region. Archives of Surgery 40: 378–381

Stillwell D L 1956 The nerve supply of the vertebral column and its associated structures in the monkey. Anatomical Record 125: 139–169

Stuck R M 1961 Cervical discography. Radiology 86: 975–982

Taveras J 1967 Is discography a useful diagnostic procedure? Journal of the Canadian Association of Radiologists 19: 294–295

Taylor J R, Twomey L T 1979 Innervation of lumbar intervertebral discs. Medical Journal of Australia 2: 701–702

Tsukada K 1938 Histologische Studien über die Zwischenwirbelscheibe des Menschen. I. Histologische Befunde des Foetus. Mitt Akademie Kioto 24: 1057, 1172

Tsukada K 1939 Histologische Studien über die Zwischenwirbelscheibe des Menschen. II. Altersveränderungen. Mitt Akademie Kioto 25: 1, 207

Van Niekerk J P de V 1979 Discography simplified. South African Medical Journal 53: 551–554

Vanharanta H, Sachs B L, Spivey M A et al 1987 The relationship of pain provocation to lumbar disc deterioration as seen by CT/discography. Spine 12: 295–298

Videman T, Malmivaara A, Mooney V 1987 The value of the axial view in assessing discograms: an experimental study with cadavers. Spine 12: 299–304

Von Luschka H 1850 Die Nerven des menschlichen Wirbelkanales. Laupp, Tübingen, The Netherlands

Walsh T R, Weinstein J N, Spratt K F et al 1990 Lumbar discography in normal subjects. Journal of Bone and Joint Surgery 72A: 1081–1088

Weinstein J, Claverie W, Gibson S 1988 The pain of discography. Spine 13: 1344–1348

Wiberg G 1949 Back pain in relation to the nerve supply of intervertebral discs. Act Orthopaedica Scandinavica 19: 211–221

Wiley J J, MacNab I, Wortzman G 1968 Lumbar discography and its clinical applications. Canadian Journal of Surgery 11: 280–289

Wilson D H, MacCarty W C 1969 Discography: its role in the diagnosis of lumbar disc protrusion. Journal of Neurosurgery 31: 520–523

Windsor M, Ingles A, Bogduk N 1985 The innervation of the cervical intervertebral discs. In Proceedings of the Anatomical Society of Australia and New Zealand. Journal of Anatomy 142: 218

Wyke B 1970 The neurological basis of thoracic spinal pain. Rheumatology and Physical Medicine 10: 356–367

Wyke B 1976 Neurological aspects of low back pain. In: Jayson M I V (ed) The lumbar spine and back pain. Grune & Stratton, New York, ch 10

Wyke B 1980 The neurology of low back pain. In: Jayson M I V (ed) The lumbar spine and back pain. 2nd edn. Pitman, Tunbridge Wells, ch 11

Yoshizawa H, O'Brien J P, Thomas-Smith W, Trumper M 1980 The neuropathology of intervertebral discs removed for low-back pain. Journal of Pathology 132: 95–104

13. Chemistry of the intervertebral disc in relation to functional requirements

J. P. Urban   S. Roberts

INTRODUCTION

The intervertebral disc has a prominent role in the structure and function of the spine. It is able to transmit load and act as a joint. Although its mechanical behaviour in compression, extension, torsion and bending has been extensively investigated, little is yet known of how the composition and structure of the disc influence its mechanical behaviour. In this chapter, current ideas on the relationship between disc mechanical function and its chemical composition will be reviewed.

GROSS STRUCTURE OF THE DISC

The intervertebral disc is generally considered to consist of two distinct regions: the outer, firm, banded annulus fibrosus and the inner, soft, gelatinous nucleus pulposus. The cartilaginous end-plates are interposed between the bony vertebral bodies and the disc itself. Some useful reviews of disc structure and the changes found with age and with degeneration are by Buckwalter (1982), Coventry et al (1945), Peacock (1952), Twomey and Taylor (1986). Figure 13.1 illustrates the regions of the disc.

The nucleus pulposus

The nucleus occupies the central region of the disc. Its composition and appearance change markedly throughout life. In children it is highly hydrated, being 85–90% water, and is white and translucent. There is a clear demarcation between it and the surrounding annulus fibrosus. In adults the hydration drops markedly, and as the tissue becomes firmer and loses its translucency the boundary between nucleus and annulus becomes more difficult to distinguish. In old age the hydration of the nucleus approaches that of the annulus.

The annulus fibrosus

To the naked eye, the annulus fibrosus appears to consist

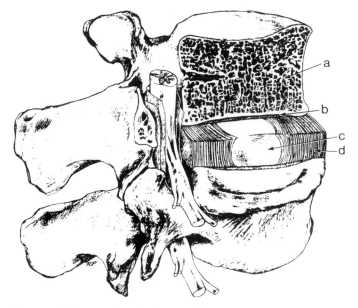

Fig. 13.1 Diagram showing location of (a) vertebral body, (b) cartilage end-plate, (c) nucleus pulposus and (d) annulus fibrosus.

of a series of concentric layers surrounding the nucleus pulposus. This banded appearance results from an intricate arrangement of fibrous lamellae which will be discussed in more detail later. The annulus is firmer and less hydrated than the nucleus, and changes with age in this structure are not so apparent.

The cartilage end-plate

In children this region acts as a growth plate until skeletal maturity is reached, when the outer ring of 2–3 mm calcifies and fuses with the rim of the vertebral body. A plate of hyaline cartilage, approximately 1–2 mm in thickness, remains abutting the central region of the disc throughout adult life. Fibres from the disc continue into the end-plate where they align horizontally. At the bony interface there is a region of calcified cartilage. The composition of the end-plate resembles that of the disc, but with less water and a greater fibrous component (Roberts et al 1989).

THE CONSTITUENTS OF THE DISC

The matrix of the intervertebral disc is very similar in composition to that of articular cartilage. It consists of collagen fibres embedded in a proteoglycan–water gel (see Fig. 13.2). Contained within this matrix are cells, the chondrocytes, which are actively maintaining and repairing it. The mean cell density in the disc is very low so that cells occupy only about 1–5% of the tissue volume. Because of the low cellularity, the mechanical properties of the disc depend chiefly on the constituents of the matrix. However, activity of the cells is vital for maintaining the integrity of the tissue.

Proteoglycans

Proteoglycans are found in many tissues and cells apart from those of the connective tissues. They are thought to have many possible functions, e.g. binding growth factors (Ruoslahti & Yamaguchi 1991), cell matrix interactions (Sommarin et al 1989). However, in this chapter only the biophysical functions of the proteoglycans will be discussed. These are principally connected with the response of the disc to mechanical load. As in all load-bearing cartilages, proteoglycans endow the matrix with a high osmotic pressure and a low hydraulic permeability and hence constitute the compression-resisting component of the disc.

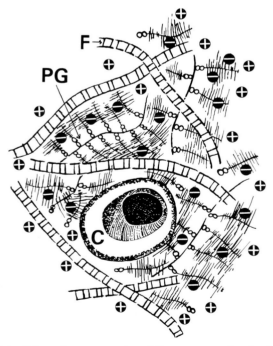

Fig. 13.2 Schematic representation of disc structure, showing banded collagen fibres (F), interspersed with numerous bottle-brush-like proteoglycan molecules (PG). These have a very high density of negative charges which are responsible for many of the physiological properties in the matrix. The average diameter of a cell (C) is approximately 10 μm and of a collagen fibril is 0.05 μm in the nucleus.

Proteoglycan structure

Proteoglycans (PGs) are a family of macromolecules consisting of polysaccharide chains covalently bound to a central protein core. The number of polysaccharide chains and the size of the core protein is very variable. The main PGs found in the disc are large molecules of molecular weight $3.10^5–2.10^6$, with the polysaccharide chains consisting mostly of the sulphated glycosaminoglycans (GAGs), chondroitin sulphate (CS) and keratan sulphate (KS). These two GAGs occupy different regions of the protein core, referred to as the KS-rich and variable regions of the monomer respectively. Beyond the KS-rich region, the protein core ends in two globular regions, one of which, the hyaluronic-acid-binding region, is so named because a proportion of the monomers are not free in the tissue but are attached, via this region, to long chains of hyaluronic acid to form PG aggregates. This attachment is stabilized by a protein, link-protein, which binds both to hyaluronic acid and to the hyaluronic-acid-binding region of the PG. Figure 13.3 is a schematic view of the large PG monomer and aggregate.

Disc PGs tend to be smaller than those from hyaline cartilages, possibly because the CS-rich region of the core protein is shorter, particularly in the nucleus. Only about 30% of monomers found in the disc nucleus can form aggregates compared with about 80% in hip cartilage. Moreover, the aggregates from the nucleus are smaller, having a molecular weight of about 7 million compared to 100 million for aggregates found in bovine nasal septum. There are indications that the disc PGs are able to form aggregates when newly synthesized, but that they are degraded in the tissue and that their hyaluronic-acid-binding region disappears. The functional significance of differences in degree of aggregation and of PG size are not yet understood. It has been suggested that the aggregation

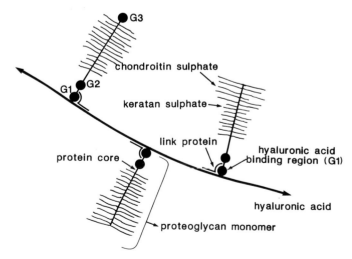

Fig. 13.3 Diagram of part of a disc proteoglycan aggregate. G1, G2 and G3 are globular, folded regions of the central core protein, though G3 is often absent, especially in the disc.

helps to keep the PGs in the tissue since there is no evidence that they are held there by any form of binding. Present knowledge of PG structure has recently been reviewed by Carney and Muir (1988).

Fixed-charge density

One important property of the GAGs is that they are charged. Both CS and KS contain charged acidic groups (SO_3^- and COO^-), which impart a net negative charge to the matrix. Figure 13.4 shows the structural formulae of these molecules; CS has two charges per disaccharide unit whereas KS has only one. The concentration of fixed negative charges, the fixed-charge density (FCD), thus depends not only on the concentration of PG in the tissue, but also on the CS/KS ratio. The FCD confers important properties on the disc since it controls the distribution of charged solutes and hence osmotic pressure, as discussed later.

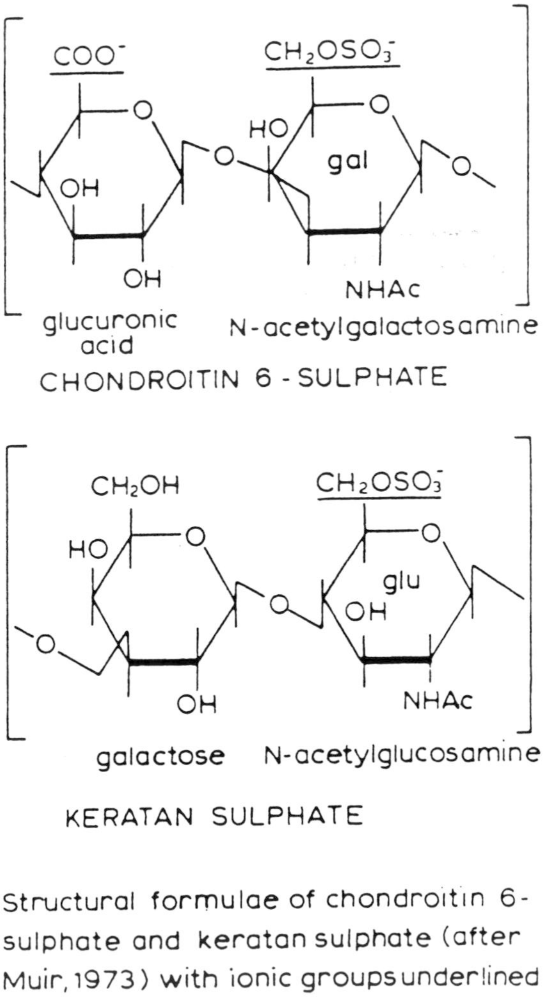

Structural formulae of chondroitin 6-sulphate and keratan sulphate (after Muir, 1973) with ionic groups underlined

Fig. 13.4 Chemical formulae of the repeating units of chondroitin and keratan sulphate, showing the charged groups (adapted from Urban & Maroudas 1980).

Collagen

Collagen is the main structural protein of the body. It is not a single substance; rather, collagen describes a family of at least 14 genetically distinct proteins. The characteristic fibrillar collagen molecule is formed from three polypeptide chains (alpha-chains), joined together in a triple helix. These molecules align in a quarter-stagger arrangement to form the collagen microfibril. Collagen fibrils are stabilized and are given their high tensile strength by inter- and intramolecular cross-links. Inherited pathologies, in which cross-linking is defective, such as Ehlers–Danlos type VI and type VII, provide insight into the important features of collagen organization and are reviewed by Levene (1978) and Eyre et al (1984).

Collagen types

The organization and type of collagen varies from tissue to tissue. The collagen found mainly in skin, bone and tendon, type I collagen, exists in fibrillar form, as does type II collagen, found in cartilage and vitreous humour. The fibrillar forms of collagen have great tensile strength, but are non-elastic and can be extended only by about 3%. Although the size of fibril varies from tissue to tissue, it is not known how far fibril formation is related to collagen type. Mechanical properties of the different collagen types are unknown. Mechanical properties of collagen are discussed in a recent general review on collagen by Nimni and Harkness (1988).

It is now clear that complex fibres, with two or more types of collagen, occur in some tissues. The fibrils of type II collagen contain a small proportion of both types IX and XI collagen. Type IX collagen is of particular interest; it is known to be covalently linked to the surface of type II collagen fibrils and since it has at least two sites for cross-linking it may serve to bind type II collagen fibrils together. It may also link the collagen fibrils to other matrix components (Wu & Eyre 1989; Van der Rest & Mayne 1988). Type I collagen fibrils similarly contain a small fraction of type V and possibly type XII collagen.

As well as these fibril-forming collagens, which make up the main structural framework of skeletal tissues, non-fibrillar collagens, in particular type VI collagen, are also found in cartilages. Type VI collagen is known to bind to cell-surface receptors and may also bind to type II collagen, thus having the potential to link the chondrocyte to the matrix. It is therefore not surprising that its concentration is highest around the cell (Poole et al 1988), although in degenerate cartilage it is also abundant throughout the matrix (McDevitt et al 1988). Table 13.1 summarizes the properties of the different collagen types.

Collagen types in the disc

The disc is unusual in that it contains fibrils of both types

Table 13.1 The properties of different types of collagen*

Type	Distribution and possible function	Present in disc
**I	Abundant and widespread, e.g. skin, bone	+
**II	Hyaline cartilage, vitreous humour, meniscus	+
**III	Widespread, e.g. skin, vascular and healing tissue	+
IV	Forms lattice, in basement membranes	
**V	Widespread in small amounts, co-distributes with type I	+
VI	Widespread, binds nerves, vessels etc. within tissues	+
VII	Anchors ectodermal basement membrane	
VIII	Anchoring, endothelial basement membrane	
IX	Controls diameter of type II fibrils, in hyaline cartilage, vitreous humour	+
X	Hypertrophic zone of ossifying cartilage	
**XI	Co-distributes with type II collagen	+
XII	Co-distributes with type I, in eye and tendon	

* Adapted from Eyre 1988.
** Fibrillar collagen, provides structural framework.

I and II collagens, the two types making up approximately 80% of the total collagen. The fine fibrils of the nucleus are virtually all type II collagen, whereas the outer annulus is predominantly type I collagen. The proportion of type I collagen in the annulus decreases towards the nucleus as the proportion of type II collagen rises (Eyre 1988). It is not known whether the fibrils of the disc are of mixed collagen types or whether each collagen type forms its own weave. The disc also contains a relatively high proportion of minor collagens. The nucleus of the bovine disc is rich in type VI collagen, but immuno-histochemical studies show that in human disc type VI collagen is found predominantly in a capsule around the cell as seen in hyaline cartilages (Roberts et al 1991). Type III and type IX collagen are also found in the capsule around the cell.

Collagen organization in the disc

The organization of collagen fibrils in the disc is highly specialized. The three-dimensional collagen framework has been described and shown in scanning electron micrographs. In the nucleus the collagen fibrils are much finer than in the annulus, mostly about 0.05 μm in diameter, and are arranged in a loose irregular meshwork. In the annulus, collagen is arranged in 15 to 25, more or less, concentric lamellae made of parallel bundles of fine fibrils 0.1–0.2 μm in diameter. These lamellae are visible to the naked eye and vary from 100 to 500 μm in width, the outer lamellae being thickest; the width varies with age and location. The lamellae in the posterior are not as wide as those in the rest of the disc. The architecture of the lamellae has been described in detail by Marchand and Ahmed (1990).

The fibre bundles of each lamella run obliquely between the adjacent vertebral bodies and are firmly anchored to them or to the cartilaginous end-plate. The resulting angle formed between the fibre bundles of the lamellae and the

vertebral bodies varies between 40 and 70°, the direction of the fibres alternating in the neighbouring lamellae. Happey (1980) has described how the angle changes with position in the annulus.

The arrangement of the collagen network in the disc has an important influence on how load is distributed. The angle between the fibre bundles of the adjacent lamellae is able to change since the lamellae are loosely interconnected. Even though collagen is only slightly extensible, the fact that the lamellae can move separately gives the structure itself considerable extensibility, especially in the vertical direction. The annulus is thus able to move and bulge outwards under the pressure evenly applied to it by the gel-like nucleus, or extend by 30% by changing the crossing angle of its fibres.

The arrangement of the collagen network in the disc and the changes that could occur under compressive load are shown schematically in Figure 13.5.

Non-collagenous proteins

In addition to collagen and PG the disc contains a considerable fraction of non-collagenous proteins. These include structural glycoproteins, such as elastin, and other less well characterized fractions (Heinegard & Oldberg 1989). Some may be associated with the cell membrane, as has been found in other cartilages, where they are strongly implicated in the interaction of the chondrocyte with the extracellular matrix. Amyloid, extravascular plasma proteins and endogenous proteinases and inhibitors are also found in disc tissue and may be involved in

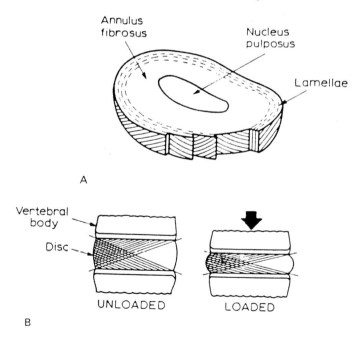

Fig. 13.5 Arrangement of the collagen network in the annulus. (**A**) Schematic view of annulus lamellae showing alternating direction of collagen bundles (after Schultz, 1974). (**B**) Change of crossing angle of collagen bundles with load (after Szirmai, 1970).

ageing and degenerative processes (Melrose & Ghosh 1988).

Cells

The disc has a low cellularity; the mean cell density of the adult human disc is about 5500 cells mm^{-3} (Maroudas et al 1975). The cell density is not uniform throughout the tissue, being highest near the end-plate and at the periphery of the annulus, i.e. in the regions nearest the blood supply. The primary function of these cells is the manufacture and maintenance of the matrix.

In adult tissue the cells are chondrocyte-like. The matrix around these is highly organized, with fine fibrils of some minor collagens forming a capsule around the cell. Cell shape varies depending on location, becoming more elongated and fibroblast-like towards the outer annulus. These differences in shape may reflect differences in function.

Water

Water, containing dissolved solutes, is the main constituent of the disc. It occupies 65–90% of the tissue volume, depending on age and region. Since the cell density is low, most of the water is extracellular. Some of it is associated with the collagen fibrils, the intrafibrillar fraction. This fraction, which is about 1.0 g water/g dry collagen, may be considerable in old or degenerate discs which have low PG concentrations. This intrafibrillar water is freely exchangeable and is accessible to small solutes such as glucose but large molecules, such as the PGs themselves, are excluded from this fraction. Their effective concentration is then often underestimated (Maroudas 1990).

Nerves

It is now well accepted that the outer region of the intervertebral disc is innervated (Yoshizawa et al 1980; Bogduk et al 1981). The type of nerves present, and their function, is less clear, although recent work has demonstrated the presence of neuropeptides in the outer annulus, which are generally considered to have a sensory function in that location (McCarthy et al 1991). Thus an injured or diseased disc has the potential to be painful. If the injury is to the innervated region of the disc, stress on that area could cause pain directly. If other, non-innervated portions were damaged, otherwise healthy and innervated regions may have to carry an increased load, and may subsequently become sources of pain.

THE RELATIVE PROPORTION OF MATRIX CONSTITUENTS

Changes across the disc

The proportions of the three main constituents of the

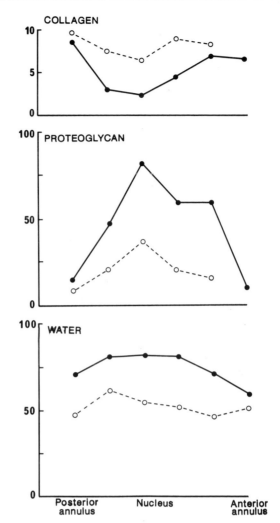

Fig. 13.6 The composition changes with location within the disc (●——●) and the endplate (○- - -○), the nucleus having the most water and proteoglycan, but least collagen content.

disc, water, collagen and PGs, vary considerably with position in the tissue. Some of the available information is summarized in Figure 13.6 where it can be seen that the nucleus is more hydrated than the annulus and has a higher concentration of PGs (expressed here as level of dye binding per unit dry weight), but a lower proportion of collagen than the annulus. The composition of the annulus is not constant; there is a gradient in the proportions of these components through the annulus, with the outer annulus having the highest collagen content and the lowest water and PG content. The composition of the inner annulus approaches that of the nucleus. The composition of the end-plate also varies with position; collagen content increases and PG and water contents decrease towards the bone.

Changes with age

The composition of the disc changes with age. The water content of the nucleus, over 85% in the juvenile disc, decreases to approach that of the annulus in mature adults. The water content of the annulus, however, stays fairly steadily at 70–76% throughout life. PG concentration falls with age in both nucleus and annulus, but the collagen content remains more or less constant. The proportion of non-collagenous protein rises with age; this rise could partly reflect an alteration in PG structure, since the KS/CS ratio also increases with age. It is clear that the composition of the disc does not remain constant throughout life.

Changes with disease

The changes in the composition of the disc have been characterized for various pathological conditions. In virtually all instances degeneration leads to loss of PG, a disorganization of the collagen network, and an ingrowth of blood vessels. In scoliosis, the discs appear to have a lower PG content than normal discs of similar age; moreover, the changes appear greatest at the apex of the curve. Collagen abnormalities in scoliosis have been reported by some authors but have not been found by others. It is now generally thought that these changes in composition are secondary and reflect changes in cell behaviour resulting from the changes in mechanical stress on the scoliotic disc (Pedrini et al 1983).

FUNCTION OF THE CONSTITUENTS OF THE DISC

The major functions of the discs are mechanical as the discs serve both to transmit load and to act as joints. These mechanical functions are directly related to the concentration and arrangement of the two major structural components of the tissue, collagen and PG.

A structural model

The functions of the macromolecular constituents of the matrix are demonstrated in a physical model built by Broom and Marra (1985) (Fig. 13.7). This model consists of a network of string enclosing balloons which inflate the network and prevent it from collapsing. The resulting structure is able to support compressive loads, though neither the string nor balloons could do so alone, as the string would collapse and the balloons would fly apart. When a load is applied to the structure, it deforms with a degree of deformation which is proportional to the magnitude of the load. Deformation also, however, depends on the extensibility of the string, on the weave of the network, particularly on the number of linkages and knots, and on how the network is anchored to its base. It depends too on the number of balloons and their degree of inflation. In general, if the network is filled with highly inflated balloons, so that the string network is taut, the network deforms less than it would if there were only a few underinflated balloons, and the network is floppy.

In cartilage, collagen forms a structural framework, which, like the string network, is strong in tension but collapses under a compressive load if unsupported. PGs are held in the matrix by the collagen network as the balloons are held in the string network. PGs imbibe water as discussed later, and inflate the collagen network, as the balloons inflate the string network, and, in so doing, give cartilage its rigidity. However, the behaviour of cartilage differs in an important respect from that of the string–balloon model. In cartilage, water is not trapped in an impermeable membrane but is expressed from the tissue when a load is applied and is re-imbibed when the load is removed. The amount of fluid lost is controlled by the osmotic and permeability properties of the PGs.

The biophysical functions of the main constituents of the disc are summarized in Table 13.2.

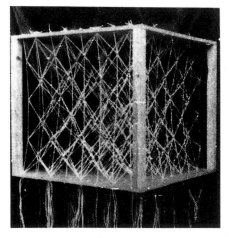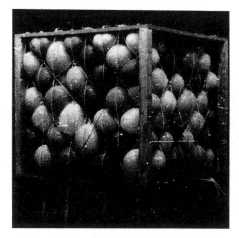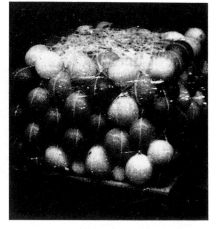

Fig. 13.7 A model of disc matrix has been developed by Broom and Marra (1985) whereby the proteoglycan molecules can be represented by inflated balloons, contained within a fibrous string network representing the collagen fibres.

Table 13.2 Functional properties of the main constituents of the disc*

Constituent	Function
Proteoglycans	1 Through their high osmotic pressure, inflate the disc and maintain its hydration in the face of high external loads
	2 Because of their close-packed interpenetrating network, impart a low hydraulic permeability to the tissue and thus slow the rate of fluid loss
	3 Because of their charge and the small pores available, exclude negatively-charged and large solutes from the matrix
Collagen	1 Acts in tension to provide the structural network which enables the disc to act as a joint and shock-absorber
	2 Anchors the disc to the vertebral bodies
	3 Entangles the proteoglycan chains and thus keeps them in the tissue
Water	1 Inflates the tissue and provides 70–80% of its volume
	2 Provides a medium for the transport of dissolved nutrients to the chondrocytes

* Adapted from Maroudas 1980.

The biophysical functions of proteoglycans

The osmotic pressure of proteoglycan solutions

The high osmotic pressure of PG solutions results mainly from the polyelectrolyte nature of the PGs, i.e. from

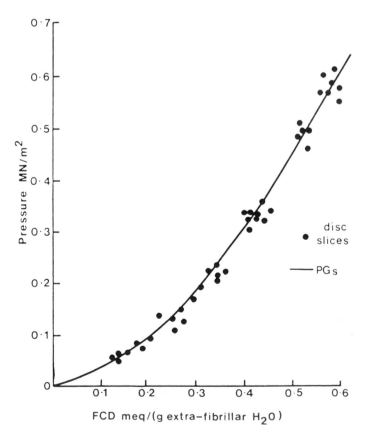

Fig. 13.8 The variation of disc proteoglycan osmotic pressure with proteoglycan concentration expressed as fixed charge density.

the fixed negative charges on the GAGs. Ions and other solutes distribute themselves between the plasma and the disc in order to maintain electrochemical equilibrium for all species. The expression which describes this equilibrium distribution, the Gibbs–Donnan equation, shows that, because of the net negative charge on the disc, the total number of ions in the disc is always greater than in the plasma. This effect is shown in Figure 13.8. Since osmotic pressure results from a difference in the number of dissolved particles between the two phases, the excess number of ions in the disc leads to a high osmotic pressure in the tissue. PG size or degree of aggregation have little influence on osmotic pressure compared with charge density (Comper and Preston 1974, Urban et al 1979).

The relationship between PG concentration expressed as fixed charge density and osmotic pressure, for PGs extracted from adult disc, is also shown in Figure 13.8. (This curve does not necessarily apply to other cartilage PGs.) In the nucleus of the resting adult disc the FCD lies between 0.2 and 0.4 mEq ml^{-1} depending on age. The osmotic pressure expressed by the PGs of these discs is consequently 0.1–0.3 MNm^{-2} (1–3 atmospheres). The FCD of the annulus, and hence its osmotic pressure, is somewhat lower, but is still considerable in comparison with that of non-weight-bearing tissues.

Hydraulic permeability

In the schematic view of the disc matrix shown in Figure 13.2, the matrix can be seen to consist of PGs densely packed in between collagen fibrils. The collagen fibrils are spaced at several hundred ångströms, whereas, because of their close packing, the distance between the GAG chains is only 20–40 Å (1 Å = 10^{-4} μm) (Byers et al 1983). The fine pore structure of the matrix is thus determined by the PG concentration rather than by the collagen network; the higher the PG concentration, the more closely packed are the GAGs and the smaller the effective 'pores' formed by the entangled GAG chains. A change in the water content of the disc alters PG concentration and thus pore size; if the tissue swells, the PG concentration falls and the effective pore size increases. Conversely, if the disc loses fluid, the pore size decreases as the same number of PG chains pack into a smaller volume of fluid.

The rate at which fluid can flow into or out of the disc under a pressure driving force depends on the hydraulic permeability of the matrix which is directly related to pore size distribution: small pores impart a low hydraulic permeability and thus restrict fluid flow. Alternatively, when the PG concentration is low and pore size is large, hydraulic permeability in high and fluid flow from the tissue is fastest. If fluid is lost from the tissue, the PG concentration increases and hence the hydraulic permeability falls; further fluid loss is thus slowed. Through this mechanism the disc limits rapid loss of hydration under

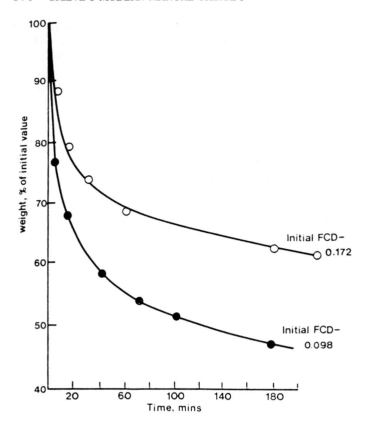

Fig. 13.9   The effect of proteoglycan content (FCD) on the rate of fluid loss from disc slices.

load. The effect of PG concentration on the hydraulic permeability coefficient is shown for two disc slices in Figure 13.9. The hydraulic permeability decreases very steeply with increase in PG concentration; at the concentrations found in the disc in vivo the hydraulic permeability is low and the amount of fluid lost under physiological loads is about 1 ml/disc in each day's activity.

Solute partitions

Proteoglycans, because they are charged and divide the extracellular spaces into small 'pores', control the concentration of dissolved solutes in the disc. The imbalance of charge in the matrix leads to the concentration of positive ions, such as calcium and sodium, being higher in the disc than in the external plasma as predicted by Gibbs–Donnan equilibrium expression (Maroudas 1980). The distribution of ions is important because it governs the osmotic pressure of the disc as discussed. Ion concentration can also influence matrix synthesis rates (Urban & Bayliss 1988, Gray et al 1988).

The concentration of large uncharged molecules in the disc is governed by the pore size distribution and this also depends on PG concentration. Many of the larger serum proteins have radii which are greater than the 20 Å radius of the 'pores' formed between the interdigitating GAG chains. Molecules such as serum albumin, haemoglobin

and immunoglobulins are virtually excluded from the matrix on account of their size. Even glucose (mol wt <200) is excluded from about 10% of the pores in a normal disc on account of its size (Urban et al 1979). It should be noted that as the PG concentration falls and pore size increases, as happens in disc degeneration or ageing, some of the pores become accessible to these large molecules. This process has not been investigated in the disc, but loss of PGs allows immunoglobulins to penetrate into the articular cartilage which might have an influence on development and progression of arthritis (Cooke 1980).

MECHANICAL BEHAVIOUR OF THE DISC IN RELATION TO ITS COMPOSITION

The disc is a composite structure consisting of PG, glycoproteins, collagen and water, and its behaviour under load, like that of Broom and Marra's model, depends both on the load and on the organization and properties of its extracellular matrix.

Swelling pressure of the disc

As discussed above, the disc contains PGs at concentrations which lead to an osmotic pressure, π, of several atmospheres in the tissue. PGs at such concentrations in contact with saline solutions would tend to imbibe water and hence cause the tissue to swell. In the disc this tendency to swell is opposed by two pressures, that arising from the combined effects of body weight and muscle tension, Pa, and that arising from the net restraining force of the collagen network of the disc, Pc. At equilibrium these effective pressures are balanced. Thus we can say:

$$Pa = (\pi - Pc) = Ps. \qquad \text{equation (1)}$$

$(\pi - Pc)$ is called the net swelling pressure of the tissue, Ps, since it describes the net potential of the tissue to swell. It can be seen that, since the swelling pressure depends on PG osmotic pressure and on the collagen network, it will vary with the composition of the disc and hence with region of the disc, with age and also with degeneration. Swelling pressure is, however, not an intrinsic property of the disc since both π and Pc vary with hydration, and hence with load.

If the load on the disc is increased, fluid will be expressed from the tissue. As fluid is expressed, the PG concentration and hence the osmotic pressure increases, but the volume of the tissue, and hence the collagen network tension, decreases. The net effect is an increase in swelling pressure (equation 1). If the load is maintained, fluid will continue to be expressed from the disc until the swelling pressure increases sufficiently to balance the applied pressure. Conversely, if the load on the disc is reduced, the disc swells. During swelling the PGs are diluted and their osmotic pressure decreases; as the disc volume increases the tension of the collagen network also increases. The swelling pressure is consequently reduced. If the load on the disc is completely removed, for instance when the disc is placed in saline solution in vitro, swelling will finally cease when the reduced osmotic pressure is balanced by the increased collagen tension. Swelling of unloaded tissue slices is considerable, especially in the nucleus where the collagen network is weakest; here the fluid content may increase 200–300% (Urban & Maroudas 1980). In such disc slices, PGs eventually escape from the swollen collagen network, π falls, and the disc slices eventually deflate. It should be noted that this behaviour has clinical relevance since sequestrated disc fragments are in effect unloaded fragments of disc, which can swell considerably.

Loads on the lumbar spine

In vivo the disc is always under load as a result of the combined effects of body weight and muscle activity. The magnitude of the load cannot be measured directly. However, it has been estimated from intradiscal pressure measurements (Nachemson 1960), and from measurements of myoelectric muscle activity and intra-abdominal pressure (reviewed by Andersson 1982). Load on the disc is very dependent on posture; Nachemson found that even in a relaxed supine subject the pressure on the lower lumbar discs was $0.1-0.2 \, \text{MNm}^{-2}$, whereas in unsupported sitting it rose to about $0.6-0.7 \, \text{MNm}^{-2}$. Peak pressures during strenuous activity may rise considerably above these values. Because of the relationship between disc pressure and posture the load on the spine tends to follow a cyclic pattern: it is at its lowest during sleep, and then increases 5- to 6-fold during the day's activities.

The deformation of the disc under load

Disc height alters with changes in load by two mechanisms. When the load on the disc is increased the disc deforms initially through a re-arrangement of the collagen network. The extent of this deformation varies from disc to disc, but the factors which govern this are not understood. No consistent pattern with age, sex or degree of degeneration has been found (Shirazi-Adl et al 1984). For changes in load of short duration this deformation is virtually constant volume. However, if the load is maintained the disc loses height or creeps, and a large part of the creep deformation results from fluid loss. Thus, for each applied load, the extent of the initial deformation will depend largely on the structure and integrity of the collagen network. In contrast, the rate and magnitude of the creep deformation is related more to the PG content, as PGs largely control swelling pressure and hence the equilibrium deformation, and also the hydraulic permeability and so the rate of water loss.

Hydration of the disc varies with load but the equilibrium hydration depends on the composition of the disc; discs with low PG concentrations will tend to lose more fluid under equivalent loads than those with high PG concentrations. The change in water content found in the nucleus of three discs when the pressure was increased from 0.1 to $0.6 \, \text{MNm}^{-2}$ is shown in Figure 13.10. The PG contents of these discs are shown in the same figure and it can be seen that the water content adjusts until the PG contents of all three discs are approximately equal at each applied pressure. Thus the 91-year, degenerate disc of low PG content is much less able to retain fluid in the face of applied pressure than the younger disc.

Schematic figure to show influence of composition on equilibrium hydration at pressure P.

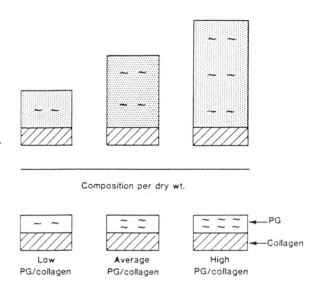

Composition per dry wt.

Low PG/collagen   Average PG/collagen   High PG/collagen

Schematic view of change in composition of disc slice with change in pressure

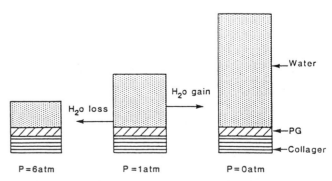

Fig. 13.10 The hydration and fixed-charge density of three nucleus slices of different ages as a function of applied pressure.

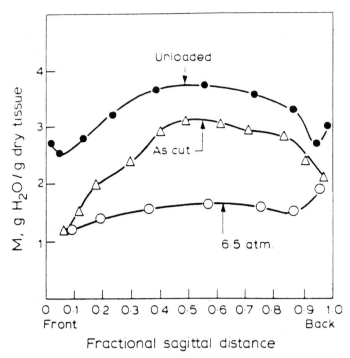

Fig. 13.11 Change in the water content profiles of two lumbar discs after applying a physiological load for 36 hours as compared with an untreated disc from the same spine.

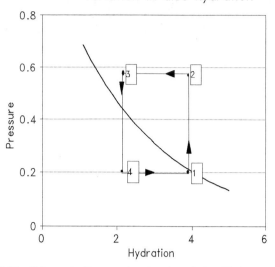

Schematic view of the diurnal variation in disc hydration

Fig. 13.12 Schematic diagram showing the relationship between the swelling pressure curve; loading history and fluid loss from the ΔP is given by (P1–P2) and by (P4–P3) and the osmotic pressure difference Δπ is given by the horizontal distance to the equilibrium curve.

The amount of water exchanged between disc and surroundings with changes in load is quite considerable. Figure 13.11 gives an indication of the extent to which water content profiles can change with alteration or variation in applied load. Adams and Hutton (1983) found that, on average, discs lost about 11% of their fluid during 4 hours loading, although the scatter was considerable. As shown in the figure, if the load is increased above the post-mortem level the disc will lose fluid and shrink; alternatively, if the load is reduced the tissue will imbibe fluid and swell. However, because the rate of fluid loss from the disc is slow, the extent of change in hydration found during the day will be far less than that necessary to reach swelling-pressure equilibrium.

The relationship between the disc swelling pressure, changes in load and fluid flow are sketched in Figure 13.12. Initially the disc is assumed to be at equilibrium at point (1), (after a night's rest). The pressure on the disc is suddenly increased to (2), (on rising, for example). The disc is no longer in equilibrium. Thus there is a driving force expressing fluid from the tissue which depends on the difference between (2) and the swelling pressure curve. While the pressure on the disc is maintained, fluid is expressed from the tissue. The rate of fluid loss depends partly on the driving force (it is fastest when the driving force is greatest) and partly on the hydraulic permeability of the tissue at point (2). Fluid loss is thus fastest initially. As fluid is expressed the PG concentration rises and the hydraulic permeability falls; also, the driving force diminishes as the equilibrium curve is approached. Both these

mechanisms help to limit the amount of fluid lost from the disc. When the pressure on the disc is released, the disc now lies under the swelling pressure curve, and thus will have a tendency to imbibe fluid in order to dilute the PGs. During swelling the hydraulic permeability increases; thus, the rate of fluid flow does not decrease drastically as equilibrium is approached. Swelling thus tends to be faster than fluid loss and hence the disc is able to replace the fluid lost in 16 hours of activity by 8 hours of rest.

Changes in height during the day are thought to result, in part, from loss of fluid from the disc. Eklund and Corlett (1984) measured loss in height of 6 mm on average during the day, and found that the rate of shrinkage depended on the load on the spine. Conversely, Thornton et al (1974) found that the sky-lab astronauts who were weightless for 85 days grew about 5 cm, in part probably through swelling of their discs under low external loads.

DISC NUTRITION AND MATRIX TURNOVER

Although the disc has a low cell density, the continued activity of the cells is vital to the health of the disc since the cells are responsible for turning over and renewing the matrix constituents.

Disc nutrition

The disc is avascular; thus, nutrients reach the cells by diffusion through the matrix of the disc from the blood vessels in contact with the annulus periphery and with the

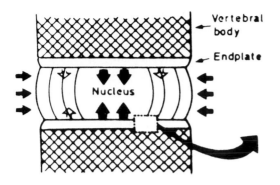
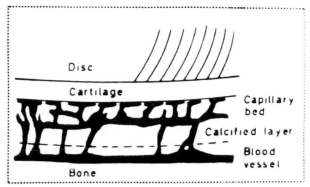

Fig. 13.13 Schematic view of the routes for transfer of nutrients into the disc and an enlarged view of the endplate (from Holm et al 1982).

cartilaginous endplate, as shown schematically in Figure 13.13. The route through the end-plate may disappear if a calcified layer forms or if the capillary bed is modified, thus putting the nucleus at risk.

Because of its size and avascularity, steep gradients in the concentration of nutrients exist in the disc. Holm et al (1982) have shown that while the outer annulus is more or less in equilibrium with the blood oxygen the interior regions of the disc are anaerobic and the oxygen concentrations are very low. The interior of the disc consequently has a high lactic acid content and hence a low pH which may lead to high activity of degradative enzymes. It has been suggested that because of the steep gradients and acid pHs the disc is in a precarious metabolic state and that instabilities could lead to cell death and disc degeneration.

The distances for diffusion of nutrients from the blood vessels to the cells are large (approximately 1 cm compared to 30 μm for most cells), and hence it has been suggested that fluid 'pumping' under changing loads may be important for the transfer of nutrients and wastes between disc chondrocytes and the surrounding blood vessels. Experimental 'pumping' has not been found to have an effect insofar as the major nutrients and metabolic products are concerned (glucose, oxygen, lactate and other molecules of similar size). In fact, theoretical calculations show that transport of these nutrients by diffusion under the concentration gradients existing in the disc is faster than transport by entrainment with the pumped fluid. However, for large molecules which diffuse more slowly (e.g. hormones), pumping may aid transport (O'Hara et al 1990).

Factors affecting the blood supply to the disc do, however, appear to have a significant effect on nutrient concentrations in the tissue. Both vibration and smoking lead to a rapid fall in oxygen concentrations in the disc nucleus and a rise in lactate concentration, which take several hours to reverse (Holm & Nachemson 1988, see Fig. 13.14). Other loading patterns have also been found to affect solute transport. Long-term exercise or lack of

it has been shown to have a permanent effect on transport of nutrients into the disc, and thus on the health of the tissue. The mechanism is not clear, but it has been suggested that exercise affects the external vascularization of the disc. Holm and Nachemson (1982, 1983) found that in dog's discs which had been fused, after 3–8 months the cellular activity decreased, PGs were lost and hence

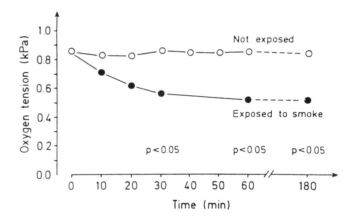

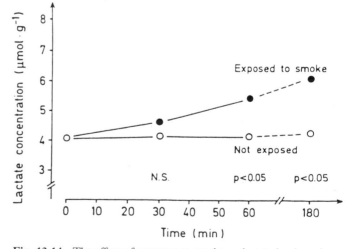

Fig. 13.14 The effect of exposure to smoke on lactate levels and oxygen tension. After 3 hours the lactate level increased by 50%, relative to the controls which were not exposed to smoke, leading to a fall in the pH of the disc matrix (Holm & Nachemson 1988).

the fluid content of the discs fell. The reverse occurred in dogs which were vigorously trained over several months.

Metabolism of matrix constituents

Little is known about matrix synthesis in the disc, but in vivo studies in animals have shown that PGs are synthesized in vivo in both adult and young animals. Turnover time was only a few weeks in 6-week-old guinea pigs, but was over 2 years in adult dogs (Lohmander et al 1973, Urban et al 1979, Holm & Nachemson 1982). In vitro measurements in human discs removed at surgery have confirmed that PG synthesis is slow. These studies also showed that the synthesis rate was not uniform across the disc, the inner annulus and nucleus were the most active regions, and also that spinal level affected results. Synthesis rates were found to differ in degenerate discs (Bayliss et al 1988).

Although these turnover times are slow, the rate of synthesis is affected by a number of factors. The loss of PGs from the pericellular environment after injury may stimulate synthesis (Hardingham & Muir 1972). Growth factors and hormones can increase the rate of synthesis in the disc and other cartilages and would have greater access to the cells after PG loss as their partition coefficient and hence concentration around the cells would increase (Maldonado et al 1991). Animal models suggest that PG replacement is possible. When dog discs were treated with chymopapain and PGs were lost from the disc and endplate, it was observed that undamaged disc cells were able to synthesize PGs and expand the disc again after several months (Garvin & Jennings 1973, Bradford et al 1983). It is not clear however whether the PGs can be replaced in damaged human discs.

While it is now known that PGs are synthesized throughout life, little is known about collagen synthesis. It is thought that once the network had been formed and cross-linked its turnover is very slow. Herbert et al (1975), however, found that in a degenerate human disc and in the disc above it, a proportion of the collagen cross-links were immature; this suggests that some form of remodelling or synthesis was occurring. In addition, Lipson (1988) found that the maturity of the cross-links in herniated disc fragments was less than it was in the bulk of the tissue. These two studies suggest that collagen can be laid down in the adult human disc under some circumstances. However, it is not clear whether this 'repair' tissue is similar to that of the original disc matrix. Whether the collagen network undergoes turnover or is capable of repair is still an unanswered question. It is clear however, that if the collagen network is injured, the mechanical function of the disc will be impaired and that full function cannot be restored without a renewal of this collagen framework.

REFERENCES

Adams M A, Hutton W 1983 The effect of posture on the fluid content of the lumbar intervertebral disc. Spine 8: 665–671

Andersson G B J 1982 Measurement of loads on the lumbar spine. In: White A A, Gordon S L (eds) Idiopathic low back pain. C V Mosby, St Louis

Bayliss M T, Johnstone B, O'Brien J P 1988 Proteoglycan synthesis in the human intervertebral disc: variation with age, region and pathology. Spine 13: 972–981

Bogduk N, Tynan, W, Wilson A S 1981 The nerve supply to the human lumbar intervertebral disc. Journal of Anatomy 132: 39–56

Bradford D S, Cooper K M, Oegema T R 1983 Chymopapain, chemonucleolysis and nucleus pulposus regeneration. Journal of Bone and Joint Surgery 65-A: 1220–1231

Broom N D, Marra D L 1985 New structural concepts of articular cartilage demonstrated with a physical model. Connective Tissue Research 14: 1–8

Buckwalter J 1982 The fine structure of the intervertebral disc. In: White A A, Gordon S L (eds) Idiopathic low back pain. C V Mosby, St Louis

Byers P D, Bayliss M T, Maroudas A, Urban J P G, Weightman B 1983 Hypothesizing about joints. In: Maroudas A, Holborrow E J (eds) Studies in joint diseases 2. Pitman Press, London

Carney S, Muir I H 1988 The structure and function of cartilage proteoglycans. Physiological Reviews 68: 858–910

Comper W, Preston B N 1974 Model connective tissue systems. Biochemistry Journal 143: 1–11

Cooke T D V 1980 The interactions and local disease manifestation of immune complexes in articular collagenous tissues. In: Maroudas A, Holborrow E J (eds) Studies in joint diseases 2. Pitman, London

Coventry M B, Ghormley R K, Kerohan T 1945 The intervertebral disc. Its microscopic anatomy and pathology. Journal of Bone and Joint Surgery 27: 233–247

Eklund J A, Corlett E N 1984 Shrinkage as a measure of the effect of load on the spine. Spine 9: 189–194

Eyre D R 1988 Collagens of the disc In: Ghosh P (ed) The biology of the intervertebral disc. CRC Press, Boca Raton, Florida

Eyre D R, Paz M A, Gallop P M 1984 Cross linking in collagen and elastin. Annual Review of Biochemistry 717–748

Garvin P J, Jennings R B 1973 Long term effects of chymopapain on the intervertebral disc of dogs. Clinical Orthopaedics 92: 281–295

Gray M L, Pizanelli A M, Grodzinsky A J, Lee R C 1988 Mechanical and physicochemical determinants of the chondrocyte biosynthetic response. Journal of Orthopaedic Research 6: 777–792

Happey P 1980 Studies of the structure of the human intervertebral disc. In: Sokoloff L (ed) Joints and synovial fluid. Academic Press, London

Hardingham T E, Muir H 1972 Biosynthesis of proteoglycans in cartilage slices. Biochemical Journal 126: 135, 905–908

Heinegard D, Oldberg A 1989 Structure and biology of cartilage and bone matrix noncollagenous macromolecules. FASEB J: 3, 2042–2051

Herbert C M, Lindberg K A, Jayson M I V, Bailey A J 1975 Changes in the collagen of human intervertebral discs during ageing and degenerative disc disease. Journal of Molecular Medicine 1: 79–91

Holm S, Nachemson A 1982 Nutritional changes in the canine intervertebral disc after fusion. Clinical Orthopaedics 169: 243–258

Holm S, Nachemson A 1983 Variation in the nutrition of the canine interverterbral disc induced by motion. Spine 8: 866–874

Holm S, Nachemson A 1988 Nutrition of the intervertebral disc: acute effects of cigarette smoking. Uppsala Journal of Medical Science 93: 91–99

Holm S, Maroudas A, Urban J P G, Selstam G, Nachemson A 1982 Nutrition of the intervertebral disc. Solute transport and metabolism. Connective Tissue Research 8: 101–119

Levene C I 1978 Diseases of the collagen molecule. In: Gardner D L (ed) Diseases of connective tissue. Journal of Clinical Pathology 31 (suppl 12): 82–94

Lipson S J 1988 Metaplastic proliferative fibrocartilage as an alternative concept to herniated intervertebral disc. Spine 13: 1055–1060

Lohmander S, Antonopoulos C A, Friberg U 1973 Chemical and metabolic heterogeneity of chondroitin sulphate and keratin sulphate in guinea pig cartilage and nucleus pulposus. Biochimica et Biophysica Acta 304: 430–448

McCarthy P, Carruthers B, Martin D, Petts P 1991 Immunohistochemical demonstration of sensory nerve fibres and endings in lumbar intervertebral discs of rat. Spine 16: 653–655

McDevitt C A, Pahl J A, Ayad A, Miller R R, Uratsuji M, Andrish J T 1988 Experimental osteoarthritic articular cartilage is enriched in guanidine-soluble type VI collagen. Biochemical and Biophysical Research Communications 157: 250–255

Maldonado B A, Comfort T, Chelberg M K, Bradfar D, Oegema T R 1991 Characterization of intervertebral disc cells in vitro. Transactions of the American Orthopedic Research Society 16: 97

Marchand F, Ahmed A M 1990 Investigation of the laminate structure of lumbar disc anulus fibrosus. Spine 15: 402–410

Maroudas A 1980 Physical chemistry of articular cartilage and the intervertebral disc. In: Sokoloff L (ed) The joints and synovial fluid. Academic Press, London

Maroudas A 1990 Different ways of expressing concentration of cartilage constituents with special reference to the tissue's organization and functional properties. In: Maroudas A, Kuettner K (eds) Methods in cartilage research. Academic Press, London

Maroudas A, Stockwell R-A, Nachemson A, Urban J P G 1975 Factors influencing the nutrition of the intervertebral disc. Journal of Anatomy 120: 113–130

Melrose J, Ghosh P 1988 The non-collagenous proteins of the intervertebral disc. In: Ghosh P (ed) The biology of the intervertebral disc. CRC Press, Boca Raton, Florida, ch 8 pp 189–237

Nachemson A 1960 Lumbar intradiscal pressures. Acta Orthopaedica Scandinavica (suppl 43)

Nimni M E, Harkness R D 1988 Molecular structure and function of collagen. In: Nimni M E (ed) Collagen I. CRC Press, Boca Raton, Florida, pp 1–77

O'Hara B, Urban J P G, Maroudas A 1990 Influence of cyclic loading on articular cartilage nutrition. Annals of Rheumatic Disease 49: 536–539

Peacock A 1952 Observations on the postnatal structure of the intervertebral disc in man. Journal of Anatomy 86: 162–179

Pedrini A M, Pedrini V A, Tudisco C, Ponseti I V, Weinstein S L,

Maynard J A 1983 Proteoglycans of human scoliotic intervertebral disc. Journal of Bone and Joint Surgery 65A: 815–823

Poole C A, Ayad S, Schofield J R 1988 Chondrons from articular cartilage: immunolocalization of type VI collagen in the pericellular capsule of isolated canine chondrons. Journal of Cell Science 90: 635–645

Roberts S, Menage J, Urban J P G 1989 Biochemical and structural properties of the cartilage end plate and its relation to the intervertebral disc. Spine 14: 166–174

Roberts S, Menage J, Duance V C, Wotton S, Ayad S 1991 Collagen types around the cells of the intervertebral discs and cartilage endplate: an immunolocalisation study. Spine 16: 1030–1038

Ruoslahti E, Yamaguchi Y 1991 Proteoglycans as modulators of growth factor activities. Cell 64: 867–869

Schultz A B 1974 Force deformation properties of human costo-sternal and costo-vertebral articulations. Journal of Biomechanics 7: 311–318

Shirazi-Adl S A, Shrivastava S C, Ahmed A M 1984 Stress analysis of the lumbar disc-body unit in compression: a three dimensional nonlinear finite element study. Spine 9: 120–133

Sommarin Y, Larsson T, Heinegard D 1989 Chondrocyte matrix interactions. Experimental Cell Research 184: 181–192

Szirmai 1970

Thornton W, Hoffler W, Rummel J 1974 Anthropometric changes and fluid shifts on skylab. Presented at the Skylab Symposium, Aug 28

Twomey L T, Taylor J R 1986 The effects of ageing on the lumbar intervertebral discs. In: Grieve G P (ed) Modern manual therapy of the vertebral column. Churchill Livingstone, Edinburgh

Urban J P G, Bayliss M T 1988 Regulation of proteoglycan synthesis rate in cartilage in vitro: influence of extracellular ionic composition. Biochimica et Biophysica Acta 992: 59–65

Urban J P G, Maroudas A 1980 The chemistry of the intervertebral disc in relation to its functional requirements. Clinics in Rheumatic Diseases 6: 51–76

Urban J P G, Maroudas A, Bayliss M T, Dillon J 1979 Swelling pressure of proteoglycans at the concentrations found in cartilaginous tissues. Biorheology 16: 447–464

Van der Rest M, Mayne R 1988 Type IX collagen proteoglycan from cartilage is covalently linked to type II collagen. Journal of Biological Chemistry 267: 1615–1618

Wu J J, Eyre D R 1989 Covalent interaction of type IX collagen in cartilage. Connective Tissue Research 20: 241–246

Yoshizawa H, O'Brien J P, Smith W T, Trumper M 1980 The neuropathology of intervertebral discs removed for low back pain. Journal of Pathology 132: 95–104

14. The effects of ageing on the intervertebral discs

J. R. Taylor   L. T. Twomey

INTRODUCTION

Comparatively few studies have used quantitative methods to study age changes in the vertebral column, particularly in the intervertebral discs (IVD), and considerable confusion exists in the literature as to what constitute 'age' changes and 'pathological' changes. There is a body of opinion which appears to regard these changes as synonymous (Naylor 1962, Vernon-Roberts & Pirie 1977), but there are some areas of uncertainty, and in some instances the two can be clearly separated. Extremes of attrition with advancing age were regarded as pathological by Coventry (1969), but the ageing process itself is regarded as normal. Some descriptive studies of intervertebral discs make judgements of disc ageing and pathology in the general population, based on disc appearance in populations reviewed for various back disorders. These are appearances therefore which are not representative of the population as a whole. While pathological changes are more frequently observed in old age, they are not an essential consequence of ageing.

The decline in spinal stature in old age is usually attributed to a reduction in the height of the IVDs (Armstrong 1967, Vernon-Roberts & Pirie 1977). However, osteoporosis is also closely linked with shortening of the trunk (Dent & Watson 1966), due to a loss in vertebral body height and an increase in vertebral end-plate concavity in old age (Ericksen 1974, Twomey et al 1983). There are no measurement studies showing a general reduction in IVD heights in the elderly. Indeed, two independent studies show that average disc height is usually maintained and may even be increased in old age in 'normal', unselected populations (Nachemson et al 1979, Twomey & Taylor 1985a). The same studies also show that while the prevalence of disc degeneration increases with increasing age, it is far from universal in old age. Disc thinning is by no means an inevitable consequence of ageing.

While there are excellent descriptions of structural and biochemical age changes, particularly in IVDs, the only measurement study of vertebral and disc changes in a large number of 'normal' adults has been made for the lumbar spine (Twomey 1981, Twomey et al 1983). This chapter will provide a general description of the natural history of the whole spine, and it will demonstrate in more detail the physical changes which have been shown to occur in the lumbar spine.

General description and development

The disc provides enough strength and stiffness for stability, but, by its thickness and moderate compliance, it gives a useful movement range. Though generally described as formed by an *annulus fibrosus* and a *nucleus pulposus*, the disc should be regarded functionally as including the *cartilage plates*, which bind and unite it to the vertebral bodies above and below. It is not generally realized that the cartilage plates and the annulus fibrosus form a continuous envelope enclosing the nucleus pulposes (Fig. 14.1).

The annulus fibrosus consists of about 12 to 16 concentric lamellae, the outer lamellae being fibrous and the inner lamellae fibrocartilaginous (Taylor 1990). These have an outwardly convex arrangement around the circumference of the nucleus and are arranged in spiralling sheets. The parallel fibres of each successive sheet of collagen bundles cross the fibres of the next sheet at an interstriation angle of about 57° (Twomey & Taylor 1987). The arrangement is not unlike that of the layering of an onion. In the intervertebral disc this arrangement gives the annulus great strength. The outermost fibrous lamellae of the annulus are firmly embedded in the bony vertebral rim. The inner fibrocartilaginous lamellae of the annulus are shown by polarized light studies (see Fig. 14.1) to be directly continuous with the horizontal lamellae of the 'hyaline' cartilage plates above and below the nucleus (Taylor 1973). These lamellae are enclosed in a plentiful glycosaminoglycan-(GAG)-rich matrix. The GAGs have an intimate association with the collagen fibrils of the inner lamellae (Scott 1990), 'making space' for the water which is attracted, to fill and inflate the inter-fibrillar

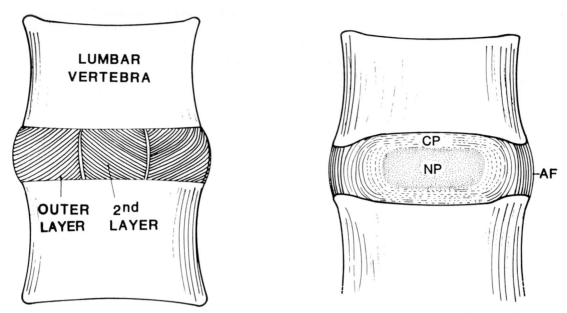

Fig. 14.1 The components of a typical intervertebral disc demonstrating the layered annulus fibrosus (AF), the nucleus pulposus (NP) and the cartilage end plates (CP).

spaces. This helps to maintain the shape of the collagen fibres in the lamellae in a manner analogous to stiff cylindrical cuffs around flexible ropes. The outer fibrous lamellae (with relatively less matrix) appear designed to resist tensile forces. The inner fibrocartilaginous lamellae (with plentiful matrix) appear to be designed to help resist compressive forces. The inextensible but deformable envelope formed by the annulus and the cartilage plates encloses the elliptical sphere, which is the nucleus pulposus.

The cartilage plates not only form an essential part of the envelope containing the nucleus, they are also firmly bound to the end-surface of the vertebral body, of which they are developmentally a part. In the growing individual, growth plates at the junction of the bony vertebral body and the cartilage plates ensure growth in vertebral height. The cartilage plates are best regarded not as belonging to the disc, or as part of the vertebra, but as the parts where the vertebra and disc interlock.

The thickest discs are the lower lumbar discs which are about 12 mm thick. Upper thoracic discs are thinnest and allow relatively little movement. Cervical discs, although only 6 mm or so thick, allow wide ranges of movement as the horizontal dimensions of the cervical vertebrae are relatively small and the facet joints are less restrictive to motion than the lumbar facet joints.

The infant nucleus pulposus is a viscous, fluid structure with a clear, watery matrix (Taylor 1973). Its appearance and consistency are quite changed in the adolescent and adult when the nucleus contains many randomly oriented collagen bundles. With increasing maturation the collagen increases, there is a reduced water content, and the nucleus becomes more difficult to dissect clear of its envelope. However, despite the increase in collagen, high

GAG and water content persists and the healthy adult nucleus still behaves hydrostatically as a viscous fluid, which is incompressible and changes shape quite freely (Nachemson 1960). By changing shape the disc acts as a joint; by receiving compressive axial loads and redistributing them outwards to produce tensile forces in the outer annulus, and vertebral rims, it acts as a shock absorber. In this way, it dissipates vertical forces in horizontal and other directions.

The outer layers of the annulus are innervated, but no nerves penetrate beyond its outer third except possibly in granulation tissue filling disc fissures (Osti et al 1990). No nerves have been demonstrated in the nucleus or the cartilage plates (Taylor & Twomey 1979, Bogduk 1983). The outer annulus and cartilage plates are quite vascular in the fetus and infant, but vascularity is progressively reduced with maturation (Taylor 1973). In the adult a few vessels penetrate the calcified cartilage layer binding the cartilage plate to the bony centrum, and a few small blood vessels persist in the surface layers of the annulus (Walmsley 1953, Maroudas et al 1975, McFadden & Taylor 1990). The avascular nucleus contains a sparse cell population in a watery matrix rich in glycosaminoglycans. The sparse cell population of the adult nucleus receives its nutrition by diffusion from the surrounding envelope, i.e. from the few vessels in the outer annulus and from the vascular buds that extend into the cartilage plates for a short distance from the vertebral marrow spaces (Maroudas et al 1975).

The nucleus is held under tension within the envelope formed by the annulus and cartilage plates. This tension, or turgor, is dependent on the inextensibility of the envelope, and is produced by the expansile chemical force resulting from the water-attracting capacity of the GAG macromolecules. These macromolecules 'imbibe' and make space for water when the disc is not mechanically compressed, e.g. in recumbent posture when the disc tends to swell. They lose some of it during the course of each day when the disc is compressed by axial loading and 'creeps' to become slightly thinner. Thus, all individuals lose height due to axial weight-bearing during the day, and regain height when recumbent at night (Taylor 1973).

Zygapophyseal (facet) joints

Further stability is provided by the guiding and restraining mechanism of the two zygapophyseal joints, which permit or restrain movement in the sagittal, coronal and horizontal planes (Twomey & Taylor 1983, 1985b, Taylor & Twomey 1986). They protect the intervertebral disc from excessive strain, particularly in the lumbar region, and also widen the weight-bearing base. In normal, erect posture they bear a significant proportion of axial loading.

CERVICAL INTERVERTEBRAL DISCS

Structure and function in cervical motion segments

The cervical region is the most mobile part of the vertebral column and it contains a more complex series of joints than does the thoracolumbar spine. The upper cervical spine has two synovial joint complexes which are unique to this region. The altanto-occipital and atlanto-axial joints are specialized for axial rotation and nodding movements respectively. These two special motion segments make very important contributions to the mobility of the cervical spine, but the structure and function of the cervical motion segments below C2 are the principal concern of this chapter.

The vertebrae from C2 to T1 are united by intervertebral discs, but the structure and function of cervical intervertebral discs are so closely affected by the particular orientation of cervical zygapophyseal joints, and by the uncovertebral joints which are unique to this region, that a brief account of the cervical motion segment as a whole is necessary. Many clinicians make the mistake of considering that the cervical motion segments are, both structurally and functionally, smaller versions of the lumbar motion segments. The six cervical motion segments between the second cervical vertebra and the first thoracic vertebra are more mobile and more complex than thoracic and lumbar motion segments. The interbody joints of lower cervical motion segments (C2–3 to C7–T1), each consist of an IVD flanked by an uncovertebral (UV) joint on each side. On average, each of these cervical motion segments allows a total of approximately 18° of axial rotation and 15° and 10° of sagittal and coronal plane motion, respectively, per individual cervical motion segment (Penning & Wilmink 1987, Dvorak et al 1988). The IVD dimensions and compliance are the most important determinants of the amount of movement possible, while the orientation and size of the zygapophyseal (Z) facets and the size of the uncinate processess forming the UV joints, control the types of movement possible. The cervical Z joints together with the UV joints (of von Luschka) are considered by many to make an important contribution to stability (White & Panjabi 1978) but the degree of stability offered is sacrificed to some extent to the need for mobility; for example, in full flexion, facet contact is reduced to only a few millimetres.

With such an arrangement the importance of the posterior muscles, ligaments and joint capsules in preventing dislocation is obvious. Both the range and the nature of cervical spinal movements make the cervical IVDs subject to more shearing and torsional strain than lumbar or thoracic discs. The lumbar zygapophyseal facets are particularly well designed to restrain torsion and translation (Taylor & Twomey 1986). On the other hand, the 45° orientation of typical cervical Z joints facilitates the translational movement which accompanies all cervical motion, with consequent shearing forces in the disc (Taylor & Milne 1988). The cervical facet orientation requires that lateral bending and axial rotation are coupled movements, accompanied by torsional strains in the cervical annulus. These movements and forces play an important role in the early fissuring observed in cervical discs. In addition, the growth of the cervical uncinate processes and the consequent narrowing of the lateral parts of the interbody space, concentrate shearing forces in this region, with the formation of clefts here, from childhood onwards, forming the uncovertebral joints.

These particular structural features of cervical motion segments, together with smaller cervical vertebral body size, compared to thoracic and lumbar vertebrae, are associated with functional differences in the relative load-bearing functions of the interbody joints and the Z joints. In normal erect standing the cervical interbody joints and the Z joints bear approximately equal compressive loads. In the lumbar spine, the IVD bears about 80% of the load and the Z joints bear the remaining 20% of the axial load. To the differences in structure of the Z joints, already described, are added obvious differences in the structure of the interbody joints which will be described below.

Cervical interbody joints

Uncovertebral joints

The cervical interbody are not flat discs in the transverse plane like thoracic and lumbar discs; the upper surface of each cervical vertebra is markedly concave in the coronal plane and the lower surface of a cervical vertebra is convex in the same plane. The lateral parts of cervical vertebral bodies are formed from the neural arch centres of ossification and not from the centra. Uncinate processes grow upwards from the upper aspects of the lateral parts of each vertebra (C3 to T1) during childhood, narrowing the lateral interbody space. In infancy, the intervertebral disc does not extend the whole way out to the lateral vertebral body margins and the uncinate processes are said to grow upwards in the loose fibrous tissue lateral to the annulus. This process or uncus rises higher in mid-cervical vertebrae than in lower cervical vertebrae and T1. Between its tip and the lower lateral surface of the vertebral body above, a cleft appears at about eight years of age, forming an uncovertebral joint (UV joint). Some doubt remains as to whether this 'joint' or pseudoarthrosis develops lateral to or within the annulus fibrosus (Penning 1968, Töndury 1972, Hayashi & Yakubi 1985). Töndury (1972) described the surfaces of the cleft as formed by the compacted split ends of fibres of the annulus. The upper UV joints lie lateral to the IVDs, and the lower UV joints occupy positions postero-lateral to the IVD. Each uncovertebral joint is enclosed laterally by a thin capsule but its medial limit is indeterminate as the cleft may project for a variable distance into the annulus. In the adolescent and young adult, the uncovertebral clefts form the lateral parts of the interbody joint and the central two-thirds of the cervical interbody space is occupied by an intervertebral disc, with a histological appearance similar in most respects to thoracic and lumbar discs.

The cervical intervertebral discs

In a child or adolescent, cervical discs, like all interverte-

bral discs, contain a central soft or gelatinous nucleus pulposus which is enclosed by a fibrocartilaginous and cartilaginous envelope, formed by the lamellae of the annulus fibrosus around the outside and by the cartilage plates above and below. The inner half of the annulus is directly continuous with the cartilage plates, completely encapsulating the nucleus. The nucleus pulposus of cervical discs is initially very small; its notochordal phase is quite short-lived in the fetus and infant, and the accumulation of collagen in the nucleus, as shown by histological and biochemical studies, is more rapid than in the cervical nucleus than in thoracic and lumbar discs (Taylor 1973). There may also be a slow loss of the soft central gel in association with the fissuring which is universal in adult cervical discs. There appears to be less 'turgor' or swelling pressure in young adult cervical discs than in young adult lumbar discs. The latter bulge and swell almost immediately on sectioning, whether cut in the fresh post mortem state or after formalin fixation. The former may swell on sectioning, but generally more slowly and less obviously than lumbar discs.

Natural history of uncovertebral joints and intervertebral discs

The UV joints are not true joints, formed like other joints during fetal development. They appear in later childhood and early adolescence, following the growth of the uncinate processes, as clefts in the lateral parts of the intervertebral discs. Within a few years, in older adolescents and young adults, the clefts begin to extend medially

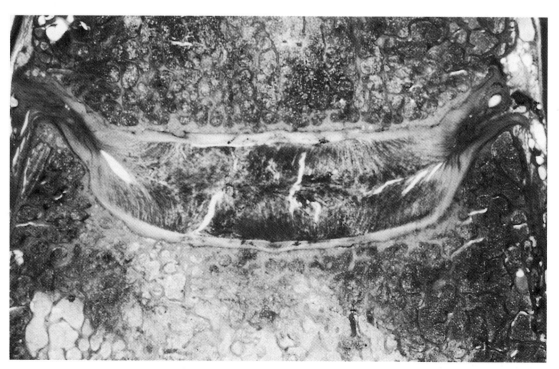

Fig. 14.2 A coronal section through the C5–6 intervertebral disc from a 59-year-old male, demonstrating the horizontal fissures extending through the disc from its postero-lateral corners.

into the intervertebral disc so that, by the age of 25 or 30 years, fine fissures extend transversely from UV joint to UV joint through the posterior and central parts of the disc (Fig. 14.2). Radio-opaque dye injected into the centre of a cervical disc usually diffuses freely out into both UV joints, and in a smaller proportion of cervical discs the dye also diffuses into the anterior epidural space of the spinal canal. After the age of 30 years, cervical discs, unlike lumbar discs, no longer contain a soft gelatinous, encapsulated nucleus pulposus (Taylor & Milne 1988, Taylor 1990, Twomey & Taylor 1990). This process of early fissuring is related to the unique combination of 45° Z joint facets and high uncinate processes.

Degenerative changes

Despite the early fissuring of cervical discs, nuclear herniation is rare, but posterior fissuring and disc bulging or protrusion into the spinal canal commonly forms a transverse osteocartilaginous bar, intruding into the anterior epidural space. The presence of uncinate processes prevents herniation of central disc material directly into the intervertebral canal, but occasionally central disc fragments are retropulsed into the spinal canal, particularly following a cervical spinal 'whiplash' injury. Isolated cervical disc degeneration and disc resorption, involving one or more discs, with marked loss of disc height compared to the other cervical discs, is common in middle-aged and elderly subjects. The lower three discs from C4–5 to C6–7 are most often affected (Kramer 1981, Taylor 1990).

With disc thinning, the UV joints bear higher compressive loads than in normal cervical interbody joints, and the cartilage lining the uncovertebral joints becomes more like articular cartilage, the whole UV joint now resembling a synovial joint with early arthritic changes. As 'arthritis' develops in these joints, large outwardly directed osteocartilaginous, uncovertebral osteophytes appear (Fig. 14.3), which may impinge on either the spinal nerves or on the vertebral artery (Balla & Langford 1967). This causes pain and paraethesiae due to nerve root irritation. The dorsal root ganglia from C5 to T1 are very large and lie just lateral to the UV joints. As they occupy a large part of the IV canal, they have little room to move out of the way. Occasionally uncovertebral osteophytes may cause circulatory problems by constricting the vertebral artery and reducing the blood supply to the cerebellum, brain stem or visual area. However, the vertebral artery has more room than the spinal nerves to curve laterally around the osteophytes. Forceful movements, for example a sudden turning of the head, a cervical spinal manipulation, or an accidental injury, like whiplash, may in these circumstances temporarily or permanently damage the artery (Livingston 1971, Lyness & Simeone 1978, Grant 1987).

Posterior disc bars, from the same degenerate discs, may project into the spinal canal to impinge on the dura and anterior spinal cord. These do not necessarily cause symptoms or signs of functional cord involvement, perhaps because the cervical spinal canal is relatively large in its antero-posterior dimensions and the cord normally occupies only 60% of its sagittal width (Penning 1968).

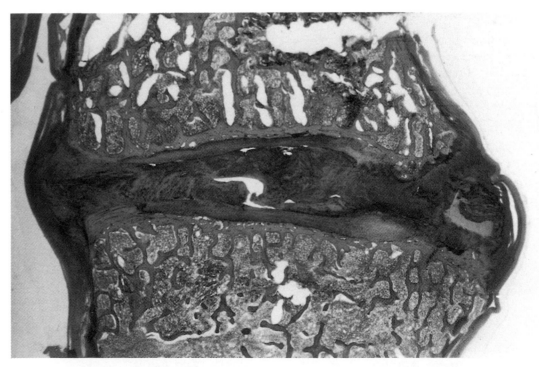

Fig. 14.3   A sagittal section through the C6–7 intervertebral disc from a 77-year-old male, indicating disc degeneration with fissuring and bony osteophytes.

THORACIC INTERVERTEBRAL DISCS

The height of thoracic discs approximates to those of cervical discs and is small in comparison to lumbar discs (Andriacchi et al 1974), while the ratio of disc diameter to height is two to three times higher in the thoracic than in the lumbar region (Kulak et al 1976). Given this geometry, thoracic discs are said to show elastic properties resembling those of solid materials (Horst & Brinckmann 1981).

In the thoracic region, the annulus fibrosus usually consists of about 8 to 12 lamellae arranged at an angle of 30° to each other (Galante 1967). The nucleus pulposus is located centrally within the disc. As it is relatively small, and given the protection afforded the IVD by the presence of the ribs, it is said to be rarely damaged by mechanical trauma. Thus, it is unusual to identify either a bulging or herniated thoracic disc (Panjabi et al 1976), but our own observations on autopsy specimens suggest that bleeding into thoracic discs may follow localized thoracic vertebral end-plate fractures resulting from motor vehicle accidents.

The relatively low mobility of thoracic motion segments, compared to cervical and lumbar motion segments, protects them from some of the degenerative changes common in the cervical and lumbar regions. However, the common growth-related deformities of scoliosis and Scheuermann's disease produce postural change in thoracic discs which predispose to early degeneration, and, at a later stage, osteoporotic bowing of thoracic vertebral end-plates which results in ballooning of thoracic discs as a compensatory change.

LUMBAR INTERVERTEBRAL DISCS

The prevailing clinical assumption that the loss of stature which occurs in ageing populations is due in large part to thinning of the lumbar intervertebral discs has been shown in recent studies to be incorrect (Nachemson et al 1979, Twomey & Taylor 1985a). Average disc height is usually maintained and may even be increased in old age (Fig. 14.4), confirming the data from earlier studies demonstrating that loss in vertebral height with associated spinal postural changes is the principal reason for loss in stature (Twomey 1981).

When the data for mid-sagittal disc heights are carefully considered, it is evident that, with increasing age, increase in central disc height is greater than the small decline in anterior and posterior disc heights. These disc changes occur in response to the primary vertebral body age changes of a decline in central height with an increase in end-plate concavity, together with an increase in peripheral osteophytosis and marginal bony hypertrophy. The peripheral changes are probably due to traction forces exerted by the annulus fibrosus on the vertebral margin (Fig. 14.5). The tough IVD is able to grow and expand centrally and adapt gradually to the change in vertebral body shape.

Disc degeneration

This is a term that is often ill-defined and variably described in the literature, where it may be used synonymously with annular fissures, disc thinning, colour change, or the presence of osteophytes at the disc margins. Such 'degenerative' changes are often considered to be universal in old age (Armstrong 1967). In 1966, Rolander provided a morphological classification of intervertebral discs based on their appearance on mid-line sagittal section as follows:

Grade 0   Macroscopically normal, juvenile discs
Grade 1   Normal adult discs, white in colour, the nucleus bulges on section
Grade 2   Age changes; less distinct boundary between nucleus and annulus; yellowish colour
Grade 3   Frank disc generation with desiccation, multiple fissures in nucleus and annulus, disc thinning

On the basis of this commonly accepted and utilized

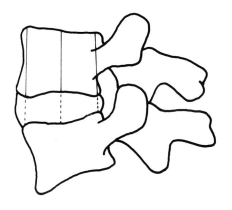
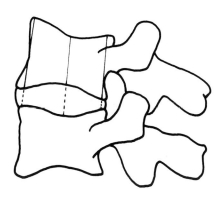

Young Adult   **Old Adult**

Fig. 14.4   A diagram demonstrating the change in lumbar disc shape which occurs in old age.

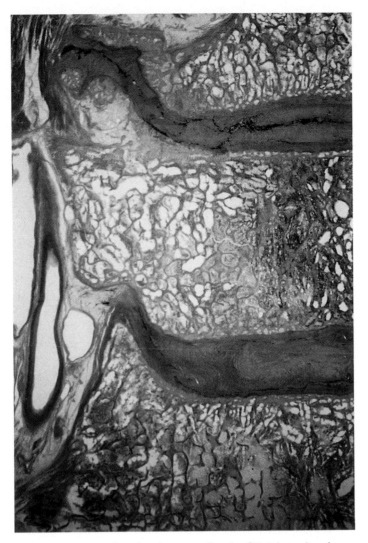

Fig. 14.5 A coronal section demonstrating the C5–6 (upper) and C6–7 (lower) intervertebral discs and uncovertebral joints. Marginal bone lipping, osteophytosis and disc fissuring are evident.

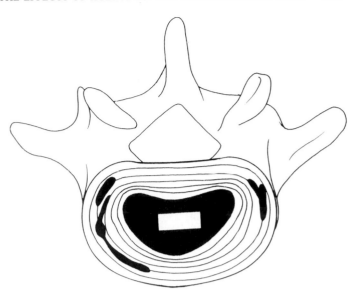

Fig. 14.6 A diagram demonstrating circumferential fissuring of a lumbar intervertebral disc.

the nucleus pulposus, which probably arise due to mechanical stress (Kramer 1981). Repeated trauma (which may include an element of sustained compression, e.g. in flexion, and may involve overstretch of annular fibres in axial rotation) may eventually result in circumferential fissures in the middle and sometimes the outer layers of the annulus (Fig. 14.6). However, repetition of high-velocity forces, particularly in association with torsional loads, is likely to result eventually in radial tears through the annulus, most often in the postero-lateral regions of the disc, as in Fig. 14.7. Since it is only the outer few lamellae of the lumbar discs which receive a nerve supply, the only fissures which are likely to result in pain from a disc are those which extend into that region (Bogduk & Twomey 1987).

classification, it is very clear that the majority of elderly discs do not suffer disc degeneration as so defined. In a previous study Twomey & Taylor (1982) demonstrated that 72% of all lumbar IVDs of elderly subjects (60+) did not show the changes classed by Rolander as grade 3, and that disc desiccation and thinning were by no means universal in old age. The common clinical misconception of the universality of disc generation with ageing arises as a result of the biased sample encountered by most clinicians involved in the treatment of low back pain and possibly 'over-reading' of minor changes in radiographs (Twomey & Taylor 1987).

The incidence of disc degeneration does increase in old age, and it is the lower two lumbar levels that are most often affected. These are the levels that are subject to the greatest physical stress. Fissuring of the annulus is seen with increasing frequency in old age. Initially, this is most often evident as one or two small central fissures close to

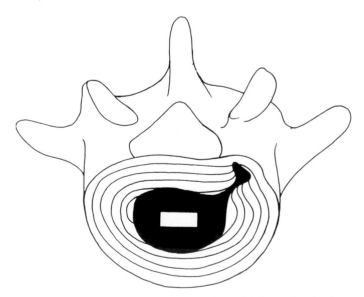

Fig. 14.7 A diagram demonstrating a major radial fissure in a lumbar intervertebral disc.

DISCOGENIC BACK PAIN

Since the peripheral parts of lumbar intervertebral discs have an excellent nerve supply they may become a potent source of low back pain. The sources of the nerve endings in lumbar discs are the lumbar sinuvertebral nerves, branches of the lumbar ventral rami and the grey rami communicantes (Bogduk & Twomey 1987). However, it is only the outer layers of the annular envelope which receive a nerve supply, so that, for a disc to become painful, any lesion must involve, directly or indirectly, the outer third of the annulus. Thus, increased intradiscal pressures following disc damage and swelling can indirectly cause discogenic pain (Bogduk & Twomey 1987).

Damage to the intervertebral discs following trauma, perhaps as a direct result of sporting activities, is well recognized. Repeated minor trauma, which may include an element of sustained compression, as in flexed rotated postures, may give rise to *circumferential fissures*, usually of the inner annulus, but also in the outer layers of the annulus (Adams & Hutton 1985a). Such damage to the outer annulus is likely to involve its nerve supply and thus be a source of back pain. The repetition of high velocity forces, particularly in association with torsional loads, may eventually result in *radial tears* through the annulus, most usually in the postero-lateral regions of the lumbar discs and often sprain the outermost lamellae (Adams & Hutton 1985a). Farfan 1973 emphasized the importance of torsional strain in annular damage. While the lumbar facets are well placed in neutral posture to resist torsion, in the flexed position some torsion is possible. In addition, with high velocity torsion, only a small range of movement may be enough to damage annular fibres.

Disc fissures also provide a potential pathway for nuclear herniation under very particular circumstances which might allow for it. In most individuals, after the third decade of life, the nucleus is not sufficiently fluid to allow itself to be expressed under normal circumstances (Crock 1986). True nuclear herniation is a condition of young people, generally up to their mid-twenties, and is rarely evident in older persons (Crock 1986, Bogduk & Twomey 1987). Acute nuclear herniation through an annular defect can thus occur only in young discs, or in older discs where the nucleus undergoes autolysis and relative liquefaction. One rationale for this to occur proposes a prior fracture of the vertebral end-plate, allowing vertebral blood to seep into the region of the avascular nucleus pulposus. Since the circulating blood has not previously been exposed directly to the nuclear protein (it is entirely avascular right through life), it reacts to it as to a foreign body, setting up an autoimmune response. Autolysis and liquefaction of the nucleus may follow, as described in Bogduk and Twomey (1987) (p. 141). Once semi-fluid, the nucleus has the ability to be expressed through a radial tear in the annulus and perhaps gain access to the spinal canal in the region of the intervertebral canal.

Thus, disc protrusion and massive disc bulging with nuclear displacement, is a phenomenon observed only in young people and in young athletes. Disc bulging, due to annular metaplasia, nuclear degeneration or annular failure, however, is seen in older persons and is usually associated with repeated minor trauma, involving sustained postures, compression and torsion. Such pathology may cause spinal canal stenosis or intervertebral foraminal stenosis and become an important source of low back pain and dysfunction. Thus, internal disc disruption (Crock 1986) is a potential source of local back pain when it is associated with disc swelling or fissuring of the outer annulus, or the leakage of pain-producing chemicals out of the disc and into the surrounding region. Many sporting and recreational activities regularly subject the lumbar spine to considerable trauma, thereby increasing the risk of internal disc damage to the participants. Similarly, the stresses involved in a single major traumatic event may be of sufficient magnitude to damage severely lumbar discs and bring about 'internal disc disruption'.

Intradiscal pressure

The nucleus of the intervertebral disc is contained under pressure within its protective fibrous and cartilaginous envelope. Intradiscal pressure has been used as an index of disc function and it has been shown to vary according to posture, movement, and age. The comprehensive study of Nachemson (1960) on lumbar intradiscal pressure in 128 discs from 38 cadavers of both sexes, from 6 to 82 years, concluded the following:

1. The loaded disc behaves hydrostatically in that the nucleus acts as a fluid, distributing external pressures equally in all outward directions to the annulus.
2. Axial loading produces lower pressure readings in children below the age of 16 years than it does in adults.
3. The level of the lumbar spine does not influence the pressures recorded in 'loaded' or resting disc (the L5–S1 disc was included in the study).
4. The posterior vertebral structures (pedicles and articular processes) absorb 16–20% of the vertical loading forces.
5. 'Moderately degenerated' discs (as suggested by disc 'thinning') show similar pressure behaviour to 'intact' discs, and the mechanical behaviour of a lumbar disc does not change appreciably, provided 'degeneration' is not advanced.

Since the original study of Nachemson (1960) it has been shown in living subjects that: intradiscal pressures are higher in the sitting than in the standing posture (Nachemson & Morris 1964, Andersson et al 1974); they are less in the physiological lordotic posture than in the straight or kyphotic posture (Andersson et al 1974); they are increased with passive lumbar flexion of 20° (Nachemson 1965); they are further increased with passive flexion exercises (Nachemson & Elfstrom 1970); and the largest increases accompany heavy lifting, particularly when the valsalva manoeuvre is performed (Andersson et al 1976). Nachemson et al (1979) and Merriam et al (1984) showed that abnormal degenerated discs did not behave in a consistent way, as they showed patterns of pressure changes in different postures often dissimilar from those shown by normal discs. Similarly, other studies have shown that the ability of the disc to withstand compressive forces depends on both the integrity of the disc envelope and the turgor of the contained nucleus pulposus (Virgin 1958, Panjabi et al 1984). This contrasts with the claim of Belytschko et al (1974) that, in a theoretical model, annular tears would reduce intradiscal pressures more than degenerative nuclear lesions.

Disc thinning

In attempting to account for the common clinical view that disc degeneration with desiccation and thinning is inevitable in old age, consideration must be given to the bias of selected clinical samples, and the method of disc assessment. Most samples cited in the literature have been drawn from patients presenting to clinicians for advice and treatment of low back pain problems. Such samples are not representative of the population as a whole, and probably contain a greater proportion of individuals with disc degeneration. In roentgenographic assessments of discs, the increased horizontal dimensions, the slight decrease in marginal disc height, and the decrease in vertebral end-plate bone density described in this study may give the mistaken impression of 'disc thinning', when in fact changes in disc shape are being observed. The large sample in the post mortem study of Twomey and Taylor (1982, 1987), with no selection for back disorders, is likely to be representative of the population as a whole. It also provides standards with which the disc dimensions of individual patients may be compared.

The study of Twomey and Taylor (1982) showed that those individuals showing disc thinning constitute a 'minority group' within the general population. In this group the lower lumbar discs are the discs most comonly affected. Possible causes of disc thinning, when it does occur, could be loss of disc material resulting from herniation, or loss of disc volume caused by loss of GAGs with disc dehydration. In most cases of intraspongious herniation (seen in 30% of cases in the series (Twomey 1981)) or of annular rupture, the loss of disc substance had an insignificant influence on disc volume because the volume lost was small (averaging 1% of total disc volume (Taylor & Twomey 1985a)). In addition, despite the increasing incidence of microfractures in the vertebral end-plates of elderly subjects, the 'stiffer' discs of old age (Twomey & Taylor 1985a) did not readily prolapse into the fractures.

A significant loss in adult disc volume by dehydration is also less common than is generally claimed, and a closer examination of the original measurements of Puschel (1930) shows that the greatest water loss in intervertebral discs occurs during childhood and adolescence. It is of interest in this context that the changes in the types of glycosaminoglycans in the disc (increase in keratan sulphate/chondroitin sulphate ratio), commonly attributed to ageing, have been shown to occur during infancy and childhood (Scott et al 1991; Taylor et al 1991). The water content of the annulus remains relatively constant throughout adult life, while that of the nucleus declines by only 6% from early adult life to old age. Furthermore, the total glycosaminoglycan content of the disc is said to be generally maintained into old age while the amount of collagen increases slightly (Adams & Muir 1976, Bushell et al 1977). This is consistent with a principal finding of the study by Twomey and Taylor (1982) that average disc height is generally maintained in old age, whereas 'pathological disc degeneration' (grade 3) applies to a minority of elderly discs.

When pathological disc degeneration and thinning do occur, the lower two disc spaces are most frequently at risk. These levels are at the apex of the lumbosacral curve, where the mobile lumbar spine abuts on the more rigid pelvis. Weight-bearing in the erect posture and more particularly in a flexed or rotated posture concentrates forces at these levels and predisposes them to a greater incidence of disc pathology (Farfan 1973).

The effects of loading in flexion on lumbar intervertebral discs

The IVDs are always under an external load that changes with posture and activity; it is highest in erect standing with the lumbar spine flexed, and lowest when recumbent (Nachemson 1960). The amount of fluid expressed from the IVDs depends both on the size of the external load and its duration of application. Fluid can interchange between the disc and adjacent tissues primarily through the vertebral end-plate. The swelling pressure of the disc arises from the difference between the expansion pressure of the proteoglycans which causes the tissue to imbibe fluid and the tensile forces of the collagen network which limit the swelling (Bayliss et al 1986). This swelling pressure is opposed by external compressive loading of the disc. In this way the disc acts as a pump for fluid and metabolite transfer. Kraemer et al (1985) suggest that, under axial load, there is an 11% fluid loss from the annulus fibrosus and an 8% loss from the nucleus pulposus. As we have previously noted, after a day's activity involving standing, fluid imbibition back into the discs occurs slowly at rest when recumbent in extension, and more rapidly when the recumbent spine rests in flexion (Tyrrell et al 1985).

Similarly, Adams and Hutton (1985b, 1986) have shown that when lumbar discs are flexed under load, fluid and metabolites are forced out of the anterior, more compressed parts of the discs and squeezed back into the posterior regions. The reverse occurs during extension movements. Thus, IVD nutrition can be significantly increased by the fluid exchanges accompanying reciprocal movements in the sagittal plane. On the other hand, sustained postures at the extremes of a movement range would deprive parts of the disc of its nutrition for a long periods of time. It is highly likely that this static loaded situation would accelerate age change and degeneration (Frank et al 1984).

High-velocity movements to end-range may take parts of the lumbar discs and their attached longitudinal ligaments beyond their normal elastic limits, causing small tears and fissures in the annulus or 'rim lesions' at the attachment of the annulus to the vertebral rim, thereby reducing its capacity to cope with the normal environmental stresses (Osti et al 1990, Taylor et al 1990). The discs are particularly vulnerable to these movements after they have been permitted to 'creep' by the prolonged maintenance of a flexed or extended posture. Repeated traumatic episodes to the disc and surrounding bony and ligamentous structures would result in loss of disc tissue,

effusion and scarring, and further reduce the ability of the disc to act efficiently as a pump.

Imaging techniques

Standard spinal radiography provides quite limited information about degenerative processess in lumbar discs. It demonstrates only the later secondary changes of osteophytosis on the margins of the vertebral body, narrowing of the disc space, and sclerosis in the vertebral end plate (Resnick 1985). Discograms, computed tomography (CT) and magnetic resonance imaging (MRI) are superior methods for demonstrating disc disruption (Crock 1986); CT scans show changes in the external shape of the discs and various aspects of disc bulging and prolapse (Quinnell 1980); CT discography (Fig. 14.8) demonstrates the anatomy of radial and circumferential fissures (Sachs et al 1987). Since MRI gives a measure of the amount of water in the disc (particularly in the nucleus pulposus), early signs of disc degeneration associated with proteoglycan and water loss are best seen by the use of this method (Gibson et al 1986). However, at present it is still not clear how closely the progressive changes seen in adolescent and young adult discs as part of the normal maturation and ageing process of the discs relate to functional and biomechanical changes and at what stage they are indicative of disc 'degeneration'.

Discography has been used as a diagnostic tool in the

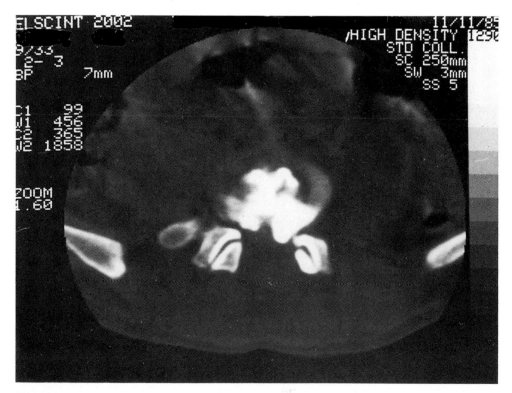

Fig. 14.8 Computed tomography of the L5–S1 intervertebral disc demonstrating disc bulging and prolapse.

assessment of disc disorders since 1948, not only to demonstrate structural changes, but to identify a painful disc. However, pain provocation discography has proved difficult to interpret clinically, particularly in the cervical spine (Quinnell 1980). In more recent times the axial discogram obtained with computer tomography has been preferred. Axial discography provides much more structural information regarding disc pathology than can be gathered from routine discography (Sachs et al 1987, Videman et al 1987). The Dallas discogram description has been devised to classify this information in a comprehensive manner and to describe the separate phenomena of disc degeneration and annular disruption. In addition, like standard discography, the technique may provide important clinical data by provoking pain in symptomatic discs (Sachs et al 1987). Pain provocation discography is a useful diagnostic tool for tracing the origin of low back pain of suspected discogenic origin (McFadden 1988).

REFERENCES

Adams M A, Hutton W C 1985a Gradual disc prolapse. Spine 10: 524–531

Adams M A, Hutton W C 1985b The effect of posture on the lumbar spine. Journal of Bone and Joint Surgery 67B: 625–629

Adams M A, Hutton W C 1986 The effect of posture on diffusion into lumbar intervertebral discs. Journal of Anatomy 147: 121–134

Adams P, Muir H 1976 Qualitative changes with age of proteoglycans of human lumbar discs. Annals of the Rheumatic Diseases 35: 289–296

Andersson G B J, Ortengren R, Nachemson A, Elfstrom G 1974 Lumbar disc pressure and myoelectric back muscle activity during sitting. Scandinavian Journal of Rehabilitation Medicine 6: 104–114

Andersson G B J, Ortengren R, Nachemson A 1976 Quantitative studies of back loads in lifting. Spine 1: 178–185

Andriacchi T, Schultz A B, Belytschko T, Galante J 1974 A model for studies of mechanical interactions between the human spine and rib cage. Journal of Biomechanics 7(6): 497–507

Armstrong J R 1967 Lumbar disc lesions. 3rd edn. E S Livingstone, Edinburgh

Balla J I, Langford K H 1967 Vertebral artery compression in cervical spondylosis. Medical Journal of Australia 1: 284–286

Bayliss M T, Urban J G, Johnstone B, Holm S 1986 In-vitro-method for measuring synthesis rates in the intervertebral disc. Journal of Orthopaedic Research 4: 10–17

Belytschko T, Kulak R F, Schultz A B, Galante J O 1974 Finite element stress analysis of an intervertebral disc. Journal of Biomechanics 4: 277–285

Bogduk N 1983 The innervation of the lumbar spine. Spine 8: 286–293

Bogduk N, Twomey L T 1987 Clinical anatomy of the lumbar spine. Churchill Livingstone, Melbourne

Bushell G R, Gosh P, Taylor T F K, Akeson W H 1977 Proteoglycan chemistry of the intervertebral disc. Clinical Orthopaedics and Related Research 129: 115–119

Coventry M D 1969 Anatomy of the intervertebral disc. Clinical Orthopaedics and Related Research 67: 9–15

Crock H V 1986 Internal disc disruption: a challenge to disc prolapse fifty years on. Spine 11: 650–653

Dent C E, Watson L 1966 Osteoporosis. Postgraduate Medical Journal suppl 42: 583–660

Dvorak J, Froehlich D, Penning L, Baumgartner H, Panjabi M M 1988 Functional radiographic diagnosis of the cervical spine: flexion/extension. Spine 13: 748–755

Ericksen M F 1974 Aging changes in the shape of human lumbar vertebrae. American Journal of Physical Anthropology 41: 477

Farfan H F 1973 Mechanical disorders of the low back. Lea & Febiger, Philadelphia

Frank C, Akeson W H, Woo, S L-Y, Amiel D, Coutts R D 1984 Physiology and therapeutic value of passive joint motion. Clinical Orthopaedics and Related Research 185: 113–125

Galante J O 1967 Tensile properties of the human lumbar annulus fibrosis. Acta Orthopaedica Scandinavica (suppl) 100: 1–19

Gibson M J, Buckley J, Mawhinney R, Mulholland R C, Worthington B S 1986 Magnetic resonance imaging and discography in the diagnosis of disc degeneration. Journal of Bone and Joint Surgery 68B: 369–373

Grant R 1987 Dizziness testing before cervical manipulation. Proceedings of the Fifth Biennial Congress of the Manipulative Therapists Association of Australia, Melbourne, pp 123–135

Hayashi K, Yakubi T 1985 Origins of the uncus and of Luschka's joint in the cervical spine. Journal of Bone and Joint Surgery 67A: 788–791

Horst M, Brinckmann P 1981 Measurement of the distribution of axial stress on the end-plate of the vertebral body. Spine 6: 217–232

Kraemer J, Kolditz D, Gowin R 1985 Water and electrolyte content of human intervertebral discs under variable load. Spine 10: 69–71

Kramer J 1981 Intervertebral disc lesions: causes, diagnosis, treatment and proplylaxis. Georg Thieme Verlag, Stuttgart

Kulak R F, Belytschko T B, Shultz A B 1976 Nonlinear behaviour of the human intervertebral disc under axial load. Journal of Biomechanics 9: 377–386

Livingston M C P 1971 Spinal manipulation causing injury. Clinical Orthopaedics and Related Research 81: 82–86

Lyness S S, Simeone F A 1978 Vascular complications of upper cervical spine injuries. Orthopaedic Clinics of North America 9: 1029–1038

Maroudas A, Nachemson A, Stockwell R A 1975 Factors involved in the nutrition of the adult human intervertebral disc. Journal of Anatomy 120: 113–130

McFadden J W 1988 The stress lumbar discogram. Spine 13: 931–937

McFadden K D, Taylor J R 1990 Axial rotation in the lumbar spine and gaping of the zygapophyseal joints. Spine 15: 295–298

Merriam W F, Quinnell R C, Stockdale H R, Willis D S 1984 The effect of postural changes on the inferred pressures within the nucleus pulposus during lumbar discography. Spine 9: 406–408

Nachemson A L 1960 Lumbar intradiscal pressure. Acta Orthopaedica Scandinavica (suppl 43)

Nachemson A L 1965 The effect of forward leaning on lumbar intradiscal pressure. Acta Orthopaedica Scandinavica XXXV: 314–328

Nachemson A L, Morris J M 1964 In vitro measurements of intradiscal pressure. Journal of Bone and Joint Surgery 46A: 1077–1092

Nachemson A L, Elfstrom G 1970 Intravital dynamic pressure measurements in lumbar discs. Scandinavian Journal of Rehabilitation Medicine (suppl 1) 1–40

Nachemson A L, Schultz A B, Berkson M H 1979 Mechanical properties of human lumbar spine motion segments. Spine 4: 1–8

Naylor A 1962 The biophysical and biochemical aspects of intervertebral disc herniation and degeneration. Annals of the Royal College of Surgery (England) 31: 91–114

Osti O L, Vernon-Roberts B, Fraser R D 1990 Anulus tears and intervertebral disc degeneration: an experimental study using an animal model. Spine 15: 762–767

Panjabi M M, Brand R A, White A A 1976 Three dimension flexibility and stiffness properties of the human thoracic spine. Journal of Biomechanics 9: 185–192

Panjabi M M, Krag M H, Chung T Q 1984 Effects of disc injury on mechanical behaviour of the human spine. Spine 9(7): 707–713

Penning L 1968 Functional pathology of the cervical spine. Williams & Wilkins, Baltimore

Penning L, Wilmink J T 1987 Posture-dependent bilateral compression of L4 or L5 nerve roots in facet hypertrophy. A dynamic CT-myelographic study. Spine 12: 488–500

Puschel J 1930 Der Wassergehalt normaler und degenerierter Zwischenwirbelscheiben. Beitr Path Anat 84: 123–130

Quinnell R C 1980 Pressure standardized discography. British Journal of Radiology 53: 1031–1036

Resnick D 1985 Degenerative diseases of the vertebral column. Radiology 156: 3–14

Rolander S D 1966 Motion of the lumbar spine with special reference to the stability effect of posterior fusion. Acta Orthopaedica Scandinavia (suppl 90) 16–23, 29–30, 64–67, 74–76, 121–126

Sachs B L, Vanharanta H, Spivey M A et al 1987 Dallas discogram description: a new classification of C/T discography in low back disorders. Spine 12: 287–294

Scott J E 1990 Proteoglycan: collagen interactions and sub-fibrillar structure in collagen fibrils. Implications in the development and ageing of connective tissues. Journal of Anatomy 169: 13–22

Scott J E, Bosworth T R, Cribb A, Taylor J R 1991 Biochemistry and ultrastructure of human intervertebral discs. Biochemical Abstracts (in press)

Taylor J R 1973 Growth and development of the human intervertebral disc. PhD thesis, University of Edinburgh pp 1–35; 149–228

Taylor J R 1990 The development and adult structure of lumbar intervertebral discs. Journal of Manual Medicine 5: 43–47

Taylor J R, Milne N 1988 The cervical mobile segments. Proceedings of Whiplash Symposium, Australian Physiotherapy Association, Adelaide, pp 21–27

Taylor J R, Twomey L T 1979 Innervation of lumbar intervertebral discs. Medical Journal of Australia 2: 701–702

Taylor J R, Twomey L T 1985 Vertebral column development and its relation to adult pathology. Australian Journal of Physiotherapy 31: 83–88

Taylor J R, Twomey L T 1986 Age changes in lumbar zygapophyseal joints. Observations on Structure and Function. Spine 11: 739–745

Taylor J R, Twomey L T 1990

Taylor J R, Twomey L T, Corker M 1990 Bone and soft tissue injuries in post-mortem lumbar spines. Paraplegia 28: 119–129

Taylor J R, Scott J E, Cribb A, Bosworth T R 1991 Maturation in human intervertebral discs. Proceedings of Combined Meeting of the Physiological Society of New Zealand, Australian Neuroscience Society and Anatomical Society of Australia and New Zealand, Auckland, January 1991, pp 18–19

Töndury G 1972 Functional anatomy of the small joints of the spine. Annales de Medecine Physique XV: 2

Twomey L T 1981 Age changes in the human lumbar spine. PhD thesis, University of Western Australia

Twomey L T, Taylor J R 1982 Flexion creep deformation and hysteresis in the lumbar vertebral column. Spine 7: 116–122

Twomey L T, Taylor J R 1983 Sagittal movements of the human lumbar vertebral column: a quantitative study of the role of the posterior vertebral elements. Archives of Physical Medicine and Rehabilitation 64: 322–325

Twomey L T, Taylor J R 1985a Age changes in the lumbar intervertebral discs. Acta Orthopaedica Scandinavica 56: 496–499

Twomey L T, Taylor J R 1985b A quantitative study of the role of the posterior vertebral elements in sagittal movements of the lumbar vertebral column. Aspects of manipulative therapy. Churchill Livingstone, Melbourne

Twomey L T, Taylor J R 1987 Physical therapy of the low back. Churchill Livingstone, New York

Twomey L T, Taylor J R 1990 Structural and mechanical disc changes with age. Journal of Manual Medicine 5: 58–61

Twomey L T, Taylor J R, Furniss B 1983 Age changes in the bone density and structure of the lumbar vertebral column. Journal of Anatomy 136: 15–25

Tyrrell A R, Reilly T, Troup J D G 1985 Circadian variation in stature and the effects of spinal loading. Spine 10: 161

Vernon-Roberts B, Pirie C J 1977 Degenerative changes in the intervertebral discs of the lumbar spine and their sequelae. Rheumatology and Rehabilitation 16: 13–21

Videman T, Malmivaara A, Mooney V 1987 The value of the axial view in assessing discograms: an experimental study with cadavers. Spine 12: 299–304

Virgin W J 1958 Anatomical and pathological aspects of the intervertebral disc. Indian Journal of Surgery 20: 113–119

Walmsley R 1953 The development and growth of the intervertebral disc. Edinburgh Medical Journal 60: 341–364

White A A, Panjabi M M 1978 The clinical biomechanics of the spine. J B Lippincott, Philadelphia

15. The anatomy and function of the lumbar back muscles

J. E. Macintosh   N. Bogduk

The lumbar spine is surrounded by muscles which, for descriptive purposes, and on functional grounds, may be divided into three groups. These are:

1. Psoas major and psoas minor, which cover the anterolateral aspects of the lumbar vertebral bodies and intervertebral discs
2. Intertransversarii laterales and quadratus lumborum, which connect and cover the transverse processes anteriorly
3. The lumbar back muscles, which lie behind and cover the posterior elements of the lumbar spine.

PSOAS MAJOR AND MINOR

The psoas major is a long muscle which arises from the anterolateral aspect of the lumbar spine and descends over the brim of the pelvis to insert into the lesser trochanter of the femur. It is essentially a muscle of the thigh whose principal action is flexion of the hip.

The psoas major has diverse, but systematic, attachments to the lumbar spine. At each segmental level it is attached to the medial half or so of the anterior surface of the transverse process, to the intervertebral disc, and to the margins of the vertebral bodies adjacent to the disc. The muscle fibres from the L5 transverse process and the L5 vertebral body form the deepest and lowest bundle of fibres within the muscle, and these fibres are systematically overlapped by fibres from the discs and transverse processes at successively higher levels. As a result, the muscle is layered in cross-section, with fibres from higher levels forming the outer surface of the muscle and those from lower levels lying sequentially, deeper within its substance.

Because the psoas major is attached to the lumber vertebrae, it has been interpreted as being a stabilizer of the lumbar spine during flexion, extension and other movements of the trunk (Nachemson 1966a, 1968). Recent anatomical and biomechanical studies have explored this proposition and found that although reasonably strong, the fascicles of psoas major lie very close to the axes of rotation the lumbar motion segments. Consequently, the maximum moments they exert are relatively small and are not able to provide any substantial stabilizing influence on the lumbar spine (Bogduk et al 1991). The morphological and biomechanical features of the psoas major indicate that it is not designed to act on the lumbar spine; rather, it is designed purely to be a hip flexor (Bogduk et al 1991).

The psoas minor is an inconstant small muscle belly which arises from the T12–L1 intervertebral disc and forms a very long narrow tendon that inserts into the region of the iliopubic eminence.

INTERTRANSVERSARII LATERALES

The intertransversarii laterales consist of two parts: the intertransversarii laterales ventrales and the intertransversarii laterales dorsales. The ventral intertransversarii connect the margins of consecutive transverse processes, while the dorsal intertransversarii each connect an accessory process to the transverse process below (Fig. 15.1). Both the ventral and dorsal intertransversarii are innervated by the ventral rami of the lumbar spine nerves (Cave 1937) and consequently cannot be classified amongst the back muscles — which are all innervated by the dorsal rami. On the basis of their attachments and their nerve supply, the ventral and dorsal intertransversarii are considered to be homologous to the intercostal and levator costae muscles of the thoracic region (Cave 1937).

The function of the intertransversarii laterales has been determined experimentally and one can only presume that on the basis of their attachments they act synergistically with the quadratus lumborum in lateral flexion of the lumbar spine.

QUADRATUS LUMBORUM

The quadratus lumborum is a wide, more or less rectangular muscle that covers the lateral two-thirds or so of the anterior surfaces of the L1 to L4 transverse processes and extends laterally a few centimetres beyond the tips of the transverse processes.

In detail, the muscle is a complex aggregation of various oblique and longitudinally running fibres that connect the lumbar transverse processes, the ilium and the 12th rib (Poirier 1912). Caudally, the muscle arises from the L5 transverse process, the trough formed by the superior and anterior ilio-lumbar ligaments, and from the iliac crest lateral to the point of attachment of the ilio-lumbar ligament. From this series of attachments the most lateral fibres pass directly towards the lower anterior surface of the 12th rib. More medial fibres pass obliquely upwards and medially to the anterior surfaces of each of the lumbar transverse processes above L5. These oblique fibres intermingle with other oblique fibres that run upwards and laterally from each of the lumbar transverse processes to the 12th rib.

The majority of the fibres of the quadratus lumborum are connected to the 12th rib, and one of the functions of this muscle is said to be to fix the 12th rib during respiration (Williams et al 1989). The remaining fibres of quadratus lumborum connect the ilium to the upper four lumbar transverse processes, and these fibres are suitably disposed to execute lateral flexion of the lumbar spine.

THE LUMBAR BACK MUSCLES

The lumbar back muscles are those muscles which lie behind the plane of the transverse processes and which exert an action on the lumbar spine. They include muscles that attach to the lumbar vertebrae and thereby act directly on the lumbar spine, and certain other muscles that, while not attaching to the lumbar vertebrae, nevertheless exert an action on the lumbar spine.

For descriptive purposes, and on morphological grounds, the lumbar back muscles may be divided into three groups:

1. The short intersegmental muscles — the interspinales and the intertransversarii mediales
2. The polysegmental muscles that attach to the lumbar vertebrae — the multifidus and the lumbar components of longissimus and iliocostalis
3. The long polysegmental muscles, represented by the thoracic components of longissimus and iliocostalis lumborum, that, in general, do not attach to the lumbar vertebrae but cross the lumbar region from thoracic levels to find attachments on the ilium and sacrum.

The descriptions of the back muscles offered in this chapter, notably those of the multifidus and erector spinae, differ substantially from those given in standard textbooks. Traditionally, these muscles have been regarded as stemming from a common origin on the sacrum

and ilium and passing upwards to assume diverse attachments to the lumbar and thoracic vertebrae and ribs. However, in the face of several recent studies of these muscles (Bogduk 1980, Macintosh & Bogduk 1986, 1987, Macintosh et al 1986) it is considered more appropriate to view these muscles in the reverse direction — from above downwards. Not only is this more consistent with the pattern of their nerve supply (Bogduk et al 1982, Macintosh et al 1986), but it clarifies the identity of certain muscles and the identity of the erector spinae aponeurosis, and it reveals the segmental biomechanical disposition of the muscles.

Interspinales

The lumbar interspinales are short paired muscles that lie on either side of the interspinous ligament and connect the spinous processes of adjacent lumbar vertebrae (Fig. 15.1). There are four pairs in the lumbar region.

Although disposed to act synergistically with the multifidus to produce posterior sagittal rotation of the vertebra above, the interspinales are quite small and would not contribute appreciably to the force required to move a vertebra. This paradox is similar to that which applies for the intertransversarii mediales and is discussed further in that context.

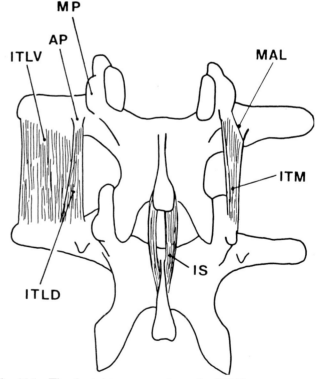

Fig. 15.1 The short, intersegmental muscles. ITLV = intertransversarii laterales ventrales; ITLD = intertransversarii laterales dorsales; ITM = intertransversarii mediales; IS = interspinales; AP = accessory process; MP = mamillary process; MAL = mamillo-accessory ligament.

Intertransversarii mediales

The intertransversarii mediales can be considered to be true back muscles for, unlike the intertransversarii laterales, they are innervated by the lumbar dorsal rami (Cave 1937, Bogduk et al 1982). The intertransversarii mediales arise from an accessory process, the adjoining mamillary process and the mamillo-accessory ligament that connects these two processes (Bogduk 1981). They insert into the superior aspect of the mamillary process of the vertebral below (Fig. 15.1).

The intertransversarii mediales lie lateral to the axis of lateral flexion and behind the axis of sagittal rotation. However, they lie very close to these axes and are very small muscles. Therefore, it is questionable whether they could contribute any appreciable force in either lateral flexion or posterior sagittal rotation. It might be argued that perhaps larger muscles might provide the bulk of the power to move the vertebrae, and the intertransversarii could act to 'fine tune' the movement. However, this suggestion is highly speculative, if not fanciful, and does not account for their small size and considerable mechanical disadvantage.

A tantalizing alternative suggestion is that the intertransversarii act as large, proprioceptive transducers — their value lying not in the force they can exert, but in the muscle spindles they contain. Placed close to the lumbar vertebral column, the intertransversarii could monitor the movements of the column and provide feed-back that influences the action of the surrounding muscles. Such a role has been suggested for the cervical intertransversarii which have been found to contain a high density of muscle spindles (Abrahams 1977, 1981, Cooper & Danial 1963). Indeed, all unisegmental muscles of the vertebral column have between two and six times the density of muscle spindles found in the longer, polysegmental muscles, and there is growing speculation that this underscores the proprioceptive function of all short, small muscles of the body (Peck et al 1984, Nitz & Peck 1986, Bastide et al 1989).

Multifidus

Multifidus is the largest and most medial of the lumbar back muscles. It consists of a repeating series of fascicles which stem from the laminae and spinous processes of the lumbar vertebrae and exhibit a constant pattern of attachments caudally (Macintosh et al 1986).

The shortest fascicles of the multifidus are the 'laminar fibres' which arise from the caudal end of the dorsal surface of each vertebral lamina and insert into the mamillary process of the vertebra two levels caudad (Fig. 15.2). The L5 laminar fibres have no mamillary process into which they can insert, and insert instead into an area on the sacrum just above the first dorsal sacral foramen. Because

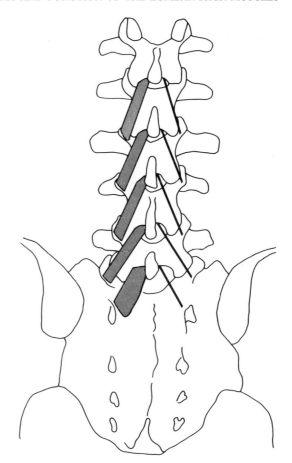

Fig. 15.2 The laminar fibres of multifidus.

of their attachments, the laminar fibres may be considered homologous to the thoracic rotatores.

The bulk of the lumbar multifidus consists of much larger fascicles that radiate from the lumbar spinous processes. These fascicles are arranged in five overlapping groups such that each lumbar vertebra gives rise to one of these groups. At each segmental level, a fascicle arises from the base and caudolateral edge of the spinous process, and several fascicles arise, by way of a common tendon, from the caudal tip of the spinous process. This tendon is referred to hereafter as 'the common tendon'. Although confluent with one another at their origin, the fascicles in each group diverge caudally to assume separate attachments to mamillary processes, the iliac crest and the sacrum.

The fascicle from the base of the L1 spinous process inserts into the L4 mamillary process, while those from the common tendon insert into the mamillary processes of L5, S1 and the posterior superior iliac spine (Fig. 15.3).

The fascicle from the base of the spinous process of L2 inserts into the mamillary process of L5, while those from the common tendon insert into the S1 mamillary process, the posterior superior iliac spine, and an area on the iliac crest just caudoventral to the posterior superior iliac spine (Fig. 15.4).

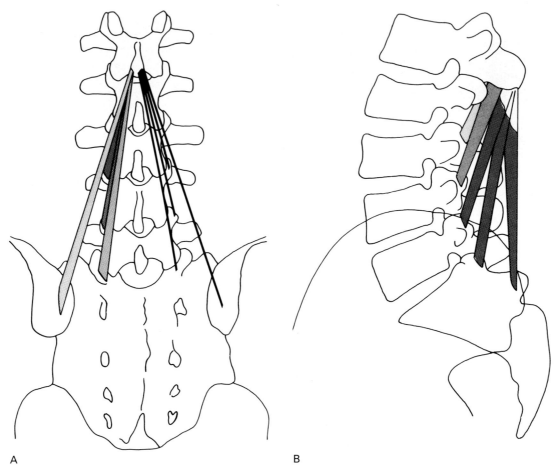

Fig. 15.3   The fascicles of multifidus from L1. **A.** Posterior view. **B.** Lateral view.

The fascicle from the base of the L3 spinous process inserts into the mamillary process of the sacrum, while those fascicles from the common tendon insert into a narrow area extending caudally from the caudal extent of the posterior superior iliac spine to the lateral edge of the third sacral segment (Fig. 15.5). The L4 fascicles insert onto the sacrum in an area medial to the L3 area of insertion, but lateral to the dorsal sacral foramina (Fig. 15.6), while those from the L5 vertebra insert onto an area medial to the dorsal sacral foramina (Fig. 15.7).

It is noteworthy that while many of the fascicles of multifidus attach to mamillary processes, some of the deeper fibres of these fascicles attach to the capsules of the zygapophysial joints next to the mamillary processes (Lewin et al 1962). This attachment allows the multifidus to protect the joint capsule from being caught inside the joint during the movements executed by the multifidus.

The key feature of the morphology of the lumbar multifidus is that its fascicles are arranged segmentally. Each lumbar vertebra is endowed with a group of fascicles that radiate from its spinous process, anchoring it below to mamillary processes, the iliac crest and the sacrum. This disposition suggests that the fibres of multifidus are arranged in such a way that their principal action is focused on individual lumbar spinous processes (Macintosh et al 1986). They are designed to act in concert on a single spinous process. This contention is supported by the pattern of innervation of the muscle. All the fascicles arising from the spinous processes of a given vertebra are innervated by the medial branch of the dorsal ramus that issues from below that vertebra (Bogduk et al 1982, Macintosh et al 1986). Thus, the muscles that directly act on a particular vertebral segment are innervated by the nerve of that segment.

In a posterior view, the fascicles of multifidus are seen to have an oblique, caudolateral orientation. Their line of action, therefore, can be resolved into two vectors: a large vertical vector, and a considerably smaller horizontal vector (Macintosh & Bogduk 1986) (Fig. 15.8).

The small horizontal vector suggests that the multifidus could pull the spinous processes sideways, and therefore produce horizontal rotation. However, horizontal rotation of lumbar vertebrae is impeded by the impaction of the contralateral zygapophysial joints. Horizontal rotation occurs after impaction of the joints only if an appropriate shear force is applied to the intervertebral discs, but

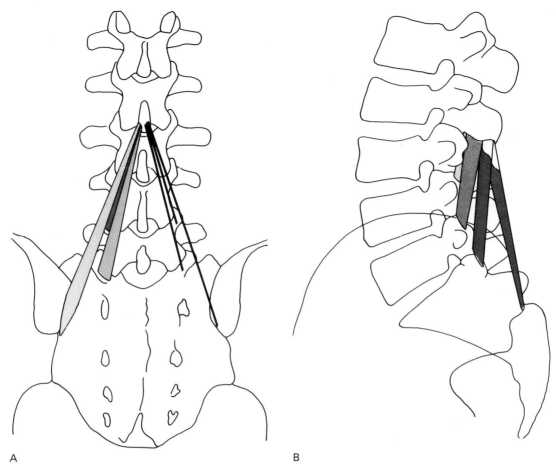

Fig. 15.4   The fascicles of multifidus from L2. **A.** Posterior view. **B.** Lateral view.

the horizontal vector of multifidus is so small that it is unlikely that multifidus would be capable of exerting such a shear force on the disc by acting on the spinous process. Indeed, electromyographic studies reveal that multifidus is inconsistently active in de-rotation and that, paradoxically, it is active in both ipsilateral and contralateral rotation (Donisch & Basmajian 1972). Rotation, therefore, cannot be inferred to be a primary action of multifidus. In this context, multifidus has been said to act only as a 'stabilizer' in rotation (Lewin et al 1962, Donsich & Basmajian 1972), but the aberrant movements which it is supposed to stabilize have not been defined (although see below).

The principal action of multifidus is expressed by its vertical vector, and further insight is gained when this vector is viewed in a lateral projection (Fig. 15.8). Each fascicle of multifidus, at every level, acts virtually at right angles to its spinous process of origin (Macintosh & Bogduk 1986). Thus, using the spinous process as a lever, every fascicle is ideally disposed to produce posterior sagittal rotation of its vertebra. The right-angle orientation, however, precluded any action as a posterior horizontal translator. Therefore, the multifidus can only exert

the 'rocking' component of extension of the lumbar spine or control this component during flexion.

Having established that multifidus is primarily a posterior sagittal rotator of the lumbar spine, it is possible to resolve the paradox about its activity during horizontal rotation of the trunk (Macintosh & Bogduk 1986). In the first instance, it should be realized that rotation of the lumbar spine is an indirect action. Active rotation of the lumbar spine occurs only if the thorax is first rotated, and is therefore secondary to thoracic rotation. Secondly, it must be realized that a muscle with two vectors of action cannot use these vectors independently. If the muscle contracts, then both vectors are exerted. Thus, multifidus cannot exert axial rotation without simultaneously exerting a much larger posterior sagittal rotation.

The principal muscles that produce rotation of the thorax are the oblique abdominal muscles. The horizontal component of their orientation is able to turn the thoracic cage in the horizontal plane and thereby impart axial rotation to the lumbar spine. However, the oblique abdominal muscles also have a vertical component to their orientation. Therefore, if they contract to produce rotation they will also simultaneously cause flexion of the trunk, and

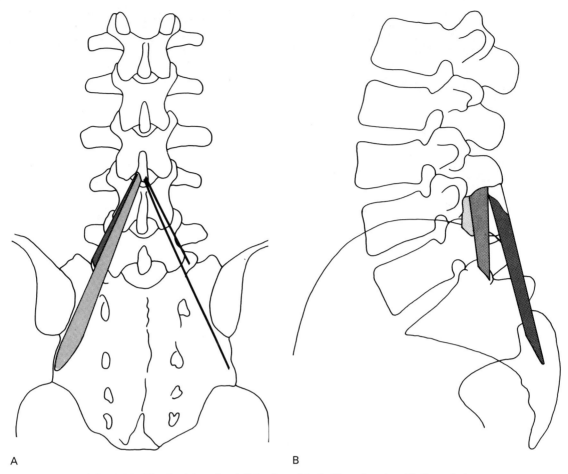

Fig. 15.5   The fascicles of multifidus from L3. **A.** Posterior view. **B.** Lateral view.

therefore, of the lumbar spine. To counteract this flexion, and maintain pure axial rotation, extensors of the lumbar spine must be recruited, and this is how multifidus becomes involved in rotation.

The role of multifidus in rotation is not to produce rotation but to oppose the flexion effect of the abdominal muscles as they produce rotation. The aberrant motion 'stabilized' by multifidus during rotation is, therefore, the unwanted flexion unavoidably produced by the abdominal muscles (Macintosh & Bogduk 1986).

Apart from its action on individual lumbar vertebrae, the multifidus, because of its polysegmental nature, can also exert indirect effects on any interposed vertebrae. Since the line of action of any long fascicle of multifidus lies behind the lordotic curve of the lumbar spine, such fascicles can act like bowstrings on those segments of the curve that intervene between the attachments of the fascicle. The bowstring effect would tend to accentuate the lumbar lordosis, resulting in compression of inter-vertebral discs posteriorly and strain of the discs and longitudinal ligament anteriorly. Thus, a secondary effect of the action of multifidus is to increase the lumbar lordosis and the compressive and tensile loads on any

vertebrae and intervertebral discs interposed between its attachments.

Lumbar erector spinae

The lumbar erector spinae lies lateral to the multifidus and forms the prominent dorsolateral contour of the back muscles in the lumbar region. It consists of two muscles — the *longissimus thoracis* and the *iliocostalis lumborum*. Furthermore, each of these muscles has two components: a lumbar part, consisting of fascicles arising from lumbar vertebrae, and a thoracic part, consisting of fascicles arising from thoracic vertebrae or ribs (Bogduk 1980, Macintosh & Bogduk 1987). These four parts may be referred to respectively as *longissimus thoracis pars lumborum, iliocostalis lumborum pars lumborum, longissimus thoracis pars lumborum* and *longissimus thoracis pars thoracis* (Macintosh & Bogduk 1987).

In the lumbar region, the longissimus and iliocostalis are separated from each other by the *lumbar intermuscular aponeurosis*, an antero-posterior continuation of the erector spinae aponeurosis (Bogduk 1980, Macintosh & Bogduk 1987). It appears as a flat sheet of collagen fibres that

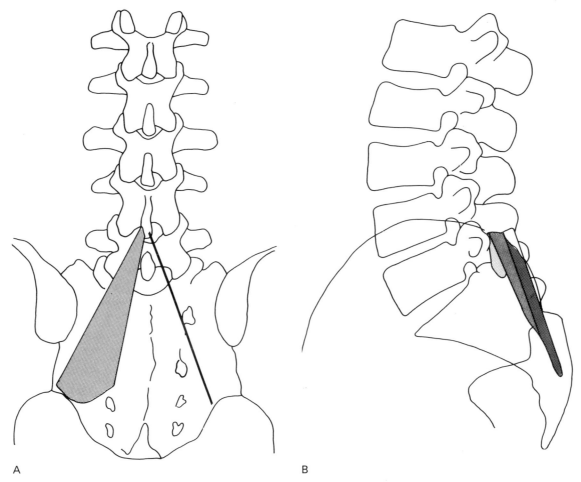

Fig. 15.6   The fascicles of multifidus from L4. **A.** Posterior view. **B.** Lateral view.

extend rostrally from the medial aspect of the posterior superior iliac spine for 6–8 cm. It is formed mainly by the caudal tendons of the rostral four fascicles of the lumbar component of longissimus (Fig. 15.9).

Longissimus thoracis pars lumborum.

The longissimus thoracis pars lumborum is composed of five fascicles, each arising from the accessory process and the adjacent medial end of the dorsal surface of the transverse process of a lumbar vertebra (Fig. 15.9).

The fascicle from the L5 vertebra is the deepest and shortest. Its fibres insert directly into the medial aspect of the posterior superior iliac spine. The fascicle from L4 also lies deeply, but lateral to that from L5. Succeeding fascicles lie progressively more dorsally so that the L3 fascicle covers those from L4 and L5, but is itself covered by the L2 fascicle, while the L1 fascicle lies most superficially.

The L1 to L4 fascicles all form tendons at their caudal ends which converge to form the lumbar intermuscular aponeurosis, which eventually attaches to a narrow area on the ilium immediately lateral to the insertion of the L5 fascicle. The lumbar intermuscular aponeurosis thus rep-resents a common tendon of insertion, or the aponeurosis, of the bulk of the lumbar fibres of longissimus.

Each fascicle of the lumbar longissimus has both a dorsoventral and a rostrocaudal orientation (Macintosh & Bogduk 1987). Therefore, the action of each fascicle can be resolved into a vertical vector and a horizontal vector, the relative sizes of which differ from L1 to L5 (Fig. 15.10). Consequently, the relative actions of longissimus differ at each segmental level. Furthermore, the action of longissimus, as a whole, will differ according to whether the muscle contracts unilaterally or bilaterally.

The large vertical vector of each fascicle lies lateral to the axis of lateral flexion and behind the axis of sagittal rotation of each vertebra. Thus, contracting unilaterally the longissimus can laterally flex the vertebral column, but acting bilaterally the various fascicles can act, like multifidus, to produce posterior sagittal rotation of their vertebra of origin. However, their attachments to the accessory and transverse processes lie close to the axes of sagittal rotation and therefore, their capacity to produce posterior sagittal rotation is less efficient than that of multifidus which acts through the long levers of the spinous processes (Macintosh & Bogduk 1987).

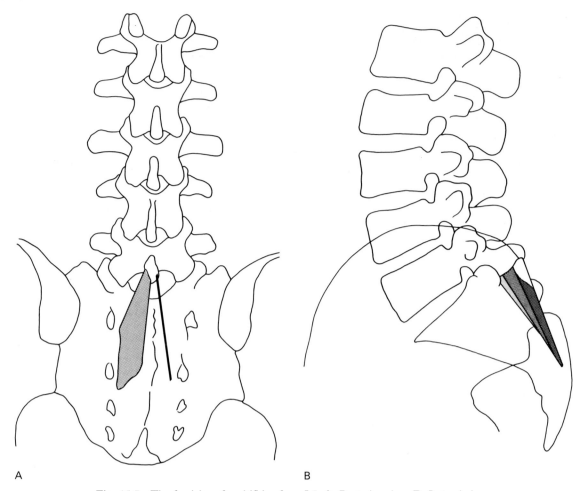

A   B

Fig. 15.7 The fascicles of multifidus from L5. **A.** Posterior view. **B.** Lateral view.

The horizontal vectors of the longissimus are directed backwards. Therefore, when contracting bilaterally the longissimus is capable of drawing the lumbar vertebrae backwards. This action of posterior translation can restore the anterior translation of the lumbar vertebrae that occurs during flexion of the lumbar column. The capacity for posterior translation is greatest at lower lumbar levels where the fascicles of longissimus assume a greater dorso-ventral orientation (Fig. 15.10).

Reviewing the horizontal and vertical actions of longissimus together, it can be seen that longissimus expresses a continuum of combined actions along the length of the lumbar vertebral column. From below upwards, its capacity as a posterior sagittal rotator increases while reciprocally, from above downwards, the fascicles are better designed to resist or restore anterior translation. It is emphasized that the longissimus cannot exert its horizontal and vertical vectors independently. Thus, whatever horizontal translation it exerts must occur simultaneously with posterior saggital rotation. The resolution into vectors simply reveals the relative amounts of simultaneous translation and sagittal rotation exerted at different segmental levels.

It might be deduced that, because of the horizontal vector of longissimus, this muscle acting unilaterally could draw the accessory and transverse processes backwards and therefore produce axial rotation. However, in this regard, the fascicles of longissimus are orientated almost directly towards the axis of axial rotation and so are at a marked mechanical disadvantage to produce axial rotation.

Iliocostalis lumborum pars lumborum

The lumbar component of iliocostalis lumborum consists of four overlying fascicles arising from the L1 through to L4 vertebrae. Rostrally, each fascicle attaches to the tip of the transverse process and to an area extending 2–3 cm laterally onto the middle layer of the thoracolumbar fascia (Fig. 15.11).

The fascicle from L4 is the deepest, and caudally it is attached directly to the iliac crest just lateral to the posterior superior iliac spine. This fascicle is covered by the fascicle from L3 that has a similar but more dorsolaterally located attachment on the iliac crest. In sequence, L2 covers L3, and L1 covers L2 with insertions on the iliac crest becoming successively more dorsal and lateral. The

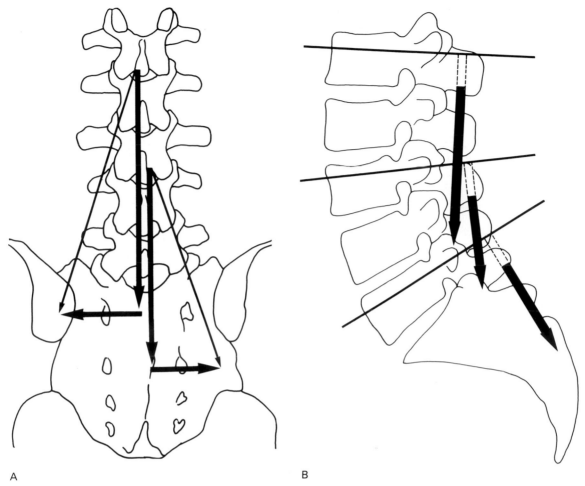

A   B

Fig. 15.8 The force vectors of multifidus. **A.** In a postero-anterior view, the oblique line of action of the multifidus at each level can be resolved into a major vertical vector and a smaller horizontal vector. **B.** In a lateral view, the vertical vectors of the multifidus are seen to be aligned at right angles to the transverse axis of their vertebra of origin.

most lateral fascicles attach to the iliac crest just medial to the attachment of the 'lateral raphe' of the thoracolumbar fascia (see below). The most medial fibres of iliocostalis contribute to the lumbar intermuscular aponeurosis, but only to a minor extent.

Although an L5 fascicle of iliocostalis lumborum is not described in the literature, it is represented in the ilio-lumbar 'ligament'. In neonates and children this 'ligament' is completely muscular in structure. By the third decade of life the muscle fibres are entirely replaced by collagen, giving rise to the familiar ilio-lumbar ligament (Luk et al 1986). On the basis of sites of attachment and relative orientation the posterior band of the ilio-lumbar ligament would appear to be derived from the L5 fascicle of iliocostalis while the anterior band of the ligament is a derivative of the quadratus lumborum.

The disposition of the lumbar fascicles of iliocostalis is similar to that of the lumbar longissimus, except that the fascicles are situated more laterally. Like that of the lumbar longissimus, their action can be resolved into horizontal and vertical vectors (Fig. 15.12).

The vertical vector is still predominant, and therefore, the lumbar fascicles of iliocostalis contracting bilaterally can act as posterior sagittal rotators (Fig. 15.12), but, because of the horizontal vector, a posterior translation will be exerted simultaneously, principally at lower lumbar levels where the fascicles of iliocostalis have a greater forward orientation. Contracting unilaterally, the lumbar fascicles of iliocostalis can act as lateral flexors of the lumbar vertebrae, for which action the transverse processes provide very substantial levers.

Contracting unilaterally, the fibres of iliocostalis are better suited to exert axial rotation than the fascicles of lumbar longissimus, for their attachment to the tips of the transverse processes displaces them from the axis of horizontal rotation and provides them with substantial levers for this action. Because of this leverage, the lower fascicles of iliocostalis are the only intrinsic muscles of the lumbar spine reasonably disposed to produce horizontal rotation. Their effectiveness as rotators, however, is dwarfed by the oblique abdominal muscles that act on the ribs and produce lumbar rotation indirectly by rotating the

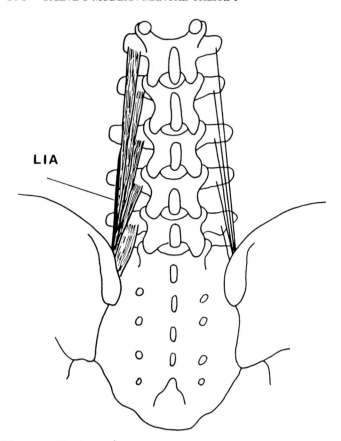

LIA

Fig. 15.9 The lumbar fibres of longissimus (longissimus thoracis pars lumborum). On the left, the five fascicles of the intact muscle are drawn. The formation of the lumbar intermuscular aponeurosis (LIA) by the lumbar fascicles of longissimus is depicted. On the right, the lines indicate the attachments and span of the fascicles.

thoracic cage. However, because iliocostalis cannot exert axial rotation without simultaneously exerting posterior sagittal rotation, the muscle is well suited to co-operate with multifidus to oppose the flexion effect of the abdominal muscles when they act to rotate the trunk.

Longissimus thoracic pars thoracis

The thoracic fibres of longissimus thoracis typically consists of 11 or 12 pairs of small fascicles arising from the ribs and transverse processes of T1 or T2 down to T12 (Fig. 15.13). At each level, two tendons can usually be recognized, a medial one from the tip of the transverse process, and a lateral one from the rib, although in the upper 3 or 4 levels, the latter may merge medially with the fascicle from the transverse process. Each rostral tendon extends 3–4 cm before forming a small muscle belly measuring 7–8 cm in length. The muscle bellies from the higher levels overlap those from lower levels. Each muscle belly eventually forms a caudal tendon that extends into the lumbar region. The tendons run in parallel, with those from higher levels being most medial. The fascicles from the T2 level attach to the L3 spinous process, while the fascicles from the remaining levels insert

into spinous processes at progressively lower levels. For example those from T5 attach to L5 and those from T7 to S2 or S3. Those from T8 to T12 diverge from the midline to find attachment to the sacrum along a line extending from the S3 spinous process to the caudal extent of the posterior superior iliac spine (Macintosh & Bogduk 1987). The lateral edge of the caudal tendon of T12 lies alongside the dorsal edge of the lumbar intermuscular aponeurosis formed by the caudal tendon of the L1 longissimus bundle.

The side to side aggregation of the caudal tendons of longissimus thoracis pars thoracis forms much of what is termed the erector spinae aponeurosis which covers the lumbar fibres of longissimus and iliocostalis, but affords no attachment to them.

The longissimus thoracis pars thoracis is designed to act on thoracic vertebrae and ribs. Nonetheless, when contracting bilaterally it acts indirectly on the lumbar vertebral column, and uses the erector spinae aponeurosis to produce an increase in the lumbar lordosis. However, not all of the fascicles of longissimus thoracis span the entire lumbar vertebral column. Those from the second rib and T2 reach only as far as L3, and only those fascicles arising between the T6 or 7 and the T12 levels actually span the entire lumbar region. Consequently, only a portion of the whole thoracic longissimus acts on all the lumbar vertebrae.

The oblique orientation of the longissimus thoracis pars thoracis also permits it to flex laterally the thoracic vertebral column and thereby indirectly flex the lumbar vertebral column laterally.

Iliocostalis lumborum pars thoracis

The iliocostalis lumborum pars thoracis consists of fascicles from the lower seven or eight ribs that attach caudally to the ilium and sacrum (Fig. 15.14). These fascicles represents the thoracic component of iliocostalis lumborum, and should not be confused with the iliocostalis thoracis which is restricted to the thoracic region between the upper six and lower six ribs.

Each fascicle of the iliocostalis lumborum pars thoracis arises from the angle of the rib via a ribbon-like tendon measuring some 9–10 cm in length. It then forms a muscle belly of 8–10 cm in length. Thereafter, each fascicle continues as a tendon, contributing to the erector spinae aponeurosis, and ultimately attaching to the posterior superior iliac spine. The most medial tendons, from the more rostral fascicles, often attach more medially to the dorsal surface of the sacrum, caudal to the insertion of multifidus.

The thoracic fascicles of iliocostalis lumborum have no attachment to lumbar vertebrae. They attach to the iliac crest and thereby span the lumbar region. Consequently, by acting bilaterally, it is possible for them to exert an

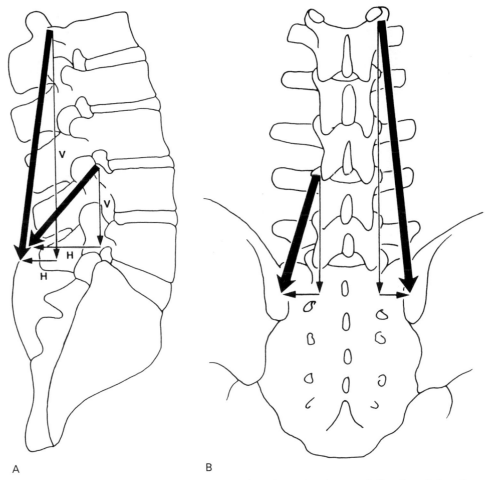

Fig. 15.10   The force vectors of the longissimus thoracis pars lumborum. **A.** In a lateral view, the oblique line of action of each fascicle of longissimus can be resolved into a vertical (V) and a horizontal (H) vector. The horizontal vectors of lower lumbar fascicles are larger. **B.** In a postero-anterior view, the line of action of the fascicles can be resolved into a major vertical vector and a much smaller horizontal vector.

indirect 'bowstring' effect on the vertebral column causing an increase in the lordosis of the lumbar spine. Acting unilaterally, the iliocostalis lumborum pars thoracis can use the leverage afforded by the ribs to laterally flex the thoracic cage and thereby laterally flex the lumbar vertebral column indirectly. The distance between the ribs and ilium does not shorten greatly during rotation of the trunk, and therefore the iliocostalis lumborum pars thoracis can have little action as an axial rotator. However, contralateral rotation greatly increases this distance, and the iliocostalis lumborum pars thoracis can serve to derotate the thoracic cage and, therefore, the lumbar spine.

ERECTOR SPINAE APONEUROSIS

One of the cardinal revelations of recent studies of the lumbar erector spinae (Bogduk 1980, Macintosh & Bogduk 1987) is that this muscle consists of both lumbar and thoracic fibres. Modern textbook descriptions largely do not recognize the lumbar fibres, especially those of

iliocostalis (Bogduk 1980). Moreover, they do not note that the lumbar fibres (of both longissimus and iliocostalis) have attachments quite separate to those of the thoracic fibres. The lumbar fibres of the longissimus and iliocostalis pass between the lumbar vertebrae and the ilium. Thus, through these muscles, the lumbar vertebrae are anchored directly to the ilium. They do not gain any attachment to the erector spinae aponeurosis, which is the implication of all modern textbook descriptions that deal with the erector spinae.

The erector spinae aponeurosis is described as a broad sheet of tendinous fibres that is attached to the ilium, the sacrum, and the lumbar and sacral spinous processes, and which forms a common origin for the lower part of erector spinae. However, as described above, the erector spinae aponeurosis is formed virtually exclusively by the tendons of the longissimus thoracis pars thoracis and iliocostalis pars thoracis (Bogduk 1980, Macintosh & Bogduk 1987). The medial half or so of the aponeurosis is formed by the tendons of longissimus thoracis, and the lateral half is formed by the iliocostalis lumborum (Fig. 15.15). The

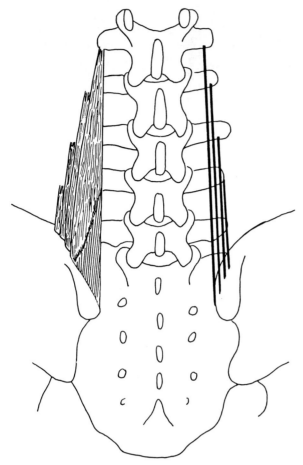

Fig. 15.11 The lumbar fibres of iliocostalis (iliocostalis lumborum pars lumborum). On the left, the four lumbar fascicles of iliocostalis are shown. On the right, their span and attachments are indicated by the lines.

only additional contribution comes from the most superficial fibres of multifidus from upper lumbar levels which contribute a small number of fibres to the aponeurosis (Macintosh et al 1986). Nonetheless, the erector spinae aponeurosis is essentially formed only by the caudal attachments of muscles acting from thoracic levels.

The lumbar fibres of erector spinae do not attach to the erector spinae aponeurosis. Indeed, the aponeurosis is free to move over the surface of the underlying lumbar fibres, and this suggests that the lumbar fibres, which form the bulk of the lumbar back musculature, can act independently from the rest of the erector spinae.

FUNCTIONS OF THE BACK MUSCLES

Each of the lumbar back muscles is capable of several possible actions. No action is unique to a muscle and no muscle has a single action. Instead, the back muscles provide a pool of possible actions that may be recruited to suit the needs of the vertebral column. Therefore, the functions of the back muscles need to be considered in terms of the observed movements of the vertebral column.

In this regard, three types of movements can be addressed: (i) minor active movements of the vertebral column, (ii) postural movements, and (iii) major movements in forward bending and lifting. In this context 'postural movements' refers to movements, usually subconscious, that occur to adjust and maintain a desired posture when this is disturbed, usually by the influence of gravity.

Minor active movements

In the upright position, the lumbar back muscles play a minor, or no active role in executing movement, for gravity provides the necessary force. During extension, the back muscles contribute to the initial tilt, drawing the line of gravity backwards (Floyd & Silver 1955, Morris et al 1962) but are unnecessary for further extension. Muscle activity is recruited when the movement is forced or resisted (Ortengren & Andersson 1977) but is restricted to muscles acting on the thorax. The lumbar multifidus, for example, shows little or no involvement (Morris et al 1961).

The lateral flexors can bend the lumbar spine sideways, but once the centre of gravity of the trunk is displaced, lateral flexion can continue under the influence of gravity. However, the ipsilateral lateral flexors are used to direct the movement, and the contralateral muscles are required to balance the action of gravity and control the rate and extent of movement. Consequently, lateral flexion is accompanied by bilateral activity of the lumbar back muscles, but the contralateral muscles are relatively more active, as it is they which must balance the load of the laterally flexing spine (Floyd & Silver 1955, Portnoy & Morin 1956, Carlsoo 1961, Morris et al 1962, Andersson et al 1977b, Ortengren et al 1978). If a weight is held in the hand on the side to which the spine is laterally flexed, a greater load is applied to the spine, and the contralateral back muscles show greater activity to balance this load (Andersson et al 1977b, Ortengren et al 1978).

Maintenance of posture

The upright vertebral column is well stabilized by its joints and ligaments, but it is still liable to displacement by gravity or when subject to asymmetrical weight-bearing. The back muscles serve to correct such displacements, and depending on the direction of any displacement, the appropriate back muscles will be recruited.

While standing at ease, the back muscles may show slight continuous activity (Allen 1948, Floyd & Silver 1955, Portnoy & Morin 1956, Carlsoo 1961, 1964, Joseph & McColl 1961, Asmussen & Klausen 1962, Morris et al 1962, De Vries 1965, Klausen 1965, Jonsson 1970, Donisch & Basmajian 1972, Andersson & Ortengren 1974, Andersson et al 1974a, Valencia & Munro 1985), intermittent activity (Floyd & Silver 1951, 1955, Portnoy

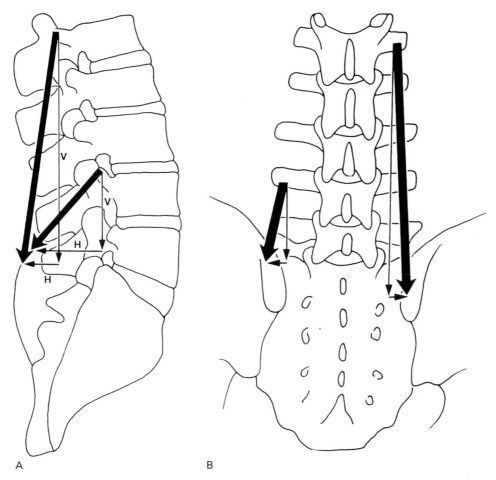

Fig. 15.12 The force vectors of the iliocostalis lumborum pars lumborum. **A.** In a lateral view, the line of action of the fascicles can be resolved into vertical (V) and horizontal (H) vectors. The horizontal vectors are larger at lower lumbar levels. **B.** In a postero-anterior view, the line of action is resolved into a vertical vector and a very small horizontal vector.

& Morin 1956, Ortengren & Andersson 1977, Valencia & Munro 1985), or no activity (Joseph & McColl 1961, Asmussen & Klausen 1962, Klausen 1965, Joseph 1970, Valencia & Munro 1985), and the amount of activity can be influenced by changing the position of the head or allowing the trunk to sway (Andersson & Ortengren 1974).

The explanation for these differences probably lies in the location of the line of gravity in relation to the lumbar spine in different individuals (Asmussen & Klausen 1962, Klausen 1965, Ortengren & Andersson 1977, Kippers & Parker 1985, Valencia & Munro 1985). In about 75% of individuals the line of gravity passes in front of the centre of the L4 vertebra, and therefore, essentially in front of the lumbar spine (Asmussen & Klausen 1962, Klausen 1965). Consequently, gravity will exert a constant tendency to pull the thorax and lumbar spine into flexion. To preserve an upright posture, a constant level of activity in the posterior sagittal rotators of the lumbar spine will be needed to oppose the tendency to flexion. Conversely, when the line of gravity passes behind the lumbar spine, gravity tends to extend it, and back muscle activity is not required. Instead abdominal muscle activity is recruited to

prevent the spine extending under gravity (Asmussen & Klausen 1962, Klausen 1965).

Activities that displace the centre of gravity of the trunk side-ways will tend to cause lateral flexion. To prevent undesired lateral flexion, the contralateral lateral flexors will contract. This occurs when weights are carried in one hand (Floyd & Silver 1955, Jonsson 1970). Carrying equal weights in both hands does not displace the line of gravity, and back muscle activity is not increased substantially on either side of the body (Floyd & Silver 1955, Jonsson 1970).

While sitting, the activity of the back muscles is similar to that during standing (Andersson & Ortengren 1974, Andersson et al 1974a, 1975), but in supported sitting, as with the elbows resting on the knees, there is no activity in the lumbar back muscles (Floyd & Silver 1955, Portnoy & Morin 1956), and with arms resting on a desk, back muscle activity is substantially decreased (Andersson & Ortengren 1974, Andersson et al 1974a). In reclined sitting, the back rest supports the weight of the thorax lessening the need for muscular support. Consequently, increasing the reclination of the back rest of a seat

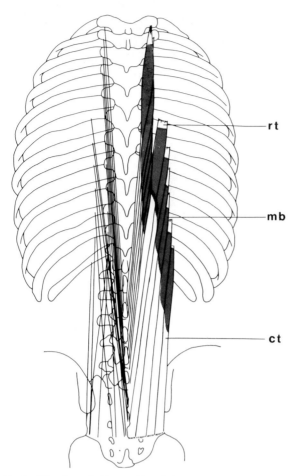

Fig. 15.13   The thoracic fibres of longissimus (longissimus thoracis pars thoracis). The intact fascicles are shown on the right, with muscles bellies (mb), short rostral tendons (rt) and long caudal tendons (ct). The span of the individual fascicles is indicated on the left. The caudal tendons of the fascicles collectively form the medial part of the erector spinae aponeurosis.

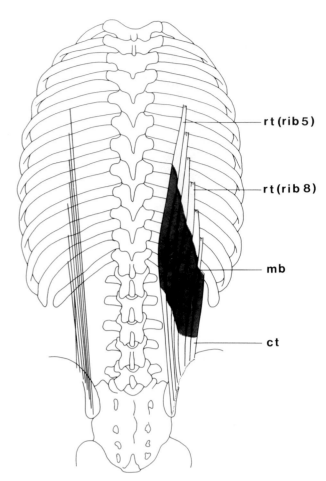

Fig. 15.14   The thoracic fibres of iliocostalis lumborum (iliocostalis lumborum pars thoracis). The intact fascicles are shown on the right, with muscle bellies (mb), rostral tendons (rt) arising the ribs, and caudal tendons (ct) attaching to the iliac crest. The span of the fascicles is shown on the right. The caudal tendons of the fascicles collectively form the lateral part of the erector spinae aponeurosis.

decreases lumbar back muscle activity (Andersson & Ortengren 1974, Andersson et al 1974a, Nachemson 1976, 1980).

Major active movements

Forward flexion and extension of the spine from the flexed position are movements during which the back muscles have their most important function. As the spine bends forward, there is an increase in the activity of the back muscles (Allen 1948, Floyd & Silver 1951, 1955, Golding 1952, Portnoy & Morin 1956, Carlsoo 1961, Morris et al 1961, Pauly 1966, Okada 1970, Donisch & Basmajian 1972, Andersson et al 1977b, Koreska et al 1977), and this increase is proportional to the angle of flexion and the size of any load carried (Andersson et al 1977a, b, Ortengren et al 1978, Schultz et al 1982). The movement of forward flexion is produced by gravity, but the extent and the rate at which it proceeds is controlled by the eccentric contraction of the back muscles. Move-

ment of the thorax on the lumbar spine is controlled by the long thoracic fibres of longissimus and iliocostalis. The long tendons of insertion allow these muscles to act around the convexity of the increasing thoracic kyphosis and anchor the thorax to the ilium and sacrum. In the lumbar region, the multifidus and the lumbar fascicles of longissimus and iliocostalis act to control the anterior sagittal rotation of the lumbar vertebrae. At the same time the lumbar fascicles of longissimus and iliocostalis also act to control the associated anterior translation of the lumbar vertebrae.

At a certain point during forward flexion, the activity in the back muscles ceases, and the vertebral column is braced by the locking of the zygapophysial joints and tension in its posterior ligaments. This phenomenon is known as 'critical point' (Floyd & Silver 1951, Morris et al 1962, Kippers & Parker 1984, 1985). However, critical point does not occur in all individuals, or in all muscles (Floyd & Silver 1955, Portnoy & Morin 1956, Donisch & Basmajian 1972, Valencia & Munro 1985). When it does

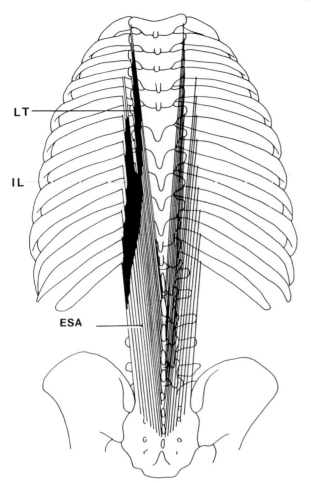

Fig. 15.15 The erector spinae aponeurosis (ESA). This broad sheet is formed by the caudal tendons of the thoracic fibres of longissimus thoracis (LT) and iliocostalis lumborum (IL).

occur, it does so when the spine has reached about 90% maximum flexion, even though at this stage the hip flexion that occurs in forward bending is still only 60% complete (Kippers & Parker 1984, 1985). Carrying weights during flexion causes the critical point to occur later in the range of vertebral flexion (Kippers & Parker 1984, 1985).

The physiological basis for critical point is still obscure. It may be due to reflex inhibition initiated by proprioceptors in the lumbar joints and ligaments, or in muscle stretch and length receptors (Kippers & Parker 1984). Whatever the mechanism, the significance of critical point is that it marks the transition of spinal load-bearing from muscles to the ligamentous system.

Extension of the trunk from the flexed position is characterized by high levels of back muscle activity (Floyd & Silver 1951, 1955, Morris et al 1962, Pauly 1966, Donisch & Basmajian 1972). In the thoracic region, the iliocostalis and longissimus, acting around the thoracic kyphosis, lift the thorax by rotating it backwards. The lumbar vertebrae are rotated backwards principally by the lumbar multifidus, causing their superior surfaces to be progressively tilted upwards to support the rising thorax.

COMPRESSIVE LOADS OF THE BACK MUSCLES

Because of the downward direction of their action, as the back muscles contract they exert a longitudinal compression of the lumbar vertebral column, and this compression raises the pressure in the lumbar intervertebral discs. Any activity that involves the back muscles, therefore, is associated with a rise in nuclear pressure. As measured in the L3–4 intervertebral disc, the nuclear pressure correlates with the degree of myoelectric activity in the back muscles (Andersson et al 1977b, Ortengren et al 1978, 1981, Nachemson 1980, Andersson 1983). As muscle activity increases, disc pressure rises.

Disc pressures and myoelectric activity of the back muscles have been used extensively to quantify the stresses applied to the lumbar spine in various postures and by various activities (Nachemson & Morris 1964, Nachemson 1966b, 1976, 1980, Nachemson & Elfstrom 1970, Andersson & Ortengren 1974, Andersson et al 1974b, c, 1975, 1978). From the standing position, forward bending causes the greatest increase in disc pressure. Lifting a weight in this position raises disc pressure even further, and the pressure is greatly increased if a load is lifted with the lumbar spine both flexed and rotated. Throughout these various manouvres, back muscle activity increases in proportion to the disc pressure.

One of the prime revelations of combined discometric and electromyographic studies of the lumbar spine during lifting relates to the comparative stresses applied to the lumbar spine by different lifting tactics. In essence, it has been shown that, on the basis of changes in disc pressure and back muscle activity, there are no differences between using a 'stoop' lift or a 'leg' lift, i.e. lifting a weight with a bent back versus lifting with a straight back (Andersson et al 1976, 1977b, Nachemson 1976, 1980). The critical factor is the distance of the load from the body. The further the load is from the chest the greater the stresses on the lumbar spine, and the greater the disc pressure and back muscle activity (Andersson et al 1976).

Strength of the back muscles

The strength of the back muscles has been determined in experiments on normal volunteers (McNeill et al 1980). Two measures of strength are available: the absolute maximum force of contraction in the upright posture and the moment generated on the lumbar spine. The absolute maximum strength of the back muscles as a whole is about 4000 N. Acting on the short moment arms provided by the spinous processes and pedicles of the lumbar vertebrae, this force converts to an extensor moment of 200 Nm. These figures apply to average males under the age of 30; young females exhibit about 60% of this strength, while individuals over the age of 30 are about 10–30% weaker, respectively (McNeill et al 1980).

Lifting

In biomechanical terms, the act of lifting constitutes a problem in balancing moments. When an individual bends forwards to execute a lift flexion occurs at the hip joint and in the lumbar spine. Indeed, most of the forward movement seen during trunk flexion occurs at the hip joint (Kippers & Parker 1984). The flexion forces are generated by gravity acting on the mass of the object to be lifted and on the mass of the trunk above the level of the hip joint and lumbar spine (Fig. 15.16). These forces exert flexion moments on both the hip joint and the lumbar spine. In each case the moment will be the product of the force and its perpendicular distance from the joint in question. The total flexion moment acting on each joint will be the sum of the moments exerted by the mass to be lifted and the mass of the trunk. For a lift to be executed these flexion moments have to be overcome by a moment acting in the opposite direction. This could be exerted by longitudinal forces acting downwards behind the hip joint and vertebral column or by forces acting upwards in front of the joints pushing the trunk upwards.

There are no doubts as to the capacity of the hip extensors to generate large moments and overcome the flexion moments exerted on the hip joint even by the heaviest of loads that might be lifted (Farfan 1975, 1978). However, the hip extensors are only able to rotate the pelvis backwards on the femurs; they do not act on the lumbar spine. Thus, regardless of what happens at the hip joint the lumbar spine still remains subject to a flexion moment that must be overcome in some other way. Without an appropriate mechanism the lumbar spine would stay flexed as the hips extended; indeed, as the pelvis rotated backwards, flexion of the lumbar spine would be accentuated as its bottom end was pulled backwards with the pelvis while its top end remained stationary under the load of the flexion moment. A mechanism is required to allow the lumbar spine to resist this deformation or to cause it to extend in unison with the hip joint.

Despite much investigation and debate, the exact nature of this mechanism remains unresolved. In various ways the back muscles, intra-abdominal pressure, the thoracolumbar fascia and the posterior ligamentous system have been believed to participate.

For light lifts the flexion moments generated are relatively small. In the case of a 70 kg man lifting a 10 kg mass in a fully stooped position, the upper trunk weights about 40 kg and acts about 30 cm in front of the lumbar spine, while the arms holding the mass to be lifted lie about 45 cm in front of the lumbar spine. The respective flexion moments are therefore $40 \times 9.8 \times 0.30 = 117.6$ Nm and $10 \times 9.8 \times 0.45 = 44.1$ Nm, a total of 161.7 Nm. This load is well within the capacity of the back muscles (200 Nm, see above). Thus, as the hips extend, the lumbar back muscles are capable of resisting further flexion of the lumbar spine and, indeed, could even actively extend it, and the weight would be lifted.

Increasing the load to be lifted to over 30 kg increases the flexion moment to 132.2 Nm which, when added to the flexion moment of the upper trunk, exceeds the capacity of the back muscles. To remain within the capacity of the back muscles such loads must be carried closer to the lumbar spine, i.e. they must be borne with a much shorter moment arm. Even so, decreasing the moment arm to about 15 cm limits the load to be carried to about 90 kg. The back muscles are simply not strong enough to raise greater loads. Such realizations have generated concepts of several additional mechanisms that serve to aid the back muscles in overcoming large flexion moments.

Bartelink (1957) raised the proposition that intra-abdominal pressure could aid the lumbar spine in resisting flexion by acting upwards on the diaphragm — the so-called intra-abdominal balloon mechanism. Bartelink

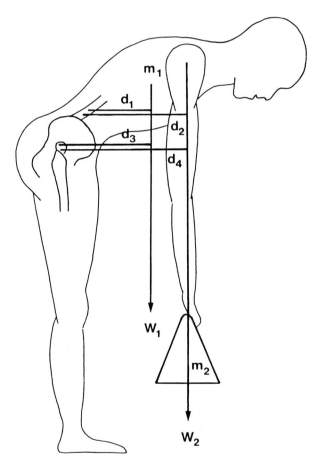

Fig. 15.16 The flexion moments exerted on a flexed trunk. Forces generated by the weight of the trunk and the load to be lifted act vertically in front of the lumbar spine and hip joint. The moments they exert on each joint are proportional to the distance between the line of action of each force and the joint in question. The mass of the trunk (m_1) exerts a force (W_1) that acts a measurable distance in front of the lumbar spine (d_1) and the hip joint (d_3). The mass to be lifted (m_2) exerts a force (W_2) that acts a measurable distance from the lumbar spine (d_2) and the hip joint (d_4). The respective moments acting on the lumbar spine will be W_1d_1 and W_1d_3; those on the hip joint will be W_2d_2 and W_2d_4.

himself was circumspect and reserved in raising this conjecture. The concept was rapidly popularized, even thought it was never validated. It received early endorsement in orthopaedic circles (Morris et al 1961), and intra-abdominal pressure was adopted by ergonomists and others as a measure of spinal stress and safe-lifting standards (Davis 1959, 1981, Davis & Troup 1964, Davis & Stubbs 1977, Troup 1977, 1979, Stubbs 1981). In more contemporary studies, intra-abdominal pressure has been monitored during various spinal movements and lifting tasks (Andersson et al 1976, 1977b, Ortengren et al 1981).

Reservations about the validity of the abdominal balloon mechanism have arisen from several quarters. Studies of lifting tasks reveal that, unlike myoelectric activity, intra-abdominal pressure does not correlate well with the size of the load being lifted or the applied stress on the vertebral column as measured by intradiscal pressure (Ortengren et al 1981, Andersson 1983, Leskinen et al 1983). Indeed, deliberately increasing intra-abdominal pressure by a Valsalva manoeuvre does not relieve the load on the lumbar spine but actually increases it (Nachemson et al 1986). Clinical studies have shown that although abdominal muscles are weaker than normal in patients with back pain, intra-abdominal pressure is not different (Hemborg & Moritz 1985). Furthermore, strengthening the abdominal muscles both in normal individuals (Hemborg et al 1983) and in patients with back pain (Hemborg et al 1985) does not influence intra-abdominal pressure during lifting.

The most strident criticism of the intra-abdominal balloon theory comes from bioengineers and others who maintain that (i) to generate any significant antiflexion moment the pressure required would exceed the maximum hoop tension of the abdominal muscles (Farfan & Gracovetsky 1983, Farfan et al 1983, Gracovetsky et al 1985); (ii) such a pressure would be so high as to obstruct the abdominal aorta (Farfan & Gracovetsky 1983), a reservation raised by Bartelink himself (Bartelink 1957); and (iii) because the abdominal muscles lie in front of the lumbar spine and connect the thorax to the pelvis, whenever they contract to generate pressure they must also exert a flexion moment on the trunk, which would negate any anti-flexion value of the intra-abdominal pressure (Bearn 1961, Farfan 1975, 1978, Gracovetsky et al 1985).

These reservations inspired an alternative explanation of the role of the abdominal muscles during lifting. Farfan, Gracovetsky and colleagues (Farfan 1975, Gracovetsky et al 1977, 1981, 1985) noted the criss-cross arrangement of the fibres in the posterior layer of thoracolumbar fascia and surmised that if lateral tension was applied to this fascia it would result in an extension moment being exerted on the lumbar spinous processes. Such tension could be exerted by the abdominal muscles that arise from the thoracolumbar fascia, and the trigonometry of the fibres in the thoracolumbar fascia was such that they could convert lateral tension into an appreciable extension moment — the so-called 'gain' of the thoracolumbar fascia (Gracovetsky et al 1985). The role of the abdominal muscles during lifting was thus to brace, if not actually extend, the lumbar spine by pulling on the thoracolumbar fascia. Any rises in intra-abdominal pressure were thereby only coincidental, occurring because of the contraction of the abdominal muscles acting on the thoracolumbar fascia.

Subsequent anatomical studies revealed several liabilities of this model (Bogduk & Macintosh 1984). First, the posterior layer of thoracolumbar fascia is well developed only in the lower lumbar region, but nevertheless its fibres are appropriately orientated to enable lateral tension exerted on the fascia to produce extension moments at least on the L2 to L5 spinous processes. However, dissection reveals that of the abdominal muscles internal oblique offers only a few fibres that irregularly attach to the thoracolumbar fascia; transversus abdominis is the only muscle that consistently attaches to the thoracolumbar fascia, but only its very middle fibres do so. The size of these fibres is such that even upon maximum contraction the force they exert is very small. Calculations revealed that the extensor moment they could exert on the lumbar spine amounted to less than 6 Nm (Macintosh et al 1987). Thus, the contribution that abdominal muscles might make to anti-flexion moments is trivial, a conclusion also borne out by subsequent, independent modelling studies (McGill & Norman 1988).

A totally different model of lifting was elaborated by Farfan and Gracovetsky (Farfan 1975, Gracovetsky et al 1981, 1985). Noting the weakness of the back muscles, these authors proposed that extension of the lumbar spine was not required to lift heavy loads or loads with long moment arms. They proposed that the lumbar spine should remain fully flexed in order to engage, i.e. maximally stretch, what they referred to as the 'posterior ligamentous system', namely, the capsules of the zygapophysial joints, the interspinous and supraspinous ligaments, and the posterior layer of thoracolumbar fascia, the latter acting passively to transmit tension between the lumbar spinous processes and ilium.

Under such conditions the active energy for a lift was provided by the powerful hip extensor muscles. These rotated the pelvis backwards. Meanwhile, the external load acting on the upper trunk kept the lumbar spine flexed. Tension would develop in the posterior ligamentous system which bridged the thorax and pelvis. With the posterior ligamentous system so engaged, as the pelvis rotated backwards the lumbar spine would be passively raised while remaining in a fully flexed position. In essence, the posterior sagittal rotation of the pelvis would be transmitted through the posterior ligaments first to the L5 vertebra, then to L4 and so on, up through the lumbar spine into the thorax. All that was required was that the posterior ligamentous system be sufficiently strong to withstand the passive tension generated in it by the movement of the pelvis at one end and the weight of the trunk and external load at the other. The lumbar spine would thereby be raised like a long, rigid arm rotating on the pelvis and raising the external load with it.

Contraction of the back muscles was not required if the ligaments could take the load. Indeed, muscle contraction was distinctly undesirable for any active extension of the lumbar spine would disengage the posterior ligaments and preclude them from transmitting tension. The back muscles could be recruited only once the trunk had been raised sufficiently to shorten the moment arm of the external load reducing its flexion moment to within the capacity of the back muscles.

The attraction of this model was that it overcame the problem of the relative weakness of the back muscles by dispensing with their need to act, which in turn was consistent with the myoelectric silence of the back muscles at full flexion of the trunk and the recruitment of muscle activity only once the trunk had been elevated and the flexion moment arm had been reduced. Support for the model also came from surgical studies which reported that if the midline ligaments and thoracolumbar fascia were conscientiously reconstructed after multi-level laminectomies, the post-operative recovery and rehabilitation of patients were enhanced (Crock & Crock 1988).

However, while attractive in a qualitative sense, the mechanism of the posterior ligamentous system was not validated quantitatively. The model requires that the ligaments be strong enough to sustain the loads applied. In this regard, data on the strength of the posterior ligaments is scant and irregular, but sufficient data is available to permit an initial appraisal of the feasibility of the posterior ligament model.

The strength of spinal ligaments varies considerably, but average values can be calculated. Table 15.1 summarizes some of the available data. It is evident that the strongest posterior 'ligaments' of the lumbar spine are the zygapophysial joint capsules and the thoracolumbar fascia forming the midline 'supraspinous ligament'. However, when the relatively short moment arms over which these ligaments act are considered, it transpires that the maximum moment they can sustain is relatively small. Even the sum total of all their moments is considerably less than that required for heavy lifting and is some four times less than the maximum strength of the back muscles. Of course, it is possible that the data quoted may not be representative of the true mean values of the strength of these ligaments, but it does not seem likely that the literature quoted underestimated their strength by a factor of four or more. Under these conditions, it is evident that posterior ligamentous system alone is not strong enough to perform the role required of it in heavy lifting. The

Table 15.1 Strength of the posterior ligamentous system[*]

Ligament	Average force at failure (N)	Moment arm (m)	Maximum moment (Nm)
PLL	90	0.02	1.8
LF	244	0.03	7.3
ZJC	672–680	0.04	27.2
ISL	107	0.05	5.4
TLF	500	0.06	30.0
Total			51.7

[*] PLL = posterior longitudinal ligament; LF = ligamentum flavum; ZJC = zygapophysial joint capsules (bilaterally); ISL = interspinous ligament; TLF = the posterior layer of thoracolumbar fascia and the erector spinae aponeurosis that forms the so-called supraspinous ligament. Average force at failure has been calculated using raw data provided in Mykelbust et al (1988) and Cyron and Hutton (1981). The moment arms are estimates based on inspection of a respresentative vertebra, and measuring the perpendicular distance between the location of the instantaneous axis of rotation and the sites of attachment of the various ligaments.

posterior ligamentous system is not strong enough to replace the back muscles as a mechanism to prevent flexion of the lumbar spine during lifting. Some other mechanism must operate.

One such mechanism is that of the *hydraulic amplifier* effect. It was originally proposed by Gracovetsky et al (1977) that because the thoracolumbar fascia surrounded the back muscles as a retinaculum it could serve to brace these muscles and enhance their power. The engineering basis for this effect is complicated, and the concept remained unexplored until very recently. A mathematical proof has been published which suggests that by investing the back muscles the thoracolumbar fascia enhances the strength of the back muscles by some 30% (Hukins et al 1990). This is an appreciable increase and an attractive mechanism for enhancing the anti-flexion capacity of the back muscles. However, the validity of this proof is still being questioned on the grounds that the principles used, while applicable to the behaviour of solids, may not be applicable to muscles; and the concept of the hydraulic amplifier mechanism still remains under scrutiny.

Quite a contrasting model has been proposed to explain the mechanics of the lumbar spine in lifting. It is based on arch theory and maintains that the behaviour, stability and strength of the lumbar spine during lifting can be explained by viewing the lumbar spine as an arch braced by intra-abdominal pressure (Aspden 1987, 1989). The intriguing concept, however, has not met with any degree of acceptance and, indeed, has been challenged from some quarters (Adams 1989).

In summary, despite much effort over recent years, the exact mechanism of heavy lifting still remains unexplained. The back muscles are too weak to extend the lumbar spine against large flexion moments; the intra-abdominal balloon has been refuted; the abdominal mechanism and thoracolumbar fascia have been refuted and the posterior ligamentous system appears too weak to replace the back muscles. Engineering models of the hydraulic amplifier effect and the arch model are still subject to debate.

What remains to be explained is what provides the missing force to sustain heavy loads, and why is intra-abdominal pressure so consistently generated during lifts if it is neither to brace the thoracolumbar fascia or to provide an intra-abdominal balloon? At present these questions can only be addressed by conjecture, but certain concepts appear worthy of consideration.

With regard to intra-abdominal pressure, one concept that has been overlooked in studies of lifting is the role of the abdominal muscles in controlling axial rotation of the trunk. Investigators have focused their attention on movements in the sagittal plane during lifting and have ignored the fact that, when bent forward to address an object to be lifted, the trunk is liable to axial rotation. Unless the external load is perfectly balanced and lies exactly in the midline, it will cause the trunk to twist to the left or the right. Thus, to keep the weight in the midline and in the sagittal plane the lifter must control any twisting effect. The oblique abdominal muscles are the principal rotators of the trunk and would be responsible for this bracing. In contracting to control axial rotation, the abdominal muscles would secondarily raise intra-abdominal pressure. This pressure rise is therefore an epiphenomenon and would reflect not the size of any external load but its tendency to twist the flexed trunk.

With regard to loads in the sagittal plane, the passive strength of the back muscles has been neglected in discussions of lifting. From the behaviour of isolated muscle fibres it is known that, as a muscle elongates, its maximum contractile force diminishes, but its passive elastic tension rises; so much so that in an elongated muscle, the total passive and active tension generated is at least equal to the maximum contractile capacity of the muscle at resting length. Thus, although they become electrically silent at full flexion, the back muscles are still capable of providing passive tension equal to their maximum contractile strength. This would allow the silent muscles to supplement the engaged posterior ligamentous system. With the back muscles providing some 200 Nm and the ligaments some 50 Nm or more, the total anti-flexion capacity of the lumbar spine rises to about 250 Nm — which would allow some 30kg to be safely lifted at 90° trunk flexion. Larger loads could be sustained by proportionally shortening the moment arm. Consequently, the mechanism of lifting may well be essentially as proposed by Farfan and Gracovetsky (Farfan 1975, Gracovetsky et al 1977, 1981), save that the passive tension in the back muscles constitutes the major component of the 'posterior ligamentous system'.

REFERENCES

Abrahams V C 1977 The physiology of neck muscles; their role in head movement and maintenance of posture. Canadian Journal of Physiology and Pharmacology 55: 332–338

Abrahams V C 1981 Sensory and motor specialization in some muscles of the neck. Trends in Neurosciences 4: 24–27

Adams M 1989 Letter to the editor. Spine 14: 1272

Allen C E L 1948 Muscle action potentials used in the study of dynamic anatomy. British Journal of Physical Medicine 11: 66–73

Andersson G B J 1983 Loads on the lumbar spine: in vivo measurements and biomechanical analyses. In: Winter D A, Norman R W, Wells R P, Hayes K C, Patla A E (eds) Biomechanics IX-B, international series on biomechanics. Human Kinetics, Champaign, p 32–37

Andersson B J G, Ortengren R 1974 Myoelectric activity during sitting. Scandinavian Journal of Rehabilitation Medicine (suppl) 3: 73–90

Andersson B J G, Jonsson B, Ortengren R 1974a Myoelectric activity in individual lumbar erector spinae muscles in sitting: a study with surface and wire electrodes. Scandinavian Journal of Rehabilitation Medicine (suppl) 3: 91–108

Andersson B J G, Ortengren R, Nachemson A, Elfstrom G 1974b Lumbar disc pressure and myoelectric activity during sitting. I. Studies on an experimental chair. Scandinavian Journal of Rehabilitation Medicine 6: 104–114

Andersson B J G, Ortengren R, Nachemson A, Elfstrom G 1974c Lumbar disc pressure and myoelectric back muscle activity during sitting. IV. Studies on a car driver's seat. Scandinavian Journal of Rehabilitation Medicine 6: 128–133

Andersson B J G, Ortengren R, Nachemson A L et al 1975 The sitting posture: an electromyographic and discometric study. Orthopaedic Clinics of North America 6: 105–120

Andersson G B J, Ortengren R, Nachemson A 1976 Quantitative studies of back loads in lifting. Spine 1: 178–184

Andersson G B J, Ortengren R, Herberts P 1977a Quantitative electromyographic studies of back muscle activity related to posture and loading. Orthopaedic Clinics of North America 8: 85–96

Andersson G B J, Ortengren R, Nachemson A 1977b Intradiscal pressure, intra-abdominal pressure and myoelectric back muscle activity related to posture and loading. Clinical Orthopaedics and Related Research 129: 156–164

Andersson G B J, Ortengren R, Nachemson A 1978 Quantitative studies of the back in different working postures. Scandinavian Journal of Rehabilitation Medicine (suppl) 6: 173–181

Asmussen E, Klausen K 1962 Form and function of the erect human spine. Clinical Orthopaedics and Related Research 25: 55–63

Aspden R M 1987 Intra-abdominal pressure and its role in spinal mechanics. Clinical Biomechanics 2: 168–174

Aspden R M 1989 The spine as an arch. A new mathematical model. Spine 14: 266–274

Bartelink D L 1957 The role of abdominal pressure in relieving the pressure on the lumbar intervertebral discs. Journal of Bone and Joint Surgery 39B: 718–725

Bastide G, Zadeh J, Lefebvre D 1989 Are the 'little muscles' what we think they are? Surgical and Radiological Anatomy 11: 255–256

Bearn J G 1961 The significance of the activity of the abdominal muscles in weight lifting. Acta Anatomica 45: 83–89

Bogduk N 1980 A reappraisal of the anatomy of the human lumbar erector spinae. Journal of Anatomy 131: 525–540

Bogduk N 1981 The lumbar mamillo-accessory ligament. Its anatomical and neurosurgical significance. Spine 6: 162–167

Bogduk N, Macintosh J 1984 The applied anatomy of the thoracolumbar fascia. Spine 9: 164–170

Bogduk N, Wilson A S, Tynan W 1982 The human lumbar dorsal rami. Journal of Anatomy 134: 383–397

Bogduk N, Pearcy M, Hadfield G 1991 The anatomy and biomechanics of psoas major. Clinical Biomechanics (submitted)

Carlsoo S 1961 The static muscle load in different work positions: an electromyographic study. Ergonomics 4: 193–211

Carlsoo S 1964 Influence of frontal and dorsal loads on muscle activity and on the weight distribution in the feet. Acta Orthopaedica Scandinavica 34: 299–309

Cave A J E 1937 The innervation and morphology of the cervical intertransverse muscles. Journal of Anatomy 71: 497–515

Cooper S, Danial P M 1963 Muscles spindles in man, their morphology in the lumbricals and the deep muscles of the neck. Brain 86: 563–594

Crock H V, Crock M C 1988 A technique for decompression of the lumbar spinal canal. Neuro-orthopaedics 5: 96–99

Cyron B M, Hutton W C 1981 The tensile strength of the capsular ligaments of the apophyseal joints. Journal of Anatomy 132: 145–150

Davis P R 1959 Posture of the trunk during the lifting of weights. British Medical Journal 1: 87–89

Davis P R 1981 The use of intra-abdominal pressure in evaluating stresses on the lumbar spine. Spine 6: 90–92

Davis P R, Stubbs D A 1977 Safe levels of manual forces for young males (1). Applied Ergonomics 8: 141–150

Davis P R, Troup J D G 1964 Pressures in the trunk cavities when pulling, pushing and lifting. Ergonomics 7: 465–474

De Vries H A 1965 Muscle tonus in postural muscles. American Journal of Physical Medicine 44: 275–291

Donisch E W, Basmajian J V 1972 Electromyography of deep back muscles in man. American Journal of Anatomy 133: 25–36

Fairbank J C T, O'Brien J P 1980 The abdominal cavity and thoracolumbar fascia as stabilisers of the lumbar spine in patients with low back pain. vol 2. Engineering aspects of the spine. Mechanical Engineering Publications, London, pp 83–88

Farfan H F 1975 Muscular mechanism of the lumbar spine and the position of power and efficiency. Orthopaedic Clinics of North America 6: 135–144

Farfan H F 1978 The biomechanical advantage of lordosis and hip extension for upright activity. Man as compared with other anthropoids. Spine 3: 336–342

Farfan H F, Gracovetsky S 1983 The abdominal mechanism. Paper presented at the International Society for the Study of the Lumbar Spine Meeting, Paris, 1981

Farfan H F, Gracovetsky S, Helleur C 1983 The role of mathematical models in the assessment of task in the workplace. In: Winter D A, Norman R W, Wells R P, Hayes K C, Patla A E (eds) Biomechanics IXB, international series in biomechanics. Human Kinetics, Champaign, pp 38–43

Floyd W F, Silver P H S 1951 Function of erectores spinae in flexion of the trunk. Lancet 1: 133–134

Floyd W F, Silver P H S 1955 The function of the erectores spinae muscles in certain movements and postures in man. Journal of Physiology 129: 184–203

Golding J S R 1952 Electromyography of the erector spinae in low back pain. Postgraduate Medical Journal 28: 401–406

Gracovetsky S, Farfan H F, Lamy C 1977 A mathematical model of the lumbar spine using an optimal system to control muscles and ligaments. Orthopaedic Clinics of North America 8: 135–153

Gracovetsky S, Farfan H F, Lamy C 1981 The mechanism of the lumbar spine. Spine 6: 249–262

Gracovetsky S, Farfan H F, Helleur C 1985 The abdominal mechanism. Spinal 10: 317–324

Hemborg B, Moritz U 1985 Intra-abdominal pressure and trunk muscle activity during lifting II: chronic low-back patients. Scandinavian Journal of Rehabilitation Medicine 17: 5–13

Hemborg B, Moritz, Hamberg J et al 1983 Intra-abdominal pressure and trunk muscle activity during lifting — effect of abdominal muscle training in healthy subjects. Scandinavian Journal of Rehabilitation Medicine 15: 183–196

Hemborg B, Moritz U, Hamberg J et al 1985 Intra-abdominal pressure and trunk muscle activity during lifting III: effects of abdominal muscle training in chronic low-back patients. Scandinavian Journal of Rehabilitation Medicine 17: 15–24

Hukins D W L, Aspden R M, Hickey D S 1990 Thoracolumbar fascia can increase the efficiency of the erector spinae muscles. Clinical Biomechanics 5: 30–34

Jonsson B 1970 The functions of the individual muscles in the lumbar part of the spinae muscle. Electromyography 10: 5–21

Joseph J 1970 Man's posture: electromyographic studies. Thomas, Springfield, Illinois

Joseph J, McColl I 1961 Electromyography of muscles of posture: posterior vertebral muscles in males. Journal of Physiology 157: 33–37

Kippers V, Parker A W 1984 Posture related to myoelectric silence of erectores spinae during trunk flexion. Spine 7: 740–745

Kippers V, Parker A W 1985 Electromyographic studies of erectores spinae: symmetrical postures and sagittal trunk motion. Australian Journal of Physiotherapy 31: 95–105

Klausen K 1965 The form and function of the loaded human spine. Acta Physiologica Scandinavica 65: 176–190

Koreska J, Robertson D, Mills R H 1977 Biomechanics of the lumbar spine and its clinical significance. Orthopaedic Clinics of North America 8: 121–123

Leskinen T P J, Stalhammar H R, Kuorinka I A A, Troup J D G 1983 Hip torque, lumbosacral compression, and intraabdominal pressure in lifting and lowering tasks. In: Winter D A, Norman R W, Wells R P, Hayes K C, Patla A E (eds) Biomechanics IXB, international series on biomechanics. Human Kinetics, Champaign, pp 55–59

Lewin T, Moffet B, Viidik A 1962 The morphology of the lumbar synovial intervertebral joints. Acta Morphologica Neerlando-Scandinavica 4: 299–319

Luk K D K, Ho H C, Leong J C Y 1986 The iliolumbar ligament. A study of its anatomy, development and clinical significance. Journal of Bone and Joint Surgery 68B: 197–200

Macintosh J E, Bogduk N 1986 The biomechanics of the lumbar multifidus. Clinical Biomechanics 1: 205–213

Macintosh J E, Bogduk N 1987 The morphology of the lumbar erector spinae. Spine 12: 658–668

Macintosh J E, Valencia F, Bogduk N, Munro R R 1986 The morphology of the lumbar multifidus muscles. Clinical Biomechanics 1: 196–204

Macintosh J E, Bogduk N, Gracovetsky S 1987 The biomechanics of the thoracolumbar fascia. Clinical Biomechanics 2: 78–83

McGill S M, Norman R W 1988 Potential of lumbodorsal fascia forces to generate back extension moments during squat lifts. Journal of Biomedical Engineering 10: 312–318

McNeill T, Warwick D, Andersson G, Schultz A 1980 Trunk strengths in attempted flexion, extension, and lateral bending in healthy subjects and patients with low-back disorders. Spine 5: 529–538

Morris J M, Lucas D B, Bresler B 1961 Role of the trunk in stability of the spine. Journal of Bone and Joint Surgery 43A: 327–351

Morris J M, Benner G, Lucas D B 1962 An electromyographic study of the intrinsic muscles of the back in man. Journal of Anatomy 96: 509–520

Mykelbust J B, Pintar F, Yoganandan N et al 1988 Tensile strength of spinal ligaments. Spine 13: 526–531

Nachemson A 1966a Electromyographic studies on the vertebral portion of the psoas muscle. Acta Orthopaedica Scandinavica 37: 177–190

Nachemson A 1966b The load on lumbar disks in different positions of the body. Clinical Orthopaedics and Related Research 45: 107–122

Nachemson A 1968 The possible importance of the psoas muscle for stabilization of the lumbar spine. Acta Orthopaedica Scandinavica 39: 47–57

Nachemson A L 1976 The lumbar spine. An orthopaedic challenge. Spine 1: 59–71

Nachemson A 1980 Lumbar intradiscal pressure. In: Jayson M I V (ed) The lumbar spine and backache, 2nd edn. Pitman, London, ch 12, pp 341–358

Nachemson A L, Elfstrom G 1970 Intravital dynamic pressure measurements in lumbar discs. A study of common movements, manoeuvers and exercises. Scandinavian Journal of Rehabilitation Medicine 2 (suppl 1): 1–40

Nachemson A, Morris J M 1964 In vivo measurments of intradiscal pressure. Journal of Bone and Joint Surgery 46: 1077–1092

Nachemson A L, Andersson G B J, Schultz A B 1986 Valsalva maneuver biomechanics. Effects on trunk load of elevated intraabdominal pressure. Spine 11: 476–479

Nitz A J, Peck D 1986 Comparison of muscle spindle concentrations in large and small human epaxial muscles acting in parallel combinations. American Surgeon 52: 273–277

Okada M 1970 Electromyographic assessment of the muscular load in forward bending postures. Journal of the Faculty of Science of the University of Tokyo 8: 311–336

Ortengren R, Andersson G B J 1977 Electromyographic studies of trunk muscles with special reference to the functional anatomy of the lumbar spine. Spine 2: 44–52

Ortengren R, Andersson G, Nachemson A 1978 Lumbar loads in fixed working postures during flexion and rotation. In: Asmussen E, Jorgensen K (eds), Biomechanics VI–B, international series on biomechanics, vol 2B, pp 159–166

Ortengren R, Andersson G B J, Nachemson A L 1981 Studies of relationships between lumbar disc pressure, myoelectric back muscle activity, and intra-abdominal (intragastric) pressure. Spine 6: 98–103

Pauly J E 1966 An electromyographic analysis of certain movements and exercises. I. Some deep muscles of the back. Anatomical Record 155: 223–234

Peck D, Buxton D F, Nitz A 1984 A comparison of spindle concentrations in large and small muscles acting in parallel combinations. Journal of Morphology 180: 243–252

Poirier P 1912 Myologie. In: Poirier P, Charpy A, Traite d'Anatomie Humaine, 3rd edn, vol 2, fasc 1. Masson, Paris, pp 139–140

Portnoy H, Morin F 1956 Electromyographic study of the postural muscles in various positions and movements. American Journal of Physiology 186: 122–126

Schulz A, Andersson G B J, Ortengren R et al 1982 Analysis and quantitative myoelectric measurements of loads on the lumbar spine when holding weights in standing postures. Spine 7: 390–397

Stubbs D A 1981 Trunk stresses in construction and other industrial workers. Spine 6: 83–89

Troup J D G 1977 Dynamic factor in the analysis of stoop and crouch lifting methods: a methodological approach to the development of safe materials handling standards. Orthopaedic Clinics of North America 8: 201–209

Troup J D G 1979 Biomechanics of the vertebral column. Physiotherapy 65: 238–244

Valencia F P, Munro R R 1985 An electromyographic study of the lumbar multifidus in man. Electromyography and Clinical Neurophysiology 25: 205–221

Williams P L, Warwick R, Dyson M, Bannister L H (eds) 1989 Gray's anatomy. 37th edn. Longman, London, p 604

16. Trunk muscle strength and endurance in the context of low-back dysfunction

G. L. Smidt

INTRODUCTION

Nachemson has stated that 80% of all adults have significant low-back pain in their lifetime (Nachemson 1971). Physicians can readily identify diagnoses of the spine such as fracture, metabolic arthritis, tumours, infections and others. However, only a small percentage of the back problems fall into these clearly identifiable diagnostic categories. Diagnosis of low-back pain seems to be difficult for a number of reasons: (i) impaired or diseased tissues in the back can cause variable symptoms; (ii) the results of available examinations and tests are frequently normal or non-contributory; and (iii) the commonly used examinations and tests do not identify most soft-tissue problems in the low back region. Soft tissues which might be implicated are the intervertebral disc, articular cartilage and capsule of the facet joints, ligaments and muscles.

The back muscles may be directly involved in back pain in cases of trauma as well as indirectly involved as a result of nerve root irritation. The strength and endurance of trunk muscles are also considered important in the prevention and treatment of low-back pain. Several authors have postulated the need for a strong protective 'corset' of muscles around the trunk to prevent back injuries (Kraus 1949, Anderson 1954, Morris et al 1961, Hambly 1967). Larson (1951) and Klausen (1965) have emphasized the proper balance of strength between the long trunk flexors and extensors for prevention and treatment of chronic low-back dysfunction. The ability of an individual to perform desired common daily functions, occupational tasks and recreational activities is influenced either directly or indirectly by the strength and endurance of the abdominal and back muscles.

Muscle weakness as a result of a sedentary life-style is believed to be a contributing factor to low-back pain. Cyriax (1970) on the other hand feels that strong muscles are undesirable because of the prospect that muscle-tension-induced loads at the spinal segments might exceed the tolerance of soft tissues. In the case of the spine the loads are imparted to the intervertebral disc, facet capsule, articular cartilage and ligament. Although clear-cut criteria for establishing muscle weakness or 'excessive' muscle strength are not available, it is empirically clear that some adequate abdominal and back muscle strength is required to initiate and control movement of the trunk. Further, muscle action provides stabilization of the lower spinal segments and distribution of forces within the abdominal and thoracic cavities. For example, during lifting, the abdominal muscles generate a stabilizing counter-balancing force to prevent the pelvis from tilting anteriorly and the spine from hyperextending. Without this abdominal muscle force, the lumbar vertebrae would tend to shift forward, potentially compromising the non-contractile soft tissues at the spinal segments. Without trunk muscle fixation of the rib cage and abdominal cavity, the forces on the lower thoracic and lumbar vertebrae have been estimated to be 30–50% greater during heavy lifting (Morris et al 1961).

MUSCLES AFFECTING TRUNK FUNCTION

For several reasons muscular control and movement of the trunk are more complex than they are for the extremities. At each vertebral level along the spinal column there is the possibility of six degrees of freedom involving movement at each of two facet joints and the intervertebral disc. Therefore, muscle testing is necessarily done across several articulations. In contrast, muscle strength testing at the extremities can be done across fewer articulations. Muscle strength testing is further complicated by respiratory muscle influence either directly through action of the abdominal muscles or indirectly by control of intra-abdominal pressure. Furthermore, the muscles at the anterior and lateral aspects of the trunk are multi-directional, and some of the key muscles of the back traverse several vertebrae and as a consequence are innervated by nerves from many spinal levels. Also, through fascial attachments, prime muscle movers at extremity joints such as the gluteus maximus, lower trapezii, latissimus dorsi, psoas major and psoas minor have significant potential for influencing strength output measures at the trunk.

For practical purposes it seems reasonable to categorize groups of muscles which most likely contribute to the directions of thoraco-lumbar-sacral movement. The flexor muscles are the rectus abdominis, external oblique, internal oblique, pyramidalis, psoas major and psoas minor. The extensors are the longissimus dorsi, spinalis dorsi, iliocostalis lumborum, multifidus, rotatores, interspinales and quadratus lumborum. Muscle action producing lateral trunk flexion and trunk rotation are less understood but probably involve combinations of many of the aforementioned muscles.

CONCEPT OF MUSCLE STRENGTH

A basic definition of muscle strength is the ability of a muscle or muscle group to generate a force or a moment of force about a joint or body axis (Smidt 1984). Muscle strength in the context of this chapter is intended to deal with isolated function of the muscle groups acting at the trunk. Study of the ability of isolated muscle groups to generate force or movement of force is necessary to learn the capabilities of specific muscles and ultimately the effect of treatment on their function. Assessment of isolated muscle groups with a view toward projecting this to function of the whole body might be considered an inductive approach in the study of human physical function. Studies of isolated muscle function are inductive in the sense that the strength capabilities of separate muscle groups at several joints could be corporately placed in a model for study of the interactive strength factors in carrying out a variety of human tasks. In essence, the weakest link in the kinetic chain will be the limiting strength factor for performance of a specific task.

In contradistinction to the inductive approach, the deductive approach to human functions starts with an analysis of the whole body while a human task is being performed. With this approach it is possible to determine the strength requirements for a function, but the absolute weakest physiological link in the system cannot be clearly identified. The deductive approach does not provide measures of maximum strength across joints, but rather the strength necessary to perform a particular function in the manner in which the function was performed when the evaluation was made. Evaluation of walking or lifting are good examples of functions commonly performed by humans.

More studies using both inductive and deductive approaches are needed to relate optimal motor function requirements with isolated anatomical, mechanical and physiological capabilities. Again, the thrust of this chapter is to concentrate on isolated function of the muscle groups at the trunk.

METHODS USED TO MEASURE TRUNK STRENGTH

Traditional approach

Clinically, the strength of the trunk flexors and extensors is tested in supine and prone positions respectively. For the traditional manual muscle test criteria are established for the grades of 0–5. Grade 0 simply means that the muscle is incapable of contracting. For a grade 1 there is a slight contraction of the abdominal muscles when the patient attempts to cough; the head can be raised for a grade 2; in addition, the upper borders of the scapulae can be cleared for grade 3, and for grades 4 and 5 the patient can flex the entire trunk through the range of motion. The patient is viewed as improving in strength capability when he is able to perform increasing numbers of sit-ups. Also, it is commonly thought that, if the patient is placed in the hook-lying position, with the hips flexed, the influence of the hip flexors will be reduced.

The traditional approach would appear to have a place in the initial examination of the patient or perhaps as a cursory component in screening individuals for gross abdominal weakness. A sit-up is truly not satisfactory for assessing progress in patients. For the average normal subject, how much muscle strength is required to perform a sit-up? Combining body segment parameter estimates for the weight of body parts and their centre of gravity location with objective measures of strength permits one to calculate the approximate percentage of maximal muscle strength. Using this method the author has estimated that, for men, the amount of abdominal strength required to raise the head, neck and trunk is considerably less than 100% maximal capacity. Experimentally based evidence is presented later in this chapter.

Viewed another way, the performance of either the sit-up or one trunk extension should probably be considered subnormal since less than 100% effort is required for the normal case. Furthermore, a person who is capable of performing 30 sit-ups should probably not be considered stronger than the person capable of performing 20 sit-ups because the actual resistance overcome by the muscles is the same, only the number of repetitions is different. Increases in the number of repetitions is more an index of improvement in endurance than strength. Therefore, the clinician should adapt ways of adding resistance to the trunk when the patient is able to perform a number of sit-up or back extension manoeuvres. Doing sit-ups on a negatively inclined board does not increase the maximum resistance the abdominals must overcome. Instead, the peak resistance is shifted to another point in the range of sagittal trunk movement, and the remainder of the submaximal resistance is larger through the arc of trunk movement.

Many clinicians believe that the action of the hip flexor muscles is negated when sit-ups are performed with the hips flexed. It is true that the psoas major and iliacus are shorted when in this position so that the tension-producing capabilities of these muscles are likely to be reduced. However, this reduction may very well be counterbalanced by an increase in the moment arm between hip flexor muscles and the hip joint. With the hip flexed the moment arm (the perpendicular distance from the line of action of the iliopsoas to the hip joint) for these muscles is increased so that the resultant hip flexor moment or turning effect at the hip may not be altered. Whatever the case, there is a lack of objective evidence to support clinically based convictions regarding the influence of the hip flexor muscles on performance of the sit-up. The interplay between the hip flexors and the abdominal muscles is simply not well understood.

Objective approaches

Methods used to obtain objective measures of trunk strength have been few in number, but the time span for reports on these methods is lengthy, dating back to 1942 (Mayer & Greenberg 1942). Trunk strength has been measured for action of the flexors, extensors and lateral flexors, using a variety of body positions and instrumentation. Measures for shortening (concentric), static (isometric) and lengthening (eccentric) muscle contractions have been obtained.

In 1942 Mayer and Greenberg developed an objective method for assessing the trunk strength of patients with residual paralysis from poliomyelitis. A swivel-type table was used in which the lower half of the table was stationary and the upper half rotated horizontally about the centre of the table. The lower extremities of the patient were strapped to the stationary half of the table. Trunk flexion and extension strength were measured side-lying, while lateral flexion was measured supine. A cable was attached at one end to the rotating part of the table, and to the patient at the other end. A scale, in series with the cable, measured the isometric strength in pounds. Apparently the lower body stabilization was less than adequate because the authors indicated that substitution from many muscle groups was encountered.

In 1958 Flint used a cable tensiometer to measure force generated by the trunk flexors and extensors (Flint 1955). The effectiveness of a progressive resistive exercise programme for subjects with chronic backache was studied. Around the chest of the subject a leather vest was connected to a cable which passed through an opening in the centre of the table surface. The cable was connected to a tensiometer or a set of weights. Trunk extension strength was measured with the subject prone on an inverted V-shaped table. Both static (isometric) and dynamic (isotonic) measures were obtained. In a similar fashion, Kluck obtained the strength of shortening (con-

centric) trunk flexor and extensor contractions (Kluck 1967).

In 1969 Nachemson and Lindh measured isometric extension with the subject in the standing position (Nachemson & Lindh 1969). A similar method was used by Petersen et al in the 1970s. A strap was placed around the patient's pelvis for stabilization. A harness around the subject's chest was connected to a cable, and the cable was in turn attached to a stationary spring scale. In similar fashion, trunk extension strength was also measured in the prone position.

In 1980 McNeill et al tested trunk flexors, extensors and lateral flexors in the isometric mode with the subjects in the standing position. A harness around the chest was attached to a cable. The cable was attached to strain-gauge load cells fixed to a rigid frame which surrounded the subject. The subject was strapped at the pelvis and lower extremities to a board which extended to the level of the iliac crests. Adjustable supports limited lateral excursion of the pelvis. The moment arm for the measured force was measured as the distance from the location of the cable near the subject's body to the L5–S1 spinal level. The cage surrounding the subject for this method seemingly negates the possibility of dynamic strength testing and limits the testing position to that of upright standing.

In the late 1970s and early 1980s investigators from Japan reported on studies of static and dynamic trunk strength (Suzuki et al 1977, Suzuki & Ohe 1978, Hasue et al 1980, Suzuki & Endo 1983). Trunk flexion measures were obtained with the subject supine and hips and knees flexed. Extension measurements were obtained with the subject prone. In each case the lower extremities were strapped to the table. A padded bar in contact with the subject transmitted forces to the Cybex dynamometer where measures of torque were recorded. The padded bar was positioned over the xiphoid process for trunk flexion and over the scapula for extension. In later studies the padded arm was placed over the manubrium and the 4th thoracic level when the strength measures were obtained. The dynamometer axis was aligned with the axis of the hip joint so that full influence of the hip musculature was allowed. Through the range of trunk motion, the angular velocity for the dynamic tests was constant at 12°/second for concentric flexion and 6°/second for concentric extension.

Davies and Gould (1981) also used the Cybex dynamometer to obtain trunk flexion and extension measures. With the subject in the upright standing position, the lower extremities and pelvis were strapped to a board. Torque was applied to the dynamometer through padded bars placed on the back and anterior chest wall. Dynamic measures were obtained as the subject from the hips and waist moved the trunk into flexion and returned to the upright position in extension.

Also in the early 1980s the University of Iowa reported

on the use of two different approaches. The Iowa Force Table, previously employed to measure isolated muscle strength at the hip and knee, was adapted to accommodate trunk flexor and extensor strength (Jensen et al 1971, Olson et al 1972, Smidt 1973, Smidt et al 1980, Herring 1982). The gravitational force of the upper body was eliminated by placing the subject in the side-lying position. The pelvis was stabilized. Strength measures for shortening (concentric), static (isometric) and lengthening (eccentric) contractions of both flexors and extensors were obtained.

Thorstenson and Nilsson (1982) also used the side-lying position for measuring isometric and concentric strength of the trunk flexors, extensors and lateral flexors. For all tests the rate of constant angular trunk velocity was 15 and 30°/second. The Iowa group then developed a system which embodied a number of important features: the pelvis and lower extremities were firmly stabilized, an adjustable seat permitted movement of the subject for alignment purposes, and a reflected laser beam was used to align the estimated location of the L5–S1 interspace with the axis of the dynamometer (Smidt et al 1983).

In the past few years, a number of dynametric instruments have been used for evaluation and exercise of the trunk muscles (Smidt et al 1987, Smidt & Blanpied 1988, Graves et al 1990, Parniapour et al 1990, DeLitto et al 1991; Gomez et al 1991). Most of the instruments have both static and dynamic capabilities. An example of a contemporary approach is the Kin-Com trunk testing device (Chattecx Corporation, Chattanooga, Tennessee USA) shown in Figure 16.1. Some of the systems have the capability of assessing strength for eccentric muscle contractions. With computer control inherently part of the systems, tests and exercises with constant angular velocity,

constant force and controls for other kinematic variables can be selected.

Some investigators have ostensibly measured back extensor strength by measuring a subject's ability to lift (Chaffin 1974, Chaffin et al 1977, Watson & O'Donovan 1977, Cady et al 1979). For most lifting tasks some back extensor strength is required, but essentially all the joints of the upper extremity, trunk and lower extremity are used so that an infinite number of different body positions and movements might be employed. For the task of lifting, each different joint position and upper extremity muscle action could influence the muscle effort required of the back extensor muscles. As mentioned earlier, a task such as lifting must necessarily be evaluated from a deductive perspective, that is, from the whole to its parts. A complete biomechanical analysis of the lifting function would yield an estimate of the muscle strength used but one cannot know, apart from muscle strength tests of isolated muscle groups, whether or not the estimated muscle strength presents the maximum strength capability of the back extensors.

PROS AND CONS FOR METHODS USED

First a decision must be made whether to evaluate the total muscle strength used in performing a task such as lifting. Clearly, if the interest is in knowing how muscles function and what muscle strength is required to perform a task to include common activities of daily living, that particular task should be evaluated. On the other hand, if the interest is to know maximal muscle strength then specific muscle groups must be accordingly isolated, and sound principles of muscle testing need to be applied.

Some important methodological considerations include standardized instructions to the patient, warm-up, type of muscle contraction, number of muscle contractions, angular velocity of trunk during dynamic tests, whether the measurement unit will be in terms of force or torque (moment) and patient comfort. With respect to methods that have been used for strength testing of the muscles of the trunk, selected factors bear enumeration.

Stabilization

For the previously described methods of trunk strength measurement the amount of stabilization varied considerably. Adequate stabilization of appropriate body segments is necessary to ensure isolation of the muscle or muscle group being tested. In the case of the muscles of the trunk, stabilization of the pelvis and lower extremities is needed.

Stabilization is important for at least three reasons. First, the influence of muscles one joint removed (e.g. the hip) is negated or minimized. Secondly, movement of the pelvis will in turn permit motion of the lower spine so that records of spinal position and motion become inaccurate, and thirdly, inadequate stabilization will prevent the

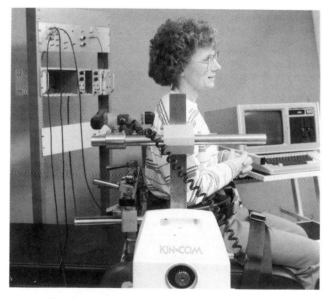

Fig. 16.1 Kin-Com trunk testing device.

patient from exerting a maximal voluntary contraction. With differing amounts of pelvic stabilization during trunk flexion and extension, Smidt et al experimentally demonstrated significant changes in the position of the upper sacrum. Strength output was altered as well. For 13 subjects, the average strength output reduction with minimal stabilization of the lower extremities and pelvis ranged from 75 to 160 Nm (Newton–metres) for the trunk extensors and from 60 to 100 Nm for the flexors. These differences are significant when viewed in the context of the average maximal strength values of approximately 300 Nm (extensors) and 150 Nm (flexors) obtained with maximal stabilization of the lower extremities and pelvis.

With the pelvis stabilized, the axis of rotation for flexion–extension influence of the trunk tends to change locations in the vicinity of the L5–S1 vertebral interspace, so the use of L5–S1 as a reference for the axis seems reasonable. As such, the axis of any dynametric instrumentation should be aligned to coincide with the estimated L5–S1 anatomical axis. Pelvic movement associated with minimal stabilization of the lower extremities and pelvis would be expected to increase the change in axis location, thus further contributing to measurement error.

Adequate stabilization also helps to assure that a right angle is maintained between the line of application of force at the anterior and posterior thoracic contact points. Regardless of transducer system, the measurement of force or torque will be reduced if a right angle of force, with respect to the vertical axis of the body, is not maintained.

Test position

Use of the prone and supine positions are convenient for manual testing in clinical work. Also, stabilization of the lower extremities can be accomplished fairly well, and the positions are comfortable for most patients. One disadvantage is the large gravitational force associated with the weight of the upper body which must be overcome during the test. This disadvantage is overcome using the side-lying position, but this position is less comfortable for patients. The side-lying positions tend to be inconvenient for test administration. For example, the patient must move from supine to prone, or vice versa, for acquisition of both flexor and extensor strength measures. Reclining positions do not simulate most functional tasks. Another disadvantage is that the prone position permits only a small portion of the available trunk motion in the sagittal plane.

Proponents of the standing position indicate that many functional tasks utilize this body orientation. The standing position permits the complete range of trunk motion. However, stabilization of body parts is difficult to accomplish. As with the supine and prone positions, the negative influence of the trunk gravitational force is large, and in fact the patient is required to bend forward with the knees straight, which is an undesirable manoeuvre from a postural mechanics vantage point. This position seems convenient to administer. Standing is comfortable to the patient for short periods of time, but patients would no doubt become uncomfortable if the strength test was lengthy.

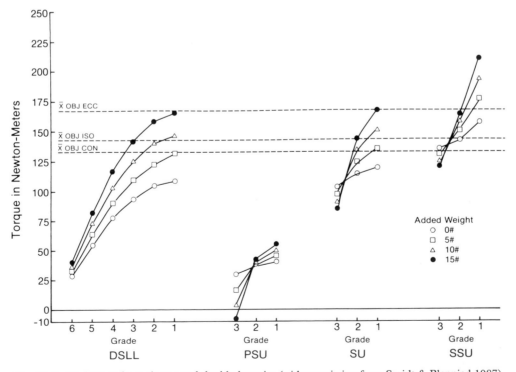

Fig. 16.2 Resistance from sit-ups and double-leg raise (with permission from Smidt & Blanpied 1987).

Table 16.1 Comparison* of various positions used in testing the strength of abdominal and back extensor muscles

Test position	Effectiveness of stabilization	Reduction of influence of trunk gravitational force	Permitted sagittal plane rotation	Comfort to patient	Convenience of test administration	Frequency used for functional tasks
Reclining						
supine–prone	Good	Fair	Fair	Excellent	Good	Fair
side-lying	Fair	Excellent	Excellent	Fair	Fair	Fair
Standing	Fair	Fair	Excellent	Good	Good	Excellent
Sitting	Excellent	Good	Good	Excellent	Excellent	Good

* The ratings included in this table are based on the author's judgement.

The sitting position has many advantages. The position is comfortable and convenient (Langrana & Lee 1984). The negative influence associated with the trunk gravitational force is compromised since trunk flexion and extension motion on either side of the vertical is more equally divided. It should be pointed out that regardless of the test position, the effect of the trunk's gravitational force can be estimated and then used appropriately to correct the recorded strength output. The gravitational effect can be estimated using body segment parameter coefficients or having the patient relax against the force application pads. Another major advantage of the sitting position is its efficacy for permitting stabilization of the pelvis. Both rotatory and translatory movement of the pelvis can be restricted by forces uniquely available in sitting. The external contact forces are applied at the ischial tuberosity, posterior superior iliac spine, top of sacrum, and anterior superior iliac spines. These forces are complemented by forces which can be transmitted to the hip joint via the femur (Fig. 16.2). The sitting position simulates the position used for some manual tasks. A disadvantage is that the range of trunk flexion may be restrictive, particularly with patients who have a pendulous abdomen. A summary of the relative advantages and disadvantages is presented in Table 16.1 The table portrays the superiority of the sitting position.

Transducers for measurement

The accuracy and range of movement capability of the transducer which provides the strength measurement is obviously important. These, transducers may measure force and may be in the form of load cells, strain gauges or other tension- or compression-sensing units. In the case of the manual test the sensors such as the Pacinian corpuscles in the fingers and other locations represent the transducers for measurement.

In general, it is desirable to have a transducer which is minimally accurate to 1% of full scale or less, and the sensitivity should accommodate the rate of force or torque produced by the trunk muscles. There is a danger in over-emphasizing the importance of the transducer and overlooking many of the other previously mentioned methodological factors involved in strength testing. The validity and reproducibility of the measurements required is contingent on these factors.

Trunk muscle strength — normal subjects

Body weight in particular, and age and height as well, have been shown to be significant influential factors in dynamic trunk muscle strength (Jerome et al 1991).

By way of comparison, studies of normal subjects (Mayer & Greenberg 1942, Kraus & Weber 1962, Petersen et al 1975, Addison & Schultz 1980; Karvonen et al 1980, Smidt et al 1980, 1983, Hemborg et al 1983) seem to indicate that the back extensors are stronger than the knee extensors and the strength of the abdominal muscles is less than that of the knee extensors. The trunk extensors are clearly the strongest muscle group in the body. As might be expected, strength in lateral trunk bending is less than the strength in trunk extension but greater than trunk flexion. As such, the back extensors must be considered among the strongest in the body.

Consistent with findings from other muscle groups, the trunk muscles generate the greatest strength when lengthening (eccentric), followed in decreasing order by static (isometric) and then to shortening (concentric) contractions. For isometric contractions the strength of the trunk flexor and extensor muscles is highest when the muscles are in the lengthened state, thus conforming to the classic physiological length–tension curve. A summary of muscle contraction characteristics is shown in Table 16.2.

Some clinicians have advocated that a particular trunk extension–flexion strength ratio is desirable for prevention or rehabilitation of low-back pain. This notion has some appeal, but, at this stage, no evidence is available to substantiate its efficacy. The data do show that the extensor–flexor strength ratio is dependent on the position of the

Table 16.2 Characteristics of muscle contraction

Type of contraction	Muscle length	Strength capability	Energy expenditure
Isometric	Constant	High	High
Concentric	Shortening	Low	High
Eccentric	Lengthening	High	Low

trunk. For example, the isometric extensor–flexor ratios have been shown to range from 1.17 with the trunk in an extended position to 3.78 with the trunk flexed. The cross-sectional area of the contributing trunk muscles and their respective moment arms are significant influential factors (Reid & Costigan 1987, Dumas et al 1991). Variability of dynamic trunk strength output was a hypothesized indicator of human effort, a hypothesis which was rejected and the need for clinical judgement was advocated (Hazard et al 1988).

In an extensive study involving 104 static and dynamic kinetics and electromyographic variables and 45 derived variables, test–retest reliability was found to be excellent for the kinetic variables and many of the desired variables (Smidt & Blanpied 1987). The reliability of the electromyographic measures in isolation were less than desirable. The angle at which peak torque occurred during the dynamic tests was also found to be unreliable.

Low-back dysfunction and correlational findings with trunk muscle strength

Most of the studies have involved patients with chronic low-back pain, and categories of symptoms have by and large not been well delineated. As presented in a previous section, the diversity of methodologies employed in trunk strength testing makes comparison between investigators problematic.

As found in a study of uninvolved subjects, trunk muscle strength in male patients with low-back problems is greater than it is for females (Smidt et al 1980). The vast majority of studies show that patients have a reduction in both abdominal and back extensor strength (Alston et al 1966, Nachemson & Lindh 1969, Hasue et al 1980, McNeill et al 1980, Nordgren et al 1980, Thorstensson & Nilsson 1982, Addison & Schultz 1980, Smidt et al 1983, Suzuki & Endo 1983). Others have reported no difference (Berkson et al 1977, Thorstensson & Arvidson 1982). The outcomes are variable, so the ratio of extensor to flexor strength has not evolved as a valuable causative discriminator for prevention or treatment of low-back dysfunction. The rate of torque development, as well as dynamic strength, also tends to be reduced in patients. Patients also seem to have hypomobility of the spinal column and a diminished ability to rotate the spinal column at a high rate of speed. In the normal case humans find it difficult to flex and extend the trunk at rates higher than 60°/second, a rate which is easily accomplished at the knee. On the other hand, many patients with back problems are unable to flex or extend the spine at 30°/second. Therefore, dynamic strength testing for patients can present some methodological problems.

The association between low-back dysfunction and trunk muscle strength is unclear. In a 5-year follow-up study of labourers, abdominal and back extensor strength did not correlate well with prospective sciatic pain symptoms (Hilkka et al 1989). With a single graded sit-up as a gauge of abdominal strength, no relationship was found with backache in pregnancy (Last et al 1990). The most difficult grade of sit-up was with the hands behind the head, for which the resistance level for the abdominals has been calculated to be approximately 80% of normal (Fig. 16.2) (Smidt & Blanpied 1987).

Further, in a study of 46 spinal surgery patients there was a statistically non-significant correlation between dynamic trunk strength and pain level (Mayer et al 1989). However, this was a cross-sectional type study. A similar result would not be expected in a longitudinal study of patients where, empirically, pain tends to have an inhibitory effect on strength output. In this study, patients who had undergone spinal fusion demonstrated greater trunk strength compared to those who had undergone disc excision. In a study of 202 girls aged 10–16, there was no difference shown between the trunk strength of the normals and those with scoliosis (average Cobb angle of 22°) (Portillo et al 1982).

From the affirmative perspective, weak trunk extensors have been shown to be associated with sciatica, and weak trunk flexors with back injuries and existing backache (Karvonen et al 1980). Trunk strength deficits are associated with physical deconditioning which, in turn, appears to be related to chronic low-back pain (Mayer et al 1985a). In a study of 46 spinal surgery patients there was a significant correlation between trunk strength and muscle density as revealed on a CT scan (Mayer et al 1989). Not only is muscle density associated with trunk strength, a relationship with bone density in post menopausal women has likewise been reported (Halle et al 1990). Thankfully, some good correlational investigations have been done. The results are mixed and insufficient to provide inclinations about using trunk strength measures to identify spinal abnormalities at risk. Perhaps more creativity is needed in the research design of these studies.

TRUNK MUSCLE ENDURANCE

Endurance, or, in contrast, fatiguability of the abdominal and back extensors, has received some investigative attention. Studies have indicated that the abdominals fatigue faster on repeated contractions than do the back extensors (Suzuki & Endo 1983, Smidt et al 1983). Typically, fatiguability is measured as the time required during repeated muscle contractions to produce a strength value which is some percentage (e.g. 25%) less than the strength value for a maximal voluntary contraction (MVC). By this criterion women have been shown to have higher endurance than men (Fig. 16.3) Two possible explanations for this finding are that women's maximum voluntary contraction is not as close to physiological maximum as is that of men, and their effort during the repeated contractions

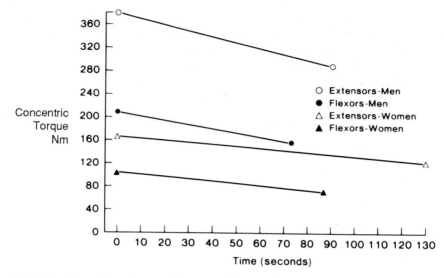

Fig. 16.3 Dynamic endurance. Time to 50% torque decrement. (Reprinted with permission from Smidt et al 1983.)

is not as intense. These explanations are supported to some degree by the fact that, in one study, repeated reciprocal trunk flexor and extensor muscle contraction yielded, at the end of the test, a heart rate increase of 78 beats/minute for men compared to only 60/minute for women. Patients tend to have greater endurance time as well probably because pain, or fear of pain, inhibit high-level muscle contractions.

Three groups (no low-back trouble, some trouble but working, and trouble and not working) of postal employees were in a study that reported a reduced isometric trunk extensor endurance time for the low-back trouble/not working group (Nicolaisen & Jorgensen 1985). These authors found superior the isometric hold approach using a dynamometer to gauge a 60% drop below an MVC level (Jorgensen & Nicolaisen 1986). Simply the maximum number of continuously repeated sit-ups at a rate of 25/minute was shown to discriminate for endurance

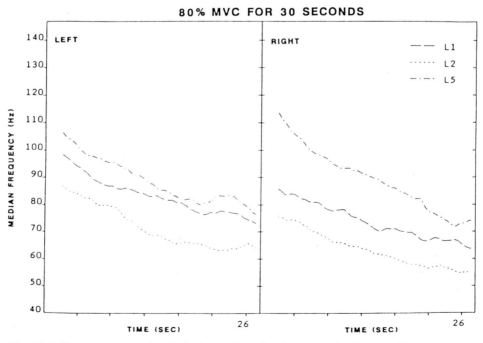

Fig. 16.4 Frequency spectral analysis. A typical median frequency plot for one subject as a function of contraction duration. The results for six concurrently active muscle sites are shown for a test conducted at 80% MVC for 30 s. Curves are arranged in groups of three, corresponding to the three lumbar electrode sites (L1, L2, L5) on the left and right sides of the back. (Reprinted with permission from Roy et al 1990.)

among 117 professional hockey players (Quinney et al 1984). Illustrative of the capability range, the players at the 5th percentile performed 20 repetitions, and those at the 90th percentile performed 100 repetitions. In a dynamic endurance study, subjects were asked to exert a force equal to 70% of their isometric maximum throughout a prescribed range of trunk motion. The velocity of sagittal trunk motion, both peak and average, decreased approximately 30% between the first three and the last three efforts within the total of 15 cycles (Parniapour et al 1988). Dynamic strength decrements with repeated MVC of the trunk muscles appears to be less striking for lateral trunk and axial trunk resisted movements (Mayer et al 1985b). Using a concentric/eccentric dynamic protocol for ten continuous flexion–extension cycles, the start-to-finish decrement was shown to be significant for all three contraction types for similar variables of torque and work (Smidt et al 1989). The decrement for the trunk flexors ranged from 16 to 23% and the extensors from 8 to 17%. The decrement in the torque rise rate (associated with rate of muscle tension development) was 32% for the flexors and 13% for the extensors.

Showing particular promise as a more definitive indicator of fatigue is the electromyograph spectral analysis. Studies (Kondraske et al 1987, Roy et al 1990) show a frequency shift with maintained submaximal contractions of the trunk flexor and extensor muscles (Fig. 16.4). Using this approach, asymmetrical trunk extensor fatigue was demonstrated in rowers (Roy et al 1990). The median frequency parameters between the rowers with and without back pain were different.

EFFECT OF EXERCISE INTERVENTION

Hemborg et al (1983) reported on the effects of a progressive resistive exercise programme on trunk strength (Table 16.2). Twenty men averaging 28 years of age exercised daily for 5 weeks. Personal instruction was given initially and the subjects kept daily records of their exercise performance. The subjects were prohibited from being involved in any other physical training during the 5-week period, and they were checked for technique twice each week. The initial position for the exercise was supine, with hips and knees flexed and feet supported. The training procedure included a sit-up in which the upper part of the body was curled up until the subject experienced 'maximal effort' without changing position of the pelvis. This sit-up position was isometrically held for a pre-set time. Each exercise was performed twice daily, with 10 repetitions at each session. The intensity of the exercise occurred by supervised increases in the holding time and varying the position of the arms. The mean reported increase (before–after exercise training) was 126 N (Newtons) for the trunk flexors and 167 N for the trunk extensors. These results are puzzling: even though the exercise programme was directed toward the trunk flexors, the greatest gains in strength were observed for the trunk extensors.

Important has been the increased number of studies reporting kinetic data reflective of trunk muscle capability under a variety of experimental conditions. Perhaps of greater interest and relevance are some interesting studies done on the effect of exercise intervention.

Kahanovitz et al (1987) compared 177 women (aged 18–49) divided into four groups, including a control. The most effective treatments in terms of the peak increases in strength of flexors and extensors were found to be the exercise and electrical stimulation groups. Treatment was administered 5 days per week for 4 weeks. The electrical stimulation was applied at the L2–L4 levels for 20 minutes at the maximum intensity which each subject could tolerate. The exercise group also performed 20 minutes of exercise consisting of prone trunk extension, prone leg lifts, prone arm lifts and a combination of 'all fours' arm and leg lifts. The gains in strength were obtained from isometric and dynametric concentric measures. On average, the concentric gains for the extensors were high for both the exercise group (range 32–48%) and electrical stimulation group (45–62%). The isometric extensor gains were less (19%) for the exercise group and 12% for the electrical stimulation group. The control group showed no change. Curiously, the gains in strength for the concentrically contracting flexors were also very high (range 27–37%) despite the fact that in neither the exercise group nor the electrical stimulation group were the trunk flexor muscles a focus.

Carpenter et al (1991) examined the effect of a dynamic resistive exercise protocol consisting of 8–12 extensor repetitions through a 72° arc of motion. The timing for each exercise cycle was 2 seconds for concentric, 1 second pause and 4 seconds for the eccentric mode. The weight load was increased by 5% when subjects could complete more than 12 repetitions. Fifty-six young normal subjects were studied. Isometric strength tests at various trunk angles were performed at baseline, 12 weeks and 20 weeks. Testing and training were done on the same device. The highest gains were shown for the fully extended position (92% at 12 weeks, and 123% at 20 weeks) with the lowest gains at the extreme flexed position (16% at 12 weeks, and 17% at 20 weeks). The gains for exercise were reported to be the same whether training occurred once per week or two to three times per week. The control group showed no change.

Smidt et al (1989) investigated the effect of a 6-week, high-intensity programme for the trunk flexors and extensors with (a) an emphasis on concentric training, and (b) an emphasis on eccentric training. A total of 45 subjects (average age 28 years) participated. The Kin-Com trunk testing device was used for both testing and training. Each subject received two sessions of orientation and practice prior to initial testing. Because some subjects experienced muscle soreness at the initial test, the training started 3–5 days later and consisted of three sessions each week for a period of 6 weeks. At each session the two exercise groups performed three sets of 10 repetitions for both the trunk flexors and extensors. The first set of 10 was performed at the subject's perceived 50% level of effort, and the last two sets were performed at 100%. The concentric group exercised only in the concentric mode, and the eccentric only in the eccentric. All subjects were tested at baseline at 2 weeks, 6 weeks, and 12 weeks post-baseline. Kinetic and EMG measures were obtained for maximal concentric/eccentric efforts for both the trunk flexors and extensors performed dynamically (constant angular velocity of 20°/second through an arc of 45°) and isometrically with the trunk upright).

Several additional results can be obtained from the study (Smidt et al 1989). In this chapter results will be limited to peak torque and specificity/transfer of exercise training. Gains in strength occurred in both concentric and eccentric groups to varying degrees in the 6-week period (Figs 16.5–16.10). The gains ranged from 17–50% with the highest gain from the eccentric training group for testing peak torque output for trunk eccentric extension. The remainder of the gains are shown in Table 16.3 where figures depict the relative occurrence of transfer of training from one type of muscle contraction to another and the specificity of training; that is, the gains for a contraction type which were above and beyond the gain yield by the other contraction type for the same muscle group (e.g. eccentric group–extensor eccentric output gain was 50%, the eccentric group–extensor concentric output gain was 18%, yielding a net 32%). These results indicate that there was considerable transfer of training for each muscle group and contraction type. The highest specificity of training effect was found for eccentric extensor exercise.

Smidt et al (1991) used 55 women with an average age of 56 years to determine the effects of a quantitatively based home exercise programme on trunk muscle strength. The same body positions were used for testing trunk strength and for the exercise programme. During the strength tests, the external forces generated by the subjects were measured using the trunk attachment of the Muscle Evaluation and Exercise Dosimeter (MEED) 3000 System. The standardized exercise programme utilized the body segments and cuff weights on the extremities to achieve the desired resistance level for the sit-up, prone trunk extension, and double-leg flexion exercises. Three sets of 10 were performed for each exercise at least three times a week over a 12-month period. Significant gains in strength (25–30%) were made by the exercise group for each exercise. The performance of the exercise group was superior to the control group. The reliability of the strength-testing method determined from interday trials using the MEED 3000 was excellent: all

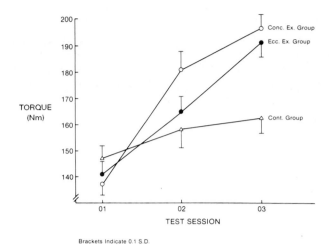

Fig. 16.5   Isometric flexor torque. 01 = baseline; 02 = 2 weeks; 03 = 6 weeks. (Reprinted with permission from Smidt et al 1989.)

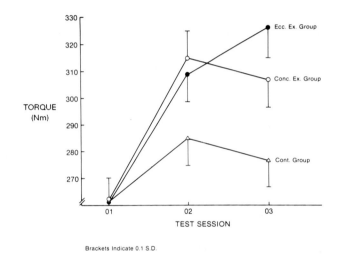

Fig. 16.6   Isometric extensor torque. 01 = baseline; 02 = 2 weeks; 03 = 6 weeks. (Reprinted with permission from Smidt et al 1989.)

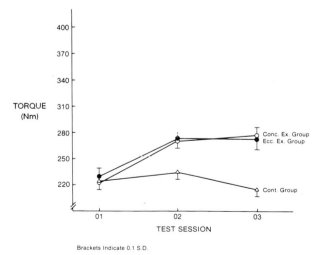

Fig. 16.7   Concentric extensor torque. 01 = baseline; 02 = 2 weeks; 03 = 6 weeks. (Reprinted with permission from Smidt et al 1989.)

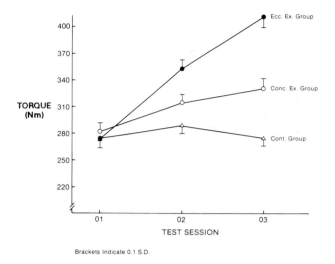

Brackets indicate 0.1 S.D.

Fig. 16.8 Eccentric extensor torque. 01 = baseline; 02 = 2 weeks; 03 = 6 weeks. (Reprinted with permission from Smidt et al 1989.)

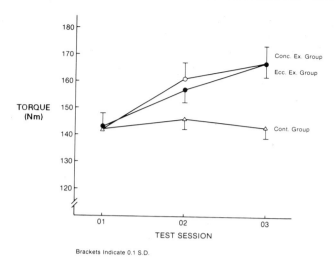

Brackets indicate 0.1 S.D.

Fig. 16.10 Eccentric flexor torque. 01 = baseline; 02 = 2 weeks; 03 = 6 weeks. (Reprinted with permission from Smidt et al 1989.)

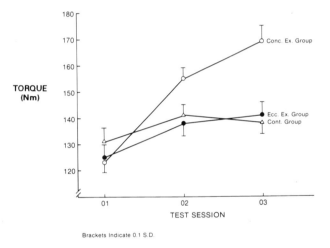

Brackets indicate 0.1 S.D.

Fig. 16.9 Concentric flexor torque. 01 = baseline; 02 = 2 weeks; 03 = 6 weeks. (Reprinted with permission from Smidt et al 1989.)

correlations were r = 0.93 or higher. This study demonstrates that older women can tolerate and increase trunk muscle strength using controlled, progressive, resistive exercise over an extended period of time. These results support the need expressed in a study of fighter pilots (Baldwin et al 1985), that is, high levels of resistance appear necessary to effect trunk muscle strength.

MUSCLE SORENESS

Particularly relevant to muscle strength testing is the amount of muscle soreness. When evaluating or treating a patient with resisted exercise, it is desirable to know the normal discomfort response for purposes of patient education and differentiation from pathologically generated symptoms. A complete treatise on muscle is beyond the scope of this chapter, so only a salient consideration will

Table 16.3 Specificity and transfer of muscle strength for trunk concentric and eccentric exercise*

	Gains in strength				Transfer to		
	Isometric output	Concentric output	Eccentric output	Specificity	Isometric	Concentric	Eccentric
Trunk flexors							
Concentric exercise group	High (30%)	High (37%)	Moderate (18%)	Moderate (19%)	Moderate (30%)		Moderate (18%)
Eccentric exercise group	High (26%)	Moderate (13%)	Moderate (17%)	Low (4%)	Moderate (26%)	Moderate (13%)	
Trunk extensors							
Concentric exercise group	Moderate (17%)	Moderate (25%)	Moderate (18%)	Low (7%)	Moderate (17%)		Moderate (18%)
Eccentric exercise group	Moderate (23%)	Moderate (18%)	High (50%)	High (32%)	Moderate (23%)	Moderate (18%)	

* Reprinted with permission from Smidt et al 1989.

be provided. Should more depth be sought the reader is invited to consider studies included in the reference list (Asmussen 1956, Abraham 1979, Friden et al 1981, Friden et al 1983a, 1983b, Newham et al 1983a, 1983b, Armstrong 1984, Friden et al 1984, Armstrong 1986, Clarkson et al 1986, Friden et al 1986, Jones et al 1986, Clarkson et al 1987, Molea et al 1987, Francis & Hoobler 1988, Friden et al 1988, Newham 1988, Smidt et al 1989, Leighton 1989, Berry et al 1990, Franklin et al 1991, Fitzgerald et al 1991).

Particularly after the first or second session of a strength or endurance test involving maximum or near maximum effort, most people subsequently develop what is now labelled as delayed-onset muscle soreness (DOMS). This dull, aching pain and stiffness typically manifests itself 24–48 hours after testing and may persist for 1–5 days thereafter, usually peaking in intensity the second or third day after the initial exercise. DOMS has also been shown to occur following electrical stimulation (Franklin et al 1991). Physiologically, elevated creatine kinase levels have been shown to be associated with DOMS, thus implicating break down of connective tissue in the muscle. Other clinical correlates associated with DOMS — such as elevation of plasma enzymes, myoglobinemia and abnormal muscle histology and ultrastructure — appear to occur only in extreme forms of DOMS (Armstrong 1984). Earlier evidence has shown that the highest strength output can be expected from an eccentric contraction, a contraction type which has now been associated with muscle soreness. Histological studies have shown that, during intensive training, muscle damage — the cause of cellular damage — is perhaps a result of metabolic and/or mechanical overload. Since eccentric contractions generate high levels of force, the precipitating factor in DOMS may be mechanical in nature.

During DOMS, a voluntary reduction in effort and inherent inability of muscles to contract vigorously affects muscular performance. However, exercise of low-level intensity is a good mode of treatment. Evidence shows that DOMS is most prevalent following eccentric muscle contractions as compared to isometric and concentric contractions. In a study by White (1987) normal subjects experienced DOMS following dynamic eccentric concentric testing of the trunk flexors and extensors. The average DOMS duration was 3 days. Thirty-one percent of the 60 subjects tested reported DOMS.

EXERCISE INTERVENTION AND LOW-BACK DYSFUNCTION

Flint (1958) evaluated the effect of resistive exercise on low-back symptoms. Nineteen female subjects performed progressive resistive exercise using the abdominal and back extensor muscles. A leather vest attached to weights by a cable was used as the exercise training method. Hook-lying and prone positions were used for the trunk flexor and extensor groups respectively. Each exercise session consisted of 20 repetitions for the flexors and 10 for the extensors. Three sessions each week for 12 weeks were conducted. The resistance was increased, on average, once per week. The trunk flexors were tested isometrically with the subject in the hook-lying position. The subjects were prone for testing the extensors.

At the end of the 12-week period 58% of the group were reported to have complete relief of back pain, 31% had partial relief and 11% reported no relief. The investigator also indicated that, for 45 patients in a previously completed pilot study, 96% of the patients experienced relief from symptoms at the conclusion of resistive exercise treatment. No control group was included so that the actual effect of the treatment programme could be open to question.

In a 5-week training programme, 20 male subjects with an average 5.5 year history of low-back pain performed maximum isometric exercise for the trunk flexors (Hemborg et al 1985). Ten repetitions were done twice daily with hold times up to 15 seconds. Gains in strength in the trunk flexors were reported as 22% for the group.

Asfour et al (1990) had patients with chronic low-back dysfunction perform prone trunk extension exercises, six times per session, while maintaining their maximum accept effort for 10 seconds. The subjects received eight treatments over a 2-week period. Auditory and visual electromyographic feedback from back extensors was included. Trunk extensor strength obtained for one position isometrically increased 45% for the subjects in the treatment group. The patients reported intensity of pain decreased over the corresponding 2-week period. This study serves to show that gains in strength, particularly when training periods are short — perhaps as short as 6 weeks or less — cannot be accounted for by morphological changes in the muscle but by other factors such as reduced pain, reduced fear and anxiety regarding physical effort, and the multiple factors that are inherently part of the neuromotor aspects of muscle contraction. Standard forms of treatment for a general group of patients with chronic low-back pain is fraught with problems incumbent on any 'shotgun' approach. For example, one study reported no difference in the gains in strength in a group of back-dysfunction patients (Martin et al 1986). The explanation was that this treatment group had high levels of pain, a rationale that appears plausible. The effort to satisfy classical research design patterns for experimental research appears to have resulted in meaningful clinical outcomes. Perhaps smaller groups — even down to a case study — whereby group homogeneity in terms of history, signs and symptoms should be considered in future intervention of studies involving low-back dysfunction. The evaluation must be standardized, but thought should be given to treatment exploration which is precedent for the type of patient and his/her condition.

CURRENT STATUS

Relatively few studies have been done on trunk strength and endurance for patients with low-back problems. Descriptive results now available must be reviewed in the contexts of the varieties of methodologies employed. Clearly, the spinal column cannot be voluntarily moved or controlled without trunk muscle action, so empirically these muscles must play a role in the prevention and treatment of low-back pain.

Authors have forwarded some ideas relative to the cause of reduced trunk strength output in patients with a history of low-back pain. Ideally, reduced measures of strength result simply because of deficient physiological function. This physiological state may be caused by a lack of physical activity performed by the patient, or local muscle inactivity may be imposed by a back brace or corset. Other potential causative factors for reduced strength output may be pain (perceived or anticipated occurrence), configuration of the spinal column, and lack of motivation.

In the area of muscle testing and exercise, high technology has emerged which permits alteration and control of multiple kinematic and kinetic variables (Table 16.4). In a testing or exercise situation these variables should be carefully considered, and when communicated verbally or in writing they need to be carefully explained. In this author's judgment, extreme caution should be exercised. If not avoided altogether, the use of 'buzz' words may not accurately convey the methodology utilized. A premiere example is the universal use of the word 'isokinetic' which, at its root, means 'same force' rather than the frequently intended meaning of constant angular velocity.

Attempts need to be made in categorizing patients with common symptoms, and the details of the symptom such as duration, intensity and frequency of pain need to be associated with the measures of strength. The influence of things such as inactivity, excessive physical activity and obesity might turn out to be risk factors for low-back pain (Karvonen et al 1980). The interrelationship between spinal segment hypermobility and hypomobility, overall

Table 16.4 Generic variables in motor performance measurements[*]

Independent variables	Dependent variables	Controlled variables	Confounding variables[**]
Muscle motions displacement velocity acceleration jerk	Muscle motions displacement velocity acceleration jerk	Individual age gender anthropometry	Motivation Fatigue Health Fitness
Mass	Mass	Environment	Skill
Repetition	Repetition	temperature	etc.
Resistance	Output:	humidity	
Body posture	force	air velocity	
etc.	torque	radiation	
	work	noise	
	power	vibration	
	etc.	Clothing	
		etc.	

[*] Reprinted with permission from Kroemer et al 1990.
[**] Should be controlled.

spinal mobility and alignment, posture, back pain symptoms and trunk muscle strength are not well understood. Seemingly, our understanding of these clinical variables in the area of the back is light-years behind our understanding of similar variables at other joints. Goals could include prospective studies of the low back involving the relationships among these variables. Further, the effects of exercise treatment on low-back pain need to be studied. Finally, we need to identify specific biological tissues responsible for sign- and symptom-based categories of low-back dysfunction. Investigations along the aforementioned lines will improve the rationale and evidence for prevention, assessment and treatment of low-back pain. In so doing, the role and potential implication of the trunk muscles should ideally be characterized by three areas: maximal strength, endurance or fatigue strength and neuromotor control (Lee 1986). Each contribute in varying degrees to functional tasks inside and outside the workplace.

Acknowledgements

The author is extremely grateful to Mrs Judy Biderman for her prompt and effective typing of the manuscript, and to Mr Anthony Allen who assisted in the acquisition of the reference materials for this chapter.

REFERENCES

Abraham W M 1979 Exercise-induced muscle soreness. Physician and Sports Medicine 7: 57–60

Addison R, Schultz A 1980 Trunk strength in patients seeking hospitalization for chronic low back disorders. Spine 5: 539–544

Alston W, Carlson K E, Feldman D J, Grim Z, Gerontinos E 1966 A quantitative study of muscle factors in the chronic low back syndrome. Journal of the American Geriatric Society 14: 1041–1047

Anderson T 1954 Physiotherapy techniques. British Journal of Physical Medicine 17: 155

Armstrong R B 1984 Mechanisms of exercise-induced delayed onset muscular soreness a brief review. Medicine and Science in Sports and Exercise 16: 529–538

Armstrong R B 1986 Muscle damage and endurance events. Sports Medicine 3: 370–381

Asfour S S, Khabl T M, Waly S M, Goldberg M L, Rosomoff R S, Rosomoff H 1990 Biofeedback in back muscle strengthening. Spine 15: 510–513

Asmussen E 1956 Observations on experimental muscle soreness. Acta Rheumatologica Scandinavica 1: 109–116

Balwin et al 1985

Berkson A, Schultz A, Nachemson A, Andersson G 1977 Voluntary strengths of male adults with acute low back syndromes. Clinical Orthopedics and Related Research 129: 84–95

Berry C B, Moritani T, Tolson H 1990 Electrical activity and soreness in muscles after exercise. American Journal of Physical Medicine and Rehabilitation 69: 60–66

Cady L D, Bischoff D P, O'Connell E R, Thomas P C, Allan J H 1979 Strength and fitness and subsequent back injuries in firefighters. Journal of Occupational Medicine 21: 269–272

Carpenter D M, Graves J E, Pollock M L, Legett S H, Foster D, Holmes B, Fulton M N 1991 Effect of 12 and 20 weeks of resistive training on lumbar extension torque production. Physical Therapy 71: 580–588

Chaffin D B 1974 Human strength capability and low back pain. Journal of Occupational Medicine 16: 248–254

Chaffin D B, Herrin G D, Keyserling W M, Garg A 1977 A method of evaluating biomechanical stresses resulting from manual materials handling jobs. American Industrial Hygiene Association Journal 38: 662–675

Clarkson P M, Byrnes W C, McCormick K M, Turcotte L P, White J S 1986 Muscle soreness and serum creatine kinase activity following isometric, eccentric, and concentric exercise. International Journal of Sports Medicine 7: 152–155

Clarkson P M, Byrnes W C, Gillisson E, Harper E 1987 Adaptation to exercise-induced muscle damage. Clinical Science 73: 383–386

Cyriax J 1970 Textbook of orthopaedic medicine, vol 1, 5 th edn. Williams & Wilkins, Baltimore

Davies P R, Gould J 1981 Prototype device tests back/trunk muscles. Physician and Sports Medicine 9: 20–21

DeLitto A, Rosie S T, Crandall C E, Strube M J 1991 Reliability of isokinetic measurements of trunk muscle performance. Spine 16: 800–803

Dumas C A, Poulin M J, Roy B, Gagnon M, Jovanovic M 1991 Orientation and moment arms of trunk muscles. Spine 16: 293–303

Fitzgerald G K, Rothstein J M, Mayhew T P, Lamb R L 1991 Exercise-induced muscle soreness after concentric and eccentric isokinetic contractions. Physical Therapy 71: 505–513

Flint M M 1958 Effect of increasing back and abdominal strength in low back pain. Research Quarterly 29: 160–171.

Francis K, Hoobler T 1988 Delayed onset muscle soreness and decreased isokinetic strength. Journal of Applied Sport Science Research 2: 20–23

Franklin M E, Currier D P, Smith S T, Mitts K K, Werrell L M, Chenier T C 1991 Effect of varying the ratio of electrically induced muscle contraction time to rest time on serum creatine kinase and perceived soreness. Journal of Orthopaedic and Sports Physical Therapy 13: 310–315

Friden J 1984 Changes in human skeletal muscle induced by long-term eccentric exercise. Cell and Tissue Research 236: 365–372

Friden J, Sjostrom M, Ekblom B 1981 Morphological study of delayed muscle soreness. Experientia 37: 506–507

Friden J, Seger J, Sjostrom M, Ekblom B 1983a Adaptive response in human skeletal muscle subjected to prolonged eccentric training. International Journal of Sports Medicine 4: 177–183

Friden J, Sjostrom M, Ekblom B 1983b Myofibrillar damage following intense eccentric exercise in man. International Journal of Sports Medicine 4: 170–176

Friden J, Kjorell U, Thornell L E 1984 Delayed muscle soreness and cytoskeletal alterations: an immunocytological study in man. International Journal of Sports Medicine 5(1): 15–18

Friden J, Sfakianos P N, Hargens A R 1986 Muscle soreness and intramuscular fluid pressure: comparison between eccentric and concentric load. Journal of Applied Physiology 61: 2175–2179

Friden J, Sfakianos P N, Hargens A R, Akeson W H 1988 Residual muscular swelling after repetitive eccentric contractions. Journal of Orthopaedic Research 6: 493–498

Gomez T, Beach G, Cooke C, Hrudey W, Goyert P 1991 Normative database for trunk range of motion, strength, velocity and endurance with the Isostation B-200 lumbar dynamometer. Spine 16: 15–21

Graves J E, Pollock M, Foster D et al 1990 Effect of training frequency and specificity on isometric lumbar extension strength. Spine 15: 504–509

Halle J S, Smidt G L, O'Dwyer K D, Lin S Y 1990 Relationship between trunk muscle strength and bone mineral content of the lumbar spine and hip in healthy postmenopausal women. Physical Therapy 70: 690–699

Hambly T 1967 Low back pain. British Medical Journal 4: 486

Hasue M, Fujiwara M, Kikuchi S 1980 A new method of quantitative measurement of abdominal and back extensor strength. Spine 5: 143–148

Hazard R G, Reid S, Fenwick J, Reeves 1988 Isokinetic trunk and lifting strength measurements: variability as an indicator of effort. Spine 13: 54–57

Hemborg B, Moritz V, Hamberg J, Lowing H, Akesson I 1983 Intra-abdominal pressure and trunk muscle activity during lifting: effect of abdominal muscle training in healthy subjects. Scandinavian Journal of Rehabilitation Medicine 15: 183–196

Hemborg B, Moritz V, Hamberg J, Holstrom E, Lowing H, Akeson I 1985 Intra abdominal pressure and trunk muscle activity during lifting III. Effect of abdominal muscle training in chronic low back patients. Journal of Rehabilitation Medicine 17: 15–24

Herring T 1982 A method for measurement of strength and dynamic endurance of flexors and extensors of normal spine. Physical therapy Master's thesis, University of Iowa, Iowa City

Jensen R H, Smidt G L, Johnston R C 1971 A technique for obtaining measurements of force generated by hip muscles. Archives of Physical Medicine and Rehabilitation 52: 207–215

Jerome J A, Hunter K, Gordon P, McKay N 1991 A new robust index for measuring isokinetic trunk flexion and extension: outcome from a regional study. Spine 16: 804–808

Jones D A, Newham D J, Round J M, Tolfree S E J 1986 Experimental human muscle damage: morphological changes in relation to other indices of damage. Journal of Physiology 375: 435–448

Jorgensen K, Nicolaisen T, 1986 Two methods for determining trunk extensor endurance. European Journal of Physiology 55: 639–644

Kahanovitz N, Nordin M, Verderame R, Yabut S, Parniapour M, Viola K, Mulvihill M 1987 Normal trunk strength and endurance in women and the effect of exercises to increase trunk muscle strength and endurance. Part 2. Comparative analysis of electrical stimulation and exercises to increase trunk muscle strength and endurance. Spine 12: 112–118

Karvonen M J, Viitasalo J T, Komi P V, Nummi J, Jarvinen T 1980 Back and leg complaints in relation to muscle strength in young men. Scandinavian Journal of Rehabilitation Medicine 12: 53–59

Klausen K 1965 The form and function of the loaded human spine. Acta Physiologica Scandinavica 65: 176–190

Kluck D J 1967 A study of strength ratios of the back extensors and trunk flexors. Physical therapy Master's thesis, University of Iowa, Iowa City

Kondraske G, Deivanayagam S, Carmichael T, Mayer T G, Mooney V, 1987 Myoelectric spectral analysis and strategies for quantifying trunk muscle fatigue. Archives of Physical Medicine and Rehabilitation 68: 103–110

Kraus H 1949 Therapeutic exercise. Thomas, Springfield

Kraus H, Weber S 1962 Back pain and tension syndromes in a sedentary profession. Archives of Environmental Health 4: 408

Kroemer K H E, Marras W S, McGlothlin J D, McIntyre D R, Nordin M 1990 On the measurement of muscle strength. International Journal of Industrial Ergonomics 6: 199–210

Langrana N A, Lee C K 1984 Isokinetic evaluation of the trunk muscles. Spine 9: 171–175

Larson C B 1951 Pathomechanics of backache. Journal of the Iowa Medical Society 51: 643–650

Lee C K 1986 The use of exercise and muscle testing in rehabilitation of spinal disorders. Clinics in Sports Medicine 5: 271–276

Leighton S 1989 Comparison of serum creatine kinase level and delayed onset muscle soreness between a high velocity and a low velocity eccentric work. Paper submitted in partial fulfillment of course requirements for 101:249 Research Practicum, University of Iowa, Iowa City

Martin P R, Rose M J, Nichols P J R, Russell P L, Hughes I G 1986 Physiotherapy exercises for low back pain: process and clinical outcome. International Rehabilitation Medicine 8: 34–38

Mayer L, Greenberg B B 1942 Measurements of the strength of trunk muscles. Journal of Bone and Joint Surgery 24: 842–856

Mayer T G, Smith S S, Keeley J, Mooney V 1985a Quantification of lumbar function. Part 2. Sagittal plane trunk strength in chronic low back pain patients. Spine 10: 765–772

Mayer T G, Smith S S, Kondraske G, Gatchel R J, Carmichael T W, Mooney V, 1985b Quantification of lumbar function. Part 3. Preliminary data on isokinetic torso rotation testing with myoelectric spectral analysis in normal and low-back pain subjects. Spine 10: 912–920

Mayer T G, Vanharanta H, Gatchell R J et al 1989 Comparison of CT scan muscle measurements and isokinetic trunk strength in post-operative patients. Spine 14: 33–36

McNeill T, Warwick D, Andersson G, Schultz A 1980 Trunk strengths in attempted flexion, extension and lateral bending in healthy subjects and patients with low back disorder s. Spine 5: 529–538

Molea D, Murcek B, Blanken C, Burns R, Chila A, Howell J 1987 Evaluation of two manipulative techniques in the treatment of postexercise muscle soreness. Journal of the American Osteopathic Association 87: 477–483

Morris J M, Lucas D B, Bresler B 1961 Role of the trunk in the stability of the spine. Journal of Bone and Joint Surgery 43A: 327–351

Nachemson A L 1971 Low back pain, its etiology and treatment. Clinical Medicine 78: 18–23

Nachemson A, Lindh M 1969 Measurement of abdominal and back extensor strength with and without low back pain. Scandinavian Journal of Rehabilitation Medicine 1: 60–65

Newham D J 1988 The consequences of eccentric contractions and their relationship to delayed onset muscle pain. European Journal of Applied Physiology 57: 353–359

Newham D J, Mills K R, Quigley B M, Edwards R H T 1983a Pain and fatigue after concentric and eccentric muscle contractions. Clinical Science 64: 55–62

Newham D J, McPhail G, Mills K R, Edwards R H T 1983b Ultrastructural changes after concentric and eccentric contractions of human muscle. Journal of the Neurological Sciences 61: 109–122

Nicolaisen T, Jorgensen K 1985, Trunk strength, back muscle endurance and low-back trouble. Scandinavian Journal of Rehabilitation Medicine 17: 121–127

Nordgren B, Schele R, Lindroth K 1980 Evaluation and prediction of back pain during military field service. Scandinavian Journal of Rehabilitation Medicine 12: 1–8

Olson V L, Smidt G L, Johnston R C 1972 The maximum torque generated by the eccentric, isometric and concentric contraction of the hip abductor muscles. Journal of the American Physical Therapy Association 52: 149–158

Parniapour M, Nordin M, Kahanovitz W, Frankel V 1988 The triaxial coupling of torque generation of trunk muscles during isometric exertions and the effect of fatiguing isoinertial movements on the motor output and movement patterns. Spine 13: 982–992

Parniapour H, Nordin M, Sheikhzadeh A 1990 The relationship of torque, velocity and power with constant resistive load during sagittal trunk movement. Spine 15: 639–643

Petersen O F, Petersen R, Stoffendt E S 1975 Back pain and isometric back strength of workers in a Danish factory. Scandinavian Journal of Rehabilitation Medicine 7: 125–128

Portillo D, Sinkora G, McNeill T, Spencer D, Schultz A 1982 Trunk strengths in structurally normal girls and girls with idiopathic scoliosis. Spine 7: 551–554

Quinney H A, Smith D J, Senges H A 1984 A field assessment of abdominal muscular endurance in professional hockey players. Journal of Orthopaedics and Sports Physical Therapy 6: 30–33

Reid J G, Costigan P A 1987 Trunk muscle balance and muscular force. Spine 12: 783–786

Roy S H, DeLuca C J, Snyder-Mackler L, Emley M S, Crenshaw R L, Lyons J P, 1990 Fatigue, recovery and low back pain in varsity rowers. Medicine and Science in Sports Medicine 22: 463–468

Smidt G L 1973 Biomechanical analysis of knee flexion and extension. Journal of Biomechanics 6: 79–92

Smidt G L 1984 Muscle strength testing: a system based on mechanics. SPARK Instruments & Academics, Coralville, IA

Smidt G L, Blanpied P R 1987 Analysis of strength tests and resistive exercises commonly used for low-back disorders. Spine 12: 1025–1034

Smidt G L, Blanpied P R 1988 Analysis of strength tests and resistive exercises commonly used for low back disorders. Spine 12: 1025–1034

Smidt G L, Amundsen L R, Dostal W F 1980 Muscle strength at the trunk. Journal of Orthopaedic and Sports Physical Therapy 1: 165–170

Smidt G L, Herring T, Amundsen L, Rogers M, Russell A, Lehmann T 1983 Assessment of abdominal and back extensor function. Spine 8: 211–219

Smidt G L, Blanpied P R, Anderson M A, White R W 1987 Comparisons of clinical and objective methods of assessing trunk muscle strength. An experimental approach. Spine 12: 1020–1024

Smidt G L, Blanpied P R, White R W 1989 Exploration of mechanical and electromyographic responses of trunk muscles to high-intensity resistive exercise. Spine 14: 815–830

Smidt G L, O'Dwyer K D, Lin S Y, Blanpied P R 1991 The effect of trunk resistive exercise on muscle strength in postmenopausal women. Journal of Orthopedic and Sports Physical Therapy 13: 300–309

Suzuki N, Endo S 1983 A quantitative study of trunk muscle strength and fatigability in the low-back-pain syndrome. Spine 8: 69–74

Suzuki N, Ohe K 1978 Abdominal and back muscle strength in patients with low back pain. Orthopaedic Surgery 29: 325–328

Suzuki N, Ohe K, Inoue H 1977 The strength of abdominal and back muscles in patients with low back pain. Central Japanese Journal of Orthopaedics and Traumatology 20: 332–334

Suzuki N E, Swiichi T, Matsuyoshi T, Suzuki Y, Teraro S 1980 A quantitative study of trunk muscle strength and fatigability in patients with low back pain. Seventeenth Annual Meeting of the Japanese Rehabilitation Medicine Association 17: 291

Thorstensson A, Arvidson A 1982 Trunk muscle strength and low back pain. Scandinavian Journal of Rehabilitation Medicine 14: 69–75

Thorstensson A, Nilsson J 1982 Trunk muscle strength during constant velocity movements. Scandinavian Journal of Rehabilitation Medicine 14: 61–69

Watson A W S, O'Donovan D J 1977 Factors relating to the strength of male adolescents. Journal of Applied Physiology 43: 834–838

White R W 1987 A comparison of concentric and eccentric resistive exercise programs utilizing the trunk flexors and extensors. Physical therapy Master's thesis, University of Iowa, Iowa City

17. Bony and soft-tissue anomalies of the vertebral column

G. P. Grieve

INTRODUCTION

There are innumerable congenital variants in the skeleton alone, and because structural variations of bone and soft tissue have considerable importance in this clinical field, and because their likelihood is always worth bearing in mind, reference should sooner or later be made to more detailed accounts, such as those by Köhler and Zimmer (1968), Schmorl and Junghanns (1971), von Torklus and Gehle (1972), Keats (1988), Epstein (1976) and Murray et al (1990). The specialist training of manual therapists continues to expand in depth and scope, hence the factor of vertebral column development, both normal and anomalous, becomes increasingly relevant; considerations of the paediatric spine (Raimondi 1987, Raimondi et al 1989) also gather importance. The work of Bagnall et al (1984) on the histochemical composition of vertebral muscle effectively disposes of nicely idealized concepts of symmetry of structure and function between vertebral sides and, by implication, chiropractic notions of 'mal-alignment'. To quote: 'These standard deviations indicate that large differences in muscle fibre characteristics can exist between the two sides of the vertebral column. Any thoughts of a balance between muscle characteristics . . . at one level would appear to be erroneous.' Similarly, the work of Wigh (1980) (see Ch. 19) highlights the fallacy that charts of dermatome distribution represent sacrosanct anatomical territories.

Clinical workers now enjoy a wide choice of excellent texts on anomalies and dysplasias, and to the books mentioned above might be added those by Beighton (1988) and Wynne-Davies et al (1986).

From a purely orthopaedic surgical standpoint, most minor skeletal anomalies are interesting but only occasionally important. Similarly, taking a neurologist's view, Spillane et al (1957) suggest, for example, that posterior spina bifida of the atlas, the commonest bony anomaly of the craniovertebral junction, is of no clinical significance. Occipitalization of the atlas may also be asymptomatic, and fusion of cervical vertebrae is usually symptomless, although the authors do also observe that patients without any anomaly other than fused cervical vertebrae may develop tetraplegia following minor trauma.

For the manual therapist, whose treatment procedures follow searching tests of movement and very careful palpation, vertebral anomalies need more consideration, particularly since the *transitional* or *junctional regions* of the spine are 'ontogenetically restless' (Schmorl & Junghanns 1971), are more subject to variations and malformation than any other part of the column and happen also to be the most common sites of the benign but painfully restrictive lesions we treat.

While it is not difficult to compile and illustrate tediously long lists of vertebral anomalies, in their infinite variety, of more value is the question: how important are they, in clinical shop-floor practice?

So far as the musculoskeletal, vascular and nervous systems are concerned, the importance of congenital anatomical deviants might be addressed on six counts:

1. The validity of the idea, particularly among chiropractors, but also among some osteopaths and physiotherapists, that 'symmetry is all' and palpable asymmetry or radiographic 'mal-alignment' must always be 'normalized', often by manipulative thrust techniques, before signs and symptoms can be expected to disappear. This questionable idea plainly underlies the philosophy of more than one school of manipulative treatment.

A radiologist (Dalseth 1973, 1974, 1976) who is familiar with manipulative theory, understands its practice and has conducted careful studies of the craniovertebral, lumbar and sacroiliac regions (Dalseth 1980, 1981), has observed that anatomical symmetry between sides is remarkably uncommon, (Fig. 17.1) if it ever exists.

Thus, while active movements of a vertebral district may appear to be quite symmetrical between sides (see lumbar spine p. 241) it does not follow that each *segmental* contribution to that range of movement bilaterally is also symmetrical, since where true structural symmetry does not exist true symmetry of segmental movement is not

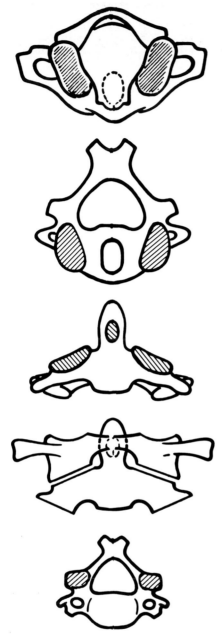

Fig. 17.1 The stylized symmetry in much illustration of vertebral structures, particularly the upper cervical spine, is a myth. Symmetry is rare.

possible. Not only the resting length of associated connective tissues, but also their degree of extensibility between sides, must be unequal, in various combinations from segment to segment.

Much of the rationalization, on biomechanical grounds, of the use of manipulative treatment could bear some inspection.

Dalseth's clinical observations of vertebral movement revealed unilaterally hypomobile joints in perfectly healthy subjects, and he suggests that the validity of this part of chiropractic or any other manipulative theory seems to be illusory. 'For the same reason, the chiropractic X-ray diagnosis of positional faults (subluxations) is as illusory as the clinical diagnosis' (Dalseth 1976).

Crelin (1973) and others (Editorial 1980, Relman 1979) have also drawn attention to this aspect of chiropractic.

2. The potential for wrong interpretation of palpation findings during assessment, for example of occipito-atlantal relationships, when aplasia or hypoplasia of the posterior arch of atlas, or its lateral dimensions, is present (Fig. 17.2).

3. The common notion, often without any demonstrable foundation, that the simple presence of a structural anomaly thereby inculpates the anomaly as responsible for pain and other symptoms emanating from that same vertebral district. While almost every congenital defect, said to be the cause of symptoms, has been demonstrated in the symptom-free population, there is nevertheless ample evidence of anomalies being the prime cause of symptoms in some (Grieve 1988).

4. The implications which abnormal segmentation, affecting the lumbosacral region, for example, in one in 20 or more, may have for theories of referred pain (see referred pain Ch. 19).

5. The effects on the nature and distribution of clinical features, particularly vagaries of referred pain, which anomalies of arterial supply may have, more especially in the neck and upper limbs. The vascular arrangement in mid-thoracic and lumbar cord segments is probably of more immediate concern to the surgeon. Jeffreys (1980) observes that the importance of abnormalities of blood supply in the causation of spinal disease is being increasingly recognized.

6. How anomalous and radiotranslucent connective tissue bands can be of much more significance than bony malformations, for example at the craniovertebral and cervicothoracic junctions, also the simulation of disc trespass, with neurological features in a lower limb, by soft-tissue anomaly in the form of a lumbar transforaminal ligament (Golub & Silverman 1969). Similarly, how anomalies of meninges and lumbosacral root formation, and the presence of cysts, may influence the distribution of neurological deficit in the lower limbs (Hanraets 1959).

Pathogenesis

Jeffreys (1980) mentions that the major cause of many congenital anomalies is recognized as being genetic transmission, with environmental factors such as drugs, irradiation, infections and metabolic factors also playing a part.

Tanaka and Uhthoff (1981) studied, in 266 human embryos and fetuses, the possible pathogenesis of malformations of the vertebral body. They concluded that most malformations occur in the early stage of definitive vertebral body anlage (primordium) formation, that the notochord does not seem to be responsible and that

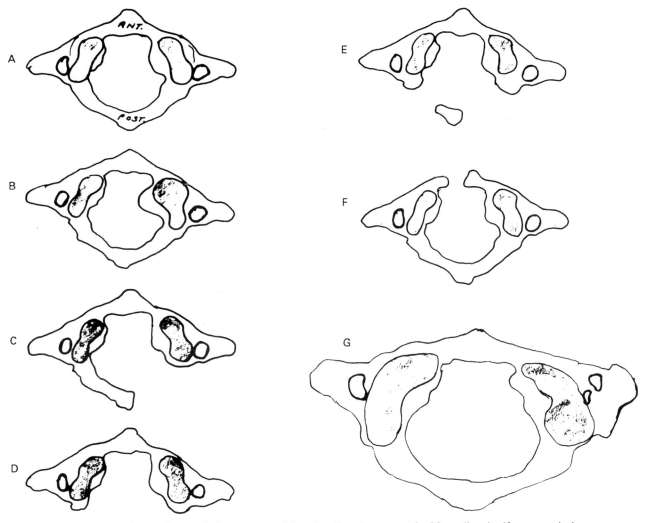

Fig. 17.2 Some possible forms of congenital asymmetry of the atlas. Superior aspect. **A.** 'Normal' — itself asymmetrical. **B.** Asymmetry of lateral mass, neural canal and superior articular surfaces. **C.** Spina bifida atlanto, aplasia of one posterior arch. **D.** Complete aplasia of posterior arch. **E.** Defective union of posterior arch. **F.** Defective union of anterior arch. **G.** This tracing of a photograph depicts the most frequent, and important, malformation, i.e. asymmetry of lateral dimensions of the atlas, besides defects of foramen transversarium and upper articular surfaces. Aggressive manipulation thrust techniques, to 'correct' this supposed 'lateralization of the atlas', would be a mistake.

malformations are likely to occur during the resegmentation stage during the earliest weeks after conception, essentially being related to an abnormal distribution of the intersegmental arteries.

Even at this very early stage, compensatory growth of other vertebral bodies is already present.

Classification

Differing categories tend to reflect the interest of the particular disciplines, e.g. geneticist, anthropologist, surgeon and radiologist.

Murray et al (1990) classify the important localized congenital anomalies as shown in Table 17.1.

The host of *generalized* congenital disorders, e.g. dysplasias and dysostoses, constitutional diseases of bone, connective tissue and other conditions are not discussed

Table 17.1 Classification of localized congenital anomalies

Type	Example
Deficient bone formation	Hemivertebra, spina bifida, aplastic sacral ala
Increased bone formation	Klippel–Feil syndrome, sacralization
Congenital dislocation	Hypoplasia of odontoid, congenital dislocation of hip
Other localized deformities	Diastematomyelia, accessory sacro-iliac joints

here, although it must be noted that many localized anomalies form part of generalized congenital disorders and these patients, too, may present with benign joint pains. In osteochondrodystrophy (Morquio–Brailsford disease), for example, there is commonly an unstable craniovertebral region due to hypoplasia of the odontoid, and extreme caution is wise.

THE CRANIOVERTEBRAL REGION

The regularity or symmetry of much anatomical illustration (Fig. 17.1) is a myth. Asymmetry is the rule and true symmetry between sides is quite rare, if it exists at all (Dalseth 1974).

Congenital malformations of the cervical spine are very common, varying from developmental failures which are incompatible with life to minor, clinically insignificant anomalies which are revealed by chance (Jeffreys 1980).

Development

Late during the embryo's third intrauterine week, some 42–44 discrete mesodermal somites have formed around the notochord, the upper unsegmented region of which is eventually incorporated as the sphenoid (Truex & Johnson 1978).

Internal specialization of each somite includes differentiation, beginning at the older, cranial end into dermatomes (precursors of the corium or true skin), myotomes (precursors of muscle) and sclerotomes, the precursors of skeletal structures (see Ch. 19, referred pain). The cranial and caudal halves of adjacent sclerotomes unite to begin forming one vertebra, albeit in more complex fashion in the upper cervical region, where the occipital bone represents three occipital somites.

The somites contribute cranial and caudal halves as indicated in Table 17.2.

The tip of the odontoid is thus derived from the mesenchymal tissue of the pro-atlas, with the odontoid as a whole being formed from the pro-atlantal segment of C1 sclerotome, the caudal part of the same sclerotome and the cranial part of C2 sclerotome.

There are five centres of ossification, and after the odontoid process has chondrified its apical and central portions ossify separately. This important blunt bony finger has been the subject of much recent study (see below) and the following scheme, suggested by von Torklus and Gehle (1972) must be taken as probably including some odontoid conditions initiated by past trauma.

1. Occipital dysplasia primary malformations of occipital bone
   { Occipital vertebra
   Basilar impression
   Condylar hypoplasia
2. Malformations of atlas
   { Assimilation of atlas
   Aplasia of arch of atlas
   Clefts in arch of atlas
3. Malformations of axis
   { Atlanto-axial fusion
   Irregular segmentation of atlas and axis
   Persistent os terminale
   Os odontoideum
   Dysplasia, hypoplasia and aplasia of dens
   Spine bifida of axis
   C1–C3 fusion

Table 17.2   Structures contributed by the somites

Sclerotome	Structure
Occipital (three)	Occiput
C1 cranial	Apex of odontoid (pro-atlas)
C1 caudal }	Base of odontoid
C2 cranial }	Atlas
C2 caudal }	Atlas
C3 cranial }	Axis

Malformations may be single or multiple in the neck, and may also be part of anomalies in other body systems. Jeffreys (1980) suggests that when the practical surgeon finds one congenital defect he should be on the lookout for others.

Basilar impression

While platybasia is an anthropological term of no clinical significance (Spillane et al 1957), *basilar impression* describes upward invagination of a variable part of the bony rim of the foramen magnum. It is frequently accompanied by osseous and non-osseous anomalies of the cervical spine, and is typically part of the Klippel–Feil deformity (Truex & Johnson 1978). This complex of malformations includes occipito-atlantal assimilation, accessory occipital vertebrae, absent articular facets, hemivertebra, spina bifida, fusion of two or more cervical vertebrae and Sprengel's shoulder. Clinically, the patient appears to have no neck and presents with a cock-robin deformity of head, a low hair-line, scoliosis and very limited neck movements. The intervertebral foramina are difficult to identify on X-ray. Milder evidence of its presence, i.e. block vertebrae, usually in the upper half of the neck, is seen, although the mere presence of block vertebrae does not justify a diagnosis of Klippel–Feil syndrome. Associated skeletal and visceral abnormalities may occur. The writer recently encountered a cheerful and durable little 54-year-old lady whose transient neck discomfort was relieved by one very gentle cervical traction treatment, in the axis of the postural deformity.

There are two types of basilar impression, i.e. (i) primary basilar impression, a congenital abnormality often associated with a variety of vertebral defects (as above) and/or skeletal dysplasias such as achondroplasia, and (ii) secondary basilar impression, usually attributed to softening of the basal osseous structures, with the deformity developing later in life. It is sometimes seen in severe osteoporosis, osteomalacia, rickets, renal osteodystrophy, osteitis deformans, osteogenesis imperfecta, rheumatoid arthritis and neurofibromatosis.

Clinical presentation

Hensinger (1986) mentions that many patients with congenital basilar impression do not develop symptoms until the second or third decade of life, and symptoms are generally due to the crowding of the neural structures at the foramen magnum level, particularly the medulla oblongata.

In patients with basilar impression or occipito-atlantal fusion, the clinical findings suggest that the major neurological damage is occurring anteriorly from the odontoid. The features of pyramidal tract irritation, muscle weakness and wasting, ataxia, spasticity, hyperreflexia and pathological reflexes are commonly found. If the primary site of impingement or trespass is posterior to the rim of the foramen magnum, dural band or posterior arch of the atlas (common in odontoid anomalies) symptoms are referable to the dorsal columns, with alteration of deep pressure sensibility, vibration and proprioception.

If cerebellar herniation is present, nystagmus, ataxia and incoordination will be seen.

Symptoms consequent upon vertebral artery compression — vertigo, seizures, syncope and mental deterioration — may occur alone or in combination with the features already mentioned.

Asymmetry of the craniovertebral bony and ligamentous structures is the rule rather than the exception. Basilar impression may be sometimes slight and occasionally marked. Absolute values do not exist, and the condition may be unilateral or bilateral.

Other anomalies

Basilar impression may occur with remnants of the occipital vertebra, and is often combined with other occipito-cervical malformations, particularly with varying degrees of assimilation of atlas. Fused or separate accessory bony elements may be in apposition to or united with the edge of the foramen magnum, and scattered islets of bone may be embedded in connective tissue around the foramen magnum. A third occipital condyle may be present (Grieve 1988). The last occipital sclerotome sometimes forms a separate entity.

The various irregularities may occur together or in isolated form. Sometimes a bony arch or a complete bony tunnel (ponticulus ponticus) is formed around the vertebral artery on the superior surface of atlas. Regarded by some as negligible, it is said by others (Jeffreys 1980) to render the atheromatous vertebral artery more likely to compression during rotation of the head.

While the frequency of frank craniovertebral malformations is small, minor asymmetry is very common indeed. For example, one occipital condyle is frequently smaller than its fellow, and may project further from the basiocciput, or the two condyles may not lie in the same coronal plane (Dalseth 1974). Wood (1972) describes an atlas vertebra in which there was an absent anterior arch, a failure of the posterior arch to unite (spina bifida atlanto) (Fig. 17.2) and a bilateral costal element defect in that the foramen transversarium was just a deep notch, open anteriorly. The superior facets of atlas commonly show the same

asymmetrical disposition, as well as difference in size; the inferior facets articulating with the axis often show similar differences. Congenital atlanto-axial fusion may occur, with a separate odontoid remnant fused to the anterior arch of atlas, only revealed on clinical examination following trauma. Again, a congenitally unfused lateral mass of atlas, dysplasia of the spinous process of axis and fusion of C2–C3, described by Hirsh (1982) were found only after trauma.

While some individuals with congenital malformations of the craniovertebral region may lead a somewhat precarious existence, Weisz (1983) describes a 27-year-old female with an aplastic arch of atlas in which the posterior arch was represented only by an island of bone, i.e. the posterior tubercle (Keller's type). Following a head-on road traffic collision, in which the force of cervical injury was sufficient to produce a compression fracture of the body of C7, besides other injuries to chest and lower limbs, the ligamentous attachments at the anomalous region were strong enough to withstand the impact of flexion and extension strain.

There appeared no residual instability or other late complication seven months after the road accident.

Os odontoideum

Infrequently, there may be congenital absence of the odontoid — the lateral mass of C1 and the body of C2 retaining their normal relationships.

Both hypoplasia of the dens and true os odontoideum are not as common as was believed, most being revealed either by radiography following injury or the spontaneous onset of complaints requiring clinical analysis. Because of increased awareness, these lesions are being discerned with a frequency which belies past observations in the literature; they are also being recognized earlier, as increasing numbers of children turn up with craniovertebral defects. Hesinger et al (1978) question the 'failure of fusion' theory. While aplasia can be recognized by standard X-rays at birth, the later radiographic appearances of os odontoideum (Murray et al 1990) may be quite similar to that of traumatic non-union.

Congenital anomalies of the odontoid are uncommon. True aplasia of the odontoid, associated with complete absence of its base, is an extremely rare anomaly (Hensinger 1986).

Since (i) in the majority of patients the history reveals a significant traumatic episode, and (ii) increasingly cases are being reported (Hukuda et al 1980) as developing os odontoideum several years after trauma when the presence of a normal odontoid had been established, it appears that os odontoideum and hypoplasia are often secondary to trauma (Fig. 17.3) and more rarely to infection. The weight of evidence suggests unrecognized fracture of the odontoid base as being a cause more common than congenital malformations. The precarious blood

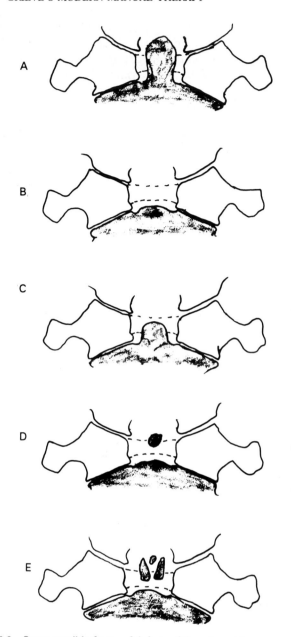

Fig. 17.3 Some possible forms of defects of the odontoid.
A. 'Normal'. **B.** Absent odontoid, which may be aplasia, which is uncommon, or secondary to trauma in childhood. **C.** Hypoplastic odontoid. **D.** Os odontoideum, in which the bony ossicle will be of varying size. **E.** Tripartite odontoid.

supply to the dens favours comparison with fracture of the carpal scaphoid (Fig. 17.4).

Murray (1988) describes traumatic displacement of an odontoid peg: that of a 2-year-old child involved in a road traffic accident while a back-seat passenger. The injury appeared to be a fracture separation of the epiphysis, and it occasioned anterior displacement of the skull and C1 on C2. Reduction in hyperextension was maintained in a Minerva plaster. He suggests that the os odontoideum seen in children may be due to a similar injury.

In passing, congenital laxity of the transverse ligament of atlas is unexpectedly common in patients with Down's syndrome (mongolism) — a reported incidence of 20% — and the defective atlanto-axial articulation constitutes a hazard if intubation for a general anaesthetic is contemplated.

While some clinicians suggest that the asymptomatic patient need not come to harm, patients with congenital or acquired odontoid defects lead a precarious life and trivial insults imposed upon already compromised structures may have disastrous consequences. Atlanto-axial instability, whether congenital or secondary to non-union of a fracture, requires surgical stabilization, since minimal trauma could lead to serious neurological insult.

Clinical features

Sensory loss is less common than weakness and ataxia, but loss of proprioception has been described, as has spasticity, exaggerated deep tendon reflexes, clonus and sphincter disturbances. Syncope, vertigo and visual disturbances, with a paucity of cervical cord signs and symptoms, may simulate vertebrobasilar ischaemia. Patients may present with no symptoms, with persistent neck complaints, with transient or permanent neurological deficits or with sudden death.

The Arnold-Chiari malformation (Schut & Bruce 1978)

A congenital elongation of the hindbrain is inevitably associated with a greater or lesser degree of hydrocephalus, bony defects such as an enlarged foramen magnum, basilar impression, assimilation of atlas and cervical spina bifida; all varying widely in form. There are anomalies of the lower cerebellum, the fourth ventricle and cervical spinal cord, with cervical nerve roots crowded down-wards and thus having to ascend to reach the foramen. Myelomeningocele is often present, with cerebellar herniation through the bony defect.

An anomalous dural band may be present, compressing the neuraxis and manifesting its presence by the clinical features of syringomyelia. Surgical decompression, repair of the spina bifida and shunting devices for hydrocephalus are the basis of treatment. While the malformation is detected early, patients with a mild degree of this complex anomaly may remain asymptomatic until later life, when they may initially present as simulated cervical spondylosis.

CERVICAL SPINE

Below C2, there may be accessory articulations of spinous processes, and marked asymmetry of the normally bifid spines very commonly occurs. Cleavage of the cervical spinous processes has been frequently described. Congenital block vertebra (synostosis) is sometimes seen at C2 and C3, and, less frequently, at any level between C2

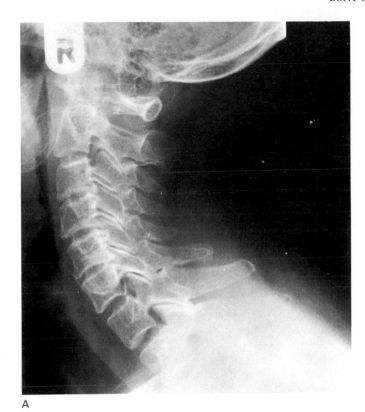
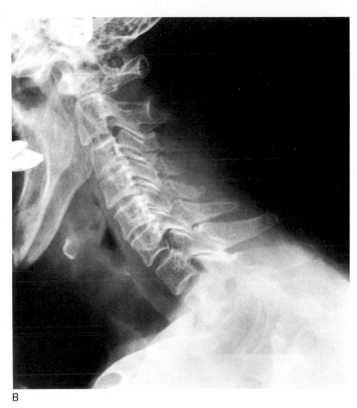

A   B

Fig. 17.4   The (**A**) neutral and (**B**) flexion films (23.9.76) of a 67-year-old lady, presenting on 22.2.80 with a history of significant trauma which included aggressive manipulation of the neck. The corticated margins of the odontoid discontinuity are plain, as is the range of sagittal movement, occurring almost entirely at the adventitious joint at the base of the odontoid. She suffers regular bouts of severe occipitofrontal pain, on one or other side.

and C7. While Lee and Weiss (1981) reviewed 13 cases of symptomatic congenital block vertebrae in the English literature, continental descriptions include others, and Keuter (1970) described a synostosis of C5–C6. All of the above 14 cases presented with the neurological symptoms of radiculopathy and/or myelopathy. The patients gave no history of trauma or of only minor trauma. Pathogenesis of symptoms was considered to be due to degenerative changes in adjacent hypermobile segments, spinal stenosis, subluxation of adjacent segments and vertebral artery occlusion.

The writer recalls two patients who, to his knowledge, have not appeared in the literature, and no doubt there are others. *While manual testing of movement will quickly detect lack of mobility at a segment, it cannot uncover the cause of that 'stiffness' with certainty, and patients may not be enthusiastic about manipulative attempts, willy nilly, to 'improve range' at such segments. Suspected ankylosis must always be approached with care and the suitability of physical methods confirmed before treatment by movement, however moderate, is employed.*

Jeffreys (1980) cautioned that synostosis may also be acquired, of course. It appears that environmental factors predisposing to the combination of cervical rheumatoid arthritis and 'block vertebra' have changed in the last 40 years (Grieve 1988).

Jeffreys also describes a spina bifida of C6, and total absence of a pedicle, unilateral pedicular defects and bilateral elongation of pedicles have also been reported. It follows that spondylolisthesis will also occur, and this is seen mostly in men.

Wilson and Norrell (1966) describe cases of congenital absence of a pedicle in the cervical spine resulting in an enlarged appearance of the IVF, which may simulate a dumbell spinal tumour (neurofibroma) or vertebral erosion.

Although bursae occur between cervical spinous processes, especially when close together, in 'normal' patients as well as those exhibiting disease processes, they are probably not congenital anomalies, although congenital malformations may initiate their development (Bywaters 1982).

Brougham et al (1989) suggest that 'sternomastoid contracture torticollis' is indeed of congenital origin and that this old hypothesis should be resurrected. They report four cases of children with torticollis secondary to congenital vertebral anomalies. Sternomastoid release considerably improved the deformity in three of them. The fourth was merely observed since the deformity was so slight.

Spinal stenosis

Since the spinal cord, its meninges and the narrow extra-

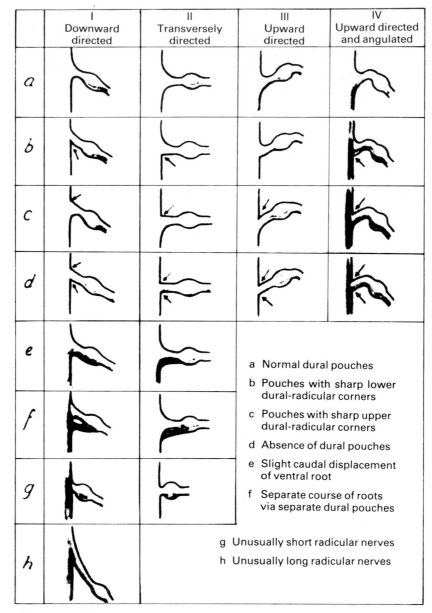

	I Downward directed	II Transversely directed	III Upward directed	IV Upward directed and angulated
a				
b				
c				
d				
e			a Normal dural pouches b Pouches with sharp lower dural-radicular corners c Pouches with sharp upper dural-radicular corners d Absence of dural pouches e Slight caudal displacement of ventral root f Separate course of roots via separate dural pouches	
f				
g				
h		g Unusually short radicular nerves h Unusually long radicular nerves		

Fig. 17.5 Different types of cervical radicular nerves observed in a long series of autopsies. Variations occur with regard to angulation and maldevelopment and/or malformation of root pouches and root sleeves. In some instances the ventral root pierces the dura at a lower level than the dorsal root. (Reproduced with permission from Frykholm 1971.)

dural space lie immediately behind the posterior longitudinal ligament, they are very easily compressed by gross bony and fibrocartilaginous projections at the level of each disc. The normal cervical vertebral canal has a sagittal diameter of about 17 mm, while that of the normal spinal cord is about 10 mm. Smaller projections are frequently present in mature people without causing serious symptoms, but a factor accentuating the likelihood of spinal cord interference is a narrow neural canal, i.e. congenital spinal stenosis, when normally insignificant backward projections at disc level may cause signs and symptoms of cord pressure reasonably associated with more marked degenerative change. These are aggravated on cervical flexion, when the length of the neural canal is increased and the neural canal contents are drawn more tightly against the prominences of degenerative, thickened tissue. The *available space* may be the decisive element in the complex of trespass by arthrotic facet joints, spondylotic spurring with osteocartilaginous bosses or bars, congenital stenosis of the spinal canal and neurological disturbances. The condition occurs in males and initially may be diagnosed as multiple sclerosis.

Anomalies of innervation

The only muscles which retain a truly segmental arrangement, and innervation, are the *intercostals*. Elsewhere in the neck, limbs and trunk each muscle is innervated by spinal cord anterior neurons which spread across two, three or more segments (Sunderland 1978).

The textbook patterns of root and plexus formation, and innervation of peripheral tissues, are subject to variation in a significant proportion of cases.

Patterns of root innervation of muscles are also subject to variations from orthodox tabulations.

Brendler (1968) electrically stimulated 56 anterior cervical roots, at open operation, in 32 patients, and examples of the pattern of innervation, on the basis of motor responses, were:

Trapezius supplied by C1, 2, 3 and 4
Deltoid supplied by C3, 4, 5, 6 and 7.

The range of the segmental contributions to the brachial plexus is not uniform, it varies from person to person and between the two sides of one individual. About 11% of brachial plexuses are prefixed, that is, receive a major contribution from the C4 root at the expense of the lower roots of the plexus, and a similar percentage are postfixed, receiving a major contribution from the T1 root with the T2 contribution always present and a very small or entirely absent contribution from C4. Frykholm (1971) has drawn attention to the wide variations of cervical root formation; in some instances the ventral root pierces the dura at a lower level than the dorsal root. He observes that nature seldom provides a completely perfect anatomy from all functional points of view, except to a small privileged group of individuals. Even in young people there are many cases of malformed root pouches, occasionally together with radicular nerves sharply angulated upwards, or nerves eccentrically located in the intervertebral foramen (Fig. 17.5).

Variations in spinal rootlet formation, roots of the plexus, distribution of the roots within trunks and cords and innervation of peripheral structures should be borne in mind, e.g. anomalous innervation of the hand occurs in at least 20% of the population. The cutaneous supply of the little finger may be derived from the sixth sensory root, for example.

Anomalies of vessels

One essential and important feature underlying clinical expression of cervical degenerative change is the great variability of the vertebrobasilar vascular system; the way patients present often depends very largely on the hand of cards nature has dealt them by way of arrangement of the intrinsic and extrinsic spinal cord blood supply. In less than 20% of individuals are the vertebral arteries of equal size.

Irritation, compression or distortion of the larger of the two vessels will be likely to have more serious effects than interference with the vessel of smaller lumen. The left artery is larger than the right in over half of the specimens examined, which may explain the greater frequency of left-sided arterial involvement.

Unilateral and even bilateral aplasia of the vertebral arteries have been described.

Variations from standard descriptions of spinal cord blood supply are so common that it is hardly possible to say what is normal. 'Segmental branches from the vertebral and cervical arteries are also subject to wide variation in number and level. There may be none, there may be paired branches at each segment' (Jeffreys 1980).

Dommisse (1980) differentiates clearly between anterior medullary feeders and the radicular branches, the latter being constant and contributing to the anastomosis on the surface of the spinal cord, while branches to the anterior spinal artery, and thus the intrinsic supply of the cord, are inconstant and irregular.

The arteries on the cord surfaces are largely immune to atheromatous changes, but this complex and *highly variable* system of spinal cord supply is especially subject to remote effects by pressure, e.g. the radicular arteries are at hazard as they traverse the intervertebral foramina with the cervical nerve roots, and despite a certain degree of collateral supply, the vertebral artery itself is subject to compression, producing a pattern of cord and nerve root ischaemia with signs and symptoms *which will depend upon the pattern of supply in particular cases*. When the ischaemia is due to vessel constriction a few segments removed, the cord areas most likely to suffer are those lying more centrally, the 'watershed areas' (Fig. 17.6) at the boundary of adjacent territories of supply of two end-artery systems.

The final intrinsic distribution of spinal cord arterial supply accounts for many discrepancies in the level of the

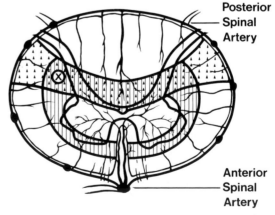

Fig. 17.6 Scheme of upper cervical cord. 'Watershed' areas between territory supplied by: ▲—anterior and posterior spinal arteries; ‖‖—peripheral and central arterial supply; ⊗—area occupied by the spinal tract of the 5th cranial nerve. (After Keuter 1970.)

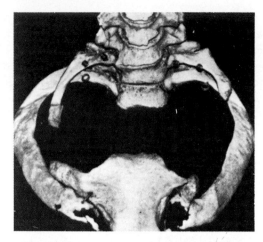

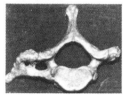 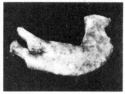

Fig. 17.7 (**Top**) Bilateral, incomplete, asymmetrical cervical ribs. The anterior end of each is represented by the spike of bone on either side of the manubrium. In life, a ligament connected the two parts of the supernumerary ribs. (**Lower left**) An anomalous first rib is fused with the first thoracic vertebra. (**Lower right**) A cervical rib is fused with the first thoracic rib to give a double-headed rib. (Reproduced from Sunderland 1978, by courtesy of author and publisher.)

lesion relative to the cause, such that arterial trespass at the level of the foramen magnum can restrict downward flow in the anterior spinal artery and cause wasting of the hands, for example (Editorial 1967).

CERVICOTHORACIC REGION

Lower in the cervical column, the foramen transversarium may be incomplete, subdivided or imperforate, and cervical ribs may be present unilaterally, or bilaterally in various forms (Fig. 17.7). A separate centre of ossification may appear as the costal element of C7 vertebra, and produce variations from an enlarged and beaked transverse process to a fully developed and sometimes quite long rib. Sometimes the tip of an incomplete cervical rib meets and articulates with the superior surface of the first rib.

A unilateral anomalous joint may be present in a normally situated first rib.

The incidence of cervical rib appears much greater than the incidence of vascular and neurological symptoms arising from its presence. The not uncommon presence of a cervical rib accords with C7 being a transitional vertebra, in that its spinous process is not bifid and is long, often longer than the spine of T1, so becoming the true 'vertebra prominens' in those cases. C7 normally lacks a foramen transversarium, and if one is present it is rarely traversed by the vertebral artery.

Supernumary fascial bands may trespass on the neurovascular bundle. A fibrous band embodied in the scalenus medius, between C7 transverse process and the first rib, frequently produces nerve trespass, the symptoms of which are often markedly relieved by division of the band. Variations in a normally situated first rib and anomalies of the scalene muscles (scalenus minimus) are common.

Sunderland (1978) clarifies the many anatomical variations at the thoracic outlet which, singly or together, may compromise normal function of the lower trunk of the brachial plexus and/or the subclavian artery. He mentions a more oblique first rib, variations in scalenus anterior muscle attachment of 2.5–6 cm from the costosternal junction, variations in the scalenus minimus and its tendon on the inner margin of the rib, a falciform connective tissue margin between scalenus anterior and medius, and variations in the attachment of Sibson's fascia (the suprapleural membrane) with narrow thickenings or ligamentous bands in the fascia. Anomalies of this junctional area attract considerable attention and much description, yet the volume of interest in anomalies is inversely proportional to clinical usefulness, in terms of revealing indications of conservative treatment for symptoms ascribed to the thoracic outlet. While not forgetting the importance of radiotranslucent fibrous bands and other soft tissue abnormalities, armies of people exhibit obvious bony anomalies on X-ray yet are sign- and symptom-free (Grieve 1988).

A puzzling feature is that sometimes gross skeletal anomalies are not necessarily associated with neurological symptoms and signs. Our understanding of symptom-causation, in this group of patients, is minimal — an island of certainty in a sea of hypothesis — '... much needs to be learnt of the dynamics and mechanics of the bones and joints and the related neural tissues and vessels' (Brain & Wilkinson 1967).

On those comparatively few occasions when the patient's distress warrants surgical attention, a surgeon (Colin 1985) comments '... one does not invariably visualize the precise nature of trespass or impingement which can reasonably be associated with the clinical features. In fact, one rarely does so.' This underlies a further comment, that resection of the first rib not only relieves such compression/trespass as might have been present, it forthwith removes some or most of the evidence, besides modifying all normal musculoskeletal strains and tensions in that district.

Wood et al (1988) mention that the thoracic outlet syndrome is incompletely understood, difficult to diagnose and often poorly managed. Some clinicians doubt the existence of the syndrome.

The very multiplicity of synonyms speaks for itself:

Shoulder–hand syndrome
Cervical rib syndrome
Scalenus anticus syndrome

Costoclavicular syndrome
Hyperabduction syndrome
Pneumatic hammer syndrome
Fractured clavicle syndrome
Effort vein thrombosis
Pectoralis minor syndrome
Subcoracoid syndrome
First thoracic rib syndrome
Brachiocephalic syndrome
Humeral head syndrome
Nocturnal paraesthetic brachialgia
Cervicobrachial neurovascular compression syndrome
Rucksack paralysis
Cervicothoracic outlet syndrome
Syndrome of the scalenus medius band

Telford and Mottershead (1947) showed, some 47 years ago, that costoclavicular compression of the neuro-muscular bundle does not occur, yet this myth continues to be perpetuated in text after text. Of the 12% of patients *who undergo surgery* for thoracic outlet syndrome, a large proportion exhibit congenital fibromuscular bands between transverse processes and the first rib (Wood et al 1988). It would be interesting to determine how many asymptomatic individuals also exhibit these anomalous bands, since resection of the first rib represents a clean sweep of the entire thoracic outlet, and ascribing subsequent relief of signs and symptoms (when achieved) to this or that factor becomes no more than a matter of opinion. Nevertheless, an awareness of the possible involvement of anomalous bands in symptom production, and of their variety, is necessary.

Roos (1979) described nine categories, illustrated by Wood et al (1988) of fibrous or fibromuscular bands in *patients who came to operation* (Figs 17.8–17.16).

Mapstone and Spetzler (1982) reported a case in which an anomalous fibrous band occluded the vertebral artery,

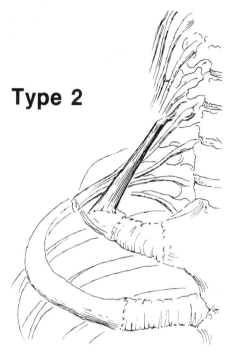

Fig. 17.9 A band similar to the above, but attached superiorly to an abnormally elongated transverse process.

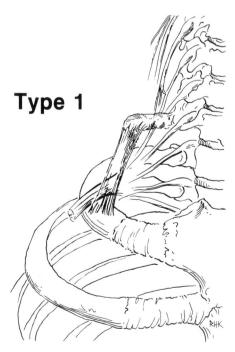

Fig. 17.8 A taut ligamentous band from a rudimentary cervical rib, attaching distally just posterior to the scalene tubercle of the first rib.

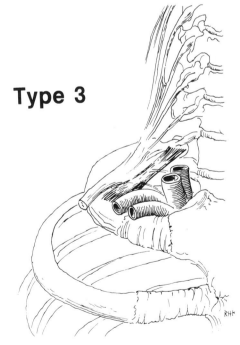

Fig. 17.10 A taut, sharp-edged, fibromuscular structure, stretching from the neck of the first rib across the outlet, to an attachment between the T1 root of the brachial plexus and the subclavian artery. This was the commonest anomaly seen.

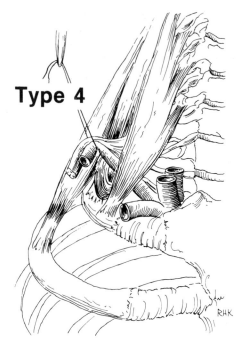

Fig. 17.11 A fibrous string-like structure looping under the plexus and subclavian artery, arising behind from the scalenus medius and attaching anteriory to the tendon of scalenus anterior.

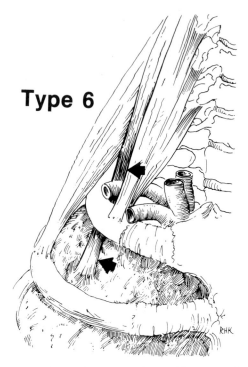

Fig. 17.13 A scalenus minimus muscle attaching not to the first rib but to Sibson's fascia (the suprapleural membrane). It may survive first rib section.

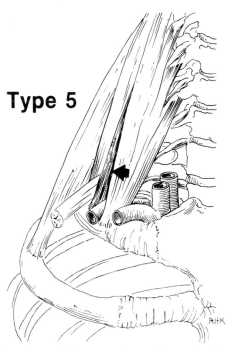

Fig. 17.12 A scalenus minimus muscle attaching to the first rib between the brachial plexus and the subclavian artery.

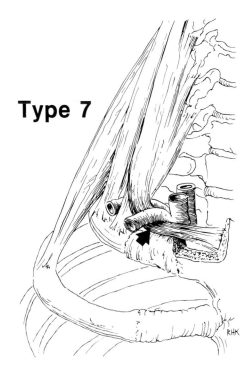

Fig. 17.14 A fibrous band, passing from the anterior surface of the scalenus anterior and under the subclavian vein to attach to the posterior surface of the sternum.

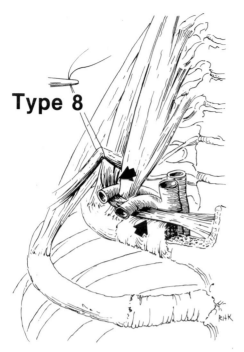

Fig. 17.15 A similar band to that depicted in Figure 17.14, arising from the anterior surface of scalenus medius and passing under the whole neurovascular bundle.

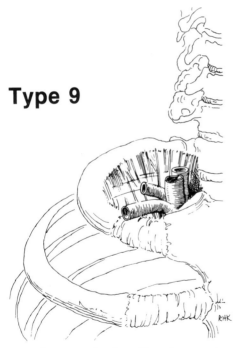

Fig. 17.16 A taut fibromuscular sheet filling the posterior concavity of the first rib. (Figures 17.8–17.16 reproduced with permission from Wood et al 1988.)

2 cm from its origin, on right head rotation. Division of the band relieved the vertigo and syncope which accompanied that movement.

Minor degrees of congenital and developmental anomalies, of bone and soft tissues of the *shoulder girdle*, may confuse examination findings when assessing joint problems of the cervicothoracic district (Samilson 1980).

Nerve roots

Besides common malformations of nerve root pouches and root sleeves which occur here as in typical cervical segments, the nerve root bundle may undergo two quite marked angulations, downward when piercing the dura and then upwards to the foramen, before emerging from it, and there is considerable variation between individuals (Nathan & Feuerstein 1970).

THORACIC REGION

Para-articular processes, as bony spicules or spurs, almost exclusively in the thoracic spine, are present on the inner surfaces of the laminae very close to the articular processes (Nathan 1959).

While not strictly anomalous, since they are found in one or more vertebrae of some 75% of all skeletons studied, their number and configuration vary quite considerably, and irregular spicules from adjacent vertebrae may almost meet to form an incomplete bony bridge in front of the apophyseal joints.

They may have some clinical significance as a factor in spinal nerve root irritation and/or compression. Developmental stenosis of a thoracic vertebra is not unknown, and in one patient severe thickening of T9 laminae was responsible for spastic paralysis of lower limbs. Congenital synostosis is occasionally seen in the thoracic spine, as a partial or complete fusion of two segments.

'Butterfly vertebra', and congenital wedge vertebra with failure of development of the anterior nucleus, may also be encountered. The latter produces a prominent postural kyphosis or gibbus, and if several vertebrae are involved an anterior deficiency of discs allows bony fusion to occur. Anomalies may be multiple, e.g. 'butterfly' vertebrae from T7–T10, together with fusion of T10–T11, without marked scoliosis.

Hemivertebra may occur at any level; in the thoracic spine a marked form of congenital scoliosis is produced. There is an extra rib on the side involved and also anomalies of ribs in that adjacent ones are fused.

Thoracic spinous processes are frequently asymmetrical, and the tips of one or more may be congenitally deviated from the midline by as much as 0.5 cm. The sternal end of the 3rd or 4th rib and its cartilage is sometimes bifid. The lowest cartilage to reach the sternum may be the 6th, 7th or 8th, therefore ribs should be counted from above downwards by their prominent angles.

Patients with congenital spinal malformations have a very high incidence of associated visceral abnormalities; frequently, cardiac and renal abnormalities occur, and there may be congenital malformations of the gastrointestinal and respiratory systems.

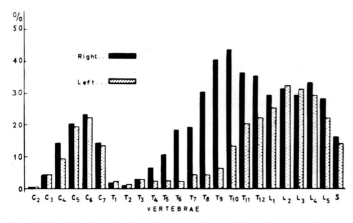

Fig. 17.17 The singular fact that osteophytes of the thoracic spine are predominantly right-sided probably underlies the predominantly right-sided referred pain of spinal origin. (Reproduced from Nathan 1962, by courtesy of author and publisher.)

In this respect, familiarity with spondylothoracic dysplasia (Herold et al 1988) and its course should prevent unjustifiably pessimistic prognoses.

Abdominal pain of spinal origin, frequently right-sided and preponderately in women (see Ch. 29) is probably due to the predominance of right-sided osteophytosis in the thoracic spine (Fig. 17.17), by reason of aortic pulsation inhibiting their development on the left side. Where the aorta descends on the right side, osteophytes will be more prominent on the left (Nathan & Schwartz 1962).

THORACOLUMBAR JUNCTION

An extra rib may attach to the 1st lumbar vertebra, and an incidence of 7.75% has been described (Schmorl & Junghanns 1971).

The lumbar rib is the most common variant at the thoracolumbar transition, is two or three times more common in men and has to be distinguished, on X-ray, from fracture of a lumbar transverse process. A large transverse process may be seen without formation of a rib. There is some variation in the segmental level at which transition from thoracic to lumbar-characteristics appears, and it may occur at segments T10–T11 or T11–12 or T12–L1 (Struthers 1875). The transition is most marked by a singular configuration of articular processes of one vertebra (Fig. 17.18) which has the effect of forming with the subjacent vertebra a mortise and tenon joint when under compression or extension.

The transitional vertebra is thoracic in type in its upper half, i.e. the superior facets face backwards, upwards and a little outwards, and begins to show lumbar characteristics in its lower half, i.e. the inferior articular processes begin to turn laterally, with facets slightly convex from side to side and facing laterally and forwards (Fig. 17.19). On extension, the lower facets of the transitional vertebra lock into the upper facets of the uppermost 'lumbar-type'

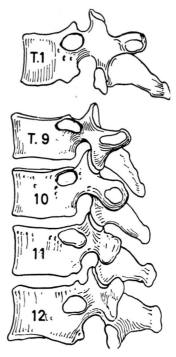

Fig. 17.18 The thoracolumbar mortise joint, in this case at T12, since the upper facet-planes of that vertebra face a little outward (thoracic characteristics) and the lower facet-planes also face outward (lumbar characteristics). See text. (Reproduced from Ellis & Feldman 1977, by courtesy of authors and publisher.)

vertebra, and no movement other than flexion is then possible.

In a series of 67 adult columns (Davis 1955) the site of the mortise joint was variously at:

T10–11	5 columns
T11–12	46 columns
T12–L1	16 columns
	67 columns

There may also be variations of articular facet-plane orientation between sides of the same vertebra, in that at one segment there exists a 'thoracic' position on one side and a 'lumbar' position on the opposite side. The importance of this characteristic is that if manual techniques of any

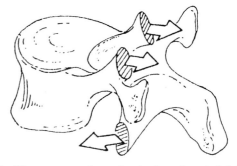

Fig. 17.19 The upper two facets face backwards and slightly outwards; the lower two facets face forward and outwards.

vigour are applied with the intention of mobilizing this junction when in extension, they will certainly be fruitless, probably painful, and if over-vigorous may even do the patient harm.

Macalister (1889) observed that the thoracolumbar junction was the point most exposed to injury.

LUMBAR AND LUMBOSACRAL

In general terms, congenital malformations of weight-bearing bones might be expected to produce wear and tear, and thus symptoms, earlier than would normal structures subjected to the same stress; this follows at times, yet as has been mentioned, many patients without symptoms exhibit a variety of skeletal abnormalities.

Asymmetry of the posterior lumbar and lumbosacral joints occurs to a varying degree in approximately one-quarter of human spines. A review (Epstein, 1976) of a long series of spinal studies in patients admitted for conditions other than back pain showed that many normal individuals have minor congenital variations at the lumbosacral junction. In a series of 3000 pre-employment X-ray examinations of the lumbosacral region over a 2-year period, a large number of asymptomatic conditions, including degenerative processes and developmental anomalies, were encountered. This part of the axial skel-

eton tends also to abnormalities of segmentation like the lumbarized first sacral segment or the sacralized fifth lumbar vertebra, which may be either partially or completely fused to the sacrum. Taylor et al (1989) studied the role of transitional vertebrae in intervertebral disc degeneration and prolapse. Four populations were investigated: 100 asymptomatic controls (group A); 142 patients with uncomplicated dorsolumbar fractures (group B); 200 patients with chronic low-back pain of more than two months' duration (group C) and 230 patients with surgically proven lumbar disc prolapse (group D). The incidence of transitional vertebrae was found to be similar in groups A, B and D, but significantly increased in group C. Narrowing of the last mobile disc in the presence of a transitional vertebra was evident in 42% of those with the anomaly in group C but only 6% of those in group A.

The age of onset of chronic low-back pain and disc prolapse was earlier in those with a transitional vertebra than in those without this structural anomaly. Also, in the presence of the anomaly, the usual distribution of prolapses at the last two interspaces was reversed. The authors concluded that transitional morphological changes predispose to disc degeneration and prolapse. Two factors might possibly be implicated in pathogenesis, (i) minor mechanical factors associated with transitional vertebra,

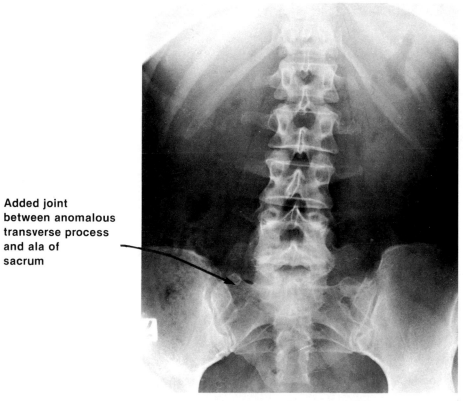

Added joint between anomalous transverse process and ala of sacrum

Fig. 17.20   The fifth lumbar vertebra is transitional and there is an adventitious joint between transverse process and sacral ala on the right side. The third lumbar spinous process is anomalous and the twelfth ribs are unusually long. This patient has a lateral pelvis tilt, up on the left, the side of her chronic low-back pain.

and (ii) the possibility of associated defective disc development, i.e. anomalies of the disc too.

MacLean et al (1990) reviewed the pre-operative lumbar spine radiographs of 200 consecutive patients who had undergone discectomy for prolapsed intervertebral disc. Measurement of the lumbar level of the interiliac line was shown to correlate with the level of disc prolapse, and the incidence of transitional vertebrae at the lumbosacral junction was significantly higher than normal. A pathological value for the lumbosacral angle could not be determined. A deep-seated L5 was associated with a higher likelihood of disc prolapse at L4/5, whereas a high-riding L5 was associated with a prolapse at L5/S1; both of these associations were highly significant (P < 0.005).

The incidence of lumbosacral transitional vertebrae in this series was compared with that observed in a population who had never been admitted to hospital for backache. The authors found a significantly higher incidence (P < 0.005) of such bony anomalies than was reported by Tini et al (1977).

Using established diagnostic criteria, the authors demonstrated a significantly increased incidence of lumbosacral transitional anomalies in patients with disc prolapse.

The large 'transverse process' of a transitional and partially sacralized L5 may form an anomalous adventitious joint (Fig. 17.20) with the ala of the sacrum on that side, the joint being subject to degenerative change like any other and perhaps more so because of the malformation. In at least two of the author's patients, mobilizing techniques for intractable backache were unavailing until movement was specifically localized to affect the adventitious joint.

Conversely, a 35-year-old lady, with a right-sided transitional L5, forming an adventitious joint with the right ala of the sacrum, required treatment for a typical left-sided disc protrusion at the L4–5 level. This combination, of anomaly on one side and clinical features on the opposite side from an adjacent segment, is common.

Hanraets (1959) regarded congenital lumbar anomalies as important in laying the groundwork for subsequent mechanical trouble. A further example of the association of an apparently asymptomatic malformation, with a second anomaly of another segment which is responsible for the clinical features, is illustrated in Figure 17.21. This patient's symptoms were relieved by mobilization localized (so far as is possible) to the left L4–L5 segment, since the lumbosacral segment appeared blameless. This not unusual circumstance may be a factor underlying the variability of opinion on the significance of skeletal anomalies.

Many with sciatica do not have a transitional L5, as many with this anomaly do not have sciatica (Grieve 1988): hence the phrase 'Bertolotti's syndrome' (sciatica associated with sacralization of the 5th lumbar vertebra) identifies only a likelihood rather than a causal link.

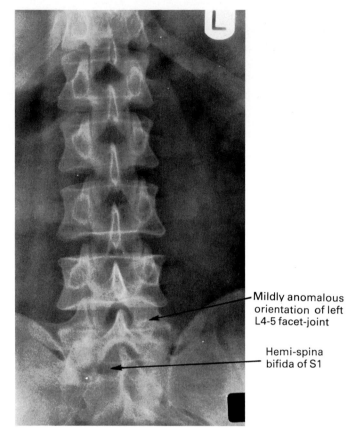

Mildly anomalous orientation of left L4-5 facet-joint

Hemi-spina bifida of S1

Fig. 17.21 A–p view of a mildly anomalous left L4–5 facet-joint and a hemi-spina bifida of Sl.

Employing CT scans and X-rays, Elster (1990) reviewed the incidence and type of pathology such as stenosis, disc protrusion and spondylolysis occurring in spines exhibiting transitional vertebrae. In these, the location of pathological change was much more commonly at the segment proximal to the transitional vertebra. This was said to indicate a mechanism of stress at the level above, leading to hypermobility and predisposing this segment to early degenerative changes of one kind or another, as has already been described. Experience teaches the worth of a clinical rule of thumb — when one anomaly is found, be on the lookout for others. In assessing a possible causal relationship between anomalies and symptoms, the issue may be clouded if only manifest or single anomalies are considered.

Rasool et al (1990) reported a series of 15 children presenting with foot deformities; each exhibited deformities of the spine, detectable clinically and radiologically. There was spina bifida occulta in 10, congenital kyphosis in three and sacral agenesis in two. Midline dorsal cutaneous lesions were noted in 10. The authors suggest that children with foot deformities and gait disorders should have careful clinical and radiological assessment of the spine, and they mention the importance of midline cutaneous abnormalities, since CT scanning and other imaging tech-

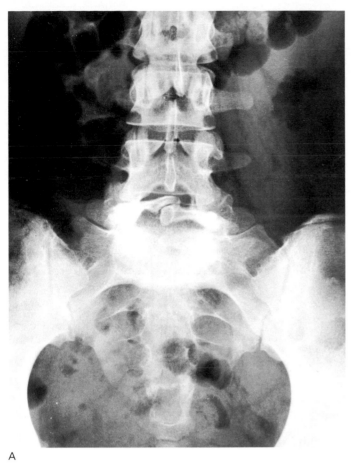
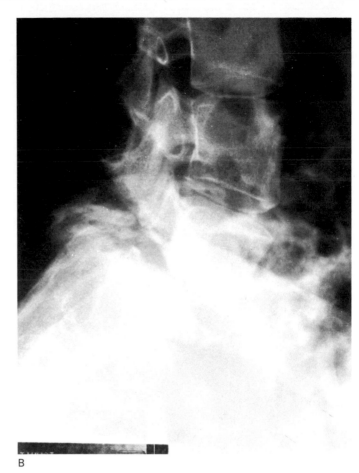

A   B

Fig. 17.22   A. The neural arch of this young female's fifth lumbar vertebra is anomalous, as is the left L4–5 facet joint, and the mid-line density overlying the S1 segment suggests spondylolisthesis. **B.** The lateral film of the same patient. Anomaly of neural arch of L5, discontinuity of the pars interarticularis and a first to second degree spondylolisthesis are plain.

niques might reveal diastematomyelia, cord tethering (James & Lassman 1972), thickened filum terminale and intraspinal lipoma.

Dysplasia of the pars interarticularis of L5 is frequently reported. These structural anomalies are often well tolerated until the additional insult of degenerative spondylosis is added to further narrow the lumbar canal. Surgical decompression may then be required. One lumbar facet-plane may be sagittally orientated, and its opposite fellow of the same segment be disposed with a slightly coronal angulation. In the segments above and below, similar asymmetry may be present, but with the sides reversed. Where evident, this alternating tropism occurs almost always as a variant in the lower half of the lumbar region. A single facet on one side may be angulated downwards and inwards, while remaining sagittal in general disposition.

Farfan (1973) draws attention to the potency of rotation strains in initiating the degenerative process, particularly on the side of the more oblique facet in asymmetrical joints, yet the shape and orientation of lumbosacral facet-planes seem to have no effect on the symmetry of *gross* lumbar rotation (Lumsden & Morris 1968). Where asymmetry exists with one joint disposed in the coronal plane

and the other more sagittally, naturally symmetrical *regional* movements of the back and pelvis may tend to exert asymmetrical forces at this segment.

Congenital absence of a pedicle, accessory laminae, osseous bridging of transverse processes, dysplasia or absence of spinous processes, clefts in pedicles of L3 and L4 and block vertebrae at L3–L4 have been reported. Incomplete segmentation, involving two or more vertebrae, may occur at multiple and separate sites in the same individual. In some cases, fused vertebrae may predispose to disc derangement in the next cranial segment and possible early apophyseal joint changes in the distal segment.

A trapezoidal-shaped fifth lumbar vertebral body may be present, albeit this does not always induce the expected mild degree of lumbar scoliosis (Grieve 1988).

The facet-planes of the lumbosacral joint frequently vary between sides, and there is also a wide variation between individuals, but excessive wear and tear with an increased likelihood of low back pain does not necessarily follow as a consequence. There are many causes for *spondylolisthesis*, and the general factor of mechanical weakness predisposes to the forward slip (Fig. 17.22).

The resisting bony mechanism can be upset, among

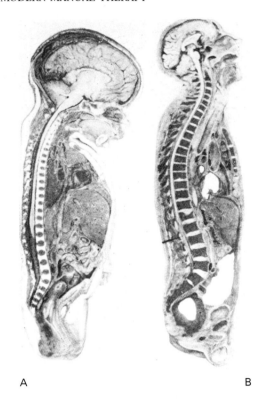

other causes, by congenital aplasia of the superior facets of the sacrum. Since the lumbosacral lordosis is present at birth (Fig. 17.23) 'abnormalities' of sacral disposition are sometimes considered, together with 'abnormalities' of sagittal spinal curvature, as conducive to joint conditions of spine, pelvic girdle and hips.

While the more horizontal sacrum would, of course, accentuate a tendency to spondylolisthesis, Schmorl and Junghanns (1971) suggest that critical evaluation of all investigative results makes it difficult to diagnose an 'abnormal' lumbosacral angle and it is even more difficult to consider it as a cause of pain (Fig. 17.24).

Spinal stenosis

Developmental reduction of the dimensions of the lumbar vertebral canal, with altered configurations of the verte-

Fig. 17.23   A. Median section of new-born child. **B.** Median section of adult. The normal lumbosacral lordosis is present in both. (Reproduced from Nassim R, Jackson Burrows H (eds) 1959 Modern advances in diseases of the vertebral column. Butterworth, London, by courtesy of Professor Walmsley and the publisher.)

A   B

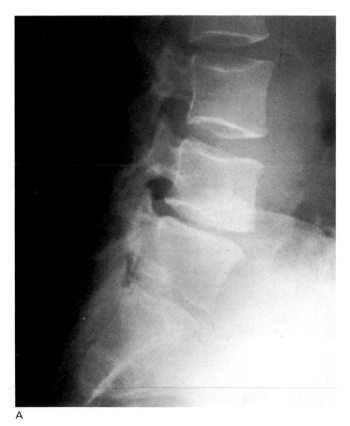

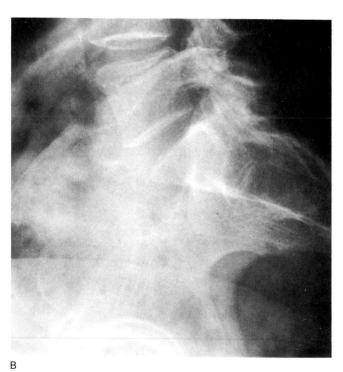

A   B

Fig. 17.24   A. The sacrum is orientated more vertically than 'normal'. Same patient as in Figure 17.9, yet it is not possible to say whether this type of sacral orientation contributed to her pain. **B.** The sacrum is more horizontal than 'normal' in this patient without low-back pain.

brae, has increasingly been recognized over the last three decades as a cause of bilateral sciatic pain, although the first account of clinical effects appeared in 1900 (Sachs & Fraenkel).

In stenotic lumbar spines the cauda equina is very frequently compressed by a degree of degenerative trespass which could easily be accommodated without symptoms by a normally roomy vertebral canal. All forms of stenosis show consistent abnormalities on a plan view of the vertebra: smaller interfacetal distance, shorter pedicles, reduced dorsoventral diameter and shallowness of the lateral recess.

The lateral recess, bounded by the medial portion of the superior articular facet and the lamina above, by the pedicle laterally and by the vertebral body, its superior lip and the adjacent disc below, contains the nerve root and it is in this limited space that the root is most vulnerable to compression.

Spinal stenosis, and anomalous lumbar and lumbo-sacral nerve root and plexus formations, are considered in much greater detail in the author's text *Common Vertebral Joint Problems* (2nd edn, 1988, Churchill Livingstone, Edinburgh).

Nerve roots

Intersegmental anastomoses between dorsal roots, uncommon in the thoracic region, are seen more frequently in the cervical (Jackson 1977) and lumbosacral regions (Pallie & Manuel 1968); no doubt these contribute to the difficulty of localizing the segmental level of root

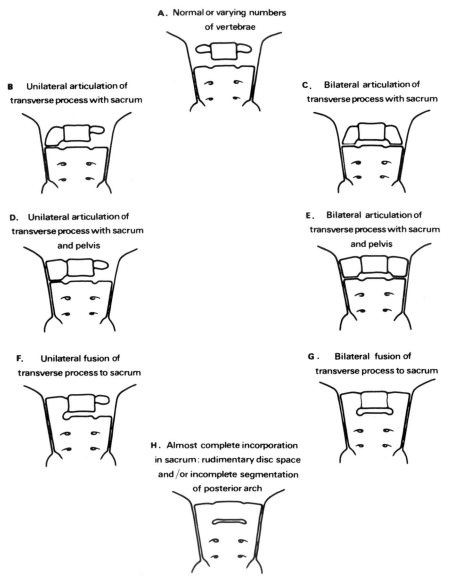

Fig. 17.25 A summary of lumbosacral segmental anomalies. (Reproduced from McCulloch & Waddell 1980, by permission of authors and publisher.)

involvement on the basis of root distribution (Lansche & Ford 1960).

Abnormal variations of lumbosacral root and plexus formation have been reported (Keon-Cohen 1968).

Hanraets (1959) described the wide dural sac, an arachnoid diverticulum, a dural diverticulum, nerve root anomalies in the form of membrana reuniens persistens, asymmetrical arrangement of nerve roots and other malformations, including anomalies of the ganglia. Agnoli (1976) reported on 20 personal observations and analysed 18 cases from the literature. The most frequent anomalies were the common dural origin of two nerve roots and the common exit of two roots via one foramen. Inter-radicular connections, and Y-shaped or horizontally disposed nerve roots, were seen in 9 of the 20, and 6 of the 18; operation revealed only the anomalies, although the history and clinical findings suggested prolapsed intervertebral disc. Decompression produced positive results.

Assessing the segmental level of nerve root involvement, on the basis of distribution of neurological symptoms and signs, may be more difficult when patients exhibit lumbar transitional vertebrae.

Following dissection of the lumbosacral plexus in 11 cadavers with lumbosacral segmental anomalies (Fig. 17.25), and electrical stimulation studies in 15 patients with the same anomalies, McCulloch and Waddell (1980) suggest that, whatever the anomaly, the 'last fully mobile level' should be identified as the most caudal one with a fully formed disc space, bilateral facet joints and two free transverse processes which have no bony articulation with any pelvic structure.

In three out of four patients with the anomalies described, the fifth lumbar nerve root emerged at the last fully mobile level (Fig. 17.26).

Wigh (1980) makes a plea for recognition of phylogenetic categories of the spine and for junctional transitional vertebrae to be properly identified and localized. Mentioning the '. . . assumption so frequently made, that all spines are in the normal mode . . .' he reports a clinical audit, involving 100 patients surgically treated for herniated lumbar disc. Speciality staff made a large number of nomenclature errors, and several laminectomies were performed at the incorrect level.

All the surgical errors occurred in those patients who had phyletic deviants, junctional bony anomalies or both, totalling 33% of the patients.

No mention was made of concomitant anomalies of lumbosacral plexus formation, which is an added source of difficulty, of course. Sixteen cases of lumbar nerve root anomalies, found at surgery, were reviewed by Neidre and Macnab (1983). All of the patients presented with radicular pain of sciatic distribution.

The authors suggest the classification:

Type I   includes those of conjoined roots, with two roots arising from a common dural sheath

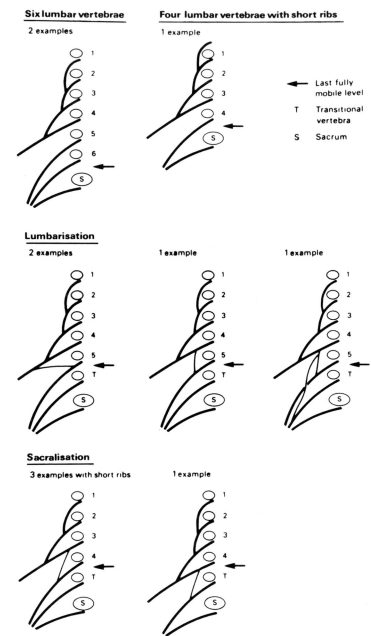

Fig. 17.26 Dissections of the lumbosacral plexus in 11 cadavers with bony lumbosacral anomalies. Key at top right of Figure. (Reproduced from McCulloch & Waddell 1980, by permission of authors and publisher.)

Type II   where two roots exit from one foramen. This may leave one root canal unoccupied, or there may be nerve roots in all foramina, one of which contains two roots

Type III   where adjacent roots are connected by an anastomotic root

Type IV   in which characteristics of types II and III are combined

and further suggest that nerve root anomalies may be found more frequently; their presence should be suspected in all cases of failed disc surgery.

Hasue et al (1983) observe that the course of a nerve root may be abnormal (i) because of a congenital deviant in the root structure, or (ii) by acquired lesions of the surrounding tissues. Anomalies of the root itself and/or other structures in the vicinity may cause radicular symptoms and signs on their own account, in addition to the effects of acquired changes. Such anomalies may also make surgical procedures more difficult. In cadavers the authors found root anomalies more frequently than expected, and they suggest that wide laminectomies for lumbar spinal stenosis might demonstrate more examples of these congenitally deviant root formations.

Connective tissue

Transforaminal ligaments (Golub & Silverman 1969) may be present. The writer recalls a patient in whom all the clinical features of discogenic lumbosacral root trespass were simulated by foraminal stenosis due to ligamentous tissue — surgery revealed that the associated intervertebral disc was innocent. Division of the anomalous band relieved the signs and symptoms.

The frequency of anomalous fibrous bands might be higher than estimated, since many soft-tissue anomalies would escape radiological detection.

The lumbosacral ligament is inconstant. Considerable variation in size and strength of this structure which, when present, helps to form an osseo-fibrous tunnel for the L5 nerve root on the ala of the sacrum, may be a factor in L5 root compression. Nathan's (1982) study of 42 lumbosacral specimens, in 26 cadavers, revealed that in some cases L5 root was flattened against the sacral ala by compressive tightness of the lumbosacral ligament. A sympathetic ramus communicans, often thicker than the sympathetic trunk, penetrates and then runs beneath the ligament, and may also be involved in compressive effects together with the root it supplies.

Spinal dysraphism

Sagittal clefts in the vertebral arches — bifid spines — are common. The vertebral anomaly, in its mildest form, is a lack of fusion of the neural arches in one or several vertebrae. The most frequent location is the fifth lumbar neural arch, and next the first sacral segment; the existence of both lesions is not rare, being a common and usually symptomless malformation. Spina magna, a much enlarged process of L5 coexisting with spina bifida of S1, may also occur (Tulsi 1974).

Abnormal splitting of the notochord can involve the central nervous system, the axial skeleton, the skin and the viscera (Sandifer 1967). The spinal abnormalities resulting from incomplete closure of a split notochord can cover a wide range from slight widening of the vertebra to a complete anterior and posterior bifida (Fig. 17.27).

At birth, occult forms of spinal dysraphism are not usually evident, and spinal cord function may not be impaired. As growth continues, occasionally the dysraphic defect begins to prevent the naturally changing relationships of spinal cord segments and vertebral segments. *The symptoms of spinal dysraphism may be delayed*, because the neurological signs vary in severity. They are often diffuse

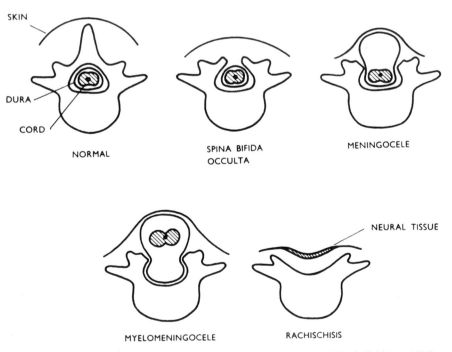

Fig. 17.27 Various forms of spinal dysraphism. (Reproduced from Ellis & Feldman 1977, by courtesy of authors and publisher.)

and complex, and difficult to interpret (James & Lassman 1972).

The spinal cord or cauda equina may be unable to 'ascend' relative to the vertebral segments during growth, and the tethering lesions may be of various kinds, including a tight filum terminale. Young people may complain of back and other spinal problems during the adolescent growth spurt (girls 12–14 years; boys 14–16 years) and the presence of mild bilateral pes cavus, shortening of the tendocalcaneous and a history of enuresis as a child, without a clear history of any neurological disease, should raise the suspicion of dysraphism as the root cause of the patient's difficulties.

Anterior spina bifida ('butterfly vertebra') is an uncommon deformity due to persistent remnants of the fetal notochord and is usually without clinical significance.

Calcification of the iliolumbar ligament is occasionally seen.

THE PELVIS

Asymmetrical sacral facet planes have been mentioned above. The sacrum may sometimes develop with its upper surface higher on one side than the other, and this can give rise to a degree of lumbar scoliosis, although not evident in every individual with the anomaly. The sacral alae may vary in height, and the sacrum is frequently asymmetrical between sides.

Of 30 sacra, Solonen (1957) found variations in width of the lateral part in 25 cases; the left lateral was wider in 19, the right in 6, and in only 5 cases were the two sides similar.

Sacroiliac joint asymmetry is so common as to be the normal state (Dalseth 1981) (Figs 17.28, 17.29). Accessory sacroiliac joints (Dalseth 1980) are not rare, and these articulations, entirely separate from the sacroiliac

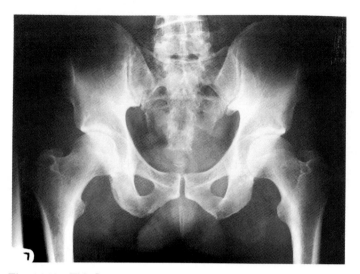

Fig. 17.29 This figure suggests the fallacy of approaching sacroiliac joint problems on the basis of assumed structural and biomechanical symmetry. The sacral ala is higher on the patient's left side, yet the lumbar spine is tilted to the left because of trapezoidal L5 vertebral body and also a trapezoidal L4–5 disc. There is a sacral scoliosis concave to the patient's left side. The sacroiliac joints, and the posterior inferior iliac spines, are clearly asymmetrical. The most casual inspection of *any* a–p view of the 'normal' pelvis will make the point of sacroiliac joint asymmetry.

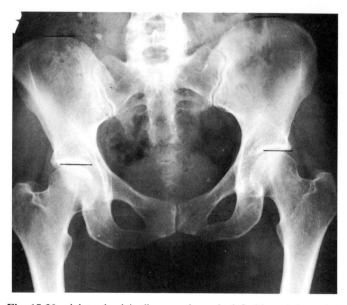

Fig. 17.30 A lateral pelvic tilt upwards on the left side and due to leg-length inequality. This commonly underlies low-back ache and other pains, which are promptly relieved by a heel lift, yet many asymptomatic people have a lateral pelvic tilt.

joint, may be associated with degenerative changes and chronic low back pain (Murray et al 1990).

Sacral agenesis may occur, in varying degrees. The iliac horn syndrome (Fong's disease) is characterized by symmetrical bony excrescences of the posterior surface of the iliac bones, these being the most consistent feature of what is a generalized hereditary syndrome.

A–p films of the pelvis may reveal a bilateral para-

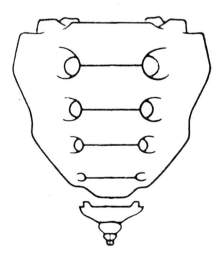

Fig. 17.28 Illustrations of true bilateral symmetry of the sacrum perpetuate a myth. True symmetry is rare.

glenoid foramen, an anomalous bony notch for the iliac artery, just lateral to the lowest margin of the sacroiliac joint. Resembling the anomalous bony arch over the vertebral artery on the superior surface of the atlas, the structure can sometimes confuse palpation findings during examination of the sacroiliac joint.

Congenital widening of the symphysis pubis (Muecke & Currarino 1968) is associated with anomalies of the genitourinary system.

Coccygeal anomalies are of practical interest when caudal anaesthesia is necessary.

Leg-length inequality, which may be congenital, developmental or the sequel of trauma, will induce a lateral pelvic tilt (Fig. 17.30). This circumstance often underlies spinal joint pain, from sacrum to occiput, in various combinations and degrees, but it need not. Its mere presence does not necessarily imply responsibility for spinal pain.

Acknowledgement

Together with my others (see Contents) this chapter is a tribute to Barbara Grieve. The first edition of this text owed its existence to her unfailing willingness to share my workload. She was wife, true friend and helpmate for 46 years. Physiotherapy owes her more than it knows.

REFERENCES

Agnoli A L 1976 Anomalies in the pattern of lumbosacral nerve roots and its clinical significance. Journal of Neurology 211: 217–228

Bagnall K M, Ford D M, McFadden K D, Greenhill B J, Raso V J 1984 The histochemical composition of human vertebral muscle. Spine 9: 470–473

Beighton P 1988 Inherited disorders of the skeleton. 2nd edn. Churchill Livingstone, Edinburgh

Brain Lord, Wilkinson M 1967 Cervical spondylosis. Heinemann, London

Brendler S J 1968 The human cervical myotomes: functional anatomy studied at operation. Journal of Neurosurgery 28: 105–111

Brougham D I, Cole W G, Dickens D R V, Menelaus N P 1989 Torticollis due to a combination of sternomastoid contracture and congenital vertebral anomalies. Journal of Bone and Joint Surgery 71B: 404–407

Bywaters E G L 1982 Rheumatoid and other diseases of the cervical interspinous bursae, and changes in the spinous processes. Annals of the Rheumatic Diseases 41: 360–370

Colin J F 1985 Personal communication

Crelin E S 1973 A scientific test of the chiropractic theory. American Scientist 61: 574–580

Dalseth I 1973 Articulations intervertebrales et symetrie. Cinésiologie 12: 19–24

Dalseth I 1974 Anatomic studies of the osseous craniovertebral joints. Manuelle Medizin 12: 130–141

Dalseth I 1976 Chiropractic and radiological diagnosis. Tidsskrift for Den norske laegeforening 11: 642–644

Dalseth I 1980 Aksessoriske iliosacralledd. Norsk Farening for Medisinsk Radiologi 1: 39–47

Dalseth I 1981 Personal communication

Davis P R 1955 The thoracolumbar mortise joint. Journal of Anatomy 89: 370–377

Dommisse G F 1980 The arteries, arterioles and capillaries of the spinal cord. Annals of the Royal College of Surgeons of England 62: 369–376

Editorial 1967 Infarction of the spinal cord. Lancet 2: 143–144

Editorial 1980 The flight from science. British Medical Journal 5 January: 1

Ellis H, Feldman S 1977 Anatomy for anaesthetists. 3rd edn. Blackwell, Oxford

Elster A 1990 Bertolotti's syndrome revisited. Spine 14: 1373–1377

Epstein B S 1976 The spine: a radiological text and atlas. 4th edn. Lea & Febiger, Philadelphia

Farfan H F 1973 Mechanical disorders of the low back. Lea & Febiger, Philadelphia, ch 4, p 83

Frykholm R 1971 The clinical picture. In: Hirsch C, Zotterman Y (eds) Cervical pain. Pergamon Press, Oxford, p 7

Golub B S, Silverman B 1969 Transforaminal ligaments of the lumbar spine. Journal of Bone and Joint Surgery 51A: 947–956

Grieve G P 1988 Common vertebral joint problems. 2nd edn. Churchill Livingstone, Edinburgh, ch 1

Hanraets P R M J 1959 The degenerative back. Elsevier, Amsterdam ch 3, p 176

Hasue M, Kikuchi S, Sakuyama Y, Tsukasa I 1983 Anatomic study of the interrelationship between lumbosacral nerve roots and their surrounding tissue. Spine 8: 50–58

Hensinger R N 1986 Osseous anomalies of the craniovertebral junction. Spine 11: 323–333

Hensinger R N, Fielding J W, Hawkins R J 1978 Congenital anomalies of the odontoid process. Orthopaedic Clinics of North America 9: 901–912

Herold H Z, Edlitz M, Baruchin A 1988 Spondylothoracic dysplasia. Spine 13: 478–481

Hirsh L F 1982 Congenital unfused lateral mass of atlas. Spine 7: 403–404

Hukuda S, Ota H, Okabe N, Tazima K 1980 Traumatic atlanto-axial dislocation causing os odontoideum in infants. Spine 5: 207–210

Jackson R 1977 The cervical syndrome. 4th edn. Charles Thomas, Springfield, ch 2, p 51

James C C, Lassman L P 1972 Spinal dysraphism. Butterworth, London, ch 4, p 25

Jeffreys E 1980 Disorders of the cervical spine. Butterworth, London, ch 3

Keats T E 1988 An atlas of normal roentgen variants that may simulate disease. 4th edn. Year Book Medical Publishers, Chicago

Keon-Cohen B 1968 Abnormal arrangement of the lower lumbar and first sacral nerves within the spinal canal. Journal of Bone and Joint Surgery 50B: 261–265

Keuter E J W 1970 Vascular origin of cranial sensory disturbances caused by pathology of the lower cervical spine. Acta Neurochirurgica 23: 229–245

Köhler A, Zimmer E A 1968 Borderlands of the normal and early pathologic in skeletal roentgenology. 3rd American edn. Grune & Stratton, New York

Lansche W E, Ford L T 1960 Correlation of the myelogram with clinical and operative findings in lumbar disc lesions. Journal of Bone and Joint Surgery 42A: 193–206

Lee C K, Weiss A B 1981 Isolated congenital cervical block vertebrae below the axis with neurological symptoms. Spine 6: 118–124

Lumsden R M, Morris J M 1968 An in vivo study of axial rotation and immobilization of the lumbosacral joint. Journal of Bone and Joint Surgery 50A: 1591–1602

Macalister A 1889 A textbook of human anatomy. Griffin, London

McCulloch J A, Waddell G 1980 Variation of the lumbosacral myotome with bony segmental anomalies. Journal of Bone and Joint Surgery 62B: 475–480

MacLean J G B, Tucker J K, Latham J B 1990 Radiographic appearances in lumbar disc prolapse. Journal of Bone & Joint Surgery 72B: 917–920

Mapstone T, Spetzier R F 1982 Vertebrobasilar insufficiency secondary to vertebral artery occlusion from a fibrous band. Journal of Neurosurgery 56: 581–583

Muecke E C, Currarino G 1968 Congenital widening of the pubic symphysis. American Journal of Röentgenology, Radium Therapy and Nuclear Medicine 103: 179–185

Murray A 1988 Traumatic displacement of the odontoid peg. Journal of Bone and Joint Surgery 70B: 856

Murray R O, Jacobson H G, Stoker D J 1990 The radiology of skeletal disorders. 3rd edn. Churchill Livingstone, Edinburgh, vol 2, ch 1

Nathan H 1959 The para-articular processes of the thoracic vertebrae. Anatomical Record 4: 605–618

Nathan H 1962 Osteophytes of the vertebral column. Journal of Bone and Joint Surgery 44A: 243

Nathan H, Feuerstein M 1970 Angulated course of spinal nerve roots. Journal of Neurosurgery 32: 349–352

Nathan H, Schwartz A 1962 Inverted pattern of development of thoracic vertebral osteophytosis in situs inversus and other instances of right descending aorta. Radiology Clinics 31: 150

Nathan H, Weizenbluth M, Halperin N 1982 The lumbosacral ligament (LSL) with special emphasis on the 'lumbosacral tunnel' and the entrapment of the 5th lumbar nerve. International Orthopaedics 6: 197–202

Neidre A, Macnab I 1983 Anomalies of the lumbosacral nerve roots. Spine 8: 294–299

Pallie W, Manuel J K 1968 Intersegmental anastomoses between dorsal spinal rootlets in some vertebrates. Acta Anatomica 70: 341–351

Raimondi A J 1987 Paedriatric neurosurgery. Springer Verlag, London

Raimondi A J, Choux M, Di Rocco C 1989 The paedriatric spine vol I Development and the dysraphic state, vol II Developmental anomalies, vol III Cysts, tumours and infections. Springer Verlag, London

Rasool M N, Govender S, Naidoo K S 1990 Foot deformities associated with congenital spinal abnormalities. Journal of Bone and Joint Surgery 72B: 744

Relman A S 1979 Chiropractic: recognized but unproved. New England Journal of Medicine 301: 659–660

Riddell D H, Smith B M 1986 Thoracic and vascular aspects of the thoracic outlet syndrome. Clinical Orthopaedics and Related Research 207: 31–36

Roos D B 1970 New concepts of thoracic outlet syndrome that explain aetiology, symptoms, diagnosis and treatment. Vascular Surgery 13: 313–318

Sachs B, Fraenkel J 1900 Progressive ankylotic rigidity of the spine. Journal of Nervous and Mental Diseases 27: 1

Samilson R L 1980 Congenital and developmental anomalies of the shoulder girdle. Orthopaedic Clinics of North America 11: 219–231

Sandifer P 1967 Neurology in orthopaedics. Butterworth, London p 38

Schmorl G, Junghanns H 1971 The human spine in health and disease. 2nd American edn. Grune & Stratton, New York

Schut L, Bruce D A 1978 The Arnold–Chiari malformation. Orthopaedic Clinics of North American 9: 913–921

Solonen K A 1957 The sacro-iliac joint in the light of anatomical röentgenological and clinical studies. Acta Orthopaedica Scandinavica suppl 26: 9–127

Spillane J D, Pallis C, Jones A M 1957 Developmental anomalies in the region of the foramen magnum. Brain 80: 11–48

Struthers J 1875 On variations of the vertebrae and ribs in man. Journal of Anatomy and Physiology 9: 17

Sunderland S 1978 Nerves and nerve injuries. 2nd edn. Churchill Livingstone, Edinburgh, ch 66

Tanaka T, Uhthoff H K 1981a Significance of resegmentation in the pathogenesis of vertebral body malformations. Acta Orthopaedica Scandinavica 52: 331–338

Tanaka T, Uhthoff H K 1981b The pathogenesis of congenital vertebral malformations. Acta Orthopaedica Scandinavica 52: 413–425

Taylor T K F, Marcucci M, Dimuria G V, Stringa G 1989 The role of transitional vertebra in intervertebral disc degeneration and prolapse. Journal of Bone and Joint Surgery 71B: 164

Telford R D, Mottershead S 1947 The costoclavicular syndrome. British Medical Journal 15: 325–328

Tini P G, Weiser C, Zinn W M 1977 The transitional vertebra of the lumbosacral spine: its radiological classification, incidence, prevalence and clinical significance. Rheumatology and Rehabilitation 16: 180–185

Truex R C, Johnson C H 1978 Congenital anomalies of the upper cervical spine. Orthopaedic Clinics of North America 9: 891–900

Tulsi R S 1974 Sacral arch defect and low backache. Australasian Radiology 18: 43–50

Von Torklus D, Gehle W 1972 The upper cervical spine. Butterworth, London, p 21

Weisz G M 1983 Trauma to anomalous cervical spine. Spine 8: 225–227

Wigh R E 1980 The thoracolumbar and lumbosacral transitional junctions. Spine 5: 215–222

Wilson C B, Norrell H A 1966 Congenital absence of a pedicle in the cervical spine. American Journal of Röentgenology, Radium Therapy and Nuclear Medicine 97: 639–647

Wood E J 1972 Anatomical aspects of some vertebral anomalies. South African Journal of Physiotherapy 28: 10–15

Wood V E, Twito R, Verska J M 1988 Thoracic outlet syndrome. Orthopaedic Clinics of North America 19: 131–146

Wynne-Davies R, Hall C M, Apley A G 1986 Atlas of skeletal dysplasias. Churchill Livingstone, Edinburgh

Clinical considerations

18. Pain and nociception: mechanisms and modulation in sensory context

R. A. Charman

INTRODUCTION

The discomfort of pain is so woven into most people's everyday experience and conversation that its sheer familiarity robs it of any strangeness. Any systematic enquiry, however, into the causes and varieties of pain, or the strange absence of pain despite very adequate cause, will soon demonstrate that everyday assumptions of cause and effect have very limited application. While much of the detailed neurophysiology underlying pain is still obscure, especially at higher centre level, a reasonably consistent outline of the main pathways and modulatory mechanisms is now known, and this knowledge forms the basis for a wide range of surgical, pharmacological, physical and psychological therapies. In the context of manual therapy this account will emphasize those aspects of pain theory and research that seem particularly relevant to musculoskeletal disorders.

Methodology

An attempt has been made to be consistent throughout the text, both in the use of pain-related terminology, and in the monistic standpoint that mental activity and brain function are one and the same. It may be helpful, therefore, if these issues are first defined and discussed.

Nociception

'Noci' is from the Latin 'noxius' or 'noxa' meaning 'harm' or 'hurt'. The terms noci stimuli, nocireceptor endings, nociceptor fibres, and nociceptive pathways related to harmful sources, will be used to refer to the non-conscious neurological activity involved in detecting, conveying, and processing such stimuli. In other words, 'noci' refers to all related peripheral and central nervous system activity occurring at non-conscious prethalamic levels up to initial entry into the thalamus.

Non-noxious or innocuous stimuli

These terms refer to stimuli arising from harmless sources, such as mechanoreceptor and thermoreceptor touch and warmth stimuli, which have not reached consciousness. Because the ever-changing input of normal stimuli and related sensation is the continuous context within which abnormal nociception occurs, the terms denoting these stimuli/sensations, such as 'touch' 'vibration' and so on, will apply at all levels unless specifically indicated.

Pain

'Pain' is from the Latin 'poena' or Greek 'poine' meaning punishment or penalty. The term 'pain' is used to indicate conscious awareness of the location and intensity of pain as an unpleasant and unwanted experience. Pain is experienced when the intensity of noci stimuli entering the thalamus activates the neuropsychic thalamocortical and thalamolimbic circuitry subserving pain. Therefore, the term 'pain pathway' will apply only at post-thalamic levels and will not be used as a generic term to refer to the pathways as a whole.

The reason for this careful distinction between non-conscious nociception and consciously experienced pain is that the two halves of the circuit do not form one sensory whole as do, for example, the retinal, optic nerve and occipital cortex activities involved in sight. Threshold sensitivities at different levels of nociception and pain vary considerably, and often quite unpredictably, in relationship to each other. For example, intense prethalamic nociceptive activity may not evoke any conscious pain. In other words, the mutual interaction of the two halves can range from synchronized correlation of nociceptor stimuli intensity and pain intensity to total disassociation between massive nociceptive barrage and no pain, or between intense pain but no nociceptive input (see Melzack & Wall 1988).

Monism as a working hypothesis

As a gross generalization there are two main philosophical

253

concepts on the structure of the universe. Dualism assumes two independent categories of substance, as in mind and matter, or, in this instance, mind and brain, which somehow interact with each other. Monism assumes one category of substance, be it materialism (that all is matter however ethereal), or idealism (that all is mind or spirit however solid). Whichever of these monisms is correct both carry the implication that knowledge of brain mechanisms means knowledge of mental mechanisms, including consciousness, because they are one and the same.

For the purpose of this discussion the monistic viewpoint is adopted as the simplest hypothesis. It is implicit in the cause and effect terminology employed in relating neurological activity to psychological processes (see Luria 1973, Cotman & McGaugh 1980, Dimond 1980, Changeux 1985, Berglund 1986, Bloom et al 1985, Walsh 1987, Kimble 1988, Nathan 1988, Gazzaniga 1989). A distinguished exception to this monistic viewpoint is Eccles (1979, 1980, 1989, Eccles & Robinson 1984) who advocates a religious concept of brain, mind and soul dualism.

The working hypothesis is that the co-ordinated hierarchy of subcortical to cortical levels of circuitry input, circuitry processing and circuitry output collectively act as multiple generators of psychological functions. The interaction of these functions in the creation of conscious self-awareness and decision making represents the highest levels of neural processing.

The evocation of conscious sensations, emotions and memories by focal electrical stimulation of specific brain areas tends to support this view. The conscious observer reports such elicited imagery as if it is projected upon an hallucinatory inner screen (Penfield 1963, 1975). The assumption, therefore, is that the brain is genetically programmed to create models of the outside world, including its own body, in terms of sensory fields and emotional intensity. The brain can 'know' the world outside the skull only by preprogrammed interpretation of the incoming sensory codes, and transformation of them into the mental world of spatial imagery, experience, meaning and response peculiar to each species, be it insect or man.

The cerebral cortex is arranged into primary reception areas specific to each incoming sensory modality, with associated secondary areas for higher level processing. The outgoing motor cortex is similarly organized. Connecting them all are the associative, tertiary areas of conscious activity, including the prefrontal, or supraorbital lobes, with strong connections to the emotional drives of the 'visceral brain' of the limbic system. Cortical organization and structure is based upon a radial mosaic of columnar microprocessing modules, each about 0.5 mm wide and 1 mm in length (cortical thickness), containing several hundred cells in complex synaptic array (Szentagothai 1983). Each module has its own input and output con-

nections and the whole mosaic is precisely organized in relation to transcortical and subcortical connections. Each module is programmed according to the level and type of processing appropriate to its position.

From birth onwards, each brain develops its sensory neural modelling by sensorimotor trial and error as it learns the rules governing the outside world. This includes gaining control of the body as a physical object for effective manipulation of its world and successful movement within it. Personal and social relationships are established on a perceptual and emotional basis, and throughout life each brain builds its own associative models of understanding, meaning and significance.

The monism/dualism debate is experientially unresolvable because conscious awareness, emotion and cognition, including the experience of pain, have no direct knowledge of the neural processing upon which they are based. This is inferential knowledge gained over the last 150 years of neurological research. To talk, therefore, of 'the brain' doing these things may be a valid inference, but each person's actual conscious experience is quite independent of such inferential knowledge. The immediacy of conscious experience precedes any theoretical speculation as to its cause.

In this account the term neuropsychical indicates non-conscious to conscious cause, and psychoneural indicates from mental neural processing to non-conscious neural effect.

Implications of the monist approach for pain theory

Pain can be considered as the primary, unpleasant, aversive, sensory and emotional model of tissue damage generated by neuropsychic nociceptive processing within the body image. In most circumstances of ordinary life, once the noci-generating source has healed so the pain disappears. Its memory is suppressed into non-consciousness. Unfortunately, nociceptor/pain processing circuits can sometimes become self-sustaining entities of unpredictable activation, and are then sources of neuropathic pain in their own right. The causalgias, migraine and postherpetic neuralgia are typical examples. Phantom limb pain is an example of pain memory, re-evoked by whatever cause, of a previous perceptual and unpleasant emotional experience which intrudes into the present with the experiential reality of hallucination.

One very important implication of the monist approach is that the high levels of neural processing related to psychological functions are based upon the same principles and mechanisms of neural processing used throughout the nervous system. The difference is one of programming and processing power. Associative area processing can be disengaged from any direct motor output, as is apparent when thinking but not acting upon the thought, but probably uses the same type of primary sensory programming for creating cognitive imagery. The psychoneural processing levels of attitudes, beliefs, self-image, social interactions, values, decision making and future planning possess inherently powerful mechanisms capable of exerting the desired facilitatory and inhibitory control over other processing activities. This view of psychoneural functioning provides a very powerful rationale for the employment of a wide range of behavioural conditioning strategies for the desired control of pain.

PAIN THRESHOLDS AND PAIN TOLERANCE

Before looking at the nociceptor-to-pain pathways, and the possible mechanisms of endogenous pain modulation systems, a little background concerning the psychophysical parameters and social context of pain may be helpful, because it is from somewhere within these considerations that the patient will have decided that his or her pain merits the necessity of obtaining professional diagnosis and treatment.

Levels of threshold

Laboratory experiments on volunteer subjects have amassed an enormous amount of verified information on the thresholds of sensory perception across all of the sensory modalities (see Barlow & Mollon 1982, Coren & Ward 1989). Carefully calibrated sources of thermal, electrical and mechanical stimuli have established that a basic sensory threshold seems common to all. From that point onwards, where stimulus intensity becomes pain, and pain becomes unbearable, differs very widely between different cultures, different individuals, and different circumstances.

Sensation threshold

Experiment has repeatedly shown that the majority of people have a uniform threshold of sensation to recognisably different stimuli. In other words, as the intensity of a stimulus is slowly increased, there is a common baseline level at which most people will say that they can just feel it. Sternbach and Tursky (1965) found, for example, no difference in the just-perceptible threshold of an electrical stimulus experienced by American-born women of Italian, Jewish, Irish and Old American origin.

Pain perception threshold

The measured level at which a steadily increasing stimulus, such as point pressure, or focal point temperature, changes from recognisable intense pressure, or heat, into a sensation of pain varies considerably between people from different cultures and lifestyles (Hardy et al 1952, Clark & Clark 1980). Those from stoic backgrounds, or in manual labour occupations, have higher thresholds that must be exceeded before intense sensation becomes pain compared to those from more vociferous cultures or sedentary lifestyles. This is not to say that a psychophysical relationship of stimulus intensity plotted against pain sensation cannot be graphed in carefully controlled circumstances, but such a graph will vary considerably between individuals.

Pain tolerance thresholds

Individual and ethnic group tolerance of pain intensity increases to unacceptable levels varies considerably, even in a stable laboratory environment. In everyday life the ability to tolerate pain, roughly defined as the ability to continue performing everyday activities despite pain, varies enormously. Factors of cultural, religious and ethnic backgrounds, and daily exposure to physical stress and incidental pain, play a major role. So does the particular circumstances and its meaning to the individual. Battle, sport and emergency situations raise pain tolerance levels to remarkable heights. So do social circumstances. Pain tolerance is somehow raised to meet an occasion where it is imperative that it must not interfere with adequate functioning. For example, acting as host to a special occasion, delivering a speech, performing in a play, holding on to a job, continuing with family duties, or nursing others.

An individual's pain tolerance is very much a learned experience. It is a compound of previous circumstances of pain and response, the accepted norms of society, social obligations, self-image, and personal goals. Animal experiments, where dogs (Melzack 1965, 1969) and monkeys (Lichstein & Sackett 1971) have been reared in complete social isolation, have shown that they have little fear of danger, or sensation of pain with injury, and seem not to learn. A flame can be investigated again and again. The rough and tumble of growing up in society, whether animal or human, seems a necessary prerequisite in learning the experience and meaning of pain, and how to avoid, endure, or ease it.

SENSORY MODALITIES — THE CONTEXT

In everyday life the sensory modalities which convey stimuli from non-harmful sources into the central nervous system (CNS) are continuously active. Mechanoreceptors monitor compressional, torsional and vibratory deformation of tissue structures, including auditory and vestibular sense, and vascular wall distension caused by blood pressure. Thermoreceptors monitor superficial and deep temperature change. Chemoreceptors monitor dissolved molecules for taste and smell, partial blood gas pressures, and blood plasma acid/alkali balance. Electromagnetic receptors monitor the pattern of light frequencies focussed onto the retina. Receptors in the viscera monitor visceral wall distension and compressive peristaltic activity. The threshold sensitivities of non-noxious sensory receptors are set to respond across the range of stimuli strength which has bodily effect short of harm.

The brain uses the combined input from all of these sources to create a non-conscious body image (brainstem, cerebellum, and related nuclei) within a three-dimensional environment, and a conscious body image (cerebral cortex) within a consciously perceived three-dimensional environment. The two images interact in everyday volitional activities. The limbic system 'visceral brain' of innate bodily drives, emotions and memory, combine with desired conscious goals and conscious decision making to provide the motive force for action.

Nociception and pain

Nociceptors tend to have a threshold of excitation that is too high to be stimulated by normal innocuous stimuli. Their function is to monitor the body for evidence of injury (noci stimuli). When this occurs they register the location, severity, duration and possible cause of tissue damage as noci reception. In a healthy and uninjured body they are mainly silent during everyday activities and contribute little to the body image. Therefore their activation by acute injury, for example, is an abrupt abnormal activity, and this abnormal input of nociceptive impulses into the CNS disrupts normal sensorimotor patterns of activity, ensuring rapid, non conscious, aversive reflex response and capturing full conscious attention. In these circumstances it is a warning that something is wrong. Chronic tissue damage, as in arthritis, is a source of sustained nociceptor input which does contribute to the body image and markedly affects the patterns of everyday movement.

One very important point concerning nocireception is that the receiving terminal branches are not just passive monitors. They may, as discussed later, actually influence the degree and duration of tissue injury by active secretion of inflammatory agents which can act as a secondary source of increased pain.

Intrinsic CNS activity

It is obvious from the preceding discussion that all incoming sensory input, be it from innocuous or noxious sources, enters a highly active CNS, which is in an ever-changing flux of sensorimotor processing and responsiveness relative to present activity and conditioned by preceding activity. The focus of conscious awareness, purpose and attention is also in a continuous state of change. The size of receptive sensory fields, and thresholds of sensitivity and response to different sources of stimuli sources, continuously vary as the synaptic patterns

of inhibitory, excitatory, and modulatory activity, underlying conscious and non-conscious functioning interact throughout the whole length of the neuroaxis from spinal cord to cerebral cortex.

Relationship of fibre type and stimuli carried

Most non-nociceptive sensation is carried by the large to medium-sized, myelinated alpha-alpha, alpha-beta and alpha-gamma fibres, ranging from 20 to 7 μm in diameter, with conduction velocities of between 120 and 20 m per second. Noci stimuli are carried mainly by the small myelinated alpha-delta (A-δ) fibres, of between 2.5 and 5 μm in diameter and velocities of 6 to 30 m per second, and unmyelinated C fibres of between 0.5 and 2 μm diameter and velocities under 2 m per second (Campbell et al 1989). A-δ fibres also carry cold stimuli (Darien-Smith et al 1973), and C fibres convey warm stimuli (Darien-Smith et al 1979).

One consequence of this difference in fibre carrying size between innocuous and noxious stimuli is that if, for example, small fibre nociceptors and large fibre touch receptors are stimulated at the same moment, the spinal cord will receive the touch stimulus in about a third of the time it would take an A-δ stimulus to arrive, and about a hundredth of the time it would take a C fibre stimulus to arrive. The same disparity of timing, of course, applies to A-δ fibres and C fibres carrying ordinary thermal stimuli.

Classification by innervation area

Sensory modalities are also classified according to the main tissue areas that they innervate. Exteroceptors supply skin and adjacent underlying tissues, proprioceptors supply the musculoskeletal system, and interoceptors the viscera. The latter organs are innervated mainly by the parasympathetic and sympathetic nervous systems (autonomic system), together with A-δ and C fibres (Bahns et al 1986) which innervate the supporting fascia such as the peritoneum. The vascular system is innervated mainly by sympathetic and A-δ and C fibres (Malliani et al 1989).

NOCICEPTORS

Nociceptor's endings

Nociceptor's endings are bare 'chicken wire' branched terminations of unmyelinated, slow-conducting C fibres, and thinly myelinated, faster-conducting A-δ fibres (Wyke 1979, Kruger et al 1981). The termination network of each C fibre innervates a three-dimensional receptive tissue field of between 6 and 15 mm in diameter and of variable depth (van Hees & Gybels 1981), with extensive field overlapping between adjacent C fibres. A-δ fields are smaller and more punctate. Relative density of innervation seems to be roughly correlated to risk of mechanical damage. The skin is highly innervated, as are joint capsules and ligaments, tendon sheaths, musculotendinous junctions, muscle attachments, bursae and periosteum. The glabrous (non-hairy) skin of body orifices is very densely innervated. Nociceptor endings have not been found in articular cartilage, synovial membranes, lung parenchyma, visceral pleura, pericardium, brain or spinal cord tissue. The membranes enclosing the CNS and peripheral nerves are, however, well innervated.

Nociceptor ending response to chemical, thermal and mechanical stimuli has been difficult to categorize as their sensitivities may alter in a rather unpredictable manner. Initial response sensitivity may undergo rapid change as the duration and type of stimuli alter according to local tissue reactions. In general terms nociceptors are classified as follows:

Unimodal

Unimodal nociceptors predictably respond to a particular type of intense stimuli, such as sharp mechanical pressure/penetration as from a pin. These receptors are mechanosensitive and are mainly A-δ endings. Some A-δ thermosensitive receptors may be unimodal in specific response to tissue temperatures of 45 °C or more.

McMahon and Koltzenburg (1990) have drawn attention to a subgroup of 'silent' C fibre nociceptors which specifically respond to inflammatory changes of a period of several hours.

Bimodal

Bimodal nociceptors respond to stimulation from one of two sources, or both combined. These are mainly A-δ mechano-heat (AMH) receptors, which are subdivided into two types (Campbell & Meyer 1986). Type I AMHs have a high thermal threshold, responding to 50 °C or more, and are found mainly in the glabrous skin of the hand and foot. Type II AMHs have a low threshold, responding across the whole range, and are widely distributed.

Polymodal

Polymodal nociceptors form the majority of receptors, particularly C fibres, and they show an increasing rate of frequency discharge as the mechanical, thermal, or chemical source of imminent tissue damage reaches potentially dangerous or actually destructive levels. Polymodal endings respond to the upper range of innocuous stimuli intensity, thus adding to normal sensory input, but, as the source of such stimuli enters the threshold of possible and actual tissue damage, their raised frequency rate is perceived and experienced as a change from intense innocuous sensation into pain. This change is probably caused by increasing temporal C fibre and A-δ fibre frequency summation in the dorsal horn of the spinal cord, or analogous trigeminal nuclei, activating the ascending noci tract systems terminating in consciousness (Campbell et al 1989). McMahon and Koltzenburg (1990) have proposed that pain intensity in non-inflamed tissue is primarily related to temporal summation, whereas pain arising from inflamed tissues superimposes a strong spatial summation.

These three categories of nociceptor responses are most clearly established at cutaneous level, but seem to apply to the deeper tissues as well, especially joint structures.

Peripheral pathway to spinal cord entry

The branched endings of unmyelinated C fibres unite to form a single nerve fibre that enters the peripheral nerve sheath alongside all the other fibres (Fig. 18.1A). They lie embedded in invaginated myelin indentations throughout the length of the nerve until it reaches the dorsal root ganglion. A-δ fibres travel individually as myelinated fibres. Sensory fibres lie in no particular relationship to one another until they have passed the T junction of their parent dorsal root ganglion cells and become the incoming dorsal root primary afferents. As the afferents cross the dorsal root entry zone into the spinal cord they separate out so that the myelinated fibres form the dorsomedial bundle and the unmyelinated fibres form the anterolateral bundle (Fig. 18.1A). The large myelinated fibres directly enter the dorsal white columns, sending collaterals into the dorsal horn to synapse onto dorsal horn cells. Most C fibre axons, and many A-δ fibres, divide into two branches as they enter the spinal cord, ascending and descending over several cord segments in small tracts, such as Lissaur's tract, adjacent to the posterolateral edge of the dorsal horn, and sending collaterals into the dorsal horn before final termination (Fitzgerald 1989).

Visceral and somatic nociceptor afferent convergence

Referred pain from visceral source to somatic site — as occurs, for example, with anginal pain extending into the left arm — is related to convergence of their afferents onto the same spinal cord neurones. The brain relocates nociceptor stimuli from the ill-defined visceral source (visceratome) to the well located somatic site of mutual embryonic innervation (Foreman et al 1981, Milne et al 1981, Beard & Pearce 1989, Blendis 1989, Bonica & Chadwick 1989, Elhilali & Winfield 1989, Procacci & Zoppi 1989). See Ness and Gebhart (1990) for a comprehensive review of experimental studies relating visceratomes to trunk and limb somatomes.

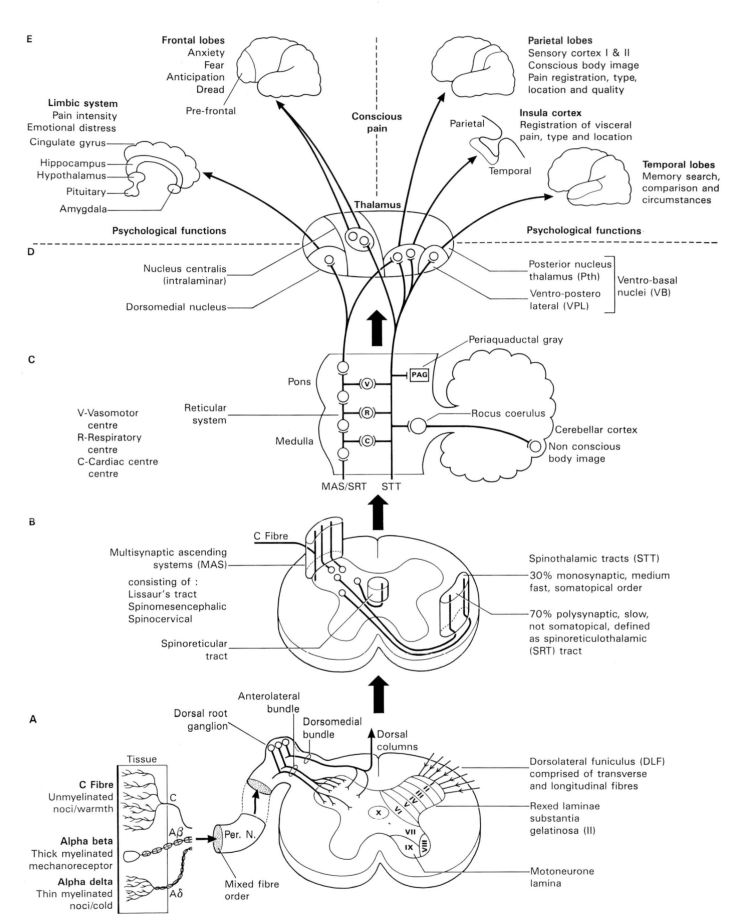

Fig. 18.1 Ascending nociceptor to pain experience pathways.

DORSAL HORN AND ASCENDING NOCICEPTOR PATHWAYS

Dorsal horn

In transverse section the grey matter of the spinal cord (SC) has been descriptively divided into 10 zones on the basis of cell type (Rexed 1952). These are known as Rexed zones, or laminae, and are extremely useful as positional reference for mapping the termination of incoming peripheral and centrally descending afferents. In reality the cell type boundaries are much less distinct than diagram lines imply, and the fields of dendritic branching, and axonal collateral terminations, spread across more than one zone.

The dorsal horn is divided into six laminae; from dorsal to ventral these are: lamina I (outermost marginal layer), lamina II (substantia gelatinosa), and laminae III, IV, V and VI (nucleus proprius), the latter forming the base of the spinal grey between the dorsal and ventral horns (Fig. 18.1A). Afferent termination into the SC from each peripheral nerve is somatopically organized; for example, the medial-to-lateral and distal-to-proximal relationships of the tissues supplied are mirrored in terminal field distribution, with no territorial overlap between nerves (Koerber & Brown 1980, Ygge & Grant 1983, Molander & Grant 1985, Swett & Woolf 1985). This somatopical organization is reflected in the arrangement of the second-order dorsal cells, and cells of origin of ascending myelinated tracts whose receptive field interacts with primary afferents. Major exceptions to the rule are muscle afferents and visceral afferents which show little somatopical order in the SC (Morgan et al 1981, Molander & Grant 1987).

A-δ fibres and C fibres form a longitudinal and transverse web of fibres which cap the outer margin of lamina I. On entering the dorsal horn A-δ fibres mainly terminate in laminae I and II (SG), with some fibres terminating in IV and V (Mense & Prabhakar 1986). The majority of C fibres terminate in laminae I and II (Lamotte 1977, Gobel et al 1981). The SG cells have very extensive dendritic fields that interlace with each other and with cells in adjacent laminae both horizontally and segmentally (Willis & Coggleshall 1978).

Collaterals from the large myelinated alpha-beta and alpha-delta fibres enter the dorsal horn from the dorsomedial side and terminate mainly in laminae III, IV and V, with some arborizations into lamina VI and a small percentage of collateral termination in lamina II (Meyer & Snow 1986). In all cases terminations are ipsilateral.

It must be emphasized that the contact between primary afferents and the cells of the laminae is not on a one-to-one basis. As Fitzgerald (1989) pointed out, a highly organized distribution of afferent collaterals from any one incoming fibre synapses onto a wide range of dendritic receptor fields. Synapses may be presynaptic, postsynaptic, axonodendritic or axosomatic. Collaterals from several C fibres may meet to form mutual clusters onto dendritic branches and cell bodies. This allows synchronous firing of presynaptic terminals onto laminal cells, causing them, in turn, to fire together (Fitzgerald & Wall 1980).

In summary, the incoming afferents from all fibre groups establish a web of synaptic contacts with the laminal cells, with C fibres terminating in the superficial laminae, myelinated A-δ somewhat deeper, and the large myelinated fibres penetrating to V and VI. Through this web they exert an everchanging pattern of excitatory and inhibitory control upon laminae cell discharge. This changing mosaic of short- or long-term inhibitory/excitatory control determines the discharge of the dorsal horn neurones that are the cells of origin of the ascending tracts which terminate in brainstem nuclei, thalamic nuclei or cerebellar cortex. They also exert control over the interneurones which relay intersegmentally, including those that synapse onto autonomic and motoneurone pools, mediating, for example, spinal reflex response to nociceptor stimuli. The complexity of interconnection is not random; there is a somatopical order, reflected in neurone arrangement and tract fibre relationships, and, in everyday life, the neuronal relay system works smoothly. However, when intense nociceptor stimuli suddenly enter the spinal cord they can, for a short while at least, dominate posture and movement, with selective reflex activation of flexor motoneurones resulting, for example, in the well known flexed posture of being 'doubled up' with pain.

ASCENDING NOCICEPTIVE PATHWAYS

The cells of origin of the ascending nociceptor tracts are not known for certain. One source of uncertainty is that while some laminal neurones are exclusively nociceptive, the majority are receptive to both nociceptive and nonnoxious stimuli. These are termed wide-dynamic-range (WDR) neurones. All laminae, from I to VIII, have been found to be represented in midbrain and thalamic nuclei terminations, with particularly detailed thalamic representation of laminae I and II (see review by Willis 1989). Noci information is also relayed via midbrain nuclei (locus coerulus) to the non-conscious body schema of the cerebellar cortex. In general terms, the deeper neurones are cells of origin for the lateral spinothalamic tract, and the superficial laminal neurones are cells of origin for the more diffuse, multisynaptic tracts to be discussed below.

The lateral spinothalamic tract

This is the classical pain and temperature tract, receiving axons which have crossed in the spinal grey commissure (Fig. 18.1B). Present opinion, based upon Boivie (1979), is that there is little functional difference between the lateral and anterior spinothalamic tracts, so the term spinothalamic tract (STT) will be used. The STT is formed mainly by myelinated, medium-fast fibres that are monosynaptic to the thalamus (Mehler 1962). Here they terminate in the ventroposterolateral nucleus (VPL) and posterior nuclear complex (Pth) which, together, form the ventral basal complex (VB), and the central lateral nucleus (CLN) of the intralaminar nuclei (Fig. 18.1D). As they pass through the brainstem they send collaterals to midbrain nuclei, including the cardiac, respiratory and vasomotor centres, and to the peri-aquaductal grey (PAG), whose modulatory function will be discussed later (Fig. 18.1C). This tract carries sharp, spatial, and discriminative noci stimuli, mainly of original A-δ origin. It is somatopically organized so that, during ascent, incoming fibres join the tract in an orderly manner. The receiving thalamic neurones are similarly organized and, in the VB nuclei, the STT and somatopical dorsal column afferents overlap.

Multisynaptic tracts

It is now known that there are several more diffuse ascending systems, some on the dorsolateral aspect of the dorsal horns at the outer edge of the dorsal columns, another, or others, that run(s) parallel with the STT in the ventrolateral column, and a central grey spinoreticular tract. Hannington-Kiff et al (1983) refers to the dorsolateral column tracts as the multisynaptic ascending system (MAS), thus indicating its complexity, and Bowsher (1988) refers to the STT-associated tract as the spinoreticulodiencephalic system (SRD), thus indicating its main relay connections (Fig. 18.1B). Neither are somatopically organized.

The multisynaptic ascending systems (MAS)

These consist mainly of relays of unmyelinated and thinly myelinated fibres that ascend in the dorsolateral fasciculus (DLF) and originate mainly from lamina I cells. They include Lissauer's tract, which is mainly intersegmental, the spinomesencephalic tract and spinocervical tract. These tracts have profuse synaptic connections with the reticular system, the respiratory, vasomotor and cardiac centres, PAG nuclei and collicular nuclei (Fig. 18.1C) before terminating mainly in intralaminal and medial thalamic nuclei, with some afferents to the VB complex (Fig. 18.1D). Related to them is the spinoreticular tract. This lies within the central spinal grey, which is considered by many to be the spinal extension of the reticular formation in the midbrain. It is concerned mainly with interspinal reflex coordination, including nociceptive motor response.

The spinoreticulodiencephalic (SRD) system

The SRD system seems analogous to the other MAS tracts, as it consists mainly of multisynaptic unmyelinated fibres originating from contralateral and unilateral laminar I cells, and runs parallel to the STT, and may well be part of it. An alternative name is the spinoreticulothalamic (SRT) system. It synapses mainly in the reticular formation and its final relays terminate in the same nuclei as the MAS systems (Willis 1985).

POST-THALAMIC NOCICEPTIVE TRANSITION INTO PAIN EXPERIENCE

Spinothalamic-tract-based thalamocortical projections (Fig. 18.1E)

The main function of the STT is to provide a monosynaptic, fairly fast, somatopically structured pattern of noci information to the thalamus. The VB thalamic nuclei then relay this pattern to the discriminative sensory cortex areas I and II (especially the latter), in the parietal lobe, to register the character and location of perceived pain within the body schema (Wyke 1981). This will be received within the context of normal (dorsal column) sensory experience which provides the circumstances in which pain is occurring. Perceived pain has little or no emotional affect as it is really for protective awareness and avoidance response. Similar information is also sent to the temporal lobe and associated deep nuclei for memory retrieval of past occurrence, or registration of the circumstance and character of pain not previously experienced. Acute noci stimuli from the viscera are relayed from the thalamus to the insula cortex gyrus between the parietal and temporal lobes. The sensory map of the viscera is much less definite than the sensory cortex body schema. The smaller relay to the intralaminal thalamic nuclei implies that some STT noci stimuli are relayed to the limbic and frontal lobe systems.

MAS/SRD-based thalamolimbic and thalamocortical projections (Fig. 18.1E)

The main ascending function of these multisynaptic tracts is to alert brainstem nuclei, especially the upper reticular nuclei which maintain cortical arousal, to the changing patterns of noci intensity before their relays terminate in the thalamus. These patterns are relayed from central intralaminal and medial nuclei to the hypothalamus and other limbic system nuclei and to the prefrontal lobes. In the limbic system they generate conscious experience of pain character and intensity with accompanying emotional distress. If really intense, as in the passage of a rough kidney stone along the ureter, pain intensity excludes any other consideration. Hypothalamic nuclei can initiate profound autonomic reactions through brainstem and spinal relays. Blood pressure can drop suddenly, causing fainting. Visceral contractions can result in nausea, vomiting and even incontinence. Respiration and heart rates can alter dramatically with pain. Raised sudomotor activity can result in running cold sweat. Voluntary muscle tone and voluntary strength can decrease markedly through motoneurone inhibition. Paradoxically, brainstem and spinal cord nocidriven reflexes can cause intense and uncontrollable writhing. Visceral interoceptor sensory feedback of nausea can intensify pain distress and result in severe prostration.

Nocidriven thalamocortical projection to the prefrontal lobe, which has strong limbic system connections, can generate intense neuropsychic anxiety, anticipation and fear. Prefrontal lobe psychoneural activity seems associated with the ability to imagine possible future scenarios and charge them with emotional affect. The high arousal effect of acute pain is probably related to the increased nocidriven cortical arousal activity of the upper reticular formation via intralaminar thalamic nuclei.

In summary, the two systems act in integrated tandem, with parietal lobe perception and analysis combining with limbic and prefrontal lobe system generation of emotional affect. The acute pain of trauma, or toothache, is highly alerting, and tends to dominate conscious attention. The dull, aching pain of chronic disorders, such as osteoarthritis and grumbling low-back pain, is carried mainly by the MAS/SRD systems, and its chronicity tends to reduce conscious alertness and induce a pain-avoidance desire to escape into solitude and sleep.

THE NEURAL BACKGROUND TO NOCICEPTOR AND PAIN MODULATION

As discussed in a previous section, the entire neuroaxis circuitry, from neocortex to spinal cord, is in a continuous state of mutual modulatory interaction between excitation or inhibition. Incoming sensory input enters into an ever-changing pattern of spinal, brainstem and diencephalic receptivity and response. This changing pattern exists at each sensory and motor reception and transmission level. The neurological locus of conscious perceptual and emotional psychoneural attention changes from moment to moment between cortical areas and related subcortical nuclei. Much of this interactive activity varies about a mean of excitatory/inhibitory values, which allows a fairly predictable constancy of sensorimotor response in everyday life, but exceptional changes of sensory input intensity, level of conscious concentration, or neuropathic pain, can dramatically alter threshold values of receptivity and response throughout the neuroaxis.

Interactive control of tract projection neurones and local circuit neurones is achieved by a wide range of mechanisms. The most decisive, and most studied, is the axonal action potential following fast transmitter depolarization of the axon hillock, resulting in synaptic depolarizing or hyperpolarizing discharge onto other neurones.

Quick motor reflex responses and voluntary movement are typical fast transmitter examples. Patterns of reflex and voluntary motor activity also includes the less obvious, but essential, component of decisive inhibition to prevent unwanted movement. Motor neurones are a special case, as they always have a depolarizing excitatory action at the neuromuscular junction of striated muscle.

Underlying the fast sensorimotor response systems is a shifting pattern of axodendritic and dendrodendritic synaptic activity. This creates changing values of electrotonic currents in dendritic branches which modify the excitator/inhibitory membrane bias across cell body and axon hillock membrane. An important factor in this shifting background of modulatory control is the changing synaptic release of neuropeptides and other neurohormones that can alter the behaviour of target cells by either binding with membrane receptors and activating intracellular activity, or effecting presynaptic control. Some classes of interneurones have no axons but interact with each other, or with projector tract neurones, by neurohormonal dendrodendritic interchange. Many neurones can alter their neurohormone synthesis profile according to the stimuli patterns they are receiving. In effect, they use incoming stimuli as a code to change what they manufacture. The brain is now recognized as the largest secreting gland in the body, and the traditional picture of on/off pulse coding is being considerably modified to include neurohormonal modulation as an essential element in information processing and neuroplasticity (Osborne 1983, Iversen 1985, Berglund 1986, Golding 1988, Noback et al 1991).

Neurones are programmed across a range of excitatory responses. They may maintain a tonic output, which is varied by incoming inhibitory or excitatory control, or fire in sustained discharge or repetitive bursts after stimulation, or, like motor neurones, they may discharge at the rate dictated by incoming synaptic depolarization.

This wide range of modulatory control mechanisms affords almost infinite scope for local and general adaptation. Neuronal memory of past patterns of input and response combine with mechanisms of neural plasticity to form new responses to changing circumstances. Neural plasticity of learning and response allows for anticipatory adaptation to possible future contingencies through the psychoneural processing of conscious imagination and future planning.

DESCENDING NOCICEPTOR AND PAIN CONTROL SYSTEMS

Endogenous nociceptor and pain modulation mechanisms

The present consensus of opinion (see reviews by Watson 1986, Fields & Basbaum 1989) is that the two major nociceptor and pain suppressor systems are the opioid mediated analgesia system (OMAS), using endogenous endorphins, such as the pentapeptides (met-encephalin and leu-encephalin), beta-endorphin and dynorphin, and the 5-hydroxytryptamine (5-HT) serotonergic system. Electrical stimulation of nuclei, such as the peri-aquaductal grey (PAG) which surrounds the aquaduct of Sylvius, containing high concentrations of these chemicals results in a considerable degree of analgesia.

In general terms their mode of action ranges from presynaptic inhibition of incoming noci afferents (particularly 5-HT), postsynaptic inhibition of polymodal cells driven by noci stimuli, or specific nocireceptive cells, and inhibition of interneurones maintaining noci activity. They may activate interneurones that effect postsynaptic inhibition of noci driven cells. Besides direct synaptic effect the stimulated activity of opioid-containing cells, for example, raises the level of free opioid molecule concentration in the cerebrospinal fluid which is therefore available to bind with membrane opioid receptors. Most research has concentrated upon the noci-suppression mechanisms of these systems in the dorsal horn, but they operate throughout the neuroaxis from noci to pain levels.

Not all noci-suppression and pain analgesia, however, can be attributed to just these two systems. Pain relief may be present following acupuncture, for example, or during meditation, which is not reversible by the opioid antagonist naloxone, or by methysergide, which is an antagonist of 5-HT. This implies that pain modulation networks may be activated by many different mechanisms.

Corticolimbic modulation (Fig. 18.2A)

Psychoneural corticolimbic circuitry may include negative feedback control of experienced pain intensity by willed motivational techniques such as transcendental meditation (TM), yoga, hypnosis and post-self-hypnotic suggestion of no pain. Positive changes of attitude towards pain, from one of helpless pain victim to one of pain manager, achieved by use of pain-relieving strategies may also be mediated through such psychoneurological mechanisms (Tan 1982, Turk & Rudy 1987, Jessup 1989, Orne & Dinges 1989, Sternbach 1989, Turk & Meichenbaum 1989). As yet there is insufficient knowledge of neuronal processing at these levels to allow more than speculative guesses, but it seems likely that mood, as a limbic function, can alter opioid levels, as there are considerable opioid cell concentrations throughout the limbic and associated nuclei systems.

As mentioned in a previous section, the higher-order processing of conscious motivation provides a rationale for the possibility of direct psychoneural suppression of pain intensity by inhibition. Willed conscious attention away from pain can suppress pain intensity, and it seems a reasonable hypothesis that the neural processes subserving

attention must also inhibit distractive stimuli. Raising the level of sensory input is a logical manoeuvre as the sensory cortex has a large cortical representation and low receptive threshold for skin stimuli. Strong input from one, or more, areas of skin can move sensory attention away from pain by competitive stimuli.

Corticofugal

Besides higher-centre modulation of pain affected by internal feedback, there are numerous descending pathways to other nuclei for modulation of noci input. Descending afferents from the sensorimotor cortex synapse in the thalamic VPL nucleus, spinoreticular and spinocervical tract nuclei, and dorsal column gracile and cuneatus nuclei in the medulla. These connections form part of a sensory feedback system whereby the cortex exerts control over the sensory (including noci) input it is about to receive in the context of information already processed (Watson 1986). The cortex can also influence the dorsal horn directly through the sensoricortex afferents which comprise about 40% of the corticospinal tract (Wyke 1981). Many of these synapse in laminae I and II and may exert presynaptic control of incoming afferents and direct postsynaptic inhibition of STT cells of origin (Fig. 18.2B).

Psychoneural prefrontal (supraorbital) cortical afferents synapse in the periaquaductal grey (PAG) with excitatory effect on noci inhibitory opioid and serotonergic neurones (Fig. 18.2C).

Diencephalic to brainstem modulation of noci pathways

Limbic system afferents, particularly from posterior nuclei in the hypothalamus, together with parafascicular nuclei outflow from the thalamus, pass directly to PAG nuclei (Reichling & Basbaum 1986), and a tract runs from the VPL to the nearby periventricular grey involved in noci modulation. Diencephalic afferents also synapse in the upper reticular formation which receives STT relays. This could be a mechanism of STT relay inhibition. The amygdala sends afferents to brainstem nuclei which may mediate aversive responses to pain.

The PAG area is one of the main afferent reception centres for efferent initiation of noci intensity modulation. The main descending system comprises PAG neurotensin afferent projection onto serotonergic nuclei in nucleus raphe magnus (NRM), whose projection fibres descend in the dorsolateral funiculus (DLF) to terminate in laminae I and II as presynaptic inhibitory endings, with some afferents terminating in laminae V and VII. PAG also has a strong input into reticular medullary nuclei which, in turn, send stimulatory 5-HT afferents to NRM nuclei which may boost its activity (Fig. 18.2C).

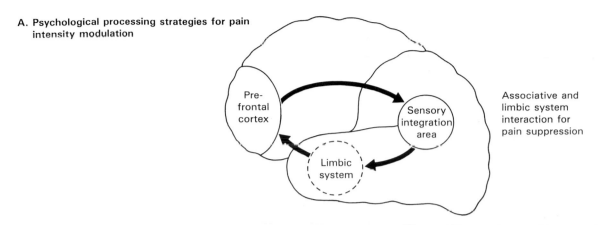

A. Psychological processing strategies for pain intensity modulation

Pre-frontal cortex

Sensory integration area

Limbic system

Associative and limbic system interaction for pain suppression

B. Corticospinal noci inhibition

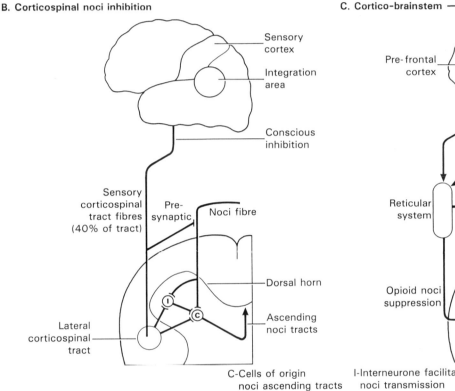

Sensory cortex

Integration area

Conscious inhibition

Sensory corticospinal tract fibres (40% of tract)

Pre-synaptic

Noci fibre

Dorsal horn

Lateral corticospinal tract

Ascending noci tracts

C-Cells of origin noci ascending tracts

C. Cortico-brainstem —spinal noci inhibition

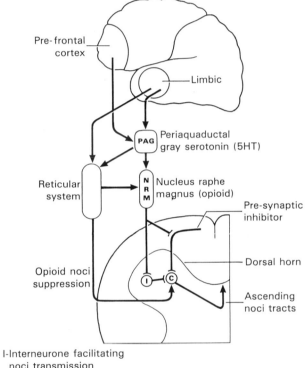

Pre-frontal cortex

Limbic

PAG Periaquaductal gray serotonin (5HT)

Reticular system

N R M Nucleus raphe magnus (opioid)

Pre-synaptic inhibitor

Opioid noci suppression

Dorsal horn

Ascending noci tracts

I-Interneurone facilitating noci transmission

D. Peripheral input gate control balance at either extreme

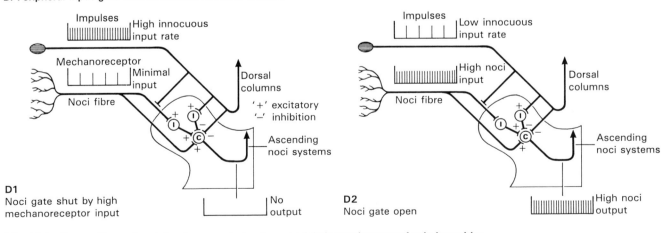

Impulses High innocuous input rate

Mechanoreceptor Minimal input

Noci fibre

Dorsal columns

'+' excitatory
'−' inhibition

Ascending noci systems

D1
Noci gate shut by high mechanoreceptor input

No output

Impulses Low innocuous input rate

High noci input

Noci fibre

Dorsal columns

Ascending noci systems

D2
Noci gate open

High noci output

Fig. 18.2 Descending and peripheral gate control systems modulating nociceptor and pain intensities.

A descending encephalinergic opioid system runs from the lower medullary reticular nuclei, via the DLF, to laminae I and II, which is thought to be postsynaptic inhibitory to noci-driven neurones (Fig. 18.2C).

The dorsal horn is rich in encephalin and dynorphin cells and terminals, and it is through these cells that much opioid nociceptive inhibition is thought to occur (Cruz & Basbaum 1985).

Wall (1989) has pointed out that, in the wider context, all the spinal cord projector neurones, and interneurone circuits, are under continuous higher-centre control and monitoring. Thus, their levels of excitation and inhibition are continually varying according to these descending influences, which include changes in emotional tension as well as postural and movement activity. Neuronal fields of receptivity to differing stimuli, and responses to different sources of input, change over time, and are particularly affected by prolonged neuropathic states which markedly affect threshold sensitivities towards nociception.

Peripheral input modulation of nociceptive intensity in the dorsal horn

Everybody has experienced the phenomenon in which acute pain is reduced by rubbing over and around a painful area. Experimental confirmation that stimulating touch mechanoreceptors reduced coincident pain was published by Wall & Cronly-Dillon in 1960. The important difference between anecdotal reportage and these experimental findings was that the latter enabled researchers to propose a working hypothesis that large-fibre afferents modulated noci intensity of small-fibre afferents by possible presynaptic inhibition in laminae I and II. This reduced the available intensity of noci afferent excitation onto the direct noci-driven, or noci-responsive polymodal cells of origin of STT and associated tracts, and therefore reduced the intensity of post-thalamic noci stimuli and level of experienced pain (Fig. 18.2, D1, D2). Thus was born the formal gate control theory of pain modulation (Melzack & Wall 1965) which has transformed the experimental and clinical approach to pain control. Dorsal column stimulation (DCS) demonstrated antidromic inhibition onto laminae I and II, and subsequent research has shown that all non-noci input, including small-fibre thermoreception, has an inhibitory effect upon dorsal horn noci activity. Stimulation of large-fibre mechano-receptors by transcutaneous electrical nerve stimulation (TENS) for pain relief stems directly from experiments in DCS during the late 1960s.

While the dorsal horn, and analogous trigeminal nucleus, are the main large-fibre sensory/small-fibre noci-gating sites, there is much evidence to show that similar gating occurs in whatever nuclei the two types of stimuli synapse. This applies particularly at the thalamus before final thalamocortical relay.

Noci modulation mechanisms in the dorsal horn

In his critique of present views on noci modulation mechanisms in the dorsal horn Wall (1989) pointed out that the attractive simplicity of the specificity theory, which proposes that a hard wire system of pain is proportional to nociceptive afferent cause relationship, accords neither with experience nor neurological findings. Research on Rexed laminae and functional connections, somadendritic morphology and receptive fields, the neurochemistry of transmitters and modulators, axonal destinations, microelectrode stimulation and cellular responses, have shown the enormous complexity of interaction. Wall's argument is that, while many experimental findings are perfectly valid, they represent 'snapshots of cells in one of the modes of operation contained in their repertoire'. Any assumption that this observed operational mode will persist in time is considered very questionable, as neuronal interaction is a living, functional relationship which alters with demand over time.

Wall considers that the neuropeptide analgesia scenario, outlined in previous sections, may be 'embarrassingly simplistic', and he comes to some cautious conclusions which can be briefly summarized as follows:

1. There is no fixed relationship between afferent input and resulting sensory, or behavioural outcome. Neither is there a fixed relationship between input and output of dorsal horn cells.

2. Dorsal horn processing of incoming afferent information, in the context of changing higher-centre information and control, leads to the following three different ways of processing the same information according to time scale:
   a. Rapid peripheral input gate control, either excitatory or inhibitory, acting over milliseconds to seconds. This is the first basis of TENS.
   b. Slow sensitivity control, over minutes or hours, during which the size of receptor field sensitivity, and threshold response to the type of stimuli, can change as the cell is exposed to unusually intense, or maybe unusually absent, stimuli. Cells may, for example, respond increasingly to light touch stimuli as a potentiation response. Intense C fibre barrage from deep tissues can have this 'wind-up' effect, which implies that cell sensitivity is very much governed by the type of rapid- or slow-firing transmitter involved.
   c. Prolonged connectivity control over days to months, especially, for example, after de-afferentation injury when previous presynaptic and postsynaptic inhibitory controls are lost and cell excitation threshold drops. In this state a cell may respond to other afferent stimuli, which were previously ineffective, and develop new receptive fields.

It can be seen from this discussion that the mechanisms

of dorsal horn response vary considerably according to different time-scales of activation, and no 'snapshot' view can give the whole story.

PERIPHERAL NOCICEPTOR AND DORSAL HORN RESPONSE TO TISSUE INJURY

Unmyelinated C fibres form about 70% of all dorsal root afferents (Willis & Coggleshall 1978) and most of them are nociceptors. If their only function is to signal injury then the majority of them will remain silent throughout life as few people manage systematically to injure their whole body. It seems an anomalous situation that so many fibres, maintained by their dorsal root cells and in good functional contact with dorsal horn cells, should have nothing to do. When they are occasionally activated by tissue damage they do not even accurately demarcate the site of pain for very long. Surrounding tissue innervation undergoes a marked change in sensory threshold response and rapidly become hyperalgesic to touch, and these tissues then become tender and painful in their own right. Again, if the role of C fibres is only nociception their slow 1 m^{-1} system seems an unnecessary back-up for the much faster A-δ fibres, which can both provide a rapid alert and register the extent and duration of injury.

Wall (1989) proposes that neurophysiological studies of C fibre activity, together with the sequence of inflammatory reactions that occur in innervated tissue, and known changes in dorsal horn circuitry and sensitivity consequent to tissue and/or peripheral nerve injury, indicate that C fibre role and function vary according to whether tissue is injured or not injured.

C fibres are in a continuous state of very active, two-way axonal transport of a wide variety of molecules. Their neurotubules convey a continuous exchange of substances between their peripheral tissue interface, their dorsal root ganglion (DRG) cells, and their dorsal horn connections. DRG cells continually synthesize a wide range of enzymes, peptides, including substance P, and monoamines (serotonin) which flow towards their peripheral endings and their spinal cord connections. These chemicals slowly leak out at either end. Axonal transport rates vary according to molecule size, the largest being the slowest, and range from about 50 mm to 400 mm per day, or 1 metre after 20 days or 2.5 days. Orthograde flow is from neurone to axon terminal, and retrograde flow is from terminal to cell. DRG cells alter the types and concentrations of transport substances they manufacture according to the chemical information arriving by retrograde flow. This information is in the form of tissue fluid molecules returned to the DRG cell by its C fibre endings. If the state of the tissue changes, as it does when inflamed, this change is signalled to the DRG cell by a change of returned molecule (McMahon & Gibson 1987). This implies that the synthesis profiles of SRG cells are, in effect, a functional map of the tissues that they innervate.

It must be noted that two-way neurotubular flow is common to all neurone bodies and their extensions, as it acts as an essential nutrient, repair and information system. Tissue state monitoring seems peculiar to C fibres and is not found, for example, in A-δ fibres.

Present views on the functions of C fibres and their SRG cells in health and injury can be summarized as follows:

1. The receptor field of each fibre continually monitors the metabolic state of the tissues in which it is embedded and returns this information to its ganglion cell and dorsal horn by orthograde neurochemical axoplasmic flow.

2. The peptide make-up of individual C fibres varies according to the type of tissue that they innervate. So the profile of DRG synthesis is tissue-specific and determined by retrograde flow.

3. Mechanical, thermal and/or chemical tissue injury is signalled to the CNS by an impulse discharge rate proportional to the severity of noxious damage. This is supplemented by increasing spatial summation as inflammatory changes develop.

4. Injury impulses travelling along axon collaterals to local blood vessels cause reflex vasodilatation.

5. The active endings leak inflammatory peptides, including substance P, and enzymes by orthograde axoplasmic expulsion pressure. These cause further vasodilatation, neurogenic oedema and sensitization of surrounding nerve endings additional to tissue cell inflammatory reactions. This effect is enhanced if unmyelinated fibres are pushed into contact with each other (ephaptic contact) so that their orthodromic impulses cause mutual contact depolarization and antidromic impulse travel back to their endings, which accelerates axon terminal leakage.

6. The inflammatory milieu reduces the sensory threshold of bimodal (mechanothermal) and polymodal nociceptive ending leading to the onset of hyperalgesic response to previously innocuous stimuli such as light touch.

7. Accelerated orthograde axoplasmic transport of chemicals from the damaged tissues informs the ganglion cells of injury. Their reactive change of synthesis profile results in different peptide concentrations being secreted at presynaptic dorsal horn connections. These substances act as synaptic modulators of laminal cell response to transmitter substances and modify receptor field sensitivities (receptor fields are the areas innervated by a particular fibre. Threshold sensitivity is usually most marked in the centre and less so at the periphery. Inflammatory agents can change this).

8. Sustained C fibre activity from deep tissues causes long-lasting, widespread sensitization of spinal cord circuits to noci stimuli and this, together with peripheral hyperalgesia, causes prolonged tenderness.

9. This prolonged tenderness extends into the repair stage of capillary revascularization, and axonal sprouting re-innervation. The latter is highly sensitive and liable to self-firing. The continuing pain and discomfort is a combination of peripheral and central changes in sensitivity.

Recent research (Woolf & Thompson 1991) has shown that repetitive low-frequency stimulation of C fibres increases spinal neurone action potential discharge and creates a state of prolonged excitability after stimulus termination. This is directly related to N-methyl-D-aspartic acid (NMDA) receptor activation, and is inhibited by NMDA antagonists. This excitatory wind-up is a result of temporal summation of slow synaptic potentials. It is thought to be the basis of spinal cord hyperalgesia by reducing receptor neurone thresholds to non-noci stimulation.

Wakisaha et al (1991) have found that unmyelinated C fibre integrity is highly resistant to disruption by peripheral nerve ligature, unlike myelinated fibres, and can maintain a high level of nociceptive activity as a response to ischaemia. This leads to a very unbalanced sensory feedback as nociceptive C fibre input into the dorsal horn is not balanced by large non-noxious fibre inhibition. These findings provide a possible mechanism for the acute pain of nerve root entrapment as the mechanical pressure, plus reactive inflammatory swelling, closely mimics experimental ligature effects.

In summary, unmyelinated C fibres play an important role in health and injury. They continually monitor their tissue environment by 'tasting' the extracellular fluid, as Wall has memorably described it, and informing their individual DRG neurone by a steady flow of chemical transport. They respond to mechanical, thermal and chemical damage by slow nociceptor impulse trains into laminae I and II. If their afferent intensity, along with A-δ activity, exceeds the ever fluctuating antinociceptor screen of large-fibre and descending control inhibition, they inevitably relay into the ascending STT and MAS/SRT systems to influence the neuroaxis up to the thalamus. Post-thalamic relays then evoke perceptual awareness and emotional experience of pain.

The role of dorsal root ganglion cells in nociceptive generation

The main function of DRG neurones is to maintain their bipolar axons and terminal endings in good repair and, in the case of C fibres, synthesize substances which act as markers to the tissues that their individual fibres innervate. They also have extra Na^+ ion channels at the soma base of the T junction to act as a signal booster for incoming depolarizing impulses as they travel into one arm of the T junction, around the soma/T junction base, and into the dorsal root afferent (see Devor & Obermeyer 1984, Matsumoto & Rosenbluth 1985, Devor review 1989).

Unlike sensory axons DRG cells are highly sensitive to mechanical distortion and can fire spontaneously (Howe et al 1976, Wall & Devor 1981, 1983) if this occurs through root traction or other cause. Chronic peripheral nerve injury makes them highly excitable and they can then become a strong source of ectopic nociceptor input. The pathophysiology of DRG infections, such as herpes zoster, can induce electrical coupling between the neurones so that they act like a syncytium. Their spontaneous volleys of impulses can then become an intense and unpredictable source of neuropathic pain (Nordin et al 1984, Mayer et al 1986).

The relationship between arthritic severity and small-fibre innervation density

An important relationship between the severity of inflammatory arthritis and density of joint innervation by efferent sympathetic fibres and afferent C fibres has been explored by Levine et al (1988). It has considerable relevance for physical therapists in the assessment and treatment of joint disorders.

DRG cells continually synthesize substance P (SP), which is transported to C fibre peripheral endings and secreted to a variable extent into adjacent tissue. SP is a strong pro-inflammatory factor which can cause vasodilatation, increased vascular permeability, mast cell degranulation and release of histamine, serotonin, leukotrienes and other inflammatory agents (Jansco et al 1967, Lembeck & Holzer 1979). Besides SP, the related peptides neurokinin A and neurokinin B have a complementary inflammatory effect, particularly upon vascular permeability. Also synthesized by the DGR cells is calcitonin gene-related peptide (CGRP) which, even at femtomole (10^{-15}) doses increases microcirculatory blood-flow for hours (Brain et al 1986). One consequence of neurogenic inflammation is the activation of efferent sympathetic terminal release of noradrenaline (norepinephrine), which increases vascular permeability and inflammatory reponse.

Raised sympathetic tone increases the availability of noradrenaline for terminal release if inflammation is present for whatever reason. Local tissue production of prostaglandins, which are strong inflammatory agents, is increased by the synergistic action of C fibres and sympathetic activity (Levine et al 1986b).

Experimental arthritis (EA) in animals closely mimics the pathological and clinical picture of rheumatoid arthritis (RA) and has been extensively used as a model for investigating the effects of drug therapy (Tsukano et al 1983). EA shows a bilateral joint involvement, and a distal-to-proximal gradient of severity. As a model for investigating the relationship between relative joint innervation density and severity of arthritic changes, EA has clearly demonstrated that high-risk joints, such as ankles in rats, are more densely innervated by C fibre afferents than low-risk joints, such as the knee in rats (Levine et al 1984, 1985, 1986a, b). The average tissue concentration of SP is higher in normal high-risk joints, correlating with innervation density, and considerably higher in the same joints when suffering from EA. The pro-inflammatory catecholamine effect of sympathetic efferents has been demonstrated by comparing the effects on EA of sympathectomy, compared to normal sympathetic activity, and raised sympathetic activity in hyperactive rats. Systemic gold therapy (sodium thiomalate), at doses which suppress EA symptoms, selectively reduces the density of unmyelinated C fibre innervation, for which it is neuropathic, but spares myelinated fibres. The concentration of joint neuropeptides and catecholamines is substantially reduced as a result (Levine et al 1985). Complementary research by Yaksh (1988) has found that a marked reduction of SP release by C fibre terminals occurs when opioids are given. There is strong evidence of direct C fibre innervation, or sympathetic fibre innervation, of mast cells which can markedly contribute to the inflammatory process (Wiesner-Menzel et al 1981, Goetzl et al 1986).

The implication of a direct link between density of innervation and joint pathology in a systemic disorder, such as RA, is strengthened by the observation that joints in limbs affected by strokes or peripheral nerve paralysis are not as severely damaged by RA as the opposite side (Glick 1967). Gout and Heberden's nodes rarely develop on the hemiplegic side following a stroke (Glynn & Clayton 1976, Helme & Andrews 1985).

Nociceptor input from joints (type IV endings; see Wyke 1979) causes long-term potentiation of dorsal horn receptive fields (Woolf & Wall 1986, Cook et al 1987) so that nocidriven cells also respond to even light touch stimulus. When joints are damaged this central effect is enhanced by the reduction in afferent nociceptor threshold resulting, in part, from increased output of neuro-inflammatory peptides and catecholamines by C fibres and sympathetic endings. They increasingly respond to the mechanical stimulus of joint movement, thus intensifying nociceptor afferent input into the already noci sensitive dorsal horn circuitry. This has two main motor effects. Firstly, the muscles controlling the joint are held in a variable state of nocidriven reflex co-contraction which acts as a physiological splint. Such sustained contraction can act as a strong source of secondary pain from muscle ischaemia through capillary compression. Secondly, these nocidriven responses are accentuated when momentarily successful attempts at voluntary movement increase nociceptor afferent input by activating joint mechanoreceptors whose input is misread as nociceptive.

Perhaps of direct physical therapy interest, and electrotherapy concern, is the fact that electrical stimulation of peripheral nerve above a critical intensity causes increased leakage of inflammatory substances from C fibre terminals in health and disease. Depolarizing electrical stimulation causes both orthodromic and antidromic impulses to travel from the site of depolarization. The resultant antidromic C fibre activity can provoke release of SP and other inflammatory mediators in sufficient quantities to cause neurogenic inflammatory responses (Jansco et al 1967, Ferrell & Russell 1986). The implications for low-frequency (LF) stimulation in the presence of arthritic and traumatic inflammatiom are unknown. So is the effect of sustained LF orthodromic stimulation on DRG cells. The main issue, however, is the sustained nociceptive sensitization that can occur when joint structures become inflamed, as it must be taken into account in manual assessment and manual therapy techniques.

SUMMARY

The working hypothesis adopted is that psychological functions, including consciousness, are the expression of preprogrammed subcortical to cortical neural network processing. The senses are the neural models of an 'outside' world which is generated within the structure of the brain. In the normally functioning brain the neural model of tissue damage is pain, which is located and superimposed upon the sensory body schema with emotional affect. Neuropathic, or pathophysiological pain, is imposed upon the body schema by self-generating abnormal pain processing, the cause of which can arise at any level of the pathways from peripheral reception, conduction, spinal cord, brainstem, thalamic, thalamo-cortical or limbocortical dysfunction.

This hypothesis provides a powerful rationale for the use of behavioural and physical therapy strategies in the modulation of pain because it assumes that the same principles of neural functioning apply at all levels. There can, therefore, be a two-way, cause and effect, interaction from non-psychological to psychological, or neuropsychical, and psychological to non-psychological, or psychoneural.

If the diencephalic level of thalamic and associated nuclei is taken as the borderline between suprathalamic psychological functioning, and prethalamic non-psychological functioning, then neural processing of tissue damage can be similarly divided between prethalamic nociception and post-thalamic pain. The two can act together as a single functioning unit, as in the normal acute pain of a sprained ankle, which subsides as the noxious source heals. At the other extreme they can act in complete disassociation, as in episodic analgesia, when no pain is experienced for about 24 hours after violent injury, such as limb avulsion or partial abdominal evisceration, and in phantom limb pain, where there is no limb to cause the pain and no peripheral stimulus (see Beecher 1959, Carlen et al 1978, Melzack & Wall 1988, Wall & Melzack 1989). An inexplicable total dysfunction exists in cases of congenital absence of pain despite apparently normal pathways (Sternbach 1968, Comings & Amromin 1974, Manfredi et al 1981).

The main peripheral nerve receptors and carriers of noci stimuli are the medium- to slow-conducting alpha-delta and C fibres. The main nocireceptive dorsal horn cells are in laminae I and II, and the main ascending tracts are the medium-fast anterolateral spinothalamic tracts, the slow multisynaptic tracts in the dorsolateral funiculus and central grey, and a similar multisynaptic tract ascending alongside the 'classical' pain tracts. Nociceptor processing occurs throughout the brainstem, including the cerebellar cortex, and noci stimuli eventually enter the ventrobasal, intralaminal and medial nuclei of the thalamus. Post-thalamic relays to the parietal, insula and temporal cortex establish the location and type of pain within the bodily schema, and relate present experience to similar previous episodes. Thalamolimbic and thalamo-frontal lobe processing generate the quality and emotional intensity of the pain. Reflexogenic motor and autonomic responses are initiated by spinal and brainstem mechanisms.

Mechanisms of nociceptive and pain intensity modulation exist throughout the neuroaxis. Descending direct corticospinal, together with brainstem opioid and serotonergic nociceptive inhibitory pathways, act at dorsal horn level, as does the noci inhibitory effects of peripheral mechanoreceptor afferent input. Reduction of ascending nociceptive intensity can occur during the multisynaptic interactions in the reticular formation, and mechano-receptor inhibition of noci stimuli can also occur at thalamic level. Willed motivational strategies may markedly inhibit the intensity of pain processing at suprathalamic levels. These endogenous modulatory controls are of very variable and unpredictable effectiveness, ranging from unaided volitional pain control within acceptable tolerance levels, to the necessity for physical therapy, pharmacology and/or surgical intervention to amplify, or substitute for, an endogenous control which does not meet tolerance level.

C fibres monitor the changing state of the tissues they innervate, both in health and injury, by 'tasting' the fluid medium and using neurotubular transport to convey tissue molecules to their DRG cells. The latter continually synthesize a range of enzymes and neuropeptides, appropriate to the type and state of the innervated tissue, which are leaked both at the periphery and at their dorsal horn contacts. Prolonged C fibre activation by tissue damage leads to leakage of neuro-inflammatory agents which exacerbate the inflammation, and leads to a reduction of nocidriven dorsal horn thresholds to innocuous stimuli. This applies particularly to joint injury, where mechano-receptor response to movement can enter the receptive field of nocidriven dorsal horn cells.

Experimental evidence indicates that there is a close link between the relative density of joint innervation and the inflammatory response of joints to systemic arthropathies such as rheumatoid arthritis. Those joints which suffer most have a greater density of innervation, and higher levels of neuro-inflammatory peptides, than those which are relatively unscathed. Strong electrical stimulation of peripheral nerves will cause a marked increase of C fibre neuropeptide leakage even in normal tissues. This may have implications for low-frequency electrotherapy but there is, as yet, no published research on the subject. The major implication of this knowledge is for musculoskeletal examination and manual therapy.

REFERENCES

Bahns E, Halsband U, Janig W, Nelke A 1986 Functional characteristics of lumbar visceral afferent fibres from the urinary bladder and the urethra of the cat. Pflügers Archiv 407: 510–518

Barlow H B, Mollon J D 1982 The senses. Cambridge University Press, Cambridge

Beard R W, Pearce S 1989 Gynaecological pain. In: Wall P D, Melzack R (eds) Textbook of pain, 2nd edn. Churchill Livingstone, Edinburgh

Beecher H K 1959 Measurement of subjective responses. Oxford University Press, Oxford

Berglund R 1986 The fabric of mind. Viking, Harmondsworth

Blendis L M 1989 Abdominal pain. In: Wall P D, Melzack R (eds) Textbook of pain, 2nd edn. Churchill Livingstone, Edinburgh

Bloom F E, Lazerson A, Hofstadter L 1985 Brain, mind and behaviour. W H Freeman, New York

Boivie J 1979 An anatomical reinvestigation of the termination of the spinothalamic tract in the monkey. Journal of Comparative Neurology 186: 343–370

Bonica J J, Chadwick H S 1989 Labour pain. In: Wall P D, Melzack R (eds) Textbook of pain, 2nd edn. Churchill Livingstone

Bowsher D 1988 Central pain mechanisms. In: Wells P E, Frampton V, Bowsher D (eds) Pain: management and control in physiotherapy. Heinemann, London

Brain S D, William T J, Tippins J R, Morris H R, MacIntyre I 1986 Calcitonin gene-related peptide is a potent vasodilator. Nature 313: 54–56

Campbell J N, Meyer R A 1986 Primary afferents and hyperalgesia. In: Yaksh T L (ed) Spinal afferent processing. Plenum Press, New York

Campbell J N, Srinivasa N, Raja R, Cohen H, Manning D C, Khan A A, Meyer R A 1989 Peripheral neural mechanisms of nociception. In: Wall P D, Melzack R (eds) Textbook of pain, 2nd edn. Churchill Livingstone, Edinburgh

Carlen P L, Wall P D, Nadvorna H, Steinbach T 1978 Phantom limbs and related phenomena in recent traumatic amputations. Neurology 28: 211–17

Changeux J P 1985 Neuronal man: the biology of mind. Oxford University Press, Oxford

Clark W C, Clark S B 1980 Pain responses in Nepalese porters. Science 209: 410–412

Comings D E, Amromin G D 1974 Autosomal dominant insensitivity to pain with hyperplastic myelinopathy and autosomal dominant indifference to pain. Neurology 24: 838–848

Cook A J, Woolf C J, Wall P D, McMahon S B 1987 Dynamic receptive field plasticity in rat spinal cord dorsal horn following C primary afferent input. Nature 325: 151–153

Coren S, Ward L M 1989 Sensation and perception. 3rd edn. Harcourt Brace Jovanovich, San Diego

Cotman C W, McGaugh J L 1980 Behavioural neuroscience. Academic Press, New York

Cruz L, Basbaum A I 1985 Multiple opioid peptides and the modulation of pain: immunohistochemical analysis of dynorphin and enkephalin in the trigeminal nucleus caudalis and spinal cord of the cat. Journal of Comparative Neurology 240: 331–338

Darien-Smith I, Johnson K O, Dykes R 1973 'Cold' fibre population innervating palmar and digital skin of the monkey: responses to cooling pulses. Journal of Neurophysiology 36: 325–346

Darien-Smith I, Johnson K O, LaMotte C, Shigenaga Y, Kenins P, Champness P 1979 Warm fibres innervating palmar and distal skin of the monkey: responses to thermal stimuli. Journal of Neurophsyiology 42: 1297–1310

Devor M 1989 The pathophysiology of damaged peripheral nerves. In: Wall P D, Melzack R (eds) Textbook of pain, 2nd edn. Churchill Livingstone, Edinburgh

Devor M, Obermeyer M L 1984 Membrane differentiation in rat dorsal root ganglia and possible consequences for back pain. Neuroscience Letters 51: 341–346

Dimond S J 1980 Neuropsychology. Butterworths, London

Eccles J 1979 The human mystery. Routledge, London

Eccles J 1980 The human psyche. Routledge, London

Eccles J 1989 Evolution of the brain. Routledge, London

Eccles J & Robinson D 1984 The wonder of being human. Routledge, London

Elhilali M M, Winfield H N 1989 Genitourinary pain. In: Wall P D, Melzack R (eds) Textbook of pain, 2nd edn. Churchill Livingstone

Ferrell W R, Russell N J W 1986 Extravasation of the knee induced by antidromic stimulation of articular C fibre afferents of the anaesthetised cat. Journal of Physiology, 379: 407–411

Fields H L, Basbaum A I 1989 Endogenous pain control mechanisms. In: Wall P D, Melzack R (eds) Textbook of pain, 2nd edn. Churchill Livingstone, Edinburgh

Fitzgerald M 1989 The course and termination of primary afferent fibres. In: Wall P D, Melzack R (eds) Textbook of pain, 2nd edn. Churchill Livingstone, Edinburgh

Fitzgerald M, Wall P D 1980 The laminar organisation of dorsal horn cells responding to peripheral C fibre stimulation. Experimental Brain Research 41: 36–44

Foreman R D, Hancock M B, Willis W D 1981 Responses of spinothalamic tract cells in the thoracic spinal cord of the monkey to cutaneous and visceral inputs. Pain 11: 149–162

Gazzaniga M 1989 Organisation of the human brain. Science 245: 947–952

Glick E N 1967 Asymmetrical rheumatoid arthritis after poliomyelitis. British Medical Journal 3: 26–29

Glynn J J, Clayton M L 1976 Sparing effect of hemiplegia on tophaceous gout. Annals of Rheumatic Diseases 35: 534–535

Gobel S, Falls W M, Humphrey E 1981 Morphology and synaptic connections of ultrafine primary axons in lamina I of the spinal dorsal horn: candidates for the terminal axonal arbors of primary neurones in unmyelinated (C) axons. Journal of Neuroscience 1: 1163–1179

Goetzl E J, Chernov-Rogan T, Furuichi K 1986 Neuromodulation of mast cell and basophil function. In: Denburgh J A (ed) Mast cell differentiation and heterogeneity. Raven Press, New York

Golding D 1988 The secret life of the neuron. New Scientist No 1626, 18 August, 52–55

Hannington-Kiff J G, Mehta M, Dudley H, Cerveco F 1983 Pain in perspective, vol 1. Dista Products, Basingstoke

Hardy J D, Wolff H G, Goodell H 1952 Pain sensations and reactions. Williams & Wilkins, Baltimore

Helme R D, Andrews P V 1985 The effect of nerve lesions on the inflammatory response to injury. Journal of Neuroscience Research 13: 453–459

Howe J F, Calvin W H, Loeser J D 1976 Impulses reflected from dorsal root ganglia and from focal nerve injuries. Brain Research 116: 139–144

Iversen L 1985 Chemicals to think by. New Scientist No 1458, 30 May, 11–14

Jansco G, Jansco-Gabor A, Szolcanyi J 1967 Direct evidence for direct neurogenic inflammation and its prevention by denervation and by pretreatment with capsaicin. British Journal of Pharmacology and Chemotherapy 31: 138

Jessup B A 1989 Relaxation and feedback. In: Wall P D, Melzack R (eds) Textbook of pain, 2nd edn. Churchill Livingstone, Edinburgh

Kimble D P 1988 Biological psychology. Holt, Rhinehart & Winston, New York

Koerber H R, Brown P B 1980 Projections of two hindlimb cutaneous nerves to cat dorsal horn. Journal of Neurophysiology 44: 259–269

Kruger L, Perl E R, Sedivec M J 1981 Fine structure of myelinated mechanical nociceptor endings in cat hairy skin. Journal of Comparative Neurology 198: 137–154

Lamotte C 1977 Distribution of the tract of Lissaur and the dorsal root fibres in the primate spinal cord. Journal of Comparative Neurology 172: 529–562

Lembeck F, Holzer P 1979 Substance P as neurogenic mediator of antidromic vasodilation and neurogenic plasma extravasation. Nauyn-Schmiedeberg's Archives of Pharmacology 310: 175–183

Levine J D, Clark R, Devor M, Helms C, Moskowitz M A, Basbaum A I 1984 Intraneuronal substance P contributes to the severity of experimental arthritis. Science 226: 547–549

Levine J D, Moskowitz M A, Basbaum A I 1985 The contribution of neurogenic inflammation in experimental arthritis. Journal of Immunology 135: 843–847

Levine J D, Dardick S J, Roizen M S, Helms C, Basbaum A I 1986a Contribution of sensory afferents and sympathetic efferents to joint injury in experimental arthritis. Journal of Neuroscience 6: 3423–3429

Levine J D, Taiwo Y O, Collins S D, Tam J K 1986b Noradrenaline hyperalgesia is mediated through interaction with sympathetic postganglionic neurone terminals rather than activation of primary afferent nociceptors. Nature 323: 158–160

Levine J D, Coderre T J, Basbaum A I 1988 The peripheral nervous system and the inflammatory process. In: Dubner R, Gebhart G F, Bond M R (eds) Proceedings of the Vth World Congress on Pain. Elsevier, New York

Lichstein L, Sackett G P 1971 Reactions by differentially raised Rhesus monkeys to noxious stimuli. Developmental Psychobiology 4: 339–352

Luria A R 1973 The working brain: an introduction to neuropsychology. Penguin Books, Harmondsworth

McMahon S B, Gibson S 1987 Peptide expression is altered when afferent nerves reinervate inappropriate tissue. Neuroscience Letters 73: 9–15

McMahon S, Koltzenburg M 1990 The changing role of primary afferent neurones in pain. Pain 43: 269–272

Malliani A, Pagani M, Lombardi F 1989 Visceral versus somatic mechanisms. In: Wall P D, Melzack R (eds) Textbook of pain, 2nd edn. Churchill Livingstone, Edinburgh

Manfredi M, Bini G, Cruccu G, Accornero N, Beradelli A, Medolago L 1981 Congenital absence of pain. Archives of Neurology 38: 507–11

Matsumoto E, Rosenbluth J 1985 Plasma membrane structure at the axon hillock, initial segment and cell body of frog dorsal root ganglion cells. Journal of Neurocytology 14: 731–747

Mayer M L, James M H, Russell R J, Kelly J S, Pasternak O A 1986 Changes in excitability induced by herpes simplex viruses in rat dorsal root ganglion neurons. Journal of Neuroscience 6: 391–402

Mehler W R 1962 The anatomy of the so-called 'pain tract' in man: an analysis of the course and distribution of the ascending fibres of the fasciculus anterolateralis. In: French J D, Porter R W (eds) Basic research in paraplegia. Thomas, Springfield, Illinois

Melzack R 1965 Effects of early experience on behaviour: experimental and conceptual considerations. In: Hoch P, Zubin J (eds) Psychopathology of perception. Grune & Stratton, New York

Melzack R 1969 The role of early experience in emotional arousal. Annals of the New York Academy of Sciences 159: 721–730

Melzack R, Wall P D 1965 Pain mechanisms: a new theory. Science 150: 971–979

Melzack R, Wall P D 1988 The challenge of pain, 2nd edn. Penguin Books, Harmondsworth

Mense S, Prabhakar N R 1986 Spinal termination of nociceptive afferent fibres from deep tissues in the cat. Neuroscience Letters 66: 169–174

Meyer D E R, Snow P J 1986 Distribution of activity in the spinal terminals of single hair follicle afferent fibres to somatopically identified regions of the cat spinal cord. Journal of Neurophysiology 56: 1022–1038

Milne R J, Foreman R D, Giesler G J, Willis W D 1981 Convergence of cutaneous and pelvic visceral nociceptor inputs onto primate spinothalamic neurones. Pain 11: 163–183

Molander C, Grant G 1985 Cutaneous projections from the rat hindlimb foot to the substantia gelatinosa of the spinal cord studied by transganglionic transport of WGA–HRP conjugate. Journal of Comparative Neurology 237: 476–484

Molander C, Grant G 1987 Spinal cord projections from hindlimb muscle nerves in the rat studied by transganglionic transport of HRP or WGA–HRP or DMSO–HRP. Journal of Comparative Neurology 260: 246–256

Morgan C, Nadelhaft I, de Groat W C 1981 The distribution of visceral primary afferents from the pelvic nerve to Lissauer's tract and the spinal grey matter and its relationship to the sacral parasympathetic nucleus. Journal of Comparative Neurology 201: 415–440

Nathan P 1988 The nervous system. 3rd edn. Oxford University Press, Oxford

Ness T J, Gebhart G F 1990 Visceral pain: a review of experimental studies. Pain 42: 167–233

Noback C R, Strominger N L, Demarest R J 1991 The human nervous system. 4th edn. Lea & Febiger, Philadelphia

Nordin M, Nystrom B, Wallin U, Hagbarth K E 1984 Ectopic sensory discharges and parasthesiae in patients with disorders of peripheral nerves, dorsal roots and dorsal columns. Pain 20: 231–245

Orne M T, Dinges D F 1989 Hypnosis. In: Wall P D, Melzack R Textbook of pain, 2nd edn. Churchill Livingstone, Edinburgh

Osborne N 1983 The brain's information technology. New Scientist 19 May, 445–447

Penfield W 1975 The mystery of the mind. Princeton University Press, Princeton

Penfield W, Perot P 1963 The brain's record of auditory and visual experience. Brain 86: 595–697

Procacci P, Zoppi M 1989 Heart pain. In: Wall P D, Melzack R (eds) Textbook of pain, 2nd edn. Churchill Livingstone, Edinburgh

Reichling D B, Basbaum A I 1986 Some periaquaductal gray neurones of the rat which project to the nucleus raphe magnus have descending collaterals. Society of Neuroscience Abstracts 12: 616

Rexed B 1952 The cytoarchitectonic organisation of the spinal cord in the cat. Journal of Comparative Neurology 96: 415–495

Sternbach R A 1968 Pain: a psychophysiological analysis. Academic Press, New York

Sternbach R A 1989 Behaviour therapy. In: Wall P D, Melzack R (eds) Textbook of pain, 2nd edn. Churchill Livingstone, Edinburgh

Sternbach R A, Tursky B 1965 Ethnic differences between housewives in psychophysical and skin potential responses to electric shock. Psychophysiology 1: 241–246

Swett J E, Woolf C J 1985 The somatopic organisation of primary afferent terminals in the superficial dorsal horn of the rat spinal cord. Journal of Comparative Neurology. 231: 66–77

Szentagothai J 1983 The modular architectonic principles of neural centers. Review of Physiology, Biochemistry and Pharmacology 98: 11–94

Tan S Y 1982 Cognitive and cognitive-behavioural methods for pain control: a selective review. Pain 12: 23–46

Tsukano M, Nawa Y, Kotani M 1983 Characterisation of low dose-induced suppressor cells in adjuvant induced arthritis in rats. Clinical and Experimental Immunology 53: 60–66

Turk D C, Meichenbaum D H 1989 A cognitive-behavioural approach to pain management. In: Wall P D, Melzack R (eds) Textbook of pain, 2nd edn. Churchill Livingstone, Edinburgh

Turk D C, Rudy T E 1987 An integrated approach to pain treatment: beyond scalpel and syringe. In: Tollinson C D (ed) Handbook of chronic pain management. Williams & Wilkins, Baltimore

van Hees J, Gybels J 1981 C nociceptor activity in human nerve during painful and non painful stimulation. Neurosurgery and Psychiatry 44: 600–607

Wakisaha S, Kajander K C, Bennett G J 1991 Abnormal skin temperature and abnormal sympathetic vasomotor innervation in an experimentally painful peripheral neuropathy. Pain 46: 299–313

Wall P D 1989 The dorsal horn. In Wall P D, Melzack R (eds) Textbook of pain 2nd edn Churchill Livingstone, Edinburgh

Wall P D, Cronly-Dillon J R 1960 Pain, itch and vibration. Archives of Neurology 2: 365–375

Wall P D, Devor M 1981 The effect of peripheral nerve injury on dorsal root potentials and on the transmission of afferent signals into the spinal cord. Brain Research 209: 95–111

Wall P D, Devor M 1983 Sensory afferent impulses originate from dorsal root ganglia as well as from the periphery in normal and nerve-injured rats. Pain 17: 321–339

Wall P D, Melzack R 1989 Textbook of pain, 2nd edn. Churchill Livingstone, Edinburgh

Walsh K 1987 Neuropsychology: a clinical approach, 2nd edn. Churchill Livingstone, Edinburgh

Watson J 1986 Pain and nociception — mechanisms and modulation. In: Grieve G P (ed) Modern manual therapy of the vertebral column. Churchill Livingstone, Edinburgh

Wiener-Menzel L, Schulz B, Vakilzadeh F, Czarnetzki B M 1981 Electron microscopical evidence for a direct contact between nerve cells and mast cells. Acta Dermatologica 61: 465–469

Willis W D 1985 Nociceptive pathways: anatomy and physiology of nociceptive ascending pathways. Philosophical Transactions of the Royal Society B308: 253–286

Willis W D 1989 The origin and destination of pathways involved in pain transmission. In: Wall P D, Melzack R (eds) Textbook of pain, 2nd edn. Churchill Livingstone, Edinburgh

Willis W D, Coggleshall R E 1978 Sensory mechanisms of the spinal cord. John Wiley, New York

Woolf C J, Thompson W N 1991 The induction and maintenance of central sensitisation is dependent upon N-methyl-D-aspartic acid receptor activation: implications for the treatment of post injury pain hypersensitivity states. Pain 44: 213–232

Woolf C J, Wall P D 1986 The relative effectiveness of C-primary afferents of different origins in evoking a prolonged facilitation on the flexor reflex of the rat. Journal of Neuroscience 6: 1433–1442

Wyke B D 1979 Neurology of the cervical spinal joints. Physiotherapy 65: 72–76

Wyke B D 1981 Neurological aspects of pain therapy. In: Swerdlow M (ed) The therapy of pain. MTP Press, Lancaster

Yaksh T L 1988 Substance P release from knee joint afferent terminals: modulation by opioids. Brain Research 458: 319–324

Ygge J, Grant G 1983 The organisation of the thoracic spinal nerve projection in the dorsal horn demonstrated with transganglionic transport of horseradish peroxidase. Journal of Comparative Neurology 216: 1–9

19. Referred pain and other clinical features

G. P. Grieve

An important requirement in effectively treating musculo-skeletal problems is a full appreciation of the behaviour and vagaries of referred pain, together with the ubiquitous problems of referred tenderness, and induced muscle spasm, often relatively remote from the site of the causative vertebral joint and limb girdle soft-tissue changes (Travell & Simons 1983).

The phenomenon of referred or projected pain is well recognized but not well understood. It is a frequent source of difficulty, in identification of the vertebral segments and soft tissues involved and in the correct localization of treatment (Grieve 1988).

Serious visceral disease and neoplastic spinal disease can produce spinal pain which mimics that of relatively innocent vertebral joint problems, and conversely, pain referred around the chest and to the abdominal wall from vertebral and rib joint involvement can easily simulate the pains of visceral disease such as pleurisy, cardiac ischaemia, gall-bladder disease and acute appendicitis (Fig. 19.1). Again, while headache arises from a variety of causes, including benign conditions of the craniovertebral joints, differential diagnosis is not assisted, alone, on the basis of the area or distribution of the head pain (Jull 1981).

'Paradoxically the more a subject is investigated the greater is the realization that our understanding of it is often based on phenomena we cannot explain.' (Sydenham 1979).

Scott-Charlton and Roebuck (1972) discussed the significance of the posterior primary divisions of spinal nerves, and mentioned in passing:

. . . the fashion of condemning a 'joint' whenever pain is felt in (spinal) musculo-tendinous structures. A very tender type of tissue in the human body, so frequently a source of pain in all sorts of conditions — traumatic, 'rheumatic', postural, occupational, etc. — is the tissue of junction between muscle, tendon, intermuscular septum, or similar structure, with periosteum and bone. . . . A great deal of pain may well be felt where muscle, tendon, ligament and capsule are attached to sensitive periosteum in the spine.

The attachments of ligaments, muscles and aponeuroses are peculiarly liable to undergo changes which are a fruitful source of musculoskeletal pain, while the true nature and genesis of these changes remain debatable.

Mooney (1983) mentioned that we still await clarification of the state of non-neural soft tissues — muscle, capsule, ligament — and that these constitute by far the most deranged aspect of anatomy in the majority of low-back disorders.

Inman and Saunders (1944) also remarked that, of ligaments and capsules, those parts in the neighbourhood of bony attachments are especially sensitive.

Significantly, the experimental injection of a 6% saline solution into facet joint cavities produces less intense pain than injection of the pericapsular tissues.

Scott-Charlton and Roebuck concluded by mentioning '. . . the still very nebulous subject of referred pain'.

'Pain' has never been satisfactorily defined (Melzack & Wall 1982). A great deal remains to be learned about the mechanisms of pain and the affective, motivational and cognitive factors of the pain experience. We can speak with more confidence about the clinical behaviour of referred pain, and its marked tendency to vary between individuals, than we knowledgeably can about the neural mechanisms underlying that behaviour.

This probably explains the common adoption of modes of thought handed down by predecessors, i.e. the beginner's error of uncritically passing on traditional views and accounts. As clinical seniority is acquired, the fog is perpetuated by continuing to trade in this limited stock of assumptions and assertions about referred pain; by habit and repetition the assumptions steadily become fossilized. 'What I say three times is probably true, is virtually true, is a fact' (Hart 1977).

Some of the popular assertions on the nature and behaviour of referred pain are copied from text to text yet have no factual basis, as clinical experience will eventually underline; a proportion of clinical writers appear to clutch at any straw sooner than admit ignorance.

Brodal (1981) observed 'In spite of all the research devoted to the nervous system our knowledge is still rather limited. On almost all points there are unresolved prob-

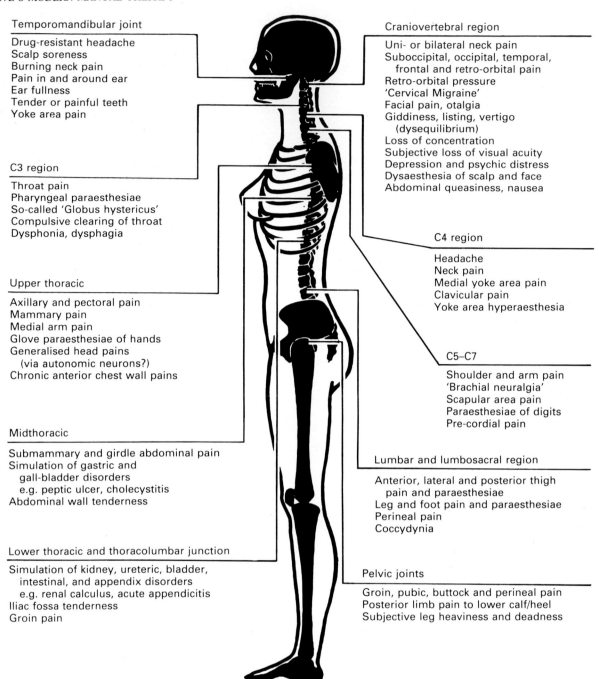

Temporomandibular joint

Drug-resistant headache
Scalp soreness
Burning neck pain
Pain in and around ear
Ear fullness
Tender or painful teeth
Yoke area pain

C3 region

Throat pain
Pharyngeal paraesthesiae
So-called 'Globus hystericus'
Compulsive clearing of throat
Dysphonia, dysphagia

Upper thoracic

Axillary and pectoral pain
Mammary pain
Medial arm pain
Glove paraesthesiae of hands
Generalised head pains
   (via autonomic neurons?)
Chronic anterior chest wall pains

Midthoracic

Submammary and girdle abdominal pain
Simulation of gastric and
   gall-bladder disorders
   e.g. peptic ulcer, cholecystitis
Abdominal wall tenderness

Lower thoracic and thoracolumbar junction

Simulation of kidney, ureteric, bladder,
   intestinal, and appendix disorders
   e.g. renal calculus, acute appendicitis
Iliac fossa tenderness
Groin pain

Craniovertebral region

Uni- or bilateral neck pain
Suboccipital, occipital, temporal,
   frontal and retro-orbital pain
Retro-orbital pressure
'Cervical Migraine'
Facial pain, otalgia
Giddiness, listing, vertigo
   (dysequilibrium)
Loss of concentration
Subjective loss of visual acuity
Depression and psychic distress
Dysaesthesia of scalp and face
Abdominal queasiness, nausea

C4 region

Headache
Neck pain
Medial yoke area pain
Clavicular pain
Yoke area hyperaesthesia

C5–C7

Shoulder and arm pain
'Brachial neuralgia'
Scapular area pain
Paraesthesiae of digits
Pre-cordial pain

Lumbar and lumbosacral region

Anterior, lateral and posterior thigh
   pain and paraesthesiae
Leg and foot pain and paraesthesiae
Perineal pain
Coccydynia

Pelvic joints

Groin, pubic, buttock and perineal pain
Posterior limb pain to lower calf/heel
Subjective leg heaviness and deadness

Fig. 19.1 A scheme of the various types of pain referral, with concomitant clinical features, commonly associated with benign musculoskeletal conditions of the spinal districts mentioned, and the temporomandibular joint. (Reproduced from Grieve 1991.)

lems. Our present-day concepts are still to a large extent based upon assumptions and hypotheses built upon a modest body of factual knowledge . . . . Working hypotheses are important and necessary tools in research, but as the history of science shows, they have a tendency to become accepted as truths and to hamper instead of promoting progress'.

REFERRED PAIN AS A CENTRAL PHENOMENON

Generally, (i) the more superficial the affected tissue the

more likely is the pain to remain localized. Hence painful lesions of the body surface hurt where the lesion is, and there is usually little spread of pain. One exception is lateral epicondylitis, of course, where a very superficial lesion often projects pain distally to the wrist region. (ii) Painful lesions of deeper tissues, musculoskeletal or visceral, hurt locally as a rule but often also refer or project pain to regions uninvolved in the primary lesion. Sometimes there is no 'local' pain but only referred pain, e.g. in arthrosis of the hip the patient may report anterior thigh pain alone. These facts are well known and need not be laboured here (Grieve 1988). It should be mentioned that because the faculty of localizing noxious stimuli to the skin surface is highly developed and very accurate, and that of perceiving the locality of deeper lesions is considerably less developed, the physiology of cutaneous sensation is of less help when considering the clinical presentation of musculoskeletal tissue damage and visceral conditions.

Almost 70 years after Smith-Petersen's (1924) account of the distribution of referred sacroiliac pain, solely on the distribution of nerve roots L4, L5, S1 and S2, it appears to remain the erroneous basis of most concepts of musculoskeletal referred pain.

Again, as recently as a decade ago, an experienced clinician (Dixon 1980) wrote ' . . . the low back pain common to nearly all disc prolapses, which the layman calls lumbago, the referred pain of which follows a pattern characteristic for each disc level . . .' thus implying that the segmental level of a disc prolapse might therefore be determined by the characteristic distribution of its referred pain. Clinical presentations as neat as this are infrequent, to say the least.

Brown (1983) remarked that neoplasms and parenchymal disease of the lung, and infections of the diaphragmatic pleura, can refer pain to the shoulder 'via the phrenic nerve'. Neoplastic disease of the lung may also refer pain to the ipsilateral ear region 'via the vagus nerve' (Bindoff & Heseltine 1988) (vide infra). There is increasing experimental evidence in support of the hypothesis that the anatomical substrate for referred pain is the convergence of afferent neurons, from one body region, onto central nervous system neurons which also receive afferents from topographically separate body regions. Sessle et al (1986) applied electrical stimuli to afferent neurons from facial skin, oral mucosa, canine and premolar tooth pulp, laryngeal mucosa, cervical skin and muscle, and jaw and tongue muscles. Their observation of the extensive convergence of different types of afferents, especially apparent in cutaneous nociceptive neurons, suggest a role for these in mediating deep pain and in the spread and referral of pain.

In a fluorescent dye double-labelling study, Laurberg and Sorensen (1985) noted that rat cervical dorsal root ganglion cells were retrogradely double-labelled with dyes following injection of one dye into a cutaneous shoulder nerve and the other into the diaphragm. The authors suggested that the peripheral dichotomization of these ganglion cells could be the substrate for referred 'phrenic' pain in the shoulder region. Similarly, Bahr et al (1981) found fibres in the inferior splanchnic nerves which could be activated by electrical stimulation of one of the lumbar white rami, as well as of a somatic nerve of the same spinal segment at stable latency. The response of these fibres followed high-frequency stimulation (20–100 Hz) of the nerves. The axons were unmyelinated, had no ongoing discharges and could not be excited by afferent stimuli via a spinal or supraspinal reflex pathway. It is likely,

therefore, that the fibres were afferent, thus supporting the hypothesis that dichotomizing afferent fibres, one branch from visceral organs and one branch from muscle or skin, may be the mechanism underlying referred pain from the viscera. Torebjörk et al (1984) found that intraneural microelectrode stimulation, of both cutaneous and muscle fascicles of the median nerve, produced pain referred to cutaneous areas within median nerve innervation territory, deep pain referred to muscles innervated by the median nerve and also to ipsilateal upper arm, axilla and chest muscles. Sensations were projected specifically to the skin if a cutaneous fascicle was stimulated, and to deep structures if a muscle fascicle was stimulated. In seven muscle fascicles in three subjects, intraneural stimulation at elbow level gave rise to pain which was clearly referred to regions *outside* the innervation territory of the median nerve. In addition to pain projected to forearm muscles, subjects felt deep pain projected as mentioned above and to the mammillary regions, hence including part of the pectoral musculature. This probably explains the mechanism of cervical angina (Brodsky 1985), when lower cervical degenerative change can refer pain to the upper limb and also to the precordium, simulating cardiac disease. Presumably the pain is referred in the distribution of myotomes of the pectoral musculature (medial and lateral pectoral nerves derived from roots C5–T1); Bogduk (1988) has also mentioned these areas of reference.

Torebjörk et al (1984) noted that the referred pain was influenced by temporal and spatial *summation* of the afferent flow (vide infra). They discussed the possible segmental organization of referred pain, postulating that convergence might also occur at peripheral level, given the existence of dichotomizing primary afferent fibres innervating separate structures.

From clinical experience the writer would suggest that, like fingerprints, each individual's 'segmental organization of referred pain' is different to others', and we should not expect to stumble upon a stereotype one day.

Bindoff and Heseltine (1988) described the pain of a lung tumour being referred to the ipsilateral ear region in eight patients. This was initially diagnosed in some as atypical face pain, and the authors urge any clinician entertaining the diagnosis of atypical face pain to consider the possibility of an underlying bronchial neoplasm. On the basis that the sympathetic outflow is restricted to between the T1 and L1 segments of the spinal cord (with which not all would agree — see Ch. 20) the authors suggest that the facial pain, non-specific and localized in or around the ear, could have been mediated via the vagus nerve. Visceral afferents from the pharynx, trachea and upper oesophagus are thought to travel in the vagus, and since the nerve contains both visceral and somatic afferents it provides both neural elements necessary for referred pain.

In seven cases, radiotherapy to the tumour rapidly

cured the facial pain; presumably the vagus nerve remained intact. In one other similar case report, the unilateral face pain was relieved after surgery, during which the vagus nerve was sectioned. Whether the surgery or the vagus nerve section relieved the pain is not established, of course. It is important to be aware of the popularity of the ear region as a site for referred pain (Al-Sheikhli 1980). In a group of 100 patients, who presented with ear pain as their main or only complaint, a study to determine the true pathology revealed that referred ear pain appears commoner than pain due to intrinsic lesions of the ear.

Much clinical teaching and writing seems to be based on the expectation that because a somatic or autonomic nerve goes to a particular anatomical district, pain in that peripheral distribution can only be due to abnormalities of the spinal segment associated with one or other of the roots of that nerve.

This may often be so — just as often, it is not.

Clinical experience of severe and distressing phantom limb pains suffered by some amputees, together with Miller's (1978) suggestion that pains do not really happen in hands or feet or heads, but in the conscious image of hands, feet and head, make the point that *pain and referred pain are essentially central phenomena*. Put another way, whereas referred pains are commonly perceived and described by the patient as lying in this or that peripheral tissue, that tissue (e.g. a limb) need not be present for very severe and disabling pain, and other symptoms, to be 'referred' to it, or rather to its very real image. Pain happens *within* the central nervous system, and does not reside 'in' the damaged locality, though it may be perceived so.

Bourdillon and Day (1987) suggest that the central mechanism involves both the spinal cord and the higher centres.

Perhaps the variable distribution of referred pain, from apparently similar segmental spinal joint problems in a group of individuals, is more an expression of organization of the cortical substrate, the representative cortical mosaic of each individual, than an anatomical distribution of a particular somatic nerve.

Yet the affective, motivational and cognitive factors mentioned above must also often be influencing the reported distribution of symptoms. Pain is *not* referred or projected down nerves to the site of reference, since 'the nerves don't know where they go' and as we note, *referred pains occur alike whether the peripheral nerves are present and functioning or whether they are not*. When the skin of a transposed end of a pedicle graft is injured, the pain is perceived at the original site, and not in the position to which the graft has been moved. Further, the technique of injecting hypertonic saline into vertebral ligaments to study the distribution of referred pains in normal subjects, also refers sharp, localized pain of short duration into the phantom limbs of amputees.

Phantom lower body pains occur in paraplegics, even when the spinal cord is known to be completely transected. Cases are reported of anginal pain being referred to a phantom upper limb (Cohen 1947). Anginal pain referred to the left arm is not abolished by a complete brachial plexus block with local anaesthesia (Harman 1951). Harman (1948) succeeded in provoking *pain* and *paraesthesiae* in phantom limbs by saline injection. Referred pain to the tip of the shoulder, initiated by phrenic nerve irritation, occurs just the same when all the cutaneous nerves to the shoulder-tip have been excised (Doran & Ratcliffe 1954). Referred pain has been experimentally evoked in areas previously anaesthetized by regional nerve block (Feinstein et al 1954).

The factor of summation

Summation is one of the important factors governing whether afferent nociceptor traffic reaches the threshold of consciousness, or whether a sensory stimulus is sufficient to fire off a motor response and/or an autonomic reaction. Similarly, summation of pain-producing factors appears to be a salient part of (a) the neural mechanism underlying the perception of pain at a distance from its origin, and (b) governing the particular distribution of the perceived pain (Brewerton 1990). If the summation component in referred pain is not appreciated, confusion may arise and precision of treatment may be compromised.

When a lesion of the pancreas (sympathetic nerve supply from segments T6–T10) coincides with a previously covert thoracic musculoskeletal problem of the segments T6–T10, this circumstance may render clinical features of the spinal condition sufficiently severe to detract attention from the more important visceral lesion. Also, it is possible that the spread or extent of the referred visceral pain may be greater when co-existing lesions (one visceral and one somatic) involve the same vertebral segments. These responses may be further heightened when premenstrual changes begin.

It would be instructive to repeat Doran's (1967) experiment (Ch. 29, p. 412), adding a careful pre-operative examination of thoracic musculoskeletal structures and then comparing both the distribution and severity of the postoperative referred torso pain, in those with and without co-existing spinal problems.

Several other factors, e.g. 'remembered pain' (see p. 286) may also summate to potentiate the clinical features presented. Anginal pain from a cardiac lesion will most likely be referred to the neck if there is a co-existing and covert cervical lesion, and into the arm if there is a co-existing mild forequarter lesion.

In short, the sites and severity of referred pain may have more to do with mild co-existing conditions of the spinal column, visceral lesions, premenstrual changes in women and the factor of summation, than they have to do with neatly-depicted territories of dermatomes and sclerotomes.

DERMATOMES, SCLEROTOMES AND MYOTOMES

Clinical bias

Because clinical features tend to occur in fairly common patterns, particularly pain and neurological changes, the patterns have a certain predictive value, so we familiarize ourselves with the territories of dermatomes and sclerotomes and the myotomes, the segmental nerve supply to skeletal muscle. Understanding their embryological development adds weight to our views of their clinical significance (Grieve 1988, 1991).

Too often, this introductory knowledge becomes inflexibly hardened; the familiar tabulations become sacrosanct. Not enough account is given to the range of variability from these conveniently neat and tidy norms. In assessing the probable segmental levels involved we may not regard each case with a sufficiently fresh eye and open mind. Unbiased assessment of clinical features, *solely as presented*, is hard.

When discussing clinical history-taking, it is useful to recall some aspects of the functions of cognition and recognition. Paul Valéry (1871–1945) remarked: 'Man sees only what he imagines'.

The scientific attitude, that of always being prepared to be surprised by facts, and to alter our preconceived ideas in relation to them, is not easy to sustain. When examining, it is necessary to strip perception of what is already known so that only virgin perception remains. This is very difficult. Modern psychology teaches that man 'is prepared for what he is going to see', recognizing what he already knows and virtually what he is seeking. Our look is just as crowded with all that we have stored in our brains as with what we receive in our vision. Receptions are unwittingly tailored in an attempt to fit previously stored patterns, as the early French impressionist painters discovered to their cost. Their 'new' way of looking, and depicting, what the eye was actually receiving initially aroused feelings of unease and sometimes anger with outright hostility.

Fodor's (1983) review of faculty psychology, and the theory of the modular organization of central nervous system input systems — vision, hearing, the initial stages of language processing and so on — makes the same point in a different way. In a work of art, we largely see what we bring to it. Alike with a set of clinical features we 'see' what we bring to them, what our minds are stored with. We see only what we look for; we recognize only what we know or can imagine.

In another context Eldevik et al (1982) have neatly revealed this pitfall. Knowledge of the patient's clinical history increased the tendency of observers to interpret questionable myelographic or computed tomography findings as positive. More studies were correctly interpreted without a knowledge of clinical history than with it. Knowledge of the clinical history increased the number of false-positive diagnoses and decreased the number of false negatives. The patient often finds it difficult to describe where their referred pain or 'root' pain may lie, and where not. It is all too easy for tidy-minded clinicians to interpret patient's sometimes vague descriptions in a somewhat arbitrary fashion, which conveniently accords with textbook tabulations and charts remembered. Even medically-qualified subjects find the distribution of experimentally induced vertebral pain difficult to describe accurately (McCall et al 1979).

The results of clinical studies, too, may unconsciously be influenced by an expectant rather than a neutral approach to findings. Cloward's (1959) study of patterns of referred pain during cervical discography prompted his assertion that pain radiated almost exclusively into the dorsal aspect of upper trunk and arm. He mentioned that 'conspicuous by their absence are pains radiating into the precordium'. Despite the fact that earlier (Phillips 1927) and subsequent reports (Holt 1964, Klafta & Collis 1969, Booth & Rothman 1976, LaBann & Meerschaert 1979, Brodsky 1985) substantially refuted Cloward's findings, his single study has been adopted by some as the clinically significant gospel for patterns of lower cervical discogenic referred pain. Many young therapists seem to begin professional life unwittingly armed with the assumption that this is how lower cervical discogenic pain *ought* to behave. Plainly, this is an inadequate basis for meaningful clinical assessment of cervical musculoskeletal problems.

The variability of pain areas

Many writers imply, if not categorically state, that it is into conceptualized anatomical territories like dermatomes and sclerotomes that pains will be referred. There is the reasonable likelihood of an approximation of this, in some of the patients for some of the time, but not in all of the patients all of the time. Observations in the literature testifying to this clinical experience are numerous enough: myofascial referred pain does not follow dermatome, myotome or sclerotome patterns of innervation (Travell & Simons 1983). The widespread and complicated attachments of the sacrospinalis muscle may refer pain radiating much more widely than the familiar knowledge of anatomy would lead us to suppose — even to the heel (Scott-Charlton & Roebuck 1972). Pain is not always distributed to the expected dermatomes, but may spread over a wider area (Brodal 1981). Pain of cervical spondylosis may be felt in myotome areas and not necessarily in dermatomes (Sandifer 1967). Pain referred from deep somatic tissues differs in location from the conventional dermatomes (Feinstein et al 1954). Pain caused by irritation of one spinal nerve root may extend in some cases more widely than the recognized distribution (Brain 1957). Referred pains are not invariably of segmental root distribution. They may miss out a segment and then spread into two adjacent segments (Hockaday & Whitty 1967). Pain from the site of lesions in patients, and from artificial 'lesions' produced in models, appears to be approximately segmental in character but does not correspond to dermatome or myotome distribution (Inman & Saunders 1944). Sensory disturbances which are not confined to dermatomal distributions should not be dismissed as hysterical (Appenzeller 1978).

Bourdillon and Day (1987) mention that previous workers described experimental referred pain as strictly segmental in distribution, but this has not been confirmed by more recent work in the same field. Some 50 years ago, Elliott (1944) noted that patterns of referred pain varied considerably from person to person — an imprecise and inconstant area of pain reference between individuals. Patients continue to report pains which neither accord with our tidy concepts nor behave in the manner confidently expected. This tendency for individuals to differ, by showing an idiosyncracy in the pattern of their pain reference, has also been shown by Hockaday and Whitty (1976) who repeated the experiments of previous workers and injected 6% saline into the interspinous ligaments of normal subjects. A response involving referred effects of some soft occurred after 94% of injections. They found that while an individual's response remained consistent there was a definite and sometimes marked variation from person to person. They concluded that because the site of reference of pain from connective-tissue lesions is quite variable between individuals, *this does not support the concept of an anatomically-fixed segmental reference like dermatomes.*

McCall et al (1979) also noted this variability of pain reference between individuals, in this case scientifically-sophisticated volunteers. In one, injection of 6% saline at the L1–2 zygapophyseal joint induced pain anteriorly alongside the umbilicus — traditionally the T10 dermatome (Fig. 19.4A). Attempts to explain this individual variation include the suggestion that threshold levels for neurotransmitter release may vary between person (Brand & Albright 1979), also that it may be necessary to study changes in cell metabolism in the affected and adjacent areas to learn more about referred pain.

Since the relief of referred pains, if not local pain too, can often be achieved in under 45 seconds, arrangements to study cell metabolism would need to be prompt.

Landmarks in the study of referred pain were the papers by Kellgren (1939) and Inman & Saunders (1944) when the concept of sclerotomes came more to the fore. Referred pain which did not accord with dermatome territo-ries was considered to lie in a sclerotome distribution. The study conducted by McCall et al (1979), on patterns of pain referral induced from the posterior elements of the lumbar spine, suggests that the considerable overlap of pain areas induced from both upper and lower lumbar spine *does not support the existence of sclerotomes.*

The need for flexibility

There is always a reason for pain; better to first be suspicious of our patchy knowledge than immediately suspect the patient's wits or motives. Our wisest course is the suspension of disbelief while we listen to *everything* the patient is telling us.

An over-reliance on dermatomes, as sacrosanct and immutable anatomical territories, may be a fruitful source of injustice to patients. Increased awareness should put an end to those extraordinary consulting-room encounters, not infrequently witnessed in times past by the writer, during which authoritarian clinicians demonstrate to patients, with the aid of diagrams of dermatomes, that they cannot possibly be suffering pain in the area reported. The patients are left puzzled and frustrated; some in unjustified doubt of their own veracity and others deeply angry.

Writing in *Physiotherapy* in times past, Parsons (1945) suggested: 'Always *listen* to a complaint of pain and remember that the pain point has the same wide individual variation as pain itself. Modify treatment according to necessity . . . failure to listen to a complaint of pain may lead to serious errors in treatment'.

Stoddard (1983) suggested: 'When all medical investigations are negative in patients whose symptoms persist, there is frequently a mechanical or structural basis for those symptoms, even though the linkage seems tenuous. It is unwise to label such patients as neurotic until the mechanics of the spine have properly been assessed'.

Referred spinal pain appears on occasion to be inadequately understood by clinicians, a minority of whom seem unacquainted with the full spectrum of its vagaries, or do not make a practice of including careful palpation of spinal segments in their clinical examinations. With depressing frequency, any clinical feature which appears bizarre, or in some way transgresses orthodox teaching as to where pain ought to be and how it ought to behave, may be regarded with the beginnings of suspicion; this is more likely to occur when the examining clinician, well-versed in his medical or surgical speciality, is not completely familiar with the behaviour of spinal musculoskeletal pain, which can simulate so many visceral conditions. (See Ch. 32.)

Brodal (1981) expressed this important point:

It is well known to critical clinical neurologists that, *more often than not,* [my italics] the symptoms observed in a patient do not correspond to the traditional schematic representation in the textbooks. But all too often, features which do not fit the scheme are disregarded as being of little importance . . . the story of medicine contains many examples of how careful investigation of a single patient has given more information of value than a collective analysis of a number of cases showing (apparently) identical symptoms.

Bond (1979) suggested:

The complaints of aching pain confined to the left side of the chest, especially in the nipple area and below and apparently linked with exercise, should be viewed with considerable suspicion especially if unaccompanied by any form of electrocardiographical evidence of heart disease. In the patient's mind the pain may not be associated with an emotional cause and therefore it arouses considerable anxiety. As he or she believes it is due to heart damage it may well be accompanied by pallor, sweating and panic, as in those who have myocardial disease. Because of its positive association with exercise the disorder is sometimes known as the effort syndrome or a cardiac neurosis. Physical investigations are negative . . .

The physical examination is not elaborated, although it is probable that thoracic segments T1–T6, and joints of the first to the sixth left ribs, were not routinely examined.

Clinical presentation of a similar but now right-sided pectoral pain would probably make an interesting diagnostic dilemma for these physicians.

THE EQUIVOCALITY OF CLINICAL FEATURES

Identification of precise level of somatic nerve root involvement, on the basis of distribution of referred pain, so-called 'root' pain and neurological deficit, is an inexact science (Fig. 19.2).

Our best attempts to correlate the cutaneous topography of dermatomes, the segmental nerve supply to muscle (myotomes), the skeletal territories of sclerotomes and the likely effects of bony and soft tissue anomalies, still leave something to be desired, in terms of accuracy of segment identification by clinical examination.

Tabulated schemes of the root values of nerve supply to muscles, of the probable localizing value of reflex changes and of the cutaneous distribution of the salient nerves (Grieve 1988, 1991), assist the newcomer to get an informed grip of the nature of the difficulty, but are not in themselves certain guides for naming the abnormal segmental level. There are many observations by clinicians about the need to recruit investigation procedures like myelography, epidurography, radiculography and sometimes electrical studies (Leyshon et al 1981) to assist in

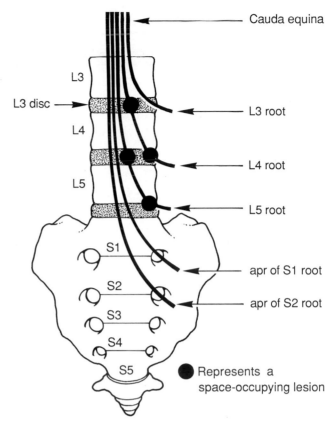

Fig. 19.2 This a–p scheme of the lower lumbar spine and pelvis illustrates one factor (see text for others) which confounds attempts to identify the segmental level of a presumed space-occupying lesion by distribution of neurological symptoms and signs. Owing to the obliquity of roots of the cauda equina, L4 root can be compromised by L3 and/or L4 disc trespass, as L5 root can be by L4 and/or L5 disc trespass. A space-occupying lesion of the L4 disc, or other tissue in that neighbourhood, can involve both L4 and L5 roots.

precise identification of the level of nerve root trespass if such exists — it sometimes does not.

When investigating lumbar syndromes, for example, Wright et al (1971) referred to the uncertain clinical localization of lesions producing 'radicular' pain and mention that the neurological findings may be identical irrespective of whether the discogenic trespass is at L3–4 or L4–5. The same may be said of referred pain, of course. In a series of 560 patients, surgically treated for disc disease, correct preoperative clinical localization was achieved in only 39.2% (Lansche & Ford 1960). This figure accords neatly with the findings reported by Leyshon et al (1981) who studied a series of 100 patients with leg pain. 70 of the patients were classed as showing evidence of a nerve root lesion, and 50 of them were treated surgically. Postoperative evaluation indicated that clinical accuracy, in detecting the segmental level of root involvement, was 40%. Radiculography scored a 52% accuracy and electrical studies a 90% accuracy. It is suggested that inaccuracy may have been due, in some patients, to variations from the orthodox patterns of segmental innervation.

The clinical features included assessment of such signs as straight-leg-raising and reflex changes, but these too were unreliable. In only 52% of the patients was the straight-leg-raising test positive, and while 18 patients had clinically reduced or absent ankle jerks, only 10 were confirmed as abnormal on the basis of ankle reflex latency findings.

Because abnormal reflex behaviour has traditionally been regarded as a valuable diagnostic and localizing sign — of both nerve root involvement and expected discogenic trespass — this clinical feature should briefly be considered. In a surgical series reported by Kirkaldy-Willis et al (1982) only one in six of the patients suffered from a pure ruptured disc syndrome.

O'Brien (1983) suggested: 'The broad basis of current clinical management of low back pain is based on the following assumptions, now known to be incorrect: (i) the disc is insensitive (ii) the main cause of pain in the leg is nerve root compression. . . . In the whole spectrum of back and leg syndromes, nerve root compression accounts for less than 10% of the total problem'.

Mooney and Robertson (1976) showed that reduced straight-leg-raising and depressed deep tendon reflexes could be normalized within minutes by the injection of local anaesthetic into lumbar facet-joint spaces. The concept that reflex changes are due primarily to aberrant neural activity of spinal cord segments, and not to root trespass only, is strongly supported by Epstein's (1976) report of four patients with bilaterally-diminished ankle jerks in whom surgically-verified unilateral disc lesions did not approach the opposite nerve root.

Davis et al (1952) reviewed the findings of sensory pattern changes in 500 patients, and found no correlation between these changes and the segmental level of the lesion. Epstein (1976) concurred with the inconstancy of clinical features in relation to the vertebral level involved, as did Hanraets (1959) who, in his comprehensive review of these difficulties, mentioned: '. . . the sensory innervation patterns of the L5 and S1 roots are not as specific as the confident interpretation of them in practice would suggest'. His review included an extended discussion of dural and nerve root anomalies (see Ch. 17, p. 246). Hasue et al (1983) also mentioned these. There may not be an identifiable lesion at all! Certainly, 'root' pain and 'root' signs for which no adequate cause can be found at operation are common enough (Grieve 1988).

Among some observations on diagnosis, Bogduk (1986) mentioned that the incidence of abnormal myelograms suggestive of disc herniation, in asymptomatic patients, is put somewhere between 24 and 50% by various workers. 'Doubt, therefore, can be raised about the validity of an abnormal finding in a symptomatic patient.' So where stands the 'disc lesion'? In the writer's opinion, much nonsense is believed and has been written and taught about disc lesions and the pains associated with them.

SEGMENTATION

Assessment of the level of nerve root involvement, particularly in the lumbosacral district, is often bedevilled by anomalies of bone and soft tissue.

Vertebral counting may be performed without full thoracic X-rays, and a lower lumbar or upper sacral root inculpated solely on the basis of lumbar and lumbosacral X-rays. Frequently, anomalies are present at both thoracolumbar and lumbosacral transitional levels, this adding a source of error.

Concerning the phylogenetic categories of the spine, Wigh (1980) observes that junctional transitional vertebrae should be properly identified and localized.

Defining a thoracic vertebra as one in which the entire costal element is a separate bone, i.e. the rib, and (among other criteria) a lumbar vertebra as one in which the costal processes are continuous with the vertebral body, the three categories are based on the number of presacral vertebrae:

Cervical section: Constant count of seven in mammals. Congenital anomalies of vertebrae do not affect the count of seven other than in rare conditions like the 'Klippel–Feil' syndrome.
Thoracic section: 11 or 12 or 13
Lumbar section: 4 or 5 or 6

Thus there may be 23, 24, or 25 *presacral* vertebrae, as shown in Table 19.1.

There is some disagreement on whether the altered appearance (when present) of the costal processes of either the last thoracic or the first lumbar vertebra are phylogenetic or congenital in type. When the lowest ribs are short, they may be confused with lumbar transverse processes; again, an anomalous transverse process may be identified as a small rib.

When a 'lumbosacral transitional vertebra' is described, it is potentially the 24th or the 25th or the 26th of the presacral number. Wigh (1980) suggests that the true lumbosacral transitional level is that next below the conventionally structured lumbar vertebra with costal processes not articulating with or fused with its subjacent

Table 19.1 The phylogenetic formulae for man and some primates*

23 presacral vertebrae	:7C :11T :5L:	man, orangutang
	:7C :12T :4L:	
24 presacral vertebrae	:7C :11T :6L:	man, gorilla, chimpanzee
	:7C :12T :5L:	
25 presacral vertebrae	:7C :13T :5L:	man, gibbon
	:7C :12T :6L:	

* The colon represents transitional levels.

neighbour. When assessing neurological symptoms, recognition of the correct phylogenetic category enhances the prospect of correct analysis of dermatome involvement; assuming that the dermatome does accord with the orthodox textbook patterns and that pain is referred in segmental distributions. He describes a clinical audit of 100 patients, diagnosed and operated on for lumbar disc protrusions. It revealed only 67 patients within the conventional human mode, 33% having anomalous spines.

There were 13 patients in the orangutang mode and 3 in the gibbon. Wigh proposed adding the first three sacral vertebrae, i.e. those articulating with the ilium, and nominating the categories as in Table 19.2.

Wigh observed: 'It is impressive that what one confidently ascribes to be an S1 root in those of us in one type subclassification of Category 26 (:7C :11T :5L :3S:) is also called an S1 root in a Category 28 subgroup (:7C :13T :5L :3S:), although these roots are two dermatome segments apart, and that this is done simply because they emerge at a fifth lumbar level.' (Fig. 19.3B).

Pheasant (1981) has noted that, with 24 presacral segments, the L5 root occupies the lumbosacral foramen, and that with a prefixed plexus this root is S1, and with a post-fixed plexus, L4. Hence anomalies of lumbosacral plexus formation are also important. McCulloch and Waddell (1980) discussed the localization of lumbar disc prolapse by clinical examination, mentioning that: '. . . A reliable knowledge of the anatomical pattern of muscles supplied by the L5 and S1 roots is a valuable aid to clinical diagnosis'. They describe a study of the foraminal exit of the L5 and S1 nerve roots in 11 cadavers with lumbosacral bony anomalies, and the evaluation by electrical stimulation of L5 and S1 roots in 5 patients with normal lumbosacral spines and in 15 with segmental anomalies.

Taking the last fully mobile level as that with a fully formed disc space, bilateral facet joints and two free, non-articulating transverse processes, the L5 root was seen to emerge at that level in three out of four patients with bony segmental anomalies. Thus about one out of four of the 'bony anomaly' population may have the involved root incorrectly localized on clinical findings as such. The authors mention that throughout the stimulation studies, and in larger series of patients undergoing both chemonucleolysis and percutaneous radio-frequency rhizolysis,

the patterns of radiation of pain and paraesthesiae were variable and inconstant. Soft-tissue anomalies, e.g. of dural sleeves, ganglia and nerve roots, were not considered.

Regarding the *thoracic* spine, Brodal (1981) suggested that even a complete lesion of a single dorsal root need not be followed by sensory loss of any degree, such is the efficiency of dermatome overlap. Sunderland (1978) mentioned that a single cutaneous spot on the trunk may be innervated by contributions from five adjacent thoracic nerve roots. It is common experience that identification of the level of an abnormal thoracic joint, solely on the basis of the distribution of pain referred around the chest wall or abdomen, is not easy. Turning to *the neck and upper limb*, Frykholm (1971) described the different effects of stimulating, under local anaesthesia for operations on the cervical spine: (a) the dorsal root, when patients immediately experienced a pain with dermatomal distribution, and (b) the ventral root, when they reported pains in muscles which preoperatively had been painful and tender to pressure. We might bear in mind that these patients were already suffering chronic pain, and therefore must have had chronically facilitated spinal cord segments, which in itself has been shown to affect significantly and enlarge the receptive field of a single dermatome (Kirk & Denny-Brown 1970).

Further, there are few pathological lesions so obliging as to apply discrete stimuli to the different components of a spinal nerve root; the phenomena observed can only

Table 19.2 Categories

Category 26	:7C :11T :5L :3S:	orangutang-type (23 presacral)
Category 27	:7C :12T :5L :3S:	human-type (24 presacral) (Fig. 19.3a)
Category 28	:7C :13T :5L :3S:	gibbon-type (25 presacral)

Tables 19.1 and 19.2 are reproduced from Wigh R. E 1980 The thoracolumbar and lumbosacral transitional junctions. Spine 5: 215–222 by kind permission of author and publisher.

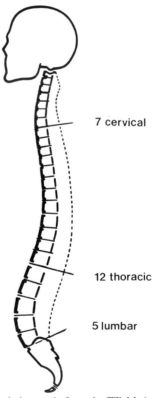

7 cervical

12 thoracic

5 lumbar

Fig. 19.3   A. The phylogenetic formula (Wigh's 'category 27') for man, gorilla and chimpanzee, i.e. 24 presacral vertebrae.

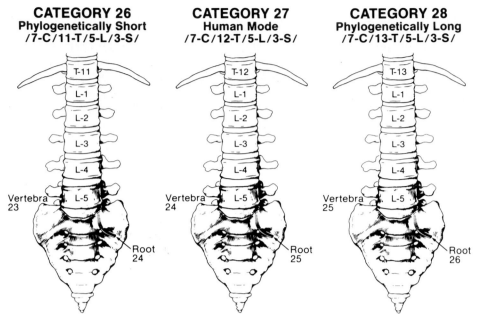

CATEGORY 26
Phylogenetically Short
/7-C/11-T/5-L/3-S/

CATEGORY 27
Human Mode
/7-C/12-T/5-L/3-S/

CATEGORY 28
Phylogenetically Long
/7-C/13-T/5-L/3-S/

Fig. 19.3 B. Illustration showing three different nerve roots that may be affected by herniation or prolapse of 'L5' disc depending upon the phyletic position of 'L5' vertebra.

(Reproduced from Wigh R E 1980 Classification of the human vertebral column: phylogenetic departures and junctional anomalies. Medical Radiography and Photography 56: 2–11 with author's and publisher's permission.)

have significance within the context of that particular experiment, in each particular patient, and extrapolation should be open-minded.

Concerning cervical spondylosis, and myelopathy, Phillips (1975) mentioned: '. . . the conclusion, reinforced by long experience, that contrary to statements of many physicians on this topic . . . neurological findings are of extremely limited use in assessment of the precise level of cord and root involvement, and may be misleading'.

The pattern of cervical spinal cord vascularity (Grieve 1988) may also take a hand in confounding snap assessments, since it is possible for vascular trespass near the foramen magnum to induce wasting of the hand, by disturbing downward flow in the anterior spinal artery. Prolonged cervicobrachial pain, for two or more years, need not involve impaired root conduction at all (Kikuchi et al 1981).

Brendler's (1968) findings, on the pattern of nerve supply to muscles of the upper limb, suggest a wider spectrum of root values than customary tabulations. Myotomes are really no more than reasonably accurate approximations in the average individual, and there is no such animal as the 'average' person, of course.

Overlap of pain areas

Referred pain can present in an exactly similar way when produced by either of two, or more, sources, and manual therapists will be familiar with the phenomenon of relieving what appears to be an identical, unilateral 'yoke' area

pain by mobilizing, on the painful side, in one patient the C1–C2 segment, in another the C4–C5 segment, in another the joints of the first rib, while in some, any two or all three sites must have attention before signs and symptoms are relieved (Grieve 1988). Injections of 6% saline into (i) lumbar apophyseal joint cavities, and (ii) the pericapsular tissues of those joints, at both the L1–L2 and the L4–L5 levels (McCall et al 1979), induced patterns of referred pain with a degree of overlap, although the injection sites were four segments apart. Individual variation, in extent of the referral, was evident. L1–L2: The effects of intracapsular injections are shown in Figure 19.4A and extracapsular injections in Figure 19.4B. L4–L5: Pain referral from intracapsular injections is shown in Figure 19.4C and extracapsular injections in Figure 19.4D.

Overlap occurred mostly over the posterior iliac crest and the upper groin. A composite distribution of pain referral, from intracapsular injection (A) at both L1–2 and L4–5 segments, and extracapsular injection (B) at the same sites, is shown in Figure 19.5 A, B. The marked similarity to pain from osteoarthrosis of the hip, at least in its proximal extent, is evident in Figure 19.6 A, B.

In 14 patients with acute low-back pain, who responded by pain relief within 5 minutes of injection of 0.5 ml of local anaesthetic into facet-joint cavities, the areas of referred pain differed (Fairbanks et al 1981). None were precisely alike, the presentations showing all manner of combinations of back, groin, haunch, thigh and calf areas. In two of the patients, the area of referred pain would have suggested the need for a meticulous examination of

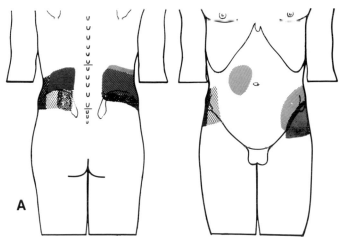

Fig. 19.4 A. The distribution of pain referral following hypertonic saline injections (intracapsular) at the L1–L2 zygapophyseal joint. Cross-hatching shows referral patterns common to all subjects; remaining patterns show individual variations.

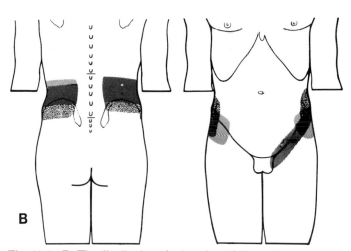

Fig. 19.4 B. The distribution of pain referral following hypertonic saline injection (pericapsular) at the L1–L2 zygapophyseal joint. Patterns as in (A).

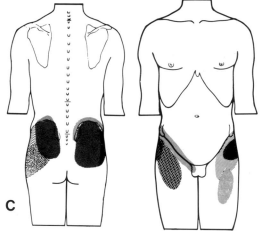

Fig. 19.4 C. Pattern of pain referral after (intracapsular) hypertonic saline injections at the L4–L5 zygapophyseal joint. Patterns as in (A).

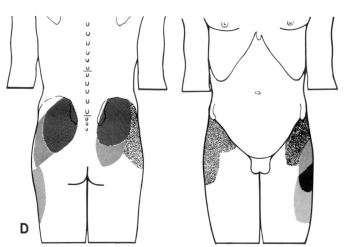

Fig. 19.4 D. Patterns of pain referral after hypertonic saline injections (pericapsular) at the L4–L5 zygapophyseal joint. Patterns as in (Λ).

(Figures 19.4 A,B and 19.5 A,B are reproduced from McCall et al 1979 by kind permission of authors and publishers.)

the ipsilateral hip joint, to exclude possible contributions from that source.

There is considerable overlapping of areas of referred pain, and two or more separate lesions may be contributing to the referred pain in a single district. Symptoms from both spine and hip may give a confusing picture, even in the absence of frank changes of the joints concerned (Offierski & Macnab 1983). Particularly careful and extensive examination is necessary when pain is reported in the suboccipital area with medial yoke pain and in mandibular, upper scapular, medial scapular, deltoid, upper pectoral, hemithoracic, groin, trochanter, anterior and posterolateral thigh and upper medial knee regions.

Because of the dire necessity for surgical attention to be directed to the right segment, the investigation procedures mentioned previously — including discography, nerve

root infiltration, CAT scan, ultrasonography, angiography and phlebography — are recruited to assist identification. Yet since only 1 in 10 000 patients (0.01%) (LeVay 1967) reaches the stage of operative treatment, a very great deal of conservative treatment has perforce to rely on interpretations of clinical examination findings.

Plain radiography is sometimes a help, but more often valueless; trying to find conservative treatment indications in X-ray appearances is like trying to recognize one's friends by the shadows they cast in the street.

Similarly, since Kirk and Denny-Brown (1970) have shown experimentally that the receptive field of a surgically-isolated dermatome can be very much widened by spinal cord segment facilitation, *the concept of dermatomes as finite and static territories is like describing an iceberg when looking only at its tip.*

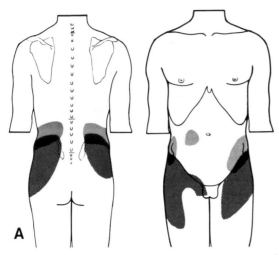

Fig. 19.5 A. Composite distribution of pain referral from intracapsular injections at L1–L2 level (diagonal lines) and L4–L5 level (cross-hatching).

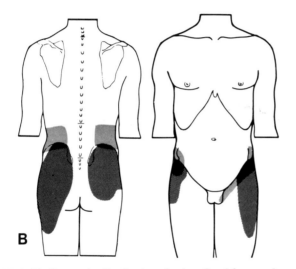

Fig. 19.5 B. Composite distribution of pain referral from pericapsular injections at L1–L2 level (diagonal lines) and L4–L5 level (cross-hatching). In (a) and (b) overlap occurs around the iliac crest and in the upper part of the groin.

An over-reliance on orthodox patterns, and on the significance and supposed immutability of dermatomes and sclerotomes, can be a source of error during manual therapy treatment for benign vertebral joint conditions.

Careful and comprehensive palpation, segment by segment, is a more valuable tool for therapists, yet there still remains opportunity for error and there is no real substitute for practised assessment — which is gained only by clinical experience. We are never relieved of the obligation to assess.

The infinite range of biological plasticity, and idiosyncratic response, continues to confound stereotyped assessments. Workers with extensive clinical experience, i.e. those who cope with 30 to 40 more benign spinal joint problems a day, every day, know that attempts to eradi-

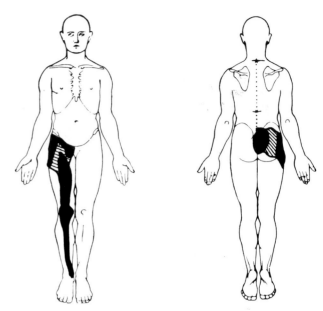

Fig. 19.6 A, B. Common areas of referred pain in osteoarthrosis of the hip. Compare proximal areas with Figures 19.4 and 19.5.

cate this annoying untidiness, by seeking to impose a spurious and artificial order and regularity where none can yet exist, have a certain futility about them. Up to five spinal segments, on either side of the main dorsal root entry zone, may be associated with the sensation from a given skin area, and it is not unreasonable to suppose that the musculoskeletal nociceptors, too, may enjoy a like measure of generosity of reception, according to their physiological requirement.

ROOT PAIN OR REFERRED PAIN

The mere naming of a thing does not explain it. Quoting Kellgren (1938) on the difference between 'root' pain and referred pain, McCulloch and Waddell (1980) mentioned that, in stimulation studies, and during rhizolysis and chemonucleolysis procedures, there was *usually* a clear distinction between the two types of pain. Stimulation of non-neural soft tissues, and of facet-joints, also the annulus and nucleus pulposus, produced dull pain referred to thigh and leg but rarely below the upper calf. Stimulation of the nerve root gave a sharper, well-localized pain, nearly always radiating to or below the ankle.

With reference to symptom-behaviour during these studies, the adjectives 'usually', 'commonly', 'nearly always', 'in general' and 'often' were used, and this accords with the common view of the broad characteristics of these pains. So prevalent is this view that writers speak of 'diffuse' pain and 'radicular' pain, as do Silversten and Christensen (1977) when describing scalenotomies, without always specifying their criteria for assuming that pain was radicular as opposed to 'ordinary' referred pain without root involvement.

We know that (i) injection of a saline irritant into the sacro-iliac joint can produce pain radiating to the heel, (ii) Kellgren (1949) also showed that injecting saline irritant alongside the spinous process of the first sacral vertebra produced pain all down the leg and (iii) Travell and Simons (1983) described pain referred down the arm to lateral digits from the proximal attachment of the subclavius muscle. Macnab and McCullough (1990) suggested that the mere complaint of pain in the leg does not indicate, by itself, root irritation or compression. Macnab (1982) also suggested that pain radiating down the arm does not necessarily indicate nerve root pressure, since it is a common manifestation of referred pain following whiplash injury. Subjective numbness at the ulnar border of the hand, and sometimes diminished sensitivity of ring and little fingers, is rarely the result of root pressure. Much more commonly, it is secondary to scalenus spasm induced by the neck injury. Travell and Simons (1983) also stress the importance of this muscle group in producing upper limb symptoms of this type.

Kikuchi et al (1981) describe the surgical fusion of a single degenerated cervical segment in 138 patients, who had suffered from cervico-brachial pain for more than two years. In none of the patients was there any evidence of impaired conduction of the root. Some 82% of the patients reported immediate post-surgical relief. The observations of Inman and Saunders (1944), Scott-Charlton and Roebuck (1972), and Mooney (1983), begin to suggest the need for a fundamental change in traditional concepts.

Distinctions between 'root' or radicular pain, and that large unspecific mass of pain which we assume to be of non-neural involvement and call 'referred' pain, become more difficult as we seek precise and reliable criteria. The very severe local and referred pain of acute sub-deltoid bursitis does not involve any nerve root, and conversely, a proportion of patients with pain to the distal parts of a limb, accompanying neurological deficit associated with that pain distribution, do not suffer nearly so severely as the phrase 'root pain' should apparently suggest. There is also the question of why 'root' pain is held to be different from other referred pains, since most assuredly it also is referred. Our customary terminology is imprecise and not always fully informative to the newcomer. In a description of the clinical features of spondylolysis and spondylolisthesis, Nelson (1980) clearly referred to 'root' pain as leg pain, sciatic pain, in one category and mentions: '. . . may be felt along the distribution of the nerve root'. A succeeding category is headed 'referred symptoms' and includes vague aching and leg heaviness, with reference to spinal stenosis, i.e. cauda equina constriction. In the same chapter, this clinical circumstance (spinal stenosis) is described as characterized by 'bilateral radicular pains, disturbance of sensation, and impairment of motor power in the legs'. As both sets of circum-

stances seem due to trespass upon neural structures comprising the cauda equina, the distinctions appear artificial. With regard to the upper limb, a cursory glance at the patterns of referred pain, induced by both contractile and inert soft tissue trigger points (Travell & Simons 1983) reveals the dichotomy which exists as to just where these pains are coming from and how we should categorize them.

Evans (1982) mentioned that skeletal muscles give diffuse pain, referred some distance, yet with a clear segmental distribution. He added: 'These segmental areas for deep pain differ from the dermatomes which form complete bands around the body'. Since the whole concept of dermatomes rests on the hypothesis of embryologically and segmentally-linked territories, which extend distally into the limbs also, of course, and referred pain from muscular trigger points very frequently invades a limb, it is difficult to see how a non-dermatomal distribution of referred pain from muscle can be regarded as 'occupying a clear segmental distribution'.

Howe (1979) observed that neither neurophysiological data nor clinical observations support the concept that repetitive firing in the mechanically compressed spinal roots produces radicular pain. Mechanical compression alone is not sufficient to account for the root pain; it is *inflammation* which probably plays the important role in its production. Also, it has been shown that irritation of the dorsal root ganglion may cause it to discharge antidromically down its afferent fibres. Triano and Luttges (1982) offer a possible model of sciatic neuritis.

Variety of clinical forms

Teachers have to summarize material for digestion, and students prefer the didactic, yet many so-called typical patterns are surprisingly uncommon (Grieve 1988). There is little justification for *diktat* when discussing referred and 'root' or 'radicular' pain. Classical descriptions of 'root' pain have been copied from text to text without discrimination. Close and unbiased attention to clinical features, and their highly variable severity, soon reveals that a good proportion of these cases do not fit classical descriptions (Brodal 1965). Spinal musculoskeletal dysfunction shows the potential for presenting in a variety of clinical forms which far exceeds that of any list of syndromes or tidy descriptions of clinical features. Some examples follow:

The pain of diabetic root involvement, verified by electromyography, is often *not* 'radicular' in character (Kikta et al 1982). The pain of chronic nerve root irritation is more aching-like than the sharply unpleasant qualities popularly associated with nerve root involvement (Ljunggren 1982). 'Root' pain may indeed 'travel into the lower limb along narrow bands' (Bogduk 1988) sometimes; on many other occasions it does not (Grieve 1988). In 94 of 100 consecutive cases of lumbosacral radiculopathy, confirmed by EMG tests, the pain was poorly localized, deep-lying and never radiating (Johnson & Fletcher 1981). So where stand classical descriptions of lumbar 'root' pain?

Discogenic cauda equina compression, producing severe disturbance of micturition with perineal pain, may occur *without* any sciatic pain (O'Ladire et al 1981). Brodsky (1985) reported the results of decompressive surgery on 88 patients for anginal chest pains of cervical origin. The levels most involved were C4–5–6–7, albeit not precisely in that order. Good relief of anginal pain was obtained in some 78% of cases. This does not support the contention (Bogduk 1988) '. . . a cardinal feature of nerve root compression is . . . for example, compression of the C6 root should be associated with sensory symptoms in the C6 dermatome . . .'. Which then is the C6 dermatome of the anterior chest wall?

Summarizing, it is suggested that:

1. All 'root' pain is referred pain, but not all referred pain is 'root' pain, i.e. *any* pain not localized to the site of its genesis is referred.

2. Severe referred pain need not be due to root trespass or root irritation or inflammation.

3. Referred pain which *is* due to root involvement need not be severe; a proportion of these patients do not suffer much.

4. Somatic root compression, as such, does not hurt; severe distortion and squashing of nerve roots, by proven bony and/or soft-tissue trespass, need not produce pain or any detectable disturbance of function.

5. The imprecise terminology, of referred pains, at present reflects traditional assumptions (often unproven) about their cause rather than their true nature, per se.

6. The topography and nature of referred pain in any one patient — whether we do or do not distinguish so-called 'true referred' pain from 'root' pain — is inadequate as a single factor in differential diagnosis, of both the tissue involved and the segmental level. Additional factors, and the recruitment of other investigation procedures, and clinical assessment, are necessary and accuracy is still not guaranteed.

Referred tenderness

Inflammation, whether infective, traumatic or the result of repetitive occupational stress, is regularly accompanied by tenderness. All of 41 patients, in a group suffering their first attack of low back pain, exhibited areas of maximum tenderness over the lower lumbar spine (Fairbanks et al 1981).

It is puzzling that an ordinarily innocuous stimulus, as touch or pressure, should become painful and sometimes exquisitely so, e.g. tender spinous and transverse processes in the region of vertebral joint problems, tender rib angles associated with lesions at thoracic levels, and tender posterior superior iliac spines in degenerative changes of the low lumbar segments and in sacro-iliac joint conditions. The abnormally enhanced sensitivity can be demonstrated (i) locally over the site of the lesion, (ii) over the surrounding area, and (iii) at times far distant.

Apart from tenderness of structures palpable within the body orifices, the word 'tenderness' by definition refers to undue sensitivity, undue reactiveness, of the surface of the body, and/or those structures available to palpation through it; muscle, superficial ligament, bony point and so on.

When positive, the sign is elicited by touch, stroking or pressure to varying degree of the skin itself, the body surface. Intra-orifice tenderness is also that via an internal surface, of course. Aside from dermatomyositis, scleroderma and the like, there is no lesion of musculoskeletal structures which physically involves the skin itself as part of the lesion. Cutaneously-evident concomitant changes — pallor, coldness, sweating, redness, warmth, altered texture, thickening and 'peau d'orange' effect — also occur, but these are reflex sequelae and not physical involvement in the changes of the deeper lesion itself.

In a real sense, therefore, most tenderness is 'referred', being elicited by palpation of the body surface, when there is no lesion of the surface of the body.

Bone

Because tenderness of a bony spinous process associated with a deep lumbar lesion feels as 'sore' to the patient as so-called 'styloiditis radii' — acute tenderness of the subcutaneous radial styloid process in tenovaginitis of thumb extensors and abductors — we note the similarity of bony point tenderness alike in deep and superficial lesions of musculoskeletal structures.

This tenderness may extend far distally, in the so-called 'innervation territory' of the segment(s) concerned, e.g. the subcutaneous head of the fibula and lateral malleolus, in sciatica.

Muscle

Travell and Simons (1983) have comprehensively investigated the acute, localized tenderness in the immediate vicinity of soft-tissue 'trigger points', when palpable tender bands in muscle give severe pain on localized pressure.

They also depict associated areas of referred pain, and referred tenderness, at some distance from these points. The distal referred tenderness disappears as soon as the trigger point is inactivated by local injection or vapo-coolant spray and stretch of the muscle concerned.

Ligament

While the precise site of a ligamentous lesion — lateral ligament of knee or anterior talofibular band of the lateral ligament of ankle — may be most tender, an area of referred tenderness also surrounds these localized points.

Skin

Bearing in mind the known phenomenon of referred abdominal tenderness, particularly manifest in vertebral joint problems at the thoracic spine, thoracolumbar junction, the upper, middle and lower lumbar region and the sacroiliac joint, the coexistence of anterior body wall tenderness in spinal pain syndromes should not be surprising. When palpating the region of the lumbosacral promontory, via the abdominal wall, O'Brien (1979) found tenderness in more than three-quarters of patients with low-back pain. Of a control group of 50 asymptomatic individuals, only two exhibited tenderness and both had experienced back pain during the previous three months. Since up to five spinal segments, *either side* of the main dorsal root entry zone, can be associated with the sensibility of a given area of the skin, it follows that the sign of anterior abdominal wall tenderness is not specific to particular levels, but generally indicative of thoracic and/or lumbar abnormality. This clinical finding is not new, of course. More than 70 years ago, Baer (1917) described acute tenderness 'anteriorly over the lesion' in what were taken to be unilateral sacro-iliac joint strains. Tenderness over 'Baer's point', described by him as 'just to the side and just below the umbilicus' had often led to an erroneous diagnosis of appendicitis and subsequent unnecessary surgery.

Even in those days, Baer mentioned: 'this point of pain (tenderness), which is invariably present in all cases of sacro-iliac strain of this type, as well as in inflammatory conditions involving the sacro-iliac joint. It is most constant and is elicited at a fixed point, owing to the structures which cause it, whereas as we know in cases of appendicitis, the pain at McBurney's point may be entirely absent, owing to the wandering proclivities of the appendix'.

Carnett (1927) clearly makes this point (Fig. 19.7). Baer describes a further diagnostic sign — the flat back or the obliterated lumbar lordosis — and it is plain from illustrations accompanying his paper that he very probably was describing a different lesion of the lumbar spine. It also seems that *any* spinal lesion, from the lower cervical region to the pelvic joints, may refer tenderness anteriorly on the surface of the body wall, producing 'counterfeit' symptoms and often inducing notions of visceral disorder. While these may indeed be present, frequently they are not, and in any case the segmental association is not precise.

Recently, the writer completely relieved acute unilateral groin tenderness, within three minutes of treatment localized to L2, in a large building labourer who was disabled by 'low' back pain (Grieve 1991). Fairbanks and O'Brien (1983) proposed an 'iliac crest syndrome' in which a small area of referred pain, unilaterally around the posterior iliac crest and upper buttock, is accompanied by a point of maximum tenderness; this is located on the posterior part of the iliac crest where it is joined by the posterior gluteal

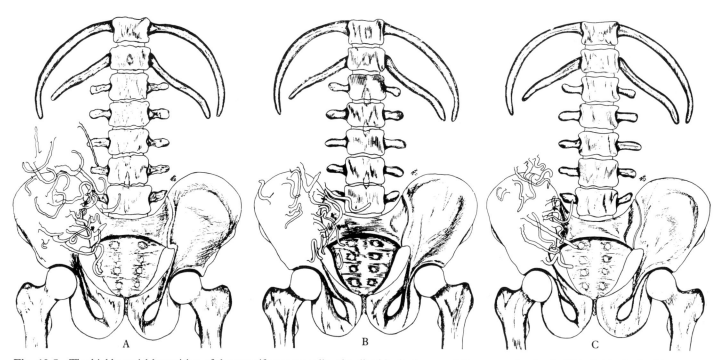

Fig. 19.7   The highly-variable position of the vermiform appendix, visualized by barium meal X-ray examination in 56 individuals. **A.** 24 appendices. **B.** 16 appendices. **C.** 16 appendices. (Reproduced from Carnett 1927 by kind permission of the publisher.)

line. Injection of local anaesthetic at the point of maximum tenderness relieved the symptoms of the seven patients comprising the group reported. Travell and Simon (1983) discuss the controversial aspects of 'trigger point' injection, as do the above authors.

Macnab and McCullough (1990) mentioned the upper outer quadrant of the buttock as a normally tender point, which becomes acutely so after injection of hypertonic saline into the supraspinous ligament of L5–S1. Why do tissues, sometimes peripherally far distant, exhibit tenderness, sometimes exquisitely so, in districts classically associated with spinal segments? Proposals that there is some actual change in the tissues which are tender are sometimes made, yet it is highly unlikely that such changes could be normalized within two minutes, or less, of the more proximal central lesion considered responsible for them.

Melzack and Wall (1982) suggested that: '. . . it is impossible to propose that there are shared nerve endings between the distant and damaged area, or that chemicals could spread or be transported to the distant tender area . . . the explanation . . . has to lie within the central nervous system, where the activity triggered by the primary lesion *excites neighbouring areas in the central nervous system to produce heightened sensitivity*'.

An important feature of somatic sensibility is that any single spot on the trunk, for example, is innervated by fibres which run into many neighbouring posterior roots. Sunderland (1978) observed: 'The nature of the fibre branching in human cutaneous nerve trunks is such that, though the individual branches of a single fibre cannot be traced to their destination, there is justification for the belief that the territory served by a posterior root ganglion neurone is greater than is generally acknowledged to be the case'.

The T-cells of dorsal horn Lamina V normally have a restricted field of reception which governs the degree of their basal activity, so that the arrival of diffuse afferent traffic from the territory of several *neighbouring segments* is inhibited and effectively negated. Full, normal sensibility, and especially adequate *spatial* sensibility, depends on this great overlap of fibres from posterior roots, and at the primary posterior horn synapses of afferent fibres, there is a convergence of input from these neighbouring roots. The threshold of T-cells is not reached by input arriving in only one root; there has to be a background polysynaptic facilitation derived from stimulation of the same sensory field arriving via two or more nerve roots (Grieve 1988).

Should inhibitory mechanisms be overcome by tissue abnormalities, initiating summation of afferent input exceeding the T-cell threshold, two things have happened:

1. Any single dorsal horn, and perhaps more than one, is 'receiving' through a gate which freely transmits stimuli from a wider region.

2. The area of neighbouring roots, including their distal extent, is effectively in a state of what may be conceived as peripheral facilitation, whereby the normally innocuous mechanical stimuli of touch and pressure, in the absence of normal inhibition, now become pain. The degree or intensity of these events will depend upon central nervous system modulation activity.

If, in an experimental animal, many neighbouring dorsal roots are sectioned either side of a single root left intact, and the normal T-cell inhibition of the intact root is removed by giving a subconvulsive dose of strychnine, the now facilitated single dorsal horn remaining will effectively transmit nociceptor stimuli from a wide area of supposedly denervated territory of neighbouring segments (Kirk & Denny-Brown 1970). Thus, dermatomes are not immutably fixed anatomical territories, but variable *neurophysiological* entities, their size and boundaries at a particular instant being an expression of the rising and falling levels of facilitation, and thus an *index* of the efficiency of sensory transmission, in the dorsal horns of spinal segments. It is upon this basis that tenderness, and referred tenderness, might reasonably be explained.

'Remembered' pain theory

In general terms, the amount of pain referred distally into a limb from vertebral joint problems governs the duration of treatment needed for its relief, and the further distal the pain the longer will be the treatment. Assessment of a patient's treatment needs may be inaccurate if history-taking is not sufficiently thorough.

A complication is the factor of what might be called the 'remembered' component of pain. Wall (1989) suggested that pain 'memories' may exist. Some factor in nerves could convey signals of *what used to be there*, superimposed upon what was currently happening. Pain 'memories' may be a potential for increased excitability, for greater sensitivity, stored in the cell and reactivated by subsequent stimuli, perhaps years later.

Patients with a history of previous shingles, boils and carbuncles in the limb girdle regions and especially painful lacerations, sprains or fractures of limbs, may present with excessive pain, or pain reasonably out of proportion with coexisting signs, proximally or more distally in the associated limb (Grieve 1988).

It is important to note that the site of a previous and painful limb injury will be disproportionately painful if referred pain of vertebral degenerative disease later invades that limb. The central nervous system appears to retain a memory for previously well-trodden neuron pathways, and pain at the old site is easily rekindled in later years, even if the limb subsequently be amputated for other reasons (Nathan 1973).

The site of a previously very painful Colles fracture

may, some 10 or more years afterwards, be the most painful part of a painful upper limb, secondary to cervical spondylosis and/or glenohumeral capsulitis.

A common clinical observation is that weather changes affect symptoms more than signs (Watson 1984). Climatic influences could affect the human body by various mechanisms; these include stimulation of thermoreceptors resulting in changes in dermal blood-flow and sweat secretion, disturbances of biological circadian rhythms and changes in the viscosity of the blood. The low-threshold type I mechanoreceptors in joint capsules are very sensitive to *changes* of capsular stress, including that initiated by changes of atmospheric pressure (Wyke 1972). The same phenomenon of remembered pain frequently occurs during particular combinations of barometric pressure and prevailing weather, e.g. on an especially cold day a patient may report unexpectedly severe pain at the site of a previously painful fracture, the clinical presentation thus very closely simulating pain referred from a coexisting but actually well-localized vertebral joint condition. It is tempting to dwell on theories of 'storage of latent-facilitation in the computer-programme memory of the c.n.s.', and this may be speculative, yet there is plainly the registration of an experience, its storage and then its recall by the neural mechanisms underlying the pain experience (Grieve 1988). Also, there may be an electrophysiological explanation for continuation of pain over a long period, and nerve cells could *remain sensitized or facilitated* for some time after the exciting cause had ceased to exert its effect. This response could depend upon the release of peptides or the transport of trophic chemical substances in unmyelinated nerves. These might, for example, explain the continued pain of postherpetic neuralgia. Again, those complaining of back pain over a long period may unjustly be considered as malingerers when there was a neurological mechanism underlying their chronic distress.

SOME CLINICAL EXAMPLES

Cervical headache

The occurrence of referred head and face pain, secondary to abnormalities of the somatic structures of the neck and particularly those of the craniovertebral district (Grieve 1988) is familiar to all manual therapists (see Chs 18, 22, 23 and 24).

Unilateral suboccipital pain

A fit athletic rugby player reported right suboccipital pain, and 35° of restriction of right rotation; the movement was limited by pain but also resistance. He had no other symptoms. Mobilization of the upper cervical spine achieved little; similar attention to the ipsilateral first rib achieved full pain-free rotation within a minute.

Acromioclavicular and rib joint

An elderly lady presented with unilateral clavicular region, yoke area and sub-clavicular fossa pain, together with articular signs at the acromioclavicular and glenohumeral joints and mild tenderness of ipsilateral upper rib joints. (Fig. 19.8).

All of her pain and restriction improved steadily in five successive treatments, except the pain in the sub-clavicular fossa, which remained persistent and unchanging until the third rib on that side had been mobilized.

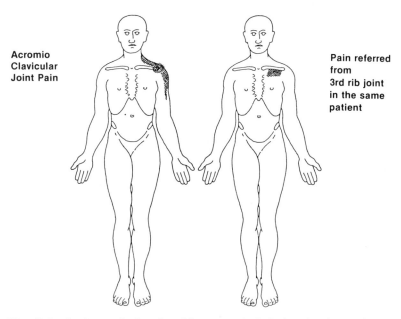

Acromio Clavicular Joint Pain

Pain referred from 3rd rib joint in the same patient

Fig. 19.8 A scheme of pain referred from acromioclavicular, glenohumeral and ipsilateral upper rib joint in an elderly patient (see text).

Breast pain

Chronic breast pain in women may be an expression of low cervical radiculopathy. LaBann et al (1979) reported a group of 18 women with this condition who, after extensive but uninformative investigations which included mammograms and biopsies in some, were successfully treated by cervical traction.

Scapular and periscapular pain

The proximal distribution of referred symptoms from the low cervical spine is not as predictable as often suggested. Since 1959, Cloward's patterns of referred pain during cervical discography have been described repetitively, yet subsequent discography studies by Klafta and Collis (1969), which substantially refuted Cloward's patterns, have hardly been mentioned.

Thorocic viscera

Not all dorsal backache is of musculoskeletal origin. In addition to pain referred to the dorsal aspect of the trunk, from visceral lesions involving the gall-bladder, pain in the back may also be the presenting symptom in a patient with a leaking aortic aneurysm or a dissecting aneurysm.

Lindahl and Hamberg (1981) mentioned the term 'angiotome', i.e. those body areas in which pain will be felt and sudomotor activity increased on stimulation of sympathetic nerves. The areas do not correspond to the segmental distribution of somatic nerve roots.

The upper lumbar region

Pain from acute lesions in the L1–L2 district can be very severe indeed (Grieve 1991) and it is noteworthy that McCall et al (1979) experimentally found that the upper lumbar region was noticeably more sensitive than the lower.

Lower lumbar and sacro-iliac pain

Before jumping to conclusions about sacro-iliac joint pain, it is of value to remember the attachments of the iliolumbar ligament. This single structure has probably confounded more snap decisions than we know.

So much referred pain involves the buttock, haunch and groin area, and so much of it emanates from what essentially are lesions of the lumbar spine and/or the hip joint. Similarly, with the 'Piriformis Syndrome' — the writer has collected various descriptions of this syndrome, dating back more than 30 years.

Yet while this particular muscle and the sacro-iliac joint may have suffered an embarrassment of attentions, lesions plainly involving them are common enough and they cannot be dismissed as being of no consequence.

Pelvic joint conditions

Some 77 years ago, Baer (1917) mentioned that symptoms from the sacro-iliac joint resembled those of certain pelvic conditions: '... The symptoms at times so closely correspond that the gynaecologist may not realise his mistake until an exploratory laparotomy is done, and no cause for symptoms is found.'.

More recently, Jeffcoats (1962) suggested that low backache in women often leads to the assumption that its cause lies in the female pelvic organs: 'In the majority of cases of low backache in women a gross lesion is not found and an obvious cause is not demonstrated. Patients tend therefore to be handed from physician to gynaecologist to orthopaedic surgeon, and back again'.

Adams (1981) suggested that the importance of gynaecological disorders as a cause of back pain has been exaggerated. Unless a major intrapelvic disorder is demonstrable, there are no reasonable grounds for attributing back symptoms to gynaecological conditions. The low back and sacro-iliac joints, as a vertebral district, are much like the cervicothoracic region, in that several quite distinct lesions frequently initiate much the same symptom complex (Kirkaldy-Willis & Hill 1979).

Discussion

With regard to assessment of the root level involved (p. 277), it is important to bear in mind differences in the number of presacral vertebrae, and the relatively high frequency of bony anomalies at the lumbosacral junction. Anomalous root innervation often accompanies skeletal variations, apart from occurring in its own right.

Young et al (1983) reported three separate studies comprising (i) electrical stimulation during surgery, when eight (16%) of 50 patients showed a marked departure from normal patterns; (ii) a prospective study of 100 patients, when half the failures (also 16%) in prediction of root level were thought due to innervation anomalies; and (iii) a study of 12 patients, with bony segmentation disorders among seven of whom anomalous innervation was demonstrated.

Farfan (1977) well makes the point: 'The surgeon forced to depend on the neurological signs leans on a broken reed. In 60 to 65% of instances the neurological signs indicate only the "neurologic area" in which to seek the problematic joint'.

Some 57 years ago, Barr (1937) mentioned that the distribution of pain and the pattern of neurological deficit bore no relation to the segmental level of the lesion.

Tile (1984) quoted Macnab's opinion that 'the dynasty of the disc' is over, and underlines his point by the CT scan of a massive disc protrusion, at L5–S1 level, in a 40-year-old woman. Despite this gross space-occupying lesion the patient's pain disappeared, as did the neurological deficit, in six weeks of conservative treatment. Similarly, chemonucleolysis relieves pain, alike with negligible change in the size of the space-occupying lesion.

Hitselberger and Witten (1968) and Chrissman et al (1964) also drew attention to this clinical feature. Not only is the pain mechanism per se ill-understood, but so-called 'root pain' must be accounted for by something other than the disc lesion. O'Brien (1984) suggested that the concept of disc prolapse had held up progress in solving the conundrums of low-back pain; he inclines increasingly to conservative treatment. In many cases, pain persists after discectomy and fusion.

Rightly, attention is being directed to the several anatomical sites, other than the single disc/root relationship, where root trespass may occur (Wiltse et al 1984). *Yet the perennial determination to link 'root pain' and mechanical 'root trespass' persists unabated; we continue to conceptualize only like mechanical engineers, when more than sufficient evidence exists to suggest investigation with more emphasis on aberrant neurophysiology and radiculitis.*

As has been mentioned (p. 282) it is quite common for surgeons to find nothing to account for the cause of so-called 'root' pain. Some 23 years ago, Brown (1971) observed '. . . perplexing is the process by which surgical ablation of an intervertebral disc relieves the syndrome of low-back pain and sciatica when true mechanical impingement of the nerve root is not found at the time of surgery'.

There is some evidence that the cause of severe sciatic pain is probably a radiculitis rather than the herniation per se — the nature of the relationship (if any) between the herniation and the radiculitis being the essential conundrum. This has been considered so for some years (Lindahl 1966), and the findings of Takata et al (1988) provide some support for this view. The authors used computed tomographic myelography to identify cauda equina root swellings corresponding to the root affected in 17 of 28 patients with proven herniation of a lumbar disc. This group of 17 patients had severe sciatic pain, while the 11 others without severe sciatica, not quite half of the total, did not exhibit swollen nerve root elements. Following surgical decompression, the nerve root swelling gradually returned to normal; likewise the sciatic pain gradually regressed.

Thus in this 'proven lumbar disc herniation' context, there may or may not be an associated radiculitis and a swollen nerve root. When manual and/or mechanical treatment techniques — massage, mobilization, stretching, posturing techniques, traction, combined movements, sustained pressure techniques and so on — are employed, what is it we believe we are doing? Despite more than two decades of scientific evidence that disc lesions and sciatic pain are not synonymous, a proportion of manipulators continue to speak of relieving low-back and sciatic pain by 'putting the disc back'.

When true radiculitis can be identified routinely by computed tomographic myelography, the terms 'radicular' or 'root' pain can be used with the confidence that they mean something identifiable. Yet whether there is radiculitis present or not, the pain in the limb is still *referred* there, in the true sense of the word. We could, with advantage, tidy up our nomenclature and dispense with the notion that 'root' pain and 'referred' pain are somehow different animals.

Of the patients who had sciatic pain without root swelling, two were 11-year-old boys. Their severely-restricted straight-leg-raising was due to marked hamstring tightness rather than sciatic pain as such. It is known that the severity of signs of disc involvement, in youngsters, are invariably more marked than the symptoms (Grieve 1988). The authors suggest that the pathology of the affected root(s), in children with tight hamstrings, may differ from adult pathology.

There are many unanswered questions, and the causal relationship between disc herniation, observed radiculitis, pain and referred pain, and relief after some weeks following surgical intervention, remains open to debate.

This brings us full circle back to Brown's (1971) observation above.

O'Brien (1984) confirmed that hypertonic saline injected into superficial ligaments at L5 level will produce pain spreading down the posterior thigh to foot. The pain is indistinguishable from sciatica said to be due to disc prolapse. On the other hand a deep and less localized pain, of no particular segmental distribution, often underestimated in severity and therefore significance, can arise in the discogenic syndrome but may nevertheless be diagnosed as psychogenic pain. Again, the belief that 'discogenic sciatica' is a self-limiting condition, of about six weeks' duration, is applied much too generally, resulting in insufficient treatment or neglect of some of these patients whose clinical features may not accord with expectations.

For manual therapists, the quality of so-called 'root pain' is a matter of some importance, and Ljunggren (1982) mentions that the pain of chronic root irritation is much more aching-like than the sharply unpleasant qualities popularly associated with nerve root involvement. The quality of pain differs with the duration of the sciatica.

As a doorbell sounds the same whether the bell-push is used or the wires short-circuited, so there need not always be a qualitative difference between pain due to nociceptor stimulation and that due to stimulation somewhere along the course of a nerve.

Lindahl and Hamberg (1981) make the point that angina pectoris, for example, is not a diagnosis but a symptom, and since it can be initiated by pathological changes in the mediastinum, oesophagus or thoracic spine, illustrates the important circumstance that similar symptoms may arise from changes in diverse and unrelated structures.

One of the writer's patients, with nocturnal bilateral paraesthesiae of median nerve distribution, right anterior axillary pain and right medial elbow pain, reported prompt exacerbation of her hand symptoms on a–p pressures applied to the spinous process of C6, and only C6. A week later, when her symptoms had satisfactorily diminished, C6 pressures did not reproduce her distal paraesthesiae, but similar pressures on T345 smartly provoked the same bilateral symptoms — they had not done so before.

Shifting patterns of spinal cord facilitation may have more to do with neurological signs and symptoms than we have recognized. It is much too early in the day to try and impose artificial order on the vagaries and causes of referred pain behaviour. We simply do not know enough about the enormous plasticity of the nervous system, or of the individual differences which make each respond to the world in unique and idiosyncratic ways (Melzack & Wall 1982).

For those whose best energies are devoted to acquiring competence at the point of sale, i.e. the clinical shop floor, there is no escaping a sustained effort to understand the vagaries of referred musculoskeletal pain and other symptoms, together with a workmanlike grasp of the great variety of more serious conditions which may masquerade, at least initially, as benign locomotor problems. Francis Bacon (1561–1626) mentioned that 'If a man will begin with certainties, he shall end in doubts; but if he will be content to begin with doubts, he shall end in certainties'.

REFERENCES

Adams J C 1981 Outline of orthopaedics. Churchill Livingstone, Edinburgh, ch 4

Al-Sheikhli A R 1980 Pain in the ear — with special reference to referred pain. Journal of Laryngology and Otology 94: 1433–1440

Appenzeller O 1978 Somato-autonomic reflexology: normal and abnormal. In: Korr I (ed) Neurobiologic mechanisms in manipulative therapy. Plenum Press, London, p 217

Baer W S 1917 Sacro-iliac strain. Bulletin of the Johns Hopkins Hospital 28: 159–163

Bahr R, Blumberg H, Janig W 1981 Do dichotomising afferent fibres exist which supply visceral organs as well as somatic structures? A contribution to the problem of referred pain. Neuroscience Letters 24: 25–28

Barr J S 1937 'Sciatica' caused by intervertebral disc lesions: a report of 40 cases. Journal of Bone and Joint Surgery 19: 323–342

Bindoff L A, Heseltine D 1988 Unilateral facial pain in patients with lung cancer: a referred pain via the vagus? Lancet 1: 812–815

Bogduk N 1986 The reliability of diagnosis. New Zealand Journal of Physiotherapy 14: 25–30

Bogduk N 1988 Innervation and pain patterns of the cervical spine. In: Grant R (ed) Physical therapy of the cervical and thoracic spine. Churchill Livingstone, New York, ch 1

Bond M R 1979 Pain: its nature, analysis and treatment. Churchill Livingstone, Edinburgh, p 68

Booth R E, Rothman R H 1976 Cervical angina. Spine 1: 28–32

Bourdillon J F, Day E A 1987 Spinal manipulation. 4th edn. Heinemann, London

Brain Lord 1957 The treatment of pain. South African Medical Journal 31: 973–975

Brand R A, Albright J (eds) 1979 The scientific basis of orthopaedics. Appleton-Century-Crofts, New York

Brendler S J 1968 The human cervical myotomes: functional anatomy studied at operation. Journal of Neurosurgery 28: 105–111

Brewerton D A 1990 Personal communication

Brodal A 1965 The cranial nerves. 2nd edn. Blackwell Scientific, Oxford, p 88

Brodal A 1981 Neurological anatomy in relation to clinical medicine. 3rd edn. Oxford University Press, Oxford, ch 11, p 775; epilogue

Brodsky A E 1985 Cervical angina. Spine 10: 699–709

Brown M D 1971 The pathophysiology of disc disease. Orthopaedic Clinics of North America 2: 359–370

Brown C 1983 Compressive, invasive referred pain to the shoulder. Clinical Orthopaedics and Related Research 173: 55–62

Carnett J B 1927 Acute and recurrent pseudo-appendicitis due to intercostal neuralgia. Americal Journal of Medical Science 174: 833–851

Chrissman O D, Mittnacht A, Snook G A 1964 A study of results following rotatory manipulation in the lumbar intervertebral disc syndrome. Journal of Bone and Joint Surgery 46A: 517–524

Cloward R B 1959 Cervical discography: a contribution to the aetiology and mechanism of neck, shoulder and arm pain. Annals of Surgery 150: 1052–1064

Cohen H 1947 Visceral Pain. Lancet 2: 933–934

Cyriax J 1982 Textbook of orthopaedic medicine. vol I, 8th edn. Baillière Tindall, London

Davis L, Martin J, Goldstein S L 1952 Sensory changes with herniated nucleus pulposus. Journal of Neurosurgery 9: 133–138

Dixon A S J 1980 Diagnosis of low back pain — sorting the complainers. In: Jayson M I V (ed) The lumbar spine and back pain. 2nd edn. Pitman Medical, Tunbridge Wells, p 140

Doran F S A, Ratcliffe A H 1954 Physiological mechanisms of referred shoulder-tip pain. Brain 77: 427

Doran F S A 1967 The sites to which pain is referred from the common bile duct in man and its implications for the theory of referred pain. British Journal of Surgery 54: 599

Eldevick O P, Dugstad G, Orrison W W, Houghton V M 1982 The effect of clinical bias on the interpretation of myelography and computed tomography. Radiology 145: 85–89

Elliott F A 1944 Tender muscles in sciatica: EMG studies. Lancet 1: 47–49

Epstein B S 1976 The spine: a radiological text and atlas. 4th edn. Lea & Febiger, Philadelphia, ch 7

Evans D P 1982 Backache: its evolution and conservative treatment. MTP Press, Lancaster, ch 19

Fairbanks J C T, Park W M, McCall I W 1981 Apophyseal injection of local anaesthetic as a diagnostic aid in primary low-back pain syndromes. Spine 6: 598–605

Fairbanks J C T, O'Brien J P 1983 The iliac crest syndrome: a treatable cause of low back pain. Spine 8: 220–224

Farfan H F 1977 A reorientation in the surgical approach of degenerative lumbar intervertebral joint disease. Orthopaedic Clinics of North America 8: 9–21

Feinstein B, Langton J N K, Jameson R M, Schiller F 1954 Experiments on pain referred from deep somatic tissues. Journal of Bone and Joint Surgery 36A: 981–997

Fodor J A 1983 The modularity of mind. MIT Press, London

Frykholm R 1971 The clinical picture. In: Hirsch C, Zotterman Y (eds) Cervical pain. Pergamon Press, Oxford, p 13

Grieve G P 1988 Common vertebral joint problems. 2nd edn. Churchill Livingstone, Edinburgh, ch 7

Grieve G P 1991 Mobilisation of the spine. 5th edn. Churchill Livingstone, Edinburgh, ch 5

Hanraets P R M J 1959 The degenerative back and its differential diagnosis. Elsevier, Amsterdam, pp 382–3

Harman J B 1948 The localisation of deep pain. British Medical Journal 1: 188–192

Harman J B 1951 Angina in the analgesic limb. British Medical Journal 2: 521–522

Hart F D 1977 Nice, simple revealed truth. World Medicine August 10: 24

Hasue M, Kikuchi S, Sakuyama Y, Tsukasa I 1983 Anatomic study of the interrelationship between lumbosacral nerve roots and their surrounding tissue. Spine 8: 50–58

Hitselberger W E, Witten R M 1968 Abnormal myelograms in asymptomatic patients. Journal of Neurosurgery 28: 204–206

Hockaday J M, Whitty C W M 1967 Patterns of referred pain in the normal subject. Brain 90: 481–496

Holt E P 1964 Fallacy of cervical discography: report of 50 cases in normal subjects. Journal of American Medical Association 188: 799–801

Howe J F 1979 A neurophysiological basis for the radicular pain of nerve root compression. In: Bonica J J (ed) Advances in pain research and therapy. Raven Press, New York

Inman V T, Saunders J B 1944 Referred pain from skeletal structures. Journal of Nervous and Mental Disease 90: 660–667

Jeffcoats T N A 1962 Principles of gynaecology. 2nd edn. Butterworth, London, ch 26

Johnson E W, Fletcher F R 1981 Lumbosacral radiculopathy: a review of 100 consecutive cases. Archives of Physical Medicine and Rehabilitation 62: 321–323

Jull G A 1981 Clinical manifestations of cervical headache. In: Proceedings MTAA symposium: cervical spine and headache. Brisbane, pp 28–44

Kellgren J H 1938 Observations on referred pain arising from muscle. Clinical Science 3: 175–190

Kellgren J H 1939 On the distribution of pain arising from deep somatic structures with charts of segmental pain areas. Clinical Science 4: 35–46

Kellgren J H 1949 Deep pain sensibility. Lancet 1: 943–949

Kikta D G, Brever A C, Wilburn A J 1982 Thoracic root pain in diabetes: the spectrum of clinical and electromyographic findings. Annals of Neurology 11: 80–85

Kikuchi S, Macnab I, Moreau P 1981 Localisation of the level of symptomatic cervical disc degeneration. Journal of Bone and Joint Surgery 63B: 272–277

Kirk E J, Denny-Brown D 1970 Functional variation in dermatomes in the macaque monkey following dorsal root lesions. Journal of Comparative Neurology 139: 307–320

Kirkaldy-Willis W H, Hill R J 1979 A more precise diagnosis for low back pain. Spine 4: 102–109

Kirkaldy-Willis W H, Wedge J H, Yong-Hing A, Tchang S, Korompay V de, Shannon R 1982 Lumbar spinal nerve lateral entrapment. Clinical Orthopaedics 169: 171–178

Klafta L A, Collis J S 1969 The diagnostic inaccuracy of the pain response in cervical discography. Cleveland Clinical Quarterly 36: 35–39

LaBann M M, Meerschaert J R, Taylor R S 1979 Breast pain: a symptom of cervical radiculopathy. Archives of Physical Medicine and Rehabilitation 60: 315–317

Lansche W E, Ford L T 1960 Correlation of the myelogram with clinical and operative findings in lumbar disc lesions. Journal of Bone and Joint Surgery 42A: 193–206

Laurberg S, Sorensen K E 1985 Cervical dorsal root ganglion cells with collaterals to both shoulder skin and the diaphragm. A fluorescent double labelling study in the rat: a model for referred pain? Brain Research 331: 160–163

LeVay D 1967 A survey of surgical management of lumbar disc prolapse in the United Kingdom and Eire. Lancet June 3: 1211–1213

Leyshon A, Kirwan E O'G, Wynn-Parry L 1981 Electrical studies in the diagnosis of compression of the lumbar root. Journal of Bone and Joint Surgery 63B: 71–75

Lindahl O 1966 Hyperalgesia of the lumbar nerve roots in sciatica. Acta Orthopaedica Scandinavica 37: 367–371

Lindahl O, Hamberg J 1981 Angina pectoris symptoms caused by thoracic spine disorders: neuro-anatomical considerations. Acta Medica Scandinavica suppl 644: 81–83

Ljunggren A E 1982 Pain quality in patients with herniated intervertebral discs. In: Proceedings, 9th International Congress, World Confederation for Physical Therapy, Stockholm, pp 333–340

McCall I W, Park W M, O'Brien J P 1979 Induced pain referral from posterior lumbar elements in normal subjects. Spine 4: 441–446

McCulloch J A, Waddell G 1980 Variation of the lumbosacral myotomes with bony segment anomalies. Journal of Bone and Joint Surgery 62B: 475–480

Macnab I 1982 Acceleration extension injuries of the cervical spine. In: Rothman R H, Simeone F A (eds) The spine. W B Saunders, Philadelphia, ch 10

Macnab I, McCullough J A 1990 Backache. Williams & Wilkins, Baltimore

Melzack R, Wall P D 1982 The challenge of pain. Penguin, Harmondsworth, ch 3, ch 5

Miller J 1978 How do you feel? The Listener 100: 665–666

Mooney V 1983 The syndromes of low back disease. Orthopaedic Clinics of North America 14: 505–515

Mooney V, Robertson J 1976 The facet syndrome. Clinical Orthopaedics and Related Research 115: 149–156

Nathan P W 1973 The nervous system. Penguin, London, p 73

Nelson A 1980 Surgery of the spine. In: Jayson M I V (ed) The lumbar spine and back pain. 2nd edn. Pitman Medical, Tunbridge Wells, ch 17, p 487

O'Brien J P 1979 Anterior spinal tenderness in low back pain syndromes. Spine 4: 85–88

O'Brien J P 1983 The role of fusion for chronic low back pain. Orthopaedic Clinics of North America 14: 639–647

O'Brien J P 1984 Mechanisms of spinal pain. British Association of Manipulative Medicine Newsletter May: 4–5

Offierski C M, Macnab I 1983 Hip-spine syndrome. Spine 8: 316–321

O'Ladire S A, Crockard H A, Thomas D G 1981 Prognosis for sphincter recovery after operation for cauda equina compression owing to lumbar disc prolapse. British Medical Journal 282: 1852–1854

Parsons K O 1945 Pain: its significance and assessment. Physiotherapy 30: 71–73

Pheasant H C 1981 Letter: The thoracolumbar and lumbosacral transitional junctions. Spine 6: 49

Phillips J 1927 The importance of examining the spine in the presence of intrathoracic or abdominal pain. Proceedings of the Interstate Postgraduate Medical Association of North America 3: 70–74

Phillips D G 1975 Upper limb involvement in cervical spondylosis. Journal of Neurology Neurosurgery and Psychiatry 38: 386–390

Sandifer P 1967 Neurology in orthopaedics. Butterworth, London, p 50

Scott-Charlton W, Roebuck D J 1972 The significance of posterior primary divisions of spinal nerves in pain syndromes. Medical Journal of Australia 2: 945–948

Sessle B J, Hu J W, Amano N, Zhong G 1986 Convergence of cutaneous tooth pulp, visceral, neck and muscle afferents onto nociceptive and non-nociceptive neurons in the trigeminal subnucleus caudalis (medullary dorsal horn) and its implications for referred pain. Pain 27: 219–235

Silversten B, Christensen J H 1977 Pain relieving effect of scalenotomy. Acta Orthopaedica Scandinavica 48: 158–160

Smith-Petersen M N 1924 Clinical diagnosis of common sacroiliac conditions. American Journal Roentgenology 12: 546–550

Stoddard A 1983 Manual of osteopathic practice. 2nd edn. Hutchinson, London, ch 1, p 16

Sunderland S 1978 Nerves and nerve injuries, 2nd edn. Churchill Livingstone, Edinburgh

Sydenham P H 1979 Measuring instruments: tools of knowledge and control. Peter Peregrinus, Stevenage, ch 1

Takata K, Inone S-I, Takahashi K, Ohtsuka Y 1988 Swelling of the cauda equina in patients who have herniation of a lumbar disc. Journal of Bone and Joint Surgery 70A: 361–368

Tile M 1984 The role of surgery in nerve root compression. Spine 9: 57–64

Torebjörk H E, Ochoa J L, Schady W 1984 Referred pain from intraneural stimulation of muscle fascicles in the median nerve. Pain 18: 145–156

Travell J G, Simons D G 1983 Myofascial pain and dysfunction: the trigger point manual. Williams & Wilkins, Baltimore, ch 2

Triano J J, Luttges M W 1982 Nerve irritation: a possible model of sciatic neuritis. Spine 7: 129–136

Wall P D 1989 Pain memories. Proceedings of the International Back Pain Society Conference, Amsterdam

Watson L 1984 Heaven's breath: a natural history of the wind. Hodder & Stoughton, London, p 209

Wigh R E 1980 The thoracolumbar and lumbosacral transitional junctions. Spine 5: 215–222

Wiltse L L, Guyer R D, Spencer C W, Glenn W V, Porter I S 1984 Alar transverse process impingement of the L5 spinal nerve: the far-out syndrome. Spine 9: 31–41

Wright F W, Sanders R C, Steel W M, O'Connor B T 1971 Some observations on the value and techniques of myelography in lumbar disc lesions: the results over a five-year period at the Nuffield Orthopaedic Centre, Oxford. Clinical Radiology 22: 33–43

Wyke B D 1972 Articular neurology — a review. Physiotherapy 58: 94–99

Young A, Getty J, Jackson A, Kirwan E O'G, Sullivan M, Wynn Parry C 1983 Variations in the pattern of muscle innervation by the L5 and S1 nerve roots. Spine 8: 616–624

20. The autonomic nervous system in vertebral pain syndromes

G. P. Grieve

INTRODUCTION

The greatest difficulty in trying to reason your way scientifically through the problems of human disease is that there are so few solid facts to reason with. It is not a science like physics or even biology, where the data have been accumulated in great mounds and the problem is to sort through them and make the connections on which theory can be based (Lewis Thomas, 1984)

Autonomic can mean operating in isolation — not accountable to other systems — but this is a misnomer since there is the greatest possible integration between autonomic and somatic divisions of the nervous system. The nervous system is a continuum and the *autonomy* of this section of the nervous system is illusory, as it is intimately responsive to changes in somatic activities. Although its connections with somatic elements are not always structurally clear, there is abundant functional evidence for visceral reflex activity stimulated by somatic events, including trauma, of course (Williams et al 1989). The term peripheral nervous system includes cranial and somatic spinal nerves, together with the entire complex of visceral or splanchnic nerves (Figs 20.1–20.5). Although useful for descriptive purposes, division into somatic and autonomic components is artificial; they are neither separate nor disparate. Williams et al (1989) suggested that the word 'autonomic', proposed by Langley (1898), is more convenient than appropriate. 'Visceral' or 'involuntary' is a better term (Gaskell 1916).

Originating from common primordial cells and developing together, autonomic and somatic divisions are formed from the same basic units or neurons associated in similar reflex arcs (Day 1979). Comprising central and peripheral pairs, they are invariably related structurally and are often closely connected (Mitchell 1954). The two systems are not different animals but complementary and co-ordinated parts of the same animal. In the past it was considered that the two systems — sympathetic and parasympathetic — differed physiologically, in that parasympathetic reactions are generally localized whereas sympathetic reactions are mass responses. Yet even though widespread activation of the sympathetic system may occur, accompanying for example, fear or rage, it is now recognised that the sympathetic system is also capable of discrete activation; many different patterns of activation of sympathetic nerves, throughout the body, occur in response to a wide variety of stimuli (Williams et al 1989). Taken as a whole, somatic and autonomic components have more similarities than differences; for example:

1. The essential morphology and arrangement of afferent neurons is similar in somatic and visceral systems, yet it is incorrect to speak of 'afferent autonomic neurons' since the sympathetic and parasympathetic systems are purely 'outflow' systems and are thus entirely efferent (Wyke 1990). The phrase 'visceral afferent neurons' is employed by Williams et al (1989).

2. The dorsal spine roots convey afferent traffic from soma and viscera alike; the dorsal spinal ganglia contain nerve cell bodies of visceral as well as somatic afferents.

3. It has been shown (Pomeranz et al 1968) that the small-fibre nociceptive afferents from both somatic tissues and viscera converge in the substantia gelatinosa cells. Somatic and visceral afferent fibres conveying nociceptive impulses have the same histological appearance, being mainly unmyelinated neurons with diameters of 0.2–1.5 μm (although some somatic nociceptive afferents may be up to 4.0 μm in diameter) (Williams et al 1989).

4. There are further similarities between the two systems in that axon reflexes can be elicited at terminals of autonomic postganglionic fibres (Williams et al 1989).

5. The phenomenon of peripheral axonal sprouting occurs in sympathetic nerve fibres as in somatic nerves (Shafar 1966).

6. Degenerative changes in the autonomic system are the same as in the somatic system (Williams et al 1989). After injury, autonomic nerves demonstrate great regenerative capacities (Brodal 1981).

Musculoskeletal pain and associated symptoms cannot be considered in isolation from concomitant changes in autonomic neuron activity. The essential continuity and interdependence of all parts of the nervous system should never be overlooked.

SOMATOVISCERAL/VISCEROSOMATIC REFLEXES

Gaskell (1961) perceived that much autonomic activity was reflexly initiated. Because similar basic neural elements are involved in autonomic reflexes controlling smooth muscle and in somatic reflexes controlling striated muscle, he suggested it was profitable to study the autonomic system in terms of reflex behaviour.

There is ample evidence of visceral reflex activities initiated by somatic events, and vice versa (Kuntz 1945, Travell & Rinzler 1946, Kennard & Haugen 1955, Eble 1960, Sato & Schmidt 1973, Sato 1975, Coote 1978), and evidence suggesting that the same visceral afferent fibres subserve both normal visceral sensation and pain (Iggo 1955).

The principle of metameric segmentation, linking vertebral segment to the spinal cord segment, spinal roots and sympathetic trunk, includes the innervation of internal organs (Kunert 1965). The skin areas of the body wall which have the same segmental innervation as a particular viscus, one somatic, the other autonomic, and which show changes in visceral disease, are Head's 'zones of secondary hyperalgesia' (Head 1920).

Both visceral and somatic afferents are capable of acting on common spinal cord pools of neurons, with summation, facilitation and inhibition effects (Doran 1967), hence the concept of 'the facilitated segment' (Denslow et al 1947). The relation between input at the posterior horns from soma and viscera (Sturge 1883, Ross 1888, McKenzie 1900, Hinsey & Phillips 1940) was confirmed by Kostyuk (1968), who demonstrated that afferents from the viscera can cause presynaptic inhibition upon somatic afferent impulse traffic, and also exert postsynaptic inhibition which is under supraspinal modulatory control from the bulbar reticular formation. It was also shown (Pomeranz et al 1968) that visceral afferents inhibit the effect of converging afferents from the skin and conversely, stimuli to the skin can cause inhibition of neurons on which visceral afferents terminate. There was the same mutual inhibition exhibited by group III afferents from skeletal muscles and skin. Generally, the thicker the nerve fibre the deeper the penetration before termination in the dorsal horn. Unmyelinated C fibres terminate in laminae I and II. Some small myelinated A-delta fibres, which mostly end in layers I and II, may reach layer V. Large myelinated cutaneous afferent fibres end in layers III, IV and V. The largest sensory afferents from muscle reach lamina VI.

The major layers of nociceptor reception are laminae I and II; nociceptive collaterals in deeper layers are polysynaptic and are active in initiating visceral and somatic efferent traffic, producing changes in autonomic function and skeletal muscle as a consequence of nociceptor output.

Impulses arising in painful conditions of the viscera travel in splanchnic nerves and almost certainly enter the spinal cord via *white rami communicantes* and *dorsal spinal roots*. Whatever their subsequent path, evidence suggests that they then occupy the lateral spinothalamic tract (Williams et al 1989).

Autonomic activity is further recruited by collaterals of the spinothalamic tract relaying in the periaqueductal grey matter and projecting to the nuclear cuneiformis — projections from these mid-brain sites to the hypothalamus are further pathways for initiating autonomic reactions.

While viscera are insensitive to cutting, burning or crushing, excessive tension on smooth (non-striated) muscle and some pathological conditions produce visceral pain. At times, the distinction between mere exaggeration of normal activity and that which is pathological is not always easy. Abdominal pain due to strong intestinal contraction is common. In diseases of the viscera vague pains, in the general vicinity of the viscus, will be felt. They may also, or only, be felt in a cutaneous area or other tissue whose somatic afferents enter the spinal segments which also receive the afferent neurons from the viscus concerned. This is referred pain (see Chapter 19). If inflammation spreads from a diseased viscus to the adjacent peritoneum, somatic afferents will be stimulated, causing local somatic and often spasmodic pain in the region involved (Williams et al 1989).

Thus in disease of a viscus, the patient will very frequently experience cutaneous pain; this painful skin area will often be acutely tender and cutaneous vasoconstriction may also be evident. Further, the underlying muscle will show a greater or lesser degree of hypertonus or spasm.

Conversely, pain *unaccompanied* by a greater or lesser degree of visceral reflex activity, e.g. one or more of changes in pulse rate, blood pressure, vasomotor and temperature changes, sudomotor activity and pupilliary diameter, has not been described.

It should be mentioned that autonomic reflex activity is not initiated solely by general visceral afferent pathways. In most instances demanding general sympathetic activity for effort, the afferent element is usually somatic, from the special senses or the skin. Rises in heart rate, blood pressure and pupillary dilatation may result from somatic receptors in the skin and other tissues. Conversely, contraction of the muscular abdominal wall — a somatic structure — often results from irritation of abdominal viscera. Also, axon reflexes may be evoked by stimulation at the terminals of autonomic postganglionic fibres (Williams et al 1989).

Musculoskeletal pain and concomitant features

Irritation of spinal joint nociceptors simultaneously evokes a large number of reflex alterations, including paravertebral muscle spasm and alterations in cardiovascular, respiratory and endocrine function (Wyke 1970). Feinstein et al (1954, 1977) by 6% saline injections into thoracic paravertebral muscle tissues, induced referred pain together with pallor, sweating, bradycardia, fall in blood pressure, subjective 'faintness' and nausea. Hamberg and Lindahl (1981) described six patients with simple thoracic joint lesions initiating not only anterior body wall pain (angina pectoris) but ECG changes, syncope, sweating, dyspnoea, acid regurgitation and vomiting. *All were relieved of these symptoms by manual treatment to the T5–6 segment and adjacent structures.* Most described one or more previous cardiac care unit admissions.

Manual therapists know that borborygmus is commonly initiated, in the prone patient, by gentle repetitive pressure on the spinous process of T5 vertebra, and are familiar with the cold sciatic leg, the impending syncope which accompanies over-vigorous correction of the laterally-deviated lumbar spine, the chronic and diffuse musculoskeletal thoracic joint conditions which accompany or follow cardiac abnormality and the sphincter disturbances which may accompany lower lumbar disc trespass (Grieve 1988). Occult bladder dysfunction appears to be a major clinical feature or lumbar nerve root compression (Rosomoff et al 1970). In 100 patients with a provisional diagnosis of lumbar root involvement, cystometry revealed the characteristics of bladder dysfunction in 83%. Lindahl and Hamberg (1981) mentioned that manual treatment of the thoracic spine can momentarily modify an electrocardiogram reading, and draw attention to the fact of exercise — for example, bicycling — which may provoke typical angina pectoris, a symptom, not a diagnosis. The cardiologist inculpates the heart, while it is self-evident to the orthopaedist and manual therapist that the effort also stresses the thoracic spine.

Similarly, the pain clinic physician may regard provocation of anterior abdominal pain by a sit-up exercise as clear proof of an abdominal attachment-tissue lesion, when it is plain that this exercise also stresses the thoracic spine. Careful palpation of it very frequently reveals a localized thoracic joint condition, which when treated promptly relieves the referred abdominal pain. That palpation of the anterolateral abdominal wall elicits tenderness is an all-too-common example of spinal referred tenderness, of course — a rich source of confusion. While these comments do not exclusively concern autonomic nerves, they do concern important aspects of examination in this field, and may help to clarify diagnostic dilemmas.

Concerning the soft tissues, Travell and Simons (1983) suggest that active myofascial 'trigger points' in abdominal wall muscles can disturb visceral function — a somatovisceral effect.

Conversely, visceral disease may refer pain not only to cutaneous areas but also to skeletal muscle, activating trigger points therein. Myofascial pain may initiate vascular changes, e.g. variation of skin temperature, reddening of the conjunctiva and secretory changes like coryza, lacrimation, localized sweating and pilomotor changes as 'gooseflesh'.

The close association of the trigeminal nerve with autonomic ganglia — ciliary, pterygopalatine (sphenopalatine), otic and submandibular — may be the substrate for concomitant features accompanying facial pain, i.e. lacrimation, conjunctival injection, salivation and flushing (Smith 1969). Disturbance of vestibular function and space perception may originate in trigger points of the clavicular division of the sternocleidomastoid muscle, causing disorientation and postural dizziness (Sola & Kuitert 1955, Travell 1957). Others suggest the opposite, i.e. overactivity of sympathetic nerves inducing hypertonicity (spasm) of the neck muscles (Langley 1898). Bogduk (Ch. 22) reviews the literature on irritation of the sympathetic plexus which accompanies the vertebral artery, and suggests this is not a cause of vertebrobasilar ischaemia, regarded in the past by some as the probable basis of dysequilibrium (Hinoki & Niki 1975, Eadie 1967, Milne 1968). Dizziness can be initiated by needling the soft tissues of the occipito-atlantal joints, for example (see later) (Campbell & Parsons 1944, Raney et al 1949). Many osteopaths and chiropractors no longer believe that musculoskeletal vertebral lesions can *produce* visceral disease (Kunert 1965, Krahe 1974, Stoddard 1983), but may frequently simulate, accentuate or decisively influence visceral conditions (Greenman 1978). Approved lists of osteopathic literature (Vyas 1979) which include, for example, titles on osteopathic techniques designed to influence the function of the pituitary–hypothalamus system, osteopathy in cardiology and pulmonary disease and management of the fluctuation of cerebrospinal fluid, do suggest the need for re-iteration that the prime impulse for physical treatment of the vertebral column is properly vertebral column disorder and not visceral disorder.

Some of the more euphoric lay writers on these matters reach the wilder shores of speculation (Grieve 1988), suggesting the need for rigorous scrutiny of their somewhat unbuttoned notions, and their claims for manipulation as a sovereign remedy for all ills, visceral as well as musculoskeletal (Greenman 1978) (see also Ch. 49).

SO-CALLED AUTONOMIC PAIN

Kellgren's (1949) comments — on 'pricking pain', 'burning pain', 'aching pain' — include the suggestion that an appalling confusion has arisen through careless and inaccurate translation of sensory experience into words. A further example is, of course, 'true visceral pain' (Grieve 1988) which invites questions of what is 'untrue' visceral pain and what is the difference. He mentions that the more ambitious investigators have introduced terms to suit their special theories, e.g. 'sympathetic pain', 'vasospastic pain', 'peculiarly unpleasant pain'. Giving coined and arbitrary clinical meanings to ordinary clinical words, without general agreement, is unhelpful, yet new and pioneering concepts need expression by new words or phrases. The whole field of science is rich in examples, e.g. Brownian movement, Doppler effect, quasar, scintigraphy, computed tomography, magnetic resonance imaging and so on. Kellgren may not have foreseen that descriptions of pain may indeed have some diagnostic value (Melzack & Torgenson 1971, Leavitt et al 1978, Melzack & Wall 1982).

Hence the phrase 'autonomic pain' may be attractive, particularly when causalgic states, reflex sympathetic dystrophy (Bogduk 1983) and phantom limb pains are being considered.

Experimental evidence has been quoted to provide some support for a concept of 'autonomic pain'. Gross (1974) describes electrical and mechanical stimulation of the cervical sympathetic trunk during surgery under local anaesthesia — pronounced pain and much-increased anxiety were produced, the painful regions not corresponding to spinal somatic nerve distribution. Direct stimulation of the upper cervical ganglion produced severe pain in the ipsilateral mandibular teeth and postauricular area. Pinching the adventitia of the common carotid artery produced the same effect. During complete lumbar anaesthesia, cutting of the splanchnic nerves induced cries of pain from the patient. Haugen (1968) mentions that (i) stimulation of the central (proximal) cut ends of splanchnic nerves above the diaphragm results in pain felt unmistakeably in the abdomen or dorsal trunk on the side of stimulation; (ii) stimulation of the vagus nerve above the diaphragm caused patients under spinal anaesthesia to complain of 'heartburn' and neck pain; (iii) by sectioning the vagus nerve below its recurrent laryngeal branch, the pain of bronchial carcinoma can be relieved.

Nathan (1976) refers to visceral afferent fibres conveying both visceral sensation and pain. Whether this is called 'autonomic pain' seems a matter of semantics.

Gross (1974) further recounts how a topographically well-defined pain, such as a neuralgia of the ulnar nerve, may be successfully affected by local anaesthesia of sympathetic nerves.

Yet if we propose an identifiable clinical feature such as 'autonomic pain', we are then bound to propose a like entity, 'somatic pain' — and to satisfactorily establish the difference between them, reviving semantic issues about the existence of so-called autonomic nociceptive afferent neurons. So far as the limbs are concerned, afferent sympathetic fibres have not been demonstrated. Visceral afferent neurons in splanchnic nerve trunks are correctly so-named. Johnson and Spalding (1974) regarded the autonomic nervous system as wholly and only efferent, as does Wyke (1990).

Bogduk (1983) reviewed the clinical features of causalgia and reflex sympathetic dystrophy and remarked that in sympathetic pain syndromes affecting the limbs, the mechanism of pain lies in the somatic and central nervous systems — 'whatever sympathetic features occur are only epiphenomena superimposed on this pain.'.

The mechanism underlying Gross' account of relieving ulnar nerve neuralgia by anaesthesia of sympathetic nerves is perhaps explained by Melzack and Wall (1982) who suggested that fibre diameter alone is not enough, or may be completely irrelevant, in explaining the origin of pain in the neuropathies. They described the crucial role of sympathetic *effector neurons* in exciting *somatic afferent* sensory fibres. Richards (1967) had previously proposed this likelihood. An example of nerve injury is the neuroma which forms following transection of a nerve. The new axon sprouts forming the neuroma show marked spontaneous ongoing activity — without apparent stimulus. A clue is their extraordinary sensitivity to noradrenalin (the neurotransmitter released by sympathetic effector endings), either applied locally or in blood vessels supplying the neuroma. A mixed nerve inevitably contains sympathetic efferent fibres, and since new axon sprouts are temporarily devoid of the tubular insulating myelin sheath small numbers of adjacent neurons begin to excite each other i.e. ephaptic transmission or 'cross talk between fibres' (Melzack & Wall 1982). Thus sympathetic neuron *effector* traffic, at the site of injury, is transposed to adjacent afferent neurons as sensory stimulation. This superimposed afferent traffic reflexly triggers even more sympathetic neuron output, so that the limb is not only painful but glossy and moist. Sympathectomy, or sympathetic ganglion block, are effective in abolishing causalgia.

The drug guanethidine (Day 1979) prevents release of noradrenalin by sympathetic effector endings, while having no effect on sensory fibres. Hannington-Kiff (1974) demonstrated that after preventing venous return by an inflatable cuff around the upper arm, intravenous injection of guanethidine produced a sympathetic block of the entire limb. Although sensory fibres remain unaffected, pain is relieved. Yet some patients respond only temporarily, and it is suggested that changes occur centrally in that cord cells are set into new, highly abnormal conduct in the handling of afferent neuron traffic (Fig. 20.6). Melzack and Wall (1982) described the anatomical, biochemical and bizarre physiological changes underlying this restricted response to sympathetic block. This is probably the mechanism of persistent pain (deafferentation pain) (Loeser 1984) after brachial plexus avulsions and after dorsal root lesions, spinal cord injury, tabes dorsalis and some cases of syringomyelia and multiple sclerosis. So-called central pain after some cases of stroke, and the thalamic pain syndrome, are not well-understood yet Loh et al (1981) demonstrated that pains initiated by lesions of spinal cord and brain are somehow reduced or abolished by blocks of sympathetic effector traffic to the periphery. Perhaps the phrases 'autonomic pain', 'sympathetic pain' or 'parasympathetic pain' have about as much validity as the phrase 'somatic pain', Perhaps there is only *pain*, with the inescapable degree of autonomic reflex activity sometimes overwhelmingly and disastrously to the fore.

THE POSSIBLE BASIS OF SOME CLINICAL FEATURES

Aside from familiar somatovisceral/viscerosomatic reflex changes which have been well documented (Appenzeller 1978, Koizumi 1978, Korr 1978, Stoddard 1983) there are some aspects of autonomic nerve involvement which particularly concern the manual therapist, viz:

1. Dissemination and amplification of autonomic effects.
2. Cranial symptoms after cervical injury of secondary to upper cervical arthrosis.
3. Musculoskeletal changes as lesions of trespass.
4. Autonomic nerve involvement in referred pain and other symptoms.

1. Dissemination and amplification of autonomic effects

When examining and treating patients, reliance on the classical anatomical facts of autonomic nerve arrangement, and the older physiology of neural traffic in autonomic ganglia and at effector endings, may be insufficient in terms of appreciating the possible basis of clinical features.

Structural and functional examples of dissemination and amplification of autonomic effects

Structure

The classically-described distribution of autonomic nerves is sketched in Figures 20.1–20.5, yet the segmental levels of outflow for sympathetic efferent neurons (Johnson & Spalding 1974, Williams et al 1989) are not universally agreed. Some authors place the sympathetic supply to the heart beginning as high as C3 (Lindahl & Hamberg 1981). Continental anatomists (Tinel 1937, Laruelle 1940, Guerrier 1944, Delmas et al 1947) reported the cell bodies of preganglionic sympathetic neurons in the cervical segments C5–C6–C7–C8 and joining these somatic roots, although many give the uppermost as T1. The French authors stated that the rami communicans from these neurons also make synaptic junctions with the small sympathetic ganglia developed around the vertebral artery in the foramen transversarium between C4 and C6.

On the other hand, Bogduk (Ch. 22) observes that: 'the

so-called "vertebral nerve" consists of no more than grey rami communicantes accompanying the vertebral artery — stimulation of those nerves in the monkey failed to influence vertebral (artery) blood flow'.

Variations, between a purely preganglionic and postganglionic arrangement, are described. In addition to white and grey rami, mixed types occur. In the cervical region, bundles of thick myelinated fibres join the grey ramus to reach the prevertebral muscles, and at thoracic segments grey and white rami may be fused (Williams et al 1989).

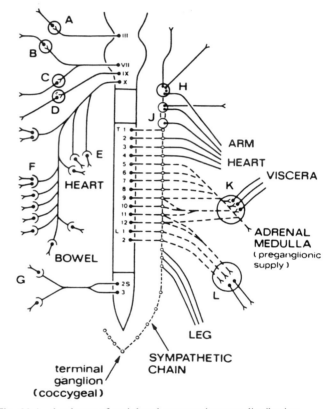

Fig. 20.1 A scheme of peripheral autonomic nerve distribution. Parasympathetic on the left, sympathetic on the right.
Parasympathetic system from cranial nerves III, VII, IX, X and from sacral nerves 2 and 3:
A ciliary ganglion
B sphenopalatine (pterygopalatine) ganglion
C submandibular ganglion
D otic ganglion
E vagal ganglion cells in heart wall
F vagal ganglion cells in bowel wall
G pelvic ganglia

Sympathetic system from T1 to L2:
preganglionic fibres — — — — — —
postganglionic fibres —————————
H superior cervical ganglion
J middle cervical ganglion and inferior cervical (stellate) ganglion including T1 ganglion
K coeliac and other abdominal ganglia
L lower abdominal sympathetic ganglia

(After Keele & Neil 1971 with permission.)

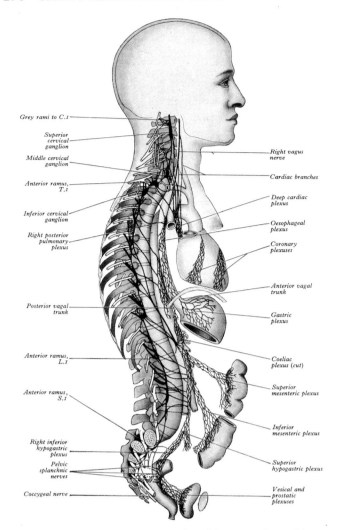

Grey rami to C.1
Superior cervical ganglion
Middle cervical ganglion
Anterior ramus, T.1
Inferior cervical ganglion
Right posterior pulmonary plexus
Posterior vagal trunk
Anterior ramus, L.1
Anterior ramus, S.1
Right inferior hypogastric plexus
Pelvic splanchnic nerves
Coccygeal nerve

Right vagus nerve
Cardiac branches
Deep cardiac plexus
Oesophageal plexus
Coronary plexuses
Anterior vagal trunk
Gastric plexus
Coeliac plexus (cut)
Superior mesenteric plexus
Inferior mesenteric plexus
Superior hypogastric plexus
Vesical and prostatic plexuses

Fig. 20.2 The right sympathetic trunk and its connections with thoracic, abdominal and pelvic plexuses. Parasympathetic contributions to the named plexuses of the viscera depicted are derived from the 10th cranial (vagus) nerve and the pelvic splanchnic nerves. (Reproduced from Williams et al 1989 with permission.)

Day (1979) mentioned that it is difficult to state precisely the source of all the nerve fibres (particularly sympathetic) supplying a particular tissue.

Peripherally, the extent of segmental areas innervated is variable. There is considerable overlap of supply by adjacent nerves. The innervation by different effector systems, e.g. vasomotor and sudomotor, of a particular nerve are not necessarily the same. Textbook descriptions of autonomic innervation differ considerably. There are special differences, as well as variations between individuals.

Schemes such as these shown in Figures 20.1–20.5 are no more than simplified summaries. It is probable that the full detail of distribution is much more complex. Williams et al (1989) allow the possibility of a limited outflow of preganglionic fibres in other spinal nerves, and mention the certainty that 'nerve cells of the same type as those in the lateral grey column also exist at other levels, above and below the thoracolumbar outflow, (Mitchell 1953),

and that small numbers of their fibres issue in corresponding ventral roots'. Operative findings indicate that many individuals do not have a symmetrical arrangement to the upper limb, and it is known that prefixation and postfixation occurs, as in the somatic limb plexuses (Johnson & Spalding 1974). Increasing deterioration of autonomic nerve function in ageing reflects the increasing occurrence of Wallerian degeneration and segmental demyelination. Regeneration does not keep pace with successive degenerative events. Appenzeller and Ogin (1973) suggested that functional deterioration may in part be attributed to changes in the myelinated fibres (white rami communicantes) of the paravertebral sympathetic chain.

Function

The presence of intermediate sympathetic ganglia, (Boyd 1957) and independent sympathetic connections, implies a multiplicity (Erhlich & Alexander 1951) of neural pathways much richer than classically described (see also Fig. 20.12). Some 50 years ago, van Buskirk (1941) described ascending sympathetic neurons from as far caudal as the seventh thoracic segment. He quotes the work of Smithwick (1936) who reported that complete sympathetic denervation of the upper extremity in the monkey, by section of the anterior roots of thoracic nerves, requires section of all the roots down as far as the twelfth thoracic segment.

The earlier concept of autonomic ganglia as mere relay stations has been much broadened by work in the fields of electron microscopy, neurohistochemistry and electrophysiology (Williams et al 1989).

The variety of neuron types in autonomic ganglia is known to be much greater than previously implied by the simple, dualistic terminology of 'preganglionic' and 'postganglionic'. In the superior cervical sympathetic ganglion, the ratio of preganglionic to postganglionic neurons may be 1:175, for example (Ebbesson 1968). There are wide variations in individuals of the same species (Gabella 1976), e.g. from 1:63 to 1:196 in man — a substrate for the wider dissemination of sympathetic effects than a simple 1:1 relationship. This characteristic is not exhibited to such a degree by parasympathetic ganglia. New knowledge also suggests the phenomenon of amplification of sympathetic effects, and mechanisms underlying this characteristic may be (a) widespread terminal arborisation of preganglionic neurons, (b) the mediation of interneurons, (c) the paracrine effect, i.e. intraganglionic diffusion of locally produced transmitter substances and/or endocrine effect, intraganglionic diffusion of substances conveyed from elsewhere.

All of these mechanisms may amplify effector activity.

Vascular channels. The vascular connective tissue stroma of ganglia is linked to perineural spaces by minute

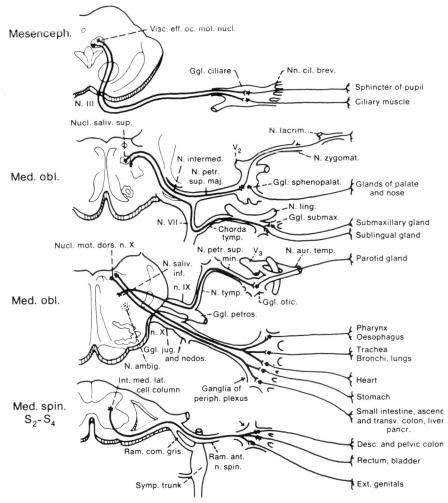

Fig. 20.3 Diagram of the craniosacral division of the autonomic nervous system. Preganglionic fibres are indicated by heavy lines, postganglionic with light lines. The preganglionic fibres, their endings in the ganglia, and the distribution of the postganglionic fibres are indicated. (Modified from Rasmussen 1952.)

channels, possible avenues for movement of neuro-transmitter and hormone substances between neurons, and between these and bloodvessels.

Synapses. In the nervous system as a whole, synapses between neurons involve the junction of almost any part of the neuronal surface. Electron microscopy reveals many types, classified by neuronal processes involved or direction of transmission, e.g. the most frequent axo-dendritic, the quite common axosomatic, and also axoaxonic, dendroaxonic, dendrodendritic, somatodendritic and somatosomatic types. The terms reflect the morphology of the junctions. Axodendritic and axosomatic synapses are found in autonomic ganglia (Williams et al 1989). While axosomatic synapses are less numerous, sympathetic ganglion neurons receive great numbers of axodendritic synapses from preganglionic fibres, forming several synapses with numerous separate dendrites — perhaps representing the mechanism for dissemination

or amplification or both. The mode of termination of preganglionic axons is highly variable (Brodal 1981).

Interneurons. Most ganglion cells are large (25–50 µm diameter) and multipolar. Smaller and less numerous cells (15–20 µm), clustered in groups and less multipolar in shape, have been identified in sympathetic ganglia and are probably interneurons. These 'small intensely fluorescent' (SIF) cells (Evänkö 1978) contain catecholamine neurotransmitters, their supposed action being the release of dopamine which unites with the surface receptors of ganglionic neurons and modifies impulse transmission patterns. Types I and II SIF cells have been described, and there is evidence that type II cells pass their secretions into local blood vessels (see above), thus exerting more diffuse and distant effects.

Brodal (1981) mentioned the many unsolved problems relating to structure and functional organization of autonomic ganglia.

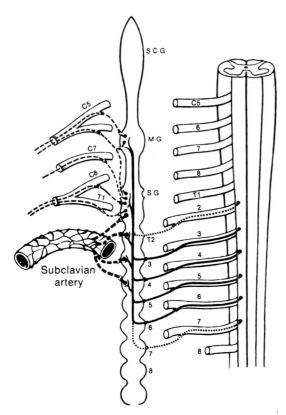

Fig. 20.4 Diagram of the origin and course of the sympathetic fibres to the upper extremity. The dotted preganglionic fibres are somewhat equivocal. Postganglionic fibres are indicated by broken lines. SCG: superior cervical ganglion; MG: middle cervical ganglion; SG: stellate ganglion. (From Haymaker & Woodhall 1945, after Foerster.)

2. Cranial symptoms after cervical injury or secondary to upper cervical arthrosis

The Barré–Lieou syndrome, initially described in 1926 (Barré), comprises a group of symptoms including headache, vertigo, tinnitus and ocular problems. This minimal list of clinical features was reported by Barré in conjunction with evidence of cervical arthrotic changes, and indeed there is sometimes little to choose between the symptom-complex of troublesome upper cervical arthrosis and that of traumatic injury to the neck. The growth of motor traffic and thus road traffic accidents is reflected in the increasing frequency of these injuries (Ch. 49). Their aetiology, diagnosis and management are to a degree still controversial, partly because no simple and characteristic radiographic findings have been reported and despite manifest evidence that manual therapists (of all persuasions) are very well acquainted with the natural history and careful physical treatment of these lesions. A significant proportion of these injuries are rear-end collisions. The magnitude of the collision forces is determined by the mass of the occupant's vehicle and the rate of change of velocity or acceleration of the colliding vehicle. The shorter the impact time the greater the rate of change of velocity or acceleration. Neck pain occurs after impact

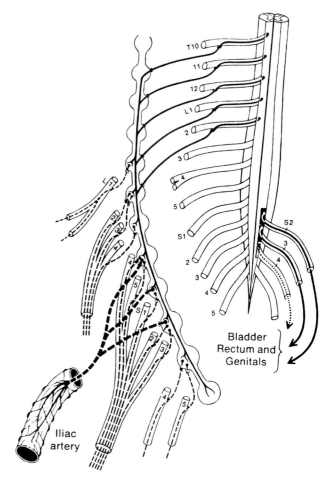

Fig. 20.5 Diagram of the sympathetic supply of the lower extremity following the principle as in Figure 20.4. The parasympathetic fibres to the pelvic organs are included on the right side. (From Haymaker and Woodhall 1945, after Foerster.)

(Figures 20.3, 20.4 and 20.5 are reproduced from Brodal 1981 with permission.)

from any direction, but is disproportionately more common after impact from the rear; the incidence is some 84% (Deans et al 1986).

Injury to the cervical spine is almost without exception due to indirect violence (von Torklus & Gehle 1972), the force being applied to head or rump and the neck sustaining a considerable proportion of it.

The direction of the force, the position and relationship of the head and spine, and the state of tension of the neck muscles determine the localization of stress. When injury has been severe, these patients suffer what might be regarded as multiple 'sprained ankles' in the neck, with all the added complications of nerve root and plexus traction injuries; meningeal traction; tearing of ligaments and probably muscle; trauma to blood vessels and lymphatics; upset to sensitive structures and delicately balanced functions (Grieve 1988).

Chusid (1985) mentioned that so-called chronic post-traumatic headache may arise from one of several mechanisms. The 'post-concussional syndrome' (Coppola 1968) may not be entirely due to intracranial changes and further, a moment's thought may show that a sideways fall on the outstretched hand can produce a lateral whiplash effect on the cervical spine besides a Colles fracture. Patients need not have been in a motor car to have suffered acceleration or deceleration trauma to the neck, many of these injuries occurring during athletics or on the sports field.

In a group of patients described by Roca (1972) one developed the acute traumatic cervical syndrome after a fall in a shower.

Depending upon the nature and magnitude of the violence applied, these cases present (Grieve 1988) with one or more of the following:

Suboccipital, neck and yoke area pains, unilaterally or bilaterally, with bouts of frontal headache which may be periodic and transient or remain as a dull and constant background ache
Facial and anterolateral throat pain
Patches of subjective facial numbness
Otalgia
Retro-orbital pain — sometimes paraesthesiae 'in' the eye
Subjective laryngeal disturbances, with compulsive clearing of the throat
Upper pectoral area and axillary pain
Feelings of instability or dysequilibrium, with sometimes a tendency to list to one side
Disturbances of hearing and/or vision
Depression, and feelings of fatigue
A belief that they are becoming neurotic and 'should pull themselves together'
Irritability, insomnia and light-headedness

Roca (1972) described 15 patients with ocular manifestations after whiplash injury, mentioning that blurred vision, strain, fatigue, diplopia, photophobia and inability to read may occur, with anxiety and a degree of depression soon to follow. Among the clinical features were included amaurotic episodes, decreased accommodation and convergence, anisocoria, possible vitreous detachment, hyperphoria, hypertropia, ptosis and inability to focus.

When the full complexity of the nervous anatomy of the cervical spine is appreciated, the bizarre symptoms reported by these patients become credible (Downs & Twomey 1979). They tend to move the neck cautiously and apprehensively, and are glad to return to a neutral position in which they feel most comfortable.

Worth's (1985) investigation, of the kinematic differences between normal cervical spines and those of road accident victims, noted that both rear-end and head-on collision victims had significantly less sagittal segmental mobility than normal subjects, at the occipitoatlantal segments — yet almost all of the post-accident X-rays had been reported as normal. For further consideration of these acceleration and deceleration injuries, and upper cervical arthrosis, see Grieve 1988, Chs 6, 7 and 8.

Radiographic investigation

Tamura (1989) and his colleagues attempted to determine the optimum oblique vertical angle at which cervical metrizamide myelography would satisfactorily demonstrate the fine anatomical details of the cervical nerve root sleeves. Views were taken at different angles, and it was determined that the most informative images of the root sleeves were obtained at 40° from the vertical plane, using metrizamide of 280 mg/Iml.

Cervical myelography was performed in patients with and without the Barré–Lieou syndrome, and the results compared.

(i) The Barré–Lieou syndrome group (40 patients) were so diagnosed because of the persistence of three or more of the main clinical features of headache, vertigo (dysequilibrium), tinnitus and ocular problems. Of these, 35 (16 female and 19 male) had developed the symptoms after cervical trauma. Their mean age was 42.2 years (range 14–67) and their neck injuries resulted from rear-end collisions in 19 cases, head-on collisions in two, side-on collisions in four and from other accidents in 10 cases. The five patients (4 female and 1 male) without trauma were aged 31 to 68 (mean age 47). Sadly, about 40% of the whole series were referred after unsuccessful treatment at other hospitals. Plain radiography showed no abnormalities in 18 cases; degenerative change of the middle and lower cervical spine was seen in eight cases. Only two showed upper cervical abnormalities: a teardrop fracture of C2 in one and ossification of the posterior longitudinal ligament at C2 and C3 in the other.

(ii) The non-Barré–Lieou syndrome group comprised 40 patients who had suffered cervical trauma but had not developed the syndrome. The group comprised 30 males and 10 females with a mean age of 39.6 years (range 14–71). The diagnoses were radiculopathy with neck pain in 27, radiculomyelopathy in seven, acute central spinal cord injury in four and brachial plexus paralysis in two. The cervical injuries resulted from rear-end collisions in 14 cases, head-on collision in seven, side-on collisions in three and other accidents in 16.

In 24 cases (60%) plain radiography showed no abnormalities; degenerative changes of the middle or lower cervical spine were seen in eight and in four cases there was disc space narrowing at C5/C6, C6/C7 or both.

Results. The special oblique views showed bilateral or unilateral defects of the nerve root sleeves of C4 in all cases of group (i) i.e. those with the Barré–Lieou syndrome, although the a–p and lateral views had presented a normal or near-normal image. In contrast, patients in group (ii), i.e. those without the Barré–Lieou syndrome, showed no defects in the C4 root sleeve, though there were defects in the root sleeves below C4 in all except five cases. No defects in the C3 root sleeves were seen in either group.

In 16 cases of group (ii) the defects in root sleeves below C4 were shown clearly only on the special oblique views. In 75% (30 cases) of group (i) there was impairment of sensibility in the C4 segmental distribution, especially the suprascapular region. Muscle testing was performed in 32 cases of this group, and revealed some weakness of combined shoulder and scapular movement; this was of MRC grade 3 in 15, and grade 4 in 14.

Prior to surgery, cervical discography at C3–4 was carried out in 16 of the patients in group (i), i.e. those with the Barré–Lieou syndrome. In the current climate of belief that segmental localization of a troublesome disc will be revealed by symptom-provocation when using this investigation procedure, it is interesting that the symptoms of the syndrome were not provoked in any of the 16 patients. Twenty-one patients (15 male and six female) of group (i) were treated surgically; anterior cervical discectomy and fusion at C3–4 was performed in all 21 cases.

Comment. This report is described in some detail because of its salient findings, a consistent involvement of the C4 root sleeve in 'whiplash' syndrome. The findings at myelography and at operation were of lateral 'soft' disc herniations at C3–4, exerting trespass not directly on the spinal cord but on the C4 root and more so the ventral root. The author enlarges upon the C4 root communications with the superior cervical ganglion, via branches of the postganglionic fibres, and suggests that irritation of the C4 root compromises the function of these communications, thus resulting in symptoms related to the sympathetic nervous system. He also mentions, among other observations, that tinnitus might be produced by sympathetic stimulation of the caroticotympanic nerve, and that ocular symptoms may be produced by the aberrant influence of the internal carotid plexus on the ciliary muscles or by reduced flow in the ophthalmic artery.

Again, the connections between the upper cervical nerves with the vagus, accessory and hypoglossal nerves, through the superior cervical ganglion, have been postulated as the substrate for the cervical spine's ability to produce the symptoms described (Campbell & Parsons 1944, Braaf & Rosner 1975). His explanation of the production of symptoms may be speculative to a degree (see also Grieve 1988), but the segmental identification of a consistently involved nerve root sleeve is a decided step forward in management, whether by surgery or conservative treatment, of these distressing syndromes.

At follow-up, of 20 patients after surgery, symptoms had settled after an average of 3.7 months (range one to seven months). Tinnitus was the symptom which settled more slowly than others. In group (i) patients who had not had surgery, the symptoms of the syndrome had persisted, this being revealed by follow-up at an average of 24 months (range 5 months to 8 years). A relevant observation is that sensations such as giddiness, nausea and tinnitus have been experimentally produced by needle stimulation of the peri-articular tissues and ligamentous tissue intimately related to the occipitoatlantal joints

(Campbell & Parsons 1944, Raney et al 1949). It is well-known among manual therapists that partial or complete relief of these distressing symptoms can be achieved by careful mobilisation of the C0–C1 and also the C3 segments, with the exception that tinnitus is the symptom more difficult to completely relieve. Hirsch et al (1988) mentioned their conviction that the Barré–Lieou syndrome is real and is manifested by symptoms consistent with the anatomical injuries sustained, that it has the potential to cause significant impairment and distress and that it benefits from a patient, rational and enlightened approach to treatment.

It is necessary for inexperienced clinical workers to be made aware of the individual nature of the physical and psychic distress occasioned by whiplash injury, and the need for careful and gentle handling.

The most important clinical aspect is that of a highly reactive 'brittleness' of condition during the early stages. It is quite different to the irritability of a single peripheral joint, for example, where unwisely energetic handling may stir up severe pain for hours or days. If the badly injured whiplash patient is handled vigorously with careless movement, the exacerbation can be very severe, with headache of hideous intensity, bizarre visual upset, psychic distress amounting to abject misery, and cervical pain of frightening viciousness. The 'brittle' stage may last for a week or for two to three months, and may return for a few days during the following months if the patient stumbles, is badly jolted or is given unnecessarily vigorous treatment. (Grieve 1988).

A retrospective analysis (Holt 1974) of 146 patients, after five years, indicated that there was a statistically significant correlation between poor treatment results and the following findings soon after injury:

Numbness or pain, or both, in an upper limb
A sharp reversal of cervical lordosis visible on X-ray
Restricted motion at one segment on 'bending' films
The need for a collar for more than three months
The need to resume physiotherapy more than once because of a recurrence of symptoms

Prognosis remains difficult. The contention that chronic symptoms diminish promptly on settlement of litigation is not borne out by review findings. Gargan and Bannister (1990) reviewed 43 patients who had sustained soft-tissue injuries of the neck, a mean of 10.8 years previously. Of these, only 12% had recovered completely, with residual symptoms intrusive in 28% and severe in 12%. Only 48% of the group had been wearing seatbelts; 88% were involved in rear-end collisions. The residual symptoms at follow-up were tabulated (Table 20.1) with neck pain the most common symptom, followed by paraesthesia. Auditory symptoms comprised tinnitus and deafness in equal proportion.

Patients were grouped according to symptom-severity: group A (12%) considered they were completely recovered.

Table 20.1 Residual symptoms at follow-up (%)

Neck pain	74
Paraesthesia	45
Lower back pain	42
Headache	33
Dizziness	19
Auditory symptoms	14
Dysphagia	2
Visual symptoms	2

Group B (48%) had mild symptoms which did not interfere with work or leisure. Group C (28%) complained of intrusive symptoms which necessitated analgesics, orthoses or physiotherapy. Group D (12%) suffered severe problems, had lost their jobs and relied continually on orthoses or analgesics and had undergone repeated medical consultations.

The authors concurred with previous workers, in that settlement of claims does not result in resolution of symptoms, in this case even after a mean of 10 years.

3. Musculoskeletal changes: lesions of trespass

The involvement of preganglionic sympathetic neurons, in lesions of neural trespass or radiculitis in the neighbourhood of intervertebral foramina T1–L2, is virtually inevitable, with consequences which are well understood.

So far as the thoracic spine is concerned a fairly detailed review of benign and malignant forms of trespass is given in Chapter 29 together with some other forms of neuropathy.

Sympathetic neurons may be compromised in other ways, for example (a) by osteophytes (spondylophytes) of intervertebral bodies on the anterior and anterolateral aspects of thoracic and lumbar regions (Figs 20.7, 20.8), (b) by arthrotic changes of costovertebral articulations (Nathan 1984) — in the thorax the sympathetic chain lies on the heads of the ribs — (Fig. 20.2), (c) acquired and/or congenital spinal stenosis (Grieve 1988). Chronic compression of the cauda equina produces not only the vascular features of intermittent claudication but also severe bilateral leg pain, (d) Nathan et al (1982) describe an osseous–fibrous tunnel on the ala of the sacrum, and the considerable variations in size and strength of the lumbosacral ligament which helps to form it. This structure may be a factor in L5 root compression, which can include a sympathetic ramus communicans.

The greater and/or lesser splanchnic nerves, more especially on the right side in the thoracic spine (Fig. 20.7) are often stretched over bony excrescences and sometimes incorporated in fibrotic thickenings of connective tissue. They are similar to those in the lumbar spine. (Figs 20.9–20.11).

Nathan's (1969) dissections of 344 cadavers revealed predominantly right-sided thoracic osteophytic trespass involving splanchnic nerves in 60.7% of the cases studied.

Nathan (1968) also dissected 390 lumbar sympathetic trunks from 195 adult cadavers. Osteophytes (spondylophytes) were found compressing the sympathetic trunks to some degree in 153 (78.4%) of the cadavers. (Figs 20.9–20.11).

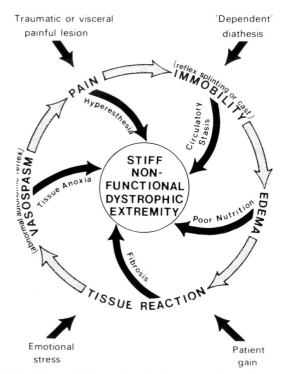

Fig. 20.6 Scheme of abnormal and self-perpetuating excitatory activity in internuncial neuron circuits of the spinal cord. (Reproduced from Lankford 1983 with permission of author and publisher.)

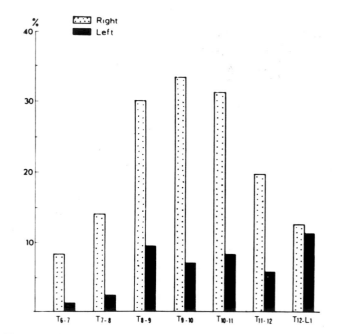

Fig. 20.7 A histogram depicting the distribution of vertebral body osteophytes trespassing upon splanchnic nerves in the lower half of the thorax. Note the greater frequency between T8–T11 and the preponderance of exostoses on the right side.

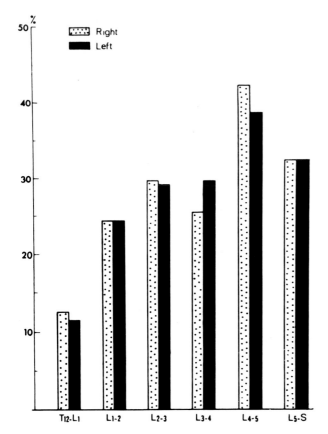

Fig. 20.8 A histogram depicting the distribution of ventral osteophytes in the lumbar spine. Note the frequency at L4–5 and L5–S1. (Figures 20.7, 20.8 reproduced from Nathan 1969 with permission.)

The macroscopic changes produced by osteophytic compression were enlargement, angulation and colour changes of the ganglia, accompanied at times by a sclerotic reaction and adhesion to the surrounding tissue.

The highest incidence (Fig. 20.8) was at the L4–L5 intervertebral joint, rather more frequently on the right side. The author speculates that symptoms of compression may be expected to appear in the lower limbs and/or pelvic viscera, since features of sympathetic dysfunction are not uncommon in adults and elderly people.

Stewart (1931) described a case of intermittent claudication, in which all the clinical features of early thromboangiitis obliterans were evident, although radiography did not reveal any arterial sclerotic change. At operation on the left lumbar sympathetic chain, extensive degenerative hypertrophy was revealed extending from L3 to L5. Between L4 and L5 the sympathetic trunk was embedded in a mass of hypertrophic tissue, and was dissected free with great difficulty. Compared with the trunk above this level, the freed section appeared to be contracted. Postoperatively, the left leg was distinctly pinker and warmer than the unoperated right leg.

4. Autonomic nerve involvement in referred pain and other symptoms

Most, if not all, peripheral branches from spinal nerves contain postganglionic sympathetic fibres (Williams et al 1989).

Bourdillon and Day (1987) suggested that the precise role of autonomic nerves in appreciation of pain remains to be clarified; so also do the precise pathways and peripheral destinations of postganglionic sympathetic neurons.

For example Keele and Neil (1971) and others, tabulated the sympathetic supply to the head and neck as follows:

Table 20.2

Head and neck	Cord segment	Ganglion	Route
Eye	T1, 2	Superior cervical	Along internal carotid artery
Face	T1, 2	Superior cervical	Along external carotid artery
Skin of head and neck	T1, 2	Superior cervical	With cervical plexus
Cerebral vessels	T1, 2	Superior and inferior cervical	Along internal carotid and vertebral arteries

The lowest somatic segmental supply to the upper limb is T3, while the sympathetic supply to upper limb may be derived as far caudally as the T8 segment (Fig. 20.12).

There is experimental evidence in man that pain afferents from the face pass back to upper thoracic segments and thus the spinal cord via the cervical sympathetic chain, i.e. in addition to the multitude of cranial nerve afferent neurons which descend in the spinal tract of the fifth cranial nerve before synapsing in the dorsal

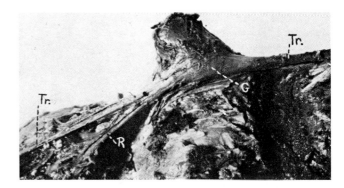

Fig. 20.9 A huge osteophyte pushing aside and compressing the right sympathetic trunk (Tr). The projecting osteophyte is seen compressing the sympathetic ganglion (G). The latter appears to be affected by a sclerotic reaction; it is enlarged, its borders are indistinct (especially in the upper part of the picture), and it was found to be tenaciously adherent to the underlying fibrotic tissues (ligaments, periosteum and intervertebral disc). A ramus communicans (R) is visible as it runs upwards from the ganglion.

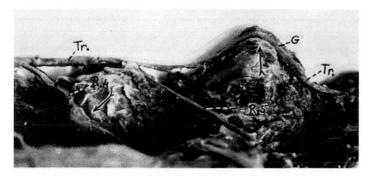

Fig. 20.10 Osteophytes impinging on the right sympathetic trunks (Tr) and on rami communicantes, right lateral view. The psoas muscles have been dissected away in order to reveal these nerves. A large osteophyte (upper arrow) impinges on and compresses a ganglion (G). Another osteophyte impinges on the ramus, which appears enlarged and angulated at the point of the compression (lower arrow) in contrast to the ramus communicans of the fifth lumbar nerve (R_5), which runs a straight course, undisturbed by osteophytes.

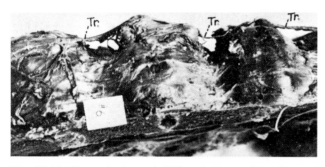

Fig. 20.11 Sympathetic trunk (Tr) pushed away from the vertebral bodies by impinging osteophytes. The trunks stretch over the depression formed by neighbouring osteophytes. The fatty connective tissue occupying the space resulting between the trunks and the vertebral bodies, as well as the lumbar vessels embedded into it, were cleaned up.

(Figures 20.9–20.11 reproduced from Nathan 1968 with permission.)

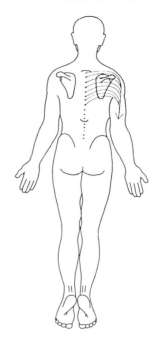

Fig. 20.12 The sympathetic supply to the upper limb may be derived as far caudally as the T8 segment.

Table 20.3

Body part	Supposed origin of pain
Head and neck	Intracranial and extracranial head lesions; temporomandibular joint; upper cervical segments
Upper limb	Lower cervical and uppermost thoracic segments; some diseases of thoracic viscera
Trunk wall	Thoracic and uppermost lumbar segments; some diseases of thoracic and abdominal viscera
Lower limb	Mid/lower lumbar segments; pelvic articulations and hip-joint

region of C1, C2 and C3 segments, as do the somatic afferents of those segments.

Electrical stimulation of the superior cervical sympathetic ganglion can produce pain in the face — precisely the same result is produced when the cervical sympathetic trunk is sectioned and the *proximal* ends are again stimulated (Smith 1969).

Pain is often referred from spinal segments to body parts which have no nerve connections other than via autonomic nerves. Unnecessary difficulty can arise because of restricted concepts about the cause of clinical features. Referred pain in the head, neck, trunk and limbs may be thought about in stereotyped ways which might briefly be tabulated as in Table 20.3.

We tend to conceive musculoskeletal referred pain in neck, trunk and limb to be a matter of somatic neurons alone, yet readily accept the phenomenon of visceral lesions referring cutaneous pain and tenderness to trunk areas and, in cardiac disease, the left upper limb. Where somatic nerve connections do not exist, e.g. (a) between mid-thoracic segments T345 and the head, and (b) be-

tween thoracic segments T4 and caudally and the upper limbs (Ch. 29), clinical familiarity and acceptance of pain referred (if that is the right word) in these ways is remarkably thin on the ground, despite the regularity with which manual therapists relieve head pain, and bilateral glove paraesthesiae of upper limbs, for example, by simple mobilization of the named thoracic segments.

Our understanding of referred pain is incomplete. Sufficient clinical experience exists to suggest that autonomic nerves may share more actively in the mechanisms underlying its vagaries.

Although much remains to be learnt of the afferent routes of impulses arising in painful pathological conditions of viscera (Williams et al 1989), visceral afferents from the heart are manifestly capable, in cardiac disease, of initiating referred pain down the left arm. Why should this known propensity not be acceptable as a central mechanism in referred musculoskeletal pain, too? There are no known visceral afferents from skeletal tissues, but might not the cortical representation of skeletal tissues include the autonomic innervation of blood vessels? Why should not the rich autonomic innervation, and thus cortical representation, have as much to do with patterns of referred somatic pain as somatic nerve representation? This may well explain the notorious untidiness of referred pains, which do *not* respect (somatic) dermatomes. The question has not yet, to my knowledge, been fully addressed by the many writers on referred musculoskeletal pain.

Stoddard (1983) mentions the considerable evidence that pain is conveyed by visceral afferent neurons — 'such pain is diffuse and poorly localised'.

Conclusion

Most autonomic components of clinical features, in the form of vasomotor, sudomotor and pupillary changes, for example, are well understood. More covert changes, sequelae of spondylosis and arthrosis in the form of collagenosis in attachment-tissues around peripheral joints (Grieve 1988, Bourdillon & Day 1987), and also the activation of painful trigger points in skeletal muscle (Travell & Simons 1983), are not so well appreciated. The phenomenon of minor pathology of attachment tissues in the limbs, secondary to spondylosis of associated spinal segments, is familiar to orthopaedists, rheumatologists and manual therapists. The common genesis of these capsular, ligamentous and tendinous lesions (a proportion due to local over-use, of course) seems less well appreciated by general practitioners and other physicians. Lateral epicondylitis (tennis elbow) is a prime example. Yet understanding the nature of the 'secondary pathology' phenomenon does not do much to improve our success rate in localized treatment of these lesions. Much is made of friction massage, mobilization, stretching, manipulation, ultrasound, acupuncture, hydrocortisone, cock-up supports and so on, yet the condition remains notoriously treatment-resistant and the passage of time is usually the one factor which helps many to recover. Labelle et al (1990) reviewed the literature, since 1966, to evaluate the best treatment of tennis elbow. Of 159 articles reviewed, 61 were analysed. Series without concurrent controls were considered doubtful because the natural history of the condition is not well documented. Articles were graded, according to a published criterion, by two orthopaedic surgeons. Of a possible 100 points, the mean score was 33 (range 11.5 to 59). Since a minimum of 70 points is necessary for a valid clinical trial, the authors concluded that there was no true scientific basis for any of the published localized treatment modalities for tennis elbow.

The case for including concomitant treatment of the relevant vertebral structures becomes undeniable (Grieve 1988), since associated spinal pain is now well recognized. Moynagh (1990) remarked on the aetiology of enthesopathies of limb girdle and more peripheral joints, observing that significant neck pain occurred in 23 out of 65 patients with tennis elbow (lateral epicondylitis), 15 of 27 with golfer's elbow (medial epicondylitis), and 17 of 42 patients with tenderness of rotator cuff insertions. Of 54 patients, mostly middle-aged women, with tenderness of the anteromedial aspect of the proximal tibia, 47 suffered low-back pain. There were no physical signs of knee pathology, and the tenderness, localized to the pes anserinus insertion, was judged not to be bursitis, medial ligament strain or fibromyalgia. There were more failures of local treatment, including surgery, in all of those conditions where spinal pain co-existed. It was concluded that although enthesopathies can have multiple causation, a neural mechanism of spinal origin is responsible for many cases, and that the work of Lewis and Kellgren on referred tenderness deserves further study. The genesis of collagenosis around peripheral joints, with aberrant vascularity possibly mediated via autonomic nerves, might also be investigated.

Of interest is the finding (Cooke et al 1989) that responses to mild cold stress, of 20 patients with reflex sympathetic dystrophy (algoneurodystrophy) and 10 patients with chronic upper limb pain, were indistinguishable; the results for these two groups were significantly ($P < 0.05$) different from a group of normal subjects. The aberrant thermo-regulation which was common to both abnormal groups is perhaps a pointer to the factor of abnormal autonomic nerve responses in the genesis of collagenosis around peripheral joints.

Similarly, Bryan et al (1990) investigated peripheral sensory function in reflex sympathetic dystrophy, noting a significant elevation of skin temperature, and a lowering of the pressure pain threshold, in the affected limb. They hypothesize that this leads to further changes in autonomic tone, thus establishing a pathological loop of activity. Sympathetic block abolished pain by allowing peripheral receptors to revert to normal thresholds in the 40 patients of their study. That sympathetic nerve distribution may be an important factor in patterns of referred pain, of musculoskeletal origin, should perhaps be more widely recognized as should the phenomenon of secondary pathology of the soft tissues in areas to which pain is commonly referred from primary axial lesions.

The effects of age, gender and physical training on the autonomic nervous system (Green 1990) are not as well understood by therapists as they might be, neither are the effects of drugs on this system. There are sound clinical reasons for the importance which dedicated lay practitioners (osteopaths, naturopaths, chiropractors) give to understanding the physiology of autonomic nerves. For the less athletic of our patients, and those who are obese, diabetic, hypertensive, atherosclerotic and possibly suffering from cardiac ischaemia, we need to appreciate the pivotal role of autonomic nerves in both the normal and disturbed functioning of body systems.

Continuing to regard autonomic and somatic components as disparate parts of the nervous system will continue to hinder our full understanding of the clinical presentation of spinal musculoskeletal conditions.

REFERENCES

Appenzeller O 1978 Somatoautonomic reflexology — normal and abnormal. In: Korr I M (ed) Neurobiologic mechanisms in manipulative therapy. Plenum Press, London, pp 179–217

Appenzeller O, Ogin G 1973 Myelinated fibres in the human paravertebral chain: quantitative studies on white rami communicantes. Journal of Neurology, Neurosurgery and Psychiatry 36: 777–785

Barré M 1926 Sur un syndrome sympathique cervical postérieur et sa cause fréquent: l'arthrite cervicale. Revue Neurologie Strasbourg 33: 1246–8

Bogduk N 1983 Sympathetic pain syndromes. Proceedings: Manipulative Therapists' Association of Australia Conference, Perth

Bourdillon J, Day E A 1987 Spinal manipulation. 4th edn. Heinemann, London

Boyd J D 1957 Intermediate sympathetic ganglia. British Medical Bulletin 13: 207–212

Braaf M M, Rosner S 1975 Trauma of the cervical spine as a cause of chronic headache. Journal of Trauma 15: 441–446

Brodal A 1981 Neurological anatomy in relation to clinical medicine. 3rd edn. University Press, Oxford, ch 11, pp 698–787

Bryan A S, Klenerman L, Bowsher D 1990 Measurement of somatic sensory modalities in reflex sympathetic dystrophy. Journal of Bone and Joint Surgery 72B: 1106–1107

Campbell D G, Parsons C M 1944 Referred head pain and its concomitants. Journal of Nervous and Mental Disorders 99: 544–551

Chusid J G 1985 Correlative neuroanatomy and functional neurology. 19th edn. Lange Medical, Los Altos

Cooke E D, Glick E N, Bowcock S A, Smith R E, Ward C, Almond N E, Beacham J H 1989 Reflex sympathetic dystrophy (algoneurodystrophy): temperature studies in the upper limb. British Journal of Rheumatology 28: 399–403

Coote J H 1978 Somatic sources of afferent input as factors in aberrant autonomic, sensory and motor function. In: Korr I M (ed) The neurobiologic mechanisms in manipulative therapy: Plenum Press, London, pp 91–127

Coppola A R 1968 Neck injury: a reappraisal. International Surgery 50: 510–515

Day M D 1979 Autonomic pharmacology: experimental and clinical aspects. Churchill Livingstone, Edinburgh, chs 1, 8, pp 5, 118

Deans G T, McGalliard J N, Rutherford W H 1986 Incidence and duration of neck pain among patients injured in car accidents. British Medical Journal 292: 94–95

Delmas J, Laux G, Guerrier Y 1947 Comment atteindre les fibres vasomotrices préganglionaires du membre supéricur. Gazette Médicale de France 54: 703–712

Denslow J S, Korr I M, Krems A D 1947 Quantitative studies of chronic facilitation in human motoneuron pools. American Journal of Physiology 105: 229–238

Doran F S A 1967 The sites to which pain is referred from the common bile-duct in man and its implications for the theory of referred pain. British Journal of Surgery 54: 599–606

Downs J, Twomey L 1979 The whiplash syndrome. Australian Journal of Physiotherapy 25: 233–241

Eadie M J 1967 Paroxysmal positional giddiness. Medical Journal of Australia 54: 1169–1173

Ebbesson S O E 1968 Quantitative studies of superior cervical sympathetic ganglia in a variety of primates including man. 11 Neuronal packing density. Journal of Morphology 124: 181–186

Eble J N 1960 Patterns of response of the paravertebral musculature to visceral stimuli. American Journal of Physiology 198: 429–433

Eränkö O 1978 Small intensely fluorescent (SIF) cells and neurotransmission in sympathetic ganglia. Annual Review of Pharmacology and Toxicology 18: 417–430

Erhlich E, Alexander W F 1951 Surgical implications of upper thoracic independent sympathetic pathways. Archives of Surgery 62: 609–614

Feinstein B 1977 Referred pain from paravertebral structures. In: Buerger A A, Tobis J F (eds) Approaches to the validation of manipulative therapy. Thomas, Springfield Illinois, pp 139–174

Feinstein B, Langton J N K, Jameson R M, Schiller F 1954 Experiments on pain referred from deep somatic tissues. Journal of Bone and Joint Surgery 36A: 981–997

Gabella G 1976 Structure of the autonomic nervous system. Chapman and Hall, London, ch 2, p 39

Gargan M F, Bannister G C 1990 Long-term prognosis of soft-tissue injuries of the neck. Journal of Bone and Joint Surgery 72B: 901–903

Gaskell W H 1916 The involuntary nervous system. Longman Green, London

Green J H 1990 The autonomic nervous system and exercise. Chapman & Hall, Andover

Greenman P E 1978 Manipulative therapy in total health care. In: Korr I M (ed) The neurobiologic mechanisms in manipulative therapy. Plenum Press, London, pp 43–52

Grieve G P 1988 Common vertebral joint problems. 2nd edn. Churchill Livingstone, Edinburgh, chs 6, 7, 8

Gross D 1974 Pain and the autonomic nervous system. In: Bonica J J (ed) Advances in neurology. Raven Press, New York, ch IV, p 92

Guerrier Y 1944 Le sympathique cervical. Imprimière de la Charité, Montpelier

Hamberg J, Lindahl O 1981 Angina pectoris symptoms caused by thoracic spine disorders: clinical examination and treatment. Acta Medica Scandinavica suppl 664: 84–86

Hannington-Kiff J G 1974 Pain relief. Heinemann, London

Haugen F P 1968 The autonomic nervous system and pain. Anaesthesiology 29: 785–792

Head H 1920 Studies in neurology. Oxford Medical Publications, London, p 653

Hinoki M, Niki H 1975 Neurotological studies in the role of the sympathetic nervous system in the formation of traumatic vertigo of cervical origin. Acta Otolaryngologica suppl 330: 185–196

Hinsey J C, Phillips R A 1940 Observations on diaphragmatic sensation. Journal of Neurophysiology 3: 175–181

Hirsch S A, Hirsch P J, Hiramoto H, Weiss A 1988 Whiplash syndrome: fact or fiction? Orthopaedic Clinics of North America 19: 791–795

Holt M 1974 Soft tissue injuries of the neck in automobile accidents: factors influencing prognosis. Journal of Bone and Joint Surgery 56A: 1675–1682

Iggo A 1955 Tension receptors in the stomach and urinary bladder. Journal of Physiology 128: 593–607

Johnson R H, Spalding J M K 1974 Diseases of the autonomic nervous system. Blackwell Scientific, Oxford, ch 1, pp 1–22

Keele C A, Neil E 1971 Samson Wright's applied physiology. 12th edn. University Press, Oxford, ch 7, p 384

Kellgren J H 1949 Deep pain sensibility. Lancet 1: 943–949

Kennard M A, Haugen F P 1955 The relation of subcutaneous focal sensitivity to referred pain of cardiac origin. Anaesthesiology 16: 297–311

Koizumi K 1978 Autonomic system reactions caused by excitation of somatic afferents. In: Korr I M (ed) Neurobiologic mechanisms in manipulative therapy. Plenum Press, London, pp 219–227

Korr I M 1978 Sustained sympathicotonia as a factor in disease. In: Korr I M (ed) Neurobiologic mechanisms in manipulative therapy. Plenum Press, London, pp 229–268

Kostyuk P G 1968 Presynaptic and postsynaptic changes produced in spinal neurones by an afferent volley from visceral afferents. In: von Euler C, Skoglund S, Söderberg U (eds) Structure and function of inhibiting neuronal mechanisms. Pergamon Press, Oxford

Krahe B 1974 Thorakal-syndrome in der differentialdiagnose der inneren medizin. Manuelle Medizin 12: 15–20

Kunert W 1965 Functional disorders of internal organs due to vertebral lesions. Ciba Symposium 13: 85–96

Kuntz A 1945 Anatomic and physiologic properties of cutaneovisceral vasomotor reflex arcs. Journal of Neurophysiology 8: 421–429

Labelle H, Fallaha M, Newman N, Rivard C-H, Guibert R 1990 The treatment of tennis elbow: a critical review of the literature. Journal of Bone and Joint Surgery 72B: 536

Langley J N 1898 On the union of cranial autonomic (visceral) fibres with the nerve cells of the superior cervical ganglion. Journal of Physiology 23: 240–270

Lankford L L 1983 Reflex sympathetic dystrophy. In: Evarts C M (ed) Surgery of the musculoskeletal system. vol 1. Churchill Livingstone, Edinburgh, p 145

Laruelle N L 1940 Les bases anatomique du système autonome cortical et bulbo-spinal. Revue Neurologie 72: 349–361

Leavitt F, Garron D C, Whisler W W, Sheinkop M B 1978 Affective and sensory dimensions in back pain. Pain 4: 273–281

Lindahl O, Hamberg J 1981 Angina pectoris symptoms caused by thoracic spine disorders: neuroanatomical consideration. Acta Medica Scandinavica Supplement 644: 81–83

Loeser J D 1984 Deafferentation pain. Proceedings: International Course on Spinal Disorders — June, Gothenburg

Loh L, Nathan P W, Schott G D 1981 Pain due to lesions of the central nervous system removed by sympathetic block. British Medical Journal 282: 1026–1028

McKenzie J 1990 Symptoms and their interpretation. Shaw, London

Melzack R, Torgenson W S 1971 On the language of pain. Anaesthesiology 34: 50–59

Melzack R, Wall P D 1982 The challenge of pain. Penguin, Harmondsworth, chs 3, 4, 8, pp 56–61, 72–86, 179–186

Milne E 1968 Giddiness in vertebro-basilar arterial insufficiency. Medical Journal of Australia 55: 417–418

Mitchell G A G 1953 Anatomy of the autonomic nervous system. Livingstone, Edinburgh

Mitchell G A G 1954 The autonomic nerve supply of the throat, nose and ear. Journal of Laryngology and Otology 68: 495–516

Moynagh P D 1990 Observations on the terminology and aetiology of enthesopathy. Journal of Bone and Joint Surgery 72B: 950

Nathan H 1968 Compression of the sympathetic trunk by osteophytes of the vertebral column in the abdomen: an anatomical study with pathological and clinical considerations. Surgery 63: 609–625

Nathan H 1969 Compression of the sympathetic trunk and its nerves by vertebral osteophytes in the thorax and abdomen. Archivos Mexicanos de Anatomia 9: 30–45

Nathan H 1984 Personal communication

Nathan H, Weizenbluth M, Halperin N 1982 The lumbosacral ligament (LSL) with special emphasis on the lumbosacral tunnel and the entrapment of the 5th lumbar nerve. International Orthopaedics 6: 197–202

Nathan P W 1976 The gate-control theory of pain: a critical review. Brain 99: 123–158

Pomeranz B, Wall P D, Weber W V 1968 Cord cells responding to fine myelinated afferents from viscera, muscle and skin. Journal of Physiology 199: 511–532

Raney A A, Raney R B, Hunter C R 1949 Chronic post-traumatic headache and the syndrome of cervical disc lesion following head trauma. Journal of Neurosurgery 6: 458–465

Rasmussen A T 1952 The principal nervous pathways. 4th edn. Macmillan

Richards R L 1967 Causalgia: a centennial review. Archives of Neurology (Chicago) 16: 399–350

Roca P D 1972 Ocular manifestations of whiplash injuries. Annals of Ophthalmology 4: 63–73

Rosomoff H L, Johnston J D H, Gallo A E, Ludmer M, Givens F T, Carney F T, Kuehn C A 1970 Cystometry as an adjunct in the evaluation of lumbar disc syndromes. Journal of Neurosurgery 33: 67–74

Ross J 1988 On the segmental distribution of sensory disorders. Brain 10: 333–361

Sato A 1975 The somatosympathetic reflexes: their physiological and clinical significance. In: Goldstein M (ed) The research status of spinal manipulative therapy. U.S. Department of Health, Bethesda. NINCDS Monograph 15: 163–172

Sato A, Schmidt R F 1973 Somatosympathetic reflexes: afferent fibres, central pathways, discharge characteristics. Physiology Review 53: 916–947

Shafar J 1966 The syndromes of the third neurone of the cervical sympathetic system. American Journal of Medicine 40: 97–109

Smith B H 1969 Anatomy of facial pain. Headache 9: 7–13

Smithwick R H 1936 Modified dorsal sympathectomy for vascular spasm (Raynaud's disease) of the upper extremity. Annals of Surgery 104: 339–350

Sola A E, Kuitert J H 1955 Myofascial trigger point pain in the neck and shoulder girdle. Northwest Medicine 54: 980–984

Stewart S F 1931 Relation of the sympathetic nervous system to hypertrophic arthritis, Journal of Bone and Joint Surgery 13: 848

Stoddard A 1983 Manual of osteopathic practice. 2nd edn. Hutchinson, London p xi

Sturge W A 1883 The phenomena of angina pectoris and their bearing upon the theory of counter irritation. Brain 5: 492–510

Tamura T 1989 Cranial symptoms after cervical injury: aetiology and treatment of the Barré-Lieou syndrome. Journal of Bone and Joint Surgery 71B: 283–287

Thomas L 1984 The youngest science: notes of a medicine-watcher. University Press, Oxford, ch 17, p 179

Tinel J 1937 Le système nerveux végétatif. Masson, Paris

Travell J G 1957 Symposium on mechanism and management of pain syndromes. Proceedings: Rudolf Virchow Medical Society 16: 128–136

Travell J, Rinzler S H 1946 Relief of cardiac pain by local block of somatic trigger areas. Proceedings of the Society of Experimental Biological Medicine 63: 480–482

Travell J G, Simons D G 1983 Myofascial pain and dysfunction: the trigger point manual. Williams & Wilkins, Baltimore, ch 2, pp 23–26

van Buskirk C 1941 Nerves in the vertebral canal: their relation to the sympathetic innervation of the upper extremities. Archives of Surgery 43: 427–432

von Torklus D, Gehle W 1972 The upper cervical spine. Butterworths, London

Vyas S H (ed) 1979 The Union List of Osteopathic Literature. College of Osteopathic Medicine, Philadelphia

Williams P L, Warwick R, Dyson M, Bannister L H 1989 Gray's anatomy. 37th edn. Churchill Livingstone, Edinburgh, pp 935, 1154–1155, 1167–1168

Worth D 1985 Cervical spine movements in normal subjects and in whiplash victims. Proceedings of the Fourth Biennial Conference of the Manipulative Therapists Association of Australia, Brisbane, p 30

Wyke B D 1970 The neurological basis of thoracic spinal pain. Rheumatology and Physical Medicine 10: 356–367

Wyke B D 1990 Personal communication

21. The assessment of chronic pain

D. Bowsher

PAIN

The International Association for the Study of Pain (IASP), the world body comprising all health professionals dealing with and researching on pain, defines pain as 'an unpleasant sensory and emotional experience associated with actual or potential tissue damage, or described in terms of such damage' (International Association for the Study of Pain 1986). This of course is a definition arrived at by a committee, and as there are more or less equal objections from all branches and specialties concerned with treatment of or research into pain, the definition is not accepted by all!

There is much greater agreement in the matter of defining thresholds, and this is most important for therapists as well as their patients. Pain threshold is defined as 'the least experience of pain which a subject can recognise' (International Association for the Study of Pain 1986). This does not vary from person to person any more than other biological thresholds — just as all individuals have a threshold for hearing and vision which can be defined in terms of the minimum amount of energy necessary to elicit conscious sensation, so it is for pain. Normal human beings feel pain when a temperature of about 44 °C is applied to the skin, or a pin is applied with a force of about 0.65 grams. No-one ever seeks therapeutic advice when their pain threshold is reached — they simply withdraw from the offending stimulus! So therapists don't know about pain thresholds, and are certainly not in a position to say that Mr Brown has a lower pain threshold than Mrs Green.

The medically important threshold is the *pain tolerance level*. This is defined as 'the greatest level of pain which a subject is prepared to tolerate' (International Association for the Study of Pain 1986). This can differ enormously from person to person, and within the same individual at different times and under different circumstances — anyone is prepared to tolerate a far greater degree of pain in a good cause such as rescuing a relative from a fire than for some trivial reason such as gratuitously inflicted pain in the laboratory, performed just to see what can be stood! In fact, of course, patients do not seek therapeutic advice about their pain until it has gone beyond tolerance level. From this point of view, it might be better to think of clinical pain in terms of *in*tolerance levels. It is the all-important tolerance level, and not the clinically unimportant threshold, which is measured by such techniques as the visual analogue scale (see below).

Chronic pain, to which the IASP classification specifically refers, is generally accepted as pain which has lasted, constantly or intermittently, for 3 or more months. This is of course an arbitrary definition, and may depend on a factor as simple as how long it is before a sufferer decides to seek professional advice. On the other side of the coin, there are many pains which therapists, if not always patients, know will become chronic if not treated early. Thus it may be best to decide that 'we know what we mean by chronic pain' without attempting to define it too closely. The rest of this chapter is devoted to the first interview, and preparation for that interview, with the chronic pain patient as understood by this very flexible definition.

In North America, Australasia, Great Britain, and much of Western Europe, there are now many pain relief clinics/services staffed by physiotherapists and physicians specializing in the relief of chronic pain, and to a lesser extent of acute pain. The therapist may see patients in the pain relief clinic, on request in other services, or in the patients' homes.

At the Centre for Pain Relief at Walton Hospital, Liverpool, one of Europe's largest pain relief clinics, seeing in excess of 3500 cases of chronic pain a year, about half the patients are referred by family physicians and half by other hospital specialists. The largest single group among the latter consists of orthopaedic surgeons, who refer 12.5% of all cases (Bowsher et al 1988). More importantly in the present context, about 25% of all chronic pain patients referred to our clinic have pains sited in or originating from the vertebral column. This means that many cases of pain originating from the vertebral column are satisfactorily dealt with elsewhere, because a population survey (Bowsher et al 1991) has shown that about 7% of the adult population of the UK suffer from chronic pain, and one-third of these locate the pain to their back or neck.

The first interview or consultation with a chronic pain patient is of capital importance. It should be carefully prepared and diligently conducted. Its primary aim is two-fold:

1. to provide the therapist with all possible information about the patient's present condition and relevant past history
2. to give the patient the confidence that he/she is in the hands of a caring, careful and competent practitioner who, during this one-to-one session, is receiving the total and undivided attention of the therapist.

Preparation

Preparation is an active process which can prepare the way for the interview, as well as persuading the patient of the therapist's interest. It is good practice to send the patient a questionnaire to be completed and returned before the first consultation. It is hoped that international agreement will soon be reached on the format of such questionnaires so that valid comparisons of core patient data can be made from most, if not all, centres.

Many questionnaires are in use in different clinics; some are so long that when completed (a task of several days for the patient!) they constitute a veritable autobiography, albeit a very stiff and formal one. This is obviously useless. A questionnaire should be designed to extract the following information in the briefest possible way:

1. Biographical details: date of birth, age of finishing education, occupation, family circumstances (number of siblings, their health, that of parents; spouse, children, their ages and health), height, weight, *handedness*; patient's health record, particularly including any chronic conditions and treatment being taken currently.

Other items differ from clinic to clinic but are usually designed to elicit personal, family, medical, social, and economic details as well as past medical history and information about the present pain. A question we have found useful is: 'What do *you* think is the cause of your pain?' Although this question may be repeated verbally at the interview, patients are often less inhibited when writing answers to a questionnaire in their own homes and in the absence of the therapist. Answers to this question can be very revealing! Another question probably better asked on paper (in case it is irrelevant) is: 'Are you engaged in litigation concerned with the cause of your pain?' It is our experience that patients are more willing to answer potentially embarrassing questions (including ones about income and effects of sexual activity on pain) on questionnaire forms than in person. By studying the patient's answers before the first consultation, the experienced therapist may glean much information and often save a considerable amount of time.

2. Pain history: when and how it started, whether constant or episodic, effects on sleep and lifestyle; pain drawing, a silhouette on which the patient shades in the distribution of the pain (this is in addition to — and may turn out to be quite different from — the pain drawing which the therapist will make after performing a physical examination; the difference may be very instructive).

It may also be found useful to ask for a list of factors which exacerbate or alleviate the pain (some therapists prefer to use a check-list, while others leave it to a free description). Finally, the pre-interview document should ask how pain affects lifestyle — sleep, ability to perform work/housework, effect on leisure activities, social relationships, etc.; these items will be cross-checked in the interview.

3. Pain description. The most important and revealing information that any therapist can glean about a pain is to determine its characteristics — what it feels *like*. Since people often mean different things by the same word, a forced-choice questionnaire is useful. This means that the patient is presented with a list of words and asked to underline only those words which apply to the pain being experienced. Most clinics use the McGill Pain Questionnaire (Melzack 1975), which is reproduced in Appendix I. There is a method of 'scoring' the McGill Questionnaire, though most practitioners find the list (and number) of words chosen to be most valuable; the lower any chosen word is in its group, the greater the intensity. The first 10 groups of words in the McGill Questionnaire are of somatic pain descriptors, and these are the ones on which subsequent physical assessment will concentrate. With experience, the answers to a McGill Pain Questionnaire become diagnostic of some types of chronic pain.

The interview/consultation

The first and golden rule of algological practice is that the patient has as much pain as he/she says he/she has. If a patient suspects that the therapist may dismiss his/her pain as 'all in the mind', the essential relationship of mutual trust will be destroyed before it starts. Thus, although the therapist will hopefully have studied not only the preparatory questionnaire and referral documents, but also earlier medical records before seeing the patient, the first thing that must be said at the initial interview is 'tell me about your pain'. Then *listen* to the response. Considering that most patients with pain originating from the vertebral column have seen several specialists and have often undergone one or more surgical procedures before visiting an algologist, there is a horrifyingly large number of patients who say 'no one has ever listened to me before'. Of course, the statement may not be true, but if the patient believes it is, that's what matters.

Following up the information obtained from the McGill Pain Questionnaire which the patient filled in before the interview, when the patient's own account has come to an end, the therapist should ask the patient the single most important question that can be put in a pain consultation: 'What does your pain feel *like*?' Get the patient to use a descriptor, not a statement of how bad (or where) the pain is; ask 'What would you have to do to me to give me the same pain?' If the patient uses several adjectives to describe what the pain feels like, it may be useful, additionally, to ask: 'If we can remove only *one* of these qualities of pain, which one would you most like taken away?' As mentioned above when discussing the McGill Pain Questionnaire, information about pain characteristics is extremely useful. Indeed, with a little experience, it becomes diagnostic in many types of pain.

Patients' answers to questions, both in a questionnaire and at interview, vary enormously according to personality, mood at the time of interview/questionnaire answering, educational and cultural background, and probably other factors. This is another way of saying that each patient must be assessed individually, not compared with other patients, even those with similar pain arising from the same cause.

Pain intensity should be measured at the first consultation, and at every subsequent session, so that there is a numerical record not only of the patient's initial pain intensity, but of progress — whether the pain is getting better or worse, or staying the same. By far the most useful measure of pain intensity is the *visual analog scale* (VAS) (Bond & Pilowsky 1966), which measures the important parameter of pain tolerance (see above). It consists of a horizontal, 10 cm line, marked 'no pain' at one end and 'the worst pain I ever felt' at the other. The patient makes a mark on the line that represents the level of pain at that moment, and its position and distance along the line is measured (in millimetres) by the therapist. (Plastic scales, with a movable cursor and a ruler on the back, can be used repeatedly; they are obtainable from: The Pain Relief Foundation, Walton Hospital, Liverpool L9 1AE, UK.) The VAS is remarkably consistent within the individual and thus may be used at successive consultations to assess the progress of the patient's pain relief, or lack of it; alternatively, the patient may be given a number of dated VAS scales to fill in at home. However, severity measurements from different patients cannot be compared; one cannot say that Mr A's pain is more severe than Mrs B's, although each individual will remain consistent. Over very large numbers, means of VAS measurements from categories of patient (e.g. low-back pain with sciatica and low-back pain without sciatica) can be compared.

Only after all this should a physical examination be undertaken. In most cases, the findings of referring physicians will be confirmed. Nevertheless, a thorough physical examination must be performed. The place and importance of the examination are somewhat paradoxical. On the one hand, it plays an important role in reassuring the patient; on the other, it may happen that the therapist is less expert in the specialist field from which the patient has been referred than the referring physician, but much more expert in others. The therapist may sometimes discover something that has been overlooked by the referring specialist. More often, the therapist, by taking a wider view, will discover parallel factors, physical or psychological, which contribute to the patient's pain. Although there are some purely 'psychological' pains, there are virtually no organic pains of long duration in which a functional overlay is lacking.

In a pain relief clinic with several therapists of differing speciality backgrounds, the choice of which person the patient will see at the first consultation is often decided after the questionnaire documents, as well as the referral letter (if any), have been studied. At other clinics the patient is seen by a panel of two or three specialists. Although there are excellent clinics where this is standard practice it is not to be recommended — on the grounds that such an experience may be rather intimidating for the patient at first interview. We prefer to send the patient to an individual colleague if another opinion is considered desirable.

THE PATIENT WITH VERTEBRAL COLUMN PAIN IN THE PAIN RELIEF CLINIC

If a patient with neck or back pain reports to a therapist soon after the onset of pain, there is usually little difficulty in arriving at a diagnosis and devising a course of therapy. This is of course even easier when the pain is of sudden rather than insidious onset.

However, it is rare for a back (as opposed to neck) pain patient to be seen at an early stage in what is to become a chronic pain history. The patient will often have consulted someone else previously for the painful condition. Even more difficult is one's own patient who has not responded to a particular treatment, and so has become chronic (regular pain tolerance level assessments with the VAS scale should give warning of this). In both instances, the patient should be assessed or re-assessed as a new patient (Bowsher 1989). Usually, one of two possibilities should be considered:

1. The patient still has the same pain for which consultation was originally undertaken, although it may be less, or occasionally more, severe than before.

2. The patient has lost the original pain but now has another pain, which may or may not be iatrogenic. In such a case, of course, it is necessary for the therapist to investigate and treat the new pain in an appropriate manner.

With the first situation, after careful examination and perhaps investigation, it is just possible that the therapist will find a previously unsuspected condition. In Great

Britain, the most common such condition in backache cases is probably facet joint pathology (Sluiter & Mehta 1981), which may be dealt with by radio-frequency or cryocoagulation if it does not yield to mobilization or manipulation. More often, however, no new pathology is discovered.

Accompanying endogenous or exogenous depression is a more important factor in continuing pain in the case of the back than of the neck. Endogenous depression may be treated by antidepressant drugs such as amitriptyline, which has the advantage of independent antalgic activity (Feinmann 1985) in cases of analgesic-resistant, often burning and/or shooting, neurogenic (i.e. caused by nerve compression rather than tissue damage) pain (Bowsher 1988). Thus, a recent survey of 50 backache patients (of whom 1 was diagnosed as having purely psychological pain) in our clinic (Madan et al 1988) revealed that amitriptyline was prescribed for 28, although determined to be the prime cause of pain relief in only 1 (organic) case. However, the important point about neurogenic pains (frequently described as burning or scalding and/or shooting or stabbing by the patient) is that they do not yield to conventional analgesics, and should be treated in the first instance with amitriptyline (Bowsher 1988).

Diazepam or chlordiazepoxide may be used primarily as muscle relaxants rather than as anxiolytics. Relaxation, supervised in the first instance by a clinical psychologist, may also be used as adjuvant therapy. Hypnosis is used for organic vertebral column pain and was the main pain-relieving factor in 2 of the 50 cases reported; interestingly, hypnosis is said to be of no value in pains of purely psychological origin.

Exogenous depression requires expert psychiatric or psychological analysis and treatment, which can sometimes be dramatically effective. The causes may be social, as in the case of a woman with an unemployed husband and five children (three of whom were delinquent and/or truant from school) who was behind with the rent and deeply in debt to back-street money-lenders. Help from the social services toward resolution of these problems led to rapid relief of her backache, although she was never aware of the connection between social problems and her pain.

CONCLUSION

This chapter attempts to stress the importance of patient assessment, particularly in the realms of (i) taking a careful and detailed history of the condition, of the patient, and of his/her family, work and social circumstances; and (ii) objective and measurable evaluation of pain intensity. The information gleaned from such assessment, coupled with the findings of physical examination, point the way to a particular type of therapeutic intervention. Some such therapeutic manoeuvres, particularly those adjuvant to physical therapy are mentioned here, but treated in more detail in other chapters in this volume. Objective measurement of pain intensity should be used as an ongoing tool, and should be used to evaluate the effect of treatment and to indicate the need for a change of strategy when necessary.

Acknowledgement

Some material in this chapter is from Bowsher (1989), with permission of the publisher.

REFERENCES

Bond M R, Pilowsky I 1966 The subjective assessment of pain and its relationship to the administration of analgesics in patients with advanced cancer. Journal of Psychosomatic Research 10: 203–207

Bowsher D 1988 Pain as a neurological emergency. In: Bowsher D (ed) Neurological emergencies in medical practice, pp 216–234. Croom Helm, Beckenham, England

Bowsher D 1989 Assessment of the chronic pain sufferer. Surgical Rounds in Orthopaedics 3: 70–73

Bowsher D, Lahuerta J, Lipton S 1987 Pain patients: a retrospective survey of 1056 cases. Pain Clinic 1: 163–170

Bowsher D, Rigge M, Sopp L 1991 Prevalence of chronic pain in the British population: a telephone survey of 1037 households (submitted for publication)

Feinmann C 1985 Pain relief by antidepressants: possible modes of action. Pain 23: 1–8

International Association for the Study of Pain 1986 Classification of chronic pain. Descriptions of chronic pain syndromes and definitions of pain terms. Pain (suppl 3)

Madan R, Ramamoorthy C, Bowsher D, Wells C 1988 A survey of intractable low back pain in a pain relief clinic and some comparisons with painful osteoarthritis and postherpetic neuralgia. Pain Schmerz Douleur 9: 116–120

Melzack R 1975 The McGill pain questionnaire: major properties and scoring methods. Pain 1: 277–299

Sluiter M E, Mehta M 1981 Treatment of chronic neck and back pain by percutaneous thermal lesions. In: Lipton S, Miles J B (eds) Persistent pain: modern methods of treatment. Grune & Stratton, New York, pp 141–180

APPENDIX I

McGill Pain Questionnaire

DIRECTIONS

Look carefully at the 20 groups of words. *If* any word in any group applies to *your* pain please circle that word — but do not circle more than one word in any one group. If more than one word in a group applies to your pain, you should circle only the most suitable word in that group.

In groups that *do not apply* to your pain there is no need to circle any word — just leave them as they are.

1.	2.	3.	4.
Flickering	Jumping	Pricking	Sharp
Quivering	Flashing	Boring	Cutting
Pulsing	Shooting	Drilling	Lacerating
Throbbing		Stabbing	
Beating		Lancinating	
Pounding			

5.	6.	7.	8.
Pinching	Tugging	Hot	Tingling
Pressing	Pulling	Burning	Itching
Gnawing	Wrenching	Scalding	Smarting
Cramping		Searing	Stinging
Crushing			

9.	10.	11.	12.
Dull	Tender	Tiring	Sickening
Sore	Taut	Exhausting	Suffocating
Hurting	Rasping		
Aching	Splitting		
Heavy			

13.	14.	15.	16.
Fearful	Punishing	Wretched	Annoying
Frightful	Gruelling	Blinding	Troublesome
Terrifying	Cruel		Miserable
	Vicious		Intense
	Killing		Unbearable

17.	18.	19.	20.
Spreading	Tight	Cool	Nagging
Radiating	Numb	Cold	Nauseating
Penetrating	Drawing	Freezing	Agonizing
Piercing	Squeezing		Dreadful
	Tearing		Torturing

Some common clinical problems

22. Cervical causes of headache and dizziness

N. Bogduk

Headache and dizziness are symptoms that can occur together or separately in a large variety of diseases. Conventional medical teaching, however, emphasizes the intracranial causes of these symptoms, almost to the exclusion of possible causes in the neck (Walton 1977, Daroff 1990, Martin 1990), but headache and dizziness are common features of cervical injury or disease, and their cervical causes are of paramount interest to manual therapists. Accordingly, it is not inappropriate, here, to redress the imbalance in the medical literature by reviewing, in detail, the cervical causes of headache and dizziness.

CERVICAL HEADACHE

Neuroanatomy

The spinal nucleus of the trigeminal nerve consists of three parts: pars oralis, pars interpolaris, and pars caudalis (Olszewski 1950). The pars caudalis starts at the level of the obex and extends caudally to merge imperceptibly with the grey matter of the spinal cord (Fig. 22.1). The spinal tract of the trigeminal nerve descends through the medulla oblongata into the upper levels of the spinal cord (Fig. 22.1). It reaches at least as far as the C2 level, and portions of it may extend as far as the C4 level (Humphrey 1952, Torvik 1956, Kerr 1961a, Taren & Kahn 1962).

Fibres from the spinal tract terminate in the pars caudalis and in the upper three segments of the spinal cord. In the cord, their terminations overlap those of the upper cervical nerves, especially at the C1 and C2 levels (Fig. 22.1). At C1, descending fibres from the trigeminal nerve end in the same nuclear groups as fibres from the C1 spinal nerve and ascending fibres from the C2 and C3 nerves (Kerr 1961a). At C2, the predominant terminals are those form the C2 nerve, but they are joined by a considerable number of trigeminal afferents and ascending fibres from the C3 nerve.

What can be perceived from this description is that terminals of the trigeminal nerve and the upper three cervical nerves ramify in a continuous column of grey

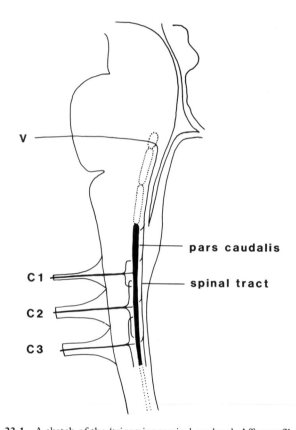

Fig. 22.1 A sketch of the 'trigeminocervical nucleus'. Afferent fibres from the trigeminal nerve (V) enter the pons and descend in the spinal tract to upper cervical levels, sending collateral branches into the pars caudalis of the spinal nucleus of the trigeminal nerve and the grey matter of the C1 to C3 spinal cord segments. Afferent fibres from the C1, C2 and C3 spinal nerves ramify in the spinal, grey matter at their segment of entry and at adjacent segments. That column of grey matter receiving both trigeminal and cervical afferents constitutes the trigeminocervical nucleus (black).

matter formed by the pars caudalis of the spinal nucleus of the trigeminal nerve and the dorsal horns of the upper three cervical segments. Within this column, that portion that receives both trigeminal and cervical afferents can be regarded as forming a single, functional nucleus which may be referred to as the trigeminocervical nucleus. This nucleus is not defined by any intrinsic features, like conventional or classical nuclei, but is defined by the afferent fibres that terminate in it.

The trigeminocervical nucleus incorporates the marginal zone, the substantia gelatinosa and the nucleus proprius of the cervical grey matter and homologous divisions of the trigeminal nucleus. In both the spinal cord and trigeminal nucleus, these regions are the principal centres involved in the transmission of nociceptive information. Consequently, since it incorporates the essential central nervous structures responsible for the transmission of pain, and since it receives afferents from the trigeminal and upper cervical nerves, the trigeminocervical nucleus can be viewed as the nociceptive nucleus for the entire head and upper neck.

The anatomical substrate for referred pain is the convergence of afferents from one region of the body onto neurons in the central nervous system that also receive afferents from topographically separate regions. The trigeminocervical nucleus provides a suitable location for this to occur in the case of head and neck pain. If units in the trigeminocervical nucleus that otherwise innervate the back of the head also receive afferents from the cervical vertebral column, then noxious vertebral stimuli could cause pain to be perceived as arising from the back of the head. Alternatively, if units that receive trigeminal afferents also receive vertebral afferents, then pain in the forehead could be generated by noxious stimuli in the vertebral column.

The overlapping pattern of the terminations of the trigeminal and cervical nerves suggests that such convergence could occur in the trigeminocervical nucleus, but to date, it has not been demonstrated anatomically. However, its existence is implied by certain physiological observations.

Physiology

By recording from various sites in the brainstem and upper spinal cord of the cat, Kerr and Olafson (1961) were able to identify units that responded to stimuli from both the trigeminal nerve and upper cervical nerves. The responses, however, included both inhibitory and facilitatory influences, and occurred throughout the grey matter, not just in the dorsal horn. Thus, whilst establishing a physiological convergence between trigeminal and cervical afferents in a general sense, these experiments did not identify the specific mechanism by which pain from the neck could be referred to the head. That some such mechanism exists, however, has been demonstrated by numerous clinical experiments in man.

Kerr (1961b) demonstrated that electrical stimulation of the rootlets of the C1 dorsal root produced pain in the orbit, frontal region and vertex.

Cyriax (1938) studying an unspecified number of patients, injected 4% saline into various cervical muscles and observed that these injections produced local pain and referred pain. Stimulation of the posterior neck muscles close to their insertions into the occiput produced pain in the forehead. Stimulating the same muscles 1–2 inches (25–50 mm) caudally produced pain in the vertex. Stimulation of the sternocleidomastoid referred pain to the temporal region.

Campbell and Parsons (1944), using 6% saline, stimulated various structures in the upper cervical regions of several normal volunteers. They stimulated the periosteum around the occipital condyles, and the paramedian tissues at the suboccipital level and the upper four cervical interspinous spaces. Each stimulation produced referred pain which, in general, was felt rostral to the site of injection. Frontal pain occurred in 85% of their basal occipital injections, in 54% of occipitocervical injections, and in 14% of C1–2 injections. Injections at successively lower levels, from C1–2 caudally, produced referred pain in successively lower regions from the parieto-occipital, through the occipital, and to the suboccipital regions.

Feinstein et al (1954) also induced referred pain to the forehead by stimulating the midline soft tissues between the occiput and C1, and occipital headache by stimulating the upper cervical interspinous spaces.

Dwyer et al (1990) showed that distending the C2–3 zygapophyseal joint in normal volunteers could produce occipital headache.

These clinical experiments clearly demonstrate the capacity of experimental painful stimuli in the upper neck to produce referred pain in the head. It is, therefore, entertainable that pathological, painful lesions of any of the structures innervated by the upper cervical nerves are equally capable of producing such referred pain.

Peripheral anatomy

The neuroanatomy of the trigeminocervical nucleus dictates that afferents from the upper three cervical nerves are the most likely to converge with trigeminal afferents. Consequently, any of the structures innervated by the first three cervical nerves would be potential sources of referred head pain. Therefore, as a prelude to examining the pathology of cervical headache, it is appropriate to review the distribution of the C1–3 spinal nerves and to determine the structures that could be affected by disease to produce referred head pain.

The C1 spinal nerve is frequently misrepresented as having no sensory distribution, but this erroneous view actually refers to the fact that usually it has no specific cutaneous branch (Bogduk 1982); it is nevertheless, sensory to deep suboccipital tissues. The C1 dorsal ramus supplies the suboccipital muscles (Bogduk 1982). The C1 ventral ramus supplies the atlanto-occipital joint (Lazorthes & Gaubert 1956), and also gives off a sinuvertebral nerve that accompanies those from C2 and C3 to innervate the median atlanto-axial joint and the paramedian dura of the posterior cranial fossa (Kimmel 1960). Through the ansa hypoglossi, fibres from the C1 ventral ramus join the hypoglossal nerve to form its recurrent meningeal branches which innervate the dura adjacent to the condylar canal (Kimmel 1960). Along with the C2, 3 ventral rami, the C1 ventral ramus innervates the upper prevertebral muscles, viz. longus capitis, longus cervicis, rectus capitis anterior, and rectus capitis lateralis.

The C2 dorsal ramus innervates the skin of the occiput and the major upper posterior neck muscles: semispinalis capitis, longissimus capitis and splenius capitis (Bogduk 1982). The C2 ventral ramus directly innervates the lateral atlanto-axial joint (Lazorthes & Gaubert 1956, Bogduk 1981b), and through its sinuvertebral branch innervates the median atlanto-axial joint and the paramedian dura of the posterior cranial fossa (Kimmel 1960). Via the cervical plexus, the C2 ventral ramus innervates the prevertebral muscles and the sternocleidomastoid and trapezius muscles (Williams et al 1989). Because their motor innervation is from the 11th cranial nerve, it is commonly forgotten that these latter two muscles belong to the sensory distribution of C2, 3. Through the cervical plexus, the C2 ventral ramus furnishes meningeal branches to the hypoglossal and vagus nerves which innervate the lateral walls of the posterior cranial fossa (Kimmel 1960).

The C3 dorsal ramus forms two medial branches: the third occipital nerve and the deep medial branch (Bogduk 1982). The latter innervates the upper fibres of multifidus while the third occipital nerve supplies the semispinalis capitis and the suboccipital skin (Bogduk 1982). Near its origin, the third occipital nerve crosses the dorsal aspect of the C2–3 zygapophyseal joint. This joint receives articular branches from the C3 dorsal ramus or from the deep communicating loop between the C2 and C3 dorsal rami (Bogduk 1982). The C3 ventral ramus joins the cervical plexus through which it innervates the prevertebral muscles and sternocleidomastoid and trapezius (Williams et al 1989).

A plexus of nerves, called the vertebral nerve, accompanies the vertebral artery and innervates its cervical portion and intracranial branches (Hovelacque 1927, Monteiro & Rodrigues 1931, Lazorthes & Cassan 1939, Laux & Guerrier 1939, 1947, Guerrier 1949, Lazorthes 1949, Bogduk et al 1981), but while most of these nerves appear to be vasomotor in nature, some of those that innervate the intracranial portion of the vertebral artery have been found to be somatic sensory fibres, for they have cell bodies in the C1 and C2 dorsal root ganglia (Kimmel 1959).

From this account, it can be concluded that the receptive field of the upper three cervical nerves includes the joints and ligaments of the upper three cervical segments, their posterior and anterior muscles, the sternocleidomastoid and trapezius muscles, the dura mater of the posterior cranial fossa, and the vertebral artery. All of these structures, therefore, become possible sources of cervical headache.

Pathology

A variety of diseases of the neck are associated with headache. Some are recognized, or accepted, causes of cervical headache because the primary source of pain is apparent. In others, the primary source is not apparent, but the clinical features of the headache implicate a cervical cause.

Rheumatoid arthritis

The literature on rheumatoid arthritis of the cervical spine tends to concentrate on the catastrophic sequelae of the disease, namely atlanto-axial subluxation and spinal cord compression. However, hidden within the case reports in this literature are frequent accounts of occipital and frontal headache associated with rheumatoid arthritis of the atlanto-axial joints (Sharp & Purser 1961, Bland et al 1963, Robinson 1966, Bland 1967, Stevens et al 1971, Cabot & Becker 1978). The pain of upper cervical rheumatoid arthritis tends to be felt locally in the suboccipital region and upper neck, but when severe it radiates to the vertex and forehead. .

The pathology of upper cervical rheumatoid arthritis is an erosive synovitis, affecting the median and lateral atlanto-axial joints, with weakening and strain of their associated ligaments. Such pathological changes are an acceptable primary source of pain. Given that these joints and ligaments are innervated by the C1–3 nerves, and given the capacity of similarly innervated structures to produce headache, it is understandable that the pain of upper cervical rheumatoid arthritis can be referred to the head.

Congenital abnormalities

Headache is a symptom frequently associated with congenital abnormalities of the craniospinal junction. It has been noted in cases of atlanto-axial dislocation, separation of the odontoid, and occipitalization of the atlas (McRae 1960, 1968). These abnormalities are not, per se, painful, but they do constitute a mechanical abnormality in the upper neck. The pain in these conditions, therefore, is most likely to arise from the ligaments and joints that are subjected to abnormal mechanical stress as a result of these abnormalities. In particular, it is apparent that in atlanto-axial dislocation and in separation of the odontoid, the atlanto-axial joints would be exposed to excessive strain. The source of pain in these conditions is thus the same as in upper cervical rheumatoid arthritis.

Atlanto-odontoid osteoarthrosis

In cases of demonstrable atlanto-odontoid osteoarthrosis,

pain is usually felt in the upper neck, but headache may be an associated feature (Fournier & Rathelot 1960). The innervation of this joint is from the C1–3 sinuvertebral nerves, and as with rheumatoid arthritis, the referral of pain to the head is understandable.

Trigger points

The pathology and cause of muscular trigger points is poorly understood (Simons 1975, 1976a, b), although recent theories are appealing (Simons & Travell 1981, Simons 1988). Nevertheless, the capacity of trigger points to produce referred pain has been repeatedly documented. In the case of headache, trigger points that caused referred pain to the head have been described in the splenius capitis (Travell & Rinzler 1952), trapezius and sternocleidomastoid (Travell & Rinzler 1952, Travell 1955, 1962), and in various suboccipital muscles (Kelly 1942, Hackett et al 1962, Kayfetz et al 1963). Relief of headache has been reported following the injection of such trigger points with local anaesthetic (Kelly 1942, Travell & Rinzler 1952, Travell 1955, 1962), or sclerosing agents (Hackett et al 1962, Kayfetz et al 1963), or simply by dry needling (Lewit 1979). Blume (1976, 1982) has reported relief by thermocoagulating such sites.

Strikingly, trigger points capable of producing headache have been reported only in muscles innervated by C1, 2, 3. Trigger points in muscles innervated by lower cervical nerves produce different referred pain patterns. This observation is consistent with the fact that it is the C1 2, 3 nerves that have access to the trigeminocervical nucleus. It is furthermore not surprising that trigger points in C1, 2, 3 muscles should produce headache for, as described above, experimental noxious stimulation of the same structures readily produces headache.

It has been argued that suboccipital trigger points represent areas of strained musculoperiosteal attachments (Hackett et al 1962, Kayfetz et al 1963) usually following neck injury. However, pathological evidence of this contention is lacking. What is questionable is whether such tender areas represent primary areas of pathology, for it is known that tender areas occur in various neck and head muscles in many forms of headache including migraine (Perelson 1947, Olesen 1978, Lous & Olesen 1982, Langemark & Olesen 1987). They are not necessarily indicative of the cause of headache, and may simply be secondary features or epiphenomena.

Neck–tongue syndrome

Neck–tongue syndrome is a disorder characterized by acute unilateral occipital pain precipitated by sudden movement of the head, usually rotation, and accompanied by a sensation of numbness in the ipsilateral half of the tongue (Lance & Anthony 1980). The mechanism of this syndrome appears to be two-fold. First, the pain is due to temporary subluxation of a lateral atlanto-axial joint. Since this joint is innervated by the C2 ventral ramus (Lazorthes & Gaubert 1956, Bogduk 1981a) the pain will be mediated by this nerve. The numbness of the tongue arises because of impingement, or stretching, of the C2 ventral ramus against the edge of the subluxated articular process (Bogduk 1981b), and indicates compression of proprioceptive afferents from the tongue which pass from the ansa hypoglossi into the C2 ventral ramus (Fitzgerald & Sachithanandan 1979, Lance & Anthony 1980). Both the pain and numbness, therefore, are mediated by the C2 ventral ramus, and the syndrome represents a fascinating condition affecting this nerve in a two-fold manner.

Studies of patients with neck–tongue syndrome reveal that it can occur in patients with rheumatoid arthritis or with congenital joint laxity (Bertoft & Westerberg 1985). Hypomobility in the contralateral lateral atlanto-axial joint may predispose to the condition (Bertoft & Westerberg 1985).

Some investigators have found immobilization by a soft collar to be adequate therapy (Fortin & Biller 1985); others have resorted to atlanto-axial fusion (Bertoft & Westerberg 1985) or resection of the C2 spinal nerves (Elisevich et al 1984). Operative findings have confirmed that the syndrome involves compression of the C2 spinal nerves by the lateral atlanto-axial joint (Elisevich et al 1984).

Third occipital headache

The C2–3 zygapophyseal joint is innervated by the third occipital nerve: the superficial medial branch of the C3 dorsal ramus (Bogduk 1982), and a number of studies have implicated this joint in the causation of headache. Being a transitional zone in the upper neck (Mestdagh 1976), this joint is particularly vulnerable in cervical trauma.

Trevor-Jones (1964) first drew attention to this region when he reported three patients with headache in whom surgical exploration revealed entrapment of the third occipital nerve by osteophytes of the C2–3 zygapophyseal joint. Release of the nerve relieved the headache.

Polletti (1983) reported one patient who suffered from occipital headache and who had post-traumatic arthritis of the C2–3 zygapophyseal joint. Her pain was relieved by resection of the joint. Maigne (1976, 1981) has written extensively on headaches arising from the C2–3 zygapophyseal joints and their diagnosis and treatment by injections of local anaesthetic and manual therapy.

Our own studies have shown that pain stemming from the C2–3 zygapophyseal joint can be referred to the occiput and as far as the frontal region and orbit (Bogduk & Marsland 1986, 1988). They can be diagnosed by anaesthetizing either the third occipital nerve or the offending joint itself (Bogduk & Marsland 1986, 1988).

Third occipital headaches exhibit no characteristic clinical features that distinguish them from other forms of headache (Bogduk & Marsland 1986, 1988) but careful manual examination can elicit pathognomonic features of a symptomatic zygapophyseal joint at C2–3 (Jull et al 1988).

Cervical spondylosis

Headaches are a well known associated feature of cervical spondylosis (Schultz & Semmes 1950, Wilkinson 1971, Peterson et al 1975, Pawl 1977, Chirls 1978), but their mechanism is not known. Where the primary abnormality is low in the neck, it has been postulated that occipital headache arises because of spasm of the posterior neck muscles which attach to the occiput (Raney & Raney 1948, Schultz & Semmes 1950, Peterson et al 1975, Pawl 1977), but this contention has never been verified electromyographically or otherwise. Treatment of lower cervical spondylosis by anterior cervical fusion can relieve the associated headache, but not in all cases (Peterson et al 1975, Pawl 1977, Chirls 1978).

Other authorities (Brain 1963, Stoddard 1970, Wilkinson 1971) consider arthrosis of the upper cervical synovial joints to be the source of headache in cervical spondylosis. Circumstantial evidence favours this view. Upper cervical osteo-arthrosis accompanies the degenerative changes of spondylosis (Holt & Yates 1966) and upper cervical joints are within the receptive field of the trigeminocervical nucleus. Therefore, they have direct access to the neuroanatomical pathways that mediate referred pain to the head. No comparable neurological link is known whereby lower cervical abnormalities could produce headache.

The belief that upper cervical synovial joints are the cause of some forms of headache prompted attempts to denervate these joints in the treatment of headache. Early reports (Sluijter & Koetsveld-Baart 1980) claimed only modest success, but more recent reports (Sluijter & Mehta 1981) claim a vastly improved success following the development of better surgical techniques.

Occipital neuralgia

Compression of the greater occipital nerve has been considered to be a cause of occipital headache or occipital neuralgia (Hunter & Mayfield 1949, Chambers 1954, Mayfield 1955, Cusson & King 1960, Hammond & Danta 1978, Murphy 1978) but recent reviews (Weinberger 1978, Bogduk 1980) have questioned this view. Anatomical studies (Bogduk 1980) show that this nerve is not susceptible to compression in the way that had been believed (Hunter & Mayfield 1949). Other interpretations which implicate arthritis of the upper cervical joints as the cause of occipital neuralgia are probably more justified (Holmes 1913, Hartsock 1940, Dugan et al 1962, Knight 1963, Trevor-Jones 1964, Sigwald & Jamet 1968, Poletti 1983).

Ehni and Benner (1984) formally addressed this contention and showed that, in patients with osteoarthrosis of the lateral atlanto-axial joints presenting with so-called occipital neuralgia, the pain could be relieved by periarticular injections of local anaesthetic around the affected joints. Similar relief, in similar patients was reported by McCormick (1987) following intra-articular anaesthetization of the lateral atlanto-axial joints.

Constant, dull aching pain in the occipital region is highly suggestive of referred pain from either the lateral atlanto-axial or C2–3 zygapophyseal joints. (Theoretically, the atlanto-occipital joints should be included, but no clinical studies have yet verified the capacity of atlanto-occipital joints to cause headaches). This quality of pain is characteristic of somatic referred pain and should not be misrepresented as 'neuralgia' (Bogduk 1989).

Neuralgic pain is characteristically lancinating in quality; associated dysaesthesias or sensory loss confirms a neurogenic basis. Occipital neuralgia cannot legitimately be ascribed to entrapment of the greater occipital nerve (see above) but it can result from disorders of the C2 ganglion. Poletti and Sweet (1990) described two patients with lancinating occipital pain in whom they found the C2 ganglion to be entrapped in a hypertrophic capsule of the lateral atlanto-axial joint. Release of the nerve relieved the symptoms.

Accessory nerve neuroma

Occipital headache may be a symptom associated with accessory nerve palsy. Cherington and Hendee (1978) reported a woman who sustained such a palsy during a lymph node biopsy and who began to suffer occipital headaches. At operation a neuroma was located on the severed nerve. Excision of the neuroma and suture of the nerve effected an almost immediate relief of pain. In this case the abnormality was topographically well displaced from the head, but it should be recalled that the sensory innervation of the sternocleidomastoid and trapezius muscles is via the C2, 3 ventral rami which join the accessory nerve. The pain from a neuroma on this nerve would, therefore, be mediated by C2, 3 nerves, giving it ready access to the trigeminocervical nucleus, and hence to the cervico-capital referred pain mechanism.

Post-traumatic headache

Headache after neck injury is a well recognized entity (Braaf & Rosner 1962a, 1962b, 1965, 1975, Hawkins 1962, Seletz 1963), but their cause and mechanism has remained controversial. As with cervical spondylosis, it is difficult to relate headaches to lower cervical injury. However, although the C5, 6 levels have been thought to be the most frequently affected by neck injury, particularly of the 'whiplash' type, there is growing awareness that the cervico-capital joints and ligaments are also vulnerable in this type of injury (Hawkins 1962, La Rocca 1978), particularly when the mid- and lower cervical levels are relatively fused by cervical spondylosis (MacNab 1969, 1973). Since the cervicocapital joints are innervated by the C1–3 nerves, it is neurologically acceptable that damage to them could be a cause of headache. Thus posttraumatic headache may be a feature of upper cervical injury concomitant with a more obvious lower cervical lesion.

Posterior fossa abnormalities

Since the dura mater of the posterior cranial fossa is innervated by the upper cervical sinuvertebral nerves and the C1–2 ventral rami (Kimmel 1960), this tissue is as much a possible source of cervical headache as structures in the neck. Head pain can be caused by traction or irritation of the posterior fossa meninges (Ray & Wolff 1949), or by traction on the C1 nerve roots exerted by brainstem or cerebellar herniation (Kerr 1961b). Intracranial abnormalities, therefore, should not be overlooked in cases of cervical headache.

Cervical migraine

French anatomists described the vertebral nerve as a branch of the stellate ganglion which runs with the vertebral artery and innervates its intracranial branches (Monteiro & Rodrigues 1931, Laux & Guerrier 1939, 1947, Lazorthes & Cassan 1939, Lazorthes 1949). Barre (1926) described a posterior cervical sympathetic syndrome which comprised headache, vertigo, tinnitus and visual disturbances, the cause of which, he proposed, was irritation of the vertebral nerve by arthritis of the cervical spine. Other authors adopted or endorsed this contention and added that a whole host of cervical lesions could cause headache in this way (Lazorthes 1949, Gayral & Neuwirth 1954, Neuwirth 1954, Kovacs 1955, Stewart 1962, Dutton & Riley 1969, Lewit 1969, Pawl 1977). By most of these authors, however, the mechanism of headache has never been more explicitly defined than 'irritation of the vertebral nerve'. Only Pawl (1977) has ventured to state that irritation of the vertebral nerve by cervical disc lesions or other lesions produces an autonomic barrage which results in spasm of the vertebrobasilar system, which produces head pain by causing ischaemia of the vessel walls.

In both man and the monkey the so-called vertebral nerve consists of no more than grey rami communicantes accompanying the vertebral artery, and moreover, stimulation of these nerves, or the cervical sympathetic trunk, in the monkey, failed to influence vertebral blood flow (Bogduk et al 1981). Thus, neither anatomical nor physiological evidence was found which could support the vertebral nerve irritation theory.

Vascular lesions

Although irritation of the vertebral nerve can be discounted as a mechanism for cervical headache, headache can occur as a result of some intrinsic, painful disorder of the vertebral artery or its branches, such as an aneurysm.

The vertebral artery has a sensory innervation, via the vertebral nerve, from the C1, 2 dorsal roots (Kimmel 1959), and experimental stimulation of the vertebral artery in humans evokes headache (Ray & Wolff 1949). Thus, the vertebral artery is a potential source of cervical headache, and, like tumours of the posterior cranial fossa, should not be overlooked or neglected because of any preoccupation with cervical skeletal abnormalities in patients with apparent cervical headache.

Similarly, the carotid arteries are innervated by cervical nerves, and lesions of these vessels may cause referred pain to the head or face. Particular examples include carotidynia (Feit 1982) and spontaneous carotid dissection (Fisher 1982).

Cluster-like headaches

In recent years, several studies and case reports have described patients in whom intermittent attacks of hemicranial pain, associated with conjunctival injection, lacrimation or rhinorrhoea, were found to be due to meningiomas or vascular irritation affecting the roots of the C2 or C3 spinal nerves (Hildebrandt & Jansen 1984, Kuritzky 1984, Jansen et al 1989b). These reports illustrate the relationship between headache and the C1–3 nerves, but indicate also that some forms of cluster-like headache may have a cervical origin.

'Cervicogenic headache' as defined by Sjaastad et al (1983) differs from simple referred pain from upper cervical osteoarthrosis in that it is said to be accompanied by lacrimation, conjunctival injection, other autonomic features, and migrainous phenomena when severe. This form of headache appears to have a cervical origin for it can be relieved by anaesthetizing the C2 and C3 nerve roots. Its cause remains unknown.

DIZZINESS AND VERTIGO

The terms 'dizziness' and 'vertigo' both refer to a false sensation of motion of the body. 'Vertigo' can be used more specifically to impart the connotation of rotation (Fisher 1967, Daroff 1990), but modern authorities define vertigo in a broader sense, as 'the consciousness of disordered orientation of the body in space' (Walton 1977). Thus, 'vertigo' and 'dizziness' can be used synonymously to describe sensations such as spinning, swaying, the subjective accompaniments of ataxia, and a variety of other colloquially described sensations (Fisher 1967).

Whereas dizziness can be a symptom of various disorders of the eyes, the parietal and temporal lobes, and cerebellum, it is most commonly due to disease affecting the labyrinth or the vestibular nuclei. Amongst these, the vestibular nuclei can be affected by disorders of the neck in two ways: either through ischaemic processes or through disturbances of the tonic neck reflexes.

Ischaemic vertigo

Anatomy

The vestibular nuclei draw their blood supply from a variety of sources. The principal artery supplying the nuclei is the anterior inferior cerebellar artery (Fisher 1967). Rostral parts of the vestibular nuclei are also supplied by direct branches of the basilar artery (Stopford 1916), while more caudal parts are supplied by direct branches of the vertebral artery (Stopford 1916, Fisher 1967), and the posterior inferior cerebellar artery via the lateral medullary or posterior spinal arteries (Stopford 1916, Fisher 1967). Despite their multiplicity, the several vessels that supply the vestibular nuclei are all derivatives of the vertebral or basilar arteries, the basilar itself being formed by the two vertebral arteries.

The vertebral arteries reach the brainstem from the subclavian arteries after a long course through the neck where they are intimately related to the cervical vertebral column. The course of the vertebral artery may be described in four parts (Williams et al 1989). The first part extends between the subclavian artery and the C6 foramen transversarium. The second part runs vertically through the foramina transversaria of the upper six cervical vertebrae. The third part turns horizontally across the atlas, and the fourth part enters the foramen magnum to join the opposite vertebral artery and form the basilar artery.

Many variations of the anatomy of the vertebral artery occur, several of which are not without clinical significance. The vertebral artery most commonly enters the C6 foramen transversarium, but may enter the C7 or any other foramen as high as C3 (Daseler & Anson 1959, Taitz et al 1978). Absence of a vertebral artery is rare (Hardin et al 1960, Faris et al 1963), but variations in the calibre of the vertebral arteries are common. Stopford (1916) studied 150 cadavers and found inequality of calibre in 92%. In 72% the difference was marked, and in 22 cadavers the vessel of one side was at least twice the size of the other. When marked inequality occurs, the basilar artery becomes supplied virtually entirely by the dominant vertebral artery.

Along its course through the neck, the vertebral artery has several important relations, each of which can become a clinically significant factor in compromising blood flow. The first part of the artery runs in the angle between the scalenus anterior and longus colli muscles and is invested by the deep cervical fascia. The second part is related to two series of bony structures: the uncinate processes of the vertebral bodies, and the superior articular processes of the zygapophyseal joints. The second and third parts of the vertebral artery are fixed within the foramina transversaria and therefore the artery must move whenever the transverse processes move. This motion is greatest at the atlanto-axial level, during rotation of the neck.

Symptomatology

If blood flow in any of the vessels supplying the vestibular nuclei is critically reduced, then vestibular function will be impaired and dizziness will occur. Although occlusion of the specific end-arteries to the vestibular nuclei is theoretically possible, such phenomena have been documented relatively infrequently (Fisher 1967). More commonly it is the basilar or vertebral arteries, or both, that are primarily compromised. Since the vertebral and basilar arteries supply more than just the vestibular nuclei, dizziness is rarely an isolated symptom in vertebrobasilar disease. It occurs in association with other symptoms, or it follows other symptoms. It may be an isolated presenting symptom initially, but in verified cases of dizziness of vascular origin other features of brainstem ischaemia have always eventually come to be associated with it (Fisher 1967).

The clinical features which can be associated with dizziness in vertebrobasilar vascular disease are disturbances in vision, diplopia, nausea, ataxia, 'drop attacks', impairment of trigeminal sensation, sympathoplegia, dysarthria, hemianaesthesia and hemiplegia, all depending on which other structures supplied by the affected artery also become ischaemic. Whatever the combination, dizziness is the most common, and usually, the predominant symptom.

Pathology

Vertebral nerve irritation

It has been claimed that symptoms of vertebrobasilar insufficiency can be produced by irritation of the vertebral nerve (the sympathetic plexus that accompanies the vertebral artery) (Barre 1926, Gayral & Neuwirth 1954, Neuwirth 1954, Kovacs 1955, Stewart 1962, Dutton & Riley 1969, Lewit 1969). Such irritation, by osteophytes or other cervical lesions, is said to produce neurally mediated spasm of the distal branches of the vertebrobasilar tree and, therefore, brainstem ischaemia.

There is some evidence consistent with this theory, at least with respect to cochlear blood flow in the cat (Romanov et al 1973), but other evidence is lacking or contradictory. As mentioned previously in the context of cervical headache, Bogduk et al (1981) undertook an investigation of the neural control of vertebral blood flow and found no anatomical evidence to support the contention that mid- or low cervical lesions could affect hindbrain blood flow, and moreover, in the monkey, they found vertebral blood flow to be profoundly unresponsive to stimulation of any component of the cervical sympathetic system. They concluded that the theory that irritation of the vertebral nerve can alter vertebral blood flow was not tenable, a conclusion in accord with modern clinical opinion (Bartschi-Rochaix 1968, Lance 1982).

Mechanical disorders

Blood flow in the vertebrobasilar arterial system can be compromised by a variety of mechanical disorders, which can be classified as either intrinsic or extrinsic.

The most common intrinsic disorder, and indeed, the most common disorder of the vertebrobasilar system, is atherosclerosis. The basilar artery is the most commonly affected component, followed by the cervical portion of the vertebral artery (Myer et al 1960). In the vertebral artery, atherosclerosis may be in the form of isolated plaques, producing focal narrowing of the lumen, or diffusely spread along the vessel, narrowing extensive lengths of its lumen (Hutchinson & Yates 1956). Although any part of the vertebrobasilar system can be affected by atherosclerosis, it has been shown that in symptomatic cases, occlusions occurred in the intracranial portion (Fisher et al 1965). Occlusions and stenoses in the extracranial portion are usually asymptomatic (Fisher & Karnes 1965).

Thrombosis of the vertebral and basilar arteries can occur, usually as a complication of atherosclerosis. Similarly, embolization from an atheromatous plaque can occur, but such emboli usually lodge in distal branches of the vertebrobasilar system, particularly the posterior cerebral artery (Fisher & Karnes 1965).

An extrinsic disorder is one which compromises blood flow in a vessel by compressing its external wall and thereby narrowing its lumen. In this respect, the vertebral artery is particularly vulnerable because of its relations in the neck, and the nature of extrinsic disorders affecting the artery is predicated by the different relations of its four parts.

Three types of anomalies can compromise the first part of the vertebral artery:

1. An anomalous origin of the vertebral artery from the posterior aspect of the subclavian, causing the vertebral artery to be kinked and occluded during rotation of the neck (Power et al 1961)
2. Bands of the deep cervical fascia which cross the vertebral artery and constrict it during rotation of the neck (Hardin & Poser 1963)
3. An anomalous course of the vertebral artery *between* fascicles of either longus colli or scalenus anterior where they attach to the C6 transverse process,

allowing the artery to be squeezed between the muscle bundles during rotation (Husni et al 1966, Husni & Storer 1967).

The second part of the vertebral artery is susceptible to compression or angulation by laterally projecting osteophytes from the uncinate processes. Attention to this phenomenon was first drawn by Hutchinson and Yates (1956). Subsequently, various investigators, using angiography, demonstrated deformation of the vertebral artery by uncinate osteophytes in cadavers (Virtama & Kivalo 1957) and in patients with symptoms of vertebro-basilar insufficiency (Hardin et al 1960, Sheehan et al 1960, Gortvai 1964, Bakay & Leslie 1965, Hardin 1965, Balla & Longford 1967, Nagashima 1970, Smith et al 1971, Pasztor 1978). Several common features were revealed in these latter clinical studies. Dizziness was by far the most frequent symptom and it was aggravated or precipitated by rotation of the neck. The common site of compression of the vertebral artery was at the C5–6 level, with a lesser incidence at the C4–5 and C6–7 levels. Distortion of the vertebral artery may or may not have been present in the neutral position of the neck, but it was produced or increased when the neck was rotated. Rotation usually compromised the ipsilateral artery. Absence or non-filling of one vertebral artery was frequently seen, with the patent artery being affected by osteophytes. In those patients who underwent operation for resection of osteophytes, dizziness was virtually always relieved, and only in a few cases were other brainstem symptoms recalcitrant. At operation, in addition to distortion of the artery by bony spurs, adhesions circumventing the vertebral artery were frequently observed. Resection of the bony spurs alone did not necessarily restore patency of the vessel. The adventitial adhesions had to be cleared as well. In those patients who underwent angiography post-operatively, distortion may or may not have been still present, but it was not produced or aggravated by rotation, and under these circumstances dizziness was no longer precipitated.

The principal pathological factors, therefore, appear to be compression of the vertebral artery by osteophytes with reactive periadventitial scar formation constricting the vessel, and rotation of the neck aggravating the obstruction to blood flow by further impaction against the osteophytes.

The second part of the vertebral artery is allegedly also susceptible to compression by subluxated osteoarthrotic superior articular processes. Osteological studies support this phenomenon as a theoretical possibility (Taitz et al 1978), but clinically it has been reported only once (Kovacs 1955), and apparently has not been seen by others. Moreover, Kovacs (1955) emphasized irritation of the vertebral nerve in this condition rather than obstruction to vertebral blood flow.

The third part of the vertebral artery is not known to

be affected by any specific focal lesion like the first and second parts. The vessel may be enclosed by an anomalous bony ring on the superior aspect of the atlas, behind the lateral atlanto-axial joint, but this anomaly occurs in about 33% of cadavers and is visible in 14% of cervical radiographs (Lamberty & Zivanovic 1973); it is not known to be pathogenetic.

In the atlanto-axial region, however, the vertebral artery is susceptible to occlusion by excursions of the atlas on the axis. In rheumatoid arthritis (Webb et al 1968, Lyness & Simeone 1978), and aplasia of the odontoid process (Ford 1952), and in os odontoideum (Lyness & Simeone 1978) the vertebral artery can be stretched by subluxation of the atlas. Post mortem studies of such cases reveal thrombosis of the atlanto-axial portion of the artery, probably initiated by the distortion imparted to it (Webb et al 1968).

In addition to vertebral subluxations affecting the atlanto-axial portion of the vertebral artery, this segment is susceptible to compromise during physiological or near physiological movements.

Tatlow and Bammer (1957) reported three patients who complained of dizziness, and in whom passive rotation of the head precipitated their symptoms. These authors then studied angiographically the vertebral arteries in a cadaver and found that rotation of the head was accompanied by narrowing of the contralateral vertebral artery in its atlanto-axial segment. They proposed that this manner of the narrowing of the vertebral artery was the cause of symptoms in the patients they described. Brown and Tatlow (1963) made further observations of this phenomenon in 41 cadavers. They found that rotation of the head occluded the contralateral vertebral artery in five specimens, and in another twelve specimens a similar occlusion occurred following rotation with traction additionally applied.

The mechanism for this manner of occlusion would appear to be stretching of the artery. The vertebral artery is relatively fixed at the end of the vertical portion of its course at the C2 foramen transversarium, and at the beginning of the horizontal part of its course at the upper opening of the C1 foramen transversarium. Combining the large range of motion between the atlas and the axis and the relative fixity of the vertebral artery at the C1–C2 level, it is quite conceivable that stretching can occur. It is, however, not a universal phenomenon, for the data of Brown and Tatlow (1963) show that 24 of their 41 specimens did not exhibit narrowing of the vertebral arteries on rotation of the head.

Despite these anatomical studies, there have been few clinical demonstrations of obstruction of the atlanto-axial segment of the vertebral artery during rotation of the head. Maslowski (1960) reported observing it, but in an unspecified number of patients; furthermore, his angiographic studies were performed on anaesthetized patients. Therefore, it is not known whether the rotatory

manoeuvre and accompanying vertebral occlusion was productive of symptoms. Okawara and Nibbelink (1974) reported one patient, a ceiling painter, who, after maintaining his head in hyper-extension and left rotation for a prolonged period, developed symptoms of a right lateral medullary syndrome; angiography revealed a thread-like narrowing of the right vertebral artery at the atlanto-axial level. Bladin and Merory (1975) described one patient in whom rotation of the head to the right induced vertigo and nystagmus. Angiography revealed a non-filling right vertebral artery and a normal left vertebral artery but one which occluded opposite C2 upon rotation to the right. Barton and Margolis (1975) described two patients who complained of dizziness and other brainstem symptoms. Angiography revealed narrowing of the contralateral vertebral artery upon rotation of the head, but in neither patient were symptoms of brainstem ischaemia reproduced by this manoeuvre.

Comment

Although the vertebral artery may be affected by a variety of disorders, the mere presence of a stenotic or occlusive lesion does not necessarily imply the presence of symptoms. Symptoms occur only when the blood supply to an area of neural tissue is critically reduced. Whether such a critical reduction occurs depends on a balance between compromising and compensating factor. A single lesion may fail to significantly reduce flow in the affected vessel, even though it may appear markedly narrow. Furthermore, proximal stenoses can be compensated for by collateral blood flow. Occlusion of one vertebral artery in the neck, for example, can be compensated for by collateral circulation from the opposite vertebral artery, the occipital artery, the ascending and deep cervical arteries, and retrograde flow from the internal carotid artery via the circle of Willis. On the other hand, symptoms are more likely to occur if these compensating mechanisms are not available either through congenital absence or because they too, are affected by concurrent disease.

In this respect, the implications made and conclusions drawn by various authors describing various causes of vertebral artery insufficiency need to be critically assessed. Although compression of the vertebral artery by uncinate osteophytes both at rest and during rotation of the head has been observed in cadavers, and had been well documented in symptomatic patients, it has also been seen in totally asymptomatic individuals (Faris et al 1963). Therefore, this phenomenon, is of itself not necessarily productive of symptoms.

Occlusion of the atlanto-axial segment of the vertebral artery during head rotation has been observed in the cadaver and has been inferred to be a cause of vertebral artery ischaemia. The anatomical studies of Brown and Tatlow (1963), however, show that such occlusions do not occur in all cadavers, and it is questionable how frequently they are causes of vertebrobasilar symptoms, clinically. The clinical data relating to this phenomenon are equivocal, and the study of Barton and Margolis (1975) shows that while such occlusions can occur they are not necessarily symptomatic.

In those cases in which occlusion of the vertebral artery does occur during head rotation, but without the production of symptoms, it would appear that vertebral blood flow is probably compromised, but not critically reduced, i.e. enough to produce symptoms.

There has been only one experimental study which attempted to quantify reduction of cerebral blood flow during neck rotation. Toole and Tucker (1960) perfused the carotid and vertebral arteries of cadavers with water and observed the reduction in flow following various movements of the head. They found that flow in the vertebral artery could be reduced to 10% of the initial rate by a variety of head positions, but rotation to less than 45° was the principal compromising manoeuvre. They did not, however, establish where the obstruction to flow occurred.

Unfortunately it is not known how accurately such cadaver studies represent the clinical situation, and whether a 90% reduction in vertebral blood flow is critical. The only comparable in vivo study provided contrasting data. Hardesty et al (1963) measured vertebral blood flow during head rotation in two patients and found only a 23% and a 9% reduction. Thus, there is a lack of adequate data defining to what extent morphological occlusion of the vertebral artery impairs actual flow in that vessel, and whether such reduction is enough to produce symptoms.

A given reduction in vertebral blood flow may, of itself, not be critical in a normal healthy vertebrobasilar tree where adequate collateral flow is available. However, the presence of intercurrent anomalies or disease may compromise overall brainstem flow to such an extent that an additional minor reduction in flow in one vertebral artery may critically reduce flow in various end-arteries. In this respect, while mechanical occlusion of the vertebral artery in the neck may alone be insufficient to cause symptoms, it is conceivable that in the presence of atherosclerosis of the vertebrobasilar tree, for example, such an occlusion could become symptomatic. Anomalies or variations in the vertebral arteries are a further example of such combined compromising lesions. It is noteworthy that in several studies which describe symptomatic extrinsic compression of the vertebral artery, the opposite vertebral artery was found to be hypoplastic or poorly filling (Husni et al 1961, Gortvai 1964, Bakay & Leslie 1965, Husni & Storer 1967, Bladin & Merory 1975, Dan 1976, Pasztor 1978). Presumably, the mechanical lesions in these patients might not have been symptomatic had the opposite vessel been large enough to provide compensating flow.

To conclude, it is evident that, in a scientific sense,

there are limitations to the various views on the cervical causes of vertebrobasilar insufficiency; various lesions may apparently compromise vertebral blood flow, but they may or may not be symptomatic. Mechanical compression alone, of the vertebral artery in the neck, may not be significant, but in the presence of intercurrent causes of reduced flow, or when compensating mechanisms are deficient, a critical or symptomatic reduction is more likely to occur.

Implications for manipulative therapy

Vertebrobasilar, cerebrovascular accidents are a potential complication of manipulation of the neck. Although relatively rare compared to the number of such manipulations that are performed, it needs to be recognized because of the seriousness of this complication. Over 100 cases of stroke following neck manipulation have been reported in the English-language literature (Pratt-Thomas & Berger 1947, Ford & Clark 1956, Schwartz et al 1956, Boshes 1959, Green & Joynt 1959, Smith & Estridge 1962, Pribek 1963, Kanshepolsky et al 1972, Lyness & Wagman 1974, Mehalic & Farhart 1974, Miller & Burton 1974, Bladin & Merory 1975, Davidson et al 1975, Mueller & Sahs 1976, Beatty 1977, Easton & Shearman 1977, Nyberg-Hansen et al 1978, Parkin et al 1978, Schellhas et al 1980, Sherman et al 1981, Simmons et al 1982, Braun et al 1983, Gutmann 1983, Daneshmend et al 1984, Fritz et al 1984, Terrett 1987) and these have been reviewed by Krueger and Okazaki (1980) and by Terrett (1987); the latter review also covers a collection of references from the European literature. A further 360 cases have been alluded to in correspondence (Robertson 1981).

Clinically, all of these patients developed features of ischaemia in some part of the vertebrobasilar distribution following forceful manipulation of the neck. Unfortunately, vertebral angiography was not performed in all cases, and autopsies were not always performed on the fatal cases. Accordingly, there is a limited amount of data from which one can determine the actual mechanism of vascular insufficiency.

From the available angiographic data, the most common level of occlusion of the vertebrobasilar tree following neck manipulation is the atlanto-axial segment of the vertebral artery, followed by the fourth part of the vertebral artery and the basilar artery. The findings at autopsy have been thrombosis of the atlanto-axial segment of the vertebral artery and of the basilar artery and its branches.

The cause of the vascular occlusion does not appear to be related to occlusion of the vertebral artery in its first part, or by uncinate osteophytes. With regard to the latter, Krueger and Okazaki (1980) appropriately pointed out that there is a poor correlation between stroke after manipulation and the incidence of cervical spondylosis. In particular, many of the patients who have suffered stroke have been quite young, at an age when uncinate osteophytes would not be expected to be present. Also, because of age factors, atheroma does not appear to be a significant factor, and indeed, has not been a feature found at autopsy.

Trauma to the atlanto-axial segment of the vertebral artery would appear to be the most plausible mechanism for stroke after manipulation. As described previously, this segment is relatively fixed, and it is entertainable that upon sudden forceful rotation, the artery is stretched and its intima torn. The damaged intimal surface then acts as a precipitant for thrombosis or allows the formation of a dissecting aneurysm. Thrombosis then occludes the artery locally, but also may propagate or embolize distally.

This hypothesis is consistent with the angiographic data and to some extent with the post mortem findings. However, detailed studies of the arterial wall have not been performed to determine whether or not intimal tearing was present.

As was discussed above, the evidence implicating occlusion of the atlanto-axial segment of the vertebral artery during head rotation as a cause of brainstem ischaemia is equivocal. So, it may seem inconsistent to postulate atlanto-axial injury to be the cause of stroke after manipulation. However, the experimental angiographic studies of atlanto-axial occlusion have all involved physiological passive rotation of the head. The circumstances are different in manipulation. Two additional factors are present: force and suddenness. All reports of stroke after manipulation refer to the speed and violence of the manoeuvre suffered by the patient. It seems probable that these two factors would increase the likelihood of intimal tearing and its sequelae.

Thus, while the atlanto-axial segment of the vertebral artery may not be clinically significant as a site of occlusion during normal movements of the neck, it may well be a potential site of injury during rapid forceful rotation of the head. A corollary of this conclusion is that the conventional tests for vertebral vascular sufficiency using passive gentle movement may in no way indicate the propensity for vascular injury upon violent rotation.

Summary

Dizziness is one of several symptoms which can occur in vertebrobasilar insufficiency, and it is frequently the predominant one.

Vertebrobasilar insufficiency can be caused by compromise of blood flow in the basilar and vertebral arteries by intrinsic and extrinsic disorders.

Intrinsic disorders are atherosclerosis and its sequelae.

Extrinsic disorders affect the cervical portion of the vertebral artery and include compression of its first party by muscles, bands, and kinks; compression of its second part by uncinate osteophytes, especially during rotation of

the head; and occlusion by stretch of the atlanto-axial segment during rotation.

Whether any of these disorders can alone produce symptoms is debatable, and the related clinical data are frequently equivocal or incomplete.

Symptoms appear more likely to occur after mechanical occlusion of a vertebral artery if vertebrobasilar blood flow or potential collateral blood flow is also compromised by other lesions like atheroma or hypoplasia of the opposite vertebral artery.

Stroke is a potential complication of cervical manipulation. The most plausible mechanism is violent tearing of the intima of the atlanto-axial segment of the vertebral artery with consequent thrombosis locally and distally.

Reflex vertigo

Along with the eyes and labyrinths, the cervical vertebral column is an important source of proprioceptive information that influences the sense of balance, and it is well known, on clinical grounds, that cervical disease or injury can be accompanied by vertigo, but of a nature that does not imply vertebrobasilar insufficiency (Stoddard 1952, Ryan & Cope 1955, Gray 1956, Newill 1972, Wing & Hargrave-Wilson 1974). In general, it is believed that in such cases the mechanism of the vertigo is a disturbance of the tonic neck reflexes. The essential difference between ischaemic and reflex vertigo is that reflex vertigo is not accompanied by other features of brainstem ischaemia or cardiovascular disease.

The tonic neck reflexes were first described when experiments in animals revealed that turning the animal's head caused appropriate postural adjustments in the limbs (Magnus & de Kleijn 1912, Magnus 1926a, b). Initially, the receptive field for these reflexes was delimited as the distribution of the first three cervical nerves. Later, the location of the receptors was found to be in the upper joints of the neck, particularly the atlanto-axial and atlanto-occipital joints (McCouch et al 1951).

More recently, there has been a move, both in the field of proprioceptive physiology in general (McCloskey 1978), and with respect to cervical proprioception in particular (Abrahams 1977, 1981, Bakker & Richmond 1980) to emphasize the role of muscle afferents in the genesis of position sense.

Regardless of whether the origin of the tonic neck reflexes is in joints or muscles of the cervical vertebral column, it is firmly established that disturbing them can produce a variety of motor and subjective abnormalities.

In monkeys, injection of the C1, 2, 3 dorsal rami with local anaesthetic, or section of these nerves, induces severe alterations of balance, orientation and motor coordination (Cohen 1961). The same effects, coupled with nystagmus can be produced by injections of local anaesthetic into the deep neck muscles of monkeys (Igarashi et al 1969, 1972, De Jong et al 1977). Positional nystagmus occurs in rabbits if their neck muscles are injected with local anaesthetic or after section of the first and second cervical dorsal roots (Biemond & de Jong 1969), while damaging the posterior neck muscles of rabbits with hypertonic saline induces muscle spasm and nystagmus (Hinoki & Niki 1975). In humans, the injection of local anaesthetic into deep neck muscles (De Jong et al 1977) or the C2 ganglion (Bogduk 1981a) produces ataxia, and a sense of light-headedness, or dizziness.

These experiments validate the contention that dizziness can be caused by a disturbance of the tonic neck reflexes. The essence of the mechanism appears to be a distortion of the normal afferent input to the vestibular nucleus from the neck. The disturbance may be either a relative decrease or an increase in the activity of certain receptors, for while in some instances anaesthetization of the neck muscles induces vertigo (De Jong et al 1977), in others similar injections can be used to relieve it (Gray 1956).

What remains unresolved is the location of the disturbance. Some contend that it is in the cervical joints (Wyke 1979), whereas others believe the offending abnormality is hypertonicity of the neck muscles induced by sympathetic over-activity (Hinoki & Niki 1975). Yet another viewpoint maintains that the lesion is strain of the intervertebral discs and cervical ligaments which recruits a diverse sympathetic response (Braaf & Rosner 1962).

Consequently, the guidelines for management have been several. Collars have been advocated (Ryan & Cope 1955) and would be applicable whether the disorder was muscular or articular. For muscular disturbances, relaxants, and heat have been advocated (Newill 1972) as have injections of local anaesthetic into tender muscles (Gray 1956, Newill 1972). For articular disorders, manipulation has been advocated (Newill 1972, Wyke 1979), and at least one preliminary communication attests to the efficacy of manipulative therapy for vertigo (Wing & Hargrave-Wilson 1974).

REFERENCES

Abrahams V C 1977 The physiology of neck muscles; their role in head movement and maintenance of posture. Canadian Journal of Physiology and Pharmacology 55: 332–338

Abrahams V C 1981 Sensory and motor specialisation in some muscles of the neck. Trends in Neurosciences, pp 24–27

Bakay L, Leslie E V 1965 Surgical treatment of vertebral artery insufficiency caused by cervical spondylosis. Journal of Neurosurgery 23: 596–602

Bakker D A, Richmond F J R 1980 Distribution of receptors around neck vertebrae in the cat. Journal of Physiology 298: 40–41

Balla J I, Longford K H 1967 Vertebral artery compression in cervical spondylosis. Medical Journal of Australia 1: 284–286

Barre N 1926 Sur un syndrome sympathique cervicale posterieure et sa cause frequente: l'arthrite cervicale. Revue du Neurologie 33: 1246–1248

Barton J W, Margolis M T 1975 Rotational obstruction of the vertebral artery at the atlanto-axial joint. Neuroradiology 9: 117–120

Bartschi-Rochaix W 1968 Headaches of cervical origin. In: Vinken P J, Bruyn G W (eds) Handbook of clinical neurology. vol 5. North Holland, Amsterdam, ch 17, pp 192–203

Beatty R A 1977 Dissecting haematoma of the internal carotid artery following chiropractic cervical manipulation. Journal of Trauma 17: 248–249

Bertoft E S, Westerberg C E 1985 Further observations on the neck–tongue syndrome. Cephalalgia 5 (suppl 3): 312–313

Biemond A, de Jong J M B V 1969 On cervical nystagmus and related disorders. Brain 92: 437–458

Bladin P F, Merory J 1975 Mechanisms in cerebral lesions in trauma to high cervical portion of the vertebral artery — rotational injury. Proceedings of the Australian Association of Neurologists 12: 35–41

Bland J H 1967 Rheumatoid arthritis of the cervical spine. Bulletin of the Rheumatic Diseases 18: 471–476

Bland J H, Davis P H, London M G et al 1963 Rheumatoid arthritis of the cervical spine. Archives of Internal Medicine 112: 892–898

Blume H G 1976 Radiofrequency denaturation in occipital pain: a new approach in 114 cases I: Bonica JJ, Albe-Fessard D (eds) Advances in pain research and therapy. vol I. Raven Press, New York, pp 691–698

Blume H G 1982 Radiofrequency denaturation in occipital pain: results in 450 cases. Applied Neurophysiology 45: 543–548

Bogduk N 1980 The anatomy of occipital neuralgia. Clinical and Experimental Neurology 17: 167–184

Bogduk N 1981a Local anaesthetic blocks of the second cervical ganglion: a technique with application in occipital headache. Cephalalgia 1: 41–50

Bogduk N 1981b An anatomical basis for neck tongue syndrome. Journal of Neurology, Neurosurgery and Psychiatry 44: 202–208

Bogduk N 1982 The clinical anatomy of the cervical dorsal rami. Spine 7: 319–330

Bogduk N 1989 Greater occipital Neuralgia. In: Lons D M (ed) Current therapy in neurological surgery — 2. Decker, Philadelphia, pp 263–267

Bogduk N, Marsland A 1986 On the concept of third occipital headache. Journal of Neurology Neurosurgery and Psychiatry 49: 775–780

Bogduk N, Marsland A 1988 The cervical zygapophysial joints as a source of neck pain. Spine 13: 610–617

Bogduk N, Lambert G, Duckworth J W 1981 The anatomy and physiology of the vertebral nerve in relation to cervical migraine. Cephalalgia 1: 1–14

Boshes L D 1959 Journal of the American Medical Association 1971: 1602

Braaf M M, Rosner S 1962a Headache following neck injuries. Headache 2: 153–159

Braaf M M, Rosner S 1962b Meniere-like syndrome following whiplash injury of the neck. Journal of Trauma 2: 494–501

Braaf M M, Rosner S 1965 More recent concepts on the treatment of headache. Headache 5: 38–44

Braaf M M, Rosner S 1975 Trauma of cervical spine as cause of chronic headache. Journal of Trauma 15: 441–446

Brain Lord 1963 Some unsolved problems of cervical spondylosis. British Medical Journal 1: 771–777

Braun I F, Pinto R S, De Filipp G J et al 1983 Brainstem infarction due to chiropractic manipulation of the cervical spine. Southern Medical Journal 76: 1199–1201

Brown B St J, Tatlow W F T 1963 Radiographic studies of the vertebral arteries in cadavers. Radiology 81: 80–88

Cabot A, Backer A 1978 The cervical spine in rheumatoid arthritis. Clinical Orthopaedics and Related research 131: 130–140

Campbell D G, Parsons C M 1944 Referred head pain and its concomitants. Journal of Nervous and Mental Diseases 99: 544–551

Chambers W R 1954 Posterior rhizotomy of the second and third cervical nerves for occipital pain. Journal of the American Medical Association 155: 431–432

Cherington M, Hendee R 1978 Accessory nerve palsy — a painful cranial neuropathy: surgical cure. Headache 18: 274–275

Chirls M 1978 Retrospective study of cervical spondylosis treated by anterior interbody fusion in 505 patients performed by the Cloward technique. Bulletin of the New York Hospital for Joint Diseases 39: 74–82

Cohen L A 1961 Role of eye and neck proprioceptive mechanisms in body orientation and motor co-ordination. Journal of Neurophysiology 24: 1–11

Cusson D, King A 1960 Cervical rhizotomy in the management of some cases of occipital neuralgia. Guthrie Clinic Bulletin 29: 198–208

Cyriax J 1938 Rheumatic headache. British Medical Journal 2: 1367–1368

Dan N G 1976 The management of vertebral artery insufficiency in cervical spondylosis: a modified technique. Australian and New Zealand Journal of Surgery 46: 164–165

Daneshmend T K, Hewer R L, Bradshaw J R 1984 Acute brainstem stroke during neck manipulation. British Medical Journal 288: 189

Daroff R B 1990 Dizziness and vertigo. In: Wilson J D, Braunwald E, Isselbacher K J, Petersdorf R G, Martin J B, Fauci A S, Root R K (eds) Harrison's principles of internal medicine. 12th edn. McGraw-Hill, New York, ch 22, pp 140–142

Daseler E H, Anson B J 1959 Surgical anatomy of the subclavian artery and its branches. Surgery Gynaecology and Obstetrics 108: 149–174

Davidson K, Weiford E C, Dixon G 1975 Traumatic vertebral artery pseudoaneurysm following chiropractic manipulation. Radiology 115: 651–652

De Jong P T V M, de Jong J M B V, Cohen B, Jongkees L B W 1977 Ataxia and nystagmus induced by injection of local anaesthetics in the neck. Annals of Neurology 1: 240–246

Dugan M C, Locke S, Gallagher J R 1962 Occipital neuralgia in adolescents and young adults. New England Medical Journal 267: 1166–1172

Dutton C D, Riley L H 1969 Cervical migraine. Not merely a pain in the neck. American Journal of Medicine 47: 141–148

Dwyer A, Aprill C, Bogduk N 1990 Cervical zygapophysial joint pair patterns I: a study in normal volunteers. Spine 15: 453–457

Easton J D, Shearman D G 1977 Cervical manipulation and stroke. Stroke 8: 594–597

Ehni G, Benner B 1984 Occipital neuralgia and the C1–2 arthrosis syndrome. Journal of Neurosurgery 61: 961–965

Elisevich K, Stratford J, Bray G, Finlayson M 1984 Neck tongue syndrome: operative management. Journal of Neurology Neurosurgery and Psychiatry 47: 407–409

Faris A A, Poser C M, Wilmore D W, Agnew C H 1963 Radiologic visualisation of neck vessels in healthy men. Neurology 13: 386–396

Feinstein B, Langton J B K, Jameson R M, Schiller F 1954 Experiments on referred pain from deep somatic tissues. Journal of Bone and Joint Surgery 36A: 981–997

Feit H 1982 Further observations on the diagnosis and management of carotidynia. Headache 25: 86–88

Fisher C M 1967 Vertigo in cerebrovascular disease. Archives of Otolaryngology 85: 529–534

Fisher C M 1982 The headache and pain of spontaneous carotid dissection. Headache 25: 60–65

Fisher C M, Karnes W E 1965 Local embolism. Journal of Neuropathology and Experimental Neurology 24: 274–175

Fisher C M, Gore I, Okabe N, White P D 1965 Atherosclerosis of the carotid and vertebral arteries — extracranial and intracranial. Journal of Neuropathology and Experimental Neurology 24: 455–476

Fitzgerald M J T, Sachithanandan S R 1979 The structure and source of lingual proprioceptors in the monkey. Journal of Anatomy 128: 523–555

Ford F R 1952 Syncope, vertigo and disturbances of vision resulting from intermittent obstruction of the vertebral arteries due to defect in the odontoid process and excessive mobility of the second cervical vertebra. Bulletin of the Johns Hopkins Hospital 91: 168–173

Ford F R, Clark D 1956 Thrombosis of the basilar artery with softenings in the cerebellum and brainstem due to manipulation of the neck. Bulletin of the Johns Hopkins Hospital 98: 37–42

Fortin C J, Biller J 1985 Neck tongue syndrome. Headache 25: 255–258

Fournier A M, Rathelot P 1960 L'arthrose atlo-odontoidienne. Presse Médicale 68: 163–165

Fritz V U, Maloon A, Tuch P 1984 Neck manipulation causing stroke. South African Medical Journal 66: 844–846

Gayral L, Neuwirth E 1954 Oto-neuro-opthalmologic manifestations of cervical origin. Posterior cervical sympathetic syndrome of Barre–Lieou. New York State Journal of Medicine 54: 1920–1926

Gortvai P 1964 Insufficiency of the vertebral artery treated by decompression of its cervical part. British Medical Journal 2: 233–234

Gray L P 1956 Extralabyrinthine vertigo due to cervical muscle lesions. Journal of Laryngology 70: 352–360

Green D, Joynt R J 1959 Vascular accidents to the brainstem associated with neck manipulation. Journal of the American Medical Association 170: 522–524

Guerrier Y 1949 Les nerfs vertebraux. Acta Anatomica 8: 62–90

Gutmann G 1983 Injuries to the vertebral artery caused by manual therapy. Manuelle Medizin 21: 2–14

Hackett G S, Huang T C, Raftery A 1962 Prolotherapy for headache. Headache 2: 20–28

Hammond S R, Danta G 1978 Occipital neuralgia. Clinical and Experimental Neurology 15: 258–270

Hardesty W H, Whitacre W B, Toole J F, Randall P, Royster H P 1963 Studies on vertebral artery blood flow in man. Surgery Gynaecology and Obstetrics 116: 662–664

Hardin C A 1965 Vertebral artery insufficiency produced by cervical osteoarthritic spurs. Archives of Surgery 90: 629–633

Hardin C A, Poser C M 1963 Rotational obstruction of the vertebral artery due to redundancy and extraluminal cervical fascial bands. Annals of Surgery 158: 133–137

Hardin C A, Williamson W P, Steegman A T 1960 Vertebral artery insufficiency produced by cervical osteoarthritic spurs. Neurology 10: 855–858

Hartsock C L 1940 Headache from arthritis of the cervical spine. Medical Clinics of North America 24: 329–333

Hawkins G W 1962 Flexion and extension injuries of the cervicocapital joints. Clinical Orthopaedics and Related Research 24: 22–33

Hildebrandt J, Jansen J 1984 Vascular compression of the C2 and C3 roots — yet another cause of chronic intermittent hemicrania? Cephalalgia 4: 167–170

Hinoki M, Niki H 1975 Neurotological studies in the role of the sympathetic nervous system in the formation of traumatic vertigo of cervical origin. Acta Otolaryngologica Supplementum 330: 185–196

Holmes G 1913 Headaches of organic origin and their treatment. Practitioner 91: 968–985

Holt S, Yates P O 1966 Cervical spondylosis and nerve root lesions. Journal of Bone and Joint Surgery 48B: 407–423

Hovelacue A 1927 Anatomie des nerfs craniens et rachidiens et du systeme grand sympathique. Doin, Paris

Humphrey T 1952 The spinal tract of the trigeminal nerve in human embryos between 71\2 and 81\2 weeks of menstrual age and its relation to early fetal behaviour. Journal of Comparative Neurology 97: 143–209

Hunter C R, Mayfield F H 1949 Role of the upper cervical roots in the production of pain in the head. American Journal of Surgery 78: 743–749

Husni E A, Storer J 1967 The syndrome of mechanical occlusion of the vertebral artery: further observations. Angiology 18: 106–116

Husni E A, Bell H S, Storer J 1966 Mechanical obstruction of the vertebral artery. Journal of the American Medical Association 196: 101–104

Hutchinson E C, Yates P O 1956 The cervical portion of the vertebral artery. A clinico-pathological study. Brain 79: 319–331

Igarashi M, Alford B R, Watanabe T, Maxian P M 1969 Role of neck proprioceptors for the maintenance of dynamic bodily equilibrium in the squirrel monkey. Laryngoscope 79: 1713–1727

Igarashi M, Miyata H, Alford B R, Wright W K 1972 Nystagmus after experimental cervical lesions. Laryngoscope 82: 1609–1621

Jansen J, Markakis E, Rama B, Hildebrandt J 1989a Hemicranial attacks or permanent hemicrania — a sequel of upper cervical root compression. Cephalalgia 9: 123–130

Jansen J, Bardosi A, Hildebrandt J, Lucke A 1989b Cervicogenic, hemicranial attacks associated with vascular irritation or compression of the cervical nerve root C2. Clinical manifestations and morphological findings. Pain 39: 203–212

Jull G, Bogduk N, Marsland A 1988 The accuracy of manual diagnosis for cervical zygapophysial joint pain syndromes. Medical Journal of Australia 148: 233–236

Kanshepolsky J, Danielson H, Flynn R E Vertebral artery insufficiency and cerebellar infarct due to manipulation of the neck. Bulletin of the Los Angeles Neurological Society 37: 62–66

Kayfetz D O, Blumenthal L S, Hackett G S, Hemwall G A, Neff F E 1963 Whiplash injury and other ligamentous headache — its management with prolotherapy. Headache 3: 24–28

Kelly M 1942 Headaches, traumatic and rheumatic: the cervical somatic lesion. Medical Journal of Australia 2: 479–483

Kerr F W L 1961a Structural relation of the trigeminal spinal tract to upper cervical roots and the solitary nucleus in the cat. Experimental Neurology 4: 134–148

Kerr F W L 1961b A mechanism to account for frontal headache in cases of posterior fossa tumors. Journal of Neurosurgery 18: 605–609

Kerr F W L, Olafson R A 1961 Trigeminal and cervical volleys. Archives of Neurology 5: 171–178

Kimmel D L 1959 The cervical sympathetic rami and the vertebral plexus in the human foetus. Journal of comparative Neurology 112: 141–161

Kimmel D L 1960 Innervation of the spine dura mater of the posterior cranial fossa. Neurology 10: 800–809

Knight G 1963 Post-traumatic occipital headache. Lancet 1: 6–8

Kovacs A 1955 Subluxation and deformation of the cervical apophyseal joints. Acta Radiologica 43: 1–16

Krueger B R, Okazaki H 1980 Vertebral-basilar distribution infarction following chiropractic cervical manipulation. Proceedings of the Mayo Clinic 55: 322–332

Kuritzky A 1984 Cluster headache-like pain caused by an upper cervical meningioma. Cephalalgia 4: 185–186

La Rocca H 1978 Acceleration injuries of the neck. Clinical Neurosurgery 25: 209–217

Lamberty B G H, Zivanovic S 1973 The retro-articular vertebral artery ring of the atlas and its significance. Acta Anatomica 85: 113–122

Lance J W 1982 Mechanism and management of headache. 4th edn. Butterworths, London

Lance J W, Anthony M 1980 Neck tongue syndrome on sudden turning of the head. Journal of Neurology Neurosurgery and Psychiatry 43: 97–101

Langemark M, Olesen J 1987 Pericranial tenderness in tension headache. Cephalalgia 7: 249–255

Laux G, Guerrier Y 1939 Innervation de l'artere vertebral. Annales d'Anatomie Pathologique et d'Anatomie Normale Medico-chirurgicale 16: 897–899

Laux G, Guerrier Y 1947 Innervation de l'artere vertebrale. Comptes Rendus de l'Association des Anatomistes vol 34: 298–300

Lazorthes G 1949 Le systeme neurovasculaire. Masson, Paris.

Lazorthes G, Cassan J 1939 Essai de schematisation des ganglions etoile et intermediare. Comptes Rendus de l'Association des Anatomistes vol 28: 193–210

Lazorthes G, Gaubert J 1956 L'innervation des articulations interapophysaire vertebrales. Comptes Rendus de l'Association des Anatomistes vol 43: 488–494

Lewit K 1969 Vertebral artery insufficiency and the cervical spine. British Journal of Geriatric Practice 6: 37–42

Lewit K 1979 The needle effect in the relief of myofascial pain. Pain 6: 83–90

Lous I, Olesen J 1982 Evaluation of pericranial tenderness and oral function in patients with common migraine, muscle contraction headache and combination headache. Pain 12: 385–393

Lyness S S, Simeone F A 1978 Vascular complications of upper cervical spine injuries. Orthopedic Clinics of North America 9: 1029–1038

Lyness S S, Wagman A D 1974 Neurological deficit following cervical manipulation. Surgical Neurology 2: 121–124

Macnab I 1969 Acceleration-extension injuries of the cervical spine. In: American Academy of Orthopaedic Surgeons Symposium on the spine. Mosby, St Louis, pp 10–17

Macnab I 1973 The whiplash syndrome. Clinical Neurosurgery 20: 232–241

Magnus R 1926a Some results of studies in the physiology of posture. Lancet 211: 531–536

Magnus R 1926b Some results of studies in the physiology of posture. Lancet 211: 585–588

Magnus R, de Kleijn a 1912 Die Abhängigkeit des Tonus der Extremitätenmuskeln von der Kopfstellung. Pflugers Archivs des Physiologie 145: 455–548

Maigne R 1976 Une signe evocateur et inattendu de cephalee cervicale: 'la douleur au pince-roule du sourcil'. Annales de Medecine Physique 19: 416–434

Maigne R 1981 Signes cliniques des cephalees cervicales: leur traitement. Medicine et Hygiene 39: 1171–1185

Martin J B 1990 Headache. In: Wilson J D, Braunwald E, Isselbacher K J, Petersdorf R G, Martin J B, Fauci A S, Root R K (eds) Harrison's principles of internal medicine. McGraw-Hill, New York, ch 18, pp 108–115

Maslowski H A 1960 The role of the vertebral artery (abstract). Journal of Neurology Neurosurgery and Psychiatry 23: 353

Mayfield F H 1955 Symposium on cervical trauma. Neurosurgical aspects. Clinical Neurosurgery 2: 83–90

McCloskey D I 1978 Kinesthetic sensibility. Physiological Reviews 58: 763–820

McCormick C C 1987 Arthrography of the atlanto-axial (C1–C2) joints: technique and results. Journal of Interventional Radiology 2: 9–13

McCouch G P, Deering I D, Ling T H 1951 Location of receptors for tonic neck reflexes. Journal of Neurophysiology 14: 191–195

McRae D L 1960 The significance of abnormalities of the cervical spine. American Journal of Roentgenology 84: 3–25

McRae D L 1968 Bony abnormalities of the cranio-spinal junction. Clinical Neurosurgery 16: 356–375

Mehalic T, Farhart S M 1974 Vertebral artery injury from chiropractic manipulation of the neck. Surgical Neurology 2: 125–129

Mestdagh H 1976 Morphological aspects and biomechanical properties of the vertebroaxial joint (C2–C3). Acta Morphologica Neerlando-Scandinavica 14: 19–30

Miller R G, Burton R 1974 Stroke following chiropractic manipulation of the spine. Journal of the American Medical Association 229: 189–190

Monteiro H, Rodrigues A 1931 Sur les variations du nerf vertebral. Comptes Rendus de l'Association des Anatomistes vol 20: 406–419

Mueller S, Sahs A L 1976 Brainstem dysfunction related to cervical manipulation. Neurology 26: 547–550

Murphy J P 1969 Occipital neurectomy in the treatment of headache. Maryland State Medical Journal 18: 62–66

Myer J S, Sheehan S, Bauer R B 1960 An arteriographic study of cerebrovascular disease in man. Archives of Neurology 2: 27–44

Nagashima C 1970 Surgical treatment of vertebral artery insufficiency caused by cervical spondylosis. Journal of Neurosurgery 35: 512–521

Neuwirth E 1954 Neurologic complications of osteoarthritis of the cervical spine. New York State Journal of Medicine 54: 2583–2590

Newill R G D 1972 Headache and giddiness of cervical origin. Journal of the Royal College of General Practitioners 1922: 51–53

Nyberg-Hansen R, Loken A C, Tenstad O 1978 Brainstem lesions with coma for five years following manipulation of the cervical spine. Journal of Neurology 218: 97–105

Okawara S, Nibbelink D 1974 Vertebral artery occlusion following hyperextension and rotation of the head. Stroke 5: 640–642

Olesen J 1978 Some clinical features of the acute migraine attack. An analysis of 750 patients. Headache 18: 268–271

Olszewski J 1950 On the anatomical and functional organization of the spinal trigeminal nucleus. Journal of Comparative Neurology 92: 401–413

Parkin P J, Wallis W E, Wilson J L 1978 Vertebral artery occlusion following manipulation of the neck. New Zealand Medical Journal 88: 441–443

Pasztor E 1978 Decompression of vertebral artery in cases of cervical spondylosis. Surgical Neurology 9: 371–377

Pawl R P 1977 Headache, cervical spondylosis, and anterior cervical fusion. Surgical Annual 9: 391–408

Perelson H N 1947 Occipital nerve tenderness: a sign of headache. Southern Medical Journal 40: 653–656

Peterson D I, Austin G M, Dayes L A 1975 Headache associated with discogenic disease of the cervical spine. Bulletin of the Los Angeles Neurological Society 40: 96–100

Poletti C E 1983 Proposed operation for occipital neuralgia: C-2 and C-3 root decompression. Neurosurgery 12: 221–224

Poletti C E, Sweet W H 1990 Entrapment of the C2 root and ganglion by the atlanto-epistrophic ligament: clinical syndrome and surgical anatomy. Neurosurgery 27: 288–291

Power S R, Drislane T M, Nevin S 1961 Intermittent vertebral artery compression: a new syndrome. Surgery 49: 257–264

Pratt-Thomas H R, Berger K E 1947 Cerebellar and spinal injuries after chiropractic manipulation. Journal of the American Medical Association 133: 600–603

Pribek R A 1963 Brainstem vascular accident following neck manipulations. Wisconsin Medical Journal 62: 141–143

Raney A A, Raney R B 1948 Headache: a common symptom of cervical disc lesions. Archives of Neurology and Psychiatry 59: 603–621

Ray B S, Wolff H G 1949 Experimental studies on headache. Archives of Surgery 41: 813–856

Robertson J T 1981 Neck manipulation as a cause of stroke. Stroke 12: 260–261

Robinson H S 1966 Rheumatoid arthritis: atlanto-axial subluxation and its clinical presentation. Canadian Medical Association Journal 94: 470–477

Romanov V A, Miller L G, Gaetvyi M D 1973 Influence of the vertebral nerve on the cochlear circulation. Bulletin of Experimental Biology and Medicine 75: 610–612

Ryan G M S, Cope S 1955 Cervical vertigo. Lancet 2: 1355–1358

Schellhas K P, Latchaw R E, Wendling L R, Gold L H A 1980 Vertebrobasilar injuries following cervical manipulation. Journal of the American Medical Association 244: 1450–1453

Schultz E C, Semmes R E 1950 Head and neck pains of cervical disc origin. Laryngoscope 60: 338–343

Schwartz G A, Geiger J K, Spano A V 1956 Posterior inferior cerebellar artery syndrome of Wallenburg after chiropractic manipulation. Archives of Internal Medicine 97: 352–354

Seletz E 1963 Trauma and the cervical portion of the spine. Journal of the International College of Surgeons 40: 47–62

Sharp J, Purser D W 1961 Spontaneous atlanto-axial dislocation in ankylosing spondylitis and rheumatoid arthritis. Annals of the Rheumatic Diseases 20: 47–77

Sheehan S, Bauer R B, Myer J S 1960 Vertebral artery compression in cervical spondylosis. Neurology 10: 968–986

Sherman D G, Hart R G, Easton J D 1981 Abrupt change in head position and cerebral infarction. Stroke 12: 2–6

Sigwald J, Jamet F 1968 Occipital neuralgia. In: Vinken P J, Bruyn G W (eds) Handbook of clinical neurology. vol 5. Elsevier, New York, ch 36, pp 368–374

Simons D G, 1975 Muscle pain syndromes — part I. American Journal of Physical Medicine 54: 289–311

Simons D G 1976a Muscle pain syndromes — part II. American Journal of Physical Medicine 55: 15–42

Simons D G 1976b Electrogenic nature of palpable bands and 'jump sign' associated with myofascial trigger points. In: Bonica J J, Albe-Fessard D (eds) Advances in pain research and therapy. vol I. Raven Press, New York, pp 913–918

Simons D G 1981 Myofascial trigger points: a need for understanding. Archives of Physical Medicine and Rehabilitation 62: 97–99

Simons D G 1988 Myofascial pain syndrome: where are we? Where are we going? Archives of Physical Medicine and Rehabilitation 69: 207–212

Simons D G, Travell J 1981 Myofascial trigger points, a possible explanation. Pain 10: 106–109

Simmons K C, Soo Y S, Walker G, Harvey P 1982 Trauma to the vertebral artery related to neck manipulation. Medical Journal of Australia 1: 187–188

Sjaastad O, Saunte C, Hovdahl H, Breivik H, Gronbaek E 1983 'Cervicogenic' headache. An hypothesis. Cephalalgia 3: 249–256

Sluijter M E, Koetsveld-Baart C C 1980 Interruption of pain pathways in the treatment of the cervical syndrome. Anaesthesia 35: 302–307

Sluijter M E, Mehta M 1981 Treatment of chronic back and neck pain by percutaneous thermal lesions. In: Lipton S, Miles J (eds) Persistent pain. Modern methods of treatment. vol 3. Academic Press, London, pp 141–179

Smith R A, Estridge M N 1962 Neurologic complications of head and neck manipulations. Journal of the American Medical Association 182: 528–531

Smith D R, Vanderark G D, Kempe L G 1971 Cervical spondylosis causing vertebrobasilar insufficiency: surgical treatment. Journal of Neurology Neurosurgery and Psychiatry 34: 388–392

Stevens J S, Cartlidge N E F, Saunders M, Appleby A, Hall M, Shaw D A 1971 Atlanto-axial subluxation and cervical myelopathy in rheumatoid arthritis. Quarterly Journal of Medicine 159: 391–408

Stewart D Y 1962 Current concepts of 'Barre Syndrome' or the 'posterior cervical sympathetic syndrome'. Clinical Orthopaedics and Related Research 24: 40–48

Stoddard A 1952 Vertigo (letter). British Medical Journal 2: 1043

Stoddard A 1970 Cervical spondylosis and cervical osteoarthritis. Manuelle Medicine 8: 31–33

Stopford J S B 1916 The arteries of the pons and medulla oblongata: part II. Journal of Anatomy and Physiology 50: 255–280

Stopford J S B 1916 The arteries of the pons and medulla oblongata: part I. Journal of Anatomy and Physiology 50: 131–164

Taitz C, Nathan H, Arensburg B 1978 Anatomical observations of the foramina transversaria. Journal of Neurology Neurosurgery and Psychiatry 41: 170–176

Taren J A, Kahn E A 1962 Anatomic pathways related to pain in face and neck. Journal of Neurosurgery 19: 116–121

Tatlow W F T, Bammer H G 1957 Syndrome of vertebral artery compression. Neurology 7: 331–340

Terrett A G J 1987 Vascular accidents from cervical spine manipulation: report on 107 cases. Journal of the Australian Chiropractors' Association 17: 15–24

Toole J F, Tucker S H 1960 Influence of head position on cerebral circulation. Archives of Neurology 2: 616–623

Torvik A 1956 Afferent connections to the sensory trigeminal nuclei, the nucleus of the solitary tract and adjacent structures. Journal of Comparative Neurology 106: 51–141

Travell J 1955 Referred pain from skeletal muscle. New York State Journal of Medicine 55: 331–340

Travell J 1962 Mechanical headache. Headache 7: 23–29

Travell J, Rinzler S H 1952 The myofascial genesis of pain. Postgraduate Medicine 11: 425–434

Trevor-Jones R 1964 Osteoarthritis of the paravertebral joints of the second and third cervical vertebrae as a cause of occipital headache. South African Medical Journal 30: 392–394

Virtama P, Kivalo E 1957 Impressions on the vertebral artery by deformations of the unco-vertebral joints. Acta Radiologica 48: 410–414

Walton J N (ed) 1977 Brain's diseases of the nervous system. 8th edn. Oxford University Press, Oxford

Warwick R, Williams P L (eds) 1973 Gray's anatomy. 35th edn. Longmans, London

Webb F W S, Hickmann J A, Brew D St J 1968 Death from vertebral artery thrombosis in rheumatoid arthritis. British Medical Journal 2: 537–538

Weinberger L M 1978 Cervico-occipital pain and its surgical treatment. American Journal of Surgery 135: 243–247

Wilkinson M 1971 Symptomatology. In: Wilkinson M (ed) Cervical spondylosis. 2nd edn. Heinemann, London, ch 4

Williams P L, Warwick R, Dyson M, Bannister L H (eds) 1989 Gray's anatomy. 37th edn. Churchill Livingstone, Edinburgh

Wing L W, Hargrave-Wilson W 1974 Cervical vertigo. Australian and New Zealand Journal of Surgery 44: 275–277

Wyke B 1979 Neurology of the cervical spinal joints. Physiotherapy 65: 72–76

23. Cervical headache: a review

G. A. Jull

INTRODUCTION

Headache is a common and often debilitating symptom (Lance 1982) (Fig. 23.1). Successful management relies on correctly identifying its origin and contributing factors.

Benign, recurrent and chronic headaches often present special problems in differential diagnosis. This is not so often the case in those associated with medical conditions such as intracranial lesions, vascular disorders, bacterial or viral infections or when there is an acute precipitating event. In these cases, there are usually definitive physical signs, laboratory test results and or radiological signs to assist diagnosis. However, there are no laboratory tests which can positively assist diagnosis of the more prevalent and chronic forms such as migraine and tension headache (Headache Classification Commmittee of the International Headache Society 1988, Rose 1988). Additionally, elementary physical examination is often apparently normal in the benign headache sufferer (Lance 1982, Biber & Warfield 1986).

Diagnosis is therefore largely made on the nature, char-

acteristics and temporal pattern of headache. While many can be successfully identified in this way, this reliance on symptomatic and historical features can lessen the accuracy and reliability of diagnosis (Sjaastad et al 1986a, Weeks & Rapoport 1987).

One reason for this is that symptoms arising from different causes of headache often overlap (Ziegler et al 1982). To compound the problem, persons may suffer from two or more forms, or different headaches may merge into a headache continuum (Olesen 1978, Fredriksen et al 1987, Pfaffenrath et al 1987, Saadah & Taylor 1987, Langemark et al 1988). The character of headaches not infrequently changes over time (Anthony 1989), and a person may suffer from a transitional form which does not possess all the characteristics of a typical and pure, readily diagnosable syndrome (Headache Classification Committee of the International Headache Society 1988). Headaches may be misdiagnosed; this distorts statistics on the frequency of particular forms of headache (Sjaastad et al 1986a, Fredriksen et al 1987). This situation could further imply that some sufferers are not receiving the appropriate management.

Headaches arising from the cervical spine are those of particular interest to the physiotherapist. There is convincing experimental and clinical evidence that the structures of the cervical spine are capable of causing headache and other associated symptoms (Campbell & Parsons 1944, Feinstein et al 1954, Kerr & Olafson 1961, Bogduk & Marsland 1986, Fredriksen et al 1987).

It would seem from the medical literature that cervical headaches share the problem of differential diagnosis from other forms of benign headache. Opinions both historically and currently vary extremely as to the frequency with which the cervical spine is the primary cause (Wolff's Headache and Other Head Pain 1972, Sjaastad et al 1983, Jamieson 1984, Peters 1984, Sjaastad et al 1986a, Edeling 1988, Saper 1989).

There is no doubt that symptoms of cervical headache can overlap with those of migraine and tension headache (Jull 1986a, Sjaastad et al 1986a, Fredriksen et al 1987,

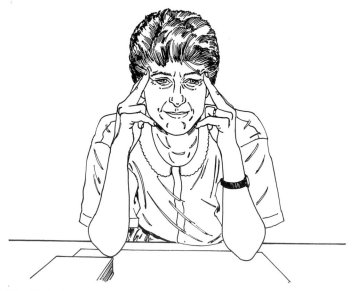

Fig. 23.1 Headache can be a debilitating symptom.

Edeling 1988, Sjaastad et al 1989a). However the predominant allocation of chronic and recurrent headache to the common migraine and tension-type categories needs to be questioned. This is especially so when it is acknowledged that tension headache is often a 'wastebasket' diagnosis used when symptoms are obviously not vascular (migraine or cluster) or associated with any readily identifiable structural disease (Saper 1989).

There is no question that the entity of tension or muscle contraction headache exists. Nevertheless, particularly in its chronic form, tension headache is poorly characterized and its mechanisms are speculative at this time (Olesen 1988, Olesen & Langemark 1988). Despite these difficulties in definition, it is regarded as the most prevalent form of headache (Olesen 1988). When it is suggested that abnormal neck postures and injury may be implicated in the cause of tension headache (Saper 1989), it is possible that the role of the cervical spine could be undervalued and underevaluated in many cases. Cervical headaches could feasibly be classified erroneously as common migraine, tension or muscle contraction headache (Bogduk & Marsland 1986, Sjaastad et al 1986a, Sluijter et al 1989).

One reason for the lack of recognition of the cervical spine's involvement could be that the physical examination of these patients is often too superficial with a misguided reliance on the results of plain X-rays of the neck. The physical examination of the neck should include a comprehensive and detailed assessment of articular, muscular and neural structures (Maitland 1986, Grieve 1988, Jull 1988). However the precise nature of the cervical musculoskeletal dysfunction has not as yet been comprehensively and adequately defined. Researchers are beginning to quantify several aspects of the physical dysfunction (Jull et al 1988, Boquet et al 1989, Jaeger 1989, Watson 1990) but this research is in its infancy.

The situation when trying to assess the aetiological role of cervical structures in either the clinical or research setting is far from simple. The cervical spine can certainly be the primary cause of headache. The area both diagnostically and clinically becomes more complex with the evidence and opinion that the cervical spine can contribute to a headache continuum or be in part responsible for the intensity of pain and frequency of attack in some migraines (Parker et al 1978, 1980, Boquet et al 1989). Although the pathophysiology is still obscure, it has also been suggested that cervical structures can be a mechanical trigger in some vascular and neurogenic headaches (Sjaastad et al 1984, Boquet et al 1989, Solomon et al 1989) and that injury to the neck may precipitate migraine (Winston 1987).

Understandably, there can be diagnostic difficulties on both symptomatic and physical bases in recognizing the cervical headache or assessing the degree of the cervical component in a headache syndrome. While physiotherapists may instinctively disagree with those current authors who contend that the cervical spine is an infrequent cause (Lance 1986, Olesen 1988), it is equally irresponsible for practitioners of any discipline to claim a 'cure all' for headache by neck manipulation (Milne 1989).

Knowledge of the role of the cervical spine in headache is far from absolute. In order to develop a better understanding, the proposed characteristics of cervical headache will be presented. The areas of symptomatic overlap with other causes of headache will be indicated as well as identifying symptoms and behaviours which should lead the practitioner to consider the cervical structures in the aetiology of headache.

The presence of relevant physical signs in the musculoskeletal system is fundamental to the diagnosis of cervical headache (Bogduk et al 1985, Headache Classification Committee of the International Headache Society 1988, Jull et al 1988). Neck pain can accompany many different headache forms. Therefore the location, nature and extent of these signs will be reviewed to provide a basis for decision making on the primary or secondary role of cervical structures in headache.

SYMPTOMATIC PROFILE OF CERVICAL HEADACHE

Headache is a symptom of many different origins and pathophysiological events. There is a common denominator to all forms of headache whether musculoskeletal, vascular or neurogenic. They share access to the head and neck region via the trigeminocervical nucleus (Bogduk 1986a, 1989a, Angus-Leppan et al 1989, Solomon et al 1989). Overlap in symptoms and indeed headache forms can be expected and this contributes to the problem of differential diagnosis.

Area and distribution of pain

Several studies of cervical headache patients have documented the reported locations of pain. Pain may be felt in any area of the head but the prevalent sites are frontal, retro-orbital, occipital and temporal areas, associated with suboccipital and neck pain (Sjaastad et al 1983, Ehni & Benner 1984, Bogduk & Marsland 1986, Jull 1986a, Fredriksen et al 1987, Edeling 1988). With knowledge that the trigeminocervical nucleus is the essential nociceptive nucleus of the head (Bogduk 1989a), it is not surprising that these distributions offer little assistance in differential diagnosis of benign headache. Similar distributions are reported for a variety of headaches including migraine (Lance 1982, Rose 1988), tension or muscle-contraction headache (Caviness & O'Brien 1980, Langemark et al 1988), chronic paroxysmal hemicrania and cluster headache (Russell 1988, Sjaastad 1988) and those associated with temporomandibular joint dysfunction (Gelb &

Bernstein 1983, Reade & Steidler 1984, Weinberg & Lapointe 1987).

The presence of neck pain associated with the head pain is considered to be one of the characteristic features of cervical headache (Edmeads 1978, Sjaastad et al 1983). In a survey of 96 headache patients presenting for physiotherapy management, occipital, suboccipital and/or mid-lower cervical pain was present in 88% of the patients (Jull 1986a). Neck pain was a feature in all patients of the smaller positively diagnosed cervical headache samples of Ehni & Benner (1984), Bogduk & Marsland (1986) and Fredriksen et al (1987). Yet neck symptoms can accompany many other headache forms, and its occurrence may not appear to be helpful in differential diagnosis. Reports from recent studies have highlighted the fact that careful questioning of the patient may still realize this aspect as important in differential diagnosis.

Sjaastad et al (1989b), recognizing the overlap in areas of head and neck symptoms in cervical headache and migraine when headaches were at their maximum intensity, conducted a study concentrating on the area of onset of pain. In 20 of the 22 subjects with classic migraine, the onset of headache occurred in the frontal or temporal region and then spread to other areas, including the neck. In only one subject did the headache begin in the neck and then radiate. In contrast, of the sample of 11 cervical headache patients, eight patients reported the focal onset of headache in the neck before it spread to other areas. In only three patients was the onset of headache in the frontal, temporal region.

Tenuous links have been made between the cervical spine and cluster or cluster-like headaches (Sjaastad et al 1982, Hildebrandt & Jansen 1984). Solomon et al (1989) studied 100 patients with cluster headaches. In all, 70% of the patients had neck pain associated with their headache but in only 10% of cases was the initial onset of pain located in the neck. Even then, this cervical pain was simultaneously accompanied by the more classical retro-orbital, temporal, frontal pain. Additionally, the type of pain in the neck was more of an ache and was of mild to moderate intensity when compared to the often excruciating pain in the orbital, temporal areas.

In relation to differential diagnosis of cervical headache, it is apparent that area of pain alone is not a criterion for diagnosis. Additionally, neck pain or aching can be present in many headache forms but there is a strong indicator that cervical structures have a primary role when headache is initiated by pain in the occipital, suboccipital or neck region.

Unilateral, bilateral headache

The unilaterality or bilaterality of headaches is regarded as a differential feature of benign, chronic or recurrent headache. Headaches such as cluster, chronic paroxysmal hemicrania, occipital neuralgia and migraine are defined predominantly as unilateral (Headache Classification Committee of the International Headache Society 1988, Rose 1988, Russell 1988, Sjaastad 1988, Anthony 1989). Unilateral headache is more common in cases of craniomandibular dysfunction (Bezuur et al 1989). Conversely, tension headache is characterized as bilateral (Lance 1982, Headache Classification Committee of the International Headache Society 1988, Olesen 1988).

In seeking to establish a diagnostic definition of cervical headache, Sjaastad et al in 1983 characterized cervicogenic headache as strictly unilateral. Since that time, several researchers have based their studies of cervical headache on the definition of Sjasstad et al (Fredriksen et al 1987, Pfaffenrath et al 1987, Boquet et al 1989, Jaeger 1989). Hence, in literature there is a strong theme of unilaterality, but other studies have indicated the not infrequent bilateral nature of cervical headache (Bogduk & Marsland 1986, Jull 1986a). There is currently a general consensus that cervical headache may be unilateral, unilateral with spread to the other side, or bilateral (Sjaastad et al 1989a). Interestingly, Bogduk and Marsland's (1986) six subjects with bilateral symptoms responded positively to unilateral nerve blocks. There appears to be no side preponderance for the cervical symptoms (Pfaffenrath et al 1987).

While unilaterality or bilaterality may contribute to headache characterization, it is not a clear criterion for cervical headache. This problem is shared by migraine for, in up to 30% of cases, this headache may be bilateral (Rose 1988) as can those arising from craniomandibular dysfunction (Bezuur et al 1989). Conversely, studies of chronic tension headache also report the occurrence of unilateral symptoms (Langemark et al 1988). However it should be questioned why 'tension' should single out one side of the head. Tension or stress can undoubtedly cause an episodic headache. It likewise has the capacity to aggravate or trigger many different forms of headache but it is suggested that when a unilateral chronic or recurrent headache is present, the diagnosis of tension headache be reserved until somatic causes located — for instance — in the cervical or craniomandibular structures are eliminated. There are problems in diagnostic terminology when it is reported that tension headaches can be unilateral in cases of imbalances of bite (Lance 1982). Should this be diagnosed as a tension headache or a headache arising from craniomandibular dysfunction?

The behaviour of the unilaterality may have diagnostic significance. If, for instance, the cause of the headache is a left C_{2-3} zygapophyseal arthropathy, then the headache will logically be on the left side. In accordance with the location of pathology, cervical headaches do not change sides (Sjaastad et al 1983, Fredriksen et al 1987). However, side alternation is not uncommon in classic migraine (Sjaastad et al 1989a). Additionally, cluster headaches can occasionally change sides between attacks (Russell 1988, Sjaastad 1988), although attacks of chronic paroxysmal hemicrania maintain a consistent laterality (Sjaastad 1988).

Quality of pain

An ache or dull boring pain is most typically described in cervical headache, although qualities such as throbbing, pulsing or pressing may be reported (Bogduk & Marsland 1986, Jull 1986a, Fredriksen & Sjaastad 1987, Pfaffenrath et al 1987, Edeling 1988). In trying to characterize uniquely the quality of pain to headache forms, throbbing in time with the pulse is the most typical description for migraine although, alternatively, the pulsing quality is not always present (Rose 1988). The feeling of the tight band or a heavy weight on the head is the common characterization of tension headache (Lance 1982, Olesen 1988) but a pressing or pulsing quality can also be reported (Langemark et al 1988). Therefore, quality of pain is not always a reliable diagnostic feature in these headache forms.

Shooting pains in the head can be reported by cervical headache sufferers (Jull 1986a) but these are far more typical of cranial neuralgias (Lance 1982). Additionally, the quality is not usually that of the superficial, shooting or lancinating pain of true neuralgia.

Pain in or behind the eye can also be associated with neck headaches (Hunter & Mayfield 1949, Gayral & Neuwirth 1954, Jull 1986a) but significant ocular symptoms and feelings such as intense pressure behind the eye alert the clinician more to the possibility of chronic paroxysmal hemicrania or cluster headache (Sjaastad 1988).

The intensity of pain can have diagnostic significance. Migraine, cervical and tension headaches can reach the moderate to severe level but they do not reach the excruciating pain heights that typify chronic paroxysmal hemicrania or cluster headache (Fredriksen et al 1987, Russell 1988). Pain of the uncontrolled migraine attack almost invariably builds to a severe and often disabling level with each attack. In contrast, the pain of a cervical headache is variable and at different times can be a dull, moderate or severe pain (Edeling 1988). Basing the severity index on factors such as the ability or inability to continue normal daily activity and sleep patterns during attacks (Jull 1986a, Fredriksen et al 1987), the cervical headache is more commonly of a moderate intensity but can reach severe levels in up to 20% of cases (Jull 1986a).

Associated symptoms

Concomitant symptoms such as nausea, vomiting and photophobia are often associated with migraine but these symptoms are not unique to any headache form and do not necessarily aid differential diagnosis (Ziegler et al 1982). They may accompany, cervical, tension, migraine

and headaches associated with craniomandibular dysfunction (Gelb & Bernstein 1983, Pfaffenrath et al 1987, Langemark et al 1988).

The associated symptoms suffered by two positively diagnosed groups of cervical headache patients are presented in Table 23.1. In addition to common symptoms such as nausea, visual disturbances, dizziness or lightheadedness, a general irritability or an inability to concentrate are often reported (Jull 1986a, Edeling 1988). From current statistics, it would appear that approximately half of the sufferers of cervical headache will present with one or more of these symptoms.

Table 23.1 Symptoms associated with cervical headache*

	Sample 1 (n = 11)	Sample 2 (n = 15)
General symptoms		
Nausea	7	5
Vomiting	6	2
Phono/Photophobia	10/5	5
Dizziness	9	6
Tinnitus	2	–
Throat symptoms	6	2
Hearing deficit	2	–
Ipsilateral symptoms		
Blurred vision	9	4
Eyelid oedema	8	5
Tearing	4	5
Redness of eye	4	5

* Adapted from Fredriksen et al (1987) (sample 1) and Pfaffenrath et al (1987) (sample 2).

Some concomitant symptoms may direct diagnosis. For example, cluster headaches can be recognized by regular autonomic disturbances including forehead sweating, tearing of the eye, ipsilateral ptosis and nasal stuffiness or secretion (Sjaastad et al 1986b, Russell 1988, Sjaastad 1988). When a patient particularly reports symptoms of stuffiness in the ear, changes in hearing, tinnitus and vertigo, in the absence of any medical disorder, craniomandibular dysfunction is suggested (Gelb & Bernstein 1983, Reade & Steidler 1984).

One interesting feature of the one-sided concomitant symptoms is that, in cervical headache, they are ipsilateral in respect to the side of pain (Sjaastad et al 1983). However, in classical migraine there is no clear correlation between the side of headache and the focal neurological features (Rose 1988). These symptoms may present opposite to the side of pain.

Neurological symptoms

Neurological signs and symptoms in the cervical musculoskeletal headache are not common, indicating that the headache is more typically a referred pain rather than that caused by irritation or compression of an upper cervical nerve (Ehni & Benner 1984, Bogduk 1985). Instances of slight sensory deficits in the distribution of the C_2 and C_3 nerves and branches of the trigeminal nerve have been reported (Fredriksen et al 1987). More overt sensory signs in the C_2 distribution were found by Dugan et al (1962) in their young patients whose chronic headache was associated with C_1–C_2 instability.

Compression of the C_2 ventral ramus caused by abnormal subluxation of the lateral atlanto-axial joint occurs in the neck–tongue syndrome (Bogduk 1981a, Bertoft & Westerberg 1985). This syndrome is characterized by the sudden onset of occipital pain radiating to the ear associated with ipsilateral numbness of the tongue on rotation of the head (Lance & Anthony 1980). The anatomical connection between the lingual nerve and the second cervical nerve is via the hypoglossal nerve (Lance & Anthony 1980).

A chronic cluster-like headache with severe unilateral frontal, retro and periorbital and occipital pain has been described in 16 patients with surgically confirmed compression of the C_2 (10), C_3 (3) or C_4 nerve root (3) (Hildebrandt & Jansen 1984, Jansen et al 1989). Of relevance to physiotherapists treating musculoskeletal dysfunction, the nerve root compression in six cases was due to spondylitic changes or scar tissue around the root. However, in nine cases there was a vascular compression of the root, surgery revealing 'varicose' veins densely interwoven around the nerve. In one patient, a neuroma was found.

Greater occipital neuralgia, which is classically defined as an entrapment neuropathy, is another potential source of cutaneous neurological symptoms. Diagnosis should be consistent with the presence of sensory changes in the distribution of the greater occipital nerve, including hyper- or hypoalgesia or dysaesthesia (Anthony 1989). Bogduk (1985) considers that the diagnosis of this condition is made far too freely and that true occipital neuralgia is rare. He advocates that the presence of occipital pain and headache in the absence of neurological symptoms necessitates a search for a musculoskeletal or non-neurogenic cause of pain.

Frequency and duration

The temporal pattern of headache is important in diagnosis (Lance 1982). Information regarding the frequency and duration of headache as well as the duration of remission periods may classify the headache.

The temporal pattern of some headaches is virtually diagnostic. Cluster headaches are characterized by attacks of head pain which last from 15 minutes to 2 hours. Attacks may occur once or twice within a 24-hour period but can range from two attacks per week up to eight in 24 hours. Cluster periods typically last from one to two months but they can be chronic and last for up to a year. Remission periods last from six months to two years but

this can be variable (Lance 1982, Russell 1988, Sjaastad 1988).

Chronic paroxysmal hemicrania is similar to cluster headaches in localization, intensity and characterization of pain. In relation to its temporal pattern, its distinction from cluster headache is that it is a chronic headache characterized by a lack of remission periods. Attacks last for a relatively short period (15 minutes) but have a high frequency — up to 15 attacks in 24 hours (Sjaastad & Dale 1974, Russell 1988, Sjaastad 1988). Despite the classical definition of chronicity, Kudrow et al (1987) believe that some cases of chronic paroxysmal hemicrania can be genuinely episodic.

The essential qualities of migraine are its episodic nature and the termination of the headache in a specified period of time (Rose 1988). Headaches may last from a few hours to days but generally they last for less than 24 hours (Lance 1982). The frequency of attack can vary from one per year to several times per week in extreme cases.

Headaches with a distinct periodicity, appropriate associated features and pain-free intervening periods are strongly suggestive of migraine. Migraine with aura is readily identified. However, the differentiation of the more prevalent migraine without aura (or common migraine) from episodic tension headache may be difficult (Headache Classification Committee of the International Headache Society 1988). Additionally, when patients suffer a high frequency of 'migrainous' headache, often in association with tension headache, separation of the two on the background of a continuous but fluctuating headache is likewise difficult (Lance 1982). The mixed headache syndrome of various proportions of migraine and tension headache has been proposed (Saper 1982).

The pattern of tension headache exemplifies the diagnostic problem. It can be episodic or chronic. Episodic headaches can last from a few hours to several days. When chronic it is often a semicontinuous headaches or at least two to three headaches are suffered per week (Langemark et al 1988, Olesen 1988). Notably, essentially the same temporal pattern has been recorded for cervical headache, and, indeed, headache associated with craniomandibular dysfunction (Sjaastad et al 1983, Reade & Steidler 1984, Bogduk & Marsland 1986, Jull 1986a, Fredriksen et al 1987, Pfaffenrath et al 1987, Edeling 1988).

In the light of these similarities it must again be questioned whether the prevalent diagnoses of common migraine and tension headache (as separate entities or as a continuum) are always accurate. It is believed that, in many cases, a cervical cause has been overlooked. Neither comprehensive studies nor accurate statistics are available. However Sjaastad et al (1986a) speculate that, if diagnosis were always accurate, cervical headache and common migraine could have approximately equal incidence within the benign chronic and recurrent headache population.

Time and mode of onset

The cervical headache is often present on waking and may worsen as the day goes on, depending on activity (Hartsock 1940, Trevor-Jones 1964, Sjaastad et al 1983, Jull 1986a). Alternatively, it may begin during or towards the end of the day. This is consistent with an arthropathy being aggravated by activity (Bogduk 1985). Patients may have a warning of onset of headache via a pain or sensation in the neck (Fredriksen et al 1987).

Waking with headache is also common in migraine (Lance 1982, Rose 1988), cluster (Russell 1988), headaches associated with craniomandibular dysfunction (Reade & Steidler 1984) and, less frequently so, tension headache (Langemark et al 1988). However, cervical headaches do not build up to excruciating attacks as occurs with cluster or trigeminal neuralgia (Lance 1982, Russell 1988). Neither is there a warning or aura of focal neurological symptoms prior to the onset of headache that distinguishes the classic migraine (Rose 1988). Premonitory symptoms such as hunger or euphoria up to 24 hours before the headache also typify migraine.

Precipitating and relieving factors

Cervical headaches are typically precipitated or aggravated by sustained neck postures or movement (Edmeads 1978, Sjaastad et al 1983, Ehni & Benner 1984, Bogduk & Marsland 1986, Jull 1986a, Fredriksen et al 1987, Pfaffenrath et al 1987). Common reports are precipitation or aggravation of headache by sustained flexion postures working at a desk, sustained extension at hairdressers, or sustained rotation postures while talking in a group. Occasionally, patients cannot nominate a particular pattern.

Although neck postures and movements are highly associated with the onset or aggravation of cervical headache, care must be taken in certain circumstances with the interpretation of such precipitants. Neck movements have been shown to trigger attacks of chronic paroxysmal hemicrania and cluster headaches (Sjaastad et al 1982, Solomon et al 1989). A trigger aggravates or provokes but it does not always represent the cause of the headache.

Stress or tension may aggravate a cervical headache (Jull 1986a) but this provocative factor is common to many headache forms. Stress induced or stress-release situations are common precipitants of migraine (Rose 1988). Surprisingly, only 23% of the sample of 148 patients of Langemark et al (1988), regarded as having chronic tension headache, identified stress as a pronounced factor in their headache pattern.

Cervical headache patients often have difficulty in identifying factors which relieve their headaches. Many take analgesics, and a few will gain relief by lying down or changing their postures. A possible differential feature is that these patients gain no relief from migrainous drugs (Sjaastad et al 1986a, Fredriksen et al 1987, Anthony 1989). Neither do they have a classic response to medication in the way, for instance, that indomethacin has for chronic paroxysmal hemicrania (Russell 1988, Sjaastad 1988). Even though a high percentage of cervical headache patients report taking some form of analgesics (Jull 1986a), once the headache has become of sufficient intensity or chronicity, analgesics and anti-inflammatory drugs often offer little relief (Edeling 1982, Mayer et al 1985).

General medical history

A thorough medical appraisal of current and past general health and a careful screen of each body system is necessary in the differential diagnosis of headache (Lance 1982). Cervical headache typically is a disorder arising from the musculoskeletal system and medical specialist examination for headache-related disorders in other systems is usually normal. The exception is that a cervical headache patient may suffer concurrently from migraine (Pfaffenrath et al 1987).

Family history

Knowledge of the patient's family history of headache can be informative. There is a reasonably strong familial tendency for migraine and tension headache (Lance 1982, Andersson 1985, Rose 1988). In contrast, a family history is virtually absent in cluster headache (Andersson 1985, Russell 1988) and this would also appear to be the case in those persons with cervical headache (Fredriksen et al 1987, Pfaffenrath et al 1987).

Age

The age of the person at onset of headache has limited diagnostic significance for many chronic benign headaches. Migraine most commonly presents in the second and third decades of life (Lance 1982, Rose 1988) and cluster and chronic paroxysmal hemicrania in the second to fourth decades (Russell 1988, Ryan & Ryan 1990). There can be variability.

The onset of cervical and tension headaches, and headaches associated with craniomandibular dysfunction, appears to be independent of age. Such headaches may begin at any time from childhood to old age (Nikiforow 1981, Gelb & Bernstein 1983, Forssell et al 1985, Wanman & Agerberg 1986, Fredriksen et al 1987, Pfaffenrath et al 1987, Langemark et al 1988). The age of presentation for management of cervical headache seems to be more common in the third, fourth and fifth decades (Jull 1986a, Jaeger 1989). When the headache is associated with arthrosis of the cervical joints, the patients are generally in the older age group (Anthony 1989).

Gender

The factor of gender is interesting. There is a clear gender association in cluster headache and chronic paroxysmal hemicrania with the former occurring predominantly in males and the latter in females (Russell 1988, Sjaastad 1988, Saper 1989). While males may suffer the other forms of headache, there is a consistent female preponderence in migraine, cervical and tension headaches, and headaches of craniomandibular dysfunction.

History of onset of headache

Patients will present with cervical headaches of weeks, months or quite commonly, several years duration (Jull 1986a, Fredriksen et al 1987, Pfaffenrath et al 1987, Jaeger 1989). A protracted history of headache can also occur with tension, migraine and headache associated with craniomandibular dysfunction (Friedman 1979, Reade & Steidler 1984). With the substantial overlap of symptoms and even temporal patterns of these benign and often chronic headaches, a careful analysis of the onset of headache is required to assist further in differential diagnosis.

The two most commonly nominated provocative causes of cervical headache are degenerative joint disease and trauma to the upper cervical articulations. The trauma may relate to a specific injury or may be of a more insidious nature resulting from accumulation of microstrain (microtrauma) (Dugan et al 1962, Treyor-Jones 1964, Braaf & Rosner 1975, Bogduk 1986b, Sjaastad et al 1986a, Fredriksen et al 1987). Classically the onset of migraine and tension headache are not related to cervical trauma or strain (Lance 1982, Langemark et al 1988). The picture is more complex in cases of headache of craniomandibular dysfunction because of the possible involvement of the temporomandibular joint in injury such as whiplash and the close interrelationship of this complex and the cervical spine in normal function and dysfunction (Weinberg & Lapointe 1987, Kraus 1988).

Studies of cervical headache patients indicate that approximately half of the patients can either directly relate headache onset to neck or head trauma or have a past history of relevant neck injury (Braaf & Rosner 1975, Jull 1986a, Fredriksen et al 1987, Pfaffenrath et al 1987). Braaf and Rosner (1975) consider that this figure is probably higher as often patients cannot recall an incident — especially when it is not directly related to their headache onset. Clinicians are very familiar with the patient who, on initial presentation, will adamantly report that there was no incident to account for their symptoms but on the second or third treatment will ask whether some past event or activity could be relevant to their condition.

For as many patients who report known trauma, there are those who have an insidious onset of headache. In middle-aged and older patients, this would be consistent with the development of degenerative joint disease (Trevor-Jones 1964). These patients often report a past history of increasingly frequent neck and shoulder aching and stiffness.

The factor of accumulation of microtrauma, not always appreciated by the patient, is probably a very relevant feature of seemingly insidious onset cervical headache. Microtrauma can be caused by poor habitual static or work postures, sustained neck positions or poor postures and movement patterns (Lewit 1977, Janda 1988, Sahrmann 1988). It is now believed that this effect of repetitive fatigue loading could be the most pertinent factor in the onset of spinogenic pain and pathology (Goel et al 1988). A careful analysis of the patient's movement patterns and work habits is essential for identifying factors causing microtrauma.

The occurrence of a headache continuum, combined headaches and the transition of migraine into a different form over time is well recognized. This associated or eventual headache is usually ascribed to the tension or muscle contraction variety (Lance 1982, Saper 1982, Langemark et al 1988). However, this blanket categorization into tension headache needs to be challenged. The reactive spasm of muscles such as the upper trapezius and other cervical paravertebral muscles, to the head pain, will induce mechanical stress and strain on the cervical articular structures. This is feasibly another mechanism of accumulation of microtrauma which over time, could set up an arthropathy in cervical joints. Indeed this situation is commonly encountered in clinical practice. Management of the cervical dysfunction can substantially influence the headache pattern.

Summary

This review has recognized that symptoms alone do not uniquely characterize cervical headache as they may resemble many other headache forms. Nevertheless, accepting variability, there is a pattern which is very suggestive of cervical headache and would direct the clinician to a thorough examination of both cervical structures and function.

Area of pain. Pain is more likely to be located in the frontal, retro-orbital, occipital and temporal areas. The head pain is usually associated with neck pain. Pain may be unilateral, unilateral with spread, or bilateral. Headache does not change sides.

Quality of pain. An ache or dull boring pain and less frequently a throbbing quality is reported. It is often of moderate intensity but can be severe. It is not excruciating.

Associated symptoms. Nausea, blurred vision and other eye symptoms, dizziness or lightheadedness are not uncommon. When symptoms are unilateral, they are ipsilateral.

Neurological signs. These are rare. Occasionally sensory deficits are present in the distribution of C_2 or C_3.

Temporal pattern. Headaches can be episodic, lasting from a few hours to several days. They can be chronic, being either semicontinuous or present at least two to three times per week.

Time and mode of onset. Headaches may be present on waking or come on during the day. Neck pain either initiates or is precursive of headache.

Precipitating and relieving factors. Sustained neck postures or movements commonly provoke headache. Relieving factors are often difficult to recognize. Simple analgesics are often ineffective in chronic cervical headache.

History of onset. A prolonged history of headache is common. Onset may be insidious, consistent with cervical degenerative joint disease or accumulation of micro-trauma. A history of definitive neck trauma will be present in approximately 50% of cases.

Age and gender. Cervical headaches are more frequent in females than in males. Onset can be at any age from childhood to old age.

Family history. There is usually no significant familial tendency.

PHYSICAL SIGNS IN CERVICAL HEADACHE

As there is considerable overlap in symptomatology between many benign and chronic headache forms, the physical examination of the neck assumes considerable importance in the diagnosis of cervical headache.

The situation is not always simple and straightforward. Concurrent and significant neck pain is one criterion highly suggestive of cervical headache. As already appreciated, neck pain and aching may accompany many headache forms (Clark et al 1987, Drummond 1987, Saadah & Taylor 1987, Solomon et al 1989). When studying 648 subjects during a work screen assessment, Henry et al (1987) found that approximately one-third suffered from chronic headache of some form. While only 8% of the non-headache subjects had neck pain, it was reported by 41% of the heterogeneous headache group.

Thus the association of neck pain with headache is quite prevalent. Its presence, although suggestive, does not necessarily indicate a primary cervical cause. Palpable tenderness around the occipital, frontal and temporal areas as well as in the neck musculature is quite common and a non-specific sign of many headaches (Drummond 1987, Saadah & Taylor 1987, Langemark & Jensen 1988). Symptoms may result from the reactive muscle spasm to the pain of headache (Boquet et al 1989, Solomon et al 1989). On a more complex level, many different forms of headache relay through the trigeminocervical nucleus (Angus-Leppan et al 1989, Bogduk 1989a, Solomon et al 1989). This shared relay system explains the overlap in distribution of pain in many headache forms but it could also directly contribute to provoking neck muscle tenderness and perhaps secondary musculo-articular dysfunction.

The situation is complex but it is necessary to establish a pathognomonic criterion on which to base a diagnosis of cervical headache. That criterion based on current knowledge is symptomatic articular dysfunction manifest as a painful motion abnormality at a relevant segment in the cervical spine.

This singular diagnostic criterion must be understood with the knowledge that the nature of musculoskeletal dysfunction is such that there is rarely an isolated lesion but rather a co-involvement of many structures in a highly interrelated neuro-muscular-articular system. A cervical headache will also involve soft-tissue tenderness and muscle and movement dysfunction which may result from, or precede, the joint abnormality. However, in the differential diagnosis of cervical headache from other headaches with associated neck tenderness, it is the presence of the articular lesion which positively diagnoses the cervical headache or a cervical component of a headache continuum. (Headache Classification Committee of the International Headache Society 1988, Jull et al 1988, Bogduk 1989b).

The cervical structures which have access to the trigeminocervical nucleus and are thus capable of causing headache are those supplied by the upper three cervical nerves (Table 23.2). These include the articular, muscular and neural structures of the area as well as the upper portion of the vertebral artery. The other musculoskeletal structure which has access to the trigeminocervical nucleus is the temporomandibular complex.

Several specific musculoskeletal signs have been investigated in cervical headache subjects but as yet there has been no comprehensive study on the full nature of physical dysfunction. This is not a deficit unique to the categorization of cervical headache, but is also the problem associated with a credible diagnosis of tension headache (Olesen 1988).

Our understanding of the nature of physical dysfunction is continuing to grow. In this atmosphere it is pertinent to draw together both known facts and empirical views on the nature and variety of physical abnormalities in cervical headache. This will reveal physical criteria which are pertinent to or need to be considered in differential diagnosis as well as identifying areas in need of further research.

Articular dysfunction

The joints of the upper cervical complex (Table 23.2) are of primary importance in the production of cervical headache as, neuroanatomically, they are the segments capable of referring pain into the head. Segments distal to C_{2-3}

Table 23.2 Structures supplied by the C_1 C_2 and C_3 nerves

Articular structures	Atlanto-occipital joints (C_{0-1})
	Lateral and medial atlanto-axial joints (C_{1-2})
	C_{2-3} zygapophyseal joints; C_{2-3} disc craniovertebral ligaments
Muscles	
Dorsal ramus	Rectus capitus posterior minor
	Rectus capitus posterior major
	Obliquus capitus inferior
	Obliquus capitus superior
	Semispinalis capitus
	Longissimus capitus
	Splenus capitus
	Multifidus (upper fibres)
	Semispinalis cervicis (upper fibres)
Ventral ramus	Rectus capitus lateralis
	Rectus capitus anterior
	Longus capitus
	Longus colli (upper fibres)
	Sternocleidomastoid
	Upper trapezius
	Scalenus medius
	Levator scapulae (C_3)
Vascular structures	Upper portion of vertebral artery
Neural structures	Dura mater of upper spinal cord and posterior cranial fossa. (These structures are supplied by the cervical sinuvertebral nerves and the meningeal branches of the 10th and 12th cranial nerves.)

have pain distributions to the neck, shoulder and upper limb (Aprill et al 1990, Dwyer et al 1990). This is not to imply that patients may not present with involvement of the lower cervical and upper thoracic levels as part of the total musculoskeletal dysfunction. However, primary diagnosis is consistent with an abnormality in the upper cervical joints. (Trevor-Jones 1964, Ehni & Benner 1984, Mayer et al 1985, Bogduk & Marsland 1986, Pfaffenrath et al 1987, Jull et al 1988, Boquet et al 1989, Jaeger 1989). It is pertinent to dismiss the results of studies that reject cervical pathology as a causative factor of headache when only the lower cervical joints have been investigated (Iansek et al 1987).

There is not one discrete pathology of these joints which is pathognomonic of cervical headache. Rather it is a symptomatic motion abnormality which characterizes the headache (Sjaastad et al 1983, Jull et al 1988, Pfaffenrath et al 1988, Bogduk 1989b). This motion abnormality may result from direct joint trauma, chronic strain or degenerative arthrosis (Dugan et al 1962, Trevor-Jones 1964, Braaf & Rosner 1975, Ehni & Benner 1984, Anthony 1986, Bogduk & Marsland 1986). Other pathologies involving the upper cervical spine, such as rheumatoid arthritis and ankylosing spondylitis, may also be instrumental in headache (Edmeads 1978). The motion abnormality may present as symptomatic joint hypomobility, hypermobility or instability (Dugan et al 1962, Lewit

1971, Mayer et al 1985, Jull 1986a, Pfaffenrath et al 1988).

The cervical joints can be assessed by active movements, radiological examination and manual examination of passive intersegmental motion (Fig. 23.2). Active motion examination should always include those movements which more selectively stress the upper cervical articulations (see Ch. 37). Examination of cervical movements in various studies of cervical headache patients has consistently revealed the presence of pain and restriction in one or more directions of motion (Sjaastad et al 1983, Bogduk & Marsland 1986, Fredriksen et al 1987, Pfaffenrath et al 1987, Jaeger 1989). Crepitus with neck motion is commonly reported (Sjaastad et al 1983, Pfaffenrath et al 1987).

While restricted neck motion with pain (especially if neck movements provoke or aggravate the headache) is highly suggestive of a cervical cause of headache, there must still be an element of caution in interpretation. Neck pain and aching have been associated with other chronic headache forms and spasm of neck muscles may limit motion (Bogduk 1987). Additionally, neck movement has been shown to provoke attacks of chronic paroxysmal hemicrania and cluster headache (Sjaastad et al 1982, Solomon et al 1988). Furthermore, in patients with a vascular compression of the C_2 nerve root as the proven cause of headache, neck motion was restricted (Jansen et al 1989). Therefore, further examination is needed to differentiate a cervical articular cause of headache from a cervical trigger or reactive association. This necessitates examination of the cervical spine at the segmental level.

Radiographic examination is the method commonly employed in medical practice. Unfortunately the routine, standard plain views of the cervical spine have been

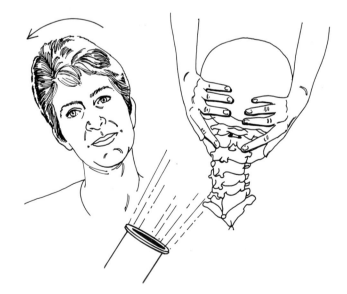

Fig. 23.2 The cervical joints are assessed actively, radiographically and by manual examination.

proven to be insensitive for positive diagnosis in cervical headache (Pfaffenrath et al 1987, 1988, Fredriksen et al 1989, Sluijter et al 1989). Likewise, computerized tomography (CT) of the neutral cervical spine in 11 confirmed cervical headache patients also failed to show any typical characteristic pathology as compared to a normal control group (Fredriksen et al 1989). A similar non-correlation between CT findings and clinical examination has been reported in a study of the temporomandibular joint (Tilds & Miller 1987).

The segmental motion abnormalities pathognomonic of cervical headache have been demonstrated on mobility radiographs of known cervical headache sufferers. Significantly, no differences were detected in segmental mobility between 15 cervical headache subjects and 18 controls when the commonly used clinical method of qualitative analysis was employed (Pfaffenrath et al 1987). However, when the axes of motion of the cervical segments were plotted using a computer-based technique, the motion abnormalities in the upper cervical joints were clearly demonstrated in the headache group (Mayer et al 1985, Pfaffenrath et al 1988).

Manual examination of intersegmental motion is the other method of assessment for painful segmental motion abnormalities. It is considered that this method could be one of the more valuable techniques in the differential diagnosis of cervical headache. This is so when recognizing that plain radiographs are valuable only as a screen against more sinister pathologies rather than a positive diagnostic aid for cervical headache. In addition, the more complex analyses of mobility radiographs will be used for selected patients only as will the other medical quantitative techniques of precise nerve blocks or intra-articular injections (Bogduk 1981b, Bogduk & Marsland 1986, Pfaffenrath et al 1987, Sluijter et al 1989). In contrast, manual examination is a low-cost, safe and non-invasive method of examination whose use can be employed on a widespread basis.

The value of a diagnostic technique is judged in terms of its sensitivity and specificity. An initial study has been undertaken investigating the accuracy of manual diagnosis for cervical zygapophyseal joint pain syndromes (Jull et al 1988). A manipulative physiotherapist's ability to judge whether or not a cervical zygapophyseal arthropathy was underlying patients' symptoms of headache, neck pain or neck and arm pain was evaluated in a single blind trial against a medical diagnosis established by radiologically-controlled diagnostic nerve blocks or intra-articular blocks. The 20 subjects were evaluated in two groups. The first group had an established medical diagnosis before later examination by the manipulative physiotherapist. The second were examined by the manipulative physiotherapist without prior medical diagnosis. The results revealed that there was complete concordance between medical and manual diagnosis with respect to segment and side of

the 15 patients with a zygapophyseal arthropathy and the one patient with a lateral atlanto-axial joint syndrome. Furthermore, in the four patients proven medically not to have a zygapophyseal joint problem causative of their pain the findings of manual diagnosis were also negative. These results are very positive but more extensive studies need to be undertaken.

In respect of manual examination, it is important to establish physical criteria on which a positive diagnosis of relevant segmental joint dysfunction is made for it has already been shown that the presence of slight joint hypomobility alone can be an asymptomatic, age-related occurrence (Jull 1986b). Those adopted and corroborated in the previous manual diagnosis study were: altered displacement, abnormal quality of physical resistance to joint motion and provocation of pain (local or referred) by the testing procedure.

As well as manually detected motion changes, positional anomalies of the atlas and axis have been noted in headache subjects. Jaeger (1989) found unilaterally tender and prominent transverse processes of the atlas in 7 of the 11 cervical headache subjects which she related to a positional rotation abnormality of C_1. Boquet et al (1989) in a radiographic study of 24 subjects (whose headaches had strong migraine traits but also some elements of cervical headache), found a contralateral rotation of C_2 with respect to the side of headache and neck tenderness. It was present in 15 of the 24 headache subjects as compared to five of the 24 control subjects. Jull (1986b) in a study of the upper cervical spine in 225 subjects of a general population, found a small incidence of rotation of C_2. When present, it was related to a motion abnormality at C_{2-3}. Asymmetrically prominent transverse processes of the atlas were also found in approximately half of the subjects but there was no significant relationship between this anomaly and movement dysfunction in the upper cervical joints. Further study is required to establish clearly the relevance of this positional deviation.

Neural tissue

Cervical headache, in the main, is a referred pain rather than one caused by compression of a nerve root or spinal nerve (Bogduk 1985). Compressive lesions do sometimes occur and are in evidence when sensory deficits are located particularly in the C_2 and C_3 distributions (Fredriksen et al 1987). Overt compressive lesions are often associated with instability at the atlanto-axial segment (Dugan et al 1962, Lance & Anthony 1980, Bertoft & Westerberg 1985).

Conventionally, neural tissue involvement is most often considered in terms of nerve irritation and compression. Over recent years there has been an explosion in knowledge of the mechanics and movements of the nervous system and the role of adverse mechanical tension as a source of musculoskeletal pain (see Chs 2, 43, 50).

Little attention to date, in research terms, has been directed towards the role of adverse mechanical tension in the neural tissues in the production of cervical headache. Clinical case histories have been presented (Rumore 1989), and with the routine inclusion of neural tissue tension tests (using the key element of upper cervical flexion) in the clinical examination of cervical headache patients, restriction of movement with reproduction of comparable head pain is not infrequently found. However, incidence data are lacking — as are descriptions of the precise neural mechanics in the upper cervical complex.

Nevertheless, when the anatomical substrates for neural tension and nerve entrapments are considered, the upper cervical, occipital complex is ripe for these disorders. The dura mater is attached to the foramen magnum and the body of C_2 (Williams et al 1989). The C_3 nerve exits through a tunnel and the nerves of the upper cervical plexus branch and penetrate through muscles and fascia. Additionally, there is surgical evidence of cervical headache being associated with fibrosis of the C_2 nerve root and fibrosis of the occipital nerve in its course before its perforation through the tendinous lamina of the upper trapezius muscle (Sjaastad et al 1986a, Jansen et al 1989). In the latter cases, an impingement of the occipital nerve seemed to have existed just at its site of penetration through the aponeurosis.

Although our knowledge of the role of adverse mechanical tension in the nervous system in cervical headache production is yet in its infancy, clinical observations suggest its presence is not rare. Current clinical research will hopefully clarify the role of this dysfunction and further add to the physical characterization of cervical headache.

Vertebral artery

The upper portion of the vertebral artery is supplied by the upper cervical nerves and arterial pathologies such as aneurysms could have a distribution of pain similar to a cervical headache. Headache is one possible symptom of vertebrobasilar insufficiency (VBI). When a patient presents with dizziness or any other possible VBI symptom associated with their headache, careful clinical screening is required before proceeding with treatment (Grant 1988, Aspinall 1989). Further medical investigation may be required.

Cervical pathology and movement can compromise the vertebral artery and be provocative of symptoms of VBI. However, earlier contentions that migraine headaches of cervical origin or 'migraine cervicale' were caused by mechanical irritation of the vertebral nerve has been challenged (Lance 1982, Sjaastad et al 1983). In this syndrome, termed posterior cervical sympathetic syndrome of Barré–Lieou, osteophytes or other cervical pathology were thought to irritate the vertebral nerve causing spasm of the vertebral artery and therefore brainstem ischaemia

(Gayral & Neuwirth 1954, Stewart 1962, Pawl 1977). However, a study of direct stimulation of the vertebral nerve in the monkey failed to show any change in blood flow in the vertebral artery (Bogduk et al 1981). As the term 'migraine cervicale' can be misleading and can confuse the entity of cervical headache, it has been recommended that it be abandoned (Sjaastad et al 1983).

Muscle dysfunction

Two issues need to be addressed when considering muscle dysfunction in cervical headache. The first is muscle as a source of local and referred pain and the second, the functional aspects of muscle and movement dysfunction.

Muscle tension and tenderness are non-specific signs of many headache forms (Langemark & Jensen 1988, Fricton 1989). Their presence should not automatically encourage a diagnosis of muscle contraction or tension headache. Electromyographic studies of muscle activity in subjects with muscle contraction headache, migraine headache and normal controls have produced conflicting results (Bakal & Kaganov 1977, Anderson & Franks 1981, Sutton & Belar 1982, Sturgis et al 1984). Increased muscle activity cannot be aligned to any headache form.

Trigger points (Travell & Simons 1983) are not uncommonly found in cervical headache subjects and are located in those muscles supplied by the C_{1-3} nerves (Table 23.2). Deep palpation of these points may produce the patient's headache (Jaeger 1989).

However it is doubtful whether trigger points are a primary pathology. Rather their pain is aggravated or perpetuated by factors which stress the muscle containing the trigger point (Graff-Radford et al 1987). These stressors may be physical — such as joint dysfunction, systemic or psychological factors.

The second aspect, that of muscle and movement dysfunction, is of primary importance when considering the full spectrum of musculoskeletal dysfunction in the pathogenesis and diagnosis of cervical headache. There is a wealth of clinical knowledge and theory on the nature of muscle and movement dysfunction and postural changes in painful disorders of the cranio-cervical, cervical and upper limb complex (Kendall et al 1952, Kendall & McCreary 1983, Janda 1986a,b, 1988, Sahrmann 1988, Richardson 1989). In common, these theories contend that imbalances in activity levels and lengths between different muscles either initiate or perpetuate (following trauma) poor movement patterns and postural changes. This imbalanced activity can alter the mechanics and load distribution on articular tissues causing adverse stress and chronic strain and pain. To compound the problem, the articular tissues often fail to receive sufficient protective support from the most appropriate muscles.

Clinical examination will reveal that some muscles (for example, upper trapezius levator scapulae, the short suboccipital extensors, the pectorals) may have become over-active and shortened. This can alter both posture and patterns of movement in the neck and shoulder girdle. Other muscles, particularly those which have an important role in cervical joint and shoulder girdle stabilization (for instance the deep cervical flexors, intrinsic neck extensors, and the mid- and lower trapezius) often lose their ability to control joint position in both static postures and movement. This has considerable influence on postural control and joint support and protection during functional activities.

The most commonly reported postural abnormality in patients with either cervical or cranio-cervical-mandibular dysfunction is that of a forward head posture (Gelb & Bernstein 1983, Ayub et al 1984, Jull 1988, Sakuta & Sakuta 1989, Watson 1990). Even though there is an ageing influence to the development of this posture (see Ch. 25), Watson (1990) in his study of 30 cervical headache subjects and 30 controls, found that the cervical headache sufferers had a significantly more forward head posture than did the non-headache group.

Weakness in the neck flexors has been found in patients with cervical pathology (Krout & Anderson 1966). In investigating other characteristics of muscle dysfunction in cervical headache patients, Watson (1990) found that the headache subjects exhibited significantly less strength and endurance in the upper cervical flexors when compared to the controls. Relevant to the clinical theory, the magnitude of the forward head posture was related to less endurance of the upper cervical flexors rather than their absolute strength.

Research into this area of movement and muscle dysfunction is difficult and comparatively, it is in its infancy. However, more controlled research is being undertaken which will hopefully further realize clinical theory. This research is also important in relation to differential diagnosis of headache. It is believed that the presence and co-existence of significant articular, muscle and movement dysfunction will most accurately characterize the true cervical headache from headaches of other causes which have neck aching and tenderness as associated symptoms.

THE COMPLEXITY OF DIAGNOSIS

The cervical spine can be a primary cause of headache. While there is symptomatic overlap with other forms, cervical headache is characterized by the presence of painful motion abnormalities in the upper three cervical joints. This joint dysfunction is accompanied by other physical signs of muscle and movement dysfunction. The incidence of cervical headache is unknown but the low frequency often reported could reflect insufficient or inadequate methods of investigation. Sluijter et al (1989) reclassified 12 of 20 patients previously diagnosed as tension headache to cervical headache based on results of nerve blocks and associated radiologically detected segmental motion abnormalities. Insufficient examination, or the 'loose' use of the term 'tension headache', has significant ramifications as the diagnostic title will influence the form of management instigated.

The complexity in diagnosis especially arises when the cervical spine has either an associated or secondary role or is a trigger for another form of headache. Migraine can change in character over time and it is considered that they often develop into a cervical headache (Pfaffenrath et al 1987). It is further believed that many of the migrainous headache continuums involve the element of cervical headache. When the cervical spine is a trigger for headaches such as migraine or chronic paroxysmal hemicrania clinically, segmental muscle spasm with associated loss of joint motion has been found on manual examination.

In such mixed headache forms, it is often difficult initially to assess or predict the contribution of the cervical spine and as yet many questions remain to be answered. In the clinical situation a key guideline would appear to be the magnitude of segmental joint signs and other signs of physical dysfunction elicited by examination. If a patient presents with a headache with clear migrainous features, and joint signs are found to be minimal, the cervical spine probably has a minor to negligible role in the headache. The reverse situation where significant joint dysfunction is present, is also encountered. When the cervical spine is considered to be a trigger rather than the cause of headache, it is wise to examine the patient in a headache-free period. At these times, often no joint dysfunction is found. While criticism is warranted against those who do not consider a cervical cause of headache, it is equally irresponsible for practitioners to treat headache patients where comparable and sufficient musculoskeletal signs are not present, or to continue treatment when beneficial changes in the headache pattern are not being achieved.

There is still much to be learnt about the precise nature of musculoskeletal dysfunction in cervical headache and, indeed, in other headache forms. As it is physiotherapists who have the knowledge and expertise in movement disorders and physical examination methods, it behoves us to meet the challenge of clearly characterizing cervical headache to assist in its future accurate diagnosis.

REFERENCES

Anderson C D, Franks R D 1981 Migraine and tension headache: is there a physiological difference. Headache 21: 63–71
Andersson P G 1985 Migraine in patients with cluster headache. Cephalalgia 5: 11–16

Angus-Leppan H, Lambert G A, Boers P, Lance J W, Zagami A S 1989 The cervical spinal cord is a relay centre for the central nervous system processing of input from the cranial vasculature. Cephalalgia 9 (suppl 10): 137–138

Anthony M 1986 Migraine and its management. Australian Family Physician 15: 643–649

Anthony M 1989 Occipital neuralgia. Cephalalgia 9 (suppl 10): 174–175

Aprill C, Dwyer A, Bogduk N 1990 Cervical zygapophyseal joint pain patterns II. A clinical evaluation. Spine 15: 458–461

Aspinall W 1989 Clinical testing for cervical mechanical disorders which produce ischemic vertigo. Journal of Orthopaedic and Sports Physical Therapy 11: 176–182

Ayub E, Glasheen-Wray M, Kraus S 1984 Head posture: a case study of the effects on rest position of the mandible. Journal of Orthopaedic and Sports Physical Therapy 5: 179–183

Bakal D A, Kaganov J A 1977 Muscle contraction and migraine headache: psychophysiological comparisons. Headache 17: 208–215

Bertoft E S, Westerberg C 1985 Further observations on the neck–tongue syndrome. Cephalalgia 5 (suppl) 312–313

Bezuur J N, Hansson Th, Wilkinson T M 1989 The recognition of craniomandibular disorders — an evaluation of the most reliable signs and symptoms when screening for CMD. Journal of Oral Rehabilitation 16: 367–372

Biber M P, Warfield C A 1986 Headache. Otolaryngologic Clinics of North America 19: 55–63

Bogduk N 1981a An anatomical basis for the neck–tongue syndrome. Journal of Neurology, Neurosurgery and Psychiatry 44: 202–208

Bogduk N 1981b Local anaesthetic blocks of the second cervical ganglion: a technique with application in occipital headache. Cephalalgia 1: 41–50

Bogduk N 1985 Greater occipital neuralgia. In: Long D M (ed) Current therapy in neurosurgery. Decker, Toronto, pp 175–180

Bogduk N 1986a Cervical causes of headache and dizziness. In: Grieve G P (ed) Modern manual therapy of the vertebral column. Churchill Livingstone, Edinburgh, pp 289–302

Bogduk N 1986b The anatomy and pathophysiology of whiplash. Clinical Biomechanics 1: 92–101

Bogduk N 1987 Headaches and cervical manipulation. A role in diagnosis. Patient Management June: 163–177

Bogduk N 1989a The anatomy of headache. In: Dalton M (ed) Proceedings of headache and face pain symposium. Manipulative Physiotherapists Association of Australia, Brisbane, pp 1–16

Bogduk N 1989b Cervical causes of headache. Cephalalgia 9 (suppl 10): 172–173

Bogduk N, Marsland A 1986 On the concept of third occipital headache. Journal of Neurology, Neurosurgery and Psychiatry 49: 775–780

Bogduk N, Lambert G, Duckworth J W 1981 The anatomy and physiology of the vertebral nerve in relation to cervical migraine. Cephalalgia 1: 1–14

Bogduk N, Corrigan B, Kelly P, Schneider G, Farr R 1985 Cervical headache. Medical Journal of Australia 143: 202–207

Boquet J, Boismare F, Payenneville G, Leclerc D, Monnier J C, Moore N 1989 Lateralisation of headache: possible role of an upper cervical trigger point. Cephalalgia 9: 15–24

Braaf M M, Rosner S 1975 Trauma of the cervical spine as a cause of chronic headache. Journal of Trauma 15: 441–446

Campbell D G, Parsons C M 1944 Referred head pain and its concomitants. Journal of Nervous and Mental Diseases 99: 544–551

Caviness V S, O'Brien P 1980 Current concepts in headache. New England Journal of Medicine 302: 446–449

Clark G T, Green E M, Dornan M R, Flack V F 1987 Craniocervical dysfunction levels in a patient sample from a temporomandibular joint clinic. Journal of American Dental Association 115: 251–256

Drummond P D 1987 Scalp tenderness and sensitivity to pain in migraine and tension headache. Headache 27: 45–50

Dugan M C, Locke S, Gallagher J R 1962 Occipital neuralgia in adolescents and young adults. The New England Journal of Medicine 267: 1166–1172

Dwyer A, Aprill C, Bogduk N 1990 Cervical zygapophyseal joint pain patterns I: a study in normal volunteers. Spine 15: 453–457

Edeling J 1982 The true cervical headache. South African Medical Journal 62: 531–534

Edeling J 1988 Manual therapy for chronic headache. Butterworths, London

Edmeads J 1978 Headache and head pain associated with diseases of the cervical spine. Medical Clinics of North America 62: 533–544

Ehni G, Benner B 1984 Occipital neuralgia and C$_1$–C$_2$ arthrosis. New England Journal of Medicine 310: 127

Feinstein B, Langton J N K, Jameson R M, Schiller F 1954 Experiments on referred pain from deep somatic tissues. Journal of Bone and Joint Surgery 36A: 981–987

Forssell H, Kirveskari P, Kangasniemi P 1985 Changes in headache after treatment of mandibular dysfunction. Cephalalgia 5: 229–236

Fredriksen T A, Sjaastad O 1987 Cervicogenic headache. A clinical entity. Cephalalgia 7 (suppl 6): 171–172

Fredriksen T A, Hovdal H, Sjaastad O 1987 'Cervicogenic headache': clinical manifestations. Cephalalgia 7: 147–160

Fredriksen T A, Fougner R, Tangerud A, Sjaastad O 1989 Cervicogenic headache. Radiographic investigations concerning head/neck. Cephalalgia 9: 139–146

Fricton J R 1989 Myofascial pain syndrome. Neurologic Clinics 7: 413–427

Friedman A P 1979 Nature of headache. Headache 19: 163–167

Gayral L, Neuwirth E 1954 Oto-neuro-opthalmologic manifestations of cervical origin. Posterior cervical sympathetic syndrome of Barre–Lieou. New York State Journal of Medicine 54: 1920–1926

Gelb H, Bernstein I 1983 Clinical evaluation of two hundred patients with temporomandibular dysfunction. Journal of Prosthetic Dentistry 49: 234–243

Goel V K, Voo L-M, Weinstein J N, Liu Y K, Okuma T, Njus G O 1988 Response to the ligamentous lumbar spine to cyclic bending loads. Spine 13: 294–300

Graaf-Radford S B, Reeves J L, Jaeger B 1987 Management of chronic headache and neck pain: effectiveness of altering factors perpetuating myofascial pain. Headache 27: 186–190

Grant R 1988 Dizziness testing and manipulation of the cervical spine. In: Grant R (ed) Physical therapy of the cervical and thoracic spine. Churchill Livingstone, New York, pp 111–124

Grieve G P 1988 Common vertebral joint problems. 2nd edn. Churchill Livingstone, Edinburgh

Hartsock C L 1940 Headache from arthritis of the cervical spine. Medical Clinics of North America 24: 329–333

Headache Classification Committee of the International Headache Society 1988 Classification and diagnostic criteria for headache disorders, cranial neuralgias and facial pain. Cephalalgia 8 (suppl 7): 1–96

Henry P, Dartigues J F, Puymirat E, Peytour P L, Lucas J 1987 The association cervicalgia–headaches: an epidemiologic study. Cephalalgia 7 (suppl 6): 189–190

Hildebrandt J, Jansen J 1984 Vascular compression of the C2 and C3 roots — yet another cause of chronic intermittent hemicrania. Cephalalgia 4: 167–170

Hunter C R, Mayfield F H 1949 Role of the upper cervical roots in the production of pain in the head. American Journal of Surgery 78: 743–751

Iansek R, Heywood J, Karnaghan J, Balla J I 1987 Cervical spondylosis and headaches. Clinical and Experimental Neurology 23: 175–178

Jaeger B 1989 Are 'cervicogenic' headaches due to myofascial pain and cervical spine dysfunction? Cephalalgia 9: 157–164

Jamieson M 1984 Headache. British Medical Journal 288: 1281–1283

Janda V 1986a Some aspects of extracranial causes of facial pain. Journal of Prosthetic Dentistry 56: 484–487

Janda V 1986b Muscle weakness and inhibition (pseudoparesis) in back pain syndromes. In: Grieve G P (ed) Modern manual therapy of the vertebral column. Churchill Livingstone, Edinburgh, pp 197–201

Janda V 1988 Muscles and cervical pain syndromes. In: Grant R (ed) Physical therapy of the cervical and thoracic spine. Churchill Livingstone, New York, pp 153–166

Jansen J, Markakis E, Rama B, Hildebrandt J 1989 Hemicranial attacks or permanent hemicrania — a sequel of upper cervical root compression. Cephalalgia 9: 123–130

Jull G A 1986a Headaches associated with the cervical spine — a clinical review. In: Grieve G P (ed) Modern manual therapy of the vertebral column. Churchill Livingstone, Edinburgh, pp 322–329

Jull G A 1986b Clinical observations of upper cervical mobility. In: Grieve G P (ed) Modern manual therapy of the vertebral column. Churchill Livingstone, Edinburgh, pp 315–321

Jull G A 1988 Headaches of cervical origin. In: Grant R (ed) Physical therapy of the cervical and thoracic spine. Churchill Livingstone, New York, pp 195–217

Jull G A, Bogduk N, Marsland A 1988 The accuracy of manual diagnosis for cervical zygapophysial joint pain syndromes. Medical Journal of Australia 148: 233–236

Kendall F P, McCreary E K 1983 Muscles, testing and function. 3rd edn. Williams & Wilkins, Baltimore

Kendall H O, Kendall F P, Boyton D A 1952 Posture and pain. Williams & Wilkins, Baltimore

Kerr F W L, Olafson R A 1961 Trigeminal and cervical volleys. Archives of Neurology 5: 171–178

Kraus S L 1988 Cervical influences on the craniomandibular region. In: Kraus S L (ed) TMJ disorders. Management of the craniomandibular complex. Churchill Livingstone, New York, pp 367–404

Krout R M, Anderson T P 1966 Role of anterior cervical muscles in production of neck pain. Archives of Physical Medicine and Rehabilitation 47: 603–611

Kudrow L, Esperanca P, Vijayan N 1987 Episodic paroxysmal hemicrania? Cephalalgia 7: 197–201

Lance J W 1982 Mechanism and management of headache. 4th edn. Butterworths, London

Lance J W 1986 Migraine and other headaches. Compass, Sydney

Lance J W, Anthony M 1980 Neck–tongue syndrome on sudden turning of the head. Journal of Neurology, Neurosurgery and Psychiatry 43: 97–101

Langemark M, Jensen K 1988 Myofascial mechanisms of pain. In: Olesen J, Edvinsson L (eds) Basic mechanisms of headache. Elsevier, Amsterdam, pp 332–341

Langemark M, Olesen J, Poulse D L, Bech P 1988 Clinical characteristics of patients with chronic tension headache. Headache 28: 590–596

Lewit K 1971 Ligament pain and antiflexion headache. European Neurology 5: 365–378

Lewit K 1977 Pain arising in the posterior arch of the atlas. European Neurology 16: 263–269

Maitland G D 1986 Vertebral manipulation. 5th edn. Butterworths, London

Mayer E Th, Herrmann G, Pfaffenrath V, Pollmann W, Auberger T 1985 Functional radiographs of the craniocervical region and the cervical spine. A new computer-aided technique. Cephalalgia 5: 237–243

Milne E 1989 The mechanism and treatment of migraine and other disorders of cervical and postural dysfunction. Cephalalgia 9 (suppl 10): 381–382

Nikiforow R C 1981 Headache in a random sample of 200 persons. A clinical study of a population in northern Finland. Cephalalgia 1: 99–107

Olesen J 1978 Some clinical features of the acute migraine attack. An analysis of 750 patients. Headache 18: 268–271

Olesen J 1988 Clinical characterisation of tension headache. In: Olesen J, Edvinsson L (eds) Basic mechanisms of headache. Elsevier, Amsterdam, pp 9–14

Olesen J, Langemark M 1988 Mechanisms of tension headache: a speculative hypothesis. In: Olesen J, Edvinsson L (eds) Basic mechanisms of headache. Elsevier, Amsterdam, pp 458–461

Parker G B, Tupling H, Pryor D S 1978 A controlled trial of cervical manipulation for migraine. Australian and New Zealand Medical Journal 8: 589–593

Parker G B, Pryor D S, Tupling H 1980 Why does migraine improve during a clinical trial? Further results from a trial of cervical manipulation for migraine. Australian and New Zealand Medical Journal 10: 192–198

Pawl R P 1977 Headache, cervical spondylosis and anterior cervical fusion. Surgery Annual 9: 391–408

Peters K S 1984 Headache-diagnosis and effective management. Western Journal of Medicine 140: 957–960

Pfaffenrath V, Dandekar R, Pollmann W 1987 Cervicogenic headache — the clinical picture, radiological findings and hypothesis on its pathophysiology. Headache 27: 495–499

Pfaffenrath V, Dandekar R, Mayer E Th, Hermann G, Pollman W 1988 Cervicogenic headache: results of computer-based measurements of cervical spine mobility in 15 patients. Cephalalgia 8: 45–48

Reade P C, Steidler N E 1984 Temporomandibular joint pain-

dysfunction syndrome: a common form of headache. Patient Management 8: 56–71

Richardson C A 1989 Rehabilitation of muscular dysfunction. In: Dalton M (ed) Proceedings of headache and face pain symposium. Manipulative Physiotherapists Association of Australia, Brisbane, pp 94–101

Rose F C 1988 Clinical characterisation of migraine. In: Olesen J, Edvinsson L (eds) Basic mechanisms of headache. Elsevier, Amsterdam, pp 3–8

Rumore A J 1989 Slump examination and treatment in a patient suffering headache. Australian Journal of Physiotherapy 35: 262–263

Russell D 1988 Clinical characterisation of the cluster headache syndrome. In: Olesen J, Edvinsson L (eds) Basic mechanisms of headache. Elsevier, Amsterdam, pp 15–23

Ryan R E, Ryan R E 1990 Cluster headaches. In: Jacobson A L, Donlon W C (eds) Headache and facial pain. Raven Press, New York, pp 109–125

Saadah H, Taylor F B 1987 Sustained headache syndrome associated with tender occipital nerve zones. Headache 27: 201–205

Sahrmann S A 1988 Postural applications in the child and adult. Neurodevelopment aspects. In: Kraus S L (ed) TMJ disorders. Management of the craniomandibular complex. Churchill Livingstone, New York, pp 295–309

Sakuta M, Sakuta Y 1989 Drooping head syndrome: significance of flexed posture and neck instability as a cause of muscle contraction headache. Cephalalgia 9 (suppl 10): 119–120

Saper J R 1982 The mixed headache syndrome: a new perspective. Headache 22: 284–286

Saper J R 1989 Chronic headache syndromes. Neurologic Clinics 7: 387–411

Sjaastad O 1988 Cluster headache and its variants. Headache 28: 667–668

Sjaastad O, Dale I 1974 Evidence for a new (?) treatable headache entity. Headache 14: 105–108

Sjaastad O, Russell D, Saunte C, Horven I 1982 Chronic paroxysmal hemicrania VI. Precipitation of attacks. Further studies on the precipitation mechanism. Cephalalgia 2: 211–214

Sjaastad O, Saunte C, Hovdahl H, Breivik H, Gronbaek E 1983 'Cervicogenic' headache. An hypothesis. Cephalalgia 3: 249–256

Sjaastad O, Saunte C, Graham J R 1984 Chronic paroxysmal hemicrania VII. Mechanical precipitation of attacks: new cases and localisation of trigger points. Cephalalgia 4: 113–118

Sjaastad O, Fredriksen T A, Stolt-Nielsen A 1986a Cervicogenic headache, C2 rhizopathy and occipital neuralgia: a connection? Cephalalgia 6: 189–195

Sjaastad O, Aasly J, Fredriksen T A, Wysocka Bokowska M 1986b Chronic paroxysmal hemicrania: on autonomic involvement. Cephalalgia 6: 113–124

Sjaastad O, Fredriksen T A, Sand T 1989a The localisation of the initial pain of attack: a comparison between classic migraine and cervicogenic headache. Functional Neurology 4: 73–78

Sjaastad O, Fredriksen T A, Sand T, Antonaci F 1989b Unilaterality of headache in classic migraine. Cephalalgia 9: 71–77

Sluijter M E, Rohof O J, Vervest A C 1989 Cervical headache — diagnosis with the aid of computerised analysis of cervical mobility. Cephalalgia 9 (suppl 10): 199–200

Solomon S, Lipton R B, Newman L 1989 Nucal features of cluster headaches. Cephalalgia 9 (suppl 10): 201–202

Stewart D Y 1962 Current concepts of 'Barre syndrome' or 'posterior cervical sympathetic syndrome'. Clinical Orthopaedics and Related Research 24: 40–48

Sturgis E T, Schaefer C A, Ahles T A, Sikora T L 1984 Effect of movement and position in the evaluation of tension headache and nonheadache control subjects. Headache 24: 88–93

Sutton E P, Belar C D 1982 Tension headache patients versus controls: a study of EMG parameters. Headache 22: 133–136

Tilds B N, Miller P R 1987 Radiographic pathology of temporomandibular joints and head pain. Headache 27: 427–430

Travell J G, Simons D G 1983 Myofascial pain and dysfunction. The trigger point manual. Williams & Wilkins, Baltimore

Trevor-Jones R 1964 Osteoarthritis of the paravertebral joints of the second and third cervical vertebrae as a cause of occipital headache. South African Medical Journal 38: 392–394

Wanman A, Agerberg G 1986 Headache and dysfunction of the masticatory system in adolescents. Cephalalgia 6: 247–255

Watson D H 1990 Cervical headache: an investigation of natural head posture and upper cervical flexor muscle performance. Thesis, South Australian Institute of Technology, Australia

Weeks R E, Rapoport A M 1987 A critical look at reliability of headache diagnosis. Annals of Neurology 22: 148–149 (abstract)

Weinberg S, Lapointe H 1987 Cervical extension–flexion injury (whiplash) and internal derangement of the temporomandibular joint. Journal of Oral and Maxillofacial Surgery 45: 653–656

Williams P L, Warwick R, Dyson M, Bennister L A (eds) 1989 Gray's anatomy. 37th edn. Churchill Livingstone, Edinburgh

Winston K R 1987 Whiplash and its relationship to migraine. Headache 27: 452–457

Wolff's headache and other head pain 1972 Revised by Dalessio D J. 3rd edn. Oxford University Press, New York

Ziegler D K, Stephenson-Hassanein R, Couch J R 1982 Headache syndromes suggested by statistical analysis of headache symptoms. Cephalalgia 2: 125–134

24. Cervical headache: an investigation of natural head posture and upper cervical flexor muscle performance

D. H. Watson

INTRODUCTION

Clinical observations suggest that forward head posture (FHP) and weakness of the upper cervical flexor musculature are associated with, and co-exist in, the cervical headache patient (Janda 1988, Jull 1988). An extensive search of the literature failed to reveal any research to support these observations.

Assessment of sagittal head and neck posture is measured in the clinical situation by observation. The subjectivity of this form of assessment and the absence of any documented range of normal values have been addressed recently (Dalton 1987, Coutts 1988) (see Ch. 25) but to the author's knowledge there were no published values for subjects with cervical headache.

The current clinical tests for assessing upper cervical flexor muscle performance involves observation of lifting the head in supine, with, and without, manual resistance (Janda 1983, Kendall & McCreary 1983). There is some doubt as to whether these tests adequately and selectively assess their performance. Furthermore, manual muscle testing introduces subjectivity to assessment, the grading of such depending on the therapist's experience and educational background.

In 1988, Janda stated that our knowledge of the deeply placed upper cervical flexor musculature was inadequate. Objective appraisal of this group of muscles until recently has been lacking, possibly because they are difficult to study in isolation from the longer, more superficially placed, neck-on-thorax flexors. Recent studies by Fulton (1988) and Barber (1989) have addressed this area by establishing normative data (in males and females respectively) for isometric strength and endurance of the upper cervical flexors using equipment designed and developed by the author in 1988.

On the basis of this information a study was designed to:

1. develop equipment capable of accurately measuring isometric strength and endurance of the upper cervical flexor musculature
2. investigate and document the relationship between a cervical headache and non-headache population with respect to:
   a. natural head posture (NHP)
   b. isometric strength of the upper cervical flexor musculature
   c. isometric endurance of the upper cervical flexor musculature
   d. determining whether a relationship exists between NHP and upper cervical flexor muscle performance.

THE STUDY

Subjects

A sample of convenience comprising 60 female subjects aged between 25 and 40 years participated in the study. They were assigned to two equal groups.

The headache group comprised subjects who were currently experiencing recurring headache which was of at least five years duration. At the time of testing they had been experiencing more than one headache per month and were not receiving treatment. The non-headache group comprised subjects without cervical pain and who either did not experience headache, or if they did, the frequency of headache was one or less per month.

While the full extent of contributory determinants of head and neck posture are not yet fully known (Vig et al 1983), the relationship between cervical posture and dysfunction of the cervical spine and temporomandibular joints, mandibular and hyoid postion, dento-alveolar and craniofacial morphology and respiration has been widely researched. Conversely, there is a paucity of studies relating cervical posture to the visual, auditory and vestibular systems. However, Vig et al (1980) have suggested that the maintenance of NHP could be expected to be influenced by the physiological requirements of these systems. Therefore, to ensure that NHP was influenced as little as possible by these factors, subjects were excluded if they had experienced, or were experiencing, one or more of the following:

- a dental prosthesis or more than four false teeth
- a history of cervical or facial fractures/trauma including cervical or temporomandibular surgery
- recurrent middle-ear infections over the previous five years
- persistent respiratory difficulties over the previous five years which had necessitated absence from work, required long-term medication, or had interfered with their daily activities
- any visual impairment not corrected by glasses
- any hearing impairment requiring the use of a hearing aid
- any bony abnormalities of the spine—for example, scoliosis
- any disease or condition of the central nervous system—for example, multiple sclerosis, meningitis
- any systemic arthritis—for example, rheumatoid arthritis

Method

The subjects were examined using the same protocol:

1. lateral photographs of NHP
2. isometric strength testing of the upper cervical flexor musculature
3. isometric endurance testing of the upper cervical flexor musculature
4. passive accessory intervertebral movement (PAIVM) examination
5. completion of a questionnaire by the headache subjects.

The headache status of each subject was not revealed until completion of the PAIVM examination, neither was the presence or absence of history of cervical pain. If a non-headache patient reported cervical pain that had necessitated absence from work, required long-term medication or had interfered with their normal daily activities in the previous five years, they were excluded from the study. Those headache subjects who had experienced mid- to low-cervical pain as above were also excluded from the study.

Natural head posture

The method used to attain NHP—the 'self balance position'—was described by Solow and Tallgren (1971) and has been used by Siersbaeck-Nielsen and Solow (1982), Goldstein et al (1984), Dalton (1987) and Coutts (1988). The 'self balance position' was achieved by the subject performing large amplitude cervical flexion and extension gradually decreasing to rest in the most comfortably balanced position.

The reference points used in this study were the same as those used by Wickens and Kiputh (1973), Cureton (1941), Goldstein et al (1984), Dalton (1987), Coutts

(1988) and Braun and Amundsen (1989). The tragus of the ear was clearly marked, and a plastic pointer taped to the skin overlying the spinous process of C7. On confirmation that the subject, who was seated, had achieved NHP, a lateral photograph was taken ensuring that a gravity-defined vertical (plumb line) was clearly visible. The subject was then asked to stand, walk around the room, resume sitting, and repeat the procedure after which another photograph was taken.

The angle between a horizontal line through the spinous process of C7 and a line from the spinous process of C7 through the tragus of the ear formed the craniovertebral (CV) angle. The CV angle of each photograph was measured using a transparent plastic overlay developed by Coutts (1988). The overlay was positioned on the photograph so that the junction of the perpendicular lines of the protractor image was directly over the base of the pointer on the spinous process of C7. At the same time, the closely arranged parallel lines were aligned parallel to, or on, the gravity-defined vertical. A transparent straight edge was then aligned to join the tragus of the ear and the base of the pointer on the C7 spinous process (Fig. 24.1). The CV angle was measured in degrees directly from the protractor image.

Performance of the upper cervical flexor musculature

The equipment to assess performance of the upper cervical flexor musculature was designed and developed for this study by the author in collaboration with Mr Phillip Walker, a Senior Technical Officer (Electronics).

During development of the equipment, isolation of the action to head-on-neck flexion was of critical importance. Other factors that required consideration were the type of contraction that would best assess the upper cervical flexor musculature, the axis of movement of head-on-neck flexion, and the influence of possible concomitant tightness of the upper cervical extensors.

The author chose to design equipment that would measure the isometric capacity of the upper cervical flexors given their predominately stabilizing, postural role (Richardson 1989). Whilst the axis of upper cervical flexion is considered to be in the vicinity of the occipital condyles (Kapandji 1974), the precise location for testing purposes is difficult, notwithstanding the changing axis as the occipital condyles roll and slide (Bogduk 1985). This source of error was minimized by testing the isometric function of the upper cervical flexors. Similarly, the affect of any tightness of the upper cervical extensors would also be minimized if it could be demonstrated that these muscles were not tight in the testing position of the subject's head.

In brief, the equipment consisted of a plinth with a moveable head section. Subjects performed head-on-neck flexion against the resistance offered by a metal bar which

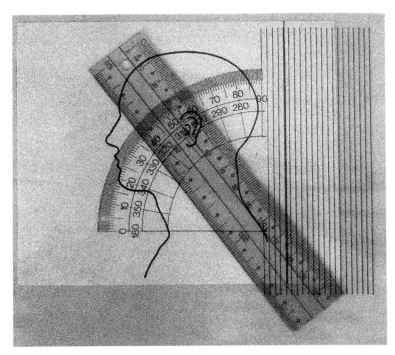

Fig. 24.1 The craniovertebral (CV) angle. The angle is read directly from a photograph using a protractor image and a straight edge. *Note.* A line diagram has been substituted for a photograph.

was rigidly attached to the plinth. Deflection of the bar, which was of the order of 1 cm or less, was detected by four strain gauges mounted 50 mm from the pivot point.

Subjects were positioned supine on the plinth with their hips and knees flexed to approximately 90°, with their legs being supported on a stool. The stool was placed on a board so that its castors could move freely. Subjects could increase the pressure on the chin bar if they combined upper cervical flexion with a caudad movement of their trunk. The latter was prevented by having their legs supported on the freely mobile stool and by placing a rolled-up towel under the sacrum to maintain a flattened lumbar spine. Similarly, to prevent subjects from using their scapulae to pull their trunk in a caudad direction they were asked to fold their arms to hold the opposite shoulder (Fig. 24.2).

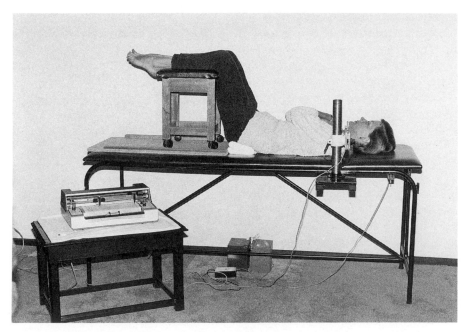

Fig. 24.2 The position of the subject for testing the upper cervical flexor musculature.

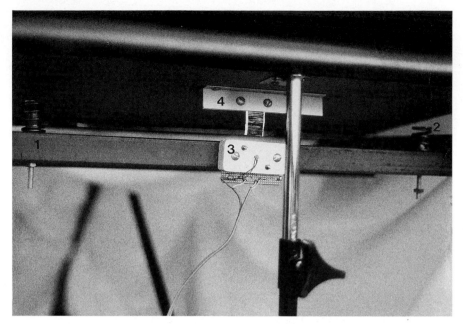

Fig. 24.3 The head support section. The hinged head support has been lifted to illustrate: 1 and 2: the spring support system; 3: the displacement sensor; 4: the clamp arrangement holding the blanking aluminium tape.

Isolation of head-on-neck flexion was ensured by constant monitoring of pressure of the subject's head on the head section of the plinth. This was monitored by a displacement sensor which was fixed to the frame of the plinth, mid-way between two springs which supported the head section (Fig. 24.3). At a corresponding point on the under surface of the head section, a piece of tape was mounted in position so that, with the subject in position, it partially blocked the light passing from the light-emitting diode (LED) to the light-dependent resistor (LDR) (Figs 24.3, 24.4). The dismantled displacement sensor illustrates the sandwich arrangement which enabled the tape to partially block light from the LED to the LDR (Fig. 24.5). If pressure on the hinged section of the plinth was increased or lessened, the blanking tape (by way of the spring support system) covered more or less of the LDR, which allowed less or more light, respectively, to pass from the LED to the LDR. The voltage from a voltage divider, of which the LDR formed a part, indicated this variation. Any variation was recorded by a dual channel chart recorder and reflected the change in pressure on the head section. If a variation was noted, subjects were requested to alter their action accordingly to maintain their initial resting head pressure.

The position of the subject's head was determined by performing large-amplitude flexion and extension movements (with their head remaining in contact with the plinth) with decreasing amplitude until they found their most comfortable position. Having attained this position the examiner passively flexed the head-on-neck to ensure that the posterior cervical musculature was not tight,

whilst simultaneously demonstrating the action required during testing. The position of comfort was then assumed once more.

Prior to testing, the subjects were given a routine set of instructions which included the maintenance of a teeth-clenched position and constant head pressure on the

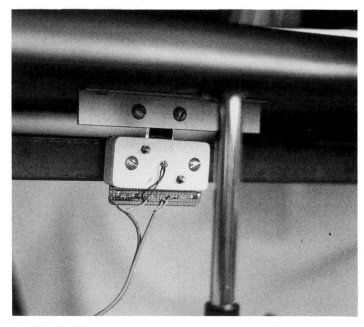

Fig. 24.4 The starting position of the blanking tape. The tape has entered the gap between LED and LDR partially blocking light from the LED to the LDR.

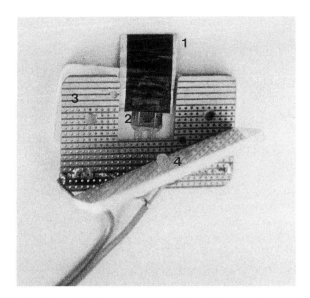

Fig. 24.5 The sandwich arrangement of the displacement sensor. The displacement sensor has been dismantled to illustrate: 1: the blanking aluminium tape; 2: the LDR; 3: the intervening veroboard; 4: the LED. Refer to the text for further explanation.

plinth, to keep the rest of the body relaxed and not to hold their breath during testing.

Strength testing was completed before endurance testing because it was considered that fatigue following endurance may have affected maximum values in the subsequent strength measurement. In order to familiarize themselves with the action required and the equipment, each subject was allowed three sub-maximal trial contractions before testing commenced. A 30-second rest interval was then taken prior to the actual testing. The subjects were then instructed to tuck their chin towards their throat as hard as they could in a smooth co-ordinated action, and, when they had completed this, to relax. Three maximum voluntary contractions (MVCs) were performed, each separated by a 30-second interval.

A rest period of 30 seconds was taken before endurance testing commenced. Instruction for endurance testing was the same as for strength except that the subject was asked to maintain the chin-tuck position for as long as possible.

In this study, uniform verbal commands and encouragement of a set volume (higher than normal conversation) were given. During endurance testing this involved encouragement to keep the chin tucked in and ongoing feedback as to head pressure status.

Those subjects unable to maintain an even head pressure were excluded from the study. Similarly, any subject who experienced neck pain, headache or facial pain during testing was also excluded.

The values for strength and endurance were calculated from the recordings of the chart recorder (Fig. 24.6). The highest value of three maximum voluntary contractions was taken as the muscle strength of the subject and was

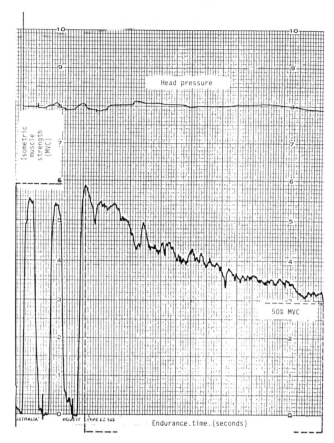

Fig. 24.6 Dual-channel chart strip recording illustrating the MVC, endurance and the monitoring of head pressure. This recording represents an MVC of 5.9 kp and an endurance value of 94 s.

measured in kiloponds (kps) from the Y axis. Endurance was deemed to be the time taken for the subject to fatigue to 50% of the commencing MVC. This was measured in seconds and was calculated from the X axis. Any alteration of the head pressure on the plinth was shown by deviation on the Y axis at the top of the recording (Fig. 24.6). This was designed to record head pressure alteration only and, as such, did not present a nominal value of the pressure on the head section of the plinth.

PAIVM examination

In relation to cervical headache, a PAIVM examination has been shown reliably to incriminate the symptomatic joint or joints (Jull & Bogduk 1985). As the symptomatic joint or joints will be located in the 0-C3 complex (Jull 1988), a PAIVM examination of the upper three cervical levels was performed to indicate whether the cervical spine was the possible cause of, or strongly implicated in, the subject's headache syndrome.

Each measurement was made by the examiner performing postero-anterior (PA) accessory gliding movements unilaterally on the left and right articular pillars of C1, C2 and centrally on the posterior tubercle of C1 and spinous processes of C2 and C3. Differentiation between the C1–2 and C2–3 joints was performed by repeating PA pressures on the articular pillar of C2 with the head in 30° of ipsilateral rotation. Transverse pressure on the tip of the transverse process of the atlas with the subject's head turned to the same side was also assessed. For a more detailed description of these procedures, the reader is referred to Maitland (1977) pages 34–41 and 88–101.

Mobility was graded on a five-point scale. Grade 3 was considered normal, while grade 4 was classified as hypomobile; very hypomobile was graded as 5. Conversely, grade 2 indicated hypermobility, and grade 1 considerably hypermobile. A symptomatic response was also recorded— no discomfort, local pain, local pain and headache, and headache only.

If on completion of the PAIVM examination, comparable joint signs, that is, altered displacement, abnormal quality of resistance, and provocation of local or referred pain, were not found in a headache subject, they were excluded from the study.

Questionnaire

The headache subjects then completed a questionnaire which provided information as to the description and behaviour of their headache. The questionnaire was designed to incorporate the features described by Edeling (1986) and Jull (1986), and included the area, quality, intensity, frequency and duration of symptoms, associated symptoms, history and precipitating and relieving (including response to analgesics) factors.

The purpose of this information was two-fold. Firstly, if the information provided suggested the presence of classic migraine, for example, the presence of any neurological prodroma or aura, or features characteristic of cluster-type headache, the subject was excluded from the study. Secondly, it is recognized that the sample population is small and for any reasonable extrapolations to be made regarding the results of this study to cervical headache patients, the profile of participating subjects should be determined and be consistent with those established by Edeling (1986) and Jull (1986) from their larger samples of 120 and 96 patients respectively.

Reliability

To calculate intra-examiner reliability for each section of the study, 12 subjects were examined on two separate occasions with 24 hours separating each examination.

The data for the CV angle was analysed using the Pearson correlation coefficient. From Table 24.1 it is evident that high correlation coefficients were obtained showing strong agreement. These significance levels were quoted on the null hypothesis H0: true correlation is 0.90, versus the one-sided alternative H1: true correlation

Table 24.1 Intra-examiner reliability for measuring the CV angle, from set up to recording CV angle, on two separate occasions using Fisher's Z transformation

CV angle	r	Significance level on HI: correlation >0.90
CV angle 1–1 and CV angle 1–2	0.982	$P < 0.005$
CV angle 2–1 and CV angle 2–2	0.989	$P < 0.0004$
CV angle 1–1 and CV angle 2–1	0.973	$P < 0.03$
CV angle 1–2 and CV angle 2–2	0.985	$P < 0.002$

exceeds 0.90. This test assumes a reasonable criterion in that 90% correlation is a requirement for reliable measurement. On this basis, the significance values presented in Table 24.1 were obtained using Fisher's Z-transformation (Kendall & Stuart 1960).

The Pearson correlation coefficient calculated for strength by strength on two occasions revealed strong agreement ($r = 0.931$). This is significantly greater than 0.7071 ($P = 0.01$). At the level of $r^2 = 0.7071$ ($r = 0.5$, coefficient of determination), 50% of the variation in one of strength 1, and strength 2, is explained by the variation in the other (the rest being due to unexplained or sampling variability). An analysis of variance performed on the values of strength by subject demonstrated that the difference in values between subjects was significantly greater than any difference between the two occasions ($F = 24.53$, $P = 0.000$). Pearson correlation coefficient and analysis of variance calculations for endurance produced similar results ($r = 0.931$; $F = 22.7, P = 0.000$).

The results of the analysis of variance and correlation coefficients demonstrated high intra-examiner reliability in muscle strength and endurance testing.

The data from the PAIVM examination was analysed using Cohen's Kappa and this revealed perfect agreement in 17 of the 22 tests ($K = 1.0$). A Kappa score of greater than 0.7 may be regarded as indicating very good agreement (Bishop et al 1975). Of the five remaining tests the lowest Kappa score was $K = 0.667$ ($P = 0.01$) which indicates good agreement. The other scores were all $K > 0.7$, the highest non-perfect score was $K = 0.8$ ($P = 0.002$) indicating very strong agreement.

In view of these results it was considered that the examiner was consistent and provided a valid measurement for comparison of the symptomatic and asymptomatic categories.

RESULTS

PAIVM examination

The subject's headache was reproduced in 12 subjects.

Table 24.2 illustrates the frequency of positive joint findings from the headache and non-headache groups. The subjects with headache clearly had more positive joint findings. Also, in both groups the incidence of positive joint findings found with central tests was much less frequent than those performed unilaterally The incidence of positive joint findings for the headache group demonstrated a greater involvement at 0–C1 (100%), when compared with C2–3, and was considerably less at C1–2.

Table 24.2 The incidence of positive joint findings in the headache (*n* = 30) and non-headache (*n* = 30) groups

PAIVM	Level	Non-headache (*n* = 30)	Headache (*n* = 30)
Central P/A	C1	1	8
	C2	7	17
	C3	5	15
Unilateral P/A	C1	16	30
	C2	15	26
	C1–2	1	2
	C2–3	14	24
Transverse	C1	12	21

Questionnaire

The profile of participating headache subjects closely resembled the larger studies of Edeling (1986) and Jull (1986). The only major discrepancy was a higher incidence (63.6%) of a throbbing/pulsating pain in the current study (Table 24.3).

Table 24.3 Quality of pain experienced by cervical headache subjects: a comparison of the findings of the present study with those of Edeling (1986) and Jull (1986)

Quality of pain	Percentage of subjects		
	Edeling (1986) (*n* = 120)	Jull (1986) (*n* = 96)	Watson (1990) (*n* = 30)
Ache	–	73.9	66.6
Throbbing/pulsating	18.3	7.0	63.6
Sharp/stabbing	27.5	5.2	20.0
Heaviness	11.0	5.2	16.6
Tightness	19.1	8.3	16.6
Thickness	–	–	3.3
Pulling	–	–	3.3

NHP/CV angle

The mean and standard deviation values of the CV angle for each subject group are presented in Table 24.4. The headache group had a smaller mean angle (44.3°) than the non-headache group (49.1°). This observation is confirmed by statistical analysis using a two-sample *t*-test

Table 24.4 The means and standard deviation (SD) of the craniovertebral (CV) angle for the headache and non-headache groups

Group	Mean (SD)	*t* Value and significance level
Headache (*n* = 30)	44.3 (5.5)	*t* = –5.98
Non-headache (*n* = 30)	49.1 (2.9)	*P* <0.00005

which revealed a highly significant difference (*t* = –5.98; *P* <0.00005). Thus, in this sample, the symptomatic group revealed a significant FHP when compared to the non-headache group. As illustrated in Figure 24.7, the values for the CV angle were lower and spread over a greater range (29.0–52.5°) in the headache group when compared with the non-headache group, in which the values were clustered over a smaller range (43.5–54.0°).

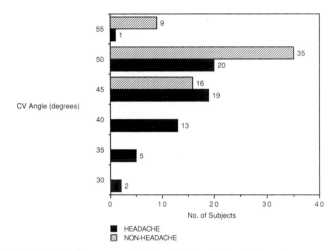

Fig. 24.7 The frequency of CV angles for the headache and non-headache groups. Note that there are two scores per subject.

Isometric strength of the upper cervical flexors

The mean and standard deviation of strength values of the upper cervical flexor muscles for the two subject groups are presented in Table 24.5. The headache group had a smaller mean strength value (5.02 kps) than the non-headache group (5.88 kps). Statistical analysis using a two-sample *t*-test revealed a significant difference in muscle strength between the two groups (*t* = 3.43; *P* <0.001). As illustrated in Figure 24.8 the values for strength were lower in the headache group (range 2.5–6.5 kps) when compared with the non-headache group (range 3.9–8.0 kps).

Table 24.5 The means and standard deviation (SD) of strength values for the headache and non-headache groups

Group	Mean (SD)	*t* Value and significance level
Headache (*n* = 30)	5.02 (0.88)	*t* = 3.43
Non-headache (*n* = 30)	5.88 (1.07)	*P* <0.001

Isometric endurance of the upper cervical flexors

The mean and standard deviation of endurance values of the upper cervical flexors are presented in Table 24.6 where it can be seen that the headache group had a much lower mean value (43.6 s) than the non-headache group (84.9 s). A two-sample *t*-test showed this difference to be

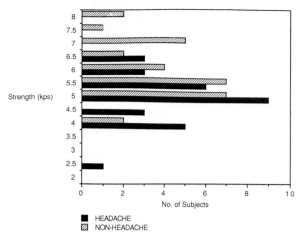

Fig. 24.8 The frequency of strength values for the headache and non-headache groups. Note that values have been taken to the nearest 0.5 kp.

Table 24.6 The means and standard deviation (SD) of endurance for the headache and non-headache groups

Group	Mean (SD)	t Value and significance level
Headache (n = 30)	43.6 (12.9)	t = 8.71
Non-headache (n = 30)	84.9 (22.6)	P <0.0005

statistically significant (t = 8.71; P <0.0005). Figure 24.9 illustrates the difference between the headache and non-headache groups in the range of individual scores for endurance. Values for the headache group ranged from 20 to 78 s whilst those of the non-headache group ranged from 42 to 145 s.

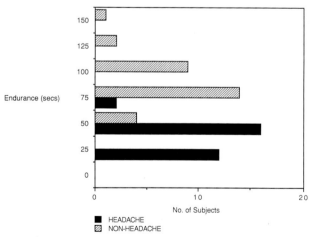

Fig. 24.9 The frequency of endurance values for the headache and non-headache groups. Note that values have been taken to the nearest 25 s.

Relationship between CV angle (NHP) and upper cervical flexor muscle performance

This chi-square test revealed that endurance was significantly related to the CV angle ($\chi^2 = 13.7$; P <0.01); that is, lower endurance values corresponded with lower CV angle values or a FHP. No relationship was found between NHP and strength of the upper cervical flexors ($\chi^2 = 8.01$; P = 0.091).

DISCUSSION

PAIVM examination

The reproduction of the subject's headache in 12 subjects confirms that the source of their headache was cervical in origin.

The higher incidence of unilateral comparable joint signs and greater involvement at 0–C1 when compared with C2–3 (and considerably less at C1–2) is in accordance with the findings of Jull (1986) in a sample of 203 patients. The 100% involvement at 0–C1 in the headache group was unexpected and may reflect the small sample size.

Questionnaire

The higher incidence of a throbbing/pulsating pain may have arisen from the fact that subjects in this study were permitted to list more than one description of their headache if it was applicable. It is unclear whether this option was available to those patients in the previous surveys (Edeling 1986, Jull 1986). Of the 30 subjects in the study, 20 used more than one description. Ten of those subjects described an aching when their headache was mild progressing to throbbing/pulsating if their headache became more severe. The description and behaviour of headaches in this sample closely resembled the larger studies of Edeling (1986) and Jull (1986).

The results of the PAIVM examination and questionnaire strongly infer that, in this sample, the cervical spine was implicated in the subjects' headaches.

CV angle/NHP

Direct comparisons cannot be made with previous studies of cervical posture using the same method of measurement because of varying and unknown ages and gender differences in the samples. However, it is interesting to note that the mean value of the CV angle of NHP in the non-headache group in this study approximates values obtained by other authors who measured NHP using the same method in asymptomatic populations (Table 24.7). The study by Dalton (1987) included 52 asymptomatic female subjects with a similar age range of 20–44 years. The mean angle of her subjects was 49°, which is virtually the same as the non-headache group in this study (49.1°) (Table 24.7). Although the sample size of both studies is small, the results demonstrate that the non-headache group of this study can be regarded as having a normal age-related value for its NHP and that the headache group presented a significantly different posture.

Table 24.7 Natural head posture (NHP): a comparison of results with previous studies

Author	NHP angle (degrees)	SD
Asymptomatic samples		
Goldstein et al (1984)		
(females *n* = 7, males *n* = 5,	49.9	3.8
mean age 27.5 years)		
Dalton (1987)		
(females, 20–34 years, *n* = 25)	49.5	4.0
(females, 35–44 years, *n* = 27)	48.6	4.6
Watson (own study, 1990)		
(females, 25–40 years, *n* = 30	49.1	2.9
mean age 30 years)		
Cureton (1941)		
(males, *n* = 644, ages unknown)	50.0	–
Coutts (1988)		
(males, 20–34 years, *n* = 24)	50.6	3.5
(males, 35–44 years, *n* = 25)	48.9	4.1
Braun & Amundsen (1989)		
(males, *n* = 20)	52.0	5.8
Headache sample		
Watson (own study, 1990)		
(females, 25–40 years, *n* = 30	44.3	5.5
mean age 31 years)		

The headache group in this study revealed a higher incidence of dysfunction of the upper cervical joints. This is particularly important when assessing postural changes because the articular capsules of the cervical spine are highly innervated by mechanoreceptors which contribute significantly to postural and kinaesthetic sensation (Wyke 1979, Lader 1983). The work of McCouch et al (1951) has demonstrated that the joint mechanoreceptors of the upper cervical spine are the origin of the tonic neck reflex (TNR). Trauma and micro-trauma are factors that influence the cervical proprioceptors, with the resultant abnormal afferent proprioceptive information affecting the TNR which subsequently alters the head-on-neck movement and position (Wyke 1979, Kraus 1988).

The centre of gravity relative to the head passes through the external auditory meatus and the odontoid process posterior to the coronal suture. This lies anterior to the transverse axis of sagittal motion for the head, and the resultant flexion moment is countered by the posterior cervical musculature. While subjects with a history of trauma were excluded from this study, the painless, insidious nature of repetitive micro-trauma in the form of abusive postural positions and abnormal movement patterns (for example, habitual flexed postures of the head and neck) may affect changes in the length–tension relationships of the cervical musculature (Darnell 1983). This forward positioning magnifies the effect of gravity, increasing the flexion moment of the head. The resultant hyperactivity or shortening of the posterior cervical musculature places the occiput in extension relative to the upper cervical spine, tipping the face upwards. To maintain the horizontal position of the otic (vestibular) and bipupular planes, the individual subconsciously flexes (relative to the thoracic spine) the lower cervical spine,

thus adopting an FHP. This conceivably results in joint dysfunction which, in turn, leads to abnormal afferent information affecting the TNR and encouraging the gradual adoption of an FHP.

Isometric performance of the upper cervical flexors

Clinical observations by Janda (1988) and Jull (1988) suggest that weakness of the upper cervical flexor musculature is frequently associated with cervical headache. This is supported by the results of this study.

The isometric strength values for both the headache and non-headache groups in this study are higher than those for asymptomatic females in the study of Barber (1989) (Table 24.8). This could be due to verbal encouragement of greater than normal conversation volume given to each subject while performing their MVCs, as an increased volume of commands has been shown to be related to greater effort (Johannson et al 1983).

Table 24.9 illustrates a considerably higher mean endurance value for the non-headache group (84.9 s) when compared with the values obtained by Barber (1989). The low mean value of the headache group (43.6 s) becomes even more striking considering the absence of verbal encouragement in the previous study.

A FHP and concomitant weakness of the upper

Table 24.8 A comparison with a previous study of isometric strength values for the upper cervical flexor musculature

Author	Mean (kps)	SD
Barber (1989)		
(asymptomatic females		
20–25 years, *n* = 28	3.8	1.0
40–45 years, *n* = 18)	3.6	0.9
Watson (own study, 1990)		
(asymptomatic females 25–40 years	5.88	1.07
mean age 30 years, *n* = 30)		
Headache sample		
Watson (own study, 1990)		
(symptomatic females 25–40 years	5.02	0.88
mean age 31 years, *n* = 30)		

Table 24.9 Endurance of the upper cervical flexor musculature: a comparison of results of studies of female subjects using the same method of measurement

Author	Mean (secs)	SD
Barber (1989)		
(asymptomatic females		
20–25 years; *n* = 18	68	60
40–45 years; *n* = 18)	59	74
Watson (own study, 1990)		
(asymptomatic females 25–40 years	84.9	22.6
mean age 30 years, *n* = 30)		
Headache sample		
Watson (own study, 1990)		
(symptomatic females 25–40 years	43.6	12.9
mean age 31 years, *n* = 30)		

cervical flexors has been commonly observed in the cervical headache patient (Janda 1988, Jull 1988). The results of this study confirm this clinical observation with respect to isometric endurance; however, isometric strength was not found to be related to NHP (CV angle). This is not surprising, for the upper cervical flexors have a predominately stabilizing role providing a holding mechanism to maintain balance and stability for the head (Richardson 1989). Whilst the upper cervical flexors also have a mobility function (Richardson 1989), that is, to initiate and perform bursts of activity, it is suggested that the mobility function (strength) of the upper cervical flexors does not play a major role in the maintenance of NHP.

Human skeletal muscle fibres have been classified according to their characteristics (Brooke & Kaiser 1970). Type I or slow twitch fibres are extremely resistant to fatigue, whilst their contraction rate is slow (Spence & Mason 1988, Tortora & Anagnostakos 1990). Type II or fast twitch fibres can be subdivided into Types IIa, IIb and IIc fibres. The Type IIb fibre fatigues easily but contracts quickly, while the IIa fibre is more resistant to fatigue than IIb (but less resistant than type I fibres) and also exhibits a rapid contraction rate. Less is known of the IIc fibres, but they appear to be an intermediate form of fast twitch fibre and usually make up only a small percentage of total fibre populations (Rose & Rothstein 1983, Spence & Mason 1988, Tortora & Anagnostakos 1990).

The upper cervical flexor muscles have been classified as postural stabilizing musculature, and, in relation to the peripheral musculature, these types of muscles have been shown to have a higher proportion of type I fibres when compared to phasic or mobility musculature (Johnson et al 1973). It has been demonstrated that the proportions of type I fibres vary considerably between individuals (Tesch & Karlsson 1978, Lexcell et al 1983). Therefore it is possible that subjects in the headache group had a lower proportion of type I fibres. This would explain the difference in the mean endurance values. However, extrapolation then leads to the possibility of an increased proportion of type II fibres. This, in effect, would provide more strength for the headache group—which is contrary to the result.

While most evidence suggests that fibre type predominance is genetically determined (Rose & Rothstein 1983, Komi 1988) it may also be influenced by environmental factors (Howald 1982, Komi 1988). The reduction of both isometric strength and endurance in the headache group could be due to an habitually FHP, which, by increasing the flexion moment arm of the head, is likely to increase tonic activity in the suboccipital muscles with a corresponding decrease in activity of the upper cervical flexors. It has been demonstrated in animal experiments that a chronic reduction in muscle activity leads to a decrease in area and number of type I fibres and a corresponding increase in number of type IIa fibres without a change in total fibre number, that is, conversion of type I fibres to type IIa fibres (Fischbach & Robbins 1969, Lieber et al 1986, Templeton et al 1988). These findings, coupled with the possibility of a lower proportion of type I fibres, could account for the considerable difference in endurance between the groups. The histochemical examination findings of Templeton et al (1988), which revealed atrophy of not only type I but also type IIa fibres, may explain the not so striking difference with respect to strength.

CONCLUSIONS AND CLINICAL IMPLICATIONS

The results of this study confirm the clinical observations that cervical headache sufferers:

- exhibit an FHP
- demonstrate weakness of the upper cervical flexor musculature
- lack endurance of the upper cervical flexor musculature
- present with an FHP and concomitant lack of isometric endurance of the upper cervical flexor musculature.

The conclusions reached can be used as starting hypotheses for future research with strictly randomized subjects over a more comprehensive age range. Nevertheless, because of the highly significant results obtained in this study, they have to be regarded as being of considerable clinical significance.

Whether FHP in cervical headache individuals causes or perpetuates their headache can be verified only by ongoing research. In the meantime, until proven otherwise, clinicians should be aware of the relationship between poor craniocervical posture and cervical headache. Postural correction and re-education should be an integral part of both prevention and management of patients with cervical headache.

The direct relationship of endurance and FHP does confirm the need for specificity in terms of rehabilitation exercises. A programme should be endurance-based because endurance training has been shown to improve the efficiency of type I fibres and convert type IIb fibres into type IIa fibres (Henriksson & Reitman 1976, Andersen & Henriksson 1977), the latter being more resistant to fatigue.

In both the headache and non-headache groups the range of strength values was considerable (3.9 and 4.0 kps respectively). Therefore, while there is a statistically significant difference between the two groups, the detection of one kp difference using the current clinical tests would be difficult and may not be meaningful owing to the large differences between individual subjects. The marked difference between the two groups with respect to endurance suggests that clinical assessment of endurance, rather than strength, may be a more realistic and reliable appraisal of the capacity of the upper cervical flexor musculature.

Acknowledgements

The author wishes to thank Associate Professor Patricia H. Trott MSc, FACP, School of Physiotherapy, University of South Australia, for supervising this study; Mr Ross A. Frick, MSc, Senior Lecturer, School of Maths and Computer Studies, University of South Australia, for assistance with statistical analyses; and Mr Phillip Walker, Senior Technical Officer (Electronics) for his perception and guidance in building the equipment for measuring upper cervical flexor muscle performance.

REFERENCES

Andersen P, Henriksson J 1977 Training induced changes in the subgroups of human Type II skeletal muscle fibres. Acta Physiologica Scandinavica 99: 123–125

Barber A 1989 The upper cervical spine flexor muscles. Unpublished thesis. Graduate diploma in manipulative therapy, South Australian Institute of Technology

Bishop Y M M, Feinberg S E, Holland P W 1975 Discrete multivariate analysis: theory and practice. MIT Press, Massachusetts p 395–397

Bogduk N 1985 The anatomical basis of coupled movements in the cervical spine. In: Proceedings of the Manipulative Therapists' Association of Australia, Fourth Biennial Conference, Brisbane

Braun B L, Amundsen L R 1989 Quantitative assessment of head and shoulder posture. Archives of Physical Medicine Rehabilitation 70: 322–329

Brooke M H, Kaiser K K 1970 Muscle fibre types: how many and what kind? Archives of Neurology 213: 369–379

Coutts A D 1988 The effects of age on cervical posture in a normal male population and comparison with a normal female population. Unpublished thesis. Graduate diploma in manipulative therapy, South Australian Institute of Technology

Cureton T K 1941 Bodily posture as an indicator of fitness. Research Quarterly 12: 348–367

Dalton M B 1987 The effect of age in cervical posture in a normal female population. Unpublished thesis. Graduate diploma in manipulative therapy, South Australian Institute of Technology

Darnell M W 1983 A proposed chronology of events for forward head posture. Physical Therapy 1(4): 50–54

Edeling J S 1986 The abandoned headache syndrome. In: Grieve G P (ed) Modern manual therapy of the vertebral column. Churchill Livingstone, Edinburgh

Fischbach G D, Robbins N 1969 Changes in contractile properties of disused muscles. Journal of Physiology 201: 305–320

Fulton I 1988 The upper cervical spine flexor muscles—do they get the nod? Unpublished thesis. Graduate diploma in manipulative therapy, South Australian Institute of Technology

Goldstein D F, Kraus S L, Williams W B, Clasheen-Wray M 1984 Influence of cervical posture in mandibular movement. Journal of Prosthetic Dentistry 52(3): 421–426

Henriksson J, Reitman J 1976 Quantitative measures of enzyme activities in type I and type II muscle fibres of man after training. Acta Physiologica Scandinavica 97: 392–397

Howald H 1982 Training induced morphological and functional changes in skeletal muscle. International Journal of Sports Medicine 3: 1–12

Janda V 1983 Muscle function testing. Butterworths, London

Janda V 1988 Muscle and cervicogenic pain syndromes. In: Grant E R (ed) Physical therapy of the cervical and thoracic spine. Churchill Livingstone, New York

Johannson C, Kent B, Shepard K 1983 Relationships between verbal command volume and magnitude of muscle contraction. Physical Therapy 63(8): 1260–1266

Johnson M, Polgar J, Seightman D, Appleton D 1973 Data on the distribution of fibre types in thirty-six human muscles. Journal of Neurological Science 18: 111–129

Jull G A 1986 Headaches associated with the cervical spine—a clinical review. In: Grieve G P (ed) Modern manual therapy of the vertebral column. Churchill Livingstone, Edinburgh

Jull G A 1988 Headaches of cervical origin. In: Grant E R (ed) Physical therapy of the cervical and thoracic spine. Churchill Livingstone, New York

Jull G A, Bogduk M 1985 Manual examination. An objective test of cervical joint dysfunction. In: Proceedings of the Fourth Biennial Conference, Manipulative Therapists' Association of Australia, Brisbane

Kapandji I 1974 The physiology of joints. Churchill Livingstone, Edinburgh, vol 3

Kendall F, McCreary E 1983 Muscles, testing and function. Williams & Wilkins, Baltimore

Kendall M G, Stuart A 1960 The advanced theory of statistics. Griffin, vol 2: 295

Komi P 1988 Physiological and biomechanical correlates of muscle function: effects of muscle structure and strength—shortening cycle on force and speed. Exercise and Sport Sciences Reviews 12: 87–121

Kraus S L 1988 Cervical spine influences on the craniomandibular region. In: Krans S L (ed) TMJ disorders. Management of the craniomandibular complex. Churchill Livingstone, Edinburgh

Lader E 1983 Cervical trauma as a factor in the development of TMJ dysfunction and facial pain. Journal of Craniomandibular Practice 1(2): 86–90

Lieber R L, Johansson C B, Vahlsing H L, Hargens A R, Feringa E R 1986 Long-term effects of spinal cord transection on fast and slow rat skeletal muscle. Experimental Neurology 91: 423–434

Lexcell J, Henriksson-Larsen K, Sjostrom M 1983 Distribution of different fibre types in human skeletal muscles. A study of cross sections of whole m. vastus lateralis. Acta Physiologica Scandinavica 117: 115–122

McCouch G P, Deering J D, Ling T H 1951 Location of receptors for tonic neck reflexes. Journal of Neurophysiology 14: 191–195

Maitland G D 1977 Vertebral manipulation, 4th edn. Butterworths, London

Richardson C 1989 Rehabilitation of muscular function of the cervical region. In: Dalton M (ed) Proceedings of headache and face pain symposium, Manipulative Therapists' Association of Australia, Brisbane

Rose S, Rothstein J 1983 Muscle mutability Part 1. General concepts and adaptations to altered patterns of use. American Physical Therapy Association

Siersbaeck-Nielsen S, Solow B 1982 Intra- and inter-examiner reliability in head posture recorded by dental auxiliaries. American Journal of Orthodontics 82(1): 50–57

Solow B, Tallgren A 1971 Natural head position in standing subjects. Acta Odontologica Scandinavica 29: 591–607

Spence A P, Mason E B 1988 Human anatomy and physiology, 3rd edn. Benjamin/Cummings, Menlo Park, CA

Templeton G H, Sweeney H L, Himson B F, Badalino M, Dudenhoeffer G A 1988 Changes in fibre composition of soleus muscle during rat hind limb suspension. Journal of Applied Physiology 65(3): 1191–1195

Tesch P, Karlsson J 1978 Isometric strength performance and muscle fibre type distribution in man. Acta Physiologica Scandinavica 98: 378–382

Tortora G J, Anagnostakos M P 1990 Principles of anatomy and physiology, 6th edn. Harper & Row, New York

Vig P S, Showfty K J, Phillips C 1980 Experimental manipulation of head posture. American Journal of Orthodontics 83(2): 138–142

Vig P S, Rirk J F, Showfty K J 1983 Adaptation of head posture in response to relocating the centre of mass: a pilot study. American Journal of Orthodontics 83(2): 138–142

Watson D H 1990 Cervical headache. An investigation of natural head posture and upper cervical flexor muscle performance. Unpublished thesis. Master of Applied Science in Manipulative Therapy. University of South Australia

Wickens J S, Kiputh O W 1937 Body mechanics analysis of Yale University freshmen. Research Quarterly 8: 37–48

Wyke B D 1979 Neurology of the cervical spinal joints. Physiotherapy 65(2): 72–80

25. The effect of age on cervical posture in a normal population

M. Dalton   A. Coutts

INTRODUCTION

Posture of the cervical spine and its potential relationship with symptoms associated with cervical dysfunction is an area of research which has been sporadically investigated this century. The dominant emphasis in posture evaluation has been in the sagittal plane where most body adjustments to gravitational forces must be made.

As early as 1928 Schwartz et al devised a series of measurements analysing various angles of the body. These measurements were made directly on lateral photographs and were an attempt to define normal sagittal posture. Since the work of Schwartz et al (1928), several authors have employed a similar measurement technique to examine cervical posture (MacEwan & Howe 1932, Cureton & Wickens 1935, Wickens & Kiputh 1937, Cureton 1941).

In dental and anthropological literature numerous radiological cephalometric studies of head and neck posture have been reported (Preiskel 1965, Daly et al 1982, Rocabado 1983, Tallgren et al 1983, Tallgren & Solow 1984, Rocabado 1986). These studies have investigated the relationship between mandibular and hyoid position, dentoalveolar and craniofacial morphology and posture of the head and neck. In addition, the physiological requirements associated with the visual, vestibular, hearing and respiratory systems and their influence on cervical posture have also been documented (Moss 1961, Ricketts 1968, Richmond et al 1976, Scranton et al 1978, Woodside & Linder-Aronson 1979, Vig et al 1980, Fjellvang & Solow 1986).

Despite these studies, the authors were unable to locate any research which has investigated 'normal' (asymptomatic) cervical posture and the alterations in this posture associated with advancing age. This is surprising since, within the clinical setting, the arbitrary grading of cervical posture as 'correct' or 'incorrect' in the absence of a recognized range of normality is unacceptable. Similarly, investigation of normal cervical posture across the years is essential if the nature of the relationship underlying postural abnormalities and cervical symptoms is to be defined.

In contrast, the active range of sagittal motion of the cervical spine and the effect of age on this motion have been extensively investigated (Buck et al 1959, Ball & Miejers 1964, Schoening & Hannan 1964, Lysell 1969, Braakman & Penning 1971, Penning 1978, Worth 1980, Ten Have & Eulderink 1981, Worth & Selvik 1986, Hayashi et al 1987).

Goldstein et al (1984) suggested that the active range of antero-posterior glide should form an additional test in the assessment of cervical mobility. Clinically, this is relevant since the reversibility of cervical posture in the sagittal plane is dependent on the antero-posterior range of motion available to an individual. However, at present there appears to be no comprehensive reports on the 'normal' antero-posterior range of motion of the cervical spine and the changes in this range associated with advancing age.

As a result, two studies were initiated to document cervical posture and the antero-posterior range of motion of the cervical spine and to identify any changes which occur with increasing age in a normal male (A.C.) and female (M.D.) population.

THE STUDY

Two samples of convenience, comprising 93 female and 97 male subjects, were measured in the studies. Subjects were drawn from several sources. The age range selected was 23–66 years, inclusive, in the female study, and 20–64 years, inclusive, in the male study. This was considered to be sufficient to reveal any changes in cervical posture and mobility with age. In both studies the subjects were grouped into four 10-year age categories.

Factors influencing cervical posture

The cranium, cervical spine, mandible, hyoid bone and shoulder girdle complex are a biomechanically functional unit. Maintenance of natural head posture is influenced by a variety of afferent stimuli arising from these structures. The full extent of the contributory determinants of head and neck posture are not yet fully known (Vig et al 1983). However, several factors which significantly influence cervical posture have been extensively researched and documented. These include mandibular and hyoid position, dentoalveolar and craniofacial morphology, respiration and dysfunction of the cervical spine and temporomandibular joints. In addition, Vig et al (1980) suggested that the maintenance of natural head posture could be expected to conform to the physiological requirements associated with sight (visual axis), the vestibular-balance system and hearing.

It is necessary, if normal cervical posture and its changes with age are to be documented accurately, that the posture of the subjects examined be influenced minimally, if at all, by these external variables. Therefore, subjects were excluded from these studies if they had suffered one or more of the following:

- Cervical, facial and/or jaw problems or pain which had necessitated absence from work, required treatment or interfered with their normal daily activities
- More than four false teeth or a dental prosthesis
- More than one headache per month
- History of cervical or facial fractures or trauma
- Cervical or temporomandibular joint surgery
- Severe recurrent middle ear infections, vertigo or dizziness over the last 5 years or longer
- Chronic obstructive airways disease or persistent (5 years or more) respiratory difficulties which had necessitated absence from work, required long-term medication, or interfered with their normal daily activities
- Visual disablement, that is, restriction or lack of ability to perform visual tasks normally (Moore 1987)
- Significant hearing impairment, indicated by the need to use amplification for comprehension of a conversation under reasonable acoustic conditions (National Acoustic Laboratory 1987 pers comm)
- Bony abnormalities of the spine, for example, scoliosis
- Any neurological disease
- Any central nervous system disease — for example, meningitis, encephalitides
- Systemic arthritides.

Experimental procedure

The examination was performed in the same order for all subjects. In both studies, lateral photographs in three test positions were taken: natural head posture, maximal forward head posture and maximal retracted head posture.

Natural head posture (NHP)

The method used to obtain a subject's NHP was that out-

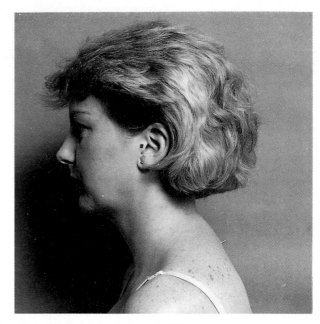

Fig. 25.1 Natural head posture (NHP).

lined by Siersbaek-Nielsen and Solow (1982). The subject was instructed to flex and extend the head continually through a progressively decreasing amplitude before eventually assuming the most neutral, comfortably relaxed position (Fig. 25.1).

Forward head posture (FHP)

The subject was instructed to poke the chin and face as far forward as possible, with back kept against the chair and with no shoulder movement. Manual guidance was given to ensure that all subjects achieved maximal anterior gliding (Fig. 25.2).

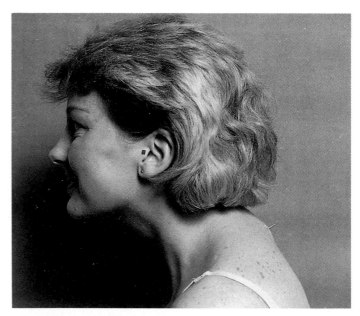

Fig. 25.2 Forward head posture (FHP).

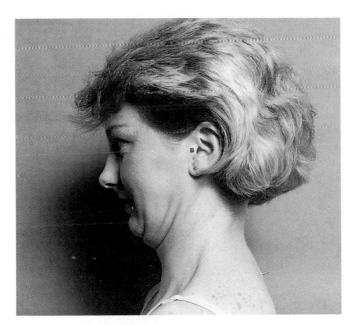

Fig. 25.3 Retracted head posture (RHP).

Retracted head posture (RHP)

The subject was instructed to tuck in the chin and to glide the head backward as far as possible without leaning backwards in the chair. Again, manual guidance assisted the subject into his or her maximally retracted head posture (Fig. 25.3).

In both FHP and RHP, verbal stimulation was also given immediately before taking the photograph, again, to facilitate maximal forward and retracted head postures.

The subjects were allowed rehearsal of each posture prior to one photograph being taken of each position. This 'warm-up' ensured that the maximum positions of FHP and RHP were achieved, and it helped to relax the subject.

The craniovertebral angle (CV) of each of the three postures was measured directly from the photographs. A plastic overlay, onto which the images of a protractor and twenty closely set parallel lines were photocopied, was used to read the CV angle. The plastic overlay was placed directly over the photograph lining a parallel line along the plumb bob line on the photograph. The point of bisection of the right angle was positioned directly over the marker on the C_7 spinous process (Fig. 25.4).

A transparent ruler was then positioned between the mid-point of a marker on the tragus of the ear and C_7, bisecting the right angle positioned at C_7 (Fig. 25.5). The CV angle was then measured in degrees directly from the protractor image.

This method of measurement was adopted in order to prevent marking the craniovertebral angle directly on the photographs. This enabled an unbiased re-measurement of the craniovertebral angle by a second observer.

EXAMINER RELIABILITY

Intra-examiner reliability for positioning of the subject, photography and measurements of the craniovertebral angle, was conducted in both studies. Nineteen female and ten male subjects ranging in age from 20 to 66 years were measured on two separate occasions one day apart. All twenty-nine subjects met the same inclusion/exclusion

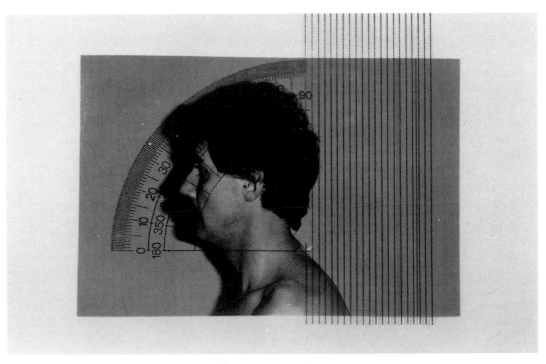

Fig. 25.4 The plastic overlay positioned over the photograph.

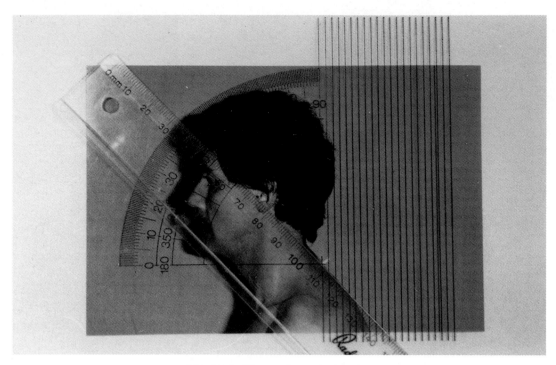

Fig. 25.5 The craniovertebral angle.

criteria employed in the studies. Analysis revealed that for each parameter tested there was no significant difference between trials ($P < 0.0001$). The correlation co-efficient (R) was no lower than 0.93 for any measurement, indicating very high repeatability.

In both studies, inter-examiner reliability was conducted with another physiotherapist on two aspects of the experimental procedure. These were: positioning of the subject, photography and measurement of the craniovertebral angles; and the procedure employed to obtain the natural head posture.

In the female study, inter-examiner reliability was conducted on nineteen subjects. In the male study, eight subjects were measured. Again, analysis revealed that, for each of the three parameters tested, there was no significant difference between trials ($P < 0.0001$). The correlation co-efficient (R) was no lower than 0.95 for any measurement.

These results demonstrate extremely high agreement between examiners for both intra- and inter-examiner reliability.

RESULTS

Changes in cervical posture with age

To document the cervical posture of a normal male and female population, and the changes in this posture associated with ageing, the means and standard deviations for each age category were computed. In addition, the relationship between each of the three test positions and age

with respect to linear and quadratic trends was also investigated using an analysis of variance.

Natural head posture

The means and standard deviations for the NHP for each gender and age group are presented in Table 25.1. The smaller the craniovertebral angle, the more forward is the head posture.

Within both the male and female populations the analysis of variance revealed that the NHP was significantly affected by age [female: F = 14.0 ($P < 0.0001$); male: F = 4.25 ($P < 0.01$)]. Further analysis revealed a significant linear trend, that is, a tendency for a forward head posture to occur with increasing age [female: F = 38.9 ($P < 0.0001$); male: F = 9.5 ($P < 0.01$)]. In addition, within the female group, there was a significant quadratic relationship between NHP and age [F = 3.6, $P = 0.05$].

Table 25.1 The means and standard deviations of the NHP CV angles with respect to age and gender (where F = female, M = male)

Age group (years)		Number of subjects	Mean ± SD (degrees)	Minimum (degrees)	Maximum (degrees)
24–34	F	25	49.5 ± 3.5	43.5	58.0
	M	24	50.6 ± 4.0	41.5	57.5
35–44	F	27	48.6 ± 4.6	37.5	57.0
	M	25	48.9 ± 4.1	41.5	56.5
45–54	F	20	46.8 ± 4.3	39.5	54.0
	M	23	49.3 ± 4.9	39.0	58.5
55–66	F	21	42.0 ± 5.0	35.5	51.0
	M	25	46.4 ± 3.8	40.5	53.5

Table 25.2 The means and standard deviations of the FHP CV angle with respect to age and gender (where F = female, M = male)

Age group (years)		Number of subjects	Mean ± SD (degrees)	Minimum (degrees)	Maximum (degrees)
23–34	F	25	32.8 ± 3.6	23.0	39.5
	M	24	30.6 ± 3.9	22.5	38.5
35–44	F	27	35.5 ± 2.9	29.0	41.0
	M	25	27.8 ± 3.4	20.0	33.0
45–54	F	20	35.2 ± 4.7	25.0	46.0
	M	23	29.7 ± 5.9	17.0	40.0
55–66	F	21	33.5 ± 3.5	27.0	41.5
	M	25	27.5 ± 5.1	18.5	39.5

Table 25.3 The means and standard deviations of the RHP CV angle with respect to age and gender (where F = female, M = male)

Age group (years)		Number of subjects	Mean ± SD (degrees)	Minimum (degrees)	Maximum (degrees)
23–34	F	25	63.0 ± 3.4	55.5	71.0
	M	24	62.7 ± 4.7	52.5	73.0
35–44	F	27	59.8 ± 3.7	54.0	68.0
	M	25	59.7 ± 3.9	52.0	69.5
45–54	F	20	57.9 ± 3.4	51.0	64.0
	M	23	57.9 ± 5.6	49.0	67.0
55–66	F	21	51.8 ± 5.8	42.0	62.5
	M	25	52.9 ± 5.7	45.0	65.5

This quadratic trend showed that the progressive decline in the NHP CV angle accelerated in the sixth decade.

Forward head posture

The means and standard deviations for each gender and age group for the FHP are presented in Table 25.2. Within both populations, it is evident that the FHP CV angle did not alter significantly with increasing age.

Retracted head posture

The relationship between age and RHP is presented in Table 25.3. The analysis of variance revealed a highly significant effect of age on the RHP in both men and women [female: F = 28.55 (P <0.0001); male: F = 16.41 (P <0.0005)].

In addition, in both populations the analysis indicated that the effect was strongly linear [female: F = 81.76 (P < 0.0001); male: F = 45.49 (P < 0.0005)]. This linear trend reflected the progressive decline in the RHP CV angle with advancing age, that is, as age increases in both men and women the ability to perform cervical retraction decreases. The major decrease occurred in the fourth and sixth decades (P = 0.05) in both populations.

An overview of the changes in the three test positions with age is presented in Fig. 25.6.

Antero-posterior mobility of the cervical spine

To document the normal antero-posterior (AP) ranges of motion of the cervical spine, the means and standard deviations of AP motion for each category were computed. The total AP range of motion (RF) was represented by the difference between the CV angles of RHP and FHP (RF = RHP – FHP). In addition, the range of posterior gliding (RN), (RN = RHP – NHP), and the range of anterior gliding (NF), (NF = NHP – FHP), were also computed. The results are presented in Table 25.4 and depicted in Fig. 25.7.

The results indicated that there was a progressive decrease in all ranges of AP mobility with increasing age in both genders. In the age span studied, females lost 40% of the total AP range of motion (an average of 0.296° per year of age), and males 8% (an average of 0.202° per year of age).

The posterior gliding range (RN) declined by 24% in females (an average of 0.181° per year of age), and in males by 47% (an average of 0.174° per year of age). The anterior gliding range (NF) decreased by 50% in the female group and by 5% in the males. Overall, the largest drop in range generally occurred in the fourth and sixth decades (P = 0.05) in both genders.

To examine the relationship between AP mobility of the cervical spine and a subject's NHP, three stepwise multiple regressions were performed. In the female populations these equations revealed that there was a significant inter-dependent relationship between AP mobility and a subject's NHP and their age. Within the male population no such relationship was found.

Therefore, on the basis of the data obtained from these stepwise multiple regressions, it may be concluded that, with advancing age, the AP ranges of motion within the female population decline in association with a more forwardly positioned NHP.

DISCUSSION

Cervical posture

These studies have presented an initial source of normal data on the CV angle in the natural head posture and the CV angle in the maximally forward and retracted head postures in normal ageing male and female populations.

The results demonstrated that there was a progressive decline in the CV angles of both NHP and RHP with increasing age. Overall, the greatest decline in the CV angles occurred during the fourth and sixth decades. In contrast, the final position of the FHP did not alter significantly with increasing age in both genders.

The decrease in the CV angle of NHP lends support to the empirically based statement of Kendall et al (1970) that, as men and women age, their natural head position tends to progress towards a more forwardly placed posi-

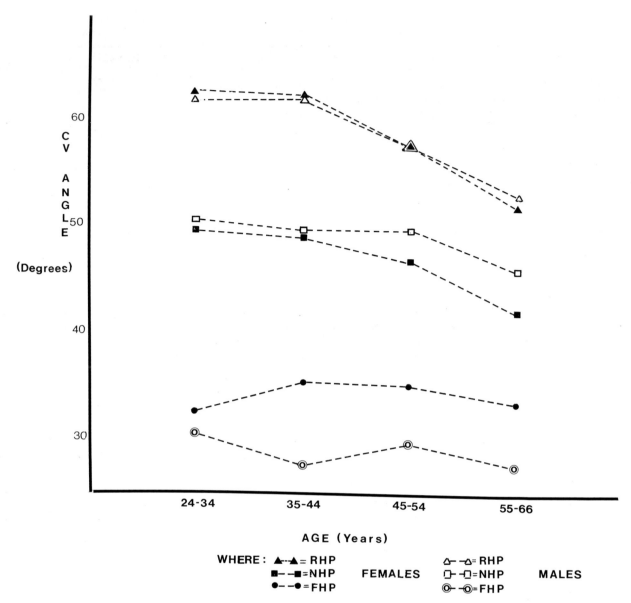

Fig. 25.6 The mean CV angle for the three test positions of NHP, FHP and RHP with respect to age and gender.

Table 25.4 The means and standard deviations of the AP mobility of the cervical spine with respect to age (measurement in degrees)

Gender	A–P Range	Age groups							
		20–34		35–44		45–54		55–66	
		Mean	SD	Mean	SD	Mean	SD	Mean	SD
Male	RF	31.9	6.1	31.9	5.6	28.5	4.7	25.4	5.2
Female	RF	30.2	5.2	24.3	3.5	22.8	5.5	18.3	5.3
Male	RN	12.3	4.6	10.8	4.5	9.3	3.8	6.5	3.5
Female	RN	13.0	2.2	11.2	3.6	11.1	4.1	9.8	3.1
Male	NF	20.0	3.8	21.1	4.5	19.8	3.7	18.9	4.6
Female	NF	17.3	5.2	13.1	3.6	11.7	5.8	8.5	4.7

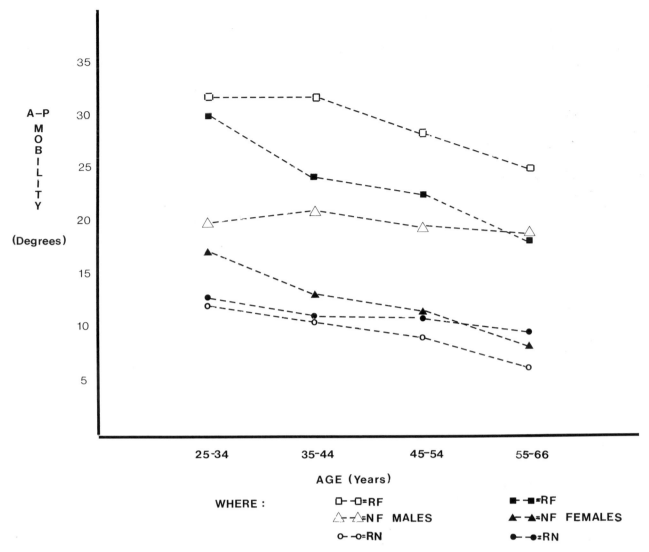

Fig. 25.7 The mean active range of antero-posterior mobility of the cervical spine with respect to age and gender.

tion. Kendall et al (1970) did not offer any reasons why this appears to occur.

It may be hypothesized that the habitual use of flexed postures of the head and neck throughout life could facilitate this progression forward of the NHP. In addition, it may be the result of gravitational forces.

The line of gravity relative to the head passes through the external auditory meatus, posterior to the coronal suture and through the odontoid process. Since this line falls anterior to the transverse axis for sagittal motion of the head, a flexion moment of the head on the neck is created. The combination of this flexion moment and the habitual use of flexed postures may gradually facilitate the adoption of a more anteriorly placed NHP, since this would provide the upper cervical extension necessary to realign the bipupilary plane with the horizontal.

Darnell (1983) has proposed that abnormal forward head postures occur due to the interaction of genetic and environmental factors. Innate genetic factors dictate to a large extent the basic body type and musculo-skeletal configuration with which a person is endowed. in terms of environment, people have always performed activities with their upper limbs anterior to their thorax. There are many occupations which necessitate having the arms and head in a more forward posture than is considered comfortable. It is possible that sustaining such postures changes the length-to-tension relationships of the muscles which control posture.

Neither of the two current studies took into account the relative changes in the upper thoracic kyphosis with increasing age. This is important since any increase or decrease in the thoracic curve may cause a compensatory change in cervical posture (Cailliet 1981). Loebl (1967) has shown that, with advancing age, women exhibit an increase in the upper thoracic incline. He reported that this occurred around forty years of age. This increase in the thoracic incline can be associated with a more anteriorly placed posture of the head and neck.

An additional potential influence which may play a role in the change in NHP with advancing age is the mechanoreceptor activity from the upper cervical articulations (Wyke 1979). This mechanoreceptor activity contributes significantly to the postural and kinaesthetic awareness of the head and neck (Wyke 1979). Therefore, the degenerative changes in the underlying upper cervical joints associated with age may interfere with this activity and consequently contribute to the change in NHP with age.

Thus, the progression forward of the NHP with increasing age may result from the complex interaction of a multitude of factors.

The ability to retract the head and neck maximally also declined significantly with age. Reasons for this change in RHP could include the age-related intrinsic changes in the tissues of the cervical spine as a causal factor. The gradual adoption of a more anteriorly placed NHP and its associated increase in upper cervical extension, may facilitate shortening of the suboccipital connective tissues and muscles. Maintenance of muscle and connective tissues in a shortened position has been shown to cause a decrease in extensibility and an increased resistance to stretching (Gutmann & Hanzlikova 1972, Schofield & Weightman 1978, Viidik 1979, Akeson et al 1980, Williams & Goldspink 1984, Frank et al 1985, St Pierre & Gardiner 1987).

Janda (1987) has also reported that the suboccipital muscles exhibit a tendency to shorten and tighten, whereas the anterior deep neck flexors are prone to hypotonia, inhibition and weakening, thereby not offering a counterbalancing force to the overactive shortened suboccipital muscles. These changes could then provide an increased resistance to the combined movement of retraction and upper cervical flexion. In addition, the ability of the deep neck flexors to flatten the cervical lordosis and achieve the RHP may also progressively deteriorate with increasing age.

Maintenance of the extensibility of the connective tissues surrounding a joint has been shown to be related to regular use of the total range of motion of that joint (Twomey & Taylor 1984). Therefore, the habitual use of forward head postures throughout life may underlie the finding that the FHP CV angle did not alter significantly with age.

Antero-posterior mobility of the cervical spine

Reduction in cervical mobility has been reported to start as early as 25 years by Schoening and Hannan (1964) and in the early forties by Ten Have and Eulderink (1981). In this study, the greatest loss of AP mobility occurred during the fourth and sixth decades.

These findings are in agreement with those of Ten Have and Eulderink (1981) since they demonstrated that the mean of the total sagittal range of motion decreased steadily from 35 to 44 years onwards. Similarly, O'Driscoll and Tomenson (1982) found that the most significant decline in cervical sagittal mobility occurred during the fourth decade and again in the seventh decade.

Based on a review of the ageing process of intervertebral tissues, it may be hypothesized that intrinsic tissue changes, such as the loss of extensibility of collagenous tissue, desiccation of the disc, the development of paradiscal and zygapophyseal joint osteophytes and muscular weakening and atrophy may play a significant role in the observed reduction in the AP range of motion of the cervical spine (Fenlin 1971, Adams et al 1977, Akeson et al 1977, Viidik 1979, Brickley-Parsons & Glimcher 1984, Ayad & Weiss 1987, Gore et al 1987, Hukins 1987, St Pierre & Gardiner 1987).

CONCLUSIONS AND THEIR CLINICAL IMPLICATIONS

Clinically, mobility of the vertebral column is judged excessive, normal or restricted on the basis of extensive documentation of the effects of age on cervical mobility. In contrast, head and neck posture in the sagittal plane is usually measured in the clinical setting purely by observation. A decision regarding normality or otherwise is then made based purely on the clinician's experience and perception of what constitutes normal or 'ideal' posture. This prompted these two studies to investigate normal cervical posture and the changes associated with ageing.

The studies measured the craniovertebral angle of the three postural positions, natural head posture (NHP), retracted head posture (RHP), and forward head posture (FHP), taken from lateral photographs.

It must be borne in mind that the CV angle is an index, reflective of only one part of the total picture of cervical posture.

The CV angle appears to be a representative measurement of a combination of an anterior or posterior position of the lower cervical spine and the associated upper cervical extension or flexion. It does not measure changes in the cervical lordosis per se, nor does it account totally for the effect of the upper thoracic incline on cervical posture. This became evident when measuring the CV angle on those subjects with an increased upper thoracic kyphosis.

Accurate measurement of complete head and neck posture requires a cephalometric radiographic analysis which was not available for this study. However, the technique employed has the advantages of producing a repeatable measurement and being non-invasive, clinically applicable and inexpensive.

The results of the studies showed that, as men and women age, their natural head position tends to progress toward a more forwardly placed position. In addition, the ability to achieve the maximally retracted head posture also significantly declined with age. In contrast, movement into the maximal forward head posture position was maintained with advancing age. It was also determined that there was a progressive decrease in the available range of antero-posterior mobility with advancing age. The average loss of range was 0.296° per year of age for women and 0.202° per year of age for men.

The results of these studies on pain-free ageing subjects do not suggest that a forward head posture is not abnormal and should not be corrected in the overall management of patients with cervical disorders. Rather, they suggest that the natural head posture has a tendency to move slightly forward with advancing age and that some shift can be tolerated in a painless state. Of further clinical importance is that the ability to correct and 'over-correct' the posture into a retracted head position declines with age and is probably associated with considerable tissue adaptations. Cervical retraction exercises, especially in the older patient, should be instituted with care in the knowledge that older persons cannot maximally retract their head, neck postures. Too vigorous exercise may overstress the ageing tissue adaptations and possibly be counterproductive in rehabilitation.

There is still much to be documented about posture and its change with age and in the pathological state. Further studies need to be undertaken on the relationships between cervico-thoracic and thoracic spinal forms and cervical posture. Indeed, total spinal postural relationships require careful documentation. From the results of these initial studies on cervical posture it could be proposed that our perception of what constitutes normal or 'optimal' posture across the years might be modified.

REFERENCES

Adams P, Eyre D, Muir H 1977 Biochemical aspects of development and ageing of human lumbar intervertebral discs. Rheumatology and Rehabilitation 16: 22–29

Akeson W H, Amiel D, Mechanic G L, Woo S L-Y, Harwood F L, Hamer M L 1977 Collagen cross-linking alterations in joint contractures: changes in reducible cross-links in periarticular connective tissue collagen after nine week of immobilization. Connective Tissue Research 5: 15–19

Akeson W H, Amiel D, Woo S L-Y 1980 Immobility effects on synovial joints. The pathomechanics of joint contracture. Biorheology 17: 95–110

Ayad S, Weiss J 1987 Biochemistry of the intervertebral disc. In: Jayson M I V (ed) The lumbar spine and back pain. Churchill Livingstone, London, pp 100–147

Ball J, Meijers K A 1964 On cervical mobility. Annals of the Rheumatic Diseases 23: 429–438

Braakman R, Penning L 1971 Injuries of the cervical spine. Excerpta Medica, Amsterdam 1, pp 3–30

Brickley-Parsons D, Glimcher M J 1984 Is the chemistry of collagen in intervertebral discs an expression of Wolff's law? A study of the human lumbar spine. Spine 9: 148–163

Buck C A, Dameron F B, Dow M J, Skowlund H V 1959 Study of normal range of motion in the neck utilizing a bubble goniometer. Archives of Physical Medicine and Rehabilitation 40: 390–392

Cailliet R 1981 Neck and arm pain. F A Davis, Philadelphia

Cureton T K 1941 Bodily posture as an indicator of fitness. Research Quarterly 12: 348–367

Cureton T K, Wickens J S 1935 The centre of gravity of the human body in the anteroposterior plane and its relation to posture, physical fitness and athletic ability. Research Quarterly (suppl) 6: 93–105

Daly P, Preston C B, Evans W G 1982 Postural response of the head to bite opening in adult males. American Journal of Orthodontics 82: 157–160

Darnell M W 1983 A proposed chronology of events for forward head posture. Physical Therapy 1: 50–54

Fenlin J M 1971 Pathology of degenerative disease of the cervical spine. Orthopaedic Clinics of North America 2: 371–387

Fjellvang H, Solow B 1986 Craniocervical postural relations and craniofacial morphology in 30 blind subjects. American Journal of Orthodontics and Dentofacial Orthopaedics 90: 327–334

Frank C, Amiel D, Woo S L-Y, Akeson W 1985 Normal ligament properties and ligament healing. Clinical Orthopaedics and Related Research 196: 15–25

Goldstein D F, Kraus S L, Williams W B, Glasheen-Wray M 1984 Influence of cervical posture on mandibular movement. Journal of Prosthetic Dentistry 52: 421–426

Gore D R, Sepic S B, Gardner G M, Murray M P 1987 Neck pain: a long term follow-up of 205 patients. Spine 12: 1–5

Gutmann E, Hanzlikova V 1972 Age changes in the neuromuscular system. Scientechnica, Bristol

Hayashi H, Okada K, Hamada M, Tada K, Ueno R 1987 Etiologic factors of myelopathy. A radiographic evaluation of the ageing changes in the cervical spine. Clinical Orthopaedics and Related Research 214: 200–209

Hukins D W L 1987 Properties of spinal materials. In: Jayson M I V (ed) The lumbar spine and back pain. Churchill Livingstone, London, pp 138–160

Janda V 1987 Muscles, central nervous motor regulation and back problems. In: Korr I M (ed) The neurobiologic mechanisms in manipulative therapy. Plenum Press, New York, pp 27–41

Kendall H O, Kendall F P, Boynton D A 1970 Posture and pain. R E Krieger, New York

Loebl W H 1967 Measurement of spinal posture and range of spinal movement. Annals of Physical Medicine 9: 103–110

Lysell E 1969 Motion in the cervical spine, an experimental study on autopsy specimens. Acta Orthopaedica Scandinavica (suppl) 123: 4–61

MacEwan C G, Howe E C 1932 An objective method of grading posture. Research Quarterly 3: 144–157

Moore L 1987 Visual disability in Australia, National telephone survey of visually disabled persons. Vol I. Issued by the Royal Guide Dogs for Blind Association of Australia. Parsifal Research, Melbourne

Moss M L 1961 Rotation of the otic capsule in bipedal rats. American Journal of Physical Anthropology 19: 301–307

National Acoustic Laboratory 1987 Personal communication

O'Driscoll S, Tomenson J 1982 The cervical spine. Clinics in Rheumatic Diseases 8: 617–630

Penning L 1978 Normal movements of the cervical spine. American Journal of Roentgenology 130: 317–326

Preiskel H W 1965 some observations of the postural position of the mandible. Journal of Prosthetic Dentistry 15: 625–633

Richmond F J, Anstee G C, Sherwin E A, Abrahams V C 1976 Motor and sensory fibres of neck muscle nerves in the cat. Canadian Journal of Physiology and Pharmacology 54: 294–304

Ricketts R M 1968 Respiratory obstruction syndrome. American Journal of Orthodontics 54: 495–503

Rocabado M 1983 Biomechanical relationship of the cranial, cervical and hyoid regions. Journal of Craniomandibular Practice 1: 62–66

Rocabado M 1986 The cranium, the spine and the mandible as a functional unit. Proceedings, Soft Tissue Conference, Hobart, pp 3–19

Schoening H A, Hannan V 1964 Factors related to cervical spine mobility. Part 1. Archives of Physical Medicine and Rehabilitation 45: 602–609

Schofield J D, Weightman B 1978 New knowledge of connective tissue ageing. Journal of Clinical Pathology (suppl 31) 12: 174–190

Schwartz L, Britten R H, Thompson L R 1928 Studies in physical development and posture. Public Health Bulletin no 179. US Public Health Service, Washington

Scranton P E, Clark M W, McClosky 1978 Musculoskeletal problems in blind children. Journal of Bone and Joint Surgery 60A: 363–365

Siersbaek-Nielsen S, Solow B 1982 Intra and interexaminer variability in head posture recorded by dental auxiliaries. American Journal of Orthodontics 82: 50–57

St Pierre D, Gardiner P F 1987 The effect of immobilization and exercise on muscle function: a review. Physiotherapy Canada 39: 24–39

Tallgren A, Solow B 1984 Long-term changes in hyoid bone position and craniocervical posture in complete denture wearers. Acta Odontologica Scandinavica 42: 257–267

Tallgren A, Lang B R, Walker G F, Ash M 1983 Changes in jaw relations, hyoid position and head posture in complete denture wearers. Journal of Prosthetic Dentistry 50: 148–156

Ten Have H A, Eulderink F 1981 Mobility and degenerative changes of the ageing cervical spine. Gerontology 27: 42–50

Twomey L, Taylor J 1984 Old age and physical capacity: use it or lose it. Australian Journal of Physiotherapy 30: 115–120

Vig P S, Showfety K J, Phillips C 1980 Experimental manipulation of head posture. American Journal of Orthodontics 77: 258–268

Vig S, Rink J F, Showfety K 1983 Adaption of head posture in response to relocating the centre of mass: a pilot study. American Journal of Orthodontics 83: 138–142

Viidik A 1979 Connective tissues — possible implications of the temporal changes for the ageing process. Mechanisms of Ageing and Development 9: 267–285

Wickens J S, Kiputh O W 1937 Body mechanics analysis of Yale University freshmen. Research Quarterly 8: 37–48

Williams P E, Goldspink G 1984 Connective tissue changes in immobilized muscle. Journal of Anatomy 138: 343–350

Woodside D, Linder-Aronson S 1979 The channelization of upper and lower anterior face heights compared to population standards in males between ages 6 to 20 years. European Journal of Orthodontics 1: 25–40

Worth D R 1980 Kinematics of the cranio-vertebral joints. In: Glasgow E F, Twomey L T, Scull E R, Kleyhans A M (eds) Aspects of manipulative therapy. Churchill Livingstone, Melbourne pp 39–44

Worth D R, Selvik G 1986 Movements of the craniovertebral joints. In: Grieve G P (ed) Modern manual therapy of the vertebral column. Churchill Livingstone, London, pp 53–63

Wyke B D 1979 Neurology of the cervical spinal joints. Physiotherapy 65: 72–80

26. Vertebral artery insufficiency: a clinical protocol for pre-manipulative testing of the cervical spine

R. Grant

Manipulative skills do not belong by right to any one profession. Treatment by manipulation is as old as mankind itself and the use of these techniques in treatment whilst a mutual inheritance is also a mutual responsibility. If we use manipulative techniques or any other treatment which may compromise the vertebral artery then it behoves us to avoid to the extent that we are able, untoward outcomes of this treatment.

In September, 1988, the Australian Physiotherapy Association (APA) formalized a protocol for pre-manipulative testing of the cervical spine and recommended its use for all patients prior to cervical manipulation. In so doing, the APA became the first professional group of any who use manipulative techniques in patient treatment in Australia (and, as far as is known, world-wide) to have such a formalized protocol. Since that time other countries' physiotherapy associations or special interest groups have developed or are about to develop similar protocols. These countries include Canada, the United Kingdom and the Netherlands.

INCIDENTS AND ACCIDENTS OF CERVICAL MANIPULATION INVOLVING THE VERTEBRAL ARTERY

It has been stated that serious consequences following cervical manipulation are rare, especially when compared with the thousands of manipulative techniques performed across the world each day. Hazards of a serious kind are much more likely to affect us as we drive (or ride our bicycles) to and from work or engage in our recreational pursuits. Hosek et al (1981) estimated that about one in a million cervical manipulations will result in a serious vertebrobasilar complication. Such an estimate may well have been based upon reports in medical journals. If indeed so, it is likely that many serious complications go unreported and that many more transient deficits or exacerbations of symptoms following manipulation do occur.

Although published case reports involving physiotherapists are very rare (Parkin et al 1978, Fritz et al 1984), the issue is not how few or how many cases can be laid at the door of any particular profession, but rather what can be learnt from all relevant reports, and what is each professional group which uses manipulation in treatment doing about the issue of quality control.

Grant (1987, 1988) reviewed 58 cases of vertebrobasilar complications following cervical manipulation, gleaned from a review of the English language literature from 1947 to 1986. Terrett (1987) reviewed 107 cases from previously published accounts which included the chiropractic literature and papers in languages other than English.

In summary, it may be deduced from these case reports that complications were experienced predominantly by young adults who often underwent multiple manipulative procedures at the incident session, who not infrequently had warning signs or symptoms of potential vertebrobasilar insufficiency (VBI) prior to the manipulation session, and who had early onset of neurological symptoms which progressed to permanent deficit or death often within minutes of the manipulative thrust techniques being applied. The most frequent description was of a rotation manipulation.

In reviewing the case reports, Grant (1988) was able to distinguish clearly between:

(a) unexpected consequences which occurred in patients, otherwise seemingly normal and healthy, in whom previous manipulative treatment had been carried out apparently without incident, and

(b) those patients in whom manipulative techniques should never have been used because signs and symptoms of vertebrobasilar insufficiency were present either following previous manipulative treatment or prior to the implicated treatment.

Further, she found that in 23 of the 26 cases where cervical spine radiographs had been taken after the incident, these were reported as normal or exhibiting minor degenerative changes only. Angiographic data were available in 32 cases, and the most commonly reported level of arterial insult was the atlanto-axial level.

371

Predisposing factors and mechanism of injury

The complications experienced following cervical manipulation were predominantly in young adults (mean age 37 years) in whose aetiology neither osseous nor vascular pathology would be expected to play a significant role.

Although the blood flow in the vertebral artery may be affected by a variety of circumstances, both intrinsic and extrinsic (George & Laurian 1987), the mere presence of a stenotic or an occlusive lesion does not necessarily imply the presence of symptoms. Symptoms occur when the blood supply to an area is critically reduced. This ultimately depends upon a balance between the compromising and the compensatory factors.

Hardesty et al (1963) noted that the vertebral arteries contributed only about 11% of the total cerebral blood flow, the remaining 89% being supplied by the carotid system. Franke et al (1980), in a review of 1256 cadaveric cases collected in the literature between 1916 and 1971, found that in only 40.8% were the two vertebral arteries equivalent in diameter. In 35.8% the left vertebral artery was the dominant (larger) artery and in the remaining 23.4% it was the right. Cavdar and Arisan (1989) also reported that the diameter of the vertebral arteries commonly showed great variation, as did their point of origin. Interruption of the flow in one vertebral artery is not necessarily accompanied by symptoms. Shintani and Zervas (1972) reviewed 100 cases of vertebral artery ligation, indicating that increases in mortality and morbidity were unlikely to occur as long as there was adequate flow through the other vertebral artery and a normal configuration of the circle of Willis.

The course of the vertebral artery is anatomically di-vided into four parts (Fig. 26.1). The extracranial portions of the vertebral artery (parts 1, 2 and 3) appear designed for movement, and in some parts designed to compensate for lack of support. This extracranial section has a well developed external elastic lamina and media (Wilkinson 1972, Winkler 1972, George & Laurian 1987). After the artery penetrates the dura (in its fourth part) the adventitia becomes much reduced, the external elastic lamina disappears and the elastic fibrils in the media become very rare.

This increased elasticity is particularly required in the atlanto-axial part of the vertebral artery (the third part, Fig. 26.1). This part of the vertebral artery is subject to stretching as a result of the large range of rotation which occurs at the C_{1-2} level, plus the relative immobility of the artery at two points, namely, at the end of its vertical path at the foramen transversarium of C_2 and after its emergence from the C_1 foramen transversarium (Fig. 26.2). As early as 1884, Gerlach (cited by George & Laurian 1987) recognized from his cadaveric studies that rotation of the neck resulted in stretching of the contralateral vertebral artery at the $C_{1/2}$ level. This observation has been reported many times since then (De Kleyn & Nieuwenhuyse 1927, Toole & Tucker 1960, Brown & Tatlow 1963, Krueger & Okazaki 1980).

Stretching and momentary occlusion of the vertebral artery occurs in normal daily activities and is asymptomatic. From the case studies, trauma to the vertebral

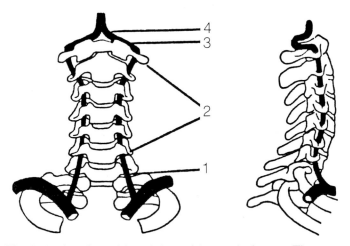

Fig. 26.1 Anterior and lateral views of the vertebral artery. The course of the vertebral artery may be described in four parts. 1. The first part extends from the subclavian artery to the C_6 foramen transversarium. 2. The second part runs vertically through the foramina transversaria of the upper six cervical vertebrae. 3. The third part passes through the foramen transversarium of the C_1 vertebra and turns horizontally across it. 4. The fourth part enters the foramen magnum to join the opposite artery to form the basilar artery. (Reproduced with permission from Bogduk 1981.)

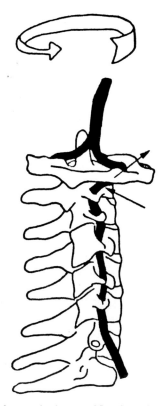

Fig. 26.2 The right vertebral artery. Note how the atlanto-axial segment (arrows) is stretched forwards by left rotation of the atlas. (Reproduced with permission from Bogduk 1981.)

artery following cervical manipulation appeared (i) to be related to a cervical rotation technique in the majority of cases, and (ii) to affect the atlanto axial segment in the majority of cases, although trauma was by no means confined to that level.

The nature of the arterial insult may be such that spasm of the artery may ensue. This may be transient or it may persist, resulting in brain stem ischaemia. If transient, it may render the affected artery irritable such that a subsequent manipulation some time later may result in a major sequela. The trauma of the manipulation may actually damage the wall, resulting in subintimal tearing, haematoma, perivascular haemorrhage, thrombosis or embolus formation. The extent of the damage may well determine the extent of the brain stem ischaemia. An understanding of the mechanism of injury highlights how concerning were the case histories in which practitioners (chiropractors in the main) continued to manipulate, in part, to relieve the additional symptoms created. Indeed Terrett's (1988) recounting of some of these case reports makes compelling reading.

Cervical extension has been less consistently reported as narrowing the vertebral artery, such compromise as was reported occurring at the atlanto-occipital and atlanto-axial levels (Lewis & Coburn 1956, Mehalic & Farhat 1974, Okawara & Nibbelink 1974). On the other hand, extension combined with cervical rotation produced occlusion of the vertebral artery, where extension alone did not (Toole & Tucker 1960, Brown & Tatlow 1963). The addition of traction to this combined position increased the number of occlusions occurring in the vertebral artery from 5 to 32 — that is, another 27 occlusions in 18 subjects (Brown & Tatlow 1963). All of these occlusions occurred at or above the level of C_2. The commonest site (in 26 out of 32 cases) was the atlanto-axial level in the vertebral artery contralateral to the direction of rotation.

Symptoms and signs of vertebrobasilar insufficiency

A wide spectrum of symptoms and signs can be referable to critical alterations in vertebrobasilar circulation. Whilst an isolated symptom is less common than a grouping of symptoms, authors agree that an isolated symptom does occur (Williams & Wilson 1962, Troost 1980, Ausman et al 1985, Bogduk 1986).

Dizziness is the most common and usually the predominant symptom of vertebrobasilar insufficiency (VBI) and may be the only presenting symptom. (It is important to remember that, whilst dizziness is usually present in VBI, other symptoms may occur without dizziness, although this is less common.)

The symptoms of VBI which may occur concomitant with dizziness, or in time come to be associated with it, or indeed be present without it, will depend upon which structures supplied by the vertebrobasilar system become ischaemic. Coman (1986) has designated the major symptoms 'the five Ds' — dizziness, diplopia, drop attacks, dysarthria and dysphagia. However, other symptoms need to be included, and a major review of cases (of what the authors termed) basilar insufficiency is worthy of consideration (Williams & Wilson 1962). These authors reviewed symptoms in 20 cases of major basilar insufficiency and 65 cases of minor syndromes of basilar insufficiency. The minor syndromes were defined as the 'occurrence of transient symptoms disturbing otherwise normal health'. The authors considered these to be not uncommon, particularly in later life, finding 65 cases in a thousand consecutive cases in their neurological practice.

Dizziness (vertigo) occurred in two-thirds of the 'minor' cases and was by far the most common harbinger of an 'attack'. The most convincing association was of vertigo with visual perceptual disturbances (including spots before the eyes, blurred vision, hallucinations, illusions and field defects), diplopia, ataxia and drop attacks. Half the patients reported visual disturbances and one-fifth visceral and vasomotor disturbances such as nausea, faintness and lightheadedness. In addition, Williams and Wilson (1962) found peri-oral dysaesthesia (tingling around the lips) to be much more common in the minor cases than the demonstrable changes in the territory of the trigeminal nerve, considered to be more typical of major syndromes of basilar insufficiency. Peri-oral changes in sensation have been reported by other authors also, including Troost (1980) and Bogduk (1986). Nystagmus, hemianaesthesia and hemiplegia are other symptoms/signs which have been described. Williams and Wilson found that the vertigo was unlikely to be associated with deafness or tinnitus in basilar insufficiency.

Dizziness may arise as a result of a distortion of the normal afferent input to the vestibular nuclei from receptors in the neck (termed cervical or reflex vertigo). These receptors are thought to be in the capsules of the upper three cervical joints, particularly the atlanto-occipital and atlanto-axial joints, and in the neck musculature (McCouch et al 1951, Cohen 1961, Norrse & Stevens 1976, De Jong et al 1977, Wyke 1979, Abrahams 1981, Reker 1985).

Whilst it may be stated that the essential difference between dizziness of vascular origin and cervical vertigo is that the latter is not accompanied by other features of brain stem ischaemia or cardiovascular disease (Bogduk 1986; Aspinall 1989) it may still be difficult to differentiate the two when dizziness is an initial unaccompanied symptom. Some authors, such as Troost (1980), considered that a latent response to a sustained position or head posture differentiates peripheral causes of vertigo (such as benign positional vertigo or cervical vertigo) from dizziness due to central causes. Others consider that dizziness occurring latently may also be a feature of brain stem ischaemia (Reker 1985, Scherer 1985). All agree, however, that fatiguability is a characteristic of peripheral causes of vertigo.

To Troost (1980, p. 415) is accorded the last word: '. . . dizziness sometimes cannot be simply classified as peripheral, central or systemic. The symptom complex may well represent a combination of abnormalities, including incomplete adaption. This is particularly true when vertebrobasilar disease is a contributing factor'.

CLINICAL PROTOCOL FOR VERTEBRAL ARTERY TESTING

This section draws heavily upon Grant (1987) and the Protocol (1988) for pre-manipulative testing of the cervical spine promulgated by the Australian Physiotherapy Association.

Clinical evaluation

In any patient for whom treatment of the cervical spine is to be undertaken, the presence or development of dizziness, or other symptoms of VBI, is carefully assessed. The four aspects of this assessment are:

- subjective examination
- physical examination
- onset of symptoms during treatment
- onset of symptoms following treatment.

Subjective examination

In every patient presenting with upper quarter dysfunction, questions are specifically asked to ascertain the presence of dizziness or other symptoms suggestive of VBI. (These symptoms were outlined in the previous section.) Should the patient respond in the affirmative then a detailed profile of each symptom is obtained. Questioning must reveal:

- the type, degree, frequency and duration of the dizziness; the occurrence, or aggravation of dizziness by head movements, and by sustained positions of the head and neck, particularly rotation, extension or combination of these movements; and any other movement, posture or position volunteered by the patient
- the nature and type of any other symptom which may or may not be associated with dizziness, but which may suggest VBI
- the history of dizziness vis-a-vis the history of neck, headache or other symptoms
- the status of the dizziness: is it improving, worsening or staying the same?
- the status of associated symptoms
- previous treatment (if any) and its effect in relieving,

exacerbating or producing dizziness and/or associated symptoms.

Physical examination

Many tests for VBI detection, or to be undertaken prior to cervical manipulation, have been described (Maitland 1968, 1973, Maigne 1972, Grant 1987, Oostendorp 1988, Terrett 1988, Aspinall 1989). In some of these reports the tests were many and/or were sustained for 40 seconds or more. There was a need to find a balance between clinical practice, literature reviewed and a knowledge that the test procedures themselves held certain risks, including a potential additive effect on the vertebral artery. On this basis the APA protocol recommended the following:

1. *Tests which are undertaken in those patients with no history of dizziness or other symptoms of VBI, but in whom cervical manipulation is the treatment of choice.* These tests are undertaken in a sitting position and/or supine (as deemed appropriate for each patient). With supine lying it is often possible to gain a greater range of movement, particularly if pain is a prominent presenting symptom.
   These tests comprise:

- sustained extension (Fig. 26.3)
- sustained rotation to left and right (Fig. 26.4)
- sustained rotation with extension to left and right (Fig. 26.5)
- simulated manipulation position; here, the patient's head and neck are held in the manipulation position as a sustained pre-manipulative procedure (Fig. 26.6).

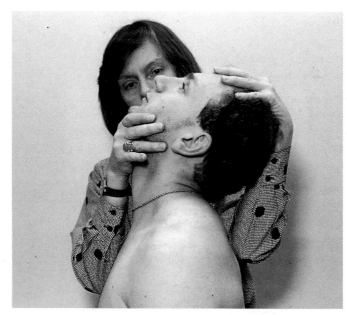

Fig. 26.3 Sustained cervical extension in the sitting position.

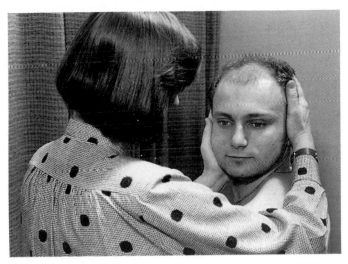

Fig. 26.4 Sustained cervical rotation in the sitting position. Whilst both rotations are carried out, only left rotation is illustrated.

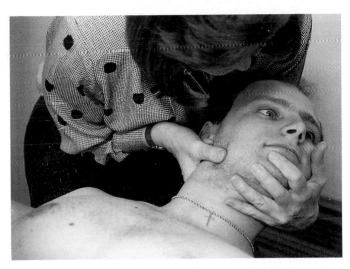

Fig. 26.6 Simulated manipulation position. (Simulation of transverse thrust technique to 'gap' the left C2–3 zygapophyseal joint.)

The patient is questioned regarding dizziness both during each test and after each test position has been released. The physiotherapist also observes the eyes for the presence of nystagmus. Each position is maintained with over-pressure for a minimum of 10 seconds (or less if symptoms are evoked) and upon release, a period of at least 10 seconds should elapse to allow for any latent response to the sustained position.

If any of these tests produce dizziness or any other symptom suggestive of VBI then cervical manipulation is not undertaken. If these tests are negative and no contraindications to manipulation have been elicited on specific overall assessment, then informed consent is obtained from the patient and the manipulative technique is carried out.

2. *Tests which are undertaken in those patients in whom dizziness is a presenting symptom.* These tests are

undertaken in a sitting position. The physiotherapist may decide to proceed to test in supine lying if all tests which follow are negative. These tests comprise:

- sustained extension (Fig. 26.3)
- sustained rotation to left and right (Fig. 26.4)
- sustained rotation with extension to left and right (Fig. 26.5)
- testing the position or movement which provokes dizziness as described by the patient (if *different* from the above)
- quick movement of the head through the available range of the relevant movement, for example, rotation; this test is carried out only where the patient relates dizziness to quick movements of the head rather than head postures or positions.

Where dizziness is provoked upon rotation, or rotation with extension, either during the sustained tests or the quick movement test, these tests are further explored in the *standing position* in order to differentiate dizziness arising from the vestibular apparatus of the inner ear from that elicited by neck movement (be it due to cervical vertigo or symptomatic compromise of the vertebral artery). The tests in the standing position are:

- head held still, sustained trunk rotation to left and right (Fig. 26.7)
- head held still, repetitive trunk rotation to left and right.

These standing tests, when positive, suggest that the patient's dizziness is not caused by labyrinth disturbance.

In all tests for this group of patients where dizziness is a presenting symptom, sustained positions are adopted for a minimum of 10 seconds or less if

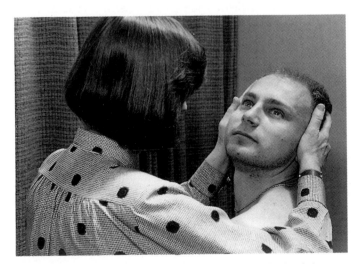

Fig. 26.5 Sustained cervical rotation with extension in the sitting position. Only left rotation is illustrated.

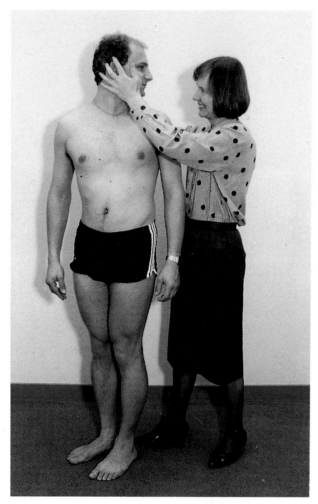

Fig. 26.7 Head held still, sustained trunk rotation in the standing position. Only trunk rotation to the right is illustrated.

symptoms are provoked, and a pause follows each test to allow for any latent responses to occur, before proceeding with the next test.

In summary, if, during the physical examination, any test is positive, that is, it produces or reproduces dizziness and/or associated symptoms suspected to be of VBI origin, then cervical manipulation is contraindicated as a treatment option.

Symptoms provoked during or following treatment procedures

Positive findings provoked whilst adopting a treatment position, during any treatment procedure or following same, are considered contraindications to cervical manipulation.

Choice of technique and method of application

For those patients who present with dizziness and/or other symptoms of possible VBI origin but in whom the tests, as outlined previously, are negative, there are some points of caution:

- Any treatment technique which provokes the dizziness should be avoided.
- Passive mobilizing techniques (or other appropriate treatment) should be used in initial treatment and their effect over a 24 hour period known, before the use of cervical manipulation is even considered.
- When manipulation is proceeded with, a single gentle manipulation should be undertaken providing all relevant tests previously described remain negative.

For any patient in whom cervical manipulation is the treatment of choice the guidelines are as follows:

- Informed consent is obtained from the patient. The patient must give verbal consent before the manipulative procedure is undertaken. It is therefore important that the patient understands what the procedure entails, that manipulation does hold certain risks, albeit very rare, and that all precautionary tests have been carried out and that little risk is deemed to be operative in their case. The Protocol (1988) of the APA advises the use of standardized wording for obtaining informed consent.
- A generalized rotary manipulation of the cervical spine is potentially dangerous and is not used. Rotation was the directional component common to almost all cases reviewed in which a major incident followed cervical manipulation (Krueger & Okazaki 1980, Grant 1988).
- The use of strong axial traction during a manipulative procedure is avoided. The reports of Brown and Tatlow (1963), Parkin et al (1978), Bourdillon (1982), and Gutmann (1983) should be considered in this light.
- At the first treatment session a single (not multiple) manipulation is performed. It is well to consider whether multiple cervical manipulations at a single treatment session are ever necessary (Krueger & Okazaki 1980, Grant 1988, Terrett 1988).
- Dizziness testing in the simulated manipulation position is performed at all subsequent attendances (not just at the initial consultation) in which cervical manipulation is used. In 13 of the 58 cases of vertebrobasilar complications following cervical manipulation reviewed by Grant in 1987, previous cervical manipulation had been carried out apparently without incident. However, it must also be remembered that whilst the pre-manipulative tests described earlier seek to simulate some of the stresses imposed on the cervical structures when a manipulation is performed, the rapid thrust component cannot be simulated. This should always be borne in mind and forceful manipulative techniques avoided.
- Recording of the pre-manipulative tests undertaken and the response to these on the part of the patient, and recording that informed consent has been obtained is necessary.

SUMMARY

The procedures outlined in this clinical protocol more than adequately meet the concerns expressed in the reported cases of vertebrobasilar symptoms reviewed. However, it is important to remember that:

- An element of unpredictability remains, and incidents do occur, even when all premanipulative tests are negative and even when the patient has responded favourably to manipulative treatment in the past (Grant 1988, Bolton et al 1990).
- The test procedures themselves hold certain risks.
- There is a need to record carefully and accurately all dizziness tests and pre-manipulative testing procedures and the responses to them on the part of the patient.
- Even when the patient is made aware of the risks attached to the manipulative procedure, that is, informed consent is obtained, the physiotherapist (or indeed any professional performing manipulative procedures) may still remain legally liable if reasonable care, that is the care expected of the average competent and prudent practitioner, is not employed.

THE APA PROTOCOL FOR PRE-MANIPULATIVE TESTING OF THE CERVICAL SPINE UNDER SCRUTINY

Survey of APA members regarding the protocol

In 1991, two and a half years after the APA developed the protocol and recommended its use with all patients prior to cervical manipulation, Grant and Trott (1991) undertook a survey of APA members.

A detailed questionnaire was formulated, and item consistency was tested in a pre-trial on a small sample of 20 physiotherapists from a variety of fields of practice.

The aim of the questionnaire was to establish the fields in which the members practised; their gender; their knowledge of the APA protocol; their attitudinal responses to statements commonly made about the protocol; whether they used manipulative techniques in treatment (defined as high-velocity localized thrust techniques); their compliance with the subjective and physical examination components of the protocol; whether informed consent was obtained prior to cervical manipulation; whether screening tests undertaken and informed consent gained were recorded and whether the format suggested in the protocol was used.

Systematic stratified random sampling of 10% of the APA membership nation-wide yielded 727 names. Questionnaires were sent to these physiotherapists and 455 (63%) responded. The fields of practice in which those who responded worked, are outlined in Table 26.1. It may be seen that a wide variety of fields of practice was represented. (It should be noted that many respondents worked in more than one field of practice.)

Table 26.1 Fields of practice of respondents

Fields of practice	Number of respondents (%)
Cardiopulmonary	183 (40)
Gerontology	153 (34)
Manipulative physiotherapy	198 (44)
Neurology	179 (39)
Occupational health	107 (24)
Orthopaedics	331 (73)
Paediatrics	106 (23)
Psychiatry	11 (2)
Sports physiotherapy	246 (54)
Women's health	123 (27)
Other fields	62 (14)

Of the respondents, 79% were female and 21% male; 89% (406) knew that there was an APA protocol.

Manipulative techniques were used occasionally, often or very frequently in the treatment of upper quarter disorders by 19% (84) of the respondents. Of these physiotherapists, 98% (82) knew that there was an APA protocol, and 92% (77) had read it.

The responses of those individuals who knew that there was an APA protocol, to statements commonly made about if follow (with the five-point scale — strongly disagree through to strongly agree — collapsed to three categories). For the whole group this comprised 406 physiotherapists, and for those respondents who used manipulative techniques in treatment the number was 82. (Missing responses to these statements were minimal.)

The APA protocol for pre-manipulative testing of the cervical spine places appropriate medico-legal restrictions upon the physiotherapy practitioner.
Whole group: disagree 8 (2%); unsure 105 (26%); agree 289 (72%).
Manip. group: disagree 5 (6%); unsure 22 (27%); agree 55 (67%).

It may be seen therefore that two-thirds of respondents in both groups agreed with this statement.

The APA protocol for pre-manipulative testing of the cervical spine is too time-consuming to be undertaken with every patient prior to cervical manipulation.
Whole group: disagree 258 (64%); unsure 79 (19%); agree 68 (17%).
Manip. group: disagree 40 (49%); unsure 8 (10%); agree 34 (41%).

For those physiotherapists who used manipulation in the treatment of upper quarter disorders, 41% considered the APA protocol to be too time-consuming for use with every patient. Approximately half of these physiotherapists (49%) disagreed with the statement.

The requirement for informed consent on the part of the patient prior to undergoing cervical manipulation will mean that fewer patients will agree to manipulation as a form of treatment, and, as a consequence, a valuable method of treatment will be used less frequently.

Whole group: disagree 191 (48%); unsure 121 (31%); agree 86 (21%).

Manip. group: disagree 33 (40%); unsure 13 (16%); agree 36 (44%).

Twice as many respondents in the whole group disagreed with this statement as compared with those in agreement, with 31% unsure. By contrast, in the group who used manipulation in treatment, a greater percentage were of the opinion that the requirement of informed consent on the part of the patient would lead to a valuable method of treatment (manipulation) being used less frequently, as compared to the percentage who disagreed.

The APA protocol for pre-manipulative testing of the cervical spine is an important initiative and should be retained.

Whole group: disagree 9 (2%); unsure 49 (12%); agree 247 (86%).

Manip. group: disagree 5 (6%); unsure 23 (28%); agree 54 (66%).

At least two-thirds of each group agreed with this statement. The manipulative group were somewhat more restrained in their support with 28% (versus 12%) being unsure with respect to this statement.

Thus, in summary, two-thirds of the group of respondents who use manipulative techniques in treatment agreed both that the APA protocol placed appropriate medicolegal restrictions on the practitioner, and that it was an important initiative and should be retained. However, many of these respondents were of the opinion that the protocol was too time-consuming and that the requirement of informed consent would mean that manipulation as a form of treatment would be used less often.

Of the 84 physiotherapists who used manipulative techniques in the treatment of upper quarter disorders, 100% complied with the subjective examination component of the protocol. Eighty-one respondents (96%) carried out some or all of the recommended screening tests prior to the first treatment using cervical manipulation, 88% (71) utilizing two or more of the tests, and 64% (52) carrying out all the tests. Prior to subsequent treatments using cervical manipulation, 89% (75) carried out screening tests, 91% of these using the simulated manipulation position (SMP). The SMP is the test recommended in the protocol to be undertaken prior to subsequent treatments using cervical manipulation. The frequency of recording of the tests carried out at the first visit was 90%, and at subsequent visits it was 60%.

Informed consent was reported as being obtained from patients by 93% (78) of respondents prior to undertaking cervical manipulation. Of these only 58% gained informed consent in every case, and only 50% recorded that such consent had been obtained. Where informed consent gained, was recorded, 33% used the wording suggested in the APA protocol, 67% either did not use this wording, or didn't know whether the wording they used was the same as that in the protocol.

In summary, it may be deduced that knowledge of the existence of the APA protocol was widespread. Amongst those physiotherapists who used manipulative techniques in the treatment of upper quarter disorders, a high percentage complied with the protocol as far as the screening procedures undertaken were concerned. However, the obtaining of informed consent, specifically the use of the wording suggested in the APA protocol, was an area where there was less compliance. This reflects the distribution of the attitudinal responses to the statement on informed consent commonly made about the APA protocol. It is proposed that this section of the protocol be modified, at least to allow practitioners to gain informed consent using phraseology of their own choice.

OTHER RESEARCH UNDERTAKEN USING THE APA PROTOCOL

Of respondents who used manipulative techniques in the treatment of upper quarter disorders, 41% felt that the APA protocol was too time-consuming to be undertaken with every patient prior to manipulation, although a very high percentage complied with most components of the protocol. It is useful, therefore, to consider the two studies to date in which the testing procedures outlined in the protocol have been investigated in patients with symptomatic disorders of the cervical spine (Hutchison 1989, Powell 1990). Both studies showed that it was important to re-test as the dizziness testing response (DTR) changed from negative to positive in some patients at the second assessment. Further, Hutchison found that the testing procedures reproduced the patients' dizziness and/or other VBI symptoms, especially when these were related to cervical movement, and also that they produced dizziness in 20% of patients in the absence of dizziness as a presenting symptom.

Whilst there was no significant difference between the sensitivity of the tests in producing a positive DTR, the combined rotation/extension test was found to be the most sensitive of the bilateral tests and more sensitive than the SMP. (The SMP is the test recommended in the protocol to be undertaken at subsequent visits prior to cervical manipulation, and, as might be expected, was the test most commonly reported to be undertaken in follow-up by respondents to the survey.) Oostendorp (1988) used a more detailed and more time-consuming screening procedure which incorporated within it the elements of the APA protocol, but also included sustained flexion, lateral flexion and lateral flexion combined with extension/rotation and flexion/rotation, in examining 90 patients with headache, dizziness and neck pain. The mean percentage of positive responses was highest for sustained extension/rotation and sustained extension/rotation/lateral flexion to either side. There was very little difference between these combined movement tests in the incidence of positive responses, suggesting perhaps that both might not need to be undertaken. The sensitivity of the bilateral extension/rotation test finds support in the later work of Hutchison (1989). Unlike Hutchison, Oostendorp found a high percentage of positive responses to rotation bilaterally as well. It must be said, however, that the mean onset of symptoms in Oostendorp's study was 55 seconds — a long time to sustain each test.

Further research is required to ascertain which of the initial screening tests need to be carried out, and which need to be carried out at each subsequent visit.

SUMMARY

Findings gleaned from cases of vertebrobasilar complications following cervical manipulation have been considered. This has included the predisposing factors and mechanism of injury to the vertebral artery. Whilst a wide spectrum of symptoms and signs may be ascribed to disorders of the vertebrobasilar system, the more common symptoms and signs of VBI and their patterns of presentation have been given. The clinical protocol for vertebral artery testing adopted by the Australian Physiotherapy Association and recommended for use by its members has been outlined, and research evaluating the APA protocol has been presented.

REFERENCES

Abrahams V C 1981 Sensory and motor specialization in some muscles of the neck. Trends in Neurosciences 24–27

Aspinall W 1989 Clinical testing for cervical mechanical disorders which produce ischemic vertigo. Journal of Orthopaedic and Sports Physical Therapy 11: 176–182

Ausman J I, Shrontz C E, Pearce J E, Diaz F G, Crecelius J L 1985 Vertebrobasilar insufficiency. A review. Archives of Neurology 42: 803–808

Bogduk N 1981 Dizziness and the vertebral artery. The cervical spine and headache symposium. Manipulative Therapists Association of Australia, Brisbane, pp 61–82

Bogduk N 1986 Cervical causes of headache and dizziness. In: Grieve G P (ed) Modern manual therapy of the vertebral column. Churchill Livingstone, Edinburgh

Bolton P S, Stick P E, Lord R S A 1990 Failure of clinical tests to predict cerebral ischemia before neck manipulation. Journal of Manipulative and Physiological Therapeutics 12: 304–307

Bourdillon J F 1982 Spinal manipulation. 3rd edn. Heinemann, London

Bourdillon J F, Day E A 1987 Spinal manipulation. 4th edn. Heinemann, London

Brown B S J, Tatlow W F T 1963 Radiographic studies of the vertebral arteries in cadavers. Radiology 81: 80–88

Cavdar S, Arisan E 1989 Variations in the extracranial origin of the human vertebral artery. Acta Anatomica 135: 236–238

Cohen L A 1961 Role of eye and neck proprioceptive mechanisms in body orientation and motor coordination. Journal of Neurophysiology 24: 1–11

Coman W B 1986 Dizziness related to ENT conditions. In: Grieve G P (ed) Modern manual therapy of the vertebral column. Churchill Livingstone, Edinburgh, ch 28

De Jong P T V M, De Jong J M B V, Cohen B, Jongkees L B W 1977 Ataxia and nystagmus induced by injection of local anaesthetics in the neck. Annals of Neurology 1: 240–246

De Kleyn A, Nieuwenhuyse P 1927 Schwindelanfaelle und nystagmus bei einer bestimmten stellung des kopfes. Acta Otolaryngolica 11: 155–157

Franke J P, Dimarina V, Pannier M, Argens C L, Libersa C L 1980 Les artéres vertébrales. Segments atlanto-axoidiens V3 et intracranien V4 collatérales. Anatomia Clinica 2: 229–242

Fritz V U, Maloon A, Tuch P 1984 Neck manipulation causing stroke. South African Medical Journal 66: 844–846

George B, Laurian C 1987 The vertebral artery. Pathology and surgery. Springer-Verlag, Vienna

Gerlach L 1984 Ueber die bewegungen in den atlasgelenken und deren beziehungen zu der blutstromung in den vertebralarterien. Beitr Morphol 1: 104–117 cited by George B, Laurian C 1987

Grant E R 1987 Clinical testing before cervical manipulation — can we recognise the patient at risk? Proceedings of the Tenth International Congress of the World Confederation for Physical Therapy, Sydney pp 192–197

Grant R 1988 Dizziness testing and manipulation of the cervical spine. In Grant R (ed) Physical therapy for the cervical and thoracic spine. Churchill Livingstone, New York, ch 7

Grant E R, Trott P H 1991 Pre-manipulative testing of the cervical spine — the APA Protocol and its aftermath. Proceedings of the Eleventh International Congress of the World Confederation for Physical Therapy, London, pp 378–380

Gutmann G 1983 Injuries to the vertebral artery caused by manual therapy. Manuelle Medizine 21: 2–14

Hardesty W H, Whitacre W B, Toole J F, Randall P, Royster H P 1963 Studies on vertebral artery blood flow in man. Surgery Gynaecology and Obstetrics 116: 662–664

Hosek R S, Schram S B, Silverman H 1981 Cervical manipulation. Journal of American Medical Association 245: 922

Hutchison M S 1989 An investigation of pre-manipulative dizziness testing. Proceedings of Sixth Biennial Conference of Manipulative Therapists Association of Australia, Adelaide, pp 104–112

Krueger B R, Okazaki H 1980 Vertebrobasilar distribution infarction following chiropractic cervical manipulation. Mayo Clinic Proceedings 55: 322–332

Lewis R C, Coburn D F 1956 The vertebral artery. Missouri Medicine 53: 1059–1063

Maigne R 1972 Orthopaedic medicine: a new approach to vertebral manipulation. Charles C Thomas, Illinois

Maitland G D 1968 Vertebral manipulation. 2nd edn. Butterworths, London

Maitland G D 1973 Vertebral manipulation. 3rd edn. Butterworths, London

McCouch G P, Deering I D, Ling T H 1951 Location of receptors for tonic neck reflexes. Journal of Neurophysiology 14: 191–195

Mehalic T, Farhat S M 1974 Vertebral artery injury from chiropractic manipulation of the neck. Surgical Neurology 2: 125–129

Norrse M, Stevens A 1976 Cervical nystagmus and functional disorders of the cervical column. Acta Otorhinolaryngolica Belgica 30: 457–462

Okawara S, Nibbelink D 1974 Vertebral artery occlusion following hyperextension and rotation of the neck. Stroke 5: 640–642

Oostendorp R A B 1988 Vertebrobasilar insufficiency. Proceedings of International Federation of Orthopaedic Manipulative Therapists Congress, Cambridge, pp 42–44

Parkin P J, Wallis W E, Wilson J L 1978 Vertebral artery occlusion following manipulation of the neck. New Zealand Medical Journal 88: 441–443

Powell V J 1990 An investigation of testing procedures for vertebrobasilar insufficiency. Australian Journal of Physiotherapy 36: 31

Protocol for pre-manipulative testing of the cervical spine. 1988 Australian Journal of Physiotherapy 34: 97–100

Reker V 1983 Cervical nystagmus caused by proprioceptors of the neck. Laryngolica Rhinol Otol Stuttgart 62: 312–314

Scherer H 1985 Neck induced vertigo. Archives Otorhinolaryngolica Supplementum 2: 107–120

Shintani A, Zervas N T 1972 Consequence of ligation of the vertebral artery. Journal of Neurosurgery 36: 447–450

Terrett A G J 1987 Vascular accidents from cervical spine manipulation: report on 107 cases. Journal of Australian Chiropractors Association 17: 15–24

Terrett A G J 1988 Vascular accidents from cervical spine manipulation: the mechanisms. ACA Journal of Chiropractic 22: 59–74

Toole J F, Tucker S H 1960 Influence of head position upon cerebral circulation. Studies on blood flow in cadavers. Archives of Neurology 2: 616–623

Troost B T 1980 Dizziness and vertigo in vertebrobasilar disease. Part 11. Central causes and vertebrobasilar disease. Stroke 11: 413–415

Wilkinson I M S 1972 The vertebral artery. Extracranial and intracranial structure. Archives of Neurology 27: 392–396

Williams D, Wilson T G 1962 The diagnosis of the major and minor syndromes of basilar insufficiency. Brain 85: 741–774

Winkler G 1972 Remarques sur la structure de l'artere vertebrale. Quad Anatomia Practica 28: 105–115

Wyke B 1979 Neurology of the cervical spinal joints. Physiotherapy 65: 72–76

27. An overview of dizziness and vertigo for the orthopaedic manual therapist

J. T. S. Meadows   D. J. Magee

INTRODUCTION

Dizziness and vertigo are terms which are often used interchangeably; however, dizziness is a more general term for a general condition and may involve one or more symptoms, including nausea, giddiness, lightheadedness, floating or swaying sensations, wooziness, unsteadiness, weakness and vertigo (Rogers 1982). Vertigo is a special case of dizziness and is more precisely defined. Vertigo may be described as a disturbed sense of relationship to space in which there is an impaired ability to orient the body in relation to surroundings, objects, space or gravity (Cecil 1947, de Weese 1950). It can imply a sensation or illusion of apparent movement either of the subject, or of the object in the line of vision (Cawthorne 1945, 1957, Ludman 1981). Taber's medical dictionary (Thomas 1979) defines vertigo as: 'Sometimes used as a synonym for dizziness, lightheadedness and giddiness. However, true vertigo is the sensation of moving around in space (subjective vertigo) or of having objects move about the person (objective vertigo) and is a result of disturbance of equilibratory apparatus'.

Dizziness, including vertigo, appears to be an increasingly frequent complaint. In 1965, one study (Elia 1968) reported that 14 million men and women in the United States suffered from dizziness to the point where it was considered to be a major complaint. In women, it was preceded only by headaches, fatigue and constipation while in men, it ranked seventh after fatigue, headaches, shortness of breath, indigestion and constipation. The incidence appears to be less in England where Berenstein (1962) found that it was as common as the duodenal ulcer and rheumatoid arthritis. A random sample of elderly people indicated that the incidence of dizziness increased with the age of the population. Some 47% of men aged over 67 years and 61% of women over 62 years experienced dizziness (Pemberton 1953). Orma and Koskenojen (1957) found in Iceland that 81% of men and 91% of women over 65 years of age had complained to their physician about dizziness.

This high and possibly increasing incidence of dizziness must be of concern to the orthopaedic therapist. While most causes of dizziness are relatively benign, the orthopaedic therapist sees many patients suffering the after-effects of a motor vehicle accident, and in this instance dizziness may be a more serious problem due to the possibility of damage to the vertebral artery. It is therefore important that the therapist be able to assess accurately the general cause of the dizziness to the point where there can be confidence that treatment will not adversely affect the patient's health.

CAUSES OF VERTIGO

A dysfunction of any of the components of the statokinetic system can produce vertigo either alone or, more usually, with other signs and symptoms. The causes which have the most impact on the orthopaedic therapist are those commonly encountered and those which, if unrecognized, can produce severe consequences for the patient's health. Table 27.1 shows the causes of vertigo and dizziness and gives examples.

EXAMINATION FOR DIZZINESS

History

A full and detailed history must be taken from patients relating any symptoms that can, in any fashion, be considered as indicative of dysfunction of the balance mechanism. The patient's age is always noted. Dizziness is not an uncommon complaint of the elderly, and, even if caused by a stenotic vertebral or basilar artery, the symptom of dizziness is not the risk it is in the younger patient. Cervical manipulation is never undertaken on the elderly patient without a very thorough evaluation and only in very exceptional circumstances. Therefore any indication that there is some danger to the patient's health should be considered as a contraindication to manipulative therapy. It is the younger patient that statistics show to be at risk

Table 27.1 Causes of dizziness and vertigo

Cause	Examples	References
Central nervous system trauma	Concussions Contusions	Gibson (1984)
Central nervous system degenerative disease	Syphilis Multiple sclerosis Parkinson's disease Syringobulbia	Finestone (1982), Toglia (1982), Pfaltz (1984)
Vertebrosbasilar and cerebellar vascular disease	Thrombosis Haemorrhage Arteriosclerosis Aneurysm	Toglia (1982), Rudge (1984), Wright(1988a)
Vertiginous epilepsy Neoplastic disease Vestibular neuronitis Acute and chronic otitis media		Toglia (1982), Wright (1988b) Toglia (1982), Luxon (1984) Harrison & Dix (1984) Wright (1988c)
Labyrinthine disease	Meniere's disease Otosclerosis Trauma	Finestone (1982), Gibson (1984), Morrison (1984), Wright (1988c, 1988d)
Iatrogenic	Drugs Surgery	Sevy (1982), Ballantyne & Ajodhia (1984)
Toxins	Alcohol Tobacco Carbon monoxide	Finestone (1982)
Migraine		Finestone (1982), Kayan (1984)
Metabolic and haematological disease	Anaemia Diabetes mellitus Hypoglycaemia Hyperventilation	Finestone (1982), Luxon (1984)
Cardiovascular disease	Postural hypotension Cardiac dysrythmias Valvular dysfunctions	Finestone (1982), Luxon (1984)
Cervical dysfunctions	Traumatic Degenerative	Wing & Hargrave-Wilson (1974), Finestone (1982), Pfaltz (1984)
Temporomandibular joint dysfunction Psychiatric		Arlen (1977), Finestone (1982) Harding (1982), Trimble (1984)

from cervical manipulation. Any patient, young or old, relating a history of dizziness needs to be fully examined by the therapist to ensure the safety of that patient.

The therapist cannot rely on the patient to offer spontaneously information concerning dizziness, visual symptoms, nausea or indeed any other symptoms. Often the patient considers these symptoms as unrelated to the cervical pain that brought him in for treatment. In order not to lead the patient's responses, initial questioning should be open-ended. Non-specific queries as to any unusual symptoms may be made, but if these are met with a negative answer more pointed questions must be asked. 'Do you ever experience dizziness?' can provide an initial response from the patient. If the patient answers 'yes', the type of dizziness must be established. Is it vertiginous? Lightheadedness? Nausea? Giddiness? To establish the presence of vertigo, the question 'Do you feel that either you or the room spins around?' should elicit an appropriate response. Inquiries must be made into disturbances of vision, parasthesia, episodes of collapsing, loss of consciousness, nausea and disturbances of gait such as veering in one direction or the other while walking.

If the patient does admit to any of these symptoms, further questions should explore the onset of the symptoms. If they coincided with the onset of the cervical pain, it is reasonable to assume that the cause of both is the same. If the symptoms coincide with severe headaches, especially in the occipital area, there is a very real possibility that the pain may be directly related to vertebrobasilar insufficiency. If the symptoms preceded the neck pain, there is a strong possibility that they are unrelated to the cervical pain. It is unlikely that an asymptomatic cervical spine could produce balance disturbances by dysfunction of its articular mechanoreceptors or by osteophytic compression of the artery. However, the vertebral artery could be the source of symptoms due to atherosclerosis. Symptoms of balance system dysfunction following cervical pain or cervical trauma may indicate that the causal factor in the cervical pain may also be causing the dysequilibrium. Causes such as discal or osteophytic compression, or dissection of the artery itself, articular dysfunction, or vestibular damage must be considered when the history is related.

The relationship of these events to the activities that precede them must be examined. Symptoms related to getting up suddenly from lying or sitting could indicate postural hypotension. From the perspective of the manual therapist, it is directional vertigo, that is, vertigo caused by head motion, that is the most important. Head movements causing dizziness may be due to the vertebral artery becoming stretched or kinked and so occluded, or to dysfunction of the vestibular apparatus or cervical articular receptors.

The quality of the vertigo is, in part, a function of the cause of the vertigo. Peripheral causes of vertigo tend to produce a very definite sensation of motion with an abrupt onset and severe associated symptoms. Neurological symptoms are less likely in vertigo of peripheral origin and the patient rarely loses consciousness. In vertigo produced by central dysfunction, the hallucination of motion is less definite, the onset is usually slower, and the intensity is generally less severe, at least initially. Ear symptoms are uncommon in central vertigo, while loss of consciousness is more frequently present than in peripheral vertigo. Nystagmus is a common feature to both but other neurological signs and symptoms frequently accompany central vertigo (Finestone 1982).

Objective tests

Because the vertebral artery indirectly supplies the vestibular labyrinth via the labyrinthine artery, vertebral artery occlusion may produce both central and peripheral vertigo.

Pulses

Consistent with the aim to be as careful as possible when testing patients who are potentially at grave risk either from craniovertebral instability or from vertebrobasilar artery insufficiency, assessing the pulses of the common carotid and the vertebral arteries is the first step in the assessment of vertigo.

Various studies have determined that a decrease in flow through the vertebral artery results in an increased flow through the common carotid artery (Hardesty et al 1963, Smith & Stern 1970). Accordingly, the carotid pulse should be taken and the sides compared for gross differences. This can be done in the rotated, and the rotated and extended positions looking for an increase in the strength of the pulse over that found in the neutral position. In children and some less well endowed adults, the vertebral artery pulse can be felt as it crosses over the posterior arch of the atlas; however, in most adults, it is not palpable. If the pulse is obtainable, it should be

assessed in the neutral and stressed positions to see whether the artery is occluded in rotation or in rotation and extension.

A side-to-side difference in either the carotid or vertebral artery pulse, or a change in pulse strength with positional change may indicate hypoplasia or occlusion. If a side-to-side difference is associated with a history of obvious neurological symptoms, or if the pulse changes with a position change, the patient should be referred back to the physician. If the patient's complaints are of a vaguer nature, and if the resting pulse is different from side to side, further testing can be carried out, but with extreme caution.

Craniovertebral ligamentous stability

In patients suffering from motor-vehicle-related, work-related or sports injury, the neck may have been subjected to sufficient force of acceleration/deceleration to damage the ligaments of the craniovertebral joints. Of particular concern are the transverse and alar ligaments of the atlanto-axial joint. There is every reason to suppose that a lesion in one of these ligaments could of itself produce dizziness (Ford 1952, Wing & Hargrave-Wilson 1974) but more importantly, for the safety of the patient, these ligaments, if previously injured, may, like any other ligament, suffer further damage when stretched as the neck is moved to its extremes of range when testing for vertebral artery function.

Insufficiency of the alar ligament will produce and increase the average contralateral rotation at the atlanto-axial joint by up to 30% or almost 11° (Dvorak et al 1987). Hypermobility of this region due to alar ligament, odontoid process, or transverse ligament insufficiency has been shown to be a factor in the production of vertigo and associated symptoms by occlusion of the vertebral artery (Ford 1952, Fielding et al 1974) or by disturbance of afferent input to the vestibular nuclei (Ford 1952, Hardesty et al 1963, Husni et al 1966, Smith & Stern 1970, Wing & Hargrave-Wilson 1974, Arlen 1977, de Jong et al 1977, Harding 1982, Trimble 1984, Dvorak et al 1987).

Many clinical tests for stability of the craniovertebral region have been developed and used for many years (Lee & Walsh 1985, Pettman 1988, Sydenham 1988, Meadows 1989). The problem, however, is that the majority of them have not been validated by research.

Transverse ligament stress test. The patient lies supine with the head supported by a pillow in the neutral position (Fig. 27.1). The examiner supports the occiput in the palms of the hands and third, fourth and fifth fingers while the two index fingers are placed in the space between the occiput and the C2 spinous process thus overlying the neural arch of the atlas. The head and C1 are then lifted as a unit anteriorly allowing no flexion or extension of the neck to occur. Gravity stabilizes the spine

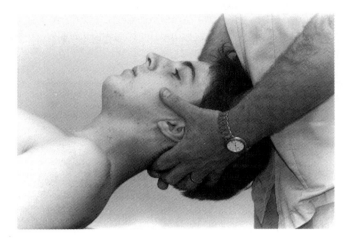

Fig. 27.1 Testing the tranverse ligament of C1.

from C2 downwards and an anterior shear force is produced at the atlanto-axial joint. This shear can be resisted only by the transverse ligament, the ligamentum nuchae being slack in the neutral starting position (Williams & Warwick 1980). This position is held until no further motion is detected or until a positive sign or symptom is produced — such as a spasm or abnormally excessively soft end-feel, dizziness, nausea, facial or limb paraesthesia, parasthesia of the lips, nystagmus, a sensation of a lump in the throat, or consistent reflex swallowing.

Most of the resulting signs and symptoms usually do not relate to transverse ligament instability but all must be taken seriously as tearing of this ligament can have serious consequences for the patient (Fielding et al 1974).

Atlanto-axial lateral shear test. There are a number of congenital conditions that may produce laxity of the craniovertebral ligaments — including adentia (absent dens), microdentia (small dens) and os odontoideum (transverse bipartitism of the dens) (Grieve 1981). In addition, osseus instability may be part of a congenital condition such as Down's syndrome (Hreidarsson et al 1982) or a result of an acquired collagen disease such as rheumatoid arthritis (Dvorak et al 1987).

The lateral shear test is designed to provide information concerning the state of the odontoid process by gently pushing it against the inside of the lateral aspect of the arch of the atlas. The patient lies supine and the examiner places the radial side of one second metacarpophalangeal joint against the transverse process of the atlas and the other metacarpophalangeal joint against the opposite transverse process of the axis (Fig. 27.2). The examiner's hands are then carefully pushed in opposite directions across the neck, thereby shearing one bone on the other.

Under normal circumstances the tendency of the dens to be pushed around the inside of the atlanteal arch is prevented by its impact with the medial tubercles of the atlas and a very hard end-feel results. However, if there is any laxity in the system, an excessive amount of motion will be felt and the end-feel will be much softer than it would be normally. In addition to the abnormal end-feel,

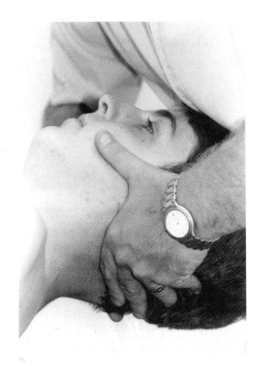

Fig. 27.2 Atlanto-axial lateral shear test.

the production of potential spinal cord or vascular symptoms may also be noted.

Alar ligament stress test. The alar ligament normally tightens with contralateral rotation of the atlanto-axial joint and contralateral side flexion of the atlano-occipital joint (Dvorak et al 1987). The patient lies supine. The examiner stabilizes the axis with a wide pinch grip around the spinous process and lamina (Fig. 27.3). The head and atlas are then side-flexed around the coronal axis of the atlanto-axial joint. The pinch grip will prevent the axis from moving as the occiput and atlas move. If the ligament is intact, no appreciable movement of side-flexion will occur and the examiner will sense a strong capsular end-feel. However, if the ligament is insufficient, some side-flexion will occur as the slack in the ligament is taken

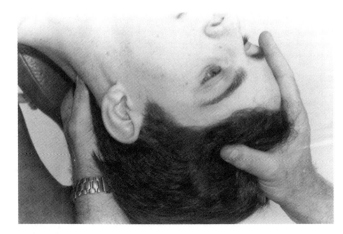

Fig. 27.3 Alar ligament stress test.

up. This motion will be felt by the examiner and considered an indicator of atlanto-axial instability. In addition to the occurrence of excessive motion, symptoms ascribable to disorders of the balance mechanism may be elicited.

Radiographs. If the orthopaedic therapist is at all concerned about the stability of the craniovertebral region, the patient should not be treated until flexion/extension and side-flexion stress radiographs are taken and found to be negative. However, it should be noted that false negatives with the radiographic results can be a potential problem. If muscle spasm is a factor when the region is moved it will splint the joints and the X-rays will appear negative. Another problem lies with the axis of the motion during the radiographic procedure. The motion must occur around the craniovertebral axis and not about a mid-cervical axis. For flexion and extension the cranio-vertebral axis is roughly through the external auditory meatus while for side-flexion, it is through the nose. If motion occurs around other axes, a false negative may result as movement may not occur at the craniovertebral joints. As a consequence of these false positives, it is essential that the examiner does not undertake any treatment that will put the patient at risk for as long as the tests appear positive. If the therapist has a good working relationship with the radiographer, positioning of the neck in stress positions should be done by the therapist, and if spasm is a factor no mechanical treatment of the region should be administered until either the clinical tests are negative or the stress X-rays have been taken correctly. It is only after negative stress tests or genuinely negative radiographs that further stress testing for dizziness should be attempted.

If these stress tests are negative for laxity but do produce dizziness, it is likely that, in part at least, the dizziness is generated by ligamentous damage. However, the remaining tests must be carried out to determine whether there is an additional contributing cause.

VESTIBULAR DIZZINESS

Possibly the best way to determine clinically and quickly the presence of vestibular vertigo is to use the observation of Cope and Ryan (1959) that the potential for the cervical spine to cause vertigo — due either to articular dysfunction or vertebral artery occlusion — is almost eliminated if the head and neck are moved as a unit while the patient wears a cervical collar.

The collar is fitted to the patient in the seated position. The head and neck are further supported by the examiner who stands beside the patient. The patient is then asked to lie down on the bed taking care not to move the head. If possible, the bed should be of the type in which the end can be dropped down so that, in the full test position, the patient's head is lower than the trunk. Dropping the patient's head over the end of the bed is not useful as this movement will result in cervical extension, despite the col-

lar, and the cervical spine cannot be excluded from any dizziness produced. If dizziness is produced during this test, the cause cannot be cervical in origin as the position of the spine has remained constant during the test. Given a negative test, amplification of the effect of the test can be achieved by removing the stabilizing effect of the eyes by repeating the test with the patient's eyes closed. The patient is asked to relate any symptomatology that occurs during the test.

To eliminate the effect of the inner ear, the head must be held still while the cervical spine is rotated beneath it (Cope & Ryan 1959, Maitland 1977, Grieve 1981). The patient sits on the edge of the bed and the examiner holds the patient's head firmly, preventing any head motion (Fig. 27.4). The patient is then asked to twist or turn the body while the head remains stationary. The labyrinthine system thus remains stationary during the test while the cervical articular receptors and the vertebral artery are moved and stressed. Therefore, any dizziness produced during the test cannot be vestibular in origin. However, because this test does stress the vertebral artery, it is suggested that it be not carried out until the general cervical stress test, which is a more controlled situation, has been done.

GENERAL CERVICAL STRESS TEST FOR DIZZINESS

The fully stressed position for the cervical structures causing dizziness is cervical extension, rotation and traction. This positioning is often called the vertebral artery

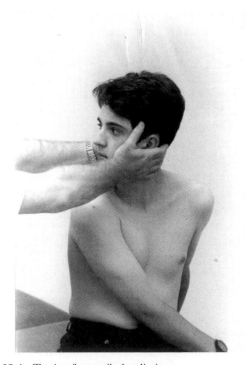

Fig. 27.4 Testing for vestibular dizziness.

stress test; however, it must be understood that, while this position is most likely to occlude the vertebral artery (Toole & Tucker 1960, Brown & Tatlow 1963, Hardesty et al 1963), it also puts under stress other tissues such as the craniovertebral and mid-cervical joints, the cervical proprioceptors and the vestibular apparatus. Therefore, the position simply tests whether or not cervical movement causes dizziness but does not in itself differentiate the specific tissues at fault. The test should not be carried out until the craniovertebral ligaments have been cleared for laxity. The test position of rotation and extension has been described in the literature for premanipulative testing of vertebrobasilar artery sufficiency (Cope & Ryan 1959, Smith & Estridge 1962, Dvorak & Orelli 1985, Grant 1987). However, it is well to note that at least one patient who had angiographic evidence of, and symptomatology ascribable to, vertebral artery occlusion did not demonstrate any signs or symptoms when the stress tests for the vertebral artery were carried out (Bolton et al 1989).

For the test to be effective, at least 30° of rotation is required for partial occlusion of the artery (Seleki 1969) and the critical angle for blood flow disturbance in the vertebral artery is required to be less than 45° with at least another 10–15° required before complete obstruction occurs in some subjects (Toole & Tucker 1960). Therefore, the patients have to have the required amount of cervical motion before they can be properly tested.

The test should be done in supine lying so that if the patient does lose consciousness there is no danger of further injury from a fall. Consistent with the practice of testing with the least risk, the full-stress position is attained in stages with progression to the next stage occurring only if the previous stage had proven negative.

The patient lies supine, and the examiner slowly rotates the head as far as possible with no extension being added. It is held in this position until the patient complains of symptoms attributable to arterial occlusion, neurological signs such as nystagmus, or loss of consciousness become apparent, or for 40 seconds (Bolton et al 1989) whichever is the sooner. If negative, the test is repeated on the other side. If this position produces dizziness or nausea, the next differential tests are carried out unless there are frank neurological signs — in which case the patient should not be treated and should be referred back to the physician.

If the tests are negative, further stress is applied by the addition of cervical extension (Fig. 27.5). This motion brings the neck into the position that maximally stresses the vertebral artery and only the addition of traction will further reduce its diameter.

It has been suggested that, for safety, the stress should be taken off the lower artery while the upper part of the artery is tested. This is done by maintaining lower cervical flexion while rotating and extending the upper spine. The

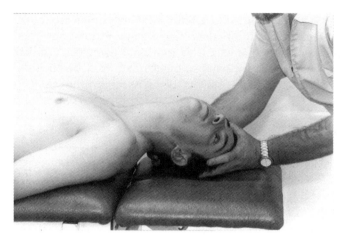

Fig. 27.5   Vertebral artery testing.

procedure can then be reversed by flexing the upper cervical spine while testing the lower (Grieve 1981, Pettman & Abbotsford 1986). The position is again held for 40 seconds or until the onset of symptoms.

While the test is being carried out the patient is asked to keep his eyes open to make sure that he retains consciousness during the test and to observe the onset of nystagmus. Near the end of the stress time period, the patient is asked to gaze in the direction to which the head is rotated to sensitize the test further (Keuter 1970).

It has been suggested that the full stress test be done with the head overhanging the bed to ensure that further stretching occurs in the aorta and subclavian artery (Aspinall 1988). However, the severe stress that is likely to be generated by stretching from top and bottom simultaneously is potentially dangerous and, in addition, the problem of repositioning the patient if loss of consciousness occurs, could be considerable.

If each of the regional tests prove negative, the neck can be taken into general full rotation and extension and traction applied, and if this also fails to be symptomatic, and the neck has a good range of motion, it can be assumed that it is safe to apply mechanical treatments. However, it is advisable to put the neck in the treatment position and maintain this position prior to any treatment actually being given for about 40 seconds (Grant 1987, Aspinall 1988). If there is considerable loss of range of motion in the neck, and the artery cannot be fully stressed, then treatment must be given only in those available ranges. High-velocity low-amplitude techniques should be carried out only very carefully with an emphasis on low amplitude. The general stress test must be repeated at every session as many of the case reports described above indicate that it is not always the first few manipulations that cause problems.

HAUTARD'S TEST

If the general stress test for the cervical spine and vertebral artery were positive, the problem now becomes one of differentiation. The vestibular system has been precluded as the cause of dizziness by the vestibular tests carried out by simultaneous head and neck displacement while the patient is wearing a collar. Hautard's test may assist with differentiating articular and vascular vertigo (Bolton et al 1989).

Hautard's test is a modification of Rhomberg's test for cerebellar disease. The principle difference between the two is that in Rhomberg's test, shutting the eyes — and thus eliminating the stabilizing effect of the eyes on balance — is sufficient to cause proprioceptive disturbance, while Hautard's test produces the disturbance by reducing the blood flow to the cerebellum. The patient sits on a treatment table and elevates both arms to 90° (Fig. 27.6). The eyes are then closed while the examiner watches for a loss of position of one or both arms. This initial phase tests for non-vascular cerebellar dysfunction. If this test is negative, the patient then stresses the vertebral artery either by rotation, or rotation with extension, whichever is the minimal head displacement necessary to produce the signs and symptoms. The arms are observed for wavering from the original position. If wavering occurs, it indicates a loss of proprioception and thus, a cerebellar dysfunction. As the dysfunction did not occur until the head was moved and the artery stressed, it must be vasculogenic. Dizziness is not a positive sign for vertebral artery occlusion. It is already known that the stress position will reproduce dizziness; it is the proprioceptive loss characterized by displacement of the arm that is important (Cyriax 1982).

CRANIOVERTEBRAL INSTABILITY

Any indication that there is a loss of integrity of the atlanto-axial osseoligamentous ring should demand immediate immobilization of the neck with the hardest collar available while the patient is left lying on the treatment table and a physician or ambulance called. No further treatment should be undertaken until either the stress tests are negative or exhaustive objective tests (for example, through mouth, flexion/extension radiographic studies, magnetic resonance imaging) have completely proven that there is no reduction in stability.

Generally, partial or complete tears of the alar ligament are not an immediate serious danger to the patient's life and a less drastic approach can be taken. Treatment can be continued but should not be such that it might transform a grade 2 to a grade 3 tear or exacerbate symptoms ascribable to damage to this ligament. The physician should be informed and side-flexion and rotation X-rays of the craniovertebral region may demonstrate the instability (Sydenham 1989). The patient should be informed that recovery will take a protracted period — which is often important for medico-legal reasons.

TREATMENT

Vestibular dysfunction

Vestibular dysfunction is not the primary concern of the orthopaedic therapist, but, of course, techniques that produce dizziness should be avoided. The physician, if unaware of the problem, should be informed. It is not, however, good enough to assume that because vestibular dysfunction has been discovered it is the sole or even main cause of the dizziness. There may be coincidental arterial occlusion or upper cervical proprioceptive dysfunction present.

Upper cervical vertigo

Upper cervical vertigo is most frequently associated with trauma, and if of recent onset, a soft collar and anti-inflammatory modalities are usually effective as treatment (Cope & Ryan 1959). If of the more chronic variety, then it is usually due to a biomechanical dysfunction and should be treated with mobilization or manipulation (Wing & Hargrave-Wilson 1974).

Vertebrobasilar insufficiency

If the examination of the patient suggests the possibility of vertebrobasilar artery insufficiency, manipulation must be considered as absolutely contraindicated (Cooper & Daniel 1949, Grieve 1981, Katirji et al 1985). Any treatment involving rotation, extension or traction of the neck is also very suspect and should be considered very carefully before being initiated. Any treatment techniques used on any patient, regardless of a negative history or examination for dizziness, should not produce dizziness or associated signs or symptoms. Cervical mechanical and manual traction in the elderly patient often produces dizziness frequently for a number of days, and manipulation should be avoided in these patients due to the danger

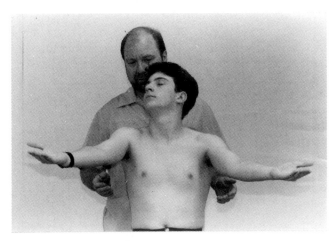

Fig. 27.6 Hautard's test.

Table 27.2 Incidence of the various symptoms related to vertebrobasilar artery insufficiency*

Symptom	Incidence (%)
Dizziness	100
Vertigo	40
Headache	30
Loss of consciousness	25
Disturbances in gait	15
Disturbances in vision	15
Nausea	10
Upper limb parasthesia	10

* Reproduced with permission from Husni et al 1966.

of stretching or kinking an already kinked and/or atherosclerotic artery.

The problem should be brought to the physician's attention and the patient should be put into a cervical collar and advised on which positions and movements should be avoided. It must be emphasized to the patient that manipulation is contraindicated until the problem has been fully investigated.

The patient who has developed signs and symptoms as a result of examination or treatment must be managed especially carefully. Due consideration must be given to the progressive nature of the signs and symptoms, and what appears immediately after the incidence as a minor bout of vertigo or nausea may develop into brain stem compression from vertebral artery haemorrhage leading to death over the following few hours. Patients with obvious neurological signs should be taken to the emergency department or their physician immediately. Those who develop less clear-cut symptoms should remain in the facility and be monitored carefully for any progression in the condition and then be referred to the emergency room if symptoms progress.

Another safety issue is the manipulative technique utilized. In every case report of vertebrobasilar artery distribution infarction where the causative technique was described, it was rotation either in neutral or in extension. The problem is seen as so pervasive that Dvorak and Orelli (1985) have suggested that manipulative techniques be abandoned totally in the neck and other less forceful manual techniques substituted. Manipulative therapy is at a point where there is no reason to use strong rotational or non-specific technique. The amplitude of the technique

can now be reduced to the point where it is measured in single degrees and specificity to one apophyseal joint at a particular level.

SUMMARY

Patients presenting with dizziness as part of their complaint are not an oddity in orthopaedic physical therapy practice. These people need to be appropriately tested to differentiate conditions that are the concern of, and a concern to, the therapist from those that fall within the physician's province.

Stringent testing must be carried out on every patient before a cervical manipulation is attempted unless testing itself is contraindicated. The examination must distinguish between drug-induced vertigo, vestibular vertigo, cervical articular vertigo and vertebrobasilar vertigo. The management of the patient depends on the cause of the dizziness, and those problems that have a potential for fatality or serious neurological consequences must be given pre-eminence in examination and treatment. The patient must always be considered to have a serious life-threatening problem until exhaustive examination has proved otherwise. The possible presence of vertebrobasilar artery insufficiency is an absolute contraindication to manipulative therapy, and patients suspected of having this problem must be referred back to the physician for definitive examination.

Treatment techniques should be specific, low-amplitude and non-rotational and should be applied only after exhaustive testing. If an injury to the vertebral artery does occur, the therapist must behave responsibly and see that the patient is either escorted to the emergency room or to the referring physician if the signs are unequivocally neurological — or monitored in the clinic for the next hour or so.

Cervical manipulation is a powerful weapon in the orthopaedic manual therapist's armory but it should be used responsibly and with some trepidation. The actual technical aspect of manipulative therapy is relatively simple. It is the knowledge of where the technique should be applied, and on whom, that is the more difficult and demanding skill. The buccaneer approach to treating the cervical spine should be a thing of the past with no place in today's treatment regimes.

REFERENCES

Arlen H 1977 The otomandibular syndrome. In: Gelb H (ed) Clinical management of head, neck and TMJ pain and dysfunction: a multidisciplinary approach to diagnosis and treatment. WB Saunders, Philadelphia, pp 181–194

Aspinall W 1988 Clinical testing for cervical mechanical disorders which produce ischemic vertigo. A presentation of the problems and solutions of spinal mobilization and manipulation. Proceedings of the Canadian Physiotherapy Association/American Physical Therapy

Association pp 12–22

Ballantyne J, Ajodhia J 1984 Iatrogenic dizziness. In: Dix M R, Hood J D (eds) Vertigo. John Wiley, Chichester, pp 217–245

Berenstein A 1962 Archives of Otolaryngology (Chicago) 76: 329–337

Bolton P S, Stick P E, Lord S A 1989 Failure of clinical tests to predict cerebral ischemia before neck manipulation. Journal of Manipulative Physiological Therapeutics 12: 304–307

Brown B S J, Tatlow W F T 1963 Radiologic studies of the vertebral artery in cadavers. Radiology 81: 80–88

Cawthorne J 1945 The physiological basis of head exercises. Journal of the Chartered Society of Physiotherapists 30: 106–107

Cawthorne J 1957 Aural vertigo. In: Modern trends in neurology. Butterworth, London, pp 193–201

Cecil R L 1947 Textbook of medicine. 7th edn. W B Saunders, Philadelphia, pp 1499–1502

Cooper S, Daniel P M 1949 Muscle spindles in human extrinsic eye muscles. Brain 72: 1–24

Cope S, Ryan G M S 1959 Cervical and otolith vertigo. Journal of Laryngology and Otology 73: 113–120

Cyriax J 1982 Textbook of orthopedic medicine. 8th edn. Baillière Tindall, Eastbourne

de Jong P T V M, de Jong J M B V, Cohen B, Jongkees B W 1977 Ataxia induced by injection of local anesthetics in the neck. Annals of Neurology 1: 240–246

de Weese D D 1950 Evaluation of dizziness. JAMA 142: 542–546

Dvorak J, Orelli F 1985 How dangerous is manipulation to the cervical spine: case report and results of a survey. Manual Medicine 2: 1–4

Dvorak J, Panjabi M, Gerber M, Wichman W 1987 CT-functional diagnostics of the rotatory instability of upper cervical spine 1. An experimental study on cadavers. Spine 12: 197–205

Elia J C 1968 The dizzy patient. Charles C Thomas, Springfield

Fielding J W, Cochron G V B, Lansing J F, Hohl M 1974 Tears of the transverse ligament of the atlas. Journal of Bone and Joint Surgery 56A: 1683–1692

Finestone A J 1982 An approach to the patient with dizziness and vertigo by the primary care physician. In: Finestone A J (ed) Dizziness and vertigo. John Wright, Boston, pp 45–68

Ford F R 1952 Syncope, vertigo and disturbances of vision resulting from intermittent obstruction of the vertebral arteries due to defect in the odontoid process and excessive mobility of the second cervical vertebra. Bulletin of the Johns Hopkins Hospital 91: 168–173

Gibson W P R 1984 Vertigo associated with trauma. In: Dix M R, Hood J D (eds) Vertigo. John Wiley, Chichester, pp 373–389

Grant R 1987 Dizziness testing before cervical manipulation: can we recognize the patient at risk? In Proceedings of the Manipulative Therapist's Association of Australia 5th Biennial Conference, pp 123–136

Grieve G P 1981 Common vertebral joint problems. Churchill Livingstone, Edinburgh, pp 12–13

Grieve G P 1981 Common vertebral joint problems. Churchill Livingstone, Edinburgh, pp 313–320

Hardesty W H, Whitacre W B, Toole J F, Randall P, Royster H P 1963 Studies on vertebral artery blood flow in man. Surgery, Gynecology & Obstetrics 116: 662–664

Harding J J 1982 Psychiatric aspects of dizziness and vertigo. In: Finestone A J (ed) Dizziness and vertigo. John Wright, Boston, pp 129–157

Harrison M S, Dix M R 1984 Vestibular neuronitis. In: Dix M R, Hood J D (eds) Vertigo. John Wiley, Chichester, pp 167–178

Hreidarsson S, Magram G, Singer H 1982 Symptomatic altanto-axial dislocation in Down's syndrome. Pediatrics 69: 568–571

Husni E A, Bell H S, Storer J 1966 Mechanical occlusion of the vertebral artery: a new clinical concept. JAMA 196: 475–478

Katirji M B, Reinmuth O M, Latchaw R E 1985 Stroke due to vertebral artery injury. Archives of Neurology 42: 244–248

Kayan A 1984 Migraine and vertigo. In: Dix M R, Hood J D (eds) Vertigo. John Wiley, Chichester, pp 249–265

Keuter E J W 1970 Vascular origin of cranial sensory disturbances caused by pathology of the lower cervical spine. Acta Neurochirurgica 23: 229–245

Lee D G, Walsh M C 1985 A workbook of manual therapy techniques for the vertebral column and pelvic girdle. Nacent Publishing, Delta, BC, pp 8–12

Ludman H 1981 Vertigo. British Medical Journal 282(6262): 454–457

Maitland G D 1977 Vertebral manipulation. 4th edn. Butterworths, London, pp 10–30

Meadows J 1989 The physical therapist's investigation and management of dizziness. Vertebral 2/3 course book (unpublished)

Morrison A W 1984 Meniere's disease. In: Dix M R, Hood J D (eds) Vertigo. John Wiley, Chichester, pp 133–152

Orma E J, Koskenojen M 1957 Postural dizziness in the aged. Geriatrics 12: 49–59

Pemberton J 1953 Vertigo in a random sample of elderly people living in their homes. Journal of Laryngology 67: 689

Pettman E, Abbotsford B C 1986 Personal communication

Pettman E 1988 Mobility and stability tests of the cranio vertebral joints. Proceedings of the 2nd Annual Orthopaedic Division, Canadian Physiotherapy Association, pp 85–100

Pfaltz C R 1984 Vertigo in disorders of the neck. In: Dix M R, Hood J D (eds) Vertigo. John Wiley, Chichester, pp 179–215

Rogers F B 1982 Historical introduction and review. In: Finestone A J (ed) Dizziness and vertigo. John Wright, Boston, pp 1–12

Rudge P 1984 Central causes of vertigo. In: Dix M R, Hood J D (eds) Vertigo. John Wiley, Chichester, pp 321–343

Seleki B R 1969 The effects of rotation of the atlas on the axis: experimental work. Medical Journal of Australia 1: 1012–1015

Sevy R W 1982 Drugs as a cause of dizziness and vertigo. In: Firestone A J (ed) Dizziness and vertigo. John Wright, Boston, pp 105–113

Smith R A, Estridge M N 1962 Neurological complications of head and neck manipulations: report of two cases. JAMA 182: 528–531

Smith G A, Stern W E 1970 Experiments on carotid artery flow increase as a result of contralateral carotid occlusion. Acta Neurochirurgica 23: 221–228

Sydenham R W 1988 Lesions of the upper cervical spine ligamentous complex. At the presentation of the problems and solutions of spinal mobilization and manipulation. Proceedings of the Canadian Physiotherapy Association/American Physical Therapy Association pp 12–22

Sydenham R W 1989 Radiographic presentation of cranio-vertebral ligament insufficiency. Presentation at the 5th Congress of the Canadian Orthopedic Manual Physiotherapists, September 1989

Thomas C L (ed) 1979 Taber's cyclopedic medical dictionary. F A Davis, Philadelphia, V22

Toglia J U 1982 Neurological aspects of vertigo and dizziness. In: Finestone A J (ed) Dizziness and vertigo. John Wright, Boston, pp 81–97

Toole J F, Tucker S H 1960 Influence of head position upon cerebral circulation: studies in blood flow in cadavers. Archives of Neurology 2: 616–621

Trimble M R 1984 Psychiatric aspects of vertigo. In: Dix M R, Hood J D (eds) Vertigo. John Wiley, Chichester, pp 345–358

Luxon L M 1984 Vertigo in old age. In: Dix M R, Hood J D (eds) Vertigo. John Wiley, Chichester, pp 291–319

Williams P L, Warwick R (eds) 1980 Gray's anatomy. 36th edn. Churchill Livingstone, Edinburgh, pp 443–449

Wing L W, Hargrave-Wilson, W 1974 Cervical vertigo. New Zealand Journal of Surgery 44: 275–277

Wright A 1988a The brainstem. In: Dizziness: a guide to disorders of balance. Croom Helm, London, pp 166–181

Wright, A 1988b The Cerebral cortex and the psyche. In: Dizziness: a guide to disorders of balance. Croom Helm, London, pp 207–226

Wright A 1988c The ear and its diseases. In: Dizziness: a guide to disorders of balance. Croom Helm, London, pp 86–98

Wright A 1988d Meniere's syndrome. In: Dizziness: a guide to disorders of balance. Croom Helm, London, 111–123

28. Cervical and lumbar pain syndromes

J. M. Moss

McKENZIE SYNDROMES OF MECHANICAL SPINAL PAIN

Over the last 30 years, Robin McKenzie has developed a unique system of examination and categorization of mechanical spinal pain. This provides manual therapists with an alternative system of diagnosis and treatment for spinal patients based on the mechanism of pain production.

This chapter deals with the spinal pain syndromes; Chapter 42 deals with repeated movement examination, and Chapter 55 with treatment of the three syndromes of non-specific mechanical spinal pain. All three chapters relate exclusively to the work of Robin McKenzie, and his texts (1981, 1990).

What is a syndrome?

A syndrome is a set of signs and symptoms that, collectively, characterize a particular disease or abnormal condition. It implies that the actual cause is unknown. Therefore, the term syndrome is extremely useful for manual therapists working in this field of spinal pain where the actual specific cause of pain for the majority of their patients is unknown.

DIFFICULTIES WITH DIAGNOSIS

Various authors (Dixon 1980, Jayson 1980, Nachemson 1980, Yates 1980) have stated the problems in arriving at a specific diagnosis of spinal pain. These diagnostic difficulties are highlighted in the Quebec Task Force (QTF) Report (Spitzer 1987). The report states:

Pain is the primordial and often the only symptom of the vast majority of spinal disorders. During the acute phase, pain is of nociceptive origin, but the influence of psychological and social factors (Beals & Hickman 1972, Fordyce et al 1986) on the continuation of pain toward a chronic phase is now increasingly recognised . . . Although there are considerably more clinical studies on patients suffering from problems of the lumbar area than there are on patients with problems in the cervical region, pain develops because of the irritation of structures sensitive to pain and these are the same for all segments of the spine. These structures are bones, discs, joints, nerves, muscles and soft tissues. They may be affected by an inflammatory, infectious, neoplastic or traumatic disease or be the site of a congenital or developmental mechanical defect.

Nevertheless, it is difficult to identify precisely the origin of the pain, because even if its characteristics may sometimes point to a given structure, the pain system remains unspecific. In addition, it is generally impossible to corroborate clinical observations through histologic studies, because on the one hand the usual benignity of spinal disorders does not justify that tissue be removed and, on the other, there is often no modification of tissue identifiable through current methods.

The QTF developed the classification system given in Table 28.1 and recommended its use universally.

The first four classes in Table 28.1 represent 90% of all patients in this table and have a striking resemblance to the McKenzie classification system (McKenzie 1981). As illustrated in Table 28.2, the McKenzie system of diagnosis actually provides further division of these four classes of pain. The McKenzie classification acknowledges the presence or absence of acute spinal deformity as this has important implications for treatment.

The QTF report recommends conservative treatment for these first four groups. These groups were labelled 'non-specific'. It is estimated that 85% of all back pain episodes are non-specific (White & Gordon 1987).

Types of pain syndrome

Mechanical spinal pain is caused by mechanical deformation of soft tissues containing nociceptive receptors (Wyke 1980). McKenzie states that all spinal mechanical pain can be classified into three syndromes: the postural, dysfunction and derangement syndromes. Each syndrome is

Table 28.1 Classification of activity-related spinal disorders (Reproduced from Spitzer 1987, with kind permission of the publisher, Harper & Row).

Classification	Symptoms	Duration of symptoms from onset	Working status at time of evaluation
1	Pain without radiation	a (< 7 days)	
2	Pain + radiation to extremity, proximally	b (7 days–7 weeks)	W (working)
3	Pain + radiation to extremity, distally*	c (> 7 weeks)	I (idle)
4	Pain + radiation to upper/lower limb, neurological signs		
5	Presumptive compression of a spinal nerve root on a simple roentgenogram (i.e. spinal instability or fracture)		
6	Compression of a spinal nerve root confirmed by: Specific imaging techniques (i.e. computerized axial tomography, myelography, or magnetic resonance imaging) Other diagnostic techniques (e.g. electromyography, venography)		
7	Spinal stenosis		
8	Postsurgical status, 1–6 months after intervention		
9	Postsurgical status, > 6 months after intervention 9.1 Asymptomatic 9.2 Symptomatic		
10	Chronic pain syndrome		W (working)
11	Other diagnoses		I (idle)

* Not applicable to the thoracic segment.

Table 28.2 Comparison of QTF and McKenzie classifications

QTF classification	McKenzie classification
Class 1	Derangement 1–4 or 7 Postural, dysfunction syndrome
Class 2	Derangement 1–4 or 7
Class 3	Derangements 5 and 6 Adherence neural tissue
Class 4	Derangements 5 and 6

a unique and separate disorder. In essence, these three classifications are separated by the location of their symptoms, the presence or absence of acute spinal deformity, and the effects of repeated movements and sustained end-range positions on their pain patterns. Briefly, the three syndromes are as follows.

The postural syndrome

Postural pain appears after prolonged static loading, which, in turn, causes overstretching and mechanical deformation of normal spinal tissue. The pain eases and then stops on removal of the loading.

The dysfunction syndrome

Dysfunctional pain appears immediately when shortened spinal tissues are mechanically deformed by overstretching. The pain eases and then stops on removal of the end-range stress.

The derangement syndrome

Derangement pain is felt immediately or eventually when there is an anatomical disruption or displacement of the intervertebral segment.

PREDISPOSING FACTORS OF MECHANICAL SPINAL PAIN

McKenzie (1981) states that there are two main predisposing factors causing mechanical spinal pain. The first and most significant factor is prolonged poor sitting posture and the second is the frequency of flexion in people's lifestyles.

Prolonged sitting

Epidemiological and laboratory studies suggest that a close connection exists between prolonged sitting and the development of back pain, especially when driving a motor vehicle (Magora 1972, Kelsey 1975a, b, Wood & Baddeley 1980, Andersson 1981). Cadaveric experiments (Hickey & Hukins 1980, Adams & Hutton 1985) caused failure of the annulus in simulated sitting and flexed postures. Wilder et al (1988) showed that one hour simulated sitting predisposes the lumbar posterior annulus to failure.

Sitting unsupported for a short period of time results in a slouched sitting posture with the lumbar spine in flexion (Andersson et al 1975, Wyke 1980) and corresponding thoracic flexion and cervical protrusion. In a study comparing the effects of two sitting postures on the low back and referred pain, Williams et al (1991) showed that sitting with lumbar kyphosis increases low back and referred pain as compared to sitting with lordosis. The lordotic posture also showed a significant shift of the most peripheral pain towards the low back.

Harms-Ringdahl (1986) studied pain provocation by end-range positioning of the head and neck in protrusion. Pain was provoked within 2–15 minutes in 10 previously asymptomatic subjects. This pain increased as the posture was maintained, and 16–57 minutes after onset of the initial pain the subjects declined to continue the protruded head posture because of the level of pain. In all subjects the pain passed off within 15 minutes, but was again experienced by four subjects that same evening or the next morning, and in some cases it lasted up to four days.

Andersson et al (1975) found the myoelectric activity in the para-vertebral lumbar muscles was reduced to zero in relaxed sitting and fully flexed postures. In these positions the intra-discal pressures were raised as compared to sitting upright (Nachemson & Morris 1964). Myoelectric activity was also found to be low in a protruded cervical posture (Harms-Ringdahl 1986).

Frequency of flexion

The second most common predisposing factor in the production of symptoms from the cervical, thoracic and lumbar region is the frequency with which spinal flexion occurs in daily living.

Adams and Hutton (1985) described gradual disc prolapse and annular failure following prolonged flexion loading on cadaveric specimens. Twomey and Taylor (1982) reported that the amount of flexion creep deformation in cadaveric lumbar spines increases with load and progresses with time irrespective of age.

Eventually, the supportive soft tissues succumb to these stresses of poor sitting and sustained flexion and fail without being subject to violent external forces (Hickey & Hukins 1980, Kramer 1981, Adams & Hutton 1985, Wilder et al 1988).

By adopting correct posture, the possibility of damage from such causes can be removed.

A detailed description of each syndrome follows.

THE POSTURAL SYNDROME

Definition

In the postural syndrome patients complain of pain because they are mechanically deforming their spinal soft tissue due to sustaining end-range postures and positions.

Mechanism of pain production

The pain of the postural syndrome is caused solely by prolonged static loading of soft tissue contained within, or adjacent to, the spinal column.

In the cervical spine this occurs most commonly with poor sitting when the neck is in end-range protrusion and with lying where end-range rotation and side-flexion occur. In the lumbar spine, postural pain occurs when the lumbar spine is kept at end-range of flexion in prolonged sitting or bending forwards, or when the low lumbar spine is in sustained extension as occurs with relaxed standing.

Sitting is the most frequent cause of postural pain. Andersson et al (1975) and Wyke (1980) stated than when sitting for a few minutes, the lumbar spine assumes the fully flexed position. The muscles that support the low back while sitting soon become tired and relax. From then on the static postural support is provided by ligamentous structures. Over-stretching of these structures leads to mechanical deformation and results in postural pain (Wyke 1980). Thus, ligamentous fatigue follows muscular fatigue.

There is no pathology present in the pure postural syndrome patient. Posture pain is most easily explained using the analogy of the 'bent finger syndrome' (McKenzie 1981). If you take a normal finger, bend it backwards and hold it there you will eventually feel pain. As long as it is held at end-range, pain will be felt. On release, the pain subsides and disappears. The same occurs in the spine when held at its end-range in a sustained fashion, as in slouched sitting.

Clinical picture

Patients with pain solely of postural origin are usually 30 years or under. They frequently have sedentary occupations and are under-exercised. The onset of postural pain is insidious, and patients describe their condition as gradually worsening.

The more often structures are stressed to the point of being painful, the more sensitive they become to mechanical stimuli. As a result, progressively less stress is required to provoke pain (Wall 1977). Thus poor sitting and standing postures maintained regularly will cause pain after the passage of less and less time and, hence, a worsening situation for the postural syndrome patient.

The pain is felt locally and symmetrically, usually adjacent to the midline of the spine in the cervico-thoracic junction and in the mid-thoracic and low-lumbar region and is often accompanied by a headache. The pain is intermittent and is felt only when the tissues are placed under prolonged stress. Therefore, there is a time factor involved. The symptoms are often worse as the day progresses. On change of the posture or position the pain subsides and disappears. Postural patients are pain-free when active or on the move.

Pain from the postural syndrome alone is never induced by movement, neither is it extensively referred, and the pain produced is never constant but always intermittent in nature. There is no pathology or loss of movement, and there are no elictable signs. There is nothing to see other than the poor posture itself.

The diagnosis is made by this absence of signs and the history.

Described simply, postural pain appears during prolonged static loading causing overstretching of normal tissue. The pain ceases immediately on removal of the loading (McKenzie 1990). The aim of the treatment is to correct the posture, thus relieving painful tension in normal tissues.

DYSFUNCTION SYNDROME

Definition

In the dysfunction syndrome patients feel pain when they mechanically deform previously shortened structures surrounding and within their spine on attempting normal end-range movement.

The term 'dysfunction' was originally coined by Mennell (1960) to describe the loss of movement known as joint play or accessory joint movement. It implies incorrect functioning without trying to state a particular pathology or pin-point a single structure. Loss of joint play (dysfunction) can be due to adaptive shortening, contracture, scarring, adherence or fibrosis.

Mechanism of pain production

In dysfunction, the soft tissues within or surrounding the involved spinal segments are shortened, have reduced elasticity or extensibility, or contain contracted scar tissue. The main reason for the development of dysfunctional changes is the absence of adequate movement while contracture of the soft tissues is occurring (Evans 1980, Hardy 1989).

The mechanism of pain production is the same as in the postural syndrome. The only difference is that the patient with dysfunction has reduced spinal mobility and, therefore, pain is produced earlier than in the patient with the postural syndrome who has full spinal mobility. Thus, in the dysfunction syndrome, normal or abnormal dynamic or static loading of the spine with spinal joints in end-range position exerts mechanical stress on the abnormal soft tissues, and mechanical deformation of these will immediately or sometimes eventually lead to pain. Dysfunction following poor posture spondylosis sometimes does not cause symptoms on end-range movement, but it may on prolonged static loading. Following trauma and derangement there is scar formation, and often immediate pain results on stressing short structures.

Dysfunction may arise as a result of poor postural habits, spondylosis, trauma or derangement. Poor postural habits maintained during the first few decades of life are the most common cause of reduced spinal mobility. The annulus, overstretched ligaments and capsular structures begin to suffer from minor tears as the flexion forces of our lifestyle 'pulls us apart'. The majority of these tears probably heal quickly, and little consequence is felt at the time. However, minor, but recurring microtraumata and repair eventually lead to a loss of elasticity and a reduction in the range of movement—dysfunction. Studies by Kelsey (1975a, b) and Shanahan & Reading (1984) show that people who habitually adopt a slouched or flexed sitting posture, especially in office and vehicular situations, have a higher incidence of neck and back pain.

A consequence of this postural neglect, especially in people who are generally unfit and under-exercised, is a loss of their extension range, not only in the lumbar spine but also in thoracic and lower cervical segments. These patients present with a loss of lumbar lordosis, an increased thoracic kyphosis and 'dowagers' hump' at the cervico-thoracic junction. A loss of lumbar extension forces the patient to live with more flexed postures and consequently with increased intradiscal pressures in their lumbar spine. This state may predispose them to developing the derangement syndrome.

Spondylosis is part of the normal ageing process of the spine. According to Dixon (1980) the term refers to the sequence of changes affecting one or more levels of disc degeneration, disc narrowing, osteophyte formation in the longitudinal ligaments, and osteo-arthrosis of the apophyseal joints. Spondylosis can be primary, in which case usually several levels are affected, or it may develop secondarily to previous trauma or disc derangement. Moll and Wright (1980) reported that age alone may reduce spinal mobility by as much as 50%.

Following trauma or intervertebral derangement, repair of damaged structures occurs by formation of fibrous scar tissue. New scar tissue will always shorten unless it is repeatedly stretched (Evans 1980).

With a lack of functional activity and exercise, not only will an inextensible scar develop and cause reduced spinal mobility, but the scar will have less strength and range (Evans 1980).

We have no way of knowing exactly what structures are affected. All we can say with confidence is that something has contracted, fibrosed or become adhered. However, when there is nerve root or dural adherence the loss of function is more readily determined and the cause can be identified more precisely.

The pain resulting from stretching adaptively shortened or contracted tissues behaves characteristically and allows manual therapists to identify the dysfunction syndrome.

Clinical picture

Patients with dysfunction syndrome are usually over 30 years of age unless there is a preceding trauma or derangement. They commonly exhibit poor posture and are under-exercised. When dysfunction follows trauma or derangement the patient will be aware of the onset and will be able to describe the progressive loss of movement. When dysfunction develops as a result of poor posture or spondylosis the onset is insidious and the patient recognizes no single cause.

Dysfunction pain is experienced intermittently, occurring only when the shortened structures are placed on full stretch, which is the patient's end-range. At this point the shortened soft tissues are mechanically deformed. Pain is felt at end-range and never during movement itself. With the exception of adherent neural tissue, pain from dysfunction is never referred into the arm or leg.

When the end-range stress is released, the pain decreases and disappears, only to return when end-range stress is applied again. The greater the loss of function the more often the pain will occur. There is always a loss of function, and certain movements have decreased range.

Dysfunction patients often suffer from early morning stiffness which eases as the day progresses. They prefer moderate activity—which can be expected, as it involves no end-range stress. Pain results when they engage in strenuous activity because they overstretch their adaptively shortened tissues causing microtraumata. This produces and increases pain—which will settle with rest—but further scarring and contracture will result and increasingly limit their available range. This becomes a vicious cycle well known to dysfunction patients.

In dysfunction patients, structural deformities may be present but poor sitting and standing postures are nearly always observed. The most common is a protruded head with 'dowagers' hump' and corresponding flattened lumbar lordosis. This highlights, in the dysfunction syndrome, the importance of examining the whole spine.

Dysfunction as a result of poor posture or spondylosis tends to exhibit a symmetrical movement loss in all directions and many segments are involved. Dysfunction as a result of trauma or derangement more often has an asymmetrical movement loss. Some movements remain full and others are partially or completely lost. The variations of movement loss are many, and the test movements will highlight these.

Described simply, the pain of dysfunction appears immediately the shortened structures are overstretched.

DERANGEMENT SYNDROME

Definition

Pain in the derangement syndrome arises as a result of disruption and or displacement within the intervertebral segment.

Mechanism of pain production

McKenzie uses disc mechanics as the basis for his conceptual model in understanding the mechanism of pain production in the derangement syndrome. There are many investigations which support his displacement or derangement conceptual model (Stahl 1977, Vogel 1977, Kramer 1981, Adams & Hutton 1982, 1985, Krag et al 1987, Schnebel & Simmons 1988), but to date there are no studies that relate displacement to the production of pain.

As the spine moves, the nucleus pulposis migrates towards the area of least load. Thus, posterior migration occurs in flexion, anterior migration occurs in extension, and lateral migration in lateral movements (Stahl 1977,

Vogel 1977, Schnebel & Simmons 1988, Shepperd et al 1990). Kramer (1981) stated:

Within the first three minutes of loading the greatest migration took place and was registered at 0.66 mm per minute. With continued asymmetric compression the registered nucleus pulposis was observed to migrate slowly, in a matter of hours toward the area of least load.

Postures involving unequal loading of the intervertebral disc cause the nucleus pulposis to become situated in an ever increasing eccentric position. This is of utmost importance in the development of discogenic discomfort and suggests its prevention.

Unequal loading was used by Adams and Hutton (1985) to produce gradual disc prolapses with off-centre loading in in vitro experiments.

Kramer (1981) describes that, on removal of asymmetrical loading, the nucleus pulposus remains in a displaced condition and will return only very slowly to its original location. This time required for relocation to a more central position can be accelerated by compression in the opposite direction, or by traction.

In the derangement syndrome the normal resting position of the articular surfaces of two adjacent vertebrae is disturbed as a result of this alteration in the position of the nucleus between these surfaces. This leads to altered mechanical stress within and around the involved disc. As long as sufficient disc disturbance is present, some structures will be subjected to increased mechanical deformation and constant pain may result.

McKenzie (1981) stated that the main predisposing factor in the derangement syndrome is flexion, especially when sustained as in prolonged slouched sitting or stooped standing.

In flexion:

1. The nucleus migrates posteriorly (Stahl 1977).
2. The mechanical stress on the posterior structures of the spine is increased, in particular the tangential stress on the posterior annulus (Stahl 1977).
3. The disc pressure is raised, compared to erect standing (Nachemson 1981). In sitting with lumbar flexion, the intradiscal pressure is higher than in any other sitting position (Andersson et al 1975, Nachemson 1980).

It appears that sufficient mechanical force, applied regularly, may lead to disc damage. In the lumbar spine, flexion—and especially the combination of flexion and rotation—are frequently stated to lead to disc damage (Farfan 1973, Hickey & Hukins 1980). Adams et al (1980) found that flexion in the lumbar spine was primarily restricted by the intervertebral discs (from 38% at half flexion to 29% at full flexion) and the capsular ligaments of the apophyseal joints (39% at full flexion). Hickey and Hukins (1980) found that bending forwards, in particular, is damaging because it concentrates stress posteriorly over a limited number of collagen fibres; the same authors also stated that the collagen fibres of the annulus possess the same mechanical properties of tendons and will be damaged irreversibly if stretched by more than 4% of their original length. Kramer (1981) stated that 'the intervertebral disc becomes susceptible to injury once the annulus fibrosis is weakened by loss of elasticity. Fissures and ruptures develop which allow the degenerated nucleus to migrate'.

The derangement syndrome is directly related to intervertebral disc pathology. With normal ageing the disc undergoes a process of degeneration. Farfan (1973) indicated that degenerative signs are evidence of the body adapting to stresses and strains and repairing damage. Vernon-Roberts (1980) demonstrated by autopsy the frequent occurrence of disc degeneration; degenerative changes were found in many spines by the age of 30 and in all spines by middle age.

Degenerative changes alone do not indicate symptomatology in the spine. Glover (1976) stated that spinal X-rays themselves are a poor indication of past, present or future pain. X-rays cannot reveal pain itself, especially in the back. La Rocca and Macnab (1969) evaluated the relationship between radiological degenerative changes and low-back pain. In a group of 150 people with no history of low-back pain, perfectly normal X-rays, without deviation of any description, were seen in only 7.3% and degenerative changes were found in 84.6%. Similar findings were made by Gore et al (1986) in the cervical spine. In their study of 200 asymptomatic men and women between the ages of 20 and 65, it was found, using lateral radiograph, that by the age of 60 to 65, 95% of men and 70% of women demonstrated at least one degenerative change. On the other hand, La Rocca and Macnab (1969) found in a group of 150 people who were all receiving compensation for a lumbar disability, degenerative changes in 98% and normal X-rays in only 2%.

Farfan (1973) stated that, with the appearance of radial fissures in the annulus, the degenerative process of the disc begins to assume clinical significance. Disc protrusion commences with a tear in the annulus which starts at the vertebral end-plate. Damage to the annulus is followed by progressive fibrosis of the nucleus and inner annulus.

Eventually, fibrotic material sequestrates and comes to lie in a cavity filled with tissue fluid. It tends to follow the path of least resistance along radial fissures where it finally may become extruded. Adams and Hutton (1982) stated that slightly degenerated discs are most vulnerable for the development of disc prolapse. In these discs some annular degeneration is present while the nucleus still exhibits hydrostatic properties and can burst through a weakened and stretched posterior annulus.

In the cervical spine the location for the initial degenerative changes in the cervical discs are the horizontal fissures normally present adjacent to the uncovertebral joints from early adolescence. The clefts are laterally closed but penetrate medially and widen towards the centre of the disc. They are in contact with the nucleus pulposus and therefore parts of the nucleus are able to escape laterally. Kramer (1981) and Tondury (1959) both considered possible that acute torticollis (derangement 4) may result from such displacement. In histological sections, Tondury (1959) observed intradiscal protrusions in the uncovertebral region in children. Tondury (1971) found only large cervical protrusions in adolescents. In the dessicated discs in older patients there was no penetration of tissue in the horizontal fissures.

The influence of disc degeneration on the site of herniation was demonstrated by Fuchioka et al (1988). These authors showed that primary postero-lateral herniation occurred only in moderately to severely degenerated discs and was not seen in groups with mild or no degeneration.

In the spine, posterior and postero-lateral fissures are often seen, but anterior and antero-lateral fissures are less common.

That the disc can be a source of pain in the cervical region was demonstrated by Cloward (1959). He reported producing pain from the scapula region to the upper arm by stimulating the lower cervical discs both externally and internally and anteriorly and posteriorly. Both antero-lateral and postero-lateral stimulations caused pain to appear unilaterally on the same side as the stimulation.

In the lumbar region, Vanharanta et al (1988) incriminate the disc as the primary source of pain in a large group of patients with non-specific back pain whose symptoms were reproduced by discography.

Types of derangement

McKenzie (1981, 1990) recognizes two different types of derangement in the spine—posterior and anterior. The posterior derangements are further divided into six categories; derangement seven is anterior. The derangements are differentiated by their history and repeated movement examination (see Table 28.3 and see Chapter 42 on repeated movements).

Posterior derangement

The posterior derangement, according to the conceptual model, is due to a posterior displacement of the nuclear/annular complex.

Derangements one and two result from postero-central migration, and derangements three to six from postero-lateral migration of the nuclear/annulus complex. Each successive derangement shows further peripheralization of pain and development of deformity.

Derangements one, three and five have no acute deformity, whereas patients with derangements two, four and six present with an acute deformity. In derangements one to four the symptoms do not extend in the extremity

Table 28.3 Lumbar (left-hand column) and cervical derangements (right-hand column)

Derangement 1 Central or symmetrical pain across low back, rarely buttock and/or pain; thigh pain; no deformity	*Derangement 1* Central or symmetrical pain about C 5–7; rarely scapula or shoulder pain; no deformity
Derangement 2 Central or symmetrical pain across low back with or without buttock and/or thigh pain; with deformity of lumbar kyphosis	*Derangement 2* Central of symmetrical pain about C 5–7 with or without scapula, shoulder or upper arm pain; with deformity of cervical kyphosis
Derangement 3 Unilateral or asymmetrical pain across low back with or without buttock and/or thigh pain; no deformity	*Derangement 3* Unilateral or asymmetrical pain about C 3–7 with or without scapula, shoulder or upper arm pain; no deformity
Derangement 4 Unilateral or asymmetrical pain across low back with or without buttock and/or thigh pain; with deformity of lumbar scoliosis	*Derangement 4* Unilateral or asymmetrical pain about C 5–6–7 with or without scapula, shoulder or upper arm pain; with deformity or acute wry neck or torticollis
Derangement 5 Unilateral or asymmetrical pain across low back with or without buttock and/or thigh pain; with sciatica extending below knee; no deformity	*Derangement 5* Unilateral or asymmetrial pain about C 5–6–7 with or without scapula or shoulder pain and with arm symptoms distal to the elbow; no deformity
Derangement 6 Unilateral or asymmetrical pain across low back with or without buttock and/or thigh pain; with sciatica extending below the knee; with deformity of lumbar scoliosis	*Derangement 6* Unilateral or asymmetrical pain about C 5–6–7 with arm symptoms distal to the elbow; with deformity of cervical kyphosis, acute wry neck or torticollis
Derangement 7 Symmetrical or asymmetrical pain across low back with or without buttock and/or thigh pain; with deformity of accentuated lumbar lordosis	*Derangement 7* Symmetrical or asymmetrical pain about C 4–5–6 with or without anterior/anterolateral neck pain; no deformity

below the elbow or knee, in contrast to derangements five and six.

The two acute deformities that may be seen in the posterior derangement are as follows.

Kyphosis

This is a flattening of the lumbar or cervical lordosis, and an inability to reverse this flattening or extend, on initial examination. Conceptually, patients in this situation have developed an obstruction to extension caused by excessive posterior flow or displacement of the fluid nucleus or sequestrum. The displacement obstructs curve reversal and locks patients in flexion.

Lateral shift deformity in the lumbar region or torticollis in the cervical region

The deformity may also be referred to as list, tilt or acute scoliosis in the lumbar spine, acute torticollis, or wry neck in the cervical spine. This is caused by a postero-lateral derangement. The disc material has moved so far postero-laterally that it forces the patient to adopt this deformity to accommodate it.

In the lumbar region, the patient with a lateral shift stands with the upper lumbar spine displaced laterally in relation to the pelvis. Side flexion away from the deviation and extension is blocked. In the cervical region the neck is fixed in lateral flexion and flexion and cannot laterally flex away from the deviation, rotate or extend normally.

There is usually a significant obstruction to curve reversal.

In a retrospective study of clinical data relating to the lumbar region, McKenzie's (1972) statistics show that:

1. Of the total number of people presenting with a lateral shift, 60% were men and 30% were women.
2. Of all patients examined, 50% had a relevant shift, i.e. alternation of the lateral shift, and produced a change in intensity and/or distribution of pain. (The retrospective study of Donelson et al (1990) of 87 patients with lumbar peripheral symptoms found similar statistics in that 46% had a relevant lateral shift.)
3. Some 90% of patients deviated away from the painful side, and the remaining 10% deviated towards it. The latter group had a higher incidence of constant sciatica, subsequent development of neurological deficit and a higher treatment failure rate.

Anterior derangement

The cause of the anterior derangement is an antero or antero-lateral migration of the nuclear/annular complex. Anterior derangements occur less frequently than posterior ones. van Wijmen (1986) states that this may be due to:

1. the anterior annulus being covered by the strong anterior longitudinal ligament
2. the fact that our flexion lifestyle places more stress on the posterior spinal structures.

This is in contrast to Farfan (1973), who stated that anterior disc extrusion does not seem to occur.

The anterior derangement may present with a deformity of acute lumbar lordosis where flexion is blocked.

Patients with anterior derangement usually state that they are worse in activities requiring sustained extension such as standing and walking in the lumbar spine or looking up in the cervical spine. Conversely, they are better with activities and postures that require some flexion, e.g. bending forwards, lying in flexion or sitting in softer rather than firm chairs.

Anterior derangements are not as disabling as posterior ones. This is presumably due to the fact that people spend so much time in flexion and this helps to reduce the anterior derangement at least in part.

Clinical picture

The majority of patients presenting with the derangement syndrome are between 20 and 55 years in the lumbar spine, and 12 to 55 years in the cervical (McKenzie 1981, 1990). The incidence of cervical derangements in the young is common, whereas in the lumbar spine it is rare to see young teenagers with the derangement syndrome. Adams and Hutton (1982) report that most people of 30 to 50 years have lumbar discs showing moderate degenerative changes. Frequently, the annulus is weakened by circumferential and radial tears but both the annular wall and the hydrostatic mechanism of the disc complex are still intact.

In the lumbar region, posterior derangements occur more frequently in men than in women (McKenzie 1972, 1979).

van Wijmen (1986) states that the contributing factors may be:

1. Traditionally, men are involved in more strenuous activity and heavy labour than women; this may enhance the development of posterior derangements.
2. The lumbar lordosis is frequently more accentuated in women than in men; this would reduce one of the predisposing factors for the development of the posterior derangements, i.e. loss of lumbar extension.

Patients presenting with derangement usually describe a sudden onset and in a matter of a few hours over a day or two they change from normal to significantly disabled beings.

Two-thirds of people with lumbar derangements state that there is no apparent reason for the onset of their pain (McKenzie 1981). McKenzie (1990) states that a similar or even greater number of patients develop cervical symptoms for no apparent reason in the cervical derangement syndrome. Regularly, patients report that they were suddenly incapacitated by the simple act of bending forwards without applying excessive mechanical stresses or turning their neck quickly in the cervical region. Further questioning, however, usually reveals that positions or movements involving prolonged flexion in the lumbar spine or protrusion in the cervical region precedes the single bending forward or rotating movement.

Commonly, the onset occurs during the first few hours of the day. Adams and Hutton (1983) demonstrated that, in the early morning, the posterior annulus is taller and the nucleus has a higher fluid content than at the end of the day. In 1987 Adams et al suggested that diurnal variations in stresses on the lumbar spine may be of clinical relevance.

Pain from derangement may alter its location. It can move distally or proximally and may intensify or diminish. The pain may move from one side of the back or neck to the other. Occasionally, overnight pain felt on one side of the spine may cease and appear on the other. This is more common in the cervical region.

When referred pain changes its location, this infers that displacement within the intervertebral disc is changing its shape and/or position. This occurs with movement or sustained positioning. Pain changing location occurs most commonly in the posterior derangement which frequently commences postero-centrally and subsequently moves postero-laterally. The findings of Cloward (1959) and Fuchioka et al (1988) support this conceptual model of why derangement pain may alter its location.

Pain from derangement is frequently constant in nature. There may be no position in which the patient can find relief. The pain is made worse by movements in certain directions, e.g. extension in an anterior derangement, but is decreased by movements in the opposite direction, e.g. flexion in an anterior derangement.

The majority of derangements—over 90% (McKenzie 1990)—are posterior, either postero-central or postero-lateral. Lumbar posterior derangement patients report that their symptoms are produced or increased when bending forwards, sitting—especially prolonged sitting—and on rising from sitting. They generally have less pain when standing, walking and prone lying. These activities allow an anterior migration of the nucleus and thus reduce the derangement. In addition, there are positions of reduced intradiscal pressure in comparison to sitting or bending forwards (Nachemson 1981); If pain is increased during both sitting and walking there is likely to be a relevant lateral shift deformity.

Cervical posterior derangement patients are similarly worse with activities involving flexion—such as slouched, sitting, and looking down—and are better when upright.

Patients with minor derangement usually state they are better when on the move. Patients with major derangements find relief only when their spine is decompressed and disc pressure reduced (Nachemson & Morris 1964) as in the lying position. Patients with a postural deformity component to their derangement find lying uncomfortable unless they accommodate their disc displacement and enhance their deformity while lying down.

Accurate and thorough examination with subsequent classification of patients' symptoms is the foundation of good treatment. The McKenzie syndromes of mechanical spinal pain provide such a framework for therapists to classify patients. More detailed descriptions of the syndromes have been reported by McKenzie (1981, 1990).

REFERENCES

Adams M A, Hutton W C 1982 Prolapsed intervertebral disc: a hyper-flexion injury. Spine 7: 184

Adams M A, Hutton W C 1983 The effect of posture on the fluid content of lumbar intervertebral discs. Spine 8: 665–671

Adams M A, Hutton W C 1985 Gradual disc prolapse. Spine 10: 524–531

Adams M A, Hutton W C, Stott J R R 1980 The resistance to flexion of the lumbar intervertebral joint. Spine 5: 245–253

Adams M A, Dolan P, Hutton W C 1987 Diurnal variations in the stresses on the lumbar spine. Spine 12: 130–137

Andersson B J G 1981 Epidemiologic aspects of low-back pain in industry. Spine 6: 53–60

Andersson B J G, Ortengren R, Nachemson A L, Elfstrom G, Broman H 1975 The sitting posture: an electromyographic and discometric study. Orthopaedic Clinics of North America 6: 105–120

Beals R K, Hickman N W 1972 Industrial injuries of the back and extremities: comprehensive evaluation—an aid in prognosis and management: a study of 180 patients. Journal of Bone and Joint Surgery 54A: 1593–1611

Cloward R B 1959 Cervical Discography: a contribution to the etiology and mechanism of neck, shoulder and arm pain. Annals of Surgery 150: 1052

Dixon A St J 1980 Introduction. In: Jayson M I V (ed) The lumbar spine and back pain, 2nd edn. Pitman Medical, Tunbridge Wells

Donelson R, Murphy K, Silva A 1990 Centralisation Phenomenon: its usefulness in evaluating and treating referred pain. Spine 15: 211–213

Evans P 1980 The healing process at cellular level. Physiotherapy 66: 8

Farfan H F 1973 Mechanical disorders of the low back. Lea & Febiger, Philadelphia

Fordyce W E, Brockway J A, Bergman J A, Spengler D 1986 Acute back pain: a control group comparison of behavioural vs traditional management methods. Journal of Behavioural Medicine 9: 127–140

Fuchioka M, Nakai O, Yamaura I 1988 A topographical study of lumbar disc herniation using CT-Discography. International Society for the Study of the Lumbar Spine, Miami, USA 13–17 April

Glover J R 1976 Prevention of back pain. In: Jayson M I V (ed) The lumbar spine and back pain, 1st edn. Pitman Medical, Tunbridge Wells

Gore D R, Sepic S B, Gardner A M 1986 Roentgenographic findings of the cervical spine in asymptomatic patients. Spine 11: 521

Hardy M A 1989 The biology of scar formation. Physical Therapy 69: 12

Harms-Ringdahl 1986 On assessment of shoulder exercises and load elicited pain in the cervical spine. Scandinavian Journal of Rehabilitative Medicine: suppl 14

Hickey D S, Hukins D W L 1980 Relationship between the structure and function of the annulus fibrosis and the function and failure of the intervertebral disc. Spine 5: 106–116

Jayson M I V (ed) 1980 The lumbar spine and back pain, 2nd edn. Pitman Medical, Tunbridge Wells

Kelsey J L 1975a An epidemiological study of the relationship between occupations and acute herniated lumbar intervertebral discs. International Journals of Epidemiology 4: 197–205

Kelsey J L 1975b An epidemiological study of acute herniated lumbar intervertebral discs. Rheumatology and Rehabilitation 14: 144–159

Krag M H, Seroussi R E, Wilder D G, Pope M H 1987 Internal displacement distribution from in vitro loading of human thoracic and lumbar spinal motion segments. Experimental results and theoretical predictions. Spine 12: 1001

Kramer J 1981 Intervertebral disc diseases. Causes, diagnosis, treatment and prophylaxis. 1981 Year Book Medical Publishers/Georg Thieme Verlag, Stuttgart

La Rocca H, Macnab I 1969 Value of pre-employment radiographic assessment of the lumbar spine. Canadian Medical Association Journal 101: 383–388

McKenzie R A 1972 Manual correction of sciatic scoliosis. New Zealand Medical Journal 76: 194–199

McKenzie R A 1979 Prophylaxis in recurrent back pain. New Zealand Medical Journal 89: 22–23

McKenzie R A 1981 The lumbar spine. Mechanical diagnosis and therapy. Spinal Publications, Waikane, New Zealand

McKenzie R A 1990 The cervical and thoracic spine: mechanical diagnosis and therapy. Spinal Publications, Waikane, New Zealand

Magora A 1972 Investigation of the relation between low back pain and occupation. Industrial Medicine 41: 5–9

Mennell J Mc M 1960 Back pain. J & A Churchill, London

Moll J, Wright V 1980 Measurement of spinal movement. In: Jayson M I V (ed) The lumbar spine and back pain, 2nd edn. Pitman Medical, Tunbridge Wells

Nachemson A 1980 A critical look at conservative treatment for low back pain. In: Jayson M I V (ed) The lumbar spine and back pain, 2nd edn. Pitman Medical, Tunbridge Wells

Nachemson A 1981 Disc presure measurements. Spine 6: 93

Nachemson A, Morris J M 1964 In vivo measurement of intradiscal pressure. Journal of Bone and Joint Surgery 46A: 1077–1092

Schnebel B, Simmons W 1988 A digitizing technique for the study of movement of intradiscal dye in response to flexion and extension of the lumbar spine. Spine 13: 3

Shah J S, Hampson W G S, Jayson M I V 1978 The distribution of the surface strain in the cadaveric lumbar spine. Journal of Bone and Joint Surgery 60B: 246–251

Shanahan D F, Reading T E 1984 Helicopter pilot back pain: a preliminary study. Aviation Space Environmental Medicine 55: 117

Shepperd J A N, Rand C, Knight G 1990 Patterns of internal disc dynamics: cadaver motion studies. International Society for the Study of the Lumbar Spine, June 13–17 1990, Boston

Spitzer W O 1987 Scientific approach to the assessment and management of activity-related spinal disorders. A monograph for clinicians. Report of the Quebec Task Force on spinal disorders. Spine 12: 7S

Stahl C 1977 Experimentelle Untersuchungen zur Biomechanik der Halswirbelsaule. Med Diss, Dusseldorf

Tondury G 1958 Entwicklungsgeschichte und Fehlbidungen der Wirbelsaule. In: Die Wirbelsaule in Forschung und Praxis, Bd 7, hrsg. von H Junghanns. Hippokrates, Stuttgart

Tondury G 1971 Cervical pain. In Hirsch C, Zotterman Y (eds) Proceedings of the International Symposium Stockholm. Pergamon Press, New York

Twomey L, Taylor J 1982 Flexion creep deformation and hysteresis in the lumbar vertebral column. Spine 7: 116–122

van Wijmen P 1986 Lumbar pain syndrome. In: Grieve G (ed) Modern manual therapy of the vertebral column. Churchill Livingstone, Edinburgh

Vanharanta H, Sachs B L, Spivey M A et al 1988 Disc deterioration in low back syndromes: a prospective multi-centre CT/discography study. Annual Meeting of the International Society for the Study of the Lumbar Spine, Miami 13–17 April

Vernon-Roberts B 1980 The pathology and interrelation of inter-vertebral disc lesions, osteoarthrosis of the apophyseal joints, lumbar spondylosis and low back pain. In: Jayson M I V (ed) The lumbar spine and back pain, 2nd edn. Pitman Medical, Tunbridge Wells

Vogel A 1977 Experimentelle Untersuchungen zur Mobilitat des nucleus pulposis in lumbalen bandscheiben. Med Diss, Dusseldorf

Wall P D 1977 Proceedings of FIMM Congress, Copenhagen

White A A, Gordon S L 1987 Synopsis: workshop on idiopathic low back pain. Spine 7: 141

Wilder D G, Pope M H, Frymoyer J W 1988 The biomechanics of lumbar disc herniation and the effects of overload and instability. Journal of Spinal Disorders 1: 16–32

Williams M, Hawley J, van Wijmen P, McKenzie R A 1991 A comparison of the effects of two sitting postures on back and referred pain. Spine 16: 1185–1191

Wood P H N, Baddeley E M 1980 Epidemiology of back pain. In: Jayson M I V (ed) The lumbar spine and back pain, 2nd edn. Pitman Medical, Tunbridge Wells

Wyke B 1980 The neurology of low back pain. In: Jayson M I V (ed) The lumbar spine and back pain, 2nd edn. Pitman Medical, Tunbridge Wells

Yates D A H 1980 Treatment of back pain. In: Jayson M I V (ed) The lumbar spine and back pain, 2nd edn. Pitman Medical, Tunbridge Wells

29. Thoracic musculoskeletal problems

G. P. Grieve

INTRODUCTION

The thoracic spine and rib joints, together with immediately adjacent cervical and lumbar segments, can give rise to a wide variety of common, benign musculoskeletal conditions; most experienced workers might promptly name two dozen or more (Grieve 1988), excluding neoplasms which are considered under 'Simulated Visceral Disease' on page 408 and in Chapters 49 and 63.

The following personal tabulation ends with the more serious of these conditions, although the relatively innocuous ones may still cause endless difficulty by way of repeated misdiagnosis and pointless treatment, even unto *unnecessary surgery thrice and six times repeated* (see p. 411). If arthrotic change in costal and zygapophyseal joints is grouped under the general heading of vertebral interbody changes, i.e. spondylosis, the tabulation might include:

— The thoracic outlet syndrome
— Acute or chronic elevation of first and/or second rib
— Chronic unilateral lesions of upper rib joints, e.g. the second rib syndrome
— Flattened interscapular region
— The scapulocostal syndrome
— The so-called T4 syndrome
— Chronic generalized upper thoracic stiffening
— Upper/mid thoracic spondylosis with stiffness
— Upper/mid thoracic spondylosis with hypermobility
— Scheuermann's disease (osteochondrosis)
— Tietze's disease (costochondrosis)
— The rib-tip syndrome
— Stress fracture of spinous processes
— Acute hemithoracic pain
— Chronic anterior chest wall pain
— Abdominal and groin pain of spinal origin
— Simulated disease of thoracic and abdominal viscera
— Acute lumbar pain of thoracic origin
— Polymyalgia rheumatica
— Ankylosing spondylitis
— Osteoporosis

— Rib erosions in rheumatoid arthritis
— Thoracic disc lesion, i.e. a segmental and acute space-occupying event as distinct from chronic regional spondylotic change.

Commonly, the genesis of clinical features in three of these conditions to be discussed:

A. the thoracic outlet syndrome
B. the so-called T4 syndrome
C. simulated disease of thoracic and/or abdominal viscera

appears to be simple spondylotic and/or minor osteochondrotic changes of thoracic segments, and associated rib joints at times. An exception is the very small handful of cases in group (A) who appear to suffer lesions of trespass, of one kind or another, at the thoracic outlet and who require surgical decompression; this is usually first rib resection but may be scalenotomy.

Steindler (1962) expressed the salient factor '... any single pathological event is bound to project itself into a number of different clinical manifestations', and the same could be said for the majority of cases listed above.

Thus, while the two ubiquitous pathological changes of thoracic spondylosis and osteochondrosis (Scheuermann's disease — in its infinite variation of degree) are discrete entities, they share the capacity to present a wide variety of clinical features. The manifestations often go by different names; excluding the last five, most of them are not so much diagnoses as a ragbag of labels of convenience.

The pathological changes tend to co-exist with the passage of time, so that lateral X-ray views in mature people often show evidence of mixed degenerative and osteochondrotic change.

A. THORACIC OUTLET SYNDROME

In presenting a fairly recent multi-author review and update of knowledge of the syndrome, editorial comment (Moore 1986a) mentioned 'This multifaceted symptom complex' (see synonyms, Ch. 17, p. 236). The update, which includes Adson's original paper (Adson 1947, Nichols 1986, Huffman 1986, Moore 1986b, Hawkes 1986, Riddell & Smith 1986) reveals that diagnostic lines of thought, for the majority of patients, have not really changed much, since, while it is recognized that women are affected twice as frequently as men, the likely reason for this is not pursued.

In management, the greatest weight of concern is surgical, although Huffman (1986) does include mention of a protocol for conservative treatment — thus perpetuating the doubtful premise (Telford & Mottershead 1947) that costoclavicular trespass commonly occurs. Nichols (1986) also contributed to the time-honoured notion that a drooping shoulder girdle may lead to costoclavicular compression. Wood et al (1988) described the results of first rib resection in 100 patients, some 12% of those presenting with the syndrome. While the results of surgery were good, manual therapists are primarily interested in conservative treatment of *the remaining 88%*. The two illustrations of cervical ribs (Figs 29.1 and 29.2) are more a nod to conformity than much else, since these X-ray appearances are very frequently of no clinical significance whatsoever. It may well be that the label 'thoracic outlet syndrome' actually describes (i) a small handful of patients who present the clinical features suggesting lesions of trespass at the thoracic outlet (or inlet), and (ii) an overwhelming majority whose clinical manifestations are secondary to scalene muscle tightness and/or covert spondylotic/osteochondrotic changes of the middle and upper thoracic segments.

It is noteworthy that Wood et al (1988) considered EMG and conduction studies through the outlet to be of little value. They asserted that there are no laboratory tests, X-rays, electrical studies, or infallible clinical tests, to establish the diagnosis.

As some soft-tissue anomalies of the thoracic outlet, and a table of 18 synonyms for this system-complex, have been included in Chapter 17, we might go on to consider the rationale of conservative treatment.

Conservative treatment

Therapists might pose the question: 'What is it that we are treating'? Gilliatt (1983) remarks on those patients with pain and sensory disturbance in the arm but without a motor deficit, who constitute a much more difficult problem in differential diagnosis and management.

Colin (1985) observed that most of the surgical patients have pain without actual vascular or neurological signs.

The genesis of symptoms is not always understood. This remains so for many surgical cases where symptoms are relieved by rib resection. Frank trespass is not invariably visualized at open operation; in fact, it rarely is (Colin 1985). Resection of the first rib not only relieves such compression as might have been present; it forthwith removes some of the evidence, besides modifying all normal musculoskeletal strains and tensions of attachment-tissues in that district.

In the much greater number of those successfully treated conservatively, the prime cause of symptoms is sel-

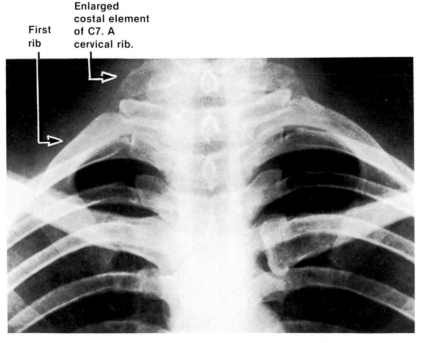

First rib

Enlarged costal element of C7. A cervical rib.

Fig. 29.1 Enlarged costal elements of C7 vertebra forming cervical ribs.

First Cervical
rib   rib

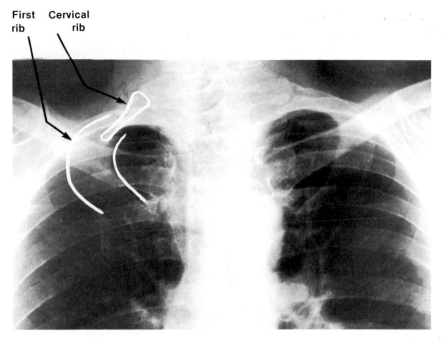

Fig. 29.2 Short cervical rib overlying the patient's right first rib.

dom clearly established. There is difficulty in confidently naming the supposed bony structure or supposed soft-tissue anomaly at fault, or in proving whether trespass exists at all. Among this larger group, a significant proportion appear not to have any overt involvement at the thoracic outlet. Carroll and Hurst (1982) made a retrospective study of 63 cases of the syndrome, together with 1000 cases of carpal tunnel syndrome. They remark that the thoracic outlet syndrome is difficult to diagnose accurately and that the signs and symptoms lack specificity. They also suggest that the carpal tunnel syndrome is still as inaccurately diagnosed as the thoracic outlet syndrome, and that these two clinical entities can be confused if the patient with carpal tunnel features presents with shoulder pain also (Rayan 1988). *Pain, besides paraesthesiae, is commonly referred to the upper limb from upper and mid-thoracic segments in patterns which have only a sketchy relationship to conventional dermatomes, and once this frequent clinical phenomenon is recognized, even if not fully understood, differential diagnosis may lead to a better outcome for many of our patients.*

Aetiology in non-surgical patients

In surgically-treated cases a variety of forms of trespass has been enumerated (Sunderland 1978, Nichols 1986, Wood et al 1988). There is no dearth of hypotheses when trespass cannot be visualized. Leffert (1983) implicates a postural descent of the scapulae on the thorax, regarded as compressing the artery and lower trunk of the plexus over the first rib and perhaps also accounting for narrowing of the costoclavicular interval, e.g. the 'drooping shoulder girdle' with 'loss of tone' in shoulder girdle elevators. Cyriax (1982) believed that pressure on the lower trunk of the brachial plexus is the cause and is of two main types: that associated either with a cervical rib or the first rib. He appeared to favour the drooping girdle hypothesis, also that the diurnal onset of the symptoms is in essence a 'release phenomenon.'

Conversely, Ingesson et al (1982) spoke of the need for relaxation therapy for contracture of, among other muscles, the upper trapezius, the levator scapulae and the scalene group. As part of a detailed postural analysis from head to lower limbs, including gait analysis, Celegin (1982) incriminated, among other faults, a high thoracic lordosis which she noted in some patients. The thoracic lordosis is said to lift the upper ribs towards the clavicle, which moves caudally and dorsally to create a scissor phenomenon — hence impingement and trespass.

The earnest search for segmental specificity of the lesion usually ends in failure. Frequently, the clinical features are merely the tip of an iceberg — of multiple covert lesions consequent upon postural and/or occupational stress of the whole upper half of the body. Considering the ordinary physical labour of housework, how can the trapezii be weak? Men might find the hard physical exertions of housecleaning, baby-care, preparation of meals, etc. more onerous than imagined. Stooping to put laden dishes into hot ovens, and remove them, is no sinecure for the trapezius or scaleni, nor is repetitively handling a heavy baby, or cleaning windows.

We seem to overlook biomechanical consequences of the anatomical fact that women have bosoms. Perhaps not 'drooping shoulder girdles' but chronically contracted pectoral soft tissues. Perhaps not costoclavicular compression but undue tightness of the scalene muscle group. Not always neurovascular trespass but wayward patterns of referred symptoms — paraesthesiae as well as pain — from chronically-stressed upper/mid thoracic segments and associated costal joints. Janda (1980, 1983) emphasized the prime importance of muscular and soft-tissue imbalance in the aetiology of musculoskeletal pain, as did Mitchell et al (1979).

Leffert (1983) mentioned that most patients are young women between their 'teens and 30s, no doubt referring to that small surgical group of patients. An alternative suggestion (Cyriax 1982) that the syndrome is an affliction of middle-aged women plainly refers to the much larger group with a more diffuse aetiology (Grieve 1991). A degree of overlap between groups is inevitable, but the distinction is clear. The fact that men suffer, too, somehow gets lost.

Many mature women exhibit a hard localized 'dowager's hump' at C7–T2, co-existing at times with a flattened or even lordotic interscapular area but more usually a stiff kyphosis, rounded shoulders, tight pectoral musculature, restricted shoulder movement (which can enjoy a different diagnosis for each day of the week depending upon the examining clinician), a forward carriage of the head and neck and a poking chin.

Frequently, upper/mid thoracic segments and rib angles are acutely sore to palpation. In other contexts, accurate diagnosis of localized shoulder lesions can be made (Watson 1978) yet the so-called frozen shoulder (Middleditch & Jarnum 1984), various forms of 'rotator cuff involvement' and 'the painful arc syndrome' are more often secondary to chronic vertebral changes than primary glenohumeral pathology (Grieve 1988).

In effect, the T4 syndrome (p. 407) may be regarded as the more caudal cousin of many cases of the thoracic outlet syndrome. After uncommon causes of frank trespass have been recognized and surgically relieved, this broader view encompasses the nature of the multifactorial involvement manifest in many of this group of patients, and in such a variety of ways.

Paraesthesiae

The nature of abnormalities of feeling is difficult to convey. 'Tingling', 'prickling', 'pins and needles', 'electric feelings', 'fizzling in the skin', 'numb feelings' and 'heaviness' probably only approximate to what the patient wishes to describe. Few patients are analytical about precise distribution unless carefully assisted to be so.

The highly subjective exchange of symptom description is underlined by Noordenbos (1984) who mentioned ' . . . Serious attempts are now undertaken to define their (abnormal sensations) meaning, though sometimes this bears more resemblance to words being in search of a syndrome than syndromes in search of a word.'

Paraesthesiae can occur from many causes, and it is clinically evident that there need be no entrapment, impingement nor irritation of somatic neural elements serving the distribution in which symptoms are reported (see Case reports p. 405).

Pectoral pain

It is notable that many workers mention pectoral pain; some seem not to have pursued questions of why this should be so. Significantly, surgeons (Dale & Levis 1975, Leffert 1983) too report that pain may be referred to chest or breast and the patient wakened at night by the troublesome symptoms in upper limbs, with tingling and deadness in fingers. Acroparaesthesia is the popular term. No broader hint is needed to suggest careful investigation of upper thoracic segments.

Clinical experience suggests that so-called rare cases of pectoral pain (Cyriax 1982), associated with upper limb symptoms, are rather more common and have more to do with lower cervical and upper thoracic segments than the costoclavicular space. Acroparaesthesia is a symptom, not a differential diagnosis — it is one form of the spectrum, and does not require reduction of 'bilateral protrusion of the seventh cervical disc' to be lastingly relieved — even in elderly people. (See case reports.)

Examination

Postural tests

Patients with frank and distressing symptoms, relieved by surgery, may have negative responses to the usual postural tests, while those with positive responses to these tests may be entirely relieved by conservative treatment, not necessarily guided by notions of trespass.

While the lynchpin of indications for seeking a surgical opinion is the presence of marked clinical features, sometimes reproduced by tests of a solely postural kind, these tests may be recruited to provide guidelines for conservative treatment. They are too often positive in healthy, asymptomatic people (Riddell & Smith 1986), and usually their performance does little more than satisfy the therapist's conscience that no examination stone has been left unturned.

There is a tendency to examine according to habit, to see only what we look for and believe in, to recognize only what we know (McLeod 1983).

By way of general principles of treatment for *any* patient, improvement of shoulder girdle posture is a good thing, but since the notion of costoclavicular compression was convincingly demonstrated some 45 years ago to be of doubtful validity (Telford & Mottershead 1947), therapists' examination of possible thoracic outlet trespass, by shoulder girdle depression tests, probably does more to clarify indications for seeking a surgical opinion — and thus more sophisticated investigation procedures — than clarify precise indications for manual therapy.

Other tests

Elvey (1988) described tests which are helpful in distinguishing between nerve root involvement and other soft-tissue abnormalities, e.g. the scalene muscle group. Lewit (1983) took up this aspect and spoke of the use of post-isometric relaxation techniques ('muscle energy') in diagnosis of what he terms the scalenus syndrome. He presented techniques for diagnosing scalene muscle tension and for inducing relaxation in those muscles. Thoracic pain occurred in 14 of 21 patients with this syndrome, headache in 8 and arm pain and/or dysaesthesia in 7. According to him there are typical painful parasternal periosteal points accompanying scalenus spasm, and a close correlation between increased tension in the pectoral and scalene muscle groups.

A glance at Figure 29.3, illustrating the long extra-sequential muscles, is relevant in this particular context. Travell and Simons (1983) described a scalene relief test, asserting that this helps to identify the sources of referred pain caused by clavicular pressure on active trigger points in the scalene muscles. Together with discussion of other factors in thoracic outlet impingement, the authors described stretch and vapocoolant spray techniques for the scalene group, and a home exercise regime for maintaining muscle extensibility.

Importance of dorsal structures

By tradition and habit, clinicians view thoracic outlet problems from the front, the anterior aspect of structures believed to be at fault. While this habit, or psychological stance almost, dies hard, it is often more productive to get *behind* the patient and give more attention to dorsal structures. Careful palpation of dorsal bony points, of the upper half of the thorax, commonly reveals varying degrees of irritability at intervertebral and costal articulations.

Just as commonly, the distal symptoms of 'lower nerve trunk irritation' are promptly reproduced on palpation — anywhere between C5 and T6 levels, with associated rib angles. With equal facility, clinical features of the thoracic outlet syndrome are often relieved by simple manual techniques applied to upper dorsal structures.

Case reports

1. The patient referred to on page 290 (Ch. 19) could well have been diagnosed as a bilateral carpal tunnel syndrome, when further questioning elicited the presence of more proximal pain, too. Her symptoms were relieved by mobilization of upper/mid thoracic segments only.

2. A 78-year-old lady (Fig. 29.4) with a manifest upper thoracic kyphosis, and symptoms which disturbed her nights, was successfully taught in four attendances how to shift for herself. A combination of gentle ligamentum nuchae stretching, manual mobilization of cervicothoracic segments and thereafter her own plodding, patient persistence with a reposturing drill (Grieve 1991) steadily cleared her pain and abnormal sensations within a month. When reviewed more than 2 years later, this 80-year-old remained asymptomatic.

3. The common co-existence of cervical spondylosis and upper/mid thoracic joint involvement creates diagnostic difficulties.

A 48-year-old rather plump lady reported left neck, yoke area, scapular and arm pain to wrist, accompanied by pins and needles of left index and middle fingers and right index finger. There were no other right arm symptoms. Her positive response to sustained wrist flexion test invited the diagnosis of carpal tunnel syndrome, at least so far as her paraesthesiae were concerned (see p. 403). She was referred for mobilization, which, at the first attendance, was confined to cervical segments and right first rib; this improved her neck movements and reduced her pain. Her paraesthesiae were unaffected. After her second attendance, when thoracic segments T1–T5 were mobilized, her pins and needles were relieved, and have remained so.

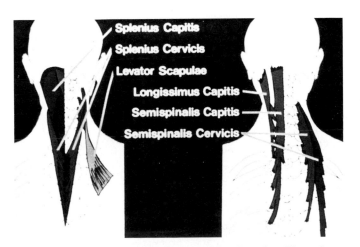

Fig. 29.3 Posterior aspect of the cervicothoracic region. These deep, long, strap-like muscles may have a tethering effect on neck movement, as well as initiating rib joint lesions by way of chronic hypertonicity.

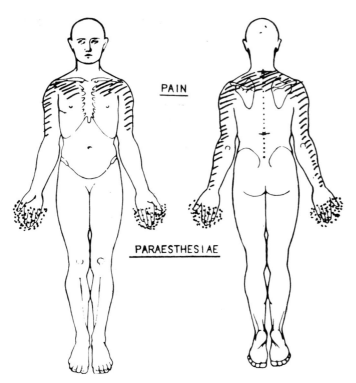

PAIN

PARAESTHESIAE

Fig. 29.4 Bilateral tingling of all digits (acroparaesthesiae) with bilateral yoke area, pectoral and upper limb pains which were cleared by a simple reposturing drill (see case-reports).

4. While it is hypothesized that shoulder girdle elevation may provoke paraesthesiae by way of a 'release phenomenon' (Cyriax 1982) this manoeuvre also disturbs upper/mid thoracic segments, of course, as *any* upper limb movement, and lying on one side in bed, must do.

An otherwise fit 57-year-old man described bilateral glove paraesthesiae, of gradual onset, which were provoked by shrugging his shoulders, gripping a steering wheel, carrying suitcases and bending his elbows, and were relieved by arm dependency. Careful examination revealed moderate cervical stiffness, slight tenderness centrally at C3–C4–C5 and a markedly sore T5 segment. On the basis of the salient clinical findings, treatment was at first restricted to mobilization of T5 only. His hand symptoms had markedly regressed after the initial treatment and were completely cleared in three attendances. Shoulder shrugging no longer provoked symptoms.

5. A bulky 39-year-old man, with once-weekly left frontal pain, more frequent left pectoral pain, medial left upper limb pain from axilla to hand, with distal tingling of predominantly C8–T1 distribution, had no neurological deficit in upper limbs and no frank articular signs at neck or thorax. Segmental palpation revealed a thickened and tender left occipito-atlantal joint, a very sore T2 segment and mildly tender segments T4–T10. The left rib angles 3, 4, and 5 were also very sore. Mobilization of the left occipito-atlantal joint relieved his head pain. Central pressures to T2 spinous process, with unilateral pressures to

the named rib angles, relieved his arm symptoms in two treatments and reduced considerably his armpit and pectoral pain.

6. It is suggested (Cyriax 1982) that the patient experiences no proximal symptoms, only those referred to the distal part of the upper limb. This need not be so. For example, one of the writer's patients, a 17-year-old girl with symptoms of spontaneous onset some 4 years previously, reported pain in the right yoke area, supraclavicular fossa, scapula, lateral forearm and palm of hand. Her muscles felt weak and her grip unreliable when her arm was dependent. There was some loss of sensibility of right index finger. The right supraclavicular fossa was definitely tender and palpation here provoked pain radiating to the hand. Peripheral pulses were good and Adson's test was negative. X-rays did not reveal a cervical rib, although her first rib appeared high-riding. Because a single exploratory treatment of sustained cervical traction, of 5 kg for 12 minutes, promptly provoked more pain and frank signs of venous congestion in the limb, she was referred for surgical opinion. Transaxillary resection of the first rib, from manubrium to the junction with transverse process, relieved her symptoms.

7. A 60-year-old male artist, who repetitively held his palette in the left hand, reported distressing left upper scapular pain spreading to medial hand, with paraesthesiae of the two medial digits. While sustained cervical extension provoked pain and mild paraesthesiae in the distribution reported, there was no neurological deficit and careful palpation revealed marked soreness only of T4 centrally and the left first rib.

Other than T4, segments C7–T5 were mildly tender but otherwise normal for his years. Paraesthesiae could not be provoked by various passive segmental testing.

The left glenohumeral joint was slightly limited with local pain on passive testing or extreme elevation.

Following central pressures to T4 (grade 11−), pain on sustained extension had moved proximally to the elbow and paraesthesiae were no longer provoked.

Unilateral first rib pressures (grade 11−) induced the pain on extension to move further proximally to the yoke area. Transverse vertebral pressures to the left, at C6–T1, were added to complete the treatment, albeit the salient source of symptoms was already manifest. At his next attendance, paraesthesiae had gone and could not be provoked by any test. Arm pain had considerably diminished. After this second treatment, all forequarter symptoms were cleared.

Conclusion

Thoracic outlet 'syndrome' might well be chased out of the literature. This foggy concept *makes* difficulties, by initiating a wild goose chase for the single site of impingement when none may exist. If the phrase 'thoracic outlet compression' is acceptable for the few with features of frank and distressing impingement, relieved by decompression, then the phrases unilateral or bilateral 'proximal forequarter lesion' or 'upper quadrant lesion' might possibly gain approval for identifying that host of patients requiring more generalised attention. Perhaps we are not so much dogged by failures of treatment as by failures to view body architecture as a whole. Comprehensively examining every structure from which symptoms could be arising is enlightening and rewarding.

The more frequently upper limb symptoms characteristic of this syndrome are relieved by scalene muscle release, simple mobilization techniques to the posterior aspects of mid/upper thoracic segments, pectoral stretching and shoulder mobilization, the more it becomes plain that an *idèe fixe*, of trespass or impingement as the sole and essential lesion in this 'syndrome' is infrequently justified. The autonomic nerve supply to the upper limb is derived from segments as far caudally as T8.

While the precise nature and extent of the underlying soft tissue changes may be arguable, their existence has been amply demonstrated on the clinical shop-floor.

B. THE T4 SYNDROME

This phrase, not a diagnosis, conveys the information that spondylotic/osteochondrotic lesions of the T345 vertebral district (sometimes T2 to T7) can initiate both a generalized headache and accompanying unilateral or bilateral upper limb pain and paraesthesiae — hence one of the synonyms in Chapter 17 (p. 237), viz. 'Nocturnal paraesthetic brachialgia'. It is difficult to avoid concluding that the autonomic nervous system (Ch. 20) provides the pathways for these seemingly bizarre projections, from the upper/mid thoracic region, of pain and aberrant sensory phenomena in arms and hands. Whatever the spread of segments involved, it always includes T4 (Fig. 29.5) and in all cases the hand is affected (Fig. 29.6). The clinical features often cause diagnostic difficulty — *all* thoracic musculoskeletal problems cause diagnostic difficulty — because carpal tunnel syndrome, thoracic outlet syndrome and lower cervical problems are considered, understandably; and sometimes cardiac disease, too. The headache component may introduce its own wild goose chase, of course. If not aware of the protean nature of the symptoms, it is easy to be misled. So far as the head pain is concerned, it is only after segmental thoracic mobilization alone has relieved it that it can be termed 'a T4 headache'.

Salient clinical features are:

—Pain, and paraesthesiae of the upper limb(s) in the distributions illustrated (Fig. 29.6); the distal limb symptoms are often worse at night and are relieved by hanging the arm out of bed. The distribution is glove-like.

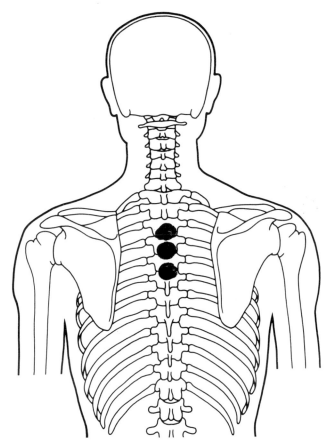

Fig. 29.5 The thoracic segments T345 are the ones most often involved in the 'T4 syndrome'. The spread of segments may be greater, and, on occasion, T4 may appear to be involved alone.

—The group of symptoms can occur alone or in combination with neck, upper thoracic and scapular pain.

—The cranial pain is often like 'a helmet of headache', although not always symmetrical.

—There are no neurological signs.

—Predisposing factors are seldom clear.

—More women are affected than men, in a ratio of more than three to one. This again raises the question of the biomechanical effects of (a) the bosom and (b) nursing a baby.

—Symptoms are usually intermittent, and are most pronounced on waking during the night or on rising in the morning.

—Besides local tenderness of bony points, palpation findings may include depression or prominence of one or more spinous processes, uneven spacing between spinous processes, pain and restriction, and occasionally elicited spasm, on accessory movement testing; occasionally, remarkable stiffness of one segment and at times thickening of interspinous soft tissues.

—Radiography is seldom rewarding and may often confuse the issue.

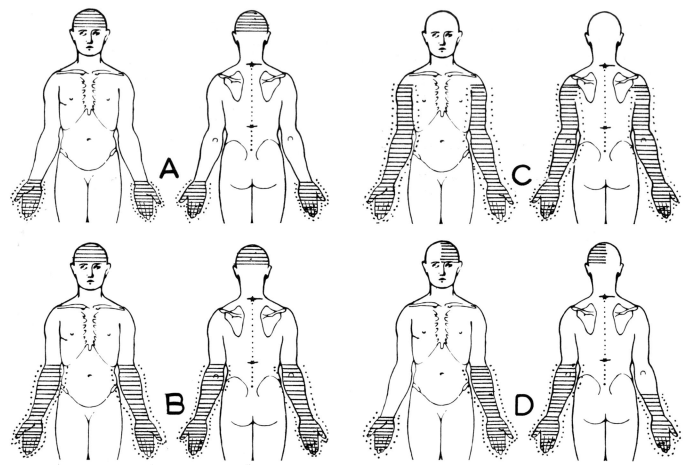

Fig. 29.6 Somewhat stylized examples of the distribution of headache, and upper limb pain and paraesthesiae. Often there is no symmetry of symptom–distribution between sides or aspects.

Treatment

Localized segmental mobilization and/or manipulation, as dictated by careful examination findings. Postural correction and localized maintenance exercises should follow. As always, patients appreciate an explanation of the genesis of their discomfort.

C. SIMULATED VISCERAL DISEASE

Introduction

Physicians and surgeons appear more familiar with body wall pain being referred from diseased viscera than with 'visceral disease' being simulated by referred pains and other clinical features, consequent upon changes in spinal musculoskeletal tissues (Bond 1979, Bourdillon & Day 1987).

Clinical experience suggests that the incidence of these changes, producing counterfeit visceral symptoms, is probably much higher than frank visceral disease. Both the cervical and the thoracic spine have a unique capacity for much mischief by way of referred pain, referred tenderness, arm and scapular pain, precordial pain,

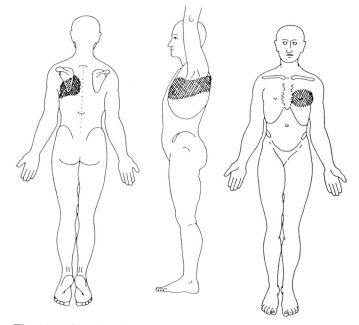

Fig. 29.7 Sites of reference of acute hemithoracic pain, which may vary from mild to severe, with stabbing pains, accompanied by dyspnoea, sweating, pallor and acute anxiety. Some will have pain in all areas depicted, others in only one or two of the three areas; scapular area pain is probably the most common.

acroparaesthesiae, spasm of the body wall musculature and even a singular type of headache together with concomitant signs and symptoms which leave no doubt of autonomic nerve involvement, and which add to the confusion — for example, sweating, dyspnoea, reduced respiratory excursion, flushing, pallor, pulse alterations, nausea and vomiting and, not infrequently, panic (Grieve 1988) (Fig. 29.7).

These ubiquitous and troublesome conditions, numerous in every general practitioner's surgery, every physiotherapy department and clinic, are recognized more often in direct relationship to increased awareness and more comprehensive clinical examination.

Stoddard (1983) observed that many types of anterior thoracic pain are referred from the back, and recommended that a consideration of spinal causes be included in the differential diagnosis of all anterior and lateral chest pain. Over forty years ago, Mennell (1945) suggested that when ordinary remedies fail to bring relief of symptoms, it is wise to examine the back in the neighbourhood of origin of the appropriate nerve roots.

' . . . One should avoid unjustifiably diagnosing coronary artery disease when it does not exist.' (Master 1964).

As McRae (1983) remarked, a frequent mistake is failure to diagnose the common. Because chest and abdominal pains engender a sense of foreboding in patients, the early clarification of simulated disease is important.

Grant and Keegan (1968) mentioned the ominous significance, until otherwise explained, of chest pain and observed that a more general recognition of musculo-skeletal chest wall pain would save unnecessary worry and invalidism.

(i) Cervical and cervicothoracic regions

Chest wall pain, of musculoskeletal origin, need not always arise from changes in thoracic segments. Recognition of the genesis of pseudoanginal pain, i.e. the counterfeit symptoms of apparent cardiac disease arising from the cervical and cervico-thoracic junctional regions, is not new (Phillips 1927, Nachlas 1934, Hanfligg 1936, Reid 1938, Semmes & Murphey 1943, Davis & Ritvo 1948, LaBan et al 1977, Godfrey et al 1983). It is plain that degenerative change in the lower neck and immediately adjacent upper dorsal segments commonly initiate precordial pain, although Cloward (1959), following his widely-reported study of cervical discography and symptoms provoked thereby, mentioned that precordial pain was conspicuous by its absence. Apart from the workers mentioned above, Cloward's findings have also been refuted by others (Meyer 1963, Holt 1964, Klafta & Collis 1969, Holt 1975).

Brodsky (1985) described a group of 438 patients, seen over a 19-year period, with pseudoangina pectoris due to a variety of causes; the majority of those were judged to be due to cervical spine pathology, with a small number attributed to the thoracic outlet. One subgroup of 30 patients comprised those who were admitted for aorto-coronary bypass surgery following a diagnosis of firmly established coronary artery insufficiency. Most were on 'cardiac' regimens including medications, activity restriction etc. for long periods, some for up to 10 years. Subsequent coronary arteriography ruled out coronary disease as the cause of their chest wall pain; in many instances this was of the classical anginal type with crushing substernal pain and concomitant autonomic symptoms.

Master (1964) studied two groups, comprising one of 200 consecutive cases of chest pain due to cardiac disease and another of 200 consecutive patients with chest pain but who were free of coronary disease. It was not possible to distinguish between the two groups using classical criteria, viz. character of pain, presence of autonomically-mediated symptoms, pain duration, response to nitrates and precipitating factors such as cold, emotions and exercise. Brodsky (1985) also noted that 25 of 33 pseudo-angina patients who had used nitroglycerin reported some degree of relief with that drug, and he suggests that many cases of chest pain can be correctly classified only with coronary arteriography; experienced manual therapists might not agree. He also refers to reproduction of arm and chest pain by the head compression test, and employed palpation of upper/middle thoracic segments — this is discussed under (ii) below.

Brodsky postulates the mechanisms of pain production as (a) radicular pain secondary to root compression, (b) motor (ventral) root compression causing deep 'protopathic' pain, (c) referred pain from degenerative changes in discs, zygapophyseal joints and ligaments, and (d) symptoms and signs mediated via the autonomic nerves, e.g. dyspnoea, nausea, diaphoresis, diplopia and pallor. This writer questions the necessity of describing three types of referred pain when all of them are, in truth, referred. As ever, the local mechanisms of pain *production* are being confused with the neural mechanisms of pain *reference*; this fundamental error virtually guarantees perpetuation of the characteristic fog surrounding the subject of referred pain (see Ch. 19).

(ii) Thoracic region

Symptoms simulating visceral disease often arise from changes in thoracic musculoskeletal tissues too, of course, and awareness of this is not new (Carnett 1926, 1927a, b, Goldthwait 1940, Smith & Kountz 1940, Davis 1948, Allison 1950, Edwards 1955, Davis 1957, Bechgaard 1981, Lindahl & Hamberg 1981, Nicholas et al 1985, Fam & Smythe 1985, Fam 1988, Benhamou et al 1988, Quast & Goldflies 1989).

It is interesting to read Brodsky's (1985) account of clinical examination of his patients. He mentions that many of them had interscapular or scapular pain and tenderness, and he regarded this 'as a common finding in cases of cervical radiculopathy due to involvement of cervical nerve roots that innervate the thoracic and scapular area, much as they do the anterior chest wall and its musculature'. While clinical features might have suggested otherwise, Brodsky (1985) seemed determined to inculpate the cervical spine, mentioning that 'cervical roots from C4 and C8 contribute to the sensory and motor innervation of the anterior chest wall' and this despite noting that some of his patients had 'varying degrees of thoracic osteoarthritis'. His remark that he was unable clearly to implicate the thoracic spine in his series does suggest a degree of rationalization; every experienced manual therapist would agree with Hamberg and Lindahl (1981) that pseudo-anginal pain is frequently initiated from thoracic segments T4 to T7. It may well be that, had Brodsky's patients' interscapular segments been carefully mobilized, treatment would have been as successful as his 78.2% success rate of surgical attention to cervical segments. Chest wall pain of musculoskeletal origin may precede, accompany or follow episodes of true cardiac disease (Prinzmetal & Nassumi 1955, Nicholas et al 1985, Brodsky 1985) although these authors disagree on the diagnostic value of response to glyceryl trinitrate.

Lindahl and Hamberg (1981) pointed out that angina pectoris merely indicates chest pain, a symptom rather than a diagnosis, and offered evidence to suggest that the link between coronary insufficiency and pain is not completely established. Bechgaard (1981) described the frequency of segmental thoracic pain in 1097 patients admitted to a medical department/coronary unit. Pains emanating from the body wall, rather than internal organs, accounted for 13% of admissions. He briefly described the simple tests which allowed differential diagnosis.

Counterfeit abdominal and low-back symptoms may often originate in thoracic segments and can cause much confusion (Carnett 1927a, Benhamou et al 1987, Monnin et al 1988, Hickey et al 1989, Mikkelsen et al 1989, Sarbandi et al 1989).

Ashby (1977) mentioned that:

Spinal root or referred pains often arise synchronously and in the same segments as visceral abnormalities, either because of summation or through visceroparietal reflexes. The latter are occasionally so marked that the visceral source of trouble is obscured. Conversely, parietal pain can cause reflex visceral symptoms . . . An acute abdomen may be simulated by aching from skeletal structures in febrile illnesses.

As an example, gall-bladder innervation is by sympathetic and parasympathetic nerves derived from the coeliac plexus; fibres from the right phrenic nerve also appear to reach the gall-bladder via the hepatic plexus, derived from communications between the phrenic and coeliac plexuses (Williams et al 1989).

This pathway is inculpated when referred shoulder pain occurs in gall-bladder disease, of course, yet this known phenomenon can mislead. Clinical experience suggests that on many occasions right scapular, right yoke area and right shoulder pain are symptoms referred from right upper/middle thoracic joint problems, in the absence of gall-bladder disease.

If vertebral segments are not routinely examined whenever visceral pathology is under consideration, presumptive diagnoses and the subsequent tests may be made on an inadequate basis.

Comprehensive screening examination of spinal structures should be included in all examinations for visceral pain, since the thoracic spine's capability for simulating visceral and other diseases is great enough to tax the most astute and experienced clinician, besides confusing very many patients. Women may be wrongly concerned that their pectoral pain is the augury of breast cancer, and men may be concerned that their pectoral pains are the ominous warnings of cardiac disease.

Despite the growth of observations on patterns of referred pain and referred tenderness, there appears a persisting lack of awareness as to where common body-wall pains may very likely be coming from.

EXAMPLES OF SIMULATED CONDITIONS

Familiar examples are:

1. The frequent employment of injections into the soft tissues of the abdominal wall because of local tenderness and supposed fascial, musculotendinous or tenoperiosteal lesions, and peripheral 'entrapment of intercostal nerves', without a comprehensive examination of their more frequent source — benign thoracic joint problems. Sunderland (1978) mentioned having examined histologically some of these peripheral points of so-called nerve entrapment, and finding surprisingly little to justify this notion.

Apart from the rib-tip syndrome (McBeath & Keene 1975, Copeland et al 1984) muscular attachment tissue and intercostal joint lesions of the anterior body wall occur less frequently than is believed. Localized intercostal muscle lesions, other than in athletes, are frequently diagnosed without sufficient examination of thoracic vertebral structures. That local anaesthetic injected at the site of referred pain will relieve the pain only adds to diagnostic difficulty.

Tietze's disease (Rawlings 1962), long considered to be an isolated and benign localized swelling, of unknown aetiology, on the anterior aspects of the second and/or third costal cartilage, is now suspected to be the secondary consequence of an extension, side-bending and rotation fixation of the related vertebral segments. Successful treatment of the vertebral component aids in reduction of swelling and anterior symptoms (Patriquin 1983), which appear to be due to covert rib torsion induced by vertebral fixation.

Barker (1983) described a patient with retrosternal pain, for which extensive cardiological investigation, including a coronary arteriogram, failed to establish a cause. 'She was depressed and tired of doctors and hospitals. She had formed the opinion that she was written off as a neurotic and would not be taken seriously again.' Manipulation of a mid-thoracic segment by the author, her general practitioner, relieved the precordial pain at once.

2. Patients being subjected to a variety of investigation procedures, extending over years, for mysterious and seemingly unaccountable abdominal symptoms, which are promptly relieved by simple measures directed to their source — the thoracic spine.

Ashby (1977) referred to one patient who had two cholecystograms, a barium meal and enema, intravenous pyelography and gastroscopy, and had also been referred to a psychosomatic clinic. Her mysterious pains were finally relieved by intercostal nerve block, of which she needed several.

3. Patients who have been subjected to needless abdominal surgery (usually laparotomy or cholecystectomy) because the segmentally-related thoracic joints and adjacent segments had not been examined, and the possible presence of referred spinal pain not considered. A patient with arthrosis of vertebral joints was subjected to *three* exploratory abdominal procedures (Marinacci & Courville 1962).

Goldthwait (1940) reported the experiences, among those of other patients, of a 45-year-old woman with abdominal pains over a period of years, for which *six* different abdominal operations were performed without relief of pain. Costovertebral joint irritability was finally recognized, and treated, with complete relief of previously intractable symptoms.

Carnett (1926, 1927b) made similar observations some 67 years ago, and mentioned: 'It is also my experience that *in the majority* [my italics] of the patients who are referred to me with a diagnosis of gall-bladder disease, the pain and tenderness are parietal rather than intra-abdominal.' Again, '. . . an average of one or two patients a week, and sometimes as many as three new patients in one day, in whom fairly competent physicians have failed to recognise the superficial neuralgia, and have referred the patients for operations for various non-existent intra-abdominal lesions.'

Experienced manual therapists would doubtless agree that, more than half a century later, unnecessary abdominal surgery appears quite as frequent.

Carnett noted the striking frequency with which tenderness is localized in the parietes, and also that in the absence of a complicating peritonitis, the great majority of true intra-abdominal lesions were free from demonstrable tenderness.

Expectations that the pain of true appendicitis will eventually be 'centred over the actual position of the appendix' (Melzack & Wall 1982), or that the initial non-localized central pain becomes 'much more precise right iliac fossa pain' (Ellis & McLarty 1969) do depend upon the appendix being where we might expect it to be (see Fig. 19).

4. Minor, successive yet fruitless surgical attentions to an intractable 'trochanteric-bursa-region' pain, without a sufficiently comprehensive examination of spinal segments T12–L1, which in the writer's experience, were found on palpation to be manifestly irritable, and probably the cause of the trouble. In this connection, intractable trochanteric pain may also persist, so long as a quadratus lumborum 'trigger point' remains unrecognized, since unsuspected and therefore unsought (Travell & Simons 1983).

Lewis and Kellgren (1939) observed that all the essential features of renal colic, pain diffused from loin to scrotum, iliac and testicular tenderness and cremasteric retraction, can be provoked by a stimulus confined to the somatic structures of the spine, i.e. injection of spinal ligaments with hypertonic saline.

Kirkaldy-Willis and Hill (1979) mentioned that lower abdominal and scrotal pain, from upper lumbar disc herniations, is not infrequently confused with renal or ureteric disorders.

Patterns of referred pain from experimental injection of interspinous tissues at the L1 and L2 segments indicate that unilateral loin pain is likely to be more frequent than groin pain, but that the latter will often occur. Since the first lumbar root provides branches for the iliohypogastric and ilioinguinal nerves, and together with the second lumbar root forms the genitofemoral nerve, a loin and groin pattern of referred pain and tenderness from lesions at the upper lumbar segments may be expected to occur in some, yet this pain does not necessarily follow the precise distribution of the nerve root.

It should be remembered that loin pain may be the feature of an upper-urinary-tract lesion in women (Fox & Saunders 1978). Of 100 consecutive female patients referred to a urology clinic with loin pain, 22% had upper-urinary-tract lesions. In the 53% of cases where the pain was provoked by movement or exercise and relieved by rest, a urinary-tract lesion was found in 21% of them. *Hence, the prior exclusion of visceral disease must take precedence over physical treatment*, yet a corollary is the need for more fruitful dialogue between general surgeons and therapists. On occasion, the cause of the confusing referred mischief is not benign. Spinal neoplastic disease is most frequent in the thoracic region (see Ch. 63).

VISCERAL SIMULATION OF SOMATIC CONDITIONS

Brain and Wilkinson (1967) mentioned that the reference of visceral pain to certain segmental somatic areas is well-

Table 29.1

Number of patients	Area of pain	Segments
20	Pain in epigastric region	T6–T10 (Fig. 29.8)
10	Pain in (R) hypochondrium	T7–T11 (Fig. 29.9)
6	Pain in epigastrium *and* across back	T6–T10 (Fig. 29.10 A,B)
5	Pain *only* in the back, bilaterally	T7–T9 (Fig. 29.11)
4	Pain only in the back, but on one side	T7–T9 (Fig. 29.12)
11	Had no pain at all	
56		

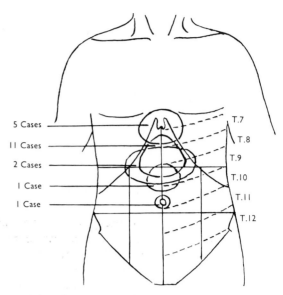

Fig. 29.8 Pain referred to both sides of the midline from xiphoid to umbilicus. Twenty cases (T6–T10 dermatomes).

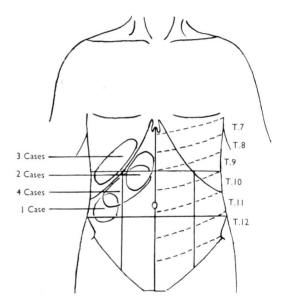

Fig. 29.9 Pain referred to right costal margin and right upper abdominal quadrant. Ten cases (T7–T11 dermatomes).

recognized, being related to the segmental level of neural traffic from visceral afferent neurons. Because of the importance of this circumstance, an example should be considered. Doran (1967) reported clinical findings on the pattern of pain reference in 56 patients who, after cholecystectomy, had the balloon of a Foley catheter left in the common bile duct. The balloon was inflated on the 12th postoperative day, when the patients had recovered sufficiently after the operation, were well orientated and able to report on the pain experienced on artificial distension of the bile duct.

Reference of pain was as shown in Table 29.1. That is, with an identical intra-abdominal lesion, only 10 out of 56 individuals experienced pain 'where it ought to be', and 11 had no pain at all.

In those patients who did feel pain, this spread across the area represented by *six* adjacent dermatomes, i.e. T6 to T11 inclusive, in various distributions. Forty-nine of the patients were women, 7 were men.

Doran suggests that: 'There is practical as well as theoretical value in banishing for ever the ambiguous notion of 'true visceral pain'. Fewer diagnostic mistakes will be made if it is clearly understood that there are no qualitative properties of a pain able to suggest its origin.'.

The spinal segments which are thrown into activity by distending the common bile duct have been enumerated. The same segments can be stimulated in other ways, and similar pain will result. For example, it can be mimicked by injecting 6% saline into the paravertebral tissues to the right of the eighth to ninth vertebrae (Kellgren 1949).

One of the most regrettably misleading signs, for the inexperienced or over-enthusiastic, is that of referred tenderness of spinal origin; to the extent that exploratory laparotomy may be performed on this basis.

Some questions might be:

1. What is the nature of the vertebral lesions causing these confusing referred pains overlying the thoracic and abdominal viscera?

2. What are the neurological mechanisms responsible, both for the size of the painful area and also its particular distribution?

3. In what way might the nature of the lesion itself govern the behaviour of the referred symptoms?

While it is easier to pose these questions than to give true and therefore satisfactory answers, there is nevertheless much to say about these problems.

1. THE NATURE OF THE LESIONS

Degenerative changes. The study of Nathan et al (1964) of 346 skeletons revealed an incidence of costovertebral joint *arthrosis* of 48% with peaks at T1, T6–7–8 and T11–12 (Fig. 29.13). The inferior hemifacets appeared to be

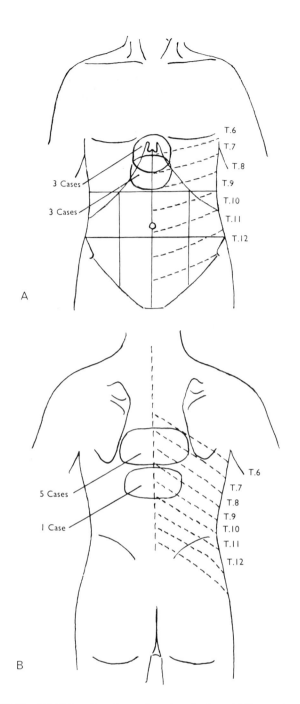

Fig. 29.10 (**A**) Pain referred to epigastrium in the mid-line; and (**B**) across the back. Six cases (T6–T10 dermatomes).

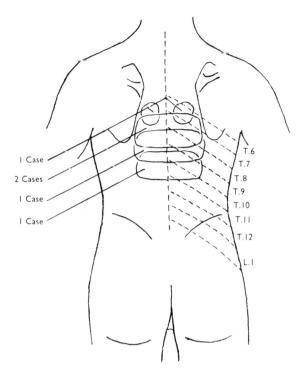

Fig. 29.11 Pain referred only to the back, on both sides of the vertebral column. Five cases (T6–T10 dermatomes).

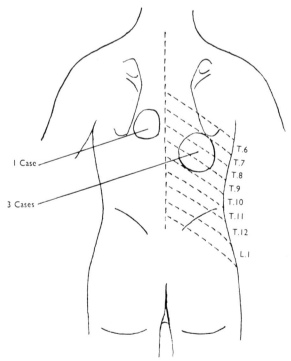

Fig. 29.12 Pain referred only to the back but confined to one side. Four cases (T7–T9 dermatomes).

(Figures 29.8 to 29.12 are reproduced from Doran 1967 with permission of author and publisher.)

more frequently affected than the superior hemifacets (Figs 29.14–29.16).

The concurrent radiological study of a random group of 100 X-rays revealed manifest arthrotic changes in 17. In no case had the presence of the changes been reported by radiologists. Nathan mentions the clinical history of three of these patients, in whom localized injections of hydrocortisone to costovertebral joints relieved intractable body-wall pains, the cause of which had remained un-elucidated by various investigation procedures.

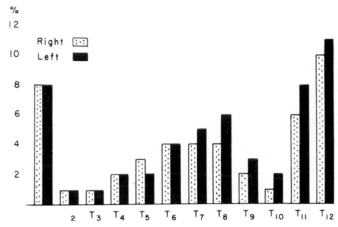

Fig. 29.13 Distribution of costovertebral arthrosis along the left and right sides of the thoracic vertebrae. No significant difference between the two sides is present.

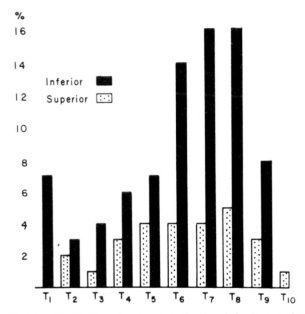

Fig. 29.14 Distribution of costovertebral arthrosis in the superior and inferior hemifacets of the thoracic vertebrae. The inferior hemifacets appear to be more frequently affected, particularly between T6 and T8.

With regard to *rib lesions*, correlations between the degree of arthrosis and/or spondylosis (demonstrated either radiologically or at autopsy), and the severity or even the presence of pain, are known to be sketchy. Many patients who are temporarily in severe unilateral thoracic pain have perfectly normal X-rays; others with marked X-ray changes enjoy free and painless function.

Whether common and easily reversible lesions of rib fixation essentially involve the costovertebral or costo-transverse joint, or both, or are due mainly to inter-segmental muscle spasm or hypaxial muscle tightness, seems more opinion than proven fact. That muscle spasm or tightness, at least in those accessible to palpation, can easily be demonstrated does not thereby prove the true genesis of the fixation.

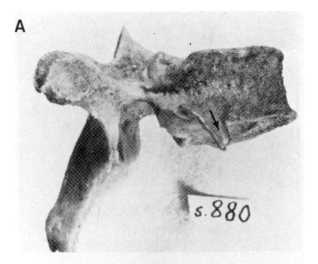

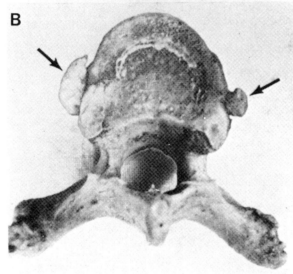

Fig. 29.15 A. The sixth thoracic vertebra shows a large spur (arrowed) projecting downwards from the inferior hemifacet. **B.** Inferior view of the eighth thoracic vertebra, showing spurs (arrowed) on both sides, projecting from the inferior costovertebral hemifacets.

The distinction between expiration and inspiration lesions seems largely academic, since the same simple techniques effectively relieve both, and incidentally cannot help but move or disturb both rib joints as well as all soft tissues attached (see Fig. 29.3).

Shore's (1935) review of arthrosis in the facet (zygapophyseal) joints of the whole vertebral column suggested peaks of incidence at the cervicothoracic junction, a smaller peak at T2–T6 and then a steadily rising frequency from T10 to the mid-lumbar spine (Fig. 29.17).

Before considering spondylotic change of the interbody joints, we may note a singular type of bony outgrowth which is almost exclusive to the thoracic spine (Shore 1931, Nathan 1959). They appear to be a normal anatomical feature of thoracic vertebrae, yet their variety borders on the anomalous (Figs 29.18, 29.19).

These *para-articular processes*, as bony spicules or spurs,

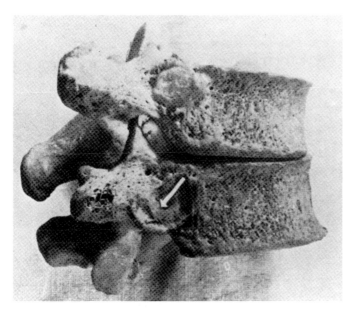

Fig. 29.16 Articulated 11th and 12th thoracic vertebrae. The articular facet of T11 is smooth and clean, while that of T12 (arrowed) is irregular, with distinct arthrotic lipping of borders.

(Figures 29.13 to 29.16 are reproduced from Nathan et al 1964 with permission of authors and publisher.)

are located on the inner surfaces of the laminae very close to the articular processes, and they may have some clinical significance as a factor in spinal nerve root compression or irritation. Their incidence is high between T6 and T11, with a peak at T9–T10 (Fig. 29.20).

With regard to *spondylotic changes*, the uncommon true thoracic disc prolapse usually occurs below the T6 level, but the phrase 'thoracic disc lesion' is too grandiose a term for the ubiquitous spondylotic changes seen in lateral thoracic spine X-rays.

Figure 29.21 illustrates predominantly spondylotic

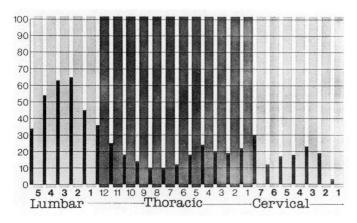

Fig. 29.17 Graph of the distribution of arthrosis of zygapophyseal joints of the vertebral column. The ordinates show the proportional incidence as percentages. Peaks of thoracic incidence at the cervicothoracic junction, at T4–T5 and T11–L1. (Reproduced from Shore 1935 with permission.)

changes in a tall man with kyphosis, probably secondary to his height and sedentary occupation.

Lawrence (1977) observed that the disc most frequently affected in United Kingdom populations, as judged by X-ray findings, was the 7th thoracic in females and the 8th thoracic in males, although the pattern of distribution also showed peaks at the 6th cervical and 3rd lumbar (Fig. 29.22). Note that T7 involvement is highest in females. Ashby (1977) remarked that counterfeit 'gall-bladder' symptoms tend to occur most frequently in women. In 53 patients with abdominal pain of spinal origin, almost 70% (37 patients) were women, so it appears that the T7 segment may be a favourite site for initiation of these clinical features in female patients, although in the writer's experience these referred pains by no means respect the T7 dermatome area of the trunk (Fig. 29.23).

Nathan (1962) drew attention to the striking predominance of osteophytes on the right side of the thoracic spine (the gall-bladder side) and their peak incidence at middle and lower thoracic levels, T5–T12. Suggesting that left-sided aortic pulsation may be a factor in this singular circumstance, he provides evidence to support this concept (Nathan & Schwartz 1962).

Almost as common as arthrosis and spondylosis is *osteochondrosis* (or Scheuermann's disease) (Stoddard 1983) identified radiologically by narrowed disc spaces, irregular contours of the anterior third of affected vertebral bodies, with deficient ossification and even destruction of upper and lower surfaces. End-plate lesions of trespass (Schmorl's nodes) are common, and the 'ring' epiphyses may be fragmented to produce in adults a residual 'limbus vertebra' or bony ossicle between chamfered anterior margins (Murray et al 1990).

A proportion of individuals with the radiological stigmata have no symptoms, and while a cause-and-effect relationship between spinal osteochondrosis and pain has not been clearly established, very many adult spines exhibit a mixture of spondylotic and osteochondrotic lesions (Figs 29.24–29.26).

Stoddard (1983) suggested that osteochondrosis is the commonest cause of spinal group lesions and a significant cause of spondylosis in maturity.

Hamberg and Lindahl (1981) urged that the thoracic spine be examined in all cases of angina pectoris, and mentioned that pains identical to angina pectoris can be initiated from thoracic discs T4–5, 5–6 and 6–7. They provided six case reports of 'anginal' pain being totally relieved by manipulation of a mid-thoracic segment, but did not indicate their method of ascertaining that the disc as such is responsible for the pain. Because signs and symptoms, when present, can occur in a variety of forms (Grieve 1988) we should add to the foregoing general diagnoses: oedema, congestion, thickening, contracture, diminished or increased movement, intrinsic muscle

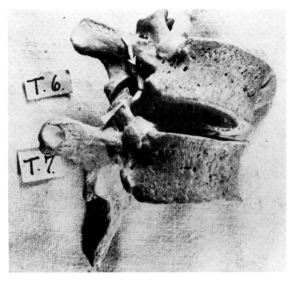

Fig. 29.18   Para-articular process of the 6th thoracic vertebra (upper arrow) is seen descending in front of inferior articular process of its own vertebra, coming into contact with a similar spur (lower arrow) arising from the superior articular process of the 7th thoracic vertebra.

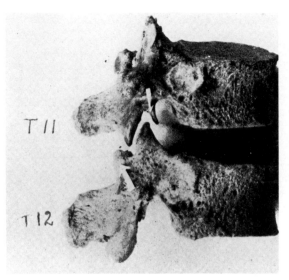

Fig. 29.19   A para-articular process of the 11th thoracic vertebra (upper arrow) is seen projecting forward and downward, in front of the interior articular process of its own vertebra and forming with it an angle open downward. The superior articular process of the 12th thoracic vertebra occupies the angle.

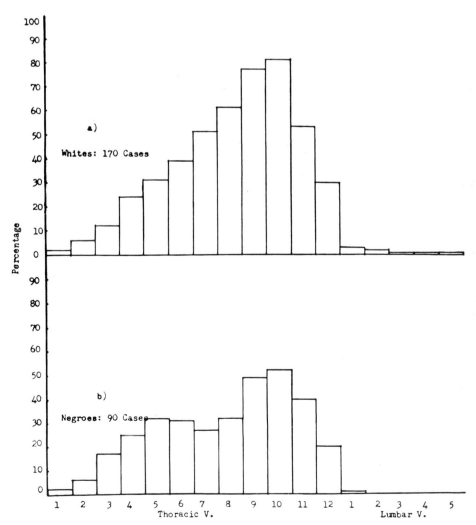

Fig. 29.20   Histograms of the distribution of thoracic para-articular processes in the various vertebrae: (a) White, and (b) Negro skeletons.

(Figures 29.18 to 29.20 reproduced from Nathan 1959 by permission of author and publishers.)

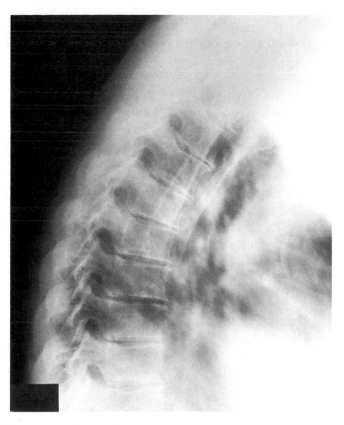

Fig. 29.21 Mild spondylotic changes in the upper mid thoracic region in a tall, kyphotic man with a sedentary occupation.

spasm and simple physical trespass. Yet trespass is not always due to minor pathology or benign processes (Longstreth & Newcomer 1977, Jooma et al 1983).

Kikta et al (1982) analysed 15 cases of *diabetic thoracic radiculopathy*, in whom severe abdominal and anterior chest pain was sometimes accompanied by back pain. Electromyography confirmed the presence of nerve root involvement, also evidenced by dysaesthesia and other abnormal sensory findings.

Primary spinal bone tumours are uncommon. Their early manifestations, particularly pain, are easily confused with the clinical features of non-neoplastic disease (Freidlander & Southwick 1982).

Spinal metastases are most frequent in the thoracic spine, especially at the T4 and T11 regions. A likely explanation is the greater number of thoracic vertebrae and the proximity of thoracic segments to lung and breast, the common organs of origin of spinal secondary deposits (Simeone & Lawner 1982).

In 1932, Craig reviewed 312 cases of proven spinal cord tumours, and it came to light that 10% of these patients had previously been subjected to various operations in the hope of relieving the pain — among the structures most frequently attacked were the gall-bladder, the appendix, the fallopian tubes and the uterus. Occasionally, pathological changes were found but the *pain*, for which this surgery was performed, was not relieved.

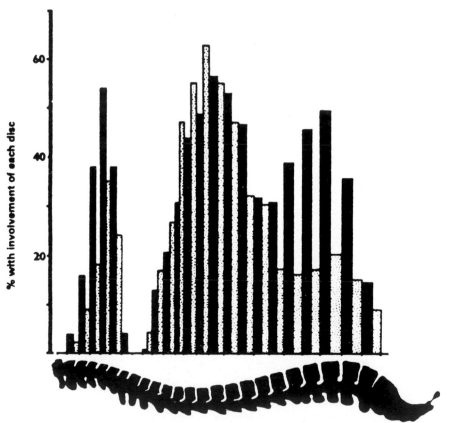

Males = block columns; Females = stippled columns

Fig. 29.22 The distribution of disc degeneration in a population sample. As judged by X-ray findings, the disc most frequently affected is T7 in females and T8 in males. (Reproduced from Lawrence 1977 by permission of author and publishers.)

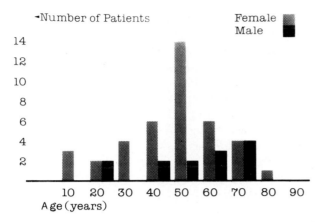

Fig. 29.23 Age and sex incidence in 53 confirmed cases of abdominal pain of spinal origin. (After Ashby 1977.)

Black (1944) reported a case of simulated gall-bladder disease which was caused by an intraspinal neurofibroma, masquerading as 'gall-bladder' disease for 3½ years. During this time the patient complained of no symptoms other than abdominal pain. The 'gall-bladder' symptoms were relieved only when the tumour, at T8, was removed. It is wise to bear in mind that the majority of spinal tumours involve the thoracic spine (Tables 29.2 and 29.3), and the possible significance of severe intractable night pain. It is unwise to rely on the notion that musculo-

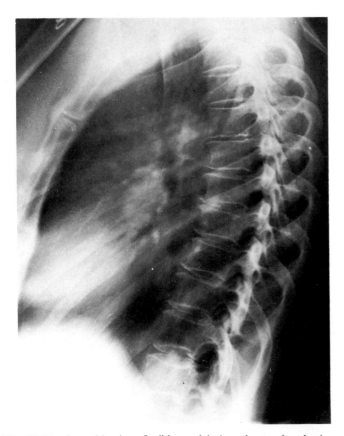

Fig. 29.24 A combination of mild spondylotic and osteochondrotic lesions in a 55-year-old woman.

Table 29.2 Summary of nature and regional incidence of 557 spinal cord tumours (after Black 1944)

Nature and distribution of tumour	Tumours	(%)
Classification		
Neurofibromas	163	29
Meningiomas	140	25
Intramedullary tumours	64	11.5
Sarcomas	55	10
Extramedullary hemangio-endotheliomas	47	8.5
Extramedullary ependymomas	32	6
Chordomas	23	4
Miscellaneous extramedullary tumours	33	6
	557	
Distribution		
Cervical	100	18
Thoracic	304	54
Lumbar	117	21
Sacral	35	7
Multiple levels	1	
	557	

Table 29.3 Regional incidence of 163 neurofibromas (after Black 1944)

Spinal region	Tumours	(%)
Cervical	35	22
Thoracic	70	43
Lumbar	55	33.5
Sacral	2	1
Multiple levels	1	0.5
	163	

skeletal pain is provoked by some postures and exercises, but relieved by others, whereas visceral and neoplastic pain is neither relieved nor provoked by these factors. This is not always so. In upper-urinary-tract lesions in women the pain is provoked by exercise and relieved by rest, and in the neurofibroma reported above, bending, coughing and sneezing provoked the pain and exercise relieved it. Similarly, the pain of a perinephric abscess, or a retrocacael appendix, can be provoked by movement (Kellgren 1940). The pain of an intradural tumour may be walked off, yet provoked by sneezing or lying down. Continuing a list of more serious conditions, Motley (1948) enumerated meningioma, perineural fibroma, chondroma, chronic arachnoiditis, pachymeningitis and spinal metastases, to which Marinacci and Courville (1962) add virus infection, compression fractures and vascular tumours.

Thus, while simple joint problems are very common — and referred to by Doran (1967) as 'those mysterious processes which go on in the paravertebral tissues' — more serious pathology is not rare. Doran mentioned being duped by herpes zoster, and one of these is included in the case reports.

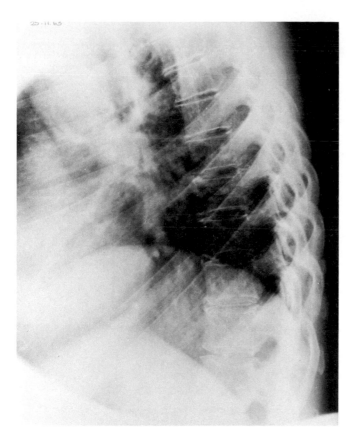

Fig. 29.25 The common presence of both spondylotic lesions (upper region) and osteochondrotic lesions (lower region) in a 60-year-old woman.

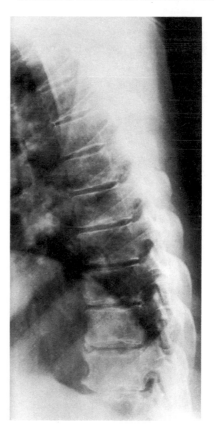

Fig. 29.26 A 44-year-old man with minimal spondylosis of upper thoracic segments and more marked osteochondrosis of lower thoracic segments, where an end-plate lesion and a limbus vertebra are evident. His lumbar segments were more markedly affected by osteochondrotic changes, and he suffered episodes of severe low-back pain.

It is worth mentioning that thoracic intervertebral discitis, in rheumatoid arthritis, has been shown to derive and spread from primary rheumatoid involvement of the costovertebral joints (Bywaters 1981). There are few symptoms, because of the limited function of the patients, and it may not be wise to manually test vertebrae and associated structures if enthusiastically searching for the genesis of chest or abdominal pain in these afflicted people.

2. NEUROLOGICAL MECHANISMS

What are the neurological mechanisms responsible, both for the size of the painful area and also its particular distribution?

Bogduk (1983) mentioned that:

The physiological basis of referred pain is convergence. Afferent fibres from topographically separate regions of the body converge on common neurons in the central nervous system. Activation of the common neuron by one set of afferents permits the pain to be perceived as arising in the area innervated by the other set of afferents. The simplest pattern of convergence is at the segmental level . . . .

Convergence of nociceptive afferents is discussed by Charman (Ch. 22).

Doran (1967) has re-stated and enlarged upon Cohen's (1947) (Fig. 29.27) helpful hypothesis, which does much to clarify our conceptions of these phenomena, i.e.:

Let the threshold of a particular group of connector neurons in a segment of the spinal cord be the constant K. Let the normal stream of subliminal impulses from the skin be A, let the impulses from the deep somatic structures be B, and let the splanchnic impulses from the disease viscus be represented by C. Let summation now occur on the common pool of neurons between these three sets of afferent impulses. If A+B+C > K, then pain will be experienced and, because the splanchnic impulses have needed the help of A+B to cross the threshold, local anaesthesia of the skin will abolish the pain because B+C will be < K.

If B+C > K, then the pain will not be abolished by injecting local anaesthetic into the skin, but it will be if the whole thickness of the abdominal wall is infiltrated because C < K.

Lastly, if C > K, the splanchnic afferents from the diseased viscus alone will cause pain and it will not be relieved by anaesthetizing the skin and the full thickness of the underlying abdominal wall.

Referring to dermatomes of the torso (Fig. 29.28), the expectation that involvement of one somatic thoracic nerve root (assuming that we know a nerve root is involved) will produce so-called root pain, within the dermatome territory of that root, could bear inspection.

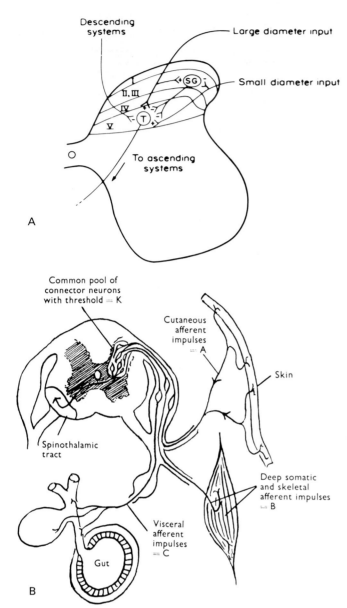

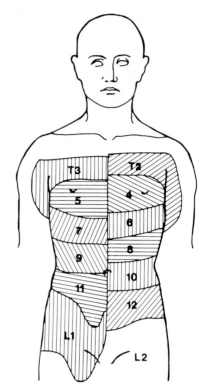

Fig. 29.28 The dermatomes of the trunk. (Reproduced from Grieve 1984 with permission.)

Fig. 29.27 **A.** A scheme of the 'pain gate' system of the posterior horn of the spinal cord. I–V are the Rexed layers of the substantia gelatinosa, and SG represents the interneurons which receive axon collaterals from afferent fibres synapsing with the T transmission cells; — is an inhibitory synapse and + a facilitatory synapse. (Reproduced from Wolf 1977 with permission of author and publisher.) **B.** The physiological mechanism of the 'irritable focus' in the grey matter of the spinal cord. (Reproduced from Doran 1967 with permission of author and publisher.)

Denny-Brown et al (1973) showed that at least five nerve roots may contribute to the innervation of any one point in the ventral segments of the trunk dermatomes. The intraspinal distribution of dorsal root fibres is such that their afferent impulses can influence the activity of dorsal horn neurons over five segments above and five segments below the segmental level of entry.

Kirk and Denny-Brown (1970) used the 'remaining sensibility' method when investigating and dermatomes of

the Macaque monkey. Section of neighbouring dorsal roots proximal to their ganglia produced patterns of dermatomes observed previously by Sherrington (1893).

However, if, in other animals, the roots were sectioned distal to their ganglia, the isolated dermatome became twice the size and additionally showed persistent hyperaesthesia. Resectioning the same dorsal roots proximal to the ganglia reduced the isolated root territories to their conventional or 'classical' size — but not immediately, only after 3 or 4 days.

Injection of small doses of strychnine sulphate, to depress inhibition and thus increase facilitation at synapses in the spinal cord, produced enormous expansion of an isolated dermatome area, irrespective of where the dorsal root had been sectioned. The conclusion is that the experimentally-observed size of an isolated dermatome is a variable quantity, and at any one moment is more of an index of the efficiency of sensory transmission in the same and neighbouring segments of the spinal cord, than an anatomically-fixed cutaneous territory.

It is for this reason, of course, that experimental delineation of dermatomes, i.e. producing lesions by hypertonic saline injections in previously intact, normal volunteers, is not quite the same thing as patients in acute or chronic pain, who have facilitated cord segments and thus whose referred pain patterns are going to be a bit wider and a bit more extensive. The experimental and the clinical are not the same. We know, for example, from the work of Hockaday and Whitty (1967) that the site of pain reference from connective-tissue lesions is quite variable between individuals, and that their findings do not support the concept of an anatomically-fixed segmental reference like dermatomes, as has already been shown in Doran's experiment.

Head's zones of cutaneous hyperalgesia.

As Head (1920) described, these zones are garland-shaped territories of the trunk which are segmentally-linked to the somatic spinal roots. In short, they are skin areas of the body wall which have the same segmental innervation as a particular viscus — one somatic, the other autonomic. For example, the heart receives autonomic innervation from the segments T1 to T5, and in cardiac disease the patient is very likely to also feel pain in the somatic distribution of these segments, the upper two of which (T1 and T2) also supply the upper limb.

So pain from cardiac lesions is substernal, and spreading into the left upper thoracic region, the axilla and down the left arm, of course, in a proportion of patients.

Willams et al (1989) tabulate the zones in full and only a proportion, of particular concern in this context, is given here:

Heart	T1–T5
Bronchi and lung	T2–T4
Oesophagus	T5–T6
Stomach	T6–T10
Liver and gall-bladder	T7–T9
Spleen	T6–T10
Kidney	T10–L1
Ureter	T11–L2

The classical segmental levels of outflow for sympathetic efferent neurons are not universally agreed (Grieve 1988). Some authors (Lindahl & Hamberg 1981) place the sympathetic supply to the heart beginning as high as C3.

As shown in Doran's (1967) experiments by inflating a Foley catheter in the bile duct of his 56 cholecystectomy patients, visceral pathology may hurt in roughly these dermatomes or Head's Zones, spreading over six dermatomes. Conversely, joint problems in the thoracic spine, involving one or more of these segments, will also refer pain roughly into these segmental zones, overlying this or that viscera.

Not only pain, but also tenderness, and sometimes reflex muscle spasm, provide for mischief and diagnostic confusion.

The point for emphasis is the *spread* of dermatomes involved, and the tendency for patients to differ, quite widely, in their patterns of referred pain from a single lesion. This is plainly evident in Doran's findings — the

autonomic supply to thoracic and abdominal viscera is anything but an exact science, as dermatomes are not an exact science, and we cannot be too precise about where pain is going to be reported when a single thoracic root is involved in vertebral joint changes.

Nerve root compression does not necessarily cause pain. Conversely, the presence of referred pain (however severe) need not necessarily imply the presence of root involvement (see. Ch. 19).

Ashby (1977) suggested that pain may arise through one or more mechanisms: (i) primary root pain, (ii) referred pain from joint structures, (iii) secondary effects, i.e. referred pain due to excessive reflex effects provoking high-threshold receptors in joints and muscles, or to root pain due to compression by reflex muscle spasm.

What is not clarified is the question: 'In what way is root pain not also referred pain, and if it is held to be different, what are the criteria for deciding this, even when neurological deficit can be demonstrated?'. In the 15 cases of diabetes, with root involvement confirmed by electromyographic findings the abdominal and chest pains were often *not* radicular in character (p. 417).

We know from the work of Nathan on osteophytes of the vertebral column (1962), arthrotic change in costo-vertebral joints (1964), and his clear demonstration of the thoracic sympathetic trunks embedded in ventral osteophytes (1969) that there is ample reason to suppose that covert thoracic root involvement may occur more frequently than we are able to show in terms of circumscribed neurological deficit, and this must include the autonomic nerves.

A histogram of their incidence (Fig. 29.29) indicates the high preponderance of right-sided osteophytes in the thoracic region, the side of the gall-bladder, of course.

We begin to note a probable cause-and-effect relationship. Reports of root compression at thoracic levels are relatively sparse, probably because it is less easy to show unilateral and obvious neurological deficit in the territory supplied by a single thoracic spinal root.

This is not to ignore the literature on thoracic disc lesions, of which Benson and Byrnes (1975) have provided an excellent review, or the well-documented changes of spinal tuberculosis and thoracic neoplasms, but only that in 22 patients with surgically-proven thoracic disc prolapse, intercostal muscle wasting was not seen and paraspinous muscle spasm was not seen. While weakness of the lower abdominal muscles was frequent, nearly all other signs involved the lower limbs. Schmorl and Junghanns (1971) remarked that several forms of intercostal neuralgia in the thoracic area have been recognized as an expression of nerve root irritation from posterior disc prolapse but, again, 'neuralgia' is not neurological deficit. They also observe that after 60 years, all spines exhibit arthrotic changes involving the facet or apophyseal joints. Most frequently involved are those from the 3rd

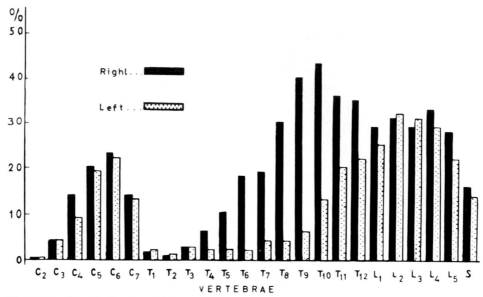

Fig. 29.29 The distribution of right- and left-sided osteophytes of the vertebral column in 346 skeletons of White and Negro races of both sexes. There is no significant difference between sides in cervical and lumbar regions, but a clear preponderance of right-sided osteophytes in the thoracic region. (Reproduced from Nathan 1962 with permission of author and publisher.)

to the 5th segment of the thoracic spine and the lower lumbar segments.

That thoracic spinal root involvement occurs is best demonstrated electromyographically. In a review describing radicular symptoms which simulate visceral disease of abdominal organs, Marinacci and Courville (1962) show that diagnostic error at times leading to unnecessary abdominal surgery is easily caused by vertebral joint problems referring pain around the trunk, and through to the abdominal wall. 'The resultant abdominal manifestations can usually be traced to stem from irritation of one or more thoracic spinal roots . . . in this group of syndromes we are concerned with the entire abdominal wall supplied by the sensory and motor roots from about T6 down to L1 level.'

Epigastric pain over stomach and pancreas produced by T6–T7 irritation, gall-bladder 'disease' by involvement of T8–T9, pain in the kidney region from T9 vertebral segment and 'physical disorders' of the urethra and bladder, are illustrative examples; also, radiculitis at T12–L1 roots will often simulate femoral and inguinal disorders.

The five examples of root involvement confirmed by electromyography of thoracic nerves were neurofibroma at T7, neuronitis at T7, 8, 9, a central disc hernia at T9, arthrotic hyperostosis at T11 and a metastatic adenocarcinoma involving T6, T7 and T8 roots. Each patient had abdominal surgery, one had two operations and the patient with facet-joint arthrosis was subjected to three exploratory operations.

Regarding precise distribution of thoracic or abdominal pain from one thoracic vertebral segment, it has been said that because of the lack of intersegmental connection between thoracic spinal roots, pain arising in any particular thoracic segment is likely to be much more localized. This notion pre-supposes then, that cervical and lumbar pain is not well-localized only because of the numerous intersegmental connections between roots, and appears to take insufficient account of the richness of the paravertebral plexus innervating all the many joints and structures of one thoracic mobility segment, including the untidy and multisegmental autonomic component of these somatic roots. We cannot, on the one hand, accept the existence of possibly autonomically-mediated headache from T345 and then virtually ignore this same phenomenon when discussing referred (or so-called root) pain in the trunk itself, emanating from one or more of those same somatic segments.

3. FACTORS GOVERNING REFERRED SYMPTOM BEHAVIOUR

In considering the third question — 'In what way might the precise nature of the vertebral lesion govern the behaviour of referred symptoms?' — we should remember that although a particular examination procedure (or manipulation technique for that matter) may indeed be moving the tissue or structure in which we are presently interested, we cannot exclude from assessment the fact of other tissue and structures simultaneously being moved by the same technique. It is sometimes suggested that:

1. Pain referred horizontally around the chest wall to the pectoral region denotes a costotransverse lesion (Fig. 29.30).

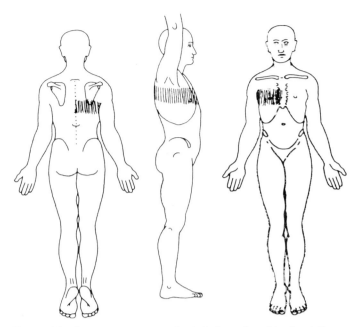

Fig. 29.30 A common pattern, of pain being referred horizontally around the chest wall to the pectoral region.

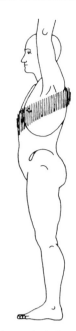

Fig. 29.31 Pain referred anteriorly in a downward sloping direction.

2. Severe pain spreading as a sloping band in an intercostal space denotes a thoracic nerve root lesion (Fig. 29.31).

3. That pain which is described as passing directly through the thorax to also involve the pectoral region, centrally or unilaterally, must be spondylotic pain (Fig. 29.32).

Whether pain felt as passing directly through the thorax in the median plane is conceived to be differently caused, and therefore distinguished, from a similar pain in the paramedian plane is not known to the writer, although these concepts appear too convenient. One thoracic vertebra takes part in 12 separate articulations, and the confident assertion, for example, 'This patient's pain is coming from the left costotransverse joint of T6' can only be intelligent guesswork.

Similarly, a sufficient number of patients with unpleasant, severe unilateral pain spreading anteriorly in a generally diagonal 'down and around' distribution, reasonably accurately in the plane of the ribs but by no stretch of the imagination occupying only one intercostal space, regularly have this pain easily relieved within minutes by localized mobilization techniques of such gentleness that it is hard to believe root trespass is being remedied.

Bearing in mind the physical interdependence of all structures of one mobility segment, we do not know enough to be quite so precise in our thinking on spinal syndromes, and should perhaps admit this.

Case reports

Having noted that osteophytes (or spondylophytes) occur

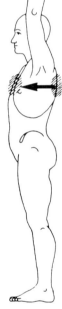

Fig. 29.32 A posterior and anterior distribution of pain, sometimes described by patients as 'shooting through' the chest, without lateral chest wall pain.

more frequently on the right side of the thoracic spine (Nathan 1962) and that their peak incidence is at T7 in females and T8 in males (Lawrence 1977) there is also the singular circumstance that while the greater proportion of patients undergoing cholecystectomy are women, the greater proportion of patients with simulated visceral disease are also women. Experienced manual therapists will be familiar with the further aspect of interest, i.e. hypochondrium pain in female patients, and the presence of gall-stones requiring surgical removal, appear to occur in-

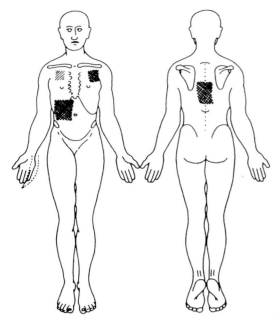

Fig. 29.33 Pain areas in a housewife of 32. Identical right hypochondrium pain preceded surgery for removal of gall-stones, and persisted after the operation (see text).

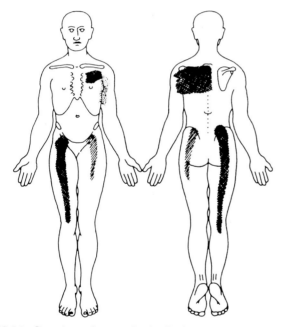

Fig. 29.34 Scapular and pectoral pain distribution in a man of 68 with shingles. The scapular pain had spread laterally to involve the posterior axilla and upper posterior arm, with left upper pectoral pain, and axilla and medial upper arm (see text).

dependently of each other. Long after the surgical procedure, patients continue to report identical pains, which are only relieved by mobilization of the appropriate thoracic segments. Some of those with pain have established gall-stones, some have not.

Therefore, do the gall-stones invariably produce the pain? If, prior to surgery, surgeons do not examine the

thoracic segments of those patients with proven gall-bladder disease, the question remains open.

1. A housewife of 32 (Fig. 29.33) works part-time as a mushroom-packer and stoops for about 5 hours a day over a conveyor-belt, which probably explains her tendency to upper and mid-thoracic problems. She presented in December, 1981, with pectoral pain, worse on the left than right, interscapular pain, right hypochondrium pain and paraesthesiae in C8 distribution of right hand.

She first consulted her general practitioner in 1970, with abdominal pain, and this grumbled on until X-ray demonstrated gall-stones which were surgically removed in Spring, 1980. In July of that year she reported the same pains — 'just like the gall-stones, doctor' — and had had recurrent episodes of the identical pain ever since. She was tender centrally at T6, 7, 8 and 9, and over the corresponding right rib angles. Her hypochondrium pain was relieved in one treatment, though her interscapular pain persisted. After her second attendance, when upper thoracic mobilizing was added, she reported feeling very much better and has remained well since.

2. Earlier, herpes zoster was mentioned and in this connection a 68-year-old man presented on 10 July 1981 with bilateral sciatic pain, worse on the right side, and bilateral mild hip arthrosis, again worse on the right side (Fig. 29.34). He also mentioned a left interscapular ache, which did not seem to be associated with any definite articular signs other than mild tenderness of T3 spinous process.

His low-back problem and hip stiffness responded well in three treatments of mobilization and exercises, during

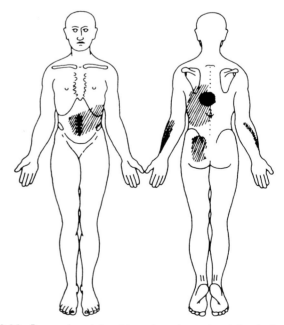

Fig. 29.35 Lower dorsal, hemithoracic and anterior abdominal pain in a 43-year-old man, with a history of surgery for a Meckel's diverticulum 10 years before (see text).

which his T3 segment was also mobilized. While his back and lower limbs remained much improved he presented again on 28 September 1981 with a recurrence of his left scapular pain, this time with posterior axillary pain as well and a feeling of prickliness of medial upper arm. He felt he'd 'lost some sensation' in the area named and could not lie on that side at night without pain. His doctor suggested that he had trapped a nerve. T2 and T3 were again tender, as were the angles of the 2nd and 3rd left ribs, but also manifest were cutaneous blebs in the left pectoral distribution of T2 and T3 nerve roots.

On suspicion of herpes zoster he was immediately referred back to his doctor who confirmed a diagnosis of shingles. The interesting point is that following gentle mobilization on 28 September 1981, he reported 2 days later that his pains and subjective sensibility changes were much improved. This is not to say that manipulation can cure posterior poliomyelitis, which is what shingles is, of course, only that in association with segmental infection by a neurotropic virus these same segments showed the signs and symptoms of a non-infective benign musculoskeletal conditon. Either this was coincidence, or there is an association we do not understand. In the light of clinical experience, the writer would suggest an association that we do not understand.

3. A tall 43-year-old man (Fig. 29.35) with a propensity for benign spinal joint problems presented in 1978 with left mid-thoracic and left hemithoracic pains, which were relieved in four attendances. He had been operated on in 1968 for a Meckel's diverticulum.

He presented again in 1980, the main item needing attention then being cervical spondylosis with bilateral 'tennis elbows', and left buttock pain.

His constant reference to abdominal pain, reminiscent of his previous operation, and his scar sensitivity, prompted further enquiry about it, when he revealed that he had undergone various investigation procedures (barium meal, X-rays etc.) over a period of 4 years (1976–1980) in fruitless endeavours to discover the cause of his chronic postoperative abdominal discomfort, which was also aggravated by isometric abdominal exercise. Segmental passive movement of T8, T9 and 10 provoked his scar sensitivity and after quite moderate mobilization of these segments he could perform his abdominal exercises without pain, although his abdominal symptoms continued to be provoked by long car drives. Modification of his car seat relieved them entirely and he had remained free of all abdominal pain for a year when last contacted, scar sensitivity included. One is left wondering whether he ever *did* have a 'Meckel's diverticulum'!

4. A 40-year-old woman (Fig. 29.36) badly bruised her right arm from shoulder to elbow at tennis, some 7 years before presenting with right hemithoracic, axillary and arm pain. While playing squash 4 years before, she had provoked a similar distribution of pain. Following consul-

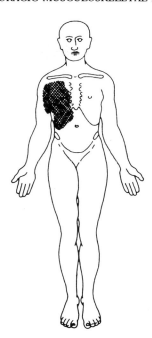

Fig. 29.36 A woman of 40 with right chest, upper arm and hypochondrium pain for some years. Abdominal surgery failed to relieve the pain, which was provoked by manual testing of vertebral segments T4–T9 (see text).

tation because of right hypochondrium pain soon after this second episode, she was given a barium meal examination which proved negative. The pain continued to trouble her for 4 years until she had abdominal surgery, some 4 months prior to presentation in the writer's clinic because of an uncomfortable operation scar. There was objective evidence of chronic segmental irritability of segments T4 to T9, more pronounced on the right side. Careful manual testing of these segments provoked her typical and perennial right hypochondrium pain.

Despite explanation, reassurance and a confident prognosis of relief, the lady was so disenchanted by her various medical experiences that she declined further treatment.

Discussion

The enigma of somatovisceral/viscerosomatic pain causes diagnostic difficulty. Our knowledge concerning visceral afferent neurons is still far from complete (Brodal 1982). Because vertebral mobilization or manipulation may reflexly modulate abdominal pain which *is* due to organic visceral disease, therapists should be aware that apparently successful manual treatment may, on occasions, transiently mask the pain of a visceral pathological process, which remains uninfluenced by attention to vertebral structures. There is also the possibility that a patient may have both visceral disease and a musculoskeletal lesion of associated segments (Bourdillon & Day 1987). Kellgren (1940) discussed these diagnostic problems, and presented nine illustrative cases; also making the point that in simulated visceral disease the normal spinal movements are often painless. Only when the spine is examined segment by segment can the typical pain be reproduced.

This leads to consideration of the suggestion, by some lay practitioners, that spinal joint conditions may actually *produce* visceral pathology. We have no evidence that musculoskeletal lesions of the vertebral column can produce visceral pathology. Stoddard (1983) regarded as ludicrous the claim that mechanical lesions are the only aetiological factor in disease. Kunert (1965) stated: 'Nothing can discredit the inherent diagnostic value of the relationship between the spine and the internal organs more than to insist on finding such a connection where none exists and to seek corroboration in threadbare hypotheses.'. However, he also asserts that there can be no doubt that the state of the spinal column does have a bearing on the *functional status* of the internal organs.

Hattersley (1983) mentioned a 52-year-old man who presented with vomiting attacks, right iliac fossa pain and tenderness, with abdominal muscle guarding. His normal temperature and pulse rate together with spinal tenderness at T11 suggested the diagnosis, and all signs and symptoms were immediately relieved by injection of the interspinous ligaments of T10–T12 with local anaesthetic and hydrocortisone.

Ashby (1977) suggested: '. . . evidence of a visceral lesion may be sought with expensive and time-consuming laboratory and radiological investigations or even laparotomy. An alternative is to treat on the hypothesis that the pain is of spinal origin. A substantial proportion of patients will gain complete relief with an intercostal block. Should sustained relief not occur the case should be kept under review.' The prime impulse for physical treatment of the vertebral column is properly vertebral column disorder and not visceral disorder (Grieve 1988). In conclusion, the comment (Brooks 1984) of an experienced general practitioner, himself troubled by simulated visceral pain some 15 years before, is of more than passing interest: 'My experience led me to look beyond the surgical texts, since these listed only rare spinal diseases as causes of abdominal pain. Having practised for so many years without a real awareness that problems in the thoracolumbar region can mimic intra-abdominal pathology, once aware of it the problem appeared to be very common indeed'.

REFERENCES

Adson A W 1947 Surgical treatment for symptoms produced by cervical ribs and the scalenus anticus muscle. Surgery, Gynaecology and Obstetrics 85: 687–700

Allison D R 1950 Pain in the chest wall simulating heart disease. British Medical Journal 1: 332–336

Ashby E C 1977 Abdominal pain of spinal origin. Annals of the Royal College of Surgeons of England 59: 242–246

Barker M E 1983 Manipulation in general practice for thoracic pain syndromes. British Osteopathic Journal 15: 95–97

Bechgaard P 1981 Segmental thoracic pain in patients admitted to a medical department and a coronary unit. Acta Medica Scandinavica suppl 644: 87–89

Benhamou C L, Roux C, Benhamou-Mayoux A, Gauvain J B, Corlieu P, Viala J F, Amor B 1987 Lower costovertebral arthritis in rheumatic pelvispondylitis: pseudourologic manifestation. Revue Rhumatisme Maladie Osteoarthrite 54: 203–207

Benhamou C L, Roux C, Gervais T, Viala J F 1988 Costovertebral arthropathy: diagnostic and therapeutic value of arthrography. Clinique Rhumatologie 7: 220–223

Benson M K D, Byrnes D P 1975 The clinical syndromes and surgical treatment of thoracic intervertebral disc prolapse. Journal of Bone and Joint Surgery 57B: 471–477

Black W A 1944 Pain produced by intraspinal tumour simulating pain caused by gall-bladder disease. Surgical Clinics of North America 24: 893–902

Bogduk N 1983 Neurology of the neck/shoulder complex. Proceedings (October). Neck and Shoulder Symposium, Brisbane, p 20

Bond M R 1979 Pain: its nature, analysis and treatment. Churchill Livingstone, Edinburgh, ch 9, p 68

Bourdillon J, Day E A 1987 Spinal manipulation. 4th edn. Heinemann, London

Brain Lord, Wilkinson M 1967 Cervical spondylosis. Heinemann, London, ch 2, p 62

Brodal A 1982 Neurological anatomy in relation to clinical medicine. 3rd edn. University Press, Oxford, ch 11, p 773

Brodsky A E 1985 Cervical angina. Spine 10: 699–709

Brooks B J 1984 Correspondence. British Association of Manipulative Medicine Newsletter, June, pp 3–4

Bywaters E G L 1981 Thoracic intervertebral discitis in rheumatoid arthritis due to costovertebral joint involvement. Rheumatology International 1: 83–97

Carnett J B 1926 Intercostal neuralgia as a cause of abdominal pain and tenderness. Surgery Gynaecology and Obstetrics 42: 625–632

Carnett J B 1927a Acute and recurrent pseudo-appendicitis due to intercostal neuralgia. American Journal of Medical Science 174: 833–851

Carnett J B 1927b The simulation of gall-bladder disease by intercostal neuralgia of the abdominal wall. Annals of Surgery 86: 747–757

Carroll R E, Hurst L C 1982 The relationship of thoracic outlet syndrome and carpal tunnel syndrome. Clinical Orthopaedics and Related Research 164: 149–153

Celegin Z 1982 Thoracic outlet syndrome: what does it mean for physiotherapists. In: Proceedings IXth Congress World Confederation for Physical Therapy, Stockholm, pp 825–832

Cloward R B 1959 Cervical discography. Annals of Surgery 150: 1052–1064

Cohen H 1947 Visceral pain. Lancet 2: 933–934

Colin J F 1985 Personal communication

Copeland G P, Machin D G, Shennan J N 1984 Surgical treatment of the 'slipping rib syndrome'. British Journal of Surgery 71: 522–523

Craig W McK 1932 The pain of tumours of the spinal cord. Western Journal of Surgery 40: 56–63

Cyriax J 1982 Textbook of orthopaedic medicine. vol 1, 8th edn. Bailliere Tindall, London, ch 8, pp 119–123

Dale W A, Levis M R 1975 Management of the thoracic outlet syndrome. Annals of Surgery 181: 575–585

Davis D 1948 Respiratory manifestations of dorsal spine radiculitis simulating cardiac asthma. American Heart Journal 35: 954–959

Davis D 1957 Radicular syndromes with emphasis on chest pain simulating coronary disease. Year Book Publishers, London

Davis D, Ritvo M 1948 Osteoarthritis of the cervical dorsal spine (radiculitis) simulating coronary arterial disease. New England Journal of Medicine 238: 857–866

Denny-Brown D, Kirk E J, Yanagisawa N 1973 The tract of Lissauer in relation to sensory transmission in the dorsal horn of the spinal cord of the macaque. Journal of Comparative Neurology 151: 175–200

Doran F S A 1967 The sites to which pain is referred from the common bile duct in man and its implication for the theory of referred pain. British Journal of Surgery 54: 599–606

Edwards W L 1955 Musculoskeletal chest pain following myocardial infarction. American Heart Journal 49: 713–718

Ellis H, McLarty M 1969 Anatomy for anaesthetists. 2nd edn. Blackwell, Oxford, p 301

Elvey R L 1988 The clinical relevance of signs of adverse brachial plexus tension. Proceedings International Federation of Orthopaedic Manipulative Therapists Congress, Cambridge, p 15

Fam A G 1988 Approach to musculoskeletal chest wall pain. Primary Care 15: 767–782

Fam A G, Smythe H A 1985 Musculoskeletal chest wall pain. Canadian Medical Association Journal 133: 379–389

Fox M, Saunders N R 1978 The significance of loin pain in women. Lancet 1: 115–116

Freidlander G E, Southwick W O 1982 Tumours of the spine. In: Rothman R H, Simeone F A (eds) The spine. 2nd edn. W B Saunders, Philadelphia, ch 5, p 1022

Gilliatt R W 1983 Thoracic outlet syndrome (letter) British Medical Journal 287: 764

Godfrey N F, Halter D G, Minna D A, Weiss M, Lorber A 1983 Thoracic outlet syndrome mimicking angina pectoris with elevated creatine phosphokinase values. Chest 83: 461–463

Goldthwait J E 1940 The rib joints. New England Journal of Medicine 223: 568–573

Grant A P, Keegan D A J 1968 Rib pain — a neglected diagnosis. Ulster Medical Journal 37: 162–169

Grieve G P 1988 Common vertebral joint problems. 2nd edn. Churchill Livingstone, Edinburgh, p 386

Grieve G P 1991 Mobilisation of the spine. 5th edn. Churchill Livingstone, Edinburgh

Hamberg J, Lindahl O 1981 Angina pectoris symptoms caused by thoracic spine disorders: clinical examination and treatment. Acta Medica Scandinavica Supplement 644: 84–86

Hanfligg S S 1936 Pain in the shoulder girdle, arm and precordium due to cervical arthritis. Journal of the American Medical Association 106: 523–526

Hattersley D A 1983 Case report. British Association of Manipulative Medicine Newsletter, March, p 10

Hawkes C D 1986 Neurosurgical considerations in thoracic outlet syndrome. Clinical Orthopaedics and Related Research 207: 24–28

Head H 1920 Studies in neurology. Oxford Medical Publications, London, p 653

Hickey M S, Kiernan G J, Weaver K E 1989 Evaluation of abdominal pain. Emergency Medical Clinics of North America 7: 437–452

Hockaday J M Whitty C W M 1967 Patterns of referred pain in the normal subject. Brain 90: 481–496

Holt E P 1964 Fallacy of cervical discography: report of 50 cases in normal subjects. Journal of the American Medical Association 188: 799–801

Holt E P 1975 Further reflections of cervical discography. Journal of the American Medical Association 231: 613–614

Huffman J D 1986 Electrodiagnostic techniques for and conservative treatment of thoracic outlet syndrome. Clinical Orthopaedics and Related Research 207: 21–23

Ingesson E, Norgren L, Ribbe E 1982 Physiotherapy in thoracic outlet syndrome. In: Proceedings IXth Congress World Confederation for Physical Therapy, Stockholm, pp 618–619

Janda V, Schmid H J A 1980 Muscles as a pathogenic factor in back pain. In: Proceedings 4th Conference International Federation of Orthopaedic Manipulative Therapists, Christchurch pp 1–23

Janda V 1983 Muscle function testing. Butterworths, London, pp 20–24

Jooma R, Torrens M S, Veerapen R J, Griffith H B 1983 Spinal disease presenting as acute abdominal pain: a report of two cases. British Medical Journal 287: 117–118

Kellgren J H 1940 Somatic simulating visceral pain. Clinical Science 4: 303–309

Kellgren J H 1949 Deep pain sensibility. Lancet 1: 943–949

Kikta D, Breder A, Wilbourn A 1982 Thoracic root pain in diabetes: the spectrum of clinical and electromyographical findings. Annals of Neurology 11: 80–85

Kirk E J, Denny-Brown D 1970 Functional variations in the dermatomes in the macaque monkey following dorsal root lesions. Journal of Comparative Neurology 139: 307–320

Kirkaldy-Willis W H, Hill R J 1979 A more precise diagnosis for low back pain. Spine 4: 102–109

Klafta L A, Collis J S 1969 The diagnostic inaccuracy of the pain response in cervical discography. Cleveland Clinical Quarterly 36: 35–39

Kunert W 1965 Functional disorders of internal organs due to vertebral lesions. Ciba symposium 13: 85–96

LaBan M M, Meerschaert J R, Johnstone K 1977 Carotid bruits: their significance in the cervical radicular syndrome. Archives of Physical Medicine & Rehabilitation 58: 491–494

LaBan M M, Meerschaert J R, Taylor R S 1979 Breast pain: a symptom of cervical radiculopathy. Archives of Physical Medicine and Rehabilitation 60: 315–317

Lawrence S J 1977 Rheumatism in populations. Heinemann, London, ch 4, p 73

Leffert R D 1983 Thoracic outlet syndrome In: Evarts C M (ed) Surgery of the musculo-skeletal system. vol 1, section 2. Churchill Livingstone, Edinburgh, ch 15, pp 2400–2406

Lewis T, Kellgren J H 1939 Observations relating to referred pain. Clinical Science 4: 47–71

Lewit K 1983 Post-isometic relaxation in the diagnosis of the scalenus syndrome. Manuelle Medizin 21: 27–30

Lindahl O, Hamberg J 1981 Angina pectoris symptoms caused by thoracic spine disorders: neuroanatomical considerations. Acta Medica Scandinavica Supplement 644: 81–83

Longstreth G F, Newcomer A D 1977 Abdominal pain caused by diabetic neuropathy. Annals of Internal Medicine 86: 166–168

Marinacci A A, Courville C B 1962 Radicular syndromes simulating intra-abdominal surgical conditions. American Surgery 28: 59–63

Master A M 1964 The spectrum of anginal and noncardiac chest pain. Journal of the American Medical Association 187: 894–899

McBeath A A, Keene J S 1975 The rib-tip syndrome. Journal of Bone and Joint Surgery 57A: 795–797

McLeod J (ed) 1983 Clinical examination. Churchill Livingstone, Edinburgh, ch 1, p 12

McRae R 1983 Clinical orthopaedic examination. 2nd edn. Churchill Livingstone, Edinburgh, p v

Melzack R, Wall P D 1982 The challenge of pain. Penguin, Harmondsworth, p 125

Mennell J B 1945 Physical treatment by movement, manipulation and massage. 5th edn. Churchill, London

Meyer R R 1963 Cervical discography: a help or hindrance in evaluating neck, shoulder and arm pain? Americal Journal of Roentgenology 90: 1208–1215

Middleditch A, Jarnam P 1984 An investigation of frozen shoulder using thermography. Physiotherapy 70: 433–439

Mikkelsen S, Rasmussen M S, Krag E 1989 Abdominal pain precipitated by thoracic segment syndrome. Ugeskrift for Laeger 151: 1036–1038

Mitchell F L, Moran P S, Pruzzo M A 1979 An evaluation and treatment manual of osteopathic muscle energy procedures. ICEOP Inc., Valley Park, Missouri, pp 126–128, pp 253–261

Monnin J L, Pierrugues R, Bories P, Michel H 1988 Cyriax syndrome: a cause of diagnostic error in abdominal pain. Presse-Médicale 17: 25–29

Moore M 1986a Editorial: thoracic outlet syndrome update. Clinical Orthopaedics and Related Research 207: 12

Moore M 1986b Thoracic outlet syndrome: experience in a metropolitan hospital. Clinical Orthopaedics and Related Research 207: 29–30

Motley L 1948 Neurogenic pain simulating visceral disease. American Journal of Medicine 4: 539–544

Murray R O, Stokes D J, Jacobson H G 1990 The radiology of skeletal disease. 3rd edn. Churchill Livingstone, Edinburgh, vol 2

Nachlas I W 1934 Pseudoangina pectoris originating in the cervical spine. Journal of the Americal Medical Association 103: 323–325

Nathan H 1959 The para-articular processes of the thoracic vertebrae. Anatomical Record 133: 605–618

Nathan H 1962 Osteophytes of the vertebral column. Journal of Bone and Joint Surgery 44A: 243–268

Nathan H 1969 Compression of the sympathetic trunk and its nerves by vertebral osteophytes in the thorax and abdomen. Archivos Mexicanos de Anatomia 9: 30–45

Nathan H 1987 Osteophytes of the spine compressing the sympathetic trunk and splanchnic nerves in the thorax. Spine 12: 527–532

Nathan H, Schwartz A 1962 Inverted pattern of development of thoracic vertebral osteophytosis in situs inversus and in other instances of right descending aorta. Radiological Clinics 31: 150–158

Nathan H, Weinberg H, Robin G C, Aviad I 1964 The costovertebral joints: anatomico-clinical observations in arthritis. Arthritis and Rheumatism 7: 228–240

Nicholas A S, DeBias D A, Ehrenfeuchter W, England K M, England R W, Greene C H, Heilig, D, Kirschbaum M 1985 A somatic component to myocardial infarction. British Medical Journal 291: 13–17

Nichols H M 1986 Anatomic structures of the thoracic outlet. Clinical Orthopaedics and Related Research 207: 13–20

Noordenbos W 1984 Prologue In: Wall P D, Melzack R (eds) Textbook of pain. Churchill Livingstone, Edinburgh

Patriquin D A 1983 The mechanical aetiology of Tietze's syndrome. British Association of Manipulative Medicine Newsletter, November, p 5

Phillips J 1927 The importance of examining the spine in the presence of intrathoracic or abdominal pain. Proceedings Interstate Postgraduate Medical Association of North America 3: 70–74

Prinzmetal M, Massumi R A 1955 The anterior chest wall syndrome: chest pain resembling pain of cardiac origin. Journal of the American Medical Association 159: 177–182

Quast M S, Goldflies M L 1989 A new differential diagnosis for musculoskeletal posterior thoracic wall pain: a case report. Orthopaedic Review 18: 461–465

Rawlings M S 1962 The rib syndrome. Disease of the Chest 41: 432–441

Rayan G M 1988 Lower trunk brachial plexus compression neuropathy due to cervical rib in young athletes. American Journal of Sports Medicine 66: 77–79

Reid W D 1938 Pressure on the brachial plexus causing simulation of coronary disease. Journal of the American Medical Association 110: 1724–1726

Riddell D H, Smith B M 1986 Thoracic and vascular aspects of thoracic outlet syndrome. Clinical Orthopaedics and Related Research 207: 31–36

Sarbandi H S, Pruss-Kaddatz U, Dohmann R 1989 Abdominal intercostal nerve pain: a contribution to differential diagnosis of acute abdominal pain. Chirurgie 60: 886–889

Schmorl G, Junghanns H 1971 The human spine in health and disease, 2nd. American edn. Grune and Stratton, New York, ch 8, pp 206, 236

Semmes R E, Murphey F 1943 The syndrome of unilateral rupture of the sixth cervical intervertebral disc with compression of seventh nerve root: report of four cases with symptoms simulating coronary heart disease. Journal of the American Medical Association 121: 1200–1214

Sherrington C S 1893 Experiments in the examination of the peripheral distribution of the fibres of the posterior roots of some spinal nerves. Philosophical Transactions B 184: 641–763

Shore L R 1931 A report of the nature of certain bony spurs arising from the dorsal arches of the thoracic vertebrae. Journal of Anatomy 65: 379–387

Shore L R 1935 On osteoarthritis in the dorsal intervertebral joints: a study in morbid anatomy. British Journal of Surgery 22: 833–849

Simeone F A, Lawner P M 1982 Intraspinal neoplasms. In: Rothman R H, Simeone F A (eds) The spine. 2nd edn. W B Saunders, Philadelphia, ch 16, p 1041

Smith J R, Kountz W R 1942 Deformities of thoracic spine as a cause of anginal pain. Annals of Internal Medicine 17: 604–607

Steindler A 1962 Ilio-psoas. Thomas, Illinois

Stoddard A 1983 Manual of osteopathic practice. 2nd edn. Hutchinson, London, p xviii; ch 1, p 16; ch 3, pp 203, 277

Sunderland S 1978 Traumatized nerves, roots and ganglia: musculo-skeletal factors and neuropathological consequences. In: Korr I M (ed) Neurobiologic mechanisms in manipulative therapy. Plenum Press, London, pp 151–152

Telford E D, Mottershead S 1947 The costo-clavicular syndrome. British Medical Journal March 15: 325–328

Travell J G, Simons D G 1983 Myofascial pain and dysfunction — the trigger point manual. Williams & Wilkins, Baltimore, ch 2

Watson M 1978 The refractory painful arc syndrome. Journal of Bone and Joint Surgery 60B: 544–546

Williams P L, Warwick R, Dyson M, Bannister L H 1989 Gray's anatomy. 37th edn. Churchill Livingstone, Edinburgh, p 1168

Wood V E, Twito R, Verska J M 1988 Thoracic outlet syndrome: the results of first rib resection in 100 patients. Orthopaedic Clinics of North America 19: 131–146

30. Lumbar dorsal ramus syndromes

N. Bogduk

The term 'lumbar dorsal ramus syndrome' was introduced in 1980 (Bogduk 1980) to highlight the fact that all back pain was not due to disorders of the intervertebral discs and disc herniation. Complaints could be due to disorders of the posterior elements of the lumbar spine, which comprise the back muscles and the joints and ligaments of the vertebral arches, and which share the anatomical feature that they are all innervated by branches of the lumbar dorsal rami.

Because of this common innervation, disorders of the posterior elements are neurologically similar. Regardless of its actual origin, the pain in these disorders will be mediated by one or more of the branches of the lumbar dorsal rami and their central connections. Consequently, the symptoms of different disorders and some of their associated features will be similar. The challenge has been to identify clinical features that are specific to specific disorders, but despite quite reasonable efforts over the last 10 years this has not been achieved. Nevertheless, it still remains possible to determine whether or not a particular complaint is mediated by the lumbar dorsal rami. As a nosological entity, 'lumbar dorsal ramus syndrome' identifies the nerves that mediate the symptoms, and stipulates that the source of pain lies in the territory of these nerves. It thereby distinguishes the condition from intervertebral disc syndromes and from back pain mediated by other nerves, and can be used when the source of pain cannot be stipulated but when it clearly lies within the posterior elements.

ANATOMY

The anatomy of the lumbar dorsal rami has been described in detail (Bogduk et al 1982, Bogduk 1983), and it is inappropriate to repeat that detail here. The salient features, of clinical relevance, are that the medial branches of the lumbar dorsal rami are distributed to the lumbar zygapophyseal joints, the interspinous ligaments and muscles, and to the multifidus muscle. The lateral and intermediate branches are distributed to the iliocostalis

and longissimus muscles respectively. Of particular relevance to the diagnosis of lumbar dorsal ramus syndromes is the fact that the medial branch of each dorsal ramus has a constant course across the root of a transverse process. This allows their location to be identified on radiographs of the lumbar spine, and enables needles or electrodes to be introduced onto these nerves under fluoroscopic control.

CLINICAL FEATURES

Ideally, the clinical features of a particular condition should be established by studying patients known to have that condition and patients known not to have it, and determining those clinical features that reliably discriminate the two groups. However, by and large, this has not been achieved for any of the disorders of the posterior elements.

An alternative approach is to define the clinical features on the basis of experimental evidence. This is less satisfying for it does not provide any power to discriminate the condition from others that may resemble it, clinically. Nevertheless, such an approach serves to characterize the particular condition so that it might be recognised in the first instance. Thereafter, steps need to be taken to verify that the clinical features are not due to some other cause.

PHYSIOLOGY

Pain and referred pain

Any of the structures innervated by the lumbar dorsal rami is potentially capable of being a primary source of pain. The joints and ligaments of the vertebral arches are endowed with nociceptive, free nerve endings, as are the back muscles and their fasciae (Bogduk 1983). For pain to be produced all that is required is for these nerve endings to be activated by a pathological process.

The algogenic potential of the posterior elements of the lumbar spine has been demonstrated by two types of clinical studies: those in which low back and referred pain have been induced in normal volunteers by injections of hypertonic saline, and those in which referred pain has been relieved by anaesthetizing lumbar dorsal rami or structures supplied by these nerves.

When injected into lumbar interspinous ligaments, back muscles, or zygapophyseal joints, hypertonic saline induces low back pain in normal volunteers. This pain can be accompanied by referred pain in the lower limbs (Kellgren 1938, 1939, Feinstein et al 1954, McCall et al 1979), although this is not always the case (Sinclair et al 1948, Hockaday & Whitty 1967, Bogduk & Munro 1979). Referred pain occurs only when an adequate stimulus is delivered, which depends on the volume of hypertonic saline injected, the speed of injection, and the density of innervation of the structure stimulated.

Referred pain in the lower limbs has been produced in normal volunteers by injecting interspinous ligaments (Kellgren 1939, Hockaday & Whitty 1967), paramedian interspinous tissues (Feinstein et al 1954), the multifidus muscle (Kellgren 1938, Sinclair et al 1948, Bogduk & Munro 1979, Bogduk 1980), and the zygapophyseal joints (Hirsch et al 1963, Mooney & Robertson 1976, McCall et al 1979). In a given individual repeated stimulations of the same structure reproduce the same distribution of referred pain, but between individuals and between different studies there are considerable differences in distribution even when ostensibly the same structure is stimulated (Fig. 30.1). Moreover, the distribution of referred pain from one vertebral level overlaps that from other vertebral levels, (Fig. 30.1). Consequently, the distribution of referred pain cannot be used to determine the level of the primary source of pain in a lumbar dorsal ramus syndrome.

Complementing these experimental studies are clinical reports of the relief of low back pain and referred pain in the lower limbs by injections of local anaesthetic into structures supplied by lumbar dorsal rami. Structures that have been so injected are the interspinous ligaments (Steindler & Luck 1938, Hackett 1956), trigger points in back muscles (Travell & Travell 1946, Travell & Rinzler 1952, Bonica 1957, Berges 1973), and the zygapophyseal joints (Pawl 1974, Oudenhoven 1974, 1979, Lora & Long 1976, Mooney & Robertson 1976, Ogsbury et al 1977, Schaerer 1978, Fairbank et al 1981). Thus, the same structures, found in experimental studies to be capable of producing referred pain, have been found clinically to be the source of referred pain in patients suffering low back pain syndromes.

There is a consensus amongst workers in this field that in general, the referred pain in any lumbar dorsal ramus syndrome is generally located proximal to the knee, mostly in the gluteal region. However, this restriction is not absolute for experimental studies have shown that it is not impossible for referred pain to extend as far as the feet (Fig. 30.1), and patients with such distal radiation

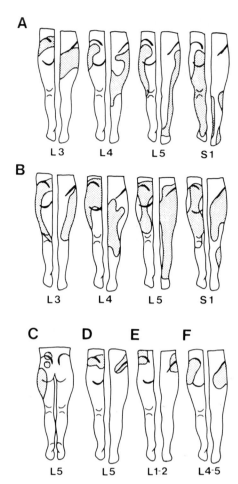

Fig. 30.1 The distribution of referred pain after the injection of 6% saline to (**A**) the L3–S1 interspinous ligaments; (**B**) the interspinous spaces at L3–S1; (**C**) (**D**) the multifidus muscle opposite L5; (**E**) the L1–2 and (**F**) L4–5 zygapophyseal joints. Based on the data of Kellgren (1938, 1939), Feinstein et al (1954), McCall et al (1979) and Bogduk (1980).

have been described (Mooney & Robertson 1976, Bogduk 1980, Fairbank et al 1981). From experimental studies, it appears that, amongst other possible factors, the extent of radiation into the lower limb is proportional to the intensity of the stimulus delivered to the back (Mooney & Robertson 1976).

Muscle spasm

Muscle spasm is a feature that may accompany pain in lumbar dorsal ramus syndromes. It has been studied both in experimental animals and in humans, and specific comments can be made about its physiology.

Pedersen et al (1956) were the first to observe that, in the spinal cat, spasm of the dorsal lumbar muscle and of the hamstrings occurred after noxious stimulation of muscles, ligaments and joints supplied by lumbosacral dorsal rami. Bogduk and Munro (1973, 1974) and Bogduk (1980) confirmed these findings, and further demonstrated that electrical stimulation of individual dorsal rami evoked reflex activity in the hamstrings. This reflex was polysynaptic and was mediated by the smaller-diameter fibres of the dorsal rami. Not all motor units in the hamstrings were activated by a given stimulus. While some units responded, others as near as 1 cm away remained silent. Some units, initially inactive, responded to sustained or more intense stimulation of the back. The reflex activity was unilateral or bilateral, but was detected only in those muscles innervated by the same spinal cord segments from which the stimulated dorsal rami were derived. Similar observations in cats have been reported following the stimulation of the articular branches to the lumbar zygapophyseal joints (Nade et al 1978).

Comparable phenomena have been observed in humans. Bogduk and Munro (1979) and Bogduk (1980) found that injections of hypertonic saline into the L5 interspinous ligament or into the multifidus muscle produced electromyographically detectable activity in the multifidus, gluteus medius and tensor fasciae latae muscles. This activity followed the onset of back pain, lasted only as long as the back pain, and occurred regardless of whether referred pain occurred or not. Mooney and Robertson (1976) found that, in normal volunteers, injections of hypertonic saline into the L4–5 or L5–S1 zygapophyseal joints produced electromyographic activity in the hamstrings, and caused a limitation of straight leg raising. Anaesthetization of the stimulated joints obliterated the increased muscle activity. In six patients presenting with limitation of straight leg raising, Mooney and Robertson (1976) were able to restore normal straight leg raising, by anaesthetizing zygapophyseal joints, revealing that the cause of limitation was spasm of the hamstrings secondary to zygapophyseal joint pain.

PATHOLOGY

The potential causes of lumbar dorsal ramus syndromes can be established by systematically reviewing the pathology of the several structures innervated by lumbar dorsal rami.

Ligaments

The interspinous ligaments can be affected by a variety of degenerative changes (Rissanen 1960), but there is no evidence that these changes are painful. Otherwise, the interspinous ligaments have been reported to be a potential source of back pain and referred pain but only in situations where the offending pathology could not be defined. On the basis of some 6000 injections of local anaesthetic, Hackett (1956) reported that the interspinous ligaments were one of many ligaments that could cause back pain. In a study of 143 patients with back pain, Steindler and Luck (1938) identified 14 in whom the source of pain could be traced to supraspinous or inter-

spinous ligaments; their back pain was associated with referred pain in the gluteal region in all cases, and in the thigh or leg in 10. Injection of the responsible ligament with local anaesthetic temporarily relieved the back pain and associated pain. However, subsequent studies have not corroborated or elaborated these findings, and it remains unclear how commonly back pain in contemporary patients can be ascribed to the interspinous ligaments.

Another condition befalling the interspinous spaces is Baastrup's disease or 'kissing spines' (Baastrup 1933, Schmorl & Junghanns 1971, Epstein 1976). In this condition, subluxation of a vertebra results in approximation of adjacent spinous processes, especially on extension, and the formation of a painful pseudoarthrosis. Clinically, Baastrup's disease poses no diagnostic problem. Focal tenderness over an interspinous space raises suspicion, and the radiological appearance of the condition is diagnostic; infiltration of the affected interspinous space with local anaesthetic should relieve the patient's pain.

Lumbar fat herniation

Herniation of fat through the thoracolumbar fascia was first described by Copeman and Ackerman (1944, 1947), and has been reiterated as a cause of low back pain and referred pain by several others (Herz 1945, Hucherson & Gandy 1948, Bonner & Kasdon 1954, Wollgast & Afeman 1961, Singewald 1966, Faille 1978). This condition is characterized by the finding of a mobile, tender nodule along the lateral border of erector spinae. Infiltration of the nodule with local anaesthetic, or its excision, relieves all symptoms. Histologically, the nodules are found to be normal fat and not lipomata. The pain in this condition is probably produced by the hernia stretching the thoracolumbar fascia or surrounding connective tissue.

Muscle pain

Theoretically, disorders of the lumbar back muscles are possible causes of lumbar dorsal ramus syndrome, but little is known of the pathology of painful muscle disorders.

Acute strains or tears of the back muscles are clinically recognized causes of pain, but because these conditions usually resolve spontaneously they have not attracted pathological study. Studies in experimental animals have shown that excessive stretching of a muscle characteristically leads to failure at its myo-tendinous junction, and the resultant injury attracts an acute inflammatory response (Garrett et al 1987, 1988, Nikolau et al 1987). It is presumable that a similar lesion befalls human back muscles following acute strains or unaccustomed exertional activity. However, no further scientific comment can be made as to how, and if, muscle trauma proceeds to cause persistent or chronic back pain.

Painful spasm of the muscles is another clinically recognized phenomenon. As described above, muscle spasm is a reflex response to noxious stimulation of structures innervated by dorsal rami, but if, and how, pain is produced in this state is unknown. A possible explanation is that continuous activity in some, or all, motor units in a muscle impairs the circulation of blood through those active units, enabling the accumulation of noxious metabolites.

The concept of the pain–spasm–pain cycle has been reviewed elsewhere (Roland 1986), but it seems that despite its clinical popularity, reliable scientific evidence is scarce, and, in particular, there are no means clinically of objectively verifying that spasm is present let alone whether or not it is causing pain. One study has shown that EMG-monitoring of back muscle during sleep reveals continuous involuntary activity in some patients with back pain (Fischer & Chang 1985). However, while this study corroborates the concept of muscle spasm secondary to pain in some patients it does not provide a practical means of diagnosing the condition.

Trigger points are said to occur in the back muscles, causing local pain, referred pain, muscle spasm and secondary trigger points in the lower limb, all of which can be relieved, at least temporarily, by infiltrating the primary trigger point with local anaesthetic (Kelly 1941, Travell & Travell 1946, Travell & Rinzler 1952, Bonica 1957, Kraft et al 1968, Berges 1973, Kraus 1973). The pathology of trigger points remains enigmatic. The results of histological studies have been equivocal (Simons 1975, 1976a, 1988), but physiological studies indicate that trigger points represent areas of hyper-irritable motor units (Simons 1976b, 1988). One theory maintains that trigger points are self-sustaining areas of muscle contraction initiated by focal tearing of sarcoplasmic reticulum (Simons & Travell 1981, Simons 1988).

What remains unstudied, however, is how frequently trigger points are the cause of low back pain. Most research studies have focused on trigger points in the cervico-scapular region. With respect to the lumbar spine, proponents of trigger point theory have simply quoted the same paper which stated that trigger points may occur in the multifidus, longissimus or iliocostalis (Travell & Rinzler 1952). While this possibility is not denied, it is not known how common this condition is. Furthermore, it is not clear the extent to which the back muscles are affected by trigger points as opposed to simple areas of tenderness near muscle attachment sites (Livingston 1941, Bauwens & Coyer 1955, Ingpen & Burry 1970, Fairbank & O'Brien 1983).

Zygapophyseal joints

Lumbar zygapophyseal joint pain, otherwise referred to as 'facet syndrome', is a form of lumbar dorsal ramus syndrome for, the nerves that innervate these joints are the medial branches of the lumbar dorsal rami (Bogduk et al 1982).

Experimental studies have shown that stimulation of the lumbar zygapophyseal joints, either with intra-articular injections of hypertonic saline (Hirsch et al 1963, Mooney & Robertson 1976, McCall et al 1979) or by electrical stimulation of their capsules or nerve supply (McCulloch & Waddell 1980, Marks 1989) can produce low back pain and referred pain. Similarly, some forms of low back pain with referred pain can be relieved by anaesthetizing either one or more lumbar zygapophyseal joints (Mooney & Robertson 1976, Glover 1977, Carrera 1979, 1980a, b, Fassio et al 1980, Dory 1981, Fairbank et al 1981, Destouet et al 1982, Pheasant & Dyck 1982, Rashbaum 1983, Carrera & Williams 1984, Lippitt 1984, Raymond & Dumas 1984, Lau et al 1985, Lewinnek & Warfield 1986, Lynch & Taylor 1986, Eisenstein & Parry 1987, Helbig & Lee 1988, Moran et al 1988, Murtagh 1988) or their nerve supply (Pawl 1974, Lora & Long 1976, Hickey & Tregonning 1977, Ogsbury et al 1977, Schaerer 1978, Mehta & Sluijter 1979, Oudenhoven 1979, Maigne 1980, Sluijter & Mehta 1981, Uyttendaele et al 1981, Rossi & Pernak 1990, Silvers 1990). For these and other reasons the concept that certain forms of back pain can stem from the lumbar zygapophyseal joints has attracted considerable support from other quarters (Rees 1971, 1975, Shealy 1974a, b, 1975, 1976, Editorial 1978, Mehta 1978, Murley 1978, Robertson 1978, Mooney 1987). However, others have not been so supportive, reporting that few patients with back pain respond unequivocally to anaesthetization of lumbar zygapophyseal joints; as few as 16% (Raymond & Dumas 1984, Moran et al 1988) or fewer than 8% (Jackson et al 1988).

The causes of pain from lumbar zygapophyseal joints, when it does occur, remain elusive. Rarely, a secondary ossification centre may occur in the tip of the inferior articular process (Schmorl & Junghanns 1971), and may fail to unite with the base of the process. Non-united epiphyses have been observed in patients with low back pain (King 1955, Pou-Serradell & Casademont 1972, Galecki 1978) but also in asymptomatic individuals (Farmer 1936, Horwitz & Smith 1940, Roche & Rowe 1951, Hadley 1964) and in mixed populations (Nichols & Schiflett 1933, Rendich & Westing 1933, Fulton & Kaltfleisch 1934, Bailey 1937, Hipps 1939). Consequently, there is no clear relationship between the presence of non-united epiphyses and pain, and this condition may be only incidental to the actual cause of back pain.

Fractures of either the inferior or superior articular process may occur (Mitchell 1933, Bailey 1937, Hadley 1964, Sims-Williams et al 1978, Twomey et al 1989, Taylor et al 1990), and, like fractures elsewhere, may be presumed to be a source of pain, if not stable. Such fractures may have been under-diagnosed to date because they are not readily demonstrated by plain radiography (Twomey et al 1989, Taylor et al 1990). They require tomography or stereoscopic radiography for proper resolution (Sims-Williams et al 1978). However, to date, the presence of fractures of the articular processes has not been correlated with the presence of pain or with the relief of pain following injection of local anaesthetic into the affected joint. Consequently, it is not yet known the extent to which such fractures may account for back pain stemming from zygapophyseal joints.

Being synovial joints, the lumbar zygapophyseal joints are theoretically susceptible to all forms of arthritides. Various uncommon arthritides such as ochronosis, and haemophilia have not been specifically reported as affecting the lumbar zygapophyseal joints, but there have been case reports of septic arthritis (Roberts 1988, Rush & Griffiths 1989) and pigmented villonodular synovitis (Campbell & Wells 1982). Rheumatoid arthritis may affect the lumbar zygapophyseal joints (Lawrence et al 1964, Jayson 1976, Sims-Williams et al 1977), although it has been reported only in patients with rheumatoid arthritis manifest elsewhere in the body. Ankylosing spondylitis is an enthesopathy (Ball 1971), and in the zygapophyseal joints causes fibrosis and ossification of the joint capsule with little change in the articular cartilage or synovium. Ankylosing spondylitis and the related seronegative spondylarthropathies (psoriasis, ulcerative colitis, Reiter's syndrome and Behçet's disease) are attracting greater interest as differential diagnoses of low back pain, but to date, interest has focused on sacro-iliac involvement, and the zygapophyseal joints have not been specifically considered.

Degenerative joint disease or osteoarthrosis, is the most common affliction of the lumbar zygapophyseal joints. With increasing age, the prevalence of this disorder increases (Lewin 1964). In younger age groups the disease tends to be unisegmental, but later it becomes polysegmental (Lewin 1964). Early, it affects upper lumbar levels, but later it predominates at lower lumbar levels (Lewin 1964). There is still controversy as to whether zygapophyseal osteoarthrosis is a primary cartilaginous disorder, like peripheral osteoarthrosis (Lewin 1964) or a condition secondary to disc degeneration (Vernon-Roberts & Pirie 1977, Butler et al 1990). Although zygapophyseal osteoarthrosis appears to be due to disc degeneration (Harris & Macnab 1954, Vernon-Roberts & Pirie 1977, Butler et al 1990), statistical analysis of findings in post mortem material do not substantiate this (Lewin 1964). Within segments the relationship between disc degeneration and changes in the zygapophyseal joints is irregular, and in some 20% of spines, zygapophyseal osteoarthrosis may be present in the absence of any histological evidence of disc degeneration (Lewin 1964).

Eisenstein and Parry (1987) reported that zygapophyseal joints, found to be symptomatic by diagnostic intra-articular injection of local anaesthetic, exhibited changes similar to those of chondromalacia patellae. However, the strength of this report is compromised by the lack of a suitable number of control observations of asymptomatic joints. Bough et al (1990) found a strong, positive correlation between whether or not pain was reproduced from a joint when injected with contrast medium, and the presence of degenerative changes evident in the joint when excised and studied histologically. Symptom reproduction was a specific indicator and positively predictive of the presence of such changes, but was poorly sensitive. The relationship between pain and degenerative changes is, therefore, not direct; some factor other than morphological changes alone determines whether or not the joint becomes symptomatic.

Some studies suggest that inflammation is unlikely to be the factor, although joints known to be symptomatic have not been expressly studied in this regard (Konttinen et al 1990). On the other hand, there has been one study which revealed that pain occurred in lumbar zygapophyseal joints when their intra-articular pressure rose above $30g/cm^2$, and that, in the presence of disc degeneration, such pressures occur during flexion of the lumbar spine (Nakajima 1969). Thus, mechanical changes, rather than inflammatory changes, may be the determining factor in whether or not an osteoarthritic zygapophyseal joint becomes symptomatic.

Subluxations of the lumbar zygapophyseal joints have been alleged to be causes of back pain (Hadley 1935, 1936). However, the lumbar zygapophyseal joints normally subluxate some 5–7 mm during flexion and extension (Lewin 1968) and the appearance on normal radiographs of over-riding articular processes can occur in normal joints (Lewin 1968). Criteria for the diagnosis of pathological and symptomatic subluxation of the zygapophyseal joints have not been defined. Consequently, until such criteria are established, the diagnosis can at best remain only an imaginary one.

There has been speculation on what might be considered physiological subluxation. The theory is that subtle changes in the position of the joint, or simply changes in capsule tension, alter the mechanoreceptor discharge from the joint. While not necessarily causing pain directly, this altered mechanoreceptor discharge has been portrayed as in some way altering central gate-control mechanisms to allow pain to be perceived (Wyke 1979). However, as with pathological subluxation, criteria for the diagnosis of this condition have not been established and so it must remain only a speculative diagnosis.

The theory of meniscus entrapment has been popularized by European manipulative therapists (Kos & Wolf 1972a, b, Wolf 1975). The theory proposes that the meniscoid structures of the zygapophyseal joints may become trapped between the articular surfaces and cause pain by capsular traction. Anatomical studies, however, argue against this theory in its original form (Engel &

Bogduk 1982, Bogduk & Engel 1984, Bogduk & Jull 1985). Persisting controversy about this entity (Lewit 1987) centres around the definition of the term 'joint locking'. In the European literature this pertains to what is known in the British and Australian literature as joint stiffness or hypomobility. For this condition, it is quite entertainable that intra-articular meniscoids constitute a nidus around which fibrous tissue can precipitate and cause intra-articular adhesions which restrict the mobility of a joint. On the other hand, a condition identified in British and Australian clinical practice is that of 'acute locked back' which is characterized by a patient being locked in a flexed position, unable to extend the lumbar spine because of the aggravation of pain. For this condition it has been proposed that rather than being trapped inside the zygapophyseal joint, meniscoids may dislocate from the joint cavity and become extrapped outside the joint space where they produce pain by acting effectively as a loose body underneath the joint capsule (Bogduk & Jull 1985).

Apart from extrapped meniscoids, loose bodies have been found in lumbar zygapophyseal joints at post mortem (Harris & Macnab 1954). By analogy with the knee joint, it would appear acceptable that such loose bodies could be a cause of low back pain. However, this contention has not been verified clinically.

Theoretically, the lumbar zygapophyseal joint capsules could be strained by excessive movements in flexion or rotation. Pathological studies of post mortem lumbar spines have identified such lesions in the form of disruption of the joint capsule or of the ligamentum flavum, some associated with intra-articular haemorrhage (Twomey et al 1989, Taylor et al 1990). What are now required are clinical studies that verify whether or not such lesions constitute a basis for zygapophyseal joint pain.

Iatrogenic disorders

Whereas all the above conditions occur naturally, there are iatrogenic disorders of the posterior elements of the lumbar spine. Prominent amongst these is graft impingement. Following posterior interlaminar fusion, patients may complain of a new pain, aggravated particularly by extension movements. The offending pathology in such cases seems to be impingement of the rostral or caudal edge of the graft mass against the adjacent vertebral lamina, for infiltrating this region with local anaesthetic relieves the symptoms, as does resection of the fusion mass (Terry et al 1981). An analogous condition, not yet formally reported in the literature, but one which has been receiving attention is pain stemming from the location of the heads of pedicle screws used to immobilize the lumbar spine.

Other unexplored, yet theoretically possible disorders, include entrapment of branches of the lumbar dorsal rami in fusions, and neuroma formation in these nerves if they are severed during spinal surgery. The latter relates particularly to the lateral branches of the lumbar dorsal rami that cross the transverse processes, and which typically are transected during intertransverse fusions. These entities, however, can only remain speculative because the nerves allegedly affected lie deep to the fusion mass and are inaccessible for diagnostic blocks or other studies.

DIAGNOSIS

The diagnosis of lumbar dorsal ramus syndromes cannot be made on clinical features alone, for none of these features is unique to any particular variant of the syndrome. This is particularly evident with respect to lumbar zygapophyseal joint pain.

Some investigators have failed to identify any clinical features that could be construed as indicative of lumbar zygapophyseal joint pain (Jackson et al 1988, Lilius et al 1990). However, certain insights were provided by Fairbank et al (1981). These investigators studied patients presenting with their first attack of back pain. Each was subjected to intra-articular injections of local anaesthetic into putatively symptomatic zygapophyseal joints, and those whose pain was relieved were compared to those whose pain was not. Responders tended to have a more acute onset of pain, and their back pain was aggravated by sitting, flexion and straight leg raising; their referred pain tended to localize over the gluteal region and thigh. However, although statistically significant, these differences were only relative; none was absolute.

Helbig and Lee (1988) attempted to overcome this lack of discrimination by developing a point scoring system with weightings for particular features, such as back pain associated with groin or thigh pain, paraspinal tenderness, pain on extension-rotation, and no pain below the knee. A score of 40 or more on their scale discriminated between responders and non-responders to anaesthetization of the offending joint, but although the positive predictive value was high, the sensitivity and specificity were only modest. Increasing the threshold score to 60 points improved the specificity of clinical assessment but decreased the sensitivity.

Collectively, the studies of Fairbank et al (1981) and of Helbig and Lee (1988) suggest that discriminating clinical criteria for zygapophyseal joint pain might be discernible, but none have yet been validated. The study of Helbig and Lee (1988) is encouraging, and suggests that a discriminating point-score system could be developed if additional clinical features were to be included and if different weightings were to be adopted.

Although clinical features do not permit the diagnosis of lumbar dorsal ramus syndromes, they do allow the distinction of other syndromes. Intervertebral disc herniation and spinal stenosis, for example, both involve spinal nerve compression and the consequent objective motor and sensory, neurological signs. Dermatomal sensory loss and myotomal muscle weakness are not features of lumbar dorsal ramus syndrome. These signs indicate an alternative diagnosis. Nevertheless, it is important to recognise that lumbar dorsal ramus syndromes may co-exist with other back pain syndromes (Bogduk 1980).

The diagnosis of lumbar dorsal ramus syndromes requires some form of objective confirmation. Either the primary source of pain must be identified, or the lumbar dorsal rami must be shown to mediate the symptoms.

With respect to the former approach, radiological examination is insufficient. The radiological presence of a morphological abnormality does not necessarily prove that the abnormality is the source of pain. This is particularly relevant in the case of zygapophyseal osteoarthrosis. Radiological surveys have shown that only about half of all patients with radiological evidence of zygapophyseal osteoarthrosis have a history of pain (Lawrence et al 1966, Magora & Schwartz 1976).

That a particular structure is responsible for a given patient's pain can be established most reliably if the pain is relieved by anaesthetizing that structure. Ideally, this should be complemented by reproducing the pain by aggravating the structure. In the case of certain accessible structures this can be done easily.

Disorders of the interspinous ligaments can be diagnosed by anaesthetizing the suspected ligament (Steindler & Luck 1938), as can fatty herniae (Copeman & Ackerman 1944, 1947, Herz 1945, Hucherson & Gandy 1948, Bonner & Kasdan 1954, Wollgast & Afeman 1961, Singewald 1966, Faille 1978) and trigger points in the back muscles (Kelly 1941, Travell & Travell 1946, Travell & Rinzler 1952, Bonica 1957, Kraft et al 1968, Berges 1973, Kraus 1973). Since these disorders are essentially subcutaneous, the pain they cause can be provoked by palpation.

Zygapophyseal joints lie too deeply to be accurately anaesthetized without radiological control. Under fluoroscopic control, however, zygapophyseal joint pain can be relieved by intra-articular injections of local anaesthetic, and provoked by intra-articular injections of hypertonic saline (Mooney & Robertson 1976). Consequently, facet arthrography and facet blocks have been popularized as diagnostic procedures for suspected zygapophyseal disorders (Carrera 1979, 1980a, b, Dory 1981, Destouet et al 1982, Pheasant & Dyck 1982, Rashbaum 1983, Carrera & Williams 1984, Lau et al 1985, Lewinnek & Warfield 1966, Lippitt 1984, Lynch & Taylor 1986, Moran et al 1988, Murtagh 1988). However, certain technical limitations prejudice this approach.

In the first instance, it is difficult to localize an injection of local anaesthetic strictly to the joint. Care must be taken to avoid rupture of the joint capsule and leakage of the local anaesthetic into surrounding tissues, whereupon anaesthetization of periarticular tissues cannot be excluded as the reason for any pain relief (Fairbank et al 1981). In the second instance, zygapophyseal joint blocks are technically difficult to perform, are painful to the patient, and in the search for a responsible joint, many normal joints might have to be punctured. Zygapophyseal joint blocks, therefore, are not a convenient screening procedure. They are probably justified only when there is strong suspicion that a particular joint is responsible. That way, the incidence of unnecessary puncture and possible damage to normal joints can be reduced.

A more convenient method of diagnosing a lumbar dorsal ramus syndrome is to identify the nerves responsible for mediating the symptoms. In this regard, most of the posterior elements of the lumbar spine are innervated by the medial branches of the lumbar dorsal rami, and the constant anatomy of these nerves allows radiological target points to be defined (Fox & Rizzoli 1976, Bogduk & Long 1979, 1980). The L1–L4 medial branches cross the medial end of the superior border of the sub-adjacent transverse process, and the L5 medial branch crosses the medial end of the ala of the sacrum. Needles or electrodes introduced onto these points under fluoroscopic control can be used, respectively, to anaesthetize or stimulate individual medial branches. The nerve (or nerves) responsible for mediating a patient's symptoms can be identified if stimulating a particular nerve reproduces the patient's pain, and if anaesthetization of that nerve relieves it. This approach establishes unequivocally whether or not the source of pain lies within the territory of one or more of the medial branches of the lumbar dorsal rami. As a screening procedure, lumbar medial branch blocks are easier to perform than intra-articular blocks, and are more comfortable for the patient.

TREATMENT

Conservative

Most published trials of conservative therapy for low pain have used heterogenous populations of patients; none have specifically addressed any of those conditions that constitute lumbar dorsal ramus syndromes. Thus, there are no formal data upon which to base any reliable recommendations for conservative therapy of lumbar dorsal ramus syndromes. Nevertheless, there are brief clinical reports that attest to the efficacy of certain conservative modalities.

Pain due to fat herniation may be relieved by injections of local anaesthetic, thereby obviating the need for surgery. Similarly, trigger points in the back muscles may be treated with injections of local anaesthetic, but the long-term benefits of this approach have not been established. In the case of zygapophyseal joint pain, prolonged relief of pain has been reported following the injection of the joint with local anaesthetic, with and without steroids (Mooney

& Robertson 1976, Carrera 1980b, Fassio et al 1980, Maigne 1980, Drevet et al 1981, Uyttendaele et al 1981, Destouet et al 1982, Lippitt 1984, Lau et al 1985, Lewinnek & Warfield 1986, Lynch & Taylor 1986, Helbig & Lee 1988, Moran et al 1988, Murtagh 1988). Manipulation of the offending joint, in cases of thoracolumbar pain, is reportedly successful (Maigne 1974, 1980, 1981).

The response to intra-articular injections of corticosteroids is unpredictable and variable. Some studies report complete relief of symptoms for over 6 months in only 15–30% of patients (Carrera 1980b, Destouet et al 1982, Lynch & Taylor 1986); others report complete relief in 17–54% of patients, but only for one to three months (Lippitt 1984, Lau et al 1985, Lewinnek & Warfield 1986, Murtagh 1988).

These low response rates suggest that intra-articular steroids may not be a particularly beneficial treatment for zygapophyseal joint pain, any may represent little more than placebo responses. One study (Lilius et al 1989) which purported to be a controlled study of intra-articular steroids for lumbar facet joint syndrome was clearly not. Although steroids and local anaesthetic were compared, they were injected into undiagnosed patients, none of whom were at all shown to have symptomatic zygapophyseal joints or not. A proper controlled trial is still required to determine the true efficacy of intra-articular steroids for zygapophyseal joint pain.

Surgical

There are two surgical approaches to lumbar dorsal ramus syndromes: either the offending lesion can be excised or it can be denervated.

The former approach encompasses the excision of fatty herniae (Copeman & Ackeman 1944, 1947, Herz 1945, Hucherson & Gandy 1948, Bonner & Kasdon 1954, Wollgast & Afeman 1961, Singewald 1966, Faille 1978), the resection of the pseudoarthrosis of Baastrup's disease (Franck 1943), and the resection of impinging posterior grafts (Terry et al 1981). A recent study, however, found that, despite adequate preoperative diagnosis, excision of Kissing's spines did not reliably lead to complete relief of the patients' presenting pain (Beks 1989).

Although facetectomy is performed to decompress spinal nerves, there have been no reports of resection of lumbar zygapophyseal joints simply for zygapophyseal joint pain. However, zygapophyseal capsulectomy has been reported, in a small number of cases, to be a successful procedure for otherwise intractable zygapophyseal joint pain (Maigne et al 1978, Maigne 1980).

Denervation procedures have been reported only in the context of zygapophyseal joint pain, and three types of procedure have been used to denervate these joints.

Rees (1971, 1975) proposed that lumbar zygapophyseal joints could be denervated using a single stab incision through the back muscles, and several investigators adopted this procedure (Brenner 1973, Toakley 1973, Houston 1975, Collier 1979), but anatomical and radiographic studies proved this operation could not possibly succeed in denervating the target joints (King & Lagger 1976, Bogduk et al 1977). Any therapeutic effect it may have had could not be ascribed to joint denervation (Bogduk 1977).

Originally, Hickey and Tregonning (1977) and more recently Silvers (1990) treated zygapophyseal joint pain by injecting phenol onto the nerves that supplied the symptomatic joint. The former authors reported excellent results lasting two to 12 months in 18 out of 30 patients; the latter reported excellent results lasting one to 10 years in 42% of 223 patients. This form of therapy would seem to warrant further exploration to determine why all patients do not respond so well and whether or not the procedure is confounded by placebo responses.

By far the greatest volume of literature on denervating lumbar zygapophyseal joints has addressed so-called 'facet denervation' a procedure in which the nerves supplying a symptomatic joint are coagulated using radiofrequency electrodes. The target nerves for this procedure are the medial branches of the lumbar dorsal rami that supply the target joint, and the procedure is properly known as lumbar medial branch neurotomy (Bogduk & Long 1980). 'Facet denervation' is in fact a misleading term for the medial branches of the lumbar dorsal rami supply more than just the zygapophyseal joints; by coagulating these nerves the procedure denervates not only the zygapophyseal joints but components of the multifidus muscle as well.

The indications for lumbar medial branch neurotomy are reproduction of the patient's pain upon electrical stimulation of the target nerves, and complete relief of pain upon anaesthetizing these nerves (Bogduk & Long 1980). In this regard, the procedure is neurosurgical in nature and consonant with the concept of lumbar dorsal ramus syndrome. The actual source of pain is immaterial. Although it is believed to arise in the zygapophyseal joints, all that is relevant is that the pain can be stopped by anaesthetizing the nerves that mediate the pain; whereupon, radiofrequency neurotomy offers a means of providing prolonged relief of this pain.

Reported success rates for lumbar medial branch neurotomy, or facet denervation as it was previously known, have varied from 90% to 25%, and appear to depend on the criteria for patient selection and the location and extent of lesions made (Pawl 1974, Oudenhoven 1974, 1977, 1979, Shealy 1974a, b, 1975, 1976, Banerjee & Pittman 1976, Burton 1976/1977, Lora & Long 1976, McCulloch 1976/1977, Florez et al 1977, McCulloch & Organ 1977, Ogsbury et al 1977, Fuentes 1978, Schaerer 1978, Mehta & Sluijter 1979, Fassio et al 1980, Drevet et al 1981, Sluijter & Mehta 1981, Uyttendaele at al 1981,

Rashbaum 1983, Andersen et al 1987, Rossi & Pernak 1990). However, laboratory studies have shown that the conventional use of the radiofrequency electrodes has been inaccurate (Bogduk et al 1987). The lesion formed by the electrodes does not extend beyond their tip; instead, it spreads radially. Consequently, electrodes introduced orthogonally onto the target nerves cannot reliably coagulate them; and the results of all previous studies using this approach must now be viewed with caution. It is more appropriate to introduce electrodes parallel to the nerves, but, to date, there have been no clinical studies of this technique. Thus, despite the enthusiasm accorded to 'facet denervation' in the past, any definitive treatment of lumbar zygapophyseal pain has still to be validated.

REFERENCES

Andersen K H, Mosdal C, Vaernet K 1987 Percutaneous radiofrequency facet denervation in low-back and extremity pain. Acta Neurochirugica 87: 48–51

Baastrup C I 1933 Proc. Spin. vert. Lumb. und einige zwischen diesen liegende Gelenkbildungen mit pathologischen Prozessen in dieser Region. Fortschritte auf dem Gebiete der Röntgenstrahlen 48: 430–435

Bailey W 1937 Anomalies and fractures of the vertebral articular processes. Journal of the American Medical Association 108: 266–270

Ball J 1971 Enthesopathy of rheumatoid and ankylosing spondylitis. Annals of the Rheumatic Diseases 30: 213–223

Banerjee T, Pittman H H 1976 Facet rhizotomy. Another armamentarium for treatment of low backache. North Carolina Medical Journal 37: 354–360

Bauwens P, Coyer A B 1955 The 'multifidus triangle' syndrome as a cause of recurrent low-back pain. British Medical Journal 2: 1306–1307

Beks J W F 1989 Kissing spines — a fact or fancy! Acta Neurochirurgica 100: 134–135

Berges P U 1973 Myofascial pain syndromes. Postgraduate Medicine 53: 161–168

Bogduk N 1977 'Rhizolysis' and low back pain (letter). Medical Journal of Australia 1: 504

Bogduk N 1980 Lumbar dorsal ramus syndrome. Medical Journal of Australia 2: 537–541

Bogduk N 1983 The innervation of the lumbar spine. Spine 8: 286–293

Bogduk N, Engel R 1984 The lumbar zygapophyseal menisci. A review of their anatomy and clinical significance. Spine 9: 454–460

Bogduk N, Jull G 1985 The theoretical pathology of acute locked back. Manual Medicine 1: 78–82

Bogduk N, Long D M 1979 The anatomy of the so-called 'articular nerves' and their relationship to facet denervation in the treatment of low back pain. Journal of Neurosurgery 51: 172–177

Bogduk N, Long D M 1980 Percutaneous lumbar medial branch neurotomy. A modification of facet denervation. Spine 5: 193–200

Bogduk N, Munro R R 1973 Posterior ramus–anterior ramus reflexes (abstract). Proceedings of the Australian Physiological and Pharmacological Society 4: 183–184

Bogduk N, Munro R R 1974 Dorsal ramus–ventral ramus reflexes in the cat and man (abstract). Journal of Anatomy 118: 394

Bogduk N, Munro R R 1979 Experimental low back pain, referred pain and muscle spasm (abstract). Journal of Anatomy 128: 661

Bogduk N, Colman R R S, Winer C E R 1977 An anatomical assessment of the 'percutaneous rhizolysis' procedure. Medical Journal of Australia 1: 397–399

Bogduk N, Wilson A S, Tynan W 1982 The human lumbar dorsal rami. Journal of Anatomy 134: 383–397

Bogduk N, Macintosh J, Marsland A 1987 Technical limitations to the efficacy of radiofrequency neurotomy for spinal pain. Neurosurgery 20: 529–535

Bonica J J 1957 Management of myofascial pain syndromes in general practice. Journal of the American Medical Association 164: 732–738

Bonner C D, Kasdon S C 1954 Herniation of fat through lumbodorsal fascia as a cause of low-back pain. New England Journal of Medicine 251: 1102–1104

Bough B, Thakore J, Davies M, Dowling F 1990 Degeneration of the lumbar facet joints: arthrography and pathology. Journal of Bone and Joint Surgery 72B: 275–276

Brenner L 1973 Report on a pilot study of percutaneous rhizolysis. Bulletin of the Postgraduate Committee in Medicine, University of Sydney 29: 203–206

Burton C V 1976/1977 Percutaneous radiofrequency facet denervation. Applied Neurophysiology 39: 80–86

Butler D, Trafimow J H, Andersson G B J, McNeill T W, Huckman M S 1990 Discs degenerate before facets. Spine 15: 111–113

Campbell A J, Wells I P 1982 Pigmented villonodular synovitis of a lumbar vertebral facet joint. Journal of Bone and Joint Surgery 64A: 145–146

Carrera G F 1979 Lumbar facet arthrography and injection in low back pain. Wisconsin Medical Journal 78: 35–37

Carrera G F 1980a Lumbar facet joint injection in low back pain and sciatica: preliminary results. Radiology 137: 665–667

Carrera G F 1980b Lumbar facet joint injection in low back pain and sciatica: description of technique. Radiology 137: 661–664

Carrera G F, Williams A L 1984 Current concepts in evaluation of the lumbar facet joints. CRC Critical Reviews in Diagnostic Imaging 21: 85–104

Collier B B 1979 Treatment for lumbar sciatic pain in posterior articular lumbar joint pain. Anaesthesia 34: 202–209

Copeman W S C, Ackerman W L 1944 'Fibrositis' of the back. Quarterly Journal of Medicine 13: 37–52

Copeman W S C, Ackerman W L 1947 Edema or herniations of fat lobules as a cause of lumbar and gluteal 'fibrositis'. Archives of Internal Medicine 79: 22–35

Destouet J M, Gilula L A, Murphy W A, Monsees B 1982 Lumbar facet joint injection: indication, technique, clinical correlation, and preliminary results. Radiology 145: 321–325

Dory M A 1981 Arthrography of the lumbar facet joints. Radiology 140: 23–27

Drevet J G, Chirossel J P, Phelip X 1981 Lombalgies — lomboradiculalgies et articulations vertebrales posterieures. Lyon Medical 245: 781–787

Editorial 1978 Apophyseal joints and back pain. Lancet 2: 247

Eisenstein S M, Parry C R 1987 The lumbar facet arthrosis syndrome. Journal of Bone and Joint Surgery 69B: 3–7

Engel R, Bogduk N 1982 The minisci of the lumbar zygapophyseal joints. Journal of Anatomy 135: 795–809

Epstein B S 1976 The spine. A radiological text and atlas. 4th edn. Lea & Febiger, Philadelphia, pp 417–418

Faille R J 1978 Low back pain and lumbar fat herniation. American Surgeon 44: 359–361

Fairbank J C T, O'Brien J P 1983 Iliac crest syndrome: a treatable cause of low-back pain. Spine 8: 220–224

Fairbank J C T, Park W M, McCall I W, O'Brien J P 1981 Apophyseal injection of local anesthetic as a diagnostic aid in primary low-back pain syndromes. Spine 6: 598–605

Farmer H L 1936 Accessory articular processes in the lumbar spine. American Journal of Roentgenology 36: 763–767

Fassio B, Bouvier J P, Ginestie J F 1980 Denervation articulaire posterieure per-cutanee et chirurgicale. Sa place dans le traitement des lombalgies. Revue du Chirurgie Orthopedique 67 (suppl II): 131–136

Feinstein B, Langton J N K, Jameson R M, Schiller F 1954 Experiments on pain referred from deep somatic tissues. Journal of Bone and Joint Surgery 36A: 981–997

Fischer A A, Chang C H 1985 Electromyographic evidence of

paraspinal muscle spasm during sleep in patients with low back pain. Clinical Journal of Pain 1: 147–154

Florez G, Erias J, Ucar S 1977 Percutaneous rhizotomy of the articular nerve of Luschka for low back and sciatic pain. Acta Neurochirurgica Supplementum 24: 67–71

Fox J L, Rizzoli H V 1976 Identification of radiologic co-ordinates for the posterior articular nerve of Luschka in the lumbar spine. Surgical Neurology 1: 343–346

Franck S 1943 Surgical treatment of interspinal osteoarthrosis ('kissing spines'). Acta Orthopaedica Scandinavica 14: 127–152

Fuentes E 1978 La neurotomia apofisaria transcutanea en el tratamento de la lumbalgia cronica. Revista Medica de Chile 106: 440–443

Fulton W S, Kaltfleisch W K 1934 Accessory articular processes of the lumbar vertebrae. Archives of Surgery 29: 42–48

Galecki J 1978 Przetrwale jadro kostniewia wyrostkow stawowych kregow ledzwiowych. Chirurgia Narzadow Ruchu i Ortopedia Polska 43: 601–604

Garrett W E, Saffrean M R, Seaber A V et al 1987 Biomechanical comparison of stimulated and non-stimulated muscle pulled to failure. American Journal of Sports Medicine 15: 448–454

Garrett W E, Nikolau P K, Ribbeck B M et al 1988 The effect of muscle architecture on the biomechanical failure properties of skeletal muscle under passive tension. American Journal of Sports Medicine 16: 7–12

Glover J R 1977 Arthrography of the joints of the lumbar vertebral arches. Orthopaedic Clinics of North America 8: 37–42

Hackett G S 1956 Referred pain from low back ligament disability. AMA Archives of Surgery 73: 878–883

Hadley L A 1935 Subluxation of the apophyseal articulations with bony impingement as a cause of back pain. American Journal of Roentgenology 33: 209–213

Hadley L A 1936 Apophyseal subluxation. Journal of Bone and Joint Surgery 18: 428–433

Hadley L A 1964 Anatomico-roentgenological studies of the spine. Thomas, Springfield

Harris R, Macnab I 1954 Structural changes in the lumbar intervertebral disc. Journal of Bone and Joint Surgery 36B: 304–322

Helbig T, Lee C K 1988 The lumbar facet syndrome. Spine 13: 61–64

Herz R 1945 Herniation of fascial fat as a cause of low back pain. Journal of the American Medical Association 128: 921–925

Hickey R F J, Tregonning G D 1977 Denervation of spinal facets for treatment of chronic low back pain. New Zealand Medical Journal 85: 96–99

Hipps H 1939 Fissure formation in articular facets of the lumbar spine. Journal of Bone and Joint Surgery 21: 289-303

Hirsch D, Ingelmark B, Miller M 1963 The anatomical basis for low back pain. Acta Orthopaedica Scandinavica 33: 1–17

Hockaday J M, Whitty C W M 1967 Patterns of referred pain in the normal subject. Brain 90: 481–496

Horwitz T, Smith R M 1940 An anatomical, pathological and roentgenological study of the intervertebral joints of the lumbar spine and of the sacroiliac joints. American Journal of Roentgenology 43: 173–186

Houston J R 1975 A study of subcutaneous rhizolysis in the treatment of chronic backache. Journal of the Royal College of General Practitioners 25: 692–697

Hucherson D C, Gandy J R 1948 Herniation of fascial fat. A cause of low back pain. American Journal of Surgery 76: 605–609

Ingpen M L, Burry H C 1970 A lumbo-sacral strain syndrome. Annals of Physical Medicine 10: 270–274

Jackson R P, Jacobs R R, Montesano P X 1988 Facet joint injection in low-back pain: a prospective statistical study. Spine 13: 966–971

Jayson M I V 1976 Degenerative disease of the spine and back pain. Clinics in Rheumatic Diseases 2: 557–584

Kellgren J H 1938 Observations on referred pain arising from muscle. Clinical Science 3: 175–190

Kellgren J H 1939 On the distribution of referred pain arising from deep somatic structures with charts of segmental pain areas. Clinical Science 4: 35–46

Kelly M 1941 The treatment of fibrositis and allied disorders by local anaesthetics. Medical Journal of Australia 1: 294–298

King A 1955 Back pain due to loose facets of the lower lumbar vertebrae. Bulletin of the Johns Hopkins Hospital 97: 271–283

King J S, Lagger R 1976 Sciatica viewed as a referred pain syndrome. Surgical Neurology 5: 46–50

Konttinen Y T, Gronblad M, Korkala O et al 1990 Immunohistochemical demonstration of subclasses of inflammatory cells and active, collagen-producing fibroblasts in the synovial plicae of lumbar facet joints. Spine 15: 387–390

Kos J, Wolf J 1972a Die 'Menisci' der Zwischenwirbelgelenke und ihre mögliche Rolle bei wirbelblockierung. Manuelle Medizin 10: 105–114

Kos J, Wolf J 1972b Les menisques intervertébraux et leur role possible dans les blocages vertébraux. Annales de Medicine Physique 15: 203–217

Kraft G, Johnson E W, La Ban M M 1968 The fibrositis syndrome. Archives of Physical Medicine and Rehabilitation 49: 155–167

Kraus H 1973 Trigger points. New York State Journal of Medicine 73: 1310–1314

Lau L S W, Littlejohn G O, Miller M H 1985 Clinical evaluation of intra-articular injections for lumbar facet joint pain. Medical Journal of Australia 143: 563–565

Lawrence J S, Sharp J, Ball J, Bier F 1964 Rheumatoid arthritis of the lumbar spine. Annals of the Rheumatic Diseases 23: 205–217

Lawrence J S, Bremner J M, Bier F 1966 Osteoarthrosis. Prevalence in the population and relationship between symptoms and X-ray changes. Annals of the Rheumatic Diseases 25: 1–24

Lewin T 1964 Osteoarthritis in lumbar synovial joints. Acta Orthopaedica Scandinavica (suppl 73)

Lewin T 1968 Anatomical variations in lumbosacral synovial joints with particular reference to subluxation. Acta Anatomica 71: 229–248

Lewinnek G E, Warfield C A 1986 Facet joint degeneration as a cause of low back pain. Clinical Orthopaedics and Related Research 213: 216–222

Lewit K 1987 Discussion invited. Manual Medicine 1: 78–82

Lilius G, Laasonen E M, Myllynen P, Harilainen A, Gronlund G 1989 Lumbar facet joint syndrome: a randomised clinical trial. Journal of Bone and Joint Surgery 71B: 681–684

Lilius G, Harilainen A, Laasonen E M, Myllynen P 1990 Chronic unilateral back pain: predictors of outcome of facet joint injections. Spine 15: 780–782

Lippitt A B 1984 The facet joint and its role in spine pain: management with facet joint injections. Spine 9: 746–750

Livingston W K 1941 Back disabilities due to strain of the multifidus muscle. Western Journal of Surgery 49: 259–263

Lora J, Long D M 1976 So-called facet denervation in the management of intractable back pain. Spine 1: 121–126

Lynch M C, Taylor J F 1986 Facet joint injection for low back pain. Journal of Bone and Joint Surgery 68B: 138–141

Magora A, Schwartz T A 1976 Relation between the low back pain syndrome and X-ray findings. Scandinavian Journal of Rehabilitation Medicine 8: 115–125

Maigne R 1974 Origine dorso-lombaire de certaines lombalgies basses. Role des articulations interapophysaires et des branches posterieures des nerfs rachidiens. Revue du Rhumatisme 41: 781–789

Maigne R 1980 Low back pain of thoracolumbar origin. Archives of Physical Medicine and Rehabilitation 61: 389–395

Maigne R 1981 Le syndrome de la charniere dorso-lombaire. Semaines des Hopitaux de Paris 57: 545–554

Maigne R, Le Courre F, Judet H 1978 Lombalgies basses d'origine dorso-lombaires: traitement chirurgicale par excision des capsules articulaires posterieures. La Nouvelle Presse Médicale 7: 565–568

Marks R 1989 Distribution of pain provoked from lumbar facet joints and related structures during diagnostic spinal infiltration. Pain 39: 37–40

McCall I W, Park W M, O'Brien J P 1979 Induced pain referral from posterior lumbar elements in normal subjects. Spine 4: 441–446

McCulloch J A 1976/1977 Percutaneous radiofrequency lumbar rhizolysis (rhizotomy). Applied Neurophysiology 39: 87–96

McCulloch J A, Organ L W 1977 Percutaneous radiofrequency lumbar rhizolysis (rhizotomy). Canadian Medical Association Journal 116: 30–32

McCulloch J A, Waddell G 1980 Variation of the lumbosacral myotomes with bony segmental anomalies. Journal of Bone and Joint Surgery 62B: 475–480

Mehta M 1978 Facet joints and low back pain (letter). British Medical Journal 1: 1624

Mehta M, Sluijter M E 1979 The treatment of chronic back pain. Anaesthesia 34: 768–775

Mitchell C L 1933 Isolated fractures of the articular processes of the lumbar vertebrae. Journal of Bone and Joint Surgery 15: 608–614

Mooney V 1987 Facet joint syndrome. In: Jayson M I V (ed) The lumbar spine and back pain. 3rd edn. Churchill Livingstone, Edinburgh, ch 18

Mooney V, Robertson J 1976 The facet syndrome. Clinical Orthopaedics and Related Research 115: 149–156

Moran R, O'Connell D, Walsh M G 1988 The diagnostic value of facet joint injections. Spine 12: 1407–1410

Murley A H G 1978 Facet joints and low back pain (letter). British Medical Journal 1: 1283

Murtagh F R 1988 Computed tomography and fluoroscopy guided anaesthesia and steroid injection in facet syndrome. Spine 13: 686–689

Nade S, Bell E, Wyke B 1978 Articular neurology of the feline lumbar spine (abstract). Journal of Bone and Joint Surgery 60B: 292

Nakajima H 1969 A study on the dynamic aspect of facet syndrome with consideration for therapy (Japanese text, English abstract). Journal of the Japanese Orthopaedic Association 43: 629–643

Nichols B H, Schiflett E L 1933 Ununited anomalous epiphyses of the inferior articular processes of the lumbar vertebrae. Journal of Bone and Joint Surgery 15: 591–609

Nikolau P K, MacDonald B L, Glisson R R et al 1987 Biomechanical and histological evaluation of muscle after controlled strain injury. American Journal of Sports Medicine 15: 9–14

Ogsbury J S, Simon R H, Lehman R A W 1977 Facet denervation in the treatment of low back syndrome. Pain 3: 257–263

Oudenhoven R C 1974 Articular rhizotomy. Surgical Neurology 2: 275–278

Oudenhoven R C 1977 Paraspinal electromyography following facet rhizotomy, Spine 2: 299–304

Oudenhoven J C 1979 The role of laminectomy, facet rhizotomy and epidural steroids. Spine 4: 145–147

Pawl R P 1974 Results in the treatment of low back syndrome from sensory neurolysis of lumbar facets (facet rhizotomy) by thermal coagulation. Proceedings of the Institute of Medicine of Chicago 30: 150–151

Pedersen H E, Blunck C F J, Gardner E 1956 The anatomy of lumbosacral posterior rami and meningeal branches of spinal nerves (sinu-vertebral nerves): with an experimental study of their function. Journal of Bone and Joint Surgery 38A: 377–391

Pheasant H C, Dyck P 1982 Failed lumbar disk surgery: cause, assessment, treatment. Clinical Orthopaedics and Related Research 164: 93–109

Pou-Serradell A, Casademont M 1972 Syndrome de la queque de cheval et presence d'appendices apophysaires vertébraux, ou apophyses articulaires accessoires, dans la region lombaire. Revue dela Neurologic 126: 435–440

Rashbaum R F 1983 Radiofrequency facet denervation. A treatment alternative in refractory low back pain with or without leg pain. Orthopedic Clinics of North America 14: 569–575

Raymond J, Dumas J-M 1984 Intra-articular facet block: diagnostic test or therapeutic procedure? Radiology 151: 333–336

Rees W E S 1971 Multiple bilateral subcutaneous rhizolysis of segmental nerves in the treatment of the intervertebral disc syndrome. Annals of General Practice 16: 126–127

Rees W E S 1975 Multiple bilateral percutaneous rhizolysis. Medical Journal of Australia 1: 536–537

Rendich R A, Westing S W 1933 Accessory articular process of the lumbar vertebrae and its differentiation from fracture. American Journal of Roentgenology 29: 156–160

Rissanen P 1960 The surgical anatomy and pathology of the supraspinous and interspinous ligaments of the lumbar spine with special reference to ligament ruptures. Acta Orthopaedica Scandinavica (suppl 46)

Roberts W A 1988 Pyogenic vertebral osteomyelitis of a lumbar facet joint with associated epidural abscess. Spine 12: 948–952

Robertson J A 1978 Facet joints and low back pain. British Medical Journal 1: 1283

Roche M B, Rowe G G 1951 Anomalous centres of ossification for inferior articular processes of the lumbar vertebrae. Anatomical Record 109: 253–259

Roland M O 1986 A critical review of the evidence for a pain–spasm–pain cycle in spinal disorders. Clinical Biomechanics 1: 102–109

Rossi U, Pernak J 1990 Low back pain: the facet syndrome. In Lipton S et al (eds) Advances in pain research and therapy. vol 13. Raven Press, New York, pp 231–244

Rush J, Griffiths J 1989 Suppurative arthritis of a lumbar facet joint. Journal of Bone and Joint Surgery 71B: 161–162

Schaerer J P 1978 Radiofrequency facet rhizotomy in the treatment of chronic neck and low back pain. International Surgery 63: 53–59

Schmorl G, Junghanns H 1971 The human spine in health and disease. 2nd American edn. Grune & Stratton, New York

Shealy C N 1974a Facets in back and sciatic pain. Minnesota Medicine 57: 199–203

Shealy C N 1974b The role of the spinal facets in back and sciatic pain. Headache 14: 101–104

Shealy C N 1975 Percutaneous radiofrequency denervation of spinal facets. Journal of Neurosurgery 43: 448–451

Shealy C N 1976 Facet denervation in the management of back sciatic pain. Clinical Orthopaedics and Related Research 115: 157–164

Silvers H R 1990 Lumbar percutaneous facet rhizotomy. Spine 15: 36–40

Simons D G 1975 Muscle pain syndromes — Part I. American Journal of Physical Medicine 54: 289–311

Simons D G 1976a Muscle pain syndromes — Part II. American Journal of Physical Medicine 55: 15–42

Simons D G 1976b Electrogenic nature of palpable bands and 'jump sign' associated with myofascial trigger points. In: Bonica J J, Albe-Fessard D (eds) Advances in pain research and therapy. vol 1. Raven Press, New York, pp 913–918

Simons D G 1988 Myofascial pain syndromes: Where are we? Where are we going? Archives of Physical Medicine and Rehabilitation 69: 207–212

Simons D G, Travell J 1981 Myofascial trigger points, a possible explanation (letter). Pain 10: 106–109

Sims-Williams H, Jayson M I V, Baddely H 1977 Rheumatoid involvement of the lumbar spine. Annals of the Rheumatic Diseases 36: 524–531

Sims-Williams H, Jayson M I V Baddely H 1978 Small spinal fractures in back patients. Annals of the Rheumatic Diseases 37: 262–265

Sinclair D C, Feindel W H, Weddel G, Falconer M A 1948 The intervertebral ligaments as a source of segmental pain. Journal of Bone Joint Surgery 30B: 515–521

Singewald M L 1966 Sacroiliac lipomata — an often unrecognized cause of low back pain. Bulletin of the Johns Hopkins Hospital 118: 492–498

Sluijter M E, Mehta M 1981 Treatment of chronic back and neck pain by percutaneous thermal lesions. In: Lipton S, Miles J (eds) Persistent pain. Modern methods of treatment. vol 3. Academic Press, London, ch 8, pp 141–179

Steindler A, Luck J V 1938 Differential diagnosis of pain low in the back. Journal of the American Medical Association 110: 106–112

Taylor J R, Twomey L T, Corker M 1990 Bone and soft tissue injuries in post-mortem lumbar spines. Paraplegia 28: 119–129

Terry A, McCall I W, O'Brien J P, Park W M 1981 Graft impingement following posterolateral fusion. Paper presented at the Annual Meeting of the International Society for the Study of the Lumbar Spine, Paris, May 16–21

Toakley J G 1973 Subcutaneous lumbar 'rhizolysis' — an assessment of 200 cases. Medical Journal of Australia 2: 490–492

Travell J, Rinzler S H 1952 The myofascial genesis of pain. Postgraduate Medicine 11: 425–434

Travell J, Travell W 1946 Therapy of low back pain by manipulation and of referred pain in the lower extremity by procaine infiltration. Archives of Physical Medicine 27: 537–547

Twomey L T, Taylor J R, Taylor M M 1989 Unsuspected damage to lumbar zygapophyseal (facet) joints after motor vehicle accidents. Medical Journal of Australia 151: 210–217

Uyttendaele D, Verhamme J, Vercauteren M 1981 Local block of lumbar facet joints and percutaneous radiofrequency denervation. Preliminary results. Acta Orthopedica Belgica 47: 135–139

Vernon-Roberts B, Pirie C J 1977 Degenerative changes in the vertebral discs of the lumbar spine and their sequelae. Rheumatology and Rehabilitation 16: 13–21

Wolf J 1975 The reversible deformation of the joint cartilage surface and its possible role in joint blockage. Rehabilitacia 8 (suppl 10–11): 30–34

Wollgast G F, Afeman C E 1961 Sacroiliac (episacral) lipomas. Archives of Surgery 83: 925–927

Wyke B 1979 Neurology of the cervical spinal joints. Physiotherapy 65: 72–76

31. Lumbar instability

G. Schneider

INTRODUCTION

It has been proposed that the restraining structures of an individual lumbar segment may become weakened by degeneration. The process results in a loss of stiffness in the restraints, compromising their constraining and restoring forces. The affected level will offer less resistance to an applied load and it may displace through excessive range or display abnormal quality of motion. In this state the segment is described as unstable. An unstable lumbar segment is considered by some to be the cause of symptoms and a group of clinical manifestations identified as lumbar instability. The proposals relating to this syndrome remain conjectural. No correlations have yet been established between specific pathology and segment laxity or between proven instability and symptoms. Moreover, instability of a lumbar segment has yet to be reliably demonstrated radiographically or by any other means.

Before considering the syndrome identified as lumbar instability a conceptual framework of the mechanical basis for instability is presented. The restraint mechanisms which maintain stability within the vertebral column are outlined initially. Subsequently, biomechanical definitions of instability will be considered so that a model of instability may be proposed. This model will then require a pathological basis for damage to restraints. The symptoms attributed to lumbar instability may then be included. Finally, the radiographic and manual methods of detecting an unstable lumbar segment are analysed.

STABILITY

The joints of the body are designed to permit motion between two bones. The direction and range of motion which occur at individual joints is governed by the articular geometry and by the soft-tissue structures investing the joint. Tissues include the joint capsule, specific ligaments and musculotendinous organization. These components have identifiable collagen organization and mechanical properties, including stiffness, which are related to their physiological functions. One function is to act as joint constraints by resisting distorting forces, limiting excess displacement and providing restoring stresses. There is a complex interaction between the static joint components and dynamic muscular control. Each direction of motion at an individual joint has a tissue which acts as the primary restraint, and other structures which provide secondary restraint. When a joint is capable of supporting a load and not being displaced beyond its normal physiological limits, it is considered stable. These general principles of joint stability may be applied to the vertebral column after considering individual segmental motion.

In the vertebral column, movements between lumbar vertebrae occur in a three-dimensional manner (Frymoyer & Selby 1985). The motion of lumbar flexion/extension includes rotation of each vertebra about the coronal axis, coupled with forward/backward translation (Posner et al 1982). Axial rotation and lateral flexion occur simultaneously as coupled movements, and the joints are also forced to flex forward (Gracovetsky & Farfan 1986). The stresses of restraining these segmental movements are shared between the structures in the anterior and posterior columns, largely between the intervertebral disc and the zygapophyseal joints (Dunlop et al 1984, Gotfried et al 1986).

The translation component of flexion and extension is resisted by the bone impact of the zygapophyseal joints (Twomey & Taylor 1983, Oliver 1986), with the coronally oriented component of the articular facets bearing most of the load (Taylor & Twomey 1986). Anterior sagittal translation is resisted by the direct impaction of the inferior articular facets of a vertebra against the superior articular facets of the vertebra below. The intervertebral disc assists in resisting the shear resistance created by the translation motion (Cyron & Hutton 1978).

The anterior sagittal rotation component of flexion is resisted by tension in the zygapophyseal joint capsules, rather than by bony impaction of the joints. The upward sliding movement of each inferior articular process in relation to the superior articular process in each joint, tenses the joint capsule (Bogduk & Twomey 1987).

Anterior sagittal rotation results in the separation of the spinous processes and laminae, but the function of the supraspinous and interspinous ligaments is not primarily to resist flexion of the spine. Although the supraspinous ligament is highly strained during flexion, its relatively low stiffness offers negligible resistance to flexion. Similarly, the fibres of the interspinous ligament are orientated so that they do not stiffen the ligament as it is stretched during flexion (Hukins et al 1990).

Axial rotation of the lumbar spine is restrained by the zygapophyseal joints and the disc annulus. During the first few degrees of rotation, whilst the axis is in the anterior column, the compressive facet joints are the primary structure resisting torsion. The compression load is borne by the sagittally orientated component of the joint (Taylor & Twomey 1986). As the range of rotation increases the axis of rotation shifts posteriorly and the annulus becomes the primary structure resisting rotation. A recent study applied axial rotation to a model consisting of intact segments of an entire lumbar spine and allowed the column to seek its own axis of rotation under torsion (Haher et al 1989). It was found that the annulus was the most important structure resisting torsion. The compressed zygapophyseal joint, lying in the vicinity of the axis of rotation, experienced significantly less torsional stress. Progressive destruction of the annulus produced a proportional loss of torsional stiffness. Axial torque normally generates a stiffening effect in the motion segment, but with loss of disc pressure, there is a softening of the segment (Shirazi-Adl et al 1986).

The three-dimensional motions between lumbar vertebrae are restrained by compression forces through the posterior joints, and by tensile stresses in the joint capsules and disc annulus. The intersegmental muscles also contribute a major component to lumbar spinal stability after injury to other restraints. Muscle action resists vertebral displacement when a load is applied (Panjabi et al 1989). If the structural organization of these tissues is damaged, mechanical properties such as stiffness may be reduced, and they may cease to function effectively. The lumbar motion segment may then displace through a greater range of movement before resistance is encountered. The segment would then be considered unstable.

INSTABILITY

A lumbar segment has been classified as unstable if it exhibited excessive or abnormal quality of motion (Dupuis et al 1985, Gertzbein et al 1985). Assessments of displacement require measurements in more than one plane in order to account for the three-dimensional nature of segment motion. An assessment of flexion–extension requires measurement of the translation and rotational components. In this manner, instability is determined by both linear and angular motion. This concept of instability considers only range of motion.

Pope and Panjabi (1985) made the concept more precise by including considerations of force. These authors defined instability as a 'loss of stiffness', with stiffness being the ratio of the force applied to a structure and the motion that results. A structure is then relatively less stiff if a given load produces greater displacement. This definition considers force as well as range of motion, and instability is determined from the relationship between both factors

These principles were developed further by Panjabi et al (1989) who proposed that neutral zone (NZ) is a better indicator of spinal instability than range of motion (ROM). NZ is the amount of vertebral displacement which occurs early in range without a significant increase in load. This zone, therefore, represents the vertebral movement which is free or not restrained. Panjabi et al found that the NZ of lumbar functional spinal units increased with increasing injury to restraining structures. That is, as restraints are damaged the segment displaces further before resistance to motion is encountered. This NZ concept of instability is similar to Pope's load–displacement ratio. In both, displacement is being assessed relative to applied load. Pope assesses stiffness from the slope of the displacement curve once a load is applied. The NZ of Panjabi measures the amount of displacement before load increase.

The NZ concept reinforces two most important principles for determining instability. First, a segment may exhibit decreased resistance to movement early in the displacement phase before excess range of motion becomes a consideration. Secondly, ROM alone is not the only parameter by which instability should be determined. An assessment of instability should address both factors and measure ROM relative to the applied force.

This model of instability proposes that, if the restraints of a vertebral segment are weakened, then the segment will displace further before resistance is encountered to control the motion, and the segment may also displace beyond its normal range. To be complete, this model requires a pathological basis for damage to restraining structures which could cause loss of stiffness in the segment and predispose it to weakness and laxity.

PATHOLOGICAL BASIS

The concept of considering instability as a loss of stiffness is consistent with the weakening of restraint mechanisms described by Farfan and Gracovetsky (1984). These authors proposed that repeated injury to the annulus and posterior joints compromises the restraining function of these structures and allows free play in the segment. Forces acting on the segment will then produce greater displacement than would occur in a normal spine.

Kirkaldy-Willis (1983) proposed that a lumbar segment may exhibit an abnormal increase in motion during the intermediate phase of the degenerative process. The degenerative changes considered to allow segment laxity involve both the disc and the posterior joints. Tears in the disc annulus cause the outer lamellae to weaken and bulge around the circumference. Degeneration of the cartilage of the zygapophyseal joints, and tensile stresses on the joint capsules, cause joint disruption and capsular laxity. Such degenerative changes are well recognized and, in principle, one would expect that injury to one or more of the segment restraints should result in some degree of instability. However, whilst the proposal is attractive there are as yet no proven correlations between specific pathology and instability.

If instability does occur secondary to degeneration the direction of instability would be determined by the specific restraint function of the tissue which was damaged. Progressive destruction of the annulus reduced torsional stiffness and resulted in rotational instability (Haher et al 1989). Structural damage to the capsules of the posterior joints would reduce their tensile stiffness and decrease their capability to restrain the anterior sagittal rotational component of flexion. Disorganization of the structure of the articular cartilage of these joints would reduce the restraint function provided by impaction.

Furthermore, degrees of instability may occur, and be dependent on the extent of the injury. Early collagen disorganization, causing only partial compromise of mechanical properties, may cause only a mild instability. The degree of instability may also be modified by secondary restraints, such as the action of intersegmental muscles, which have been found to decrease the neutral zone of vertebral displacement after injury (Panjabi et al 1989). The authors hypothesized that muscle spasm, often observed clinicially, may indicate the body's attempt to stabilize an unstable spine.

When proposing degeneration as the pathological basis for instability, it is pertinent to note that instability of a lumbar segment has not been identified in all cases where degeneration is evident. The question remains why instability might occur in some cases and not in others. There is the possibility that a specific pathology in the degenerative spectrum, occurring only in a proportion of cases, may account for an unstable state.

CLINICAL PRESENTATION

Lumbar instability is frequently cited as a cause of low-back pain (Ogston et al 1986, Stokes & Frymoyer 1987). The symptoms which have been attributed to an unstable state have been described by several authors (Corrigan & Matiland 1983, Grieve 1986, Paris 1985). The symptoms are reported to occur most commonly in the earlier age groups of the third or fourth decades. Pain is localized to

the low back but may radiate proximally into one or both legs. Symptoms are rarely felt distal to the knee and evidence of nerve root involvement is not a feature. A purported characteristic of lumbar instability is the recurring nature of episodes of severe pain which cause temporary immobility. Typically, the episodes may be provoked by simple unguarded actions such as stooping or twisting, or even by maintaining a fixed posture in standing or sitting. During an episode the patient is unable to bend forwards more than a few degrees, or may become fixed in a flexed position and be temporarily unable to straighten. The spine may be deviated. If flexion is possible, spinal motion will be abnormal, appearing as a superimposed hitching, deviation or rolling action. An arc of pain may occur during flexion or recovery. The loss of mobility accompanying these painful episodes typically resolves relatively quickly within forty-eight hours. The patient is usually familiar with routines of exercises and posture control which restore function, but a return to a fully active lifestyle is not possible.

When these clinical manifestations occur together, they may constitute a recognizable syndrome. However, it remains a presumption that instability is the underlying cause of the condition. Correlation remains entirely conjectural. Only one study has shown a statistically significant correlation between low-back pain and excess segmental motion (Friberg 1987). This study measured the horizontal translation component of intervertebral motion. Symptoms have yet to be correlated with abnormal excess motion measured in more than one dimension.

Another difficulty with defining lumbar instability as a recognizable syndrome is that the signs which are commonly attributed to an unstable state are neither consistent findings, nor features that are unique to this condition. If a shoulder or knee joint is unstable, there are distinguishing features which occur in all cases, and which are found only if the joint is unstable. Their presence becomes diagnostic, and moreover confirms damage to specific joint restraints. No such correlation yet exists for lumbar instability as a syndrome so the features described cannot be classed as diagnostic. Until instability can be accurately and consistently demonstrated radiographically clinical correlations cannot be tested.

Nevertheless, from our present observations, an attempt should be made to identify key signs which may prove to be reliable indicators of a lumbar segment which has become unstable. These signs can then be tested against proven instability and either rejected as unreliable, or retained as diagnostic.

Criteria which may be proved to correlate with an unstable lumbar segment are:

1. History. All four aspects must apply:
   (a) age group twenties or thirties
   (b) recurring episodes of pain and loss of mobility

(c) simple onset

(d) relatively rapid resolution

2. Site of pain: lumbar region, with or without radiation into one or both buttocks or posterior thighs

3. Abnormal spinal motion during active sagittal plane movements, with or without an arc of pain. The emphasis is abnormal rather than restricted motion

4. Abnormal compliance detected on accessory palpation, indicating loss of stiffness or increased neutral zone at one segment. Compliance criteria are considered in detail under 'Manual demonstration of lumbar instability' (see later).

It is possible to theorize on how weakened restraints and segment laxity might cause these symptoms. Spasm of the intersegmental muscles, recruited to limit vertebral displacement and protect the tissues from further injury, may be a source of pain. The lesion itself may cause pain by irritating the sensitized outer layer of the annulus or the capsules of the posterior joints. Finally, the reduced capability of the segment to support a load, together with the excess vertebral displacement, may strain normal tissues and further damage previously injured structures. Excess motion could be expected to increase the tensile stresses on the annulus fibrosus and joint capsules and evoke pain. If proven instability is shown to be a cause of back pain, it is conceivable that different symptoms and clinical presentation may be found to correlate with specific types of vertebral displacement, such as anterior or posterior directions, or displacements through an increased arc of axial rotation (Frymoyer & Selby 1985). It has also been proposed that the direction and pattern of instability may relate to whether the dominant lesion is anterior or posterior restraint failure (Dupuis et al 1985).

RADIOGRAPHIC DEMONSTRATION

A model for instability has been proposed. A pathological basis has been considered, together with the probability of an unstable lumbar segment being the cause of symptoms. The means of detecting excess or abnormal segment motion are now examined.

Static and dynamic radiography

Several signs on static X-rays have been cited as indicators of instability. These include traction spurs (Macnab 1971), gas in the disc (Knuttson 1944), disc space narrowing, static spondyl- or retro-olisthetic malalignment and hypertrophied subluxed facet joints (Rosenberg 1974, Frymoyer & Selby 1985). While these features may be evidence of segment pathology and vertebral displacement, their presence does not confirm abnormal segment motion. This can be detected only by dynamic investigations. Motion studies of the lumbar spine have been carried out under research laboratory conditions using superimposition of successive exposures (Pennal et al 1972), stereo film comparisons (Suh 1974) and three-dimensional characterization of movement with computer analysis (Brown et al 1976). These methods were criticized as complex and inaccurate (Dupuis et al 1985) and were not used subsequently to evaluate abnormal motion in symptomatic individuals.

To classify segment motion as abnormal, threshold values for normal displacement were required. These were calculated using sequential transections in an experimental setting which the authors considered to correspond clinically to physiological flexion and extension movements applied to a person lying supine (Posner et al 1982). Horizontal displacement was calculated as a percentage of mid-body width of the upper vertebra, and angular displacement in degrees. The figures at the lumbosacral joint were 6% or more of anterior translation, or 9% or more of posterior translation and flexion angular displacement smaller than 1°.

Dupuis et al (1985) used a slightly modified version of the Posner technique to measure horizontal and angular displacement in symptomatic patients. Radiographic study was conducted with dynamic views obtained in the frontal and lateral planes to identify unstable states in the clinical environment. Prominences on the posterior aspect of the upper-end plates, and notches on the posterior aspect of the inferior-end plate were used as radiological markers. On film measurements of displacement between vertebrae were made from lines joining the landmarks (Fig. 31.1).

The authors reported cases of dynamic spondylolisthesis and retrolisthesis evidenced by excessive anterior or posterior translaton along the horizontal plane. In some cases the translation was pure and in others it was associated with excessive angular displacement. The anterior or posterior slip induced by one position was reduced when the opposite position was adopted. The findings were interpreted as motion segment laxity.

The validity of these findings must be considered. The number of cases reported in the study was small. The in vivo measurements from patients were compared against values from in vitro experiments. There is no normative data from living subjects for the threshold of stability using such measurements. The issue of errors using this technique, particularly relating to accurately defining vertebral body landmarks and vertebral dimensions, was not addressed. Finally the degrees of displacement found were not analysed statistically for significance. The authors contended that some loss in precision using this method was compensated for by simplicity and everyday clinical usefulness.

The studies considered above did not establish the reliability of detecting instability with biplanar radiography and the method was challenged in subsequent investigations. Cases of lytic spondylolithesis, which could be ex-

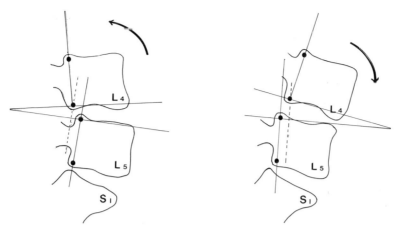

Fig. 31.1   Calculation of the percentage of horizontal displacement and angular displacement on flexion/extension views (Dupuis et al 1985). (Reproduced with permission from P. R. Dupuis, 1991.)

pected to demonstrate excess intervertebral motion, were evaluated during flexion–extension (Pearcy & Shepherd 1985) and axial traction–compression (Friberg 1987). The amount of translation and angulation computed from the sagittal motion study was not found to be significant. Translatory movement of 5 mm or more was detected with the axial method but only in 55% of cases.

Two studies examined the reliability of demonstrating excess vertebral displacement in cases of segment degeneration. Stokes and Frymoyer (1987) selected cases of degenerative instability from the radiographic criteria of disc space alterations, malaligned spinous processes, traction spurs, and a horizontal translation of at least 3 mm measured from flexion–extension radiographs. Three-dimensional co-ordinates from vertebral landmarks were computerized to measure intersegmental motion. The forward shear displacement at the degenerated segment was found to be less than at other levels. The authors concluded that flexion–extension biplanar radiography was not useful in the diagnosis of lumbar instability.

Friberg (1987) used axial traction and compression forces on the spine instead of flexion/extension to study patients with degenerative malalignments on static standing radiography. Measurements were made by superimposing vertebral silhouettes (Fig. 31.2). Translatory movement of 5 mm or more was found in all seven patients with degenerative spondylolithesis of L4, and in 57% of patients with retro-olisthetic displacements, mainly of L5. The technique did not measure angular displacements.

In summary, the studies using flexion–extension radiography have proved unreliable for detecting instability both in cases of lytic spondylolisthesis and in cases of suspected instability due to degeneration. In similar cases, the technique of axial loading detected excess translatory motion but in only a little over half of the subjects. As horizontal displacement alone is measured by this method, it is not sensitive to irregular or erratic motion.

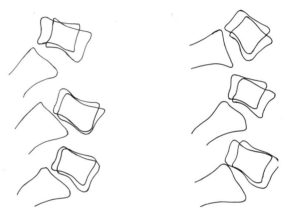

Fig. 31.2   Outlines of the body of L5 and the sacrum as plotted from traction–compression radiographs in six patients with unstable spondylolisthesis (Friberg 1987). (Reproduced with permission from O. Friberg 1991.)

A factor which must be considered in these studies is the role of secondary restraints which may hinder the detection of an unstable state. Pearcy and Shepherd (1985) hypothesized that the lytic segments in their subjects were being restrained by muscle spasm. This proposal is supported by the study investigating the role of intersegmental muscles providing stability to the spine (Panjabi et al 1989). The study found that muscle activity decreased intervertebral motions after injury, evidenced by a decreased neutral zone in flexion and extension loading.

Other investigators have proposed that erratic or abnormal segment motion may be more important factors in instability than excessive sagittal motion, and that these factors can be evaluated more accurately by plotting centrodes than by measuring displacement.

Instantaneous axes of rotation and centrode patterns

The concept of instantaneous axes or rotation (IAR) has

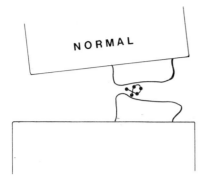

Fig. 31.3   Location of centrode pattern in normal L4–5 cadaveric segment (Gertzbein et al 1984). (Reproduced with permission from J. B. Lippincott, 1991.)

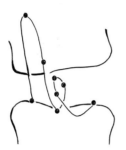

Fig. 31.4   Centrode patterns of L4–5 segment with minor degenerative disc disease (Gertzbein et al 1985). (Reproduced with permission from J. B. Lippincott, 1991.)

been used to analyse motion in the lumbar spine (Cossette & Farfan 1971, Pennal et al 1972, Dimnet & Fischer 1978, Panjabi et al 1981). As an individual lumbar vertebra rotates and translates in the sagittal plane, the motion occurs about a series of different IARs, or centrodes. The location, length and pattern of centrodes were found to be consistent in an extension–flexion study of five normal L4–5 cadaveric segments (Gertzbein et al 1984) (Fig. 31.3).

Seligman et al (1984) determined centrode patterns for 47 cadaveric L4–5 segments with minor, mild, moderate and severe disc degeneration. The segments with early degeneration, the minor and mild categories, demonstrated significantly longer loci (average 116 mm and 78 mm respectively) than the normal (average 21 mm). As degeneration progresses to a moderate degree, the centrode is still longer (average 49 mm) than normal and its position shifts inferiorly into the lower vertebra. As the segment stiffens with severe degeneration the centrode shortens (average 34 mm) and is similar to the normal centrode length. Gertzbein et al (1985) found similar results with 28 cadaveric L4–5 segments (Fig. 31.4).

Seligman et al (1984) relate these centrode patterns to instability in the segment. Unstable segments will have abnormal translation motion which in turn will 'cause a large change in the position of the centre of rotation and thus, much longer loci should be formed'. The longer,

more complex centrode patterns found in the segments with early disc degeneration indicate abnormal translation and instability. Mechanical dysfunction may cause an inconsistent distribution of the relative amounts of translation and rotation which occur through the total extension/flexion arc. This causes the centres of rotation for adjacent increment arcs to shift and increase centrode length. Excessive or erratic movement of the segment is reflected by increased centrode length.

The study of centrode patterns to assess motion in the lumbar spine was progressed to an in vivo method (Ogston et al 1986). Centrode patterns were determined at the L4–5 and L5–S1 levels in 21 normal male volunteers. From a standing position the subject moved between full extension and full flexion. Six lateral radiographs of the lumbar spine were taken, dividing the total range of motion at each level into a series of small amplitude segments. The arcs fell between 2° and 6°. Five radiographs were used to determine four centres of rotation. Vertebral motion was tracked by a method of contour matching and superimposing traced images of vertebral pairs. The co-ordinates of the centrode for each motion arc were plotted, and the cumulative length of the line that joined sequential centres of rotation was calculated to obtain the centrode length. The normal values for centrode length at the L4–5 and L5–S1 levels were defined as 43.7 mm and 55.9 mm respectively. The value for the L4–5 level is considerably longer than the 20.9 mm length reported for normal cadaver spines (Seligman et al 1984). The effects of muscle action in living subjects is one explanation given by the authors for the variations, and it was also noted that if motion arcs of smaller than 3° were used the error magnification increased and tended to lengthen the centrode. The position of the centrode at the L5–S1 level was in the posterior half of the disc, and at L4–5 it was just below the vertebral end plate in the posterior half of the L5 vertebral body.

The authors of a subsequent study have proposed that the notion of plotting centrodes to diagnose mechanical disorders is invalid (Pearcy & Bogduk 1988). The study determined the location of the instantaneous axis of rotation (IAR) of every lumbar vertebra of ten normal individuals, and quantified the errors involved in the technique to establish confidence limits for the results. The sources of error addressed were the adequacy of the digitizer, the initial tracings of the vertebrae, the superimposition of the flexion and extension tracings, and the marking of the x–y axes on each vertebra. The errors incurred at individual steps of the process used in this study were found to be acceptably small. The errors were quantified as 96% confident limits for within-observer and between-observer determination of IARs. Some features of the method will be considered to highlight the errors and practical difficulties which occur with centrode determinations in vivo.

The IAR study used three lateral radiographs: one with the subject standing upright, and one each in full flexion and full extension. Segmental motion was depicted by superimposing images of the vertebrae traced in each position. Vertebral dimensions were normalized to standardized rectangular images that reflected the mean x and y dimension of the vertebra. IARs were determined by calculating the point of intersection of the perpendicular bisectors of the vectors of motion for two points on the moving vertebral body (Fig. 31.5).

This process yielded three IARs for each segmental level but only the IAR for full extension to full flexion carries a satisfactory level of confidence. The total range of this movement at each level is approximately 13°. The potential error for calculating IARs increases greatly if the amplitude of movement is small and to reduce errors the study showed that a rotation of 10° is desirable, and one of at least 5° is required for a satisfactory level of confidence. For the movement of flexion from extension the IARs for all ten subjects fell within a well clustered scatter at each segmental level. This method of examining segmental motion revealed only a small biological variation in the location of IARs and a relatively small inter-observer error. The authors have proposed therefore that when diagnosing mechanical disorders the determination of a single extension to flexion IAR is of more value clinically than plotting centrodes. Centrodes constructed on incremental movements of less than 5° are subject to errors. Because centrodes are determined from a series of small amplitude segments, the IAR for each segment is subject to potentially large errors, and hence the centrode is also subject to large errors.

In summary, the notion of plotting centrodes to diagnose mechanical disorders has been challenged as invalid because of the large errors which arise from calculating instantaneous centres of rotation from multiple small amplitude arcs less than 5° (Pearcy & Bogduk 1988). On the other hand, the errors incurred in determining a single extension to flexion IAR were found to be acceptably small (Pearcy & Bogduk 1988). The authors have proposed, therefore, that mechanical disorders and instability of lumbar segments can be detected on the basis of abnormally located IARs, using the results from their study as normative data. Previous studies using extension to flexion loading have proved unreliable in detecting instability. However, the method of measurement to detect a single IAR, described by Pearcy and Bogduk, has much greater accuracy than previous measurement of vertebral displacement. The technique is also more sensitive to irregular or erratic motion than pure horizontal displacement, as the location of the IAR is governed by both angular and horizontal displacement. No study to date has analysed both these components, with acceptable accuracy, in symptomatic patients in an attempt to diagnose instability.

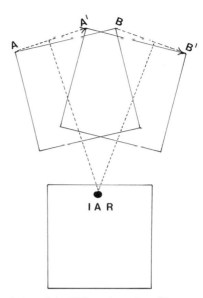

Fig. 31.5 Calculation of the IAR as the point of intersection of the perpendicular bisectors of the vectors for the motion of two points on a rigid body (Pearcy & Bogduk 1988). (Reproduced with permission from N. Bogduk, 1991.)

MANUAL DEMONSTRATION OF LUMBAR INSTABILITY

Some clinicians who use manual palpation to examine intersegmental motion consider that an unstable segment can be detected by perceiving abnormal compliance of the segment during accessory tests. Compliance assesses the relationship between ROM and the force required to produce displacement. The ratio between these two factors may be expressed as a force–displacement curve. These diagrams are used by clinicians to illustrate motion perceived by palpation, and also by biomechanists studying the compliance of cadaveric segments.

Pope and Panjabi (1985) used force–displacement relationships to define instability as a 'loss of stiffness', with stiffness being the ratio between the force applied and the motion which results. A structure is unstable if a given load produces greater displacement (Fig. 31.6) or if less force is required to produce the same displacement (Fig. 31.7). Panjabi et al (1989) also used load–displacement curves to record the findings of sequentially injured lumbar spinal units subjected to three-dimensional biomechanical tests. The neutral zone (NZ) motion parameter was determined as part of the total ROM. NZ is the amount of vertebral displacement which occurs early in range without a significant load increase before the segment enters the elastic zone (EZ) (Fig. 31.8).

NZ therefore represents the vertebral displacement which occurs before restraining structures offer resistance to the load applied. As restraints are damaged the segment displaces further before resistance to motion is encountered. Unstable segments, therefore, have an increased NZ. This concept allows an indicator of instability early in

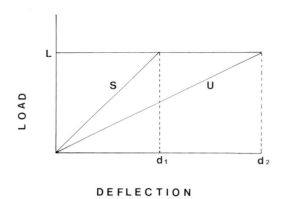

Fig. 31.6 Stiffness of material U is L/d$_2$. Structure U is unstable relative to S (Pope & Panjabi 1985). (Reproduced with permission from M. Pope, 1991.)

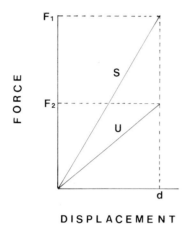

Fig. 31.7 Stiffness of material U is F$_1$/d. Half the force causes structure U to displace the same distance as S.

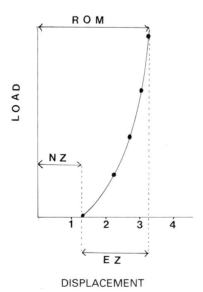

Fig. 31.8 Motion parameters documented for physiological load applications. NZ = neutral zone; EZ = elastic zone; ROM = range of motion. (Adapted from Panjabi et al 1989.) (Reproduced with permission from M. Panjabi, 1991.)

the range of movement, and is independent of assessments of excess amplitude at the end of the range. The study suggested that the NZ parameter is a better indicator of spinal instability than the ROM parameter.

There is a congruence between the force–displacement curves generated by biomechanists on cadaveric material and the movement diagrams (Maitland 1986) which manipulative physiotherapists use to record segment motion qualitatively. These compliance diagrams graphically depict the therapists' estimates of force and displacement perceived through palpation. The segment motion which is commonly palpated to detect instability is the accessory movement of postero-anterior glide (Maitland 1986). Manual pressure is exerted on a lumbar spinous process with the patient prone. Only the initial or clinical range of movement is tested, just beyond the toe phase and well before the 4% elongation at which microscopic injury occurs (Bogduk & Twomey 1987, p. 54).

The amplitude of segment displacements for postero-anterior motion is judged from the resting position of the vertebra to the limit of what is perceived to be the average normal passive clinical range. Estimates may then be made of different points in the range which indicate the early, middle and late phases of the total ROM. The force applied to the vertebra cannot be measured during clinical testing, but therapists are conscious of increasing resistance to deformation, whether the resistance is increasing gradually or rapidly, and whether the increasing resistance is occurring early or late in range. These perceptions of the relationship between resistance to deformation and displacement, which are depicted on the movement diagram, estimate the stiffness of tissues. Stiffness is indicated by the slope of the force displacement curve. Stiffer structures resist deformation and the slope of their curve will be steeper. The relationship between resistance and displacement perceived by palpation is analogous to the stiffness measurements recorded by biomechanists. Although therapists perceptions are not measured and calibrated, tissues stiffness can be estimated from the slope of the curve.

The path traced out by a vertebra when it moves in a postero-anterior direction is generally thought of as horizontal translation. Since sagittal plane movement is a combination of translation and rotation, it is probable that the vertebra also angulates when manual force is applied. The motion being palpated would then be more complex than pure horizontal translation. The range of horizontal translation of a lumbar vertebra is of the order of magnitude of 1 mm. It would be improbable to detect relative changes of compliance within this range, which attests further to the notion that what is being perceived is some form of rotation.

Another factor which may influence perceptions of compliance is intersegmental muscle activity. Asymmetrical paraxial muscle activity may induce axial rotation

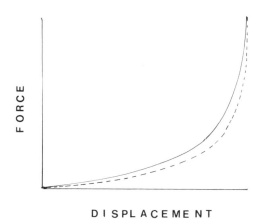

Fig. 31.9 Exponential force–displacement curves for normal lumbar segment motion. - - - - - = mechanical; ——— = manual. (Reproduced with permission from B. Lam.)

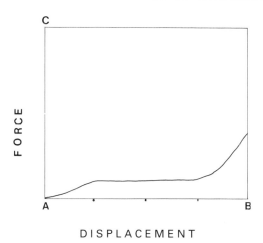

Fig. 31.10 Postero-anterior motion of abnormal lumbar segment. A = resting position of vertebra; B = limit of average normal passive ROM; C = force necessary to displace normal segment to end of normal ROM.

during sagittal plane motion (Gracovetsky & Farfan 1986) and produce coupled movements at higher levels in cases of lower lumbar instability (Pearcy & Shepherd 1985). Furthermore, intersegmental muscle forces have been found to maintain or decrease intervertebral motions after injury (Panjabi et al 1989). If this muscle activity was provoked during manual palpation it could modify the displacement of the segment.

Postero-anterior motion of the normal lumbar segment has a positively accelerating force displacement curve. The force required to effect displacement increases at an increasing rate in the second half of the range. At no point, within the range used for physical examination, is there a levelling off of force. Similarly shaped exponential curves have been found in an experiment using manual and mechanical force to move normal lumbar segments anteriorly (Lam 1985) (Fig. 31.9). Therefore, a positively accelerating curve can be regarded as normal when a lumbar segment is tested manually by postero-anterior glide.

Postero-anterior motion of the 5th lumbar vertebra was tested manually in a group of 21 patients whose clinical behaviour suggested instability (Schneider 1987). All patients were found to have similarly shaped compliance curves which differed from the positively accelerating curves found in normal subjects. After an initial increase in force, it was perceived that the segments of the symptomatic subjects continued to displace for an interval without an increase in force being necessary. This finding translated to a plateau on the compliance curve instead of the exponential increase in force necessary to displace normal segments (Fig. 31.10). Furthermore, it was estimated that the limit of normal range was reached without resistance to displacement ever increasing to normal levels.

The compliance findings in this symptomatic group can be related to the biomechanical definitions of instability, both in terms of stiffness and NZ. Force was not perceived to increase exponentially as the segments displaced, a finding which equates with Pope and Panjabi's definition of loss of stiffness. The interval early in the range in which the segments displaced further without a significant load increase equated with an increased NZ. Both loss of stiffness and increased NZ are indicators of instability. As segmental instability was not confirmed radiologically in this group, the reliability of detecting instability by palpation was not validated. Nevertheless, these observations suggest that instability may be considered in biomechanical terms by interpreting the slope of compliance curves determined by palpation.

Reliability of compliance perception

Studies have evaluated the reliability of therapists's assessment of spinal compliance when manually testing the posterio-anterior motion of lumbar segments (Matyas & Bach 1985). Different aspects were studied, including ability to select a point in range where resistance changed, the amplitude of movement, the most abnormal segments, and difference in the shape of compliance curves. Reliability scores in these studies were not high. However, any question of reliability arising out of these studies pertains to aspects of compliance curves which, although varying slope, have the common similarity of an exponential increase in force. The compliance curves of patients with suspected instability had significantly different characteristics. Whilst the normal curve rises exponentially, the curve for the unstable segment flattened out to a plateau. This more marked contrast may enhance the reliability of detection. The segments were perceived to displace for an interval without a significant force increase. During passive accessory testing therapists are conscious of increasing resistance to displacement. If there is less resistance, and no increase in force is required for further displacement, it is probable that such a variation from the normal may be reliably detected.

DISCUSSION

Lumbar instability has yet to be reliably demonstrated radiographically or by any other means. Analysis of both angular and horizontal displacement is required to assess abnormal segment motion. Determining the location of a single IAR is the most accurate method of assessing vertebral displacement, and therefore offers the highest probability of detecting movement disorders. The technique has not been tested in symptomatic patients in an attempt to diagnose instability, but normative data has been established. If joint compliance is a better indicator of instability than ROM, determinations of instability could address both factors of compliance by considering displacement relative to an applied force.

Until there is an objective measurement of instability, clinical and manual findings cannot be attributed to an unstable state, and correlations remain conjectural. There is no agreement or accurate definition of the abnormal compliance which is perceived by palpation as instability. It is probable, nevertheless, that loss of stiffness in a lumbar segment may be detected reliably by palpation and interpreted from the slope of the compliance curve. Further work is required to analyse manual perceptions once objective measurements are available for correlation. It may prove to be the case that an unstable segment will be most accurately signalled by diminished resistance to displacement early in range, rather than by judgements pertaining to ROM.

Acknowledgement

The author wishes to acknowledge the valuable assistance of Professor Nikolai Bogduk in the preparation of this work.

REFERENCES

Bogduk N, Twomey L T 1987 Clinical anatomy of the lumbar spine. Churchill Livingstone, Melbourne, p 54, 64

Brown R H, Burstein A H, Nash C L et al 1976 Spinal analysis using a three dimensional radiographic technique. Journal of Biomechanics 9: 355–365

Corrigan B, Maitland G D 1983 Vertebral instability. In: Corrigan B, Maitland G D (eds) Practical orthopaedic medicine. Butterworths, London, p 279–280

Cossette J, Farfan H F 1971 The instantaneous centre of rotation of the third lumbar intervertebral joint. Journal of Biomechanics 4: 149–153

Cyron B M, Hutton W C 1978 The fatigue strength of the lumbar neural circle in spondylolysis. Journal of Bone and Joint Surgery 60B: 234–238

Dimnet J, Fischer L 1978 Radiographic studies of lateral flexion in the lumbar spine. Journal of Biomechanics 11: 143–140

Dunlop R B, Adams M A, Hutton W C 1984 Disc space narrowing and the lumbar facet joints. Journal of Bone and Joint Surgery 66B: 706–710

Dupuis P R, Yong-Hing K, Cassidy J D, Kirkaldy-Willis W H 1985 Radiologic diagnosis of degenerative lumbar spine instability. Spine 10: 262–276

Farfan H F, Gracovetsky S 1984 The nature of instability. Spine 9: 714–719

Friberg O 1987 Lumbar instability: a dynamic approach by traction–compression radiography. Spine 12: 119–129

Frymoyer J W, Selby D J 1985 Segmental instability. Rationale for treatment. Spine 10: 280–286

Gertzbein S, Holtby R, Tile M et al 1984 Determination of the locus of instantaneous centers of rotation of the lumbar disc by moire fringes: a new technique. Spine 9: 409–413

Gertzbein S, Seligman J, Holtby R, Chan K H, Kapasouri A, Tile M, Cruickshan B 1985 Centrode patterns and segmental instability in degenerative disc disease. Spine 10: 257–261

Gotfried Y, Bradford D S, Oegema T R 1986 Facet joint changes after chemonucleolysis—induced disc space narrowing. Spine 11: 944–950

Gracovetsky S, Farfan H 1986 The optimum spine. Spine 11: 543–572

Grieve G 1986 Lumbar instability. In: Grieve G (ed) Modern manual therapy of the vertebral column. Churchill Livingstone, Edinburgh, pp 416–441

Haher T, Felmy W, Baruch H et al 1989 The contribution of the three columns of the spine to rotational stability. A biomechanical model. Spine 14: 663–669

Hukins D W, Kirby M C, Sikoryn T A, Aspden R M, Cox A J 1990 Comparison of structure, mechanical properties, and functions of lumbar spinal ligaments. Spine 15: 787–795

Kirkaldy-Willis W H 1983 Managing low back pain. Churchill Livingstone, New York, pp 23–43

Knuttson F 1944 The instability associated with disc degeneration in the lumbar spine. Acta Radiologica 25: 593–609

Lam Kui-Ping 1985 A comparison of the movement diagram with force-displacement curve of lumbar spine using PAIVM. Research project, Graduate diploma in manual therapy. School of Physiotherapy, Lincoln Institute of Health Sciences, Victoria, Australia

Macnab I 1971 The traction spur: an indication of segmental instability. Journal of Bone and Joint Surgery 53A: 663–666

Maitland G D 1986 Vertebral manipulation, 5th edn. Butterworths, London, pp 351–364

Matyas T Z, Bach T M 1985 The reliability of selected techniques in clinical arthrometrics. Australian Journal of Physiology 31: 175–199

Ogston N G, King G J, Gertzbein S D, Conn G S, McDonald G, Dale G, Garside H 1986 Centrode patterns in the lumbar spine. Baseline studies in normal subjects. Spine 11: 591–595

Oliver M 1986 Extension of the human lumbar spine. M. App. Sc. thesis, Curtin University, Western Australia

Panjabi M M 1979 Centers and angles of rotation of body joints: a study of error and optimization. Journal of Biomechanics 12: 911–920

Panjabi M, Krag M, Goel V 1981 A technique for measurement and description of three dimensional six degree of motion of a body joint with an application to the human spine. Journal of Biomechanics 14: 447–460

Panjabi M, Abumi K, Duranceau J, Oxland T 1989 Spinal stability and intersegmental muscle forces. A biomechanical model. Spine 14: 194–200

Paris S 1985 Physical signs of instability. Spine 10: 277–279

Pearcy M J, Bogduk N 1988 Instantaneous axes of rotation of the lumbar intervertebral joints. Spine 13: 1033–1041

Pearcy M, Shepherd J 1985 Is there instability in spondylolisthesis? Spine 10: 175–177

Pennal G F, Tile M, Kapasouri A, Rubenstein J D 1972 Motion studies of the lumbar spine. Journal of Bone and Joint Surgery 54B: 442–459

Pope M H, Panjabi M 1985 Biomechanical definitions of spinal instability. Spine 10: 255–256

Posner I, White A A, Edwards W T, Wilson C H 1982 A biomechanical analysis of the clinical stability of the lumbar and lumbosacral spine. Spine 7: 374–389

Rosenberg N J 1974 Degenerative spondylolisthesis, predisposing factors. Journal of Bone and Joint Surgery 57A: 467–474

Schneider G 1987 Degenerative lumbar instability. In: Dalziel B A, Snowsill J C (eds) Manipulative Therapists' Association of Australia. Proceedings of the Fifth Biennial Conference, pp 91–205

Seligman J, Gertzbein S, Tile M et al 1984 Computer analysis of spinal segment motion in degernerative disc disease with and without axial loading. Spine 9: 566–673

Shirazi-Adl A, Ahmed A M, Shrivastava S C 1986 Mechanical response of a lumbar motion segment in axial torque alone and combined with compression. Spine 11: 914–927

Stokes I A F, Frymoyer J W 1987 Segmental motion and instability. Spine 12: 688–691

Suh C H 1974 The fundamentals of computer aided X-ray analysis of the spine. Journal of Biomechanics 7: 161–169

Taylor J R, Twomey L T 1986 Age changes in lumbar zygapophyseal joints. Observations on structure and function. Spine 11: 739–745

Twomey L T, Taylor J R 1983 Sagittal movements of the human lumbar vertebral column: a quantitative study of the role of the posterior vertebral elements. Archives of Physical Medicine and Rehabilitation 64: 322–325

32. Clinical manifestations of pelvic girdle dysfunction

D. G. Lee

INTRODUCTION

A century ago, the sacro-iliac joint was thought to be the major source of sciatica, lumbago and backache (Meisenbach 1911). The aetiology included trauma, poor posture and secondary breakdown due to prolonged adaptation for faulty mechanics elsewhere.

The etiology of the pelvic joint conditions is not always clear, but there are many features of definite importance. At times the lesion apparently represents simply an excess of a normal physiological process. At other times trauma is a definite factor, 'sitting down hard', or the 'giving way' under severe strains, such as lifting, being the two most common forms of injury. Attitudes or postures are also of importance in causing or predisposing to joint weakness or displacement (Goldthwait & Osgood 1905).

The sacro-iliac joint was acquitted in the middle of this century when Mixter and Barr (1934) drew attention to the role of the intervertebral disc in low-back pain. As this century draws to a close, clinicians and researchers are once again focusing on the function of the pelvic girdle as a potential accomplice in low-back pain.

Current thoughts on the aetiology of pelvic girdle dysfunction remain the same today as they were at the turn of the century. However, aside from mechanical trauma, a number of metabolic conditions have been found to affect the pelvic girdle. These are listed in Table 32.1 and will not be described in this chapter.

This chapter will present a brief overview of a classification for mechanical pelvic girdle dysfunction, a description of the subjective and objective findings for each classification and some suggestions for treatment. The reader is referred to other sources (Lee 1989) for a more detailed exposition on this topic, as well as to Chapter 57 in this text for the specific treatment of the dysfunctions outlined.

CLASSIFICATION OF MECHANICAL PELVIC GIRDLE DYSFUNCTION

There are many classifications for mechanical pelvic girdle dysfunction, and while most describe the position of the

Table 32.1 Conditions affecting the sacro-iliac joint (Bellamy et al 1983)

Inflammatory disorders
Ankylosing spondylitis
Reiter's syndrome
Inflammatory bowel disease
Psoriatic spondylitis
Rheumatoid arthritis
Juvenile rheumatoid arthritis
Pustulotic arthro-osteitis
Familial Mediterranean fever
Behçet's syndrome
Relapsing polychondritis
Whipple disease

Joint infection
Pyogenic
Brucellosis
Tuberculosis

Metabolic disorders
Gout
Calcium pyrophosphate deposition disease
Hyperparathyroidism

Miscellaneous
Osteitis condensans ilii
Paget's disease
Acro-osteolysis in polyvinyl chloride workers
Alkaptonuria
Gaucher's disease
Tuberous sclerosis

restricted bone (i.e. innominate or sacrum), there has been little regard to standard terminology in the literature. Subsequently, diagnoses such as 'posterior innominate', 'anterior sacrum', 'forward sacral torsion' and 'upslip' have emerged. The difficulty with this method of classification arises when communication between the health disciplines is attempted.

The biomechanical classification outlined below is easily understood by all health care practitioners and has facilitated a consistent team approach to treatment. The classification includes:

1. hypomobility with or without pain
2. hypermobility with or without pain
3. normal mobility with pain.

This classification reflects the objective findings noted on mobility and stability testing of the pelvic girdle and suggests the appropriate treatment. It does not provide a reason for the faulty mobility noted, however, since mobilization and stabilization techniques are specific to restoring movement patterns, the cause is not always required for formulating treatment plans.

HYPOMOBILITY WITH OR WITHOUT PAIN

The essential objective finding for classification here is decreased motion of either the sacrum or the innominate bone (Fryette 1954, Mitchell 1965, Mitchell et al 1979, Beal 1982, Fowler 1984, 1986, Aitken 1986, Lee 1989). Sacro-iliac joint restrictions occur more often in the young given the natural history of degeneration of the joint (see Lee, this volume, Ch. 10).

Subjective findings

The onset may be either insidious or traumatic; a fall on the buttocks or a sudden lift and twist is not an uncommon finding in the patient's history. The stage of pathology and the degree of inflammation governs the degree of pain. The pain is usually localized to the sacro-iliac joint (although not necessarily the hypomobile one) and may radiate through the pelvis to the groin and/or down the buttock and thigh to the knee. Dysaesthesia is not often reported.

The activities which tend to aggravate the pain include walking, stair climbing/descent, rolling over in bed, getting in/out of chair/car and standing on one leg. They cannot tolerate one position or one activity for prolonged periods of time and will frequently alter their posture/activity for relief. The most comfortable sleeping position tends to be asymmetric.

Objective findings

Mobility

To understand the significance of the mobility findings a brief review of the normal pelvic girdle biomechanics is required (see Lee, this volume, Ch. 10).

The pelvic girdle as a unit is capable of motion in all three body planes. During forward bending of the trunk, the innominate bones rotate about an anteroposterior oblique axis such that the iliac crests and the PSISs approximate while the ischial tuberosities and the ASISs separate (see Lee, this volume, Ch. 10, Fig. 10.10). However, relative to one another there is no *intrapelvic* torsion of the innominate bones. During this motion, sacral flexion is followed by sacral extension bilaterally, i.e. without rotation. Unilateral hypomobility (with or

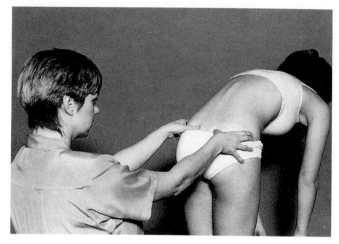

Fig. 32.1 Forward bending test in standing. The PSISs should travel an equal distance in a superior direction. The presence of intrapelvic torsion during the test (i.e. one PSIS travelling superiorly further than the other) is indicative of a positive test but does not confirm the side of the lesion. (Reproduced with permission from Lee 1989 and the publisher, Churchill Livingstone.)

without pain) produces intrapelvic torsion of the innominate bones and/or sacrum during forward bending of the trunk (see Lee, this volume, Ch. 10, Fig. 10.12). This twist is detected during the forward bending test in standing (Fig. 32.1). The presence of this finding should direct the examiner to a complete evaluation of the osteokinematic, (movement of bones) arthrokinematic (movement of joints) and myokinematic ('movement' of muscles) function of the pelvic girdle.

During backward bending of the trunk, the innominate bones simultaneously rotate about an anteroposterior oblique axis such that the iliac crests and the PSISs separate while the ischial tuberosities and the ASISs approximate. However, relative to one another there is no intrapelvic torsion of the innominate bones. Sacral flexion between the innominate bones occurs purely (i.e. without rotation).

Unilateral hypomobility (with or without pain) produces intrapelvic torsion of the innominate bones and/or sacrum during backward bending of the trunk and should direct the examiner to a further detailed evaluation of the kinematic function of the pelvic girdle.

Translation of the pelvic girdle in the coronal plane during lateral bending of the trunk normally produces intrapelvic torsion of the innominate bones and the sacrum (see Lee, this volume, Ch. 10). Unilateral hypomobility restricts lateral bending of the body and the ability to translate the pelvic girdle in the coronal plane without deviation. Consequently, the pelvic girdle is not displaced lateral to the pedal base and increased muscular effort both from the trunk and the lower extremities is required to maintain balance (Fig. 32.2).

The hypomobile sacro-iliac joint also restricts the striding tests (ipsilateral kinetic test in standing and prone

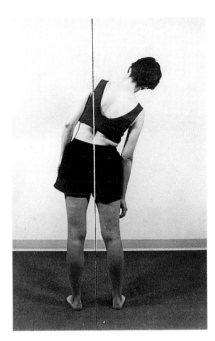

Fig. 32.2 Restricted lateral translation of the pelvic girdle in the coronal plane during right lateral bending of the trunk.

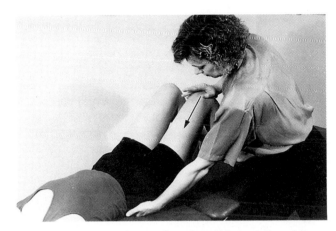

Fig. 32.4 Arthrokinematic test of craniocaudal translation of the sacro-iliac joint. The therapist's left hand is palpating the right sacral sulcus.

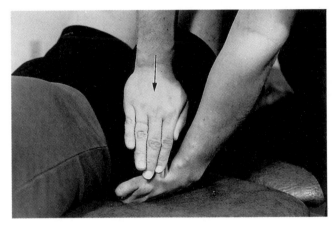

Fig. 32.5 Arthrokinematic test of anteroposterior translation of the sacro-iliac joint. The therapist's left hand is palpating the right sacral sulcus.

since treatment specificity relies on determining the system in dysfunction and not just the 'pain-generator'.

Stability

Pelvic girdle disorders in this category do not exhibit a loss of stability.

Muscle function

Muscle imbalances can influence pelvic girdle function. Janda (1976, 1978, 1986) has observed that postural muscles tighten in response to pain while phasic muscles weaken.

Relative to the pelvic girdle, the postural muscles include the erector spinae, quadratus lumborum, hamstrings, rectus femoris, iliopsoas, tensor fascia lata, adductors and piriformis. The phasic muscles include the abdominals, gluteus maximus, medius, minimus, vastus medialis, lateralis and intermedius.

Grieve (1986) noted that the more established the

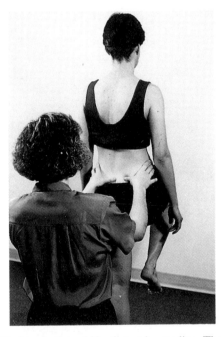

Fig. 32.3 Positive ipsilateral kinetic test in standing. The right PSIS should travel inferomedial to the median sacral crest.

lying, see Fowler, this volume, Ch. 57). The restriction becomes apparent as a reduction or total absence of relative motion between the innominate bone and the sacrum during one or both of the tests (Fig. 32.3).

If the dysfunction of the pelvic girdle is intra-articular, the arthrokinematic tests (Figs 32.4, 32.5) (craniocaudal translation, anteroposterior translation) are restricted. If the dysfunction is extra-articular, (i.e. myofascial) these tests are normal. This is a critical part of the examination altered muscle pattern, the more disturbed the functional movement pattern becomes. The long-term effect of dysfunctional movement patterns can be a painful, degenerative joint condition.

In the past, manual therapy courses have emphasized the assessment and treatment of the articular components of the pelvic girdle. Recently, attention has been directed to how the motor system functions as a whole and the effect of persistent abnormal movement patterns on the lower quadrant.

Neurological function

Impedance of neurological function and/or dural mobility can occur as a result of breakdown of the lumbosacral junction as a consequence of the pelvic girdle dysfunction.

Classification of the hypomobile dysfunction

Unilateral restrictions of the innominate bone and/or sacrum can be further classified according to the position in which the restricted bone is held. The following restrictions are commonly seen in clinical practice.

Flexed/laterally rotated innominate bone (posterior rotated/outflared) (Fig. 32.6)

Subjective findings. The patient will often report a traumatic incident such as a sudden step off a curb, a fall involving sudden flexion of one leg or an overzealous kick against a missed target. This is also a common restriction found during pregnancy.

The intensity of the pain can vary depending upon the stage of the pathology. It is often localized to the restricted sacro-iliac joint; however, if the history is long, the painful side may not be the hypomobile one. Weight-bearing on one limb, walking and supine lying with the extremity in extension often aggravate the pain.

Objective findings. The fixed flexed posture of the innominate bone restricts extension of the lower extremity. This restriction is evident during the stance phase of the gait cycle. The stance phase is shortened and a marked vertical limp can be present. The lower quadrant attempts to compensate for this loss of extension, and if the restriction is minor and the duration is long the adaptive mechanism may restore the gait pattern. Careful observation of the various components of the lower quadrant during the gait cycle will reveal the compensatory pattern.

Marked intrapelvic torsion occurs on the forward/backward bending tests both in standing (Fig. 32.1) and sitting. The ability to translate laterally the pelvic girdle in the coronal plane during lateral flexion of the trunk is unilaterally blocked (Fig. 32.2) and the ipsilateral kinetic test in prone lying (Fig. 32.7) is limited.

The innominate bone is positioned in flexion/lateral rotation relative to the innominate bone of the opposite side. The L5 vertebra and the sacrum are rotated towards the flexed innominate bone. On passive physiological mobility testing, extension/medial rotation of the innominate bone (Fig. 32.8) is restricted. If the lesion is intra-articular, the accessory arthrokinematic glides (Figs 32.4, 32.5) are restricted, whereas if the lesion is extra-articular (i.e. myofascial) the glides are normal. The lesion occurs more frequently on the left side.

Extended/medially rotated innominate bone (anterior rotated/inflared) (Fig. 32.9)

Subjective findings. Trauma rarely plays a role in the onset of this dysfunction. The onset is usually insidious

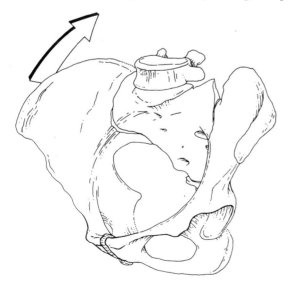

Fig. 32.6 Flexed/laterally rotated right innominate bone. (Reproduced with permission from Lee 1989 and the publisher, Churchill Livingstone.)

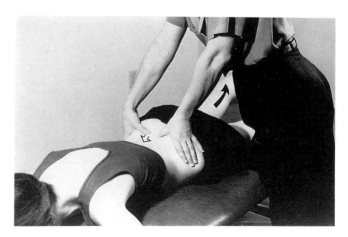

Fig. 32.7 Positive right ipsilateral kinetic test in prone lying. The relative motion between the right PSIS and the median sacral crest is reduced such that during extension of the right leg both the PSIS and the median sacral crest travel superiorly as a unit.

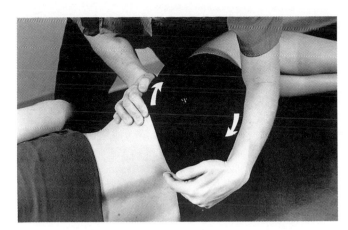

Fig. 32.8 Passive physiological mobility test for extension/medial rotation of the innominate bone. The therapist's left hand is palpating the relative motion between the innominate bone and the sacrum.

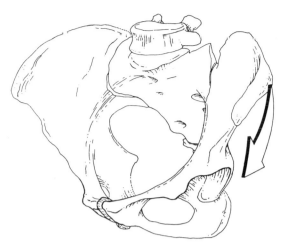

Fig. 32.9 Extended/medially rotated left innominate bone. Reproduced with permission from Lee 1989 and the publisher, Churchill Livingstone.)

and the cause is difficult to identify. The pain is rarely localized to the sacro-iliac joint and is commonly referred distally to the knee.

Objective findings. A slight shortening occurs in the swing phase of the gait cycle. It can be compensated by the lower quadrant and is easily missed even on careful observation.

Intrapelvic torsion occurs on the forward/backward bending tests both in standing (Fig. 32.1) and sitting. The ability to translate laterally the pelvic girdle in the coronal plane during lateral flexion of the trunk is unilaterally reduced (Fig. 32.2) and the ipsilateral kinetic test in standing (Fig. 32.3) is limited, although not entirely blocked.

The innominate bone is positioned in extension/medial rotation relative to the innominate bone of the opposite side. The L5 vertebra and the sacrum are rotated away from the extended innominate bone. On passive physiological mobility testing, flexion/lateral rotation (Fig. 32.10) of the innominate bone is reduced. If the lesion is intra-articular, the accessory arthrokinematic glides (Figs 32.4, 32.5) are restricted, whereas if the lesion is extra-articular (i.e. myofascial) the glides are normal. This lesion occurs more frequently on the right side.

Superiorly subluxed/extended (flexed) innominate bone (upslip in anterior rotation/posterior rotation) (Fowler 1984, 1986, Lee 1989)

Subjective findings. Trauma is always present in the aetiology of the 'upslip' although it may not have been recent. A fall on the buttocks is a common cause. If the vertical force occurs posterior to the paracornal axis of extension/flexion (Fig. 32.11), the superior subluxation will be associated with extension of the innominate bone as well. If the vertical force is anterior to this axis (Fig. 32.12), the subluxation will be associated with flexion.

The pain may be acute or chronic, localized to the

sacro-iliac joint and/or distally referred to the knee, depending upon the stage of pathology. Secondary problems at the lumbosacral junction frequently occur. Coccygodynia secondary to the altered pull of the sacrospinous ligament is a common complaint. Unilateral weight bearing, walking and sitting on the effected side aggravate the symptoms.

Objective findings. Marked intrapelvic torsion is noted on both the forward/backward bending tests in standing (Fig. 32.1) and sitting. The ability to translate laterally the pelvic girdle in the coronal plane during lateral flexion of the trunk is unilaterally blocked (Fig. 32.2) and the ipsilateral kinetic tests in both standing (Fig. 32.3) and prone lying (Fig. 32.7) are limited.

The innominate bone is positioned superiorly and is either flexed or extended relative to the innominate bone of the opposite side. The L5 vertebra and the sacrum are rotated towards the side of the flexed innominate bone. When the superior subluxation occurs in extension, the tension of the sacrotuberous ligament is markedly re-

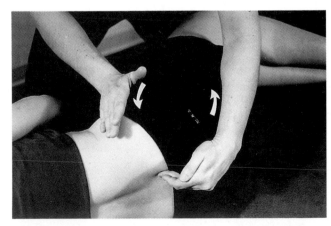

Fig. 32.10 Passive physiological mobility test for flexion/lateral rotation of the innominate bone. The therapist's left hand is palpating the relative motion between the innominate bone and the sacrum.

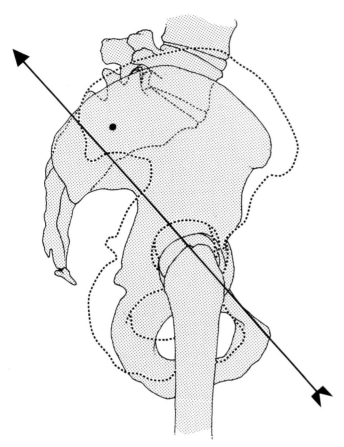

Fig. 32.11 The innominate bone will sublux superiorly and if the vertical force occurs posterior to the paracoronal axis of extension/flexion (dot). (Reproduced with permission from Lee 1989 and the publisher, Churchill Livingstone.)

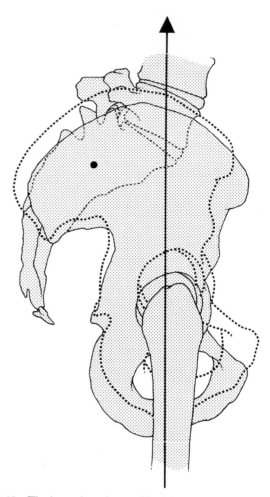

Fig. 32.12 The innominate bone will sublux superiorly and flex if the vertical force occurs anterior to the paracoronal axis of extension/flexion (dot). (Reproduced with permission from Lee 1989 and the publisher, Churchill Livingstone.)

duced. However, flexion of the innominate bone increases the tension of the sacrotuberous ligament, and when the superior subluxation occurs in flexion the tension of the sacrotuberous ligament can feel normal. On passive physiological mobility testing, marked restriction of both extension and flexion of the innominate bone (Figs 32.8, 32.10) is noted. The lesion is always intra-articular so that the accessory arthrokinematic glides (Figs 32.4, 32.5) are restricted. Following reduction of the subluxation (see Fowler, this volume, Ch. 57) repeated testing of these glides often reveals hypermobility of the sacro-iliac joint. The superiorly subluxed/extended lesion is commonly seen on the right, the superiorly subluxed/flexed lesion is commonly seen on the left.

Unilateral sacral flexion/extension

Subjective findings. A lifting/twisting episode frequently causes the unilateral sacral flexion/extension lesion. A sudden twinge of pain localized to the sacro-iliac joint may be felt at the time of the injury. The lift is commonly a horizontal one, performed without a pelvic tilt and therefore with an 'unlocked' sacrum (Fig. 32.13).

This lesion is also found following motor-vehicle rear-end collisions. Typically, the patient was wearing a three-point seat belt and had the right foot firmly planted on the brake at the time of the impact. Initially, these patients present with an acute whiplash of the cervical spine and rarely complain of low-back pain; however, as the cervical symptoms subside, the low-back pain becomes evident.

Objective findings. Intrapelvic torsion is noted during the forward bending test in standing (Fig. 32.1) but may be minimal. The torsion is magnified during forward bending in sitting. The ability to translate laterally the pelvic girdle in the coronal plane during lateral flexion of the trunk is only slightly limited (Fig. 32.2) and the ipsilateral kinetic test in standing (Fig. 32.3) is reduced.

The sacrum is positioned in unilateral flexion (i.e. a deep sacral sulcus together with an anterior sacral base) on one side and extension (i.e. a shallow sacral sulcus together with a posterior sacral base) on the other. On passive physiological mobility testing, a marked restriction of unilateral sacral flexion/extension (Fig. 32.14) is noted.

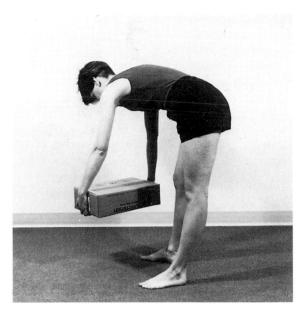

Fig. 32.13 A horizontal lift with an 'unlocked' sacrum facilitates the sacral flexion/extension lesion since the sacrotuberous ligament is slack in this position.

The accessory arthrokinematic glides (Figs 32.4, 32.5) are restricted since the dysfunction is intra-articular. This test differentiates the side of the restriction and whether the lesion is in flexion or extension.

Sacral torsion (Fig. 32.15) (Fowler 1986, Lee 1989)

Subjective findings. The mode of onset may be either insidious or traumatic. The location of pain is variable, occasionally localized to the sacro-iliac joint but not consistently. A trigger point is often found deep in the buttock within the piriformis muscle.

Objective findings. Intrapelvic torsion is noted on either the forward (Fig. 32.1) or the backward bending tests in both standing and sitting. The ability to translate

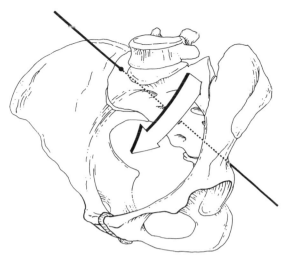

Fig. 32.15 Sacral rotation to the right. (Reproduced with permission from Lee 1989 and the publisher, Churchill Livingstone.)

laterally the pelvic girdle in the coronal plane during lateral flexion of the trunk is unilaterally restricted (Fig. 32.2) and the ipsilateral kinetic tests in both standing (Fig. 32.3) and prone lying (Fig. 32.7) are limited.

The sacrum is positioned in rotation (i.e. a deep sacral sulcus together with an anterior sacral base and a posterior inferior lateral angle on the opposite side) in one position of the trunk—hyperflexion or hyperextension. On passive physiological mobility testing, sacral rotation is reduced to the contralateral side (Fig. 32.16). The accessory arthrokinematic glides (Figs 32.4, 32.5) are not restricted since the lesion is extra-articular. The reader is referred to Fowler (this volume, Ch. 57) for a further description of the combined patterns of lumbo/sacral torsion lesions.

Treatment of the hypomobile pelvic girdle

At the turn of this century, sacro-iliac joint dysfunction was treated in one of two ways—manipulation or immobi-

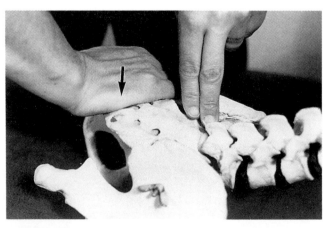

Fig. 32.14 Passive physiological mobility test for extension of the sacrum. The anterior pressure is directly over the sacral hiatus at the distal end of the median sacral crest.

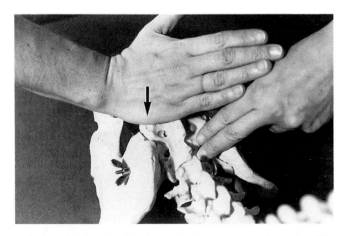

Fig. 32.16 Passive physiological mobility test for sacral rotation. The anterior pressure is over the contralateral inferior lateral angle of the sacrum.

lization (Goldthwait & Osgood 1905, Albee 1909, Meisenbach 1911, Young 1940, Fryette 1954). The manipulation techniques for the 'subluxed' sacro-iliac joints are poorly described in the literature and usually included non-specific pressure over the sacrum. Essentially, treatment of sacro-iliac joint disorders has remained unchanged. Hypomobile joints are mobilized and hypermobile joints are immobilized.

The goal of therapy is to restore the optimal biomechanics of the pelvic girdle via passive and active mobilization techniques and exercise programs (Lee 1989). The reader is referred to Fowler (this volume, Ch. 57) for a detailed description of the manual therapy techniques for the conditions outlined in this chapter.

HYPERMOBILITY WITH OR WITHOUT PAIN

Hypermobility of the pelvic girdle can occur following repeated microtrauma, one major trauma or secondary to hormonal changes such as those associated with pregnancy. The essential objective finding for classification here is increased motion of either the sacrum or the innominate bone.

Subjective findings

The mode of onset may be traumatic or insidious. A subluxation of the sacro-iliac joint will attenuate the ligamentous system. If stability is not restored during recovery, the sacro-iliac joint will remain hypermobile. Conversely, the patient may report a gradual onset of sacro-iliac joint and/or pubic symphysis pain during or after pregnancy secondary to hormonal relaxation. The symptoms may radiate into the buttock, posterior thigh and/or abdomen and groin. The aggravating activities can include unilateral weight bearing, bending forward, lifting, lying supine and rolling over from this position, fast walking and any activity for prolonged periods of time.

Clicking of the pubic symphysis and/or sacro-iliac joint is frequently reported (Harris & Murray 1974). Rest usually affords relief as long as the hypermobile joint is not under stress while in the resting position.

Objective findings

Mobility

The hypermobile pelvic girdle interferes with the normal transference of weight from the trunk to the lower extremity during unilateral weight-bearing (Fig. 32.17). This loss of kinetic stability is reflected in the gait pattern. The patient typically shifts the weight laterally during the stance phase (lateral limp). Forward bending of the trunk is achieved by walking the hands down the thighs. If the pelvic girdle is manually stabilized in the transverse plane, forward flexion is possible with less support and less pain (Goldthwait & Osgood 1905, Sweeting 1984).

The accessory arthrokinematic glides (Figs 32.4, 32.5) are the most important part of the objective examination

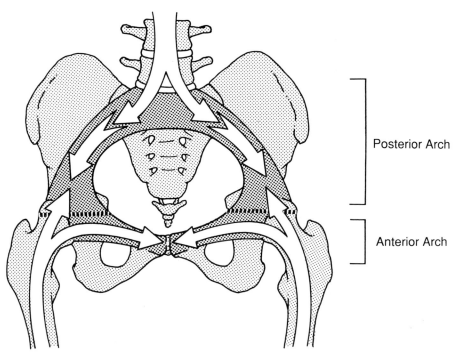

Fig. 32.17 The posterior and anterior arches of the pelvic girdle. The function of each arch is dependent upon the structural integrity of the other. (Reproduced with permission from Lee 1989 and the publisher, Churchill Livingstone.)

since the hypermobile joint can appear hypomobile when tested in weight-bearing. The passive glides are always excessive when the joint is hypermobile. According to Young (1940), hypermobility of the pubic symphysis can occur only if the sacro-iliac joint is also loose. Bellamy et al (1983) noted that 'the most reliable clinical sign of instability of disruption of the SI joint is that of disruption of the pubic symphysis. This will only occur when there is excessive movement at the SI joint and can be readily assessed by observing the relative movements of the pubic rami on weight bearing alternately on either leg'.

Stability

The transverse anterior (Fig. 32.18) and the supero-inferior pubic symphysis (Fig. 32.19) stress tests are usually painful in the symptomatic hypermobile patient.

Treatment of the hypermobile pelvic girdle

Immobilization was, and still is, the treatment of choice for hypermobile joints. At the turn of this century, the pelvic girdle was immobilized with plaster of paris for four weeks to six months followed by a four-inch elastic belt to be worn indefinitely (Albee 1909, Meisenbach 1911).

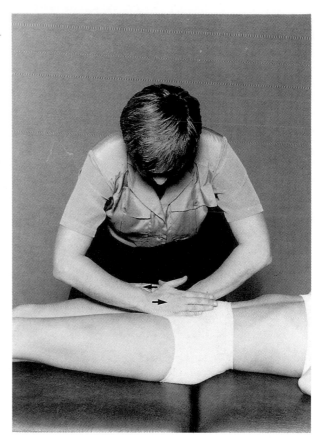

Fig. 32.19 Supero-inferior pubic symphysis stress test. (Reproduced with permission from Lee 1989 and the publisher, Churchill Livingstone.)

The loss of kinetic stability within the pelvic girdle can be debilitating, and very little can be achieved via manual therapy alone. The temporary application of an external support can be very helpful during pregnancy. The support should be worn at all times when weight-bearing. Currently, sclerosing injections into the dorsal sacro-iliac ligaments has shown some promise in affording relief for patients with permanent instability. It is critical that the pelvic girdle be sclerosed in a position of function, and therefore it is pertinent that a manual therapist familiar with treatment of the pelvic girdle be part of this team (Sweeting 1984, Schamberger 1990).

NORMAL MOBILITY WITH PAIN

Patients presenting with localized pain within the pelvic girdle in the absence of 'hard' objective findings are a challenge to treat. Clinically, several mobility tests reproduce the pain but never consistently. Careful objective evaluation of mobility reveals normal function. The only cause of a biomechanical nature for this dysfunction can be over-use of the articular and myofascial tissues secondary to altered function elsewhere. A global approach to assessment and treatment of the lower quadrant is often the only means of improving function with these patients.

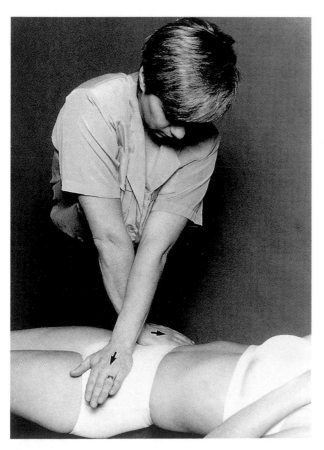

Fig. 32.18 Transverse anterior stress test of the pelvic girdle. (Reproduced with permission from Lee 1989 and the publisher, Churchill Livingstone.)

Alternatively, the patient may have a disorder which is non-mechanical in nature (Table 32.1), a possibility of which the clinician must always be aware.

CONCLUSION

The sacro-iliac joint is not the commonest cause of low-back pain. However, when present, a restriction of the innominate bone and/or sacrum can have far-reaching implications on the function of the lower quadrant. Manual therapy which follows an accurate assessment of the pelvic girdle based on the known biomechanics will yield rewarding results for the therapist who accepts the challenge.

Acknowledgements

The author would like to gratefully acknowledge the assistance of Frank Crymble for preparing the original line drawings, Janet Lowcock for modelling, and Thomas Lee for taking the clinical photographs in this chapter.

REFERENCES

Aitken G S 1986 Syndromes of lumbo-pelvic dysfunction. In: Grieve G P (ed) Modern manual therapy of the vertebral column. Churchill Livingstone, Edinburgh, Ch. 43, p 473

Albee F H 1909 A study of the anatomy and the clinical importance of the sacroiliac joint. Journal of the American Medical Association 53: 1273–1276

Beal M C 1982 The sacroiliac problem: review of anatomy, mechanics, and diagnosis. Journal of the American Osteopathic Association 81: 667

Bellamy N, Park W, Rooney P J 1983 What do we know about the sacroiliac joint? Seminars in Arthritis and Rheumatism 12: 282–312

Fowler C 1984 Superior innominate subluxation (the upslip). In: Gilraine F, Sweeting L (eds) Proceedings of the International Federation of Orthopaedic Manipulative Therapists Fifth International Seminar on Manual Therapy, Vancouver, June 25–29, pp 122–124

Fowler C 1986 Muscle energy techniques for pelvic dysfunction. In: Grieve G P (ed) Modern manual therapy of the vertebral column. Churchill Livingstone, Edinburgh

Fryette H H 1954 Principles of osteopathic technique. American Academy of Osteopathy, Colorado

Goldthwait J E, Osgood R B 1905 A consideration of the pelvic articulations from an anatomical, pathological and clinical standpoint. Boston Medical and Surgical Journal 152: 593–602

Grieve G P (ed) 1986 Modern manual therapy of the vertebral column. Churchill Livingstone, Edinburgh

Harris N H, Murray R O 1974 Lesions of the symphysis in athletes. British Medical Journal 4: 211–214

Janda V 1976 The muscular factor in the pathogenesis of back pain syndrome. Physiotherapy Symposium, Oslo

Janda V 1978 Muscles, central nervous motor regulation and back problems. In: Korr I (ed) The neurobiologic mechanisms in manipulative therapy. Plenum Press, London

Janda V 1986 Muscle weakness and inhibition (pseudoparesis) in back pain syndromes. In: Grieve G P (ed) Modern manual therapy of the vertebral column. Churchill Livingstone, Edinburgh, Ch. 19, p 197

Kapandji I A 1974 The physiology of joints III: the trunk and vertebral column 2nd edn. Churchill Livingstone, Edinburgh, p 58

Lee D 1989 The pelvic girdle: an approach to the examination and treatment of the lumbo-pelvic-hip region. Churchill Livingstone, Edinburgh

Meisenbach R O 1911 Sacro-iliac relaxation; with analysis of eighty-four cases. Surgery, Gynecology and Obstetrics 12: 411–434

Mitchell F 1965 Structural pelvic function. Year book: Academy of Applied Osteopathy. Carmel, California

Mitchell F L, Moran P S, Pruzzo N A 1979 An evaluation and treatment manual of osteopathic muscle energy procedures. Mitchell, Moran and Pruzzo, Missouri

Mixter W J, Barr J S 1934 Rupture of intervertebral disc with involvement of the spinal cord. New England Journal of Medicine 211: 210

Schamberger W 1990 Personal communication

Sweeting R S 1984 Hypermobility of the sacroiliac joints. In: Gilraine F, Sweeting L (eds) Proceedings of the International Federation of Orthopaedic Manipulative Therapists Fifth International Seminar on Manual Therapy, Vancouver, June 25–29, pp 258–267

Young J 1940 Relaxation of the pelvic joints in pregnancy: pelvic arthropathy of pregnancy. Journal of Obstetrics and Gynecology 47: 493–524

33. Bone loss and osteoporosis of the spine

L. T. Twomey   J. R. Taylor

INTRODUCTION

Bone is a dynamic tissue which is regulated by endocrine factors, nutrition and physical activity through all phases of life. In recent years, attention has focused primarily on the influence of hormonal and calcium deficiencies on bone loss and gain, particularly in women. Less emphasis has been placed on the physical activity component of this equation in spite of the long-standing appreciation of the relationship between bone density and physical activity enunciated so clearly by Wolff in 1892.

Osteoporosis is the most common and widespread of all of the degenerative processes involving bone. The term 'osteoporosis' refers more accurately to bone loss with fracture, while 'osteopenia' is used to describe bone loss without fracture. The term osteoporosis is used in this paper to include both definitions as the clinical distinction is not clear cut. It involves a loss of bone substance and it may occur as a consequence of disease (Dent & Watson 1966), a marked decrease in weight bearing (Hall 1976), or it may simply be considered as an inevitable accompaniment of ageing (Gitman & Kamholtz 1965). It is more prevalent in females after the menopause than in males, and more prevalent in white females than in black females (Boukhris & Becker 1972). At the age of 65, X-ray comparison with a 'standard' suggests that 65.8% of females and 21.5% of males have osteoporosis. In women, the incidence increases by about 8% for each additional decade, whereas in men, a large increase does not occur until after the age of 76 (Gitman & Kamholtz 1965).

Vertebrae

During childhood and early adult life, the 'cortical shell' of a vertebral body is thin and dense, while its cartilage-covered vertebral end-plates contain multiple perforations (Warwick & Williams 1973). Cancellous bone comprises about 66% of all vertebral bone, and in the vertebral bodies it is arranged in irregular plates or trabeculae 0.12 to 0.24 mm thick (Fig. 33.1). The trabecular plates are

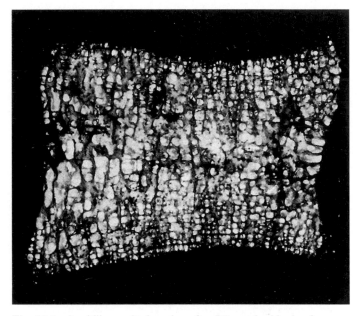

Fig. 33.1 A midline sagittal section of an L3 vertebral body of a young adult male, demonstrating the trabecular arrangement.

oriented parallel to the lines of stress with 'vertical' and 'horizontal' components. In the anterior two-thirds of the vertebral body vertical trabeculae predominate, whereas in the posterior one-third horizontal trabeculae are more evident, as in the pedicles (Singh 1978).

In Western societies, there is a significant loss of vertebral bone substance in both men and women in old age. This can be considered to be a 'normal' part of the ageing process, although the definition of the critical level when this 'sub-clinical' osteopenia becomes clinical osteoporosis remains a clinical problem (Nordin et al 1980).

Trabecular loss

While there is a reduction in the numbers of both horizontal and vertical trabeculae in the old age, as Fig. 33.2 shows, the principal and significant reduction is in the numbers of horizontal trabeculae (Twomey et al 1983,

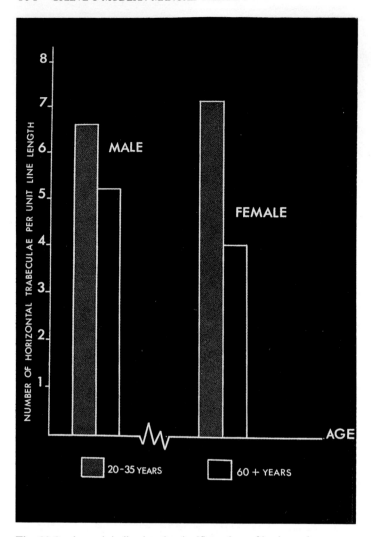

Fig. 33.2 A graph indicating the significant loss of horizontal trabeculae which occurs in old age in both men and women.

Preteux et al 1985) as in Fig. 33.2. This research confirms earlier speculation that it is the particular loss of horizontal trabeculae which plays the major role in vertebral bone loss in old age (Casuccio 1962, Atkinson 1967).

Young adult vertebral bodies are able to resist the vertical compressive forces of body weight because of their trabecular arrangement (Twomey et al 1983). Atkinson (1967) argued that the reduction in the number of horizontal trabeculae leads to fracture of weight-bearing vertical trabeculae, resulting in end-plate fracture. The consequence of this is usually an increase in the concavity of the end-plates in old age, although in extreme cases, end-plate collapse occurs. This observation is in accordance with Euler's theory, which may be used to explain the inherent strength of cancellous bone (Bell et al 1967, Doyle 1972, Twomey & Taylor 1987). It demonstrates that the rigidity of a structure depends more on its geometry than its mass. The strength of columns of bone (e.g. vertical trabeculae) is dependent on the number of reinforcing 'ties' or 'cross-braces' between them (Pugh

et al 1973). In the vertebrae, these are represented by the horizontal trabeculae, which are more effective in providing strength to the vertical struts than would be an increase in the diameters of these vertical struts (Fig. 33.3).

As in the disc, vertical compressive forces may be partly resolved in a horizontal direction. In a vertebral body these forces are partly resolved along 'cross-braces'. The selective loss of horizontal trabeculae in old age allows buckling of vertical trabeculae to the point of fracture. The collapse of vertical trabeculae tends to be most marked below the nucleus pulposus, that part of the disc most concerned with transmitting loads from one vertebra to the next (Fig. 33.4). It is the area of bone immediately adjacent to the nucleus pulposus that shows the greatest number of microfractures in old age (Vernon-Roberts & Pirie 1977, Twomey & Taylor 1987).

Thus, in old age, lumbar vertebrae are slightly shorter, wider at the 'waist' and more concave at the disc vertebral junction (Twomey et al 1983). Thus, spinal osteoporosis is also linked with a loss of stature due to shortening of the trunk, causing the crown–pubis distance to become less than the pubis–heel distance (Dent & Watson 1966). This decrease in trunk length may be due in part to the loss of bone substance and change in vertebral body shape which may in extreme cases proceed to vertebral body wedging with collapse and kyphosis (Buchanan et al 1987).

The research described briefly above poses the question as to why there is a selective loss of horizontal trabeculae in lumbar vertebral bodies. It is generally assumed that hormonal factors are of primary importance in osteo-porosis of the elderly (Nordin et al 1980) but mechanical factors are also known to influence bone structure, notably in young athletes (Jones et al 1977) but also in middle-aged men (Dalen & Olsson 1974). The effect to the forces imposed on bone by exercise, causing cancellous bone to be organized parallel to the lines of stress, is well known (Dent & Watson 1966). Exercise has also been shown to prevent osteoporosis in post menopausal women (Aloia et al 1978). Hormonal deficiencies alone would be expected to lead to a generalized loss of cancellous bone, and the selective loss of horizontal trabeculae suggests that mechanical factors are also important. It may be postulated that the reduced muscular activity of old age is responsible for the selective decline in the numbers of horizontal trabeculae, while the axial forces of body weight through the vertebrae are responsible for the persistence of vertical trabeculae.

In recent years, there has been an increasing literature on the relationship between high levels of exercise and skeletal health. Exercise appears to increase bone density mainly in areas of maximum use, while inactivity is associated with bone loss (Smith & Gilligan 1987, Twomey & Taylor 1989).

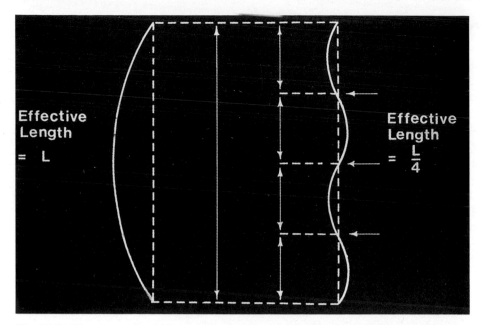

Fig. 33.3 The manner in which vertical trabeculae may buckle under load if no transverse ties are present (as on left) where effective length = L. If ties are present (right), effective length = L/4 and the buckling load must be four times greater. From Twomey et al (1983).

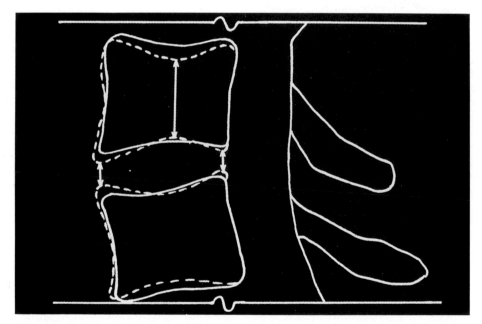

Fig. 33.4 The changes which occur in the shape of the anterior vertebral structures in old age. The young adult shape is indicated by the solid lines, and the old adult shape is indicated by the broken lines. The arrows indicate reduction in height.

Physical activities

Athletes of all ages have been shown to have greater bone density than age-matched sedentary individuals (Lane et al 1986). It is clear that in young adults, and probably to a lesser extent in the elderly, bone atrophy occurs in the absence of exercise, while bone hypertrophy follows increased levels of physical activity (Smith & Gilligan 1987).

The amount of bone density in athletes correlates closely with the levels of stress exerted, so that amongst athletes, weightlifters have the most dense bones and swimmers the least (Nilsson & Westin 1971). Despite the less obvious increase in bone density in swimmers, it is true that even elderly habitual swimmers have more dense bones in their arms and vertebrae than do their age-matched, non-exercising colleagues (Orwoll et al 1987).

Bone loss inactivity

In contrast to the bone gain evident in athletes, bone loss occurs with immobilization and inactivity. For example, it has long been known that just a few days of weightlessness in space can cause astronauts to lose massive amounts of bone (Whedon 1984). However, in recent times, Russian cosmonauts have spent in excess of 300 days aboard the space station Mir without the skeletal deterioration which might have been expected (Barringer 1988). This situation has been achieved by a combination of exercise and medication. Each cosmonaut spends an hour a day on an exercise ergometer and another on a specially adapted treadmill, while for a further 16 hours a day they are required to wear a suit criss-crossed with a web of elastic cords so that movement in any direction forces them to strain against resistance. This daily programme is described as 'constant physical therapy' and is seen as essential to the maintenance of reasonable skeletal health in space (Bailey et al 1986, Lemonick 1987).

Bone gain and exercise

The effects of exercise are site-specific, and they result in greater bone density in those body areas subjected to the higher stress levels (Bailey et al 1986). Montoye et al (1980) measured the dominant and non-dominant arms of elderly male tennis players (mean age 64 years) and showed a significant difference in the amount of hypertrophy of bone in the dominant limb, a situation which is likely to have developed over many years. Similarly, Dalen and Olsson (1974), in a study of elderly male cross-country runners, showed significantly greater bone mass in their legs (20%) and lumbar vertebrae (10%) than in their non-athletic controls. In a fascinating study, Smith (1981) examined 30 elderly women with a mean age of 84 years. The women were placed into two groups which were matched on the basis of age, weight and degree of ambulation. The experimental group participated in a 30-minute exercise programme, three days a week, for three years. At the end of this period, there was a 5.6% difference in bone mineral content, consisting of a 2.3% loss in the control group and a 3.3% gain in the exercise group. These results added substance to a previous study (Aloia et al 1978) which indicated a significant increase in total body calcium in post-menopausal females who exercised regularly for one year, in contrast with a fall in total body calcium in a matched sedentary control group. In a further study of the effects of dynamic forearm loading exercise in post-menopausal women (aged 53 to 74 years), a 3.8% increase in bone density of radius and ulna was demonstrated after five months of exercise (three 50-minute sessions per week) compared to controls, who continued to decline in bone density (Ayalon et al 1987). These and other studies demonstrate that an appropriate physical regime can be effective as a prophylactic treatment for osteoporosis.

Although the reasons for the effect which exercise has on bone are not fully understood, they may be related to the piezo-electric phenomenon (Smith & Gilligan 1987). Bone responds locally to stress by developing strain-related electrical potentials at the point of compressive stress. The bone elements align themselves in the direction of the functional force and there is local production of skeletal growth factor. Similarly, the application of electrical fields to bone stimulates osteogenesis. Thus, it is hypothesized that the strain-related potentials increase bone formation.

CLINICAL MANAGEMENT

Physiotherapy has a role in:

- Educational and preventive programmes of physical activity for the middle-aged and elderly.
- Rehabilitation of those with osteoporosis.
- Preventive programmes. The general public needs to understand that all the bones, including vertebrae, require a moderate level of stress through life if they are to remain strong and healthy. Many elderly people believe that the need for exercise declines with age, that exercise is risky for old people, that light exercise is enough, and that age itself is a barrier to exercise. Nothing could be further from the truth. All of the evidence now available demonstrates clearly that elderly bones and joints must have the continuing stresses of exercise if they are to remain strong and active.

Physiotherapists are ideally situated to convey this message to elderly people and to develop programmes of group exercise which provide activies designed to enable skeletal health to be maintained in old age (Twomey & Taylor 1984, MacKinnon 1988). The Health Department of Western Australia has been conducting regular exercise classes for the middle-aged and elderly in metropolitan and country centres since 1979. The classes are run by physiotherapists and include a component on health education, stressing the need for continuing relatively high levels of exercise activity throughout life for all elements of the musculoskeletal and cardiopulmonary systems.

The classes take the participants progressively through a careful, graded programme of interesting physical activity. There are currently in excess of 4000 participants in 50 centres, run by about 40 different physiotherapists. The activities include stretching, relaxation and mobility exercises on the one hand and dynamic exercises involving tension and impact on the other. The participants are carefully examined prior to commencement of the programme and prescription of appropriate activities. Since the incidence of degenerative pathology increases in the elderly, any one large group may consist of a number of subgroups of people whose exercise needs may differ in accordance with the particular circumstances of individuals. Physiotherapists, with their excellent knowledge of pathology and human movement (MacKinnon 1988), are ideally suited to lead these programmes.

Rehabilitation

For patients disabled by osteoporosis associated with increasing fragility of bone, possibly even compression fractures of vertebrae and often quite severe back pain, exercise programmes are important but must be introduced very carefully and slowly. Ideally, doctor and physiotherapist should consult thoroughly and at some length prior to commencing programmes for such fragile, elderly individuals, and then proceed with caution. Nevertheless, exercise remains an essential element of treatment.

Initially, exercise periods must be brief and take place in an environment where the individual feels secure and comfortable. Thus, hydrotherapy, where the person is warm and supported by both the buoyancy of water and the presence of the physiotherapist, is an ideal starting medium. It is usually recommended that the fragile elderly progress gradually from about 5 to 10 minutes exercise a day, at a rate which is congruent with their condition and physical response. The exercise should emphasize joint flexibility primarily in the early stages, and progressively aim at strengthening the trunk and limbs. Controlled back extensor movements should be encouraged rather than flexion, since flexion is in the direction of the thoracic kyphosis deformity and may increase the likelihood of vertebral microfracture and damage. The rate of progression of exercise is dependent on the response of the individuals concerned and must not be rushed. As strength and endurance improve, the time spent on activities should increase.

Exercise is also important to maintain the integrity of all joint structures throughout life. The alternative compression and relaxation of articular cartilage and the tension and relaxation of joint collagenous elements facilitate fluid transfer and aid joint nutrition. Recent evidence shows clearly that there is a valuable role for carefully progressed exercise activities in the management of degenerative and inflammatory joint disease, as well as in the maintenance of 'normal' joints (Burry 1987).

SUMMARY

Increasing age is associated with vertebral bone loss, primarily due to a significant reduction in the horizontally oriented trabecular plates. This causes the vertebrae in old age to be slightly shorter, thicker at their 'waist' and increasingly concave at their end-plates, and it also causes a loss of stature. Osteoporosis is particularly significant in women after the menopause when hormonal deficiency may compound the trend toward increasing bone loss, and the 'dowagers hump', which may become evident, is testimony to osteoporosis and to vertebral fractures and collapse (Thevanon et al 1987).

There is an increasing body of evidence supporting the value of high levels of regular exercise in elderly people in preserving skeletal health. This is true for both sexes, but is particularly the case for females after menopause, when hormonal deprivation adds considerably to involutional bone loss.

Preventive physiotherapy for the middle-aged and elderly must stress the necessity for adequate levels of physical activity into old age. There is little doubt that the incidence of osteoporotic bone fractures in elderly persons could be reduced substantially if exercise levels were generally maintained into retirement. This reduced risk of fracture may relate as much to the maintenance of muscle strength and neuromuscular co-ordination as to the associated maintenance of bone mass.

REFERENCES

Aloia J F, Cohn S H, Ostuni J A, Cane R, Elis K 1978 Prevention of involutional bone loss by exercise. Journal of Clinical Endocrinology and Metabolism 43: 992–999

Atkinson P J 1967 Variation in trabecular structure of vertebrae with age. Calcified Tissue Research 1: 24–32

Ayalon J, Simkin A, Leichter I, Raifmann S 1987 Dynamic bone exercises for postmenopausal women: effect on the density on the distal radius. Archives of Physical Medicine and Rehabilitation 68: 280–283

Bailey D A, Martin A D, Houston C S, Howie L J 1986 Physical activity nutrition, bone density and osteoporosis. Australian Journal of Science and Medicine in Sports 18: 3–7

Barringer F 1988 Soviet space prescription: artificial gravity for long flights. New York Times, Tuesday May 17, B8

Bell G H, Dunbar O, Beck J A 1967 Variations in strength of vertebrae with age and their relation to osteoporosis. Calcified Tissue Research 1: 75–86

Boukhris R, Becker K L 1972 Calcification of the aorta and osteoporosis. Journal of the American Medical Association 219: 1307–1311

Buchanan J R, Myers C, Greer R B, Lloyd T, Varano L A 1987 Assessment of the risk of vertebral fracture in menopausal women. Journal of Bone and Joint Surgery 69: 212–218

Burry H C 1987 Sports, exercise and arthritis. British Journal of Rheumatology 26: 386–388

Casuccio C 1962 An introduction to the study of osteoporosis (biochemical and biophysical research in bone ageing). Proceedings of the Royal Society of Medicine 55: 663–668

Dalen N, Olsson K E 1974 Bone mineral content and physical activity. Acta Orthopaedica Scandinavica 45: 170–174

Dent C E, Watson L 1966 Osteoporosis. Postgraduate Medical Journal (suppl) (October 1966) 583–608

Doyle F H 1972 Involutional osteoporosis. Clinics in Endocrinology and Metabolism 1: 143–167

Gitman L, Kamholtz T 1965 Incidence of radiographic osteoporosis in a large series of aged individuals. Journal of Gerontology 20: 32–33

Hall D M 1976 The ageing of connective tissue. Academic Press, London

Jones H H, Priest J D, Hayes W C, Tichenor C C, Nagel D A 1977

Humeral hypertrophy in response to exercise. Journal of Bone and Joint Surgery 59: 204–208

Lane N E, Bloch D A, Jones H H, Marshal W H, Wood P D, Fries J F 1986 Long-distance running, bone density and osteoporosis. Journal American Medical Association 255: 1147–1151

Lemonick M D 1987 Surging ahead. Time Magazine, October 5, 1987, 64–70

MacKinnon J L 1988 Osteoporosis: a review. Physical Therapy 68: 1533–1540

Montoye H J, Smith E L, Fardon D F 1980 Bone mineral in senior tennis player. Scandinavian Journal of Sports Science 2: 26–32

Nilsson B E, Westlin N E 1971 Bone density in athletes. Clinical Orthopaedics and Related Research 77: 179

Nordin B E C 1980 Treatment of postmenopausal osteoporosis. Current Therapeutics 10: 51–62

Nordin B E C, Horsman A, Crilly R G, Marshall D H, Simpson M 1980 Treatment of spinal osteoporosis in postmenopausal women. British Medical Journal 280 (6212) 451–454

Orwoll E S, Ferar J L, Ovlatt S K, Huntington K 1987 The effect of swimming on bone mineral content. Clinical Research 35: 194

Preteux F, Bergot C, Laval-Jeantet A M 1985 Automatic quantification of vertebral cancellous bone remodelling during ageing. Anatomica Clinica 7: 203–208

Pugh J W, Rose R M, Radin E L 1973 Elastic and visco-elastic properties of trabecular bone: dependence on structure. Journal of Biomechanics 6: 475–485

Singh I 1978 The architecture of cancellous bone. Journal of Anatomy 127: 305–310

Smith E L (Jr) 1981 Physical activity: a preventive and maintenance modality for bone loss with age. In: Nagle F J, Montoye H J (eds) Exercise in health and disease. Thomas, Springfield

Smith E L, Gilligan C 1987 Effects of inactivity and exercise on bone. Physician and Sports Medicine 15: 91–100

Thevenon A, Pollez B, Cantegrit F, Tison-Muchery F, Marchandise X, Duquesnoy B 1987 Relationship between kyphosis, scoliosis and osteoporosis in the elderly population. Spine 12: 744–745

Twomey L T, Taylor J R 1984 Old age and physical capacity. Australian Journal of Physiotherapy 30: 115–120

Twomey L T, Taylor J R 1987 Physical therapy of the low back. Churchill Livingstone, New York

Twomey L T, Taylor J R 1989 Physical activity and ageing bones. Patient Management (August 1989) 27–34

Twomey L T, Taylor J R, Furniss B 1983 Age changes in the bone density and structure of the lumbar vertebral column. Journal of Anatomy 136: 15–25

Vernon-Roberts B, Pirie C J 1977 Degenerative changes in the intervertebral discs of the lumbar spine and their sequela. Rheumatology and Rehabilitation 16: 13–21

Warwick R, Williams P L 1973 Gray's anatomy. 35th edn. Longman, Edinburgh

Whedon G D 1984 Disuse osteoporosis: physiological aspects. Calcified Tissue International 36: 146–150

Examination and assessment

34. Clinical reasoning process in manipulative therapy

M. A. Jones

INTRODUCTION

Greater attention to the thinking process or 'clinical reasoning' behind the examination and management of patients will improve patient outcomes. Understanding one's clinical reasoning will also facilitate improved reasoning and broaden the repertoire of clinical patterns which can be recognized. In the physiotherapy education process, attention is often given only to the teaching of examination and treatment techniques without providing the necessary reasoning behind them, exactly where they fit in, when to vary the routine and how to use the information once it has been obtained. Therefore, if clinical reasoning is to be given greater attention in education, consideration should be given to how clinical reasoning can be assessed and what teaching methods are available to improve it.

This chapter presents one perspective on the clinical reasoning process. First, the reasoning of two physiotherapists examining and treating the same patient is compared to illustrate differences in their clinical reasoning. The clinical reasoning process is then discussed in the context of the information-processing literature in medical education. This is followed by discussion of differences between experts and novices and consideration of errors in reasoning. Finally, some implications for education are put forward.

CLINICAL REASONING OF TWO PHYSIOTHERAPISTS

A physiotherapist examined and treated a 45-year-old plumber who presented with a 'hip ache'. The first treatment consisted of stretching/mobilizing the hip into flexion and flexion/adduction which improved the patient's hip mobility, and the patient came back at the second appointment feeling better with less ache when walking. Much the same treatment was given two more times with further increase in hip range of motion but no change in his ache; at his last appointment the hip was mobilized more firmly with no further improvement.

A physiotherapy colleague was asked to examine and treat the patient. His treatment consisted of postero-anterior accessory movement over the L5/S1 posterior intervertebral joint from a combined position of right rotation, extension and right lateral flexion, into resistance and provoking the patient's 'hip ache'. This treatment produced sustained improvement, and progression of the same technique rendered the patient symptom-free after four treatments.

Assuming that the decision of Therapist One to treat the hip was incorrect, why did these two therapists arrive at different treatment decisions? Was Therapist One's examination incomplete or did he misinterpret information obtained? A review of each therapist's summary of his examination findings will reveal significant differences.

Therapist One's summary of his examination findings (ET = examiner's thoughts)

The patient is a 45-year-old plumber whose main complaint was a 'hip' ache which developed three weeks earlier. He was kneeling, attempting to loosen a fitting, when a wrench suddenly slipped resulting in an immediate jab of pain in the buttock (ET: twisting injury to hip). It was very sore for a few days but then improved, although it still ached after he had been on his feet for more than 20 minutes. Sleeping had not been a problem, and he would typically feel his 'hip' first thing in the morning when getting out of bed. There was no past history of any hip or back problems, although the patient has had more difficulty over the past 5 years assuming low squat positions (ET: patient must have injured his old stiff hip).

The physical examination revealed good posture and full painless lumbar physiological movements in all directions. He was a bit sore to postero-anterior glides to the right of the L5 spinous process, but the most significant findings were his restricted hip movements which were worse on the right (ET: this stiff hip will have to be mobilized).

471

Therapist Two's summary of his examination findings (ET = examiner's thoughts)

A 45-year-old plumber presented with complaints of an ache in his 'hip' localized to just below the right iliac crest with no symptoms in any other areas. This was clarified further by asking about the depth of ache while rotating the hip for the patient to feel. He reported that the ache felt higher in the buttock and more superficial than where he felt his hip being moved. (ET: atypical for hip, must consider lumbar spine, sacro-iliac joint, local soft tissues, neural structures and the hip itself as potential sources of the symptoms). His main problem was a general ache after walking for more than 20 minutes. It was not related to any specific phase of his gait, never built up, and settled completely within 5 minutes of sitting down (ET: mechanical, non-irritable, non-inflammatory disorder). Sitting would ease the ache, and getting up from sitting was not a problem. Lying in any position but prone would settle the ache and he felt best if his knees were bent up. (ET: spinal and/or lower limb extension are more implicated). When questioned about specific activities and postures which might implicate other sources, he remembered feeling a slight ache a few times when twisting right to reverse the car. All other activities and postures which may have implicated lumbar, neural, sacro-iliac or hip sources (e.g. bending, lifting, sustained flexion, crossing legs, using stairs, stepping off curb, dressing, squatting) were negative (ET: source of symptoms is less likely to be muscle, sacro-iliac joint, hip or lumbar disc). Squatting is another action that gives him difficulty. He has found getting into a full squat position progressively more difficult over the past 5 years. He doesn't get any discomfort when squatting, but the hips feel 'stiff' and he feels certain that this hasn't been any different since having the hip ache (ET: not likely to be the direct source of his symptoms but may well be a contributing factor). Sleeping was not a problem (ET: supports disorder being non-inflammatory). This all started 3 weeks ago when he was trying to loosen a tight fitting and the wrench slipped. He was kneeling and leaning forward under a kitchen sink at the time, and as the wrench let go his body twisted quickly to the right with a sudden jab of pain. He didn't lose his kneeling position and fall backwards, and, from his demonstration, most movement occurred at the trunk (ET: this could fit with lumbar joint, neural tissue, sacro-iliac or muscle/fascia in the lumbar-pelvic area—however, the hip joint continues to be the less likely). He worked on with only slight ache and had no difficulty standing up after about 10 minutes (ET: posterior intervertebral joint not locked). It has stayed the same since and he hasn't had any other treatment or tried any tablets. There was no significant past history except the 5 years of progressive hip stiffness.

On physical examination, sitting and twisting right to simulate reversing the car was not a problem, but, when various combined movements were assessed in this position, the combination of right rotation, extension, then right lateral flexion reproduced his ache. There was no change when neck flexion, knee extension or hip movements were altered from this combined position (ET: this supported lumbar spine but not the hip joint or neural tension). He had good posture with no pelvic asymmetries, and conventional spinal movements were all full and painless, although the ache was again reproduced with the same movement combination in standing. All sacro-iliac, neural tension and resisted static contraction tests were negative (ET: lumbar joints were still highest on the list of sources). Hip examination revealed painless stiffness in all directions especially flexion, flexion/adduction and internal rotation, right being more limited than left (ET: this supports the idea that the hip is not the source of the symptoms, but it fits in with the patient's difficulty in squatting, and may be a contributing factor requiring treatment). There was marked thickening over the right L5/S1 posterior intervertebral joint which was hypomobile to posterior-anterior accessory movement testing but only produced minimal local soreness. When this was re-assessed in a combined posture to simulate the combined movement findings, the local soreness was accentuated and the right 'hip' ache was reproduced (ET: these are the local signs expected for posterior intervertebral joint involvement)

Comparison of the reasoning of Therapist One with that of Therapist Two

What is the difference between the reasoning of these two therapists? Therapist One did appear to be reasoning logically. He was not blindly following a referral, neither was he so biased as to examine only the patient's perception of the problem, the hip. Was the different conclusion of Therapist Two simply the result of a more thorough routine examination, or was Therapist Two actually reasoning differently when compared with Therapist One? That is, what factors guided the specific questions and physical tests of each therapist, and what—if any—were the deficiences in reasoning of Therapist One? Hopefully, it will become evident throughout this chapter that it was Therapist Two who applied the more skilled clinical reasoning by using an hypothesis-directed inquiry.

CLINICAL REASONING

Clinical reasoning can be defined as the thinking skills and knowledge (facts, procedures, concepts, principles and patterns) used to make clinical decisions and judgements through the evaluation, diagnosis and management of a patient problem (Jones 1987, Higgs 1990). The clinical reasoning process is a description of the actions and evolving

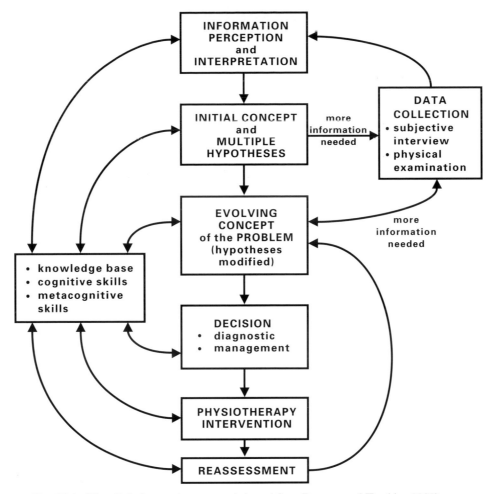

Fig. 34.1 The clinical reasoning process (adapted from Barrows and Tamblyn 1980).

thoughts used by a clinician to arrive at a diagnostic and management decision and subsequently administer and advance the patient's treatment.

Extensive research has been conducted on the topic of clinical reasoning (under numerous synonyms and related topics including problem solving, decision making, decision analysis and judgement) in diverse fields such as medicine, psychology, artificial intelligence, programming, law, mathematics, engineering and physics (Chi et al 1988, Downie & Elstein 1988). Different paradigms have been used to investigate various aspects of clinical reasoning. These range from 'information processing' studies, where the aim is to describe the intellectual processes used by clinicians examining patients and making decisions, to the approach of 'artificial intelligence' where the knowledge used by clinicians in making diagnostic and management decisions is encoded on a computer for use in simulating the 'expert', and 'decision analytic' studies, which mathematically combine data to determine the optimal strategy in a clinical situation. All these areas of research offer valuable insight into the growing understanding of clinical reasoning. They provide physiotherapy with research

methodology for conducting our own clinical reasoning investigations and hold immediate clinical and educational applications for improving our clinical reasoning skills. A principal aim of this chapter is to present a descriptive model of clinical reasoning in an attempt to portray how clinical decisions are made. For a more prescriptive approach in identifying the optimal clinical decisions the reader is referred to the 'decision analysis' literature (Weinstein et al 1980, Watts 1985, Downie & Elstein 1988, Watts 1989).

THE CLINICAL REASONING PROCESS

The early medical education studies analysed clinicians' thoughts (e.g. perceptions, interpretations, plans) either retrospectively as they thought aloud through a video or audio playback of a patient examination just completed, or concurrently as they read a patient's unfolding clinical history (Barrows et al 1978, 1980, 1982, Elstein et al 1978, Neufeld et al 1981, Gale & Marsden 1983). A general clinical reasoning process was described as hypothetico-deductive. Clinicians were seen to develop multiple diagnostic hypotheses early in the patient encounter which then served to guide their inquiry in an hypothesis-testing manner to support or refute these hypotheses. Additional information would lead to an evolving picture of the problem as working hypotheses were modified.

Clinical reasoning was investigated only through the initial examination of a patient in these medically based studies, and the only hypotheses considered were the medical clinicians' diagnostic hypotheses. Figure 34.1 illustrates the clinical reasoning process used by physiotherapists. This diagram has been adapted from one by Barrows and Tamblyn (1980) with modifications to highlight the continuation of the clinical reasoning process throughout the ongoing physiotherapy management. Diagnosis is only one category of hypothesis physiotherapists must consider. Other categories of hypothesis are discussed in detail later.

The clinical reasoning process begins with the clinician's perception and interpretation of initial cues from the patient. Even in the opening moments of greeting a patient, the clinician will perceive specific cues such as the patient's age, appearance, facial expressions, movement patterns, resting posture and any spontaneous comments.

These initial cues from the patient should elicit an initial concept of the problem that includes preliminary working hypotheses for consideration through the rest of the subjective and physical examination as well as the ongoing patient management. If the patient in the opening example limped into the treatment room with an apparent attempt to decrease weight-bearing through the right leg followed by a spontaneous comment of needing to sit to rest his hip, the therapist would naturally have already formed some idea (a working hypothesis) as to the structure(s) at fault. While the hip may be an obvious possibility, the therapist should also be considering other possible structures (e.g. lumbar joints, sacro-iliac joint, neural tension, etc.) which could give or contribute to this presentation.

Further information (data collection) is then sought throughout the subjective and physical examination with these working hypotheses in mind. Information might include site and behaviour of symptoms, specific questions pertaining to general health, investigations, medications, history, posture, behaviour of symptoms and quality of movement during active and passive physiological and passive accessory movements, muscle performance, including quality of contraction, length, strength, and endurance. The specific information sought, the order in which it is obtained, and the emphasis it is given will vary depending on the therapist's individual philosophy.

It is important to recognize here that the physical examination, like the subjective, is not a routine series of tests. There may be specific physical tests that are scanned for different areas, but these should be an extension of the

hypothesis testing performed through the subjective examination. Hypotheses regarding precautions and contraindications to physical examination and treatment will guide the extent to which the physical examination and first treatment can be performed without risk of aggravating the patient's disorder. The physical examination is then used to test hypotheses regarding potential sources of symptoms and contributing factors in such a way that each structure that could be implicated is specifically examined.

Despite differences in information obtained and the significance it holds for different therapists, the underlying reasoning process should be similar. That is, the initial working hypotheses should guide the therapist's direction of examination (questions and physical tests) within those aspects of patient information sought by the therapist. With the addition of new information through the ongoing data collection the initial hypotheses are refined, re-ranked or ruled out, or perhaps new ones are added. In this way the therapist acquires an evolving concept of the patient's problem. While area, behaviour, and history of the symptoms along with active, passive and resistive tests may be scanned with most patients, the specific questions and physical tests should vary in accordance with the evolving hypotheses. The clinical reasoning through the patient examination continues until sufficient information is obtained to make a diagnostic and/or management decision.

The clinical reasoning process does not stop when the patient has been examined. Rather, the therapist will have reached the management decisions as to whether or not to treat; whether to address the source(s), contributing factor(s) or both initially; which mode of treatment to use initially (e.g. passive movement, modalities, exercise, etc.); if passive treatment is to be used, whether to provoke symptoms, the direction of movement, grade of movement, amplitude and rhythm of movement etc. The clinical reasoning process can then be seen to continue throughout the physiotherapy intervention. Every treatment, whether it is hands-on or advice, should be a form of hypothesis testing. Continual re-assessment is essential and provides the empirical evidence on which our hypotheses are accepted or rejected. Re-assessment should contribute to the therapist's evolving concept of the patient's problem. This evolving concept should elicit clinical decisions regarding progression of treatment (e.g. continue same or modify) and may necessitate the need for additional data collection.

The clinical reasoning process portrayed in Figure 34.1 is designed to highlight the evolving thoughts which should occur through the examination of a patient and during ongoing treatment. Higgs (1990) highlights the importance of the ability to monitor conscious thoughts (metacognition) to a therapist's clinical reasoning. That is, therapists' attention to the thoughts behind their actions should facilitate more efficient and effective management of the patient. This will become more evident later when errors in clinical reasoning are discussed.

The box on the left in Figure 34.1 emphasizes the crucial relationship that exists between the therapist's knowledge base, cognitive skills (e.g. data analysis, synthesis and evaluation, and problem-solving strategies) and metacognitive skills and all aspects of the clinical reasoning process. The two-way arrows highlight the reciprocal relationship where clinical reasoning experiences, as outlined here, will, in turn, contribute to the therapist's knowledge base, cognitive and metacognitive skills. For example, each time therapists reason through a patient's problem, their current knowledge should be either supported or challenged. It is recognition of discrepancies between the therapist's existing knowledge and understanding of a patient's problem which facilitates continued learning.

Other important factors not highlighted in the clinical reasoning process illustrated in Figure 34.1 include interpersonal and clinical skills. These skills will clearly influence data collection, physiotherapy intervention and re-assessment. Thus, the success of one's clinical reasoning can be attributed to a combination of thinking, interpersonal and clinical skills combined with an organized and accessible knowledge base.

CATEGORIES OF HYPOTHESIS

The focus for the medically-based studies on clinical reasoning has been the medical clinician's diagnostic hypotheses. The physiotherapist's examination is aimed at not only identifying the source of the symptoms (i.e. diagnosis) but also identifying an appropriate management plan that often includes the therapist's own physical treatment. To achieve these aims efficiently and safely we must acquire information regarding the following categories of hypothesis:

1. source of the symptoms and/or dysfunction
2. contributing factors
3. precautions and contraindications to physical examination and treatment
4. management
5. prognosis.

That is, information regarding these categories of hypothesis should be sought with all patients regardless of their presenting complaint. The different categories of hypothesis are not necessarily pursued separately; rather, the therapist should be prepared to interpret information about the patient as it relates to any category of hypothesis, and frequently more than one category will be considered concurrently. This is not a chapter to present the content of examination; however, a diversion to describe further these categories of hypothesis will provide some insight into the 'organization of knowledge' unique to manipulative therapy, which, as will be discussed later, is critical to the nature of expertise in this speciality.

Source of the symptoms and/or dysfunction

Information regarding the different categories of hypothesis is available within each of the major aspects of the patient's presentation scanned by the therapist. For example, hypotheses regarding 'source of the symptoms and/or dysfunction' are often available in the opening moments of an encounter—as with the patient who walks in with an obvious list or stands with one knee flexed to minimize his back and leg pain. Further information regarding the source of the symptoms is available through learning the exact site of symptoms, as different structures have recognized patterns of symptoms (Trott 1985, Aprill et al 1990, Dwyer et al 1990). Naturally, any single piece of information, especially information such as site of symptoms—some of which are still only empirically recognized—makes conclusive structural differentiation at this stage impossible. Rather, each newly acquired clue should be clarified for accuracy and then considered in the light of the building clinical picture and working hypotheses. In this way, the patient's spontaneous account of what troubles he is having (i.e. behaviour of symptoms, or physical limitations) allows the therapist to interpret the specific aggravating activity or limitation as to what structures are involved and match this against the evolving list of structures considered to this point. Active consideration of the working hypotheses also allows the therapist to direct inquiry toward those structures as a further test of their involvement. For example, a patient complaining of hip pain may spontaneously describe difficulty in bending over from the upright position when working in the garden. If further questioning revealed that the patient had no difficulty squatting fully, this may be sufficient to alter the ranking of possible structures at fault—with the hip now occurring lower than others such as lumbar joints, muscles and structures of the nervous system. These hypotheses are then tested further through other aspects of symptom behaviour (e.g. relationship with other symptoms present; what eases the symptoms) as well as via the present and past history.

Contributing factors

Any predisposing or associated factor in the development and/or maintenance of the patient's problem, be it environmental, behavioural, emotional, physical or biomechanical, is a contributing factor. Examples include inadequate work stations, a change in sporting technique, stressful personal problems, poor posture and unequal leg length. As with 'sources' discussed above, initial clues may be evident in the opening moments and the therapist must continue to recognize potential contributing factors as the examination continues and, where possible, test any contributing factor hypothesis that does arise. For example, a patient may appear unusually tense and fidgety, eliciting an hypothesis that 'tension' and its predisposing factors might be contributing to the patient's complaint of headaches. This should then be pursued with hypothesis-testing questions to establish whether a relationship exists between any such predisposing factors and the patient's headaches. What is the pattern of headaches and are they associated with any stressful circumstances/situations? Equally important, can the headaches ever occur without such associated stressful circumstances such as weekends or holidays? Contributing factors should be considered separately from the source of the symptoms and specific hypotheses developed about them. The C2/3 posterior intervertebral joint may be the source of the patient's headache, but recent personal problems and an easily corrected forward head posture may be significant contributing factors. The thoracic joints may be the source of local thoracic and referred chest pain with poor posture and muscular endurance the contributing factor. Whether treatment should address the source(s), the contributing factor(s), or both, is yet another clinical decision which will be determined by the weight given to the different factors and—importantly—the continued clinical reasoning through the ongoing management.

Precautions and contradictions to physical treatment

Hypotheses formed here will dictate the extent of the physical examination (i.e. how far specific movements are performed or taken and how many movements are tested) and whether physical treatment is indicated and, if so, how much (e.g. short of pain, into pain, etc.). Factors which determine these hypotheses include the severity and irritability of the disorder, whether the disorder is progressive, its rate of impairment, the stability (i.e. predictability/variability) of the disorder, general health and the presence of any indicators such as unexplained weight loss or relevant difficulties with bowel and bladder control. Questions and physical tests here can also be described as hypothesis testing. For further information regarding definitions, examples and significance of these factors the reader is referred to Maitland (1986).

Prognosis

Hypotheses regarding prognosis enable the clinician to discuss with the patient expectations of extent and time span for recovery. All therapists will recognize the difficulty with this type of hypothesis; however, attempts to consider prognosis will serve to direct one's attention to those factors in the patient's presentation which influence the outcome. Examples of such factors include the mechanical versus inflammatory balance of the disorder, irritability of the disorder, degree of damage/injury, length of history and progression of the disorder, pre-existing disorders, patient's expectations, patient's personality and lifestyle and patient's healing potential. Prognosis is never so straightforward that all factors are positive or negative, but rather a combination of both will be present. Consideration of these positives and negatives will usually lead to a prognostic picture that is favourable or not. By attempting to judge the extent and time for recovery the therapist creates the opportunity to reflect on errors in prediction which will, in turn, assist in recognizing the relative significance of these different factors in future patient presentations.

Management

Clues that enable the formation of management hypotheses are available from the patient's chief complaint, site of symptoms, behaviour of symptoms (e.g. aggravating and easing factors, irritability, 24 hour pattern), precautionary questions, onset and progression of symptoms, mechanism of injury, past treatment, pain threshold, personality, physical examination and ongoing management. The patient in the opening example clearly had a mechanical, non-inflammatory disorder that could safely be treated with passive techniques provoking pain at the stiff symptomatic joint. A patient sitting in the waiting room in a semiflexed and right laterally flexed posture leaning off his left buttock may be demonstrating a combined movement position for use in treatment if a pain-easing/non-provoking technique was required and this proved to be his most comfortable position. Conversely, a detailed analysis of a ballet dancer's jump that causes low-back pain may provide an essential clue to the angle at which a passive technique will have to be directed. In other words, whether passive techniques, muscle re-education or work site modification are used, the clues will be found throughout the subjective examination, physical examination and ongoing management.

THE NATURE OF EXPERTISE

The superior clinical reasoning skill of the expert has been too easily explained by words such as 'intuition', 'judgement' and 'experience' which seem to discourage any further search for how the expert actually thinks and subsequently how these thinking skills should be taught. What is it that differentiates the recognized clinical 'experts' in physiotherapy? What were the errors of reasoning made by Therapist One in the opening example, and do 'experts' make errors? Extensive research has been carried out in medicine and other fields to clarify the nature of expertise.

Early expert/novice studies were conducted in chess,

comparing the thought processes and representation of knowledge of chess masters to that of novices (DeGroot 1965, Chase & Simon 1973). Short-term memory experiments revealed that experts have a remarkable ability to reconstruct a chess board almost perfectly after viewing it for only seconds. In contrast, there was a dramatic drop off of this ability below the master level. No differences were found between the expert and novice with the same experiment using randomly placed chess pieces, precluding the notion that the results could be attributed to superior memory. With experts and novices constrained by the same short-term memory, the authors concluded that experts have a superior ability to perceive patterns in chess positions and encode these as chunks in their memory. A chunk is anything that is recognized as a single unit by the familiarity acquired through previous repeated exposure. Short-term memories have the capacity of only four to seven chunks (Simon 1979, 1981), necessitating that the expert acquire larger and more elaborate chunks to manage effectively the volume of information frequently encountered.

These early chess studies influenced the pioneering investigations of medical clinical reasoning where clinicians were found to use a general hypothetico-deductive process as described in Figure 34.1. However, these early investigations of medical clinical reasoning failed to identify a consistent differentiating feature of the process between experts and novices. Students were seen to use the same hypothesis testing process as experts and no differences were found on a number of process variables, including data gathering and hypotheses-related parameters (Feltovich & Barrows 1984, Norman et al 1990). Feltovich and Barrows (1984) concluded that the best indicator of competent clinical reasoning is the clinician's conceptualization of the problem as reflected by the quality (as judged by expert standards) of hypotheses considered.

Further attempts to replicate and extend the DeGroot (1965) and Chase and Simon (1973) studies in medicine have demonstrated similar findings as to experts' and novices' representation of knowledge (Chi et al 1981, Lesgold et al 1981, Muzzin et al 1983, Feltovich et al 1984, Patel & Frederiksen 1984, Patel et al 1986, Patel & Groen 1986). Patel et al (1986) showed that expert clinicians recalled more information in patterns and made significantly more inferences about the clinically relevant information, while novices made more verbatim recall of the surface features and remembered more irrelevant details.

The search for understanding expert reasoning has continued with growing debate over the existence of the process(es) used by experts and novices and the appropriate methodology to use in research (Berner 1984, McGuire 1984, Groen & Patel 1985, Patel & Groen 1986, Barrows & Feltovich 1987, Norman 1988, Barrows 1990, Bordage et al 1990, Norman et al 1990). Descriptions of expert reasoning have ranged from purely inductive

pattern recognition to combined inductive and deductive reasoning as occurs in the hypothetico-deductive model. The only real consensus is that experts have a superior organization of knowledge (Feltovich et al 1984, Glaser 1984, Bordage & Lemieux 1986, Grant & Marsden 1987, 1988, Chi et al 1988, Bordage et al 1990, Patel et al 1990).

Patel et al (1986) portrayed the expert clinician as having a more highly developed knowledge base that includes a store of patterns that can be recognized and procedural rules that guide actions, interpretations and inferences made from information obtained.

Bordage and Lemieux (1986) added that the organization of knowledge in memory goes beyond a simple list of signs, symptoms and rules, and includes abstract qualitative relationships such as 'local–general' or 'constant–intermittent' which contribute to the expert's representation of a case.

Thus, the effectiveness of one's clinical reasoning appears largely dependent on the individual's organization of knowledge. Less experienced therapists would have less developed and fewer variations of patterns stored in their memory, causing them difficulty in selecting relevant from irrelevant information. The inexperience of the novice leaves him/her with only those patterns which have been learned through texts. The patterns recognized by novices are excessively rigid, and the inability to recognize relevant information leads them to act indiscriminately on every detail. Furthermore, the novice has a newly acquired pathophysiological knowledge base which, in traditional models of education, has not been linked with the signs and symptoms of the relevant patient presentations. Thus, when initially confronting patients, the novice actively attempts to relate the patient's symptoms to this pathophysiological knowledge base in order to understand the patient's problem. This lesser developed knowledge base and strict reliance on pathophysiological interpretations makes the novice's clinical reasoning more cognitively demanding and inefficient. In contrast, the expert has integrated the pathophysiological knowledge with the relevant clinical patterns. The expert's organization of knowledge is more highly developed, and since it is built on individual experiences, clinical patterns may be idiosyncratic and may not necessarily match the patterns of other clinicians or the textbook (Schmidt et al 1990).

The organization of knowledge relevant to physiotherapy would include the facts (e.g. anatomy, pathophysiology, etc.), procedures (e.g. examination and treatment strategies and techniques), concepts (e.g. irritability, adverse neural tension) and patterns of presentation. This knowledge is utilized with the assistance of rules or principles (e.g. selection of grade of passive movement technique, Maitland 1986, 1987) to acquire, interpret, infer, and collate patient information.

Expert physiotherapists also appear to use more efficient search strategies (e.g. advanced communication, physical examination and treatment progression skills) and more effective cognitive skills, although this is yet to be validated (Grant et al 1988).

While the medical literature has suggested that all clinicians use hypothesis testing, the author's personal experience in teaching clinical reasoning suggests that this general skill occurs with differing degrees of proficiency among students.

The expert's superior organization of knowledge allows for solution of a typical problem almost automatically through recognition of clinical patterns. However, when faced with an atypical problem, the expert, like the novice, must rely more on the hypothetico-deductive (i.e. hypotheses testing) method of reasoning to solve it.

It should be apparent that solution of a patient's problem is not derived from simple application of a clinical reasoning process, nor a vast knowledge of facts. Rather, it is dependent on the therapist's organization of knowledge and cognitive skills. Therefore, to improve clinical reasoning, therapists should attempt to improve both organization of knowledge and clinical reasoning abilities. Experience in years alone will not ensure that one's organization of knowledge and cognitive skills will grow. This requires experience using a clinical reasoning process as described here, a process that is founded in the logic of hypothesis testing while encouraging open-mindedness and lateral thinking. When features do not fit, further inquiry is indicated to understand better any discrepancies that exist. In this way we can continually test our present understanding of different patterns, and in the process, acquire new ones. The experts in our profession are such, not simply on the basis of years of experience or superior handling skills, but because they have highly developed knowledge bases acquired through advanced clinical reasoning where critical thinking has allowed them to formulate a larger repertoire of clinical patterns which they can recognize. It has been estimated that the grandmaster chess player has 50 000 familiar chunks stored in long-term memory. This appears to be consistent with experts in other domains where even the most talented individuals require approximately 10 years to achieve the highest professional proficiency (Simon 1981). Thus, there is no short cut to expertise; however, attention to one's clinical reasoning should hasten the process.

ERRORS IN REASONING

The summary of Therapist One in the opening example does not reflect the extent of reasoning errors. Surprisingly, even direct observation of Therapist One examining and treating the patient would not reveal many of the reasoning errors which become evident when attempting to gain access to the therapist's ongoing thoughts. When this was done retrospectively, Therapist One was clearly not reasoning through the patient's examination. Instead,

he was following a routine series of questions and tests, merely collecting information and making the simplest level of interpretations, with to attempt to collate information or test hypotheses. The only real extension of the subjective examination to the physical examination was the therapist's biased attention to the patient's continual reference to his 'hip'. Other potential structures at fault were inadequately examined, allowing Therapist One to be misled by the hip stiffness without truly testing its relevance to the patient's present problem. Therapist One's physical examination was a combination of routine tests not tailored to the specific patient. He over-attended to those findings (e.g. stiff hip) that supported the one hypothesis he had maintained from the opening moments of the encounter with the patient. The continued hypothesis testing which must occur through the ongoing reassessment of treatment was also lacking as only the hip mobility and subjective report were re-assessed, further supporting the therapist's misinterpretation that the hip was the source of symptoms.

In contrast, Therapist Two was actively reasoning from the start. The patient's opening description of site of symptoms elicited a working hypothesis regarding source(s) of the symptoms which included several potential structures. Further questioning can be seen to scan the same general categories of information as did Therapist One's questions; however, the search for details were tailored to this specific patient and the evolving hypotheses being considered. When information was not spontaneously forthcoming, as with aggravating factors, Therapist Two would specifically question other possible aggravating factors. This served as a test of the different potential sources and can be seen as attending to the negating as well as the supporting features of a problem. Therapist Two's physical examination was clearly an extension of the subjective where structures were examined to test the hypotheses of sources and contributing factors and not simply a routine followed with all patients. This was most apparent with his use of a functional aggravating position to differentiate the most likely source and identify a combined movement position which later proved useful as a clue to how the minimal lumbar passive accessory intervertebral movement sign could be accentuated.

Errors of reasoning can obviously occur through any stage of the clinical reasoning process, including errors of perception, interpretation, inquiry, synthesis and planning. 'Experts' also make errors, as demonstrated by the tendency, even for those clinicians who arrive at the correct conclusion, to overemphasize positive findings, ignore or misinterpret negative findings, deny findings that conflict with a favourite hypothesis and obtain redundant information (Elstein et al 1978, Lesgold et al 1981, Feltovich et al 1984, Voytovich et al 1985).

What is it that causes a clinician to misinterpret information or fail to consider a highly probable hypothesis?

Errors of interpretation and synthesis may be related less to the clinician's limited amount of medical or clinical knowledge than one might think, and more so to the clinician's inadequate organization of that knowledge limiting the ability to retrieve relevant knowledge already stored in memory (Bordage & Allen 1982, Bordage & Zacks 1984, Bordage et al 1990). Reasoning errors are often unrecognized, as even skilled therapists rarely consider their own clinical reasoning as suggested here.

Physiotherapy school provides the foundation of our clinical practice. Curricula should therefore include the thinking or clinical reasoning skills necessary to test continually our knowledge base and acquire new knowledge and new clinical patterns.

IMPLICATIONS FOR EDUCATION

The research cited throughout this chapter is principally based in medical education. As alluded to previously, the information sought in a medical examination will differ from that required by a physiotherapist. While some evidence does suggest that the medical and physiotherapy clinical reasoning processes are similar (Payton 1985, Dennis & May 1987, Thomas-Edding 1987) and theoretical reflection on physiotherapy clinical decision making is increasing (Wolf 1985, Grant et al 1988, Jones 1989, Rothstein 1989), further research clarifying the clinical reasoning process and nature of expertise in physiotherapy is necessary.

Meanwhile, attempts to teach clinical reasoning should continue—with attention given to students' organization of knowledge, the importance of which is now recognized across numerous professional domains. Glaser (1984, p 99) stated that 'Effective thinking is the result of conditionalized knowledge—the knowledge that becomes associated with the conditions and constraints of its use'. Thus the facts, procedures, concepts, principles and patterns unique to manipulative physiotherapy need to be linked with the conditions and constraints of their use, or integrated into learning experiences with patients' problems. This principle of facilitating the acquisition of knowledge through teaching centred around patients' problems is promoted throughout the health education literature (Barr 1977, May 1977a, b, Barrows & Tamblyn 1980, Willems 1981, Schmidt 1983, Schmidt & DeVolder 1984, Boud 1985, Titchen 1987a, b, Burnett & Pierson 1988, Jones 1989, Slaughter et al 1989, Walton & Matthews 1989). In this way knowledge is paired with the appropriate retrieval cues to facilitate its recall in clinical situations (Tulving & Thompson 1973, Rumelhart & Ortony 1977). While this is clearly not a new educational principle, its application to clinical reasoning still appears to be lacking in physiotherapy undergraduate and postgraduate curricula.

Physiotherapy subject content should be linked with the clinical reasoning guiding its use. That is, clinical reasoning should be incorporated into all physiotherapy subjects (e.g. orthopaedics, neurology, cardiothoracics, etc.). This, combined with the continual use of patients' problems, will facilitate the acquisition of relevant knowledge that is retrievable in clinical situations. While courses which teach thinking or problem-solving as a specific skill have existed for years (De Bono 1977, 1978, Rubinstein 1980, Tuma & Reif 1980, Nickerson et al 1985), the value and transfer ability of general domain independent problem-solving skills remain in doubt (Norman 1990). Content and clinical reasoning integrated subjects are still relatively uncommon in physiotherapy (May & Dennis 1987, Jones 1988, Higgs 1990, Carr & Scutter 1991), with further experience and evaluation needed to determine their value.

A subject incorporating clinical reasoning should give students the opportunity to encounter patients' problems with attention given to both the reasoning process and the organization of knowledge. Students should not only be taught to think, but also to think about their thinking (Schon 1983, Higgs 1990, Schon 1990). In this way, examination and management strategies are not learned as rigid routines and rules; rather, the student acquires the appropriate knowledge together with an understanding of when and why that knowledge is relevant. The student should learn a clinical reasoning process which is active throughout the patient's examination and ongoing management. This will enable the student continually to test existing knowledge and, in turn, acquire new knowledge to increase the repertoire of clinical patterns which can be recognized.

Numerous formats for presenting patients' problems are available—including both real and simulated patients. Experience with real patients is invaluable. Students can utilize all aspects of the clinical reasoning process while working under the pressures, responsibilities and rewards to the real world. No other form of problem format can match the variations and unpredictability that can occur with real patients. The principal difficulty with teaching clinical reasoning using real patients is in gaining access to students' ongoing thoughts. The interpretative and planning elements of the clinical reasoning process can only be inferred from observed behaviour. This is inadequate as a student may go through the correct motions of an examination or treatment with surprisingly incorrect reasoning. Interruptions to gain access to students' thoughts (e.g. 'What did you make of that?', 'What are you thinking now?', 'How would you summarize what you've learned thus far?', 'What are your working hypotheses at this stage?') are effective, but interruptions can be distracting to both patient and student and must be used selectively. Retrospective thoughts can be obtained by having students complete a 'clinical reasoning form' at key points through the encounter with the patient (e.g. after subjective examination, physical examination, first treatment, third treatment and discharge). Here, students must reflect on their reasoning and answer questions which will reveal their perceptions, interpretations and ongoing planning. Variations of this form are in use at each of the manipulative therapy programmes in Australia, and one example is included here in the Appendix.

Patients' problems can also be effectively presented using various forms of simulated patients, including individuals trained to role-play patients' problems, less costly teacher or student role playing, patients' problems in written form, and real patients' problems on video tape (Barrows & Tamblyn 1980, Stillman et al 1986, Jones 1988). Whichever format is used, students need to be given the opportunity to reason through the problem. The instructor should act as a facilitator, assisting students to recognize the different aspects of the clinical reasoning process while directing and reinforcing their acquisition of knowledge relevant to each problem. Role playing has the added advantage of allowing students to perform their own inquiries following their own line of reasoning. Students can work in pairs or in larger groups, alternating as patient or therapist. Video-taped encounters with patients enable students to observe more experienced therapists and additionally provide an excellent resource for a student's independent study. With each of these formats, the action should be stopped at different points, with students prompted to identify observations, interpretations (i.e. working hypotheses) and plans as well as continually to reflect on how these relate to the clinical reasoning process itself (e.g. hypothesis formation, hypothesis testing, inquiry strategies, etc.).

Modification of the teaching methods and educational materials to facilitate clinical reasoning requires that consideration also be given to the methods by which clinical reasoning is assessed. No one assessment method can assess all the knowledge, skills and personal qualities which comprise the repertoire of a competent practitioner. It is not possible in the scope of this chapter to discuss the relative merits, validity and reliability of the various assessment methods available. However, a review of the literature suggests that no single assessment method appears adequate to assess all aspects of clinical reasoning efficiently, and as such, multiple assessment formats are warranted (Jones 1989). Those considered by this author to be most effective are direct observation and the modified essay question (MEQ) in either written or video form.

Direct observation requires clearly established behavioural criteria for performance. It also requires interventions to gain access to students' thoughts, such as stimulus questions interjected either during the encounter or incorporated in a short answer interpretation form. Rater reliability should be tested and, if necessary, improved through training sessions.

The MEQ has been described in both the physiotherapy and medical education literature as a written examination format used for assessing clinical reasoning (Hodgkin and Knox 1975, Stratford & Pierce-Fenn 1985, Feletti & Smith 1986). Patients' data are provided in stages (written or video form) followed by questions which require short written (essay) answers. To simulate the natural temporal sequence of an encounter with a patient, the MEQ does not permit students to preview items, nor to turn back and change decisions on earlier items. This allows access to students' evolving reasoning as the patient's story unfolds.

SUMMARY

In reading this chapter, many therapists will recognize their own use of a reasoning process, only without the formal 'hypotheses' jargon as used here. That is, clinical reasoning is something that most clinicians practise without having thought specifically about it. Similarly, most educators would argue that they not only teach facts but also teach students to think, to know when and where such facts are relevant and provide as much clinical experience as possible. However, what proportion of the clinical experience is devoted to routine practice of what was learned in the classroom versus the use of clinical experience as a means of developing clinical reasoning skills and of acquiring the relevant knowledge in the context in which it will be used later? Therapists may well be taught to think, but should also be taught to think about their thinking. While the process(es) of clinical reasoning and differentiation of expertise in physiotherapy require further investigation, both practising therapists and students can improve their clinical reasoning through the ongoing process of reflection. By consideration of one's reasoning during and after an encounter with a patient, therapists can identify poor reasoning habits such as failure to consider negating features and overattention to those features that support a favourite hypothesis. Therapists differ in the attention and significance they give to the numerous clues available from patients. However, all therapists should consider and test multiple hypotheses throughout the examination of the patient and during ongoing management.

Clinical reasoning enhances the acquisition of new knowledge and broadens the therapist's repertoire of clinical patterns which can be recognized. The acquisition of expertise by individuals, and advancement of the whole profession, would be promoted by the broader range of knowledge and opinions that could be developed through widespread adoption of clinical reasoning by physiotherapists. The challenge should be to increase the attention given to the clinical reasoning of students and to encourage practising therapists to reflect on their clinical reasoning processes.

REFERENCES

Aprill C, Dwyer A, Bogduk N 1990 Cervical zygapophyseal joint pain Patterns II. Spine 15: 458–461

Barr J S 1977 A problem-solving curriculum design in physical therapy. Physical Therapy 57: 262–270

Barrows H S 1990 Inquiry: the pedagogical importance of a skill central to clinical practice. Medical Education 24: 3–5

Barrows H S, Feltovich P J 1987 The clinical reasoning process. Medical Education 21: 86–91

Barrows H S, Tamblyn R M 1980 Problem-based learning: an approach to medical education. Springer, New York

Barrows H S, Feightner J W, Neufeld V R, Norman G R 1978 Analysis of the clinical methods of medical students and physicians. Report to the Ontario Department of Health, McMaster University, Hamilton

Barrows H S, Norman G R, Neufeld V R, Feightner J W 1982 The clinical reasoning of randomly selected physicians in general medical practice. Clinical and Investigative Medicine 5: 49–55

Berner E S 1984 Paradigms and problem-solving: a literature review. Journal of Medical Education 59: 625–633

Bordage G, Allen T 1982 The etiology of diagnostic errors: process or content? An exploratory study. Proceedings of the 21st Conference on Research in Medical Education, Washington, pp 171–176

Bordage G, Lemieux M A 1986 Some cognitive characteristics of medical students with and without diagnostic reasoning difficulties. Proceedings of the 25th Annual Conference on Research in Medical Education, New Orleans, pp 185–190

Bordage G, Zacks R 1984 The structure of medical knowledge in the memories of medical students and general practitioners: categories and prototypes. Medical Education 18: 406–416

Bordage, G, Grant J, Marsden P 1990 Quantitative assessment of diagnostic ability. Medical Education 24: 413–425

Boud D 1985 Problem-based learning in education for the professions. Higher Education Research and Development Society of Australia, University of New South Wales, Kensington

Burnett C N, Pierson F M 1988 Developing problem-solving skills in the classroom. Physical Therapy 69: 441–447

Carr J A, Scutter S D 1991 Curriculum innovation in first year physiotherapy. Proceedings of the Eleventh International Congress of the World Confederation for Physical Therapy, London, pp 158–160

Chase W G, Simon H A 1973 Perception in chess. Cognitive Psychology 4: 55–81

Chi M T H, Feltovich P J, Glaser R 1981 Categorization and representation of physics problems by experts and novices. Cognitive Science 5: 121–152

Chi M T H, Glaser R, Farr M J 1988 The nature of expertise. Lawrence Erlbaum, Hillsdale

De Bono E 1977 Lateral thinking. Penguin Books, London

De Bono E 1978 Teaching thinking. Penguin Books, London

DeGroot A D 1965 Thought and choice in chess. Basic Books, New York

Dennis J K, May B J 1987 Practice in the year 2000: expert decision making in physical therapy. Proceedings of the 10th International Congress of the World Confederation of Physical Therapy, Sydney, pp 543–551

Downie J, Elstein A (eds) 1988 Professional judgment: a reader in clinical decision making. Cambridge University Press, Cambridge

Dwyer A, Aprill C, Bogduk N 1990 Cervical zygapophyseal joint pain patterns I: a study in normal volunteers. Spine 15: 453–457

Elstein A S, Shulman L S, Sprafka S S 1978 An analysis of clinical reasoning. Harvard University Press, Cambridge

Feletti G I, Smith E K M 1986 Modified essay questions: are they worth the effort? Medical Education 20: 126–132

Feltovich P J, Barrows H S 1984 Issues of generality in medical problem solving. In: Schmidt H G, DeVolder M L (eds) Tutorials in problem-based learning. Van Gorcum, Assen/Maastricht, pp 128–141

Feltovich P J, Johnson P E, Moller J H, Swanson D B 1984 LCS: The role and development of medical knowledge in diagnostic expertise. In: Clancey W J, Shortliffe E H (eds) Readings in medical artificial intelligence: the first decade. Addison-Wesley, Reading, pp 275–319

Gale J, Marsden P 1983 Medical diagnosis: from student to clinician.

Oxford Press, Oxford

Glaser R 1984 Education and thinking: the role of knowledge. American Psychologist 39: 93–104

Grant J, Marsden P 1987 The structure of memorized knowledge in students and clinicians: an explanation for diagnostic expertise. Medical Education 21: 92–98

Grant J, Marsden P 1988 Primary knowledge, medical education and consultant expertise. Medical Education 22: 173–179

Grant R, Jones M A, Maitland G D 1988 Clinical decision making in upper quadrant dysfunction. In: Grant R (ed) Physical therapy of the cervical and thoracic spine. Churchill Livingstone, New York, ch 5

Groen G J, Patel V L 1985 Medical problem-solving: some questionable assumptions. Medical Education 19: 95–100

Higgs J 1990 Fostering the acquisition of clinical reasoning skills. New Zealand Journal of Physiotherapy 18: 13–17

Hodgkin K, Knox J D E 1975 Problem centred learning. Churchill Livingstone, London

Jones M A 1987 The clinical reasoning process in manipulative therapy. In: Dalziel B A, Snowsill J C (eds) Proceedings, Fifth Biennial Conference of Manipulative Therapists Association of Australia, Melbourne, pp 62–69

Jones M A 1988 Clinical reasoning process in manipulative therapy. In: Proceedings of the International Federation of Orthopaedic Manipulative Therapists Congress. Cambridge, pp 29–30

Jones M A 1989 Clinical reasoning in manipulative therapy education. Master's Thesis, University of South Australia

Lesgold A, Rubinson H, Feltovich P, Glaser R, Klopfer D, Wang Y 1981 Expertise in a complex skill: diagnosing x-ray pictures. In: Chi M T H, Glaser R, Farr M (eds) The nature of expertise. Lawrence Erlbaum, Hillsdale, ch 11

McGuire C 1984 Medical problem-solving: a critique of the literature. Proceedings of the 23rd Annual Conference on Research in Medical Education, Washington, pp 3–12

Maitland G D 1986 Vertebral manipulation, 5th edn. Butterworth, London

Maitland G D 1987 The maitland concept: assessment, examination, and treatment by passive movements. In: Twomey L T, Taylor J R (eds) Physical therapy of the low back. Churchill Livingstone, New York, ch 5

May B J 1977a An integrated problem-solving curriculum design for physical therapy education. Physical Therapy 57: 807–813

May B J 1977b Evaluation in a competency-based educational system. Physical Therapy 57: 28–33

May B J, Dennis J K 1987 Clinical reasoning and clinical decision making. Post congress course, 10th International Congress of the World Confederation of Physical Therapy, Sydney

Muzzin L J, Norman G R, Feightner J W, Tugwell P, Guyatt G 1983 Expertise in recall of clinical protocols in two specialty areas. Proceedings of the 22nd Annual Conference on Research in Medical Education, Washington, pp 122–127

Neufeld V R, Norman G R, Feightner J W, Barrows H S 1981 Clinical problem-solving by medical students: a cross-sectional and longitudinal analysis. Medical Education 15: 315–322

Nickerson R S, Perkins D N, Smith E E 1985 The teaching of thinking. Lawrence Erlbaum, Hillsdale

Norman G R 1988 Problem-solving skills, solving problems and problem-based learning. Medical Education 22: 279–286

Norman G R 1990 Editorial: problem-solving skills and problem-based learning. Physiotherapy Theory and Practice 6: 53–54

Norman G R, Patel V L, Schmidt H G 1990 Clinical inquiry and scientific inquiry. Medical Education 24: 396–399

Patel V L, Frederiksen C H 1984 Cognitive processes in comprehension and knowledge acquisition by medical students and physicians. In: Schmidt H G, DeVolder M L (eds) Tutorials in problem-based learning. Van Gorcum, Assen/Maastricht, pp 143–157

Patel V L, Groen G J 1986 Knowledge-based solution strategies in medical reasoning. Cognitive Science 10: 91–108

Patel V L, Groen G J, Frederiksen C H 1986 Differences between medical students and doctors in memory for clinical cases. Medical Education 20: 3–9

Patel V L, Evans, D A, Kaufman D R 1990 Reasoning strategies and the use of biomedical knowledge by medical students. Medical Education 24: 129–136

Payton O D 1985 Clinical reasoning process in physical therapy. Physical Therapy 65: 924–928

Rubinstein M F 1980 A decade of experience in teaching an interdisciplinary problem-solving course. In: Tuma D T, Reif F (eds) Problem solving and education: issues in teaching and research. Lawrence Erlbaum, Hillsdale, ch 3

Rumelhart D E, Ortony E 1977 The representation of knowledge in memory. In: Anderson R C, Spiro R J, Montague W E (eds) Schooling and the acquisition of knowledge. Lawrence Erlbaum, Hillsdale, pp 99–135

Schmidt H G 1983 Problem-based learning: rationale and description. Medical Education 17: 11–16

Schmidt H G, DeVolder M L 1984 Tutorials in problem-based learning. Van Gorcum, Assen/Maastricht

Schmidt H G, Norman G R, Boshuizen H P A 1990 A cognitive perspective on medical expertise: theory and implications. Academic Medicine 65: 611–621

Schon D A 1983 The reflective practitioner. Basic Books, New York

Schon D A 1990 Educating the reflective practitioner. Jossey-Bass, San Francisco

Simon H A 1979 How big is a chunk? In: Simon H A (ed) Models of thought. Yale University Press, New Haven

Simon H A 1981 The sciences of the artificial. MIT Press, Cambridge

Slaughter D S, Brown D S, Garder D L, Perritt L J 1989 Improving physical therapy students' clinical problem-solving skills: an analytical questioning model. Physical Therapy 69: 441–447

Stillman P L, Swanson D B, Smee S, Stillman A E, Ebert T H, Emmel V S, Caslowitz J, Grenne H L, Hamolsky M, Hatem C, Levenson D L, Levin R, Levinson G, Ley B, Morgan G J, Parrino T, Robinson S, Willms J 1986 Assessing clinical skills of residents with standardized patients. Annals of Internal Medicine 105: 762–771

Stratford P, Pierce-Fenn H 1985 Modified essay question. Physical Therapy 65: 1075–1079

Thomas-Edding D 1987 Clinical problem solving in physical therapy and its implications for curriculum development. Proceedings of the 10th International Congress of the World Confederation of Physical Therapy, Sydney, pp 100–104

Titchen A C 1987a Design and implementation of a problem-based continuing education programme. Physiotherapy 73: 318–323

Titchen A C 1987b Problem-based learning: the rationale for a new approach to physiotherapy continuing education. Physiotherapy 73: 324–327

Trott P H 1985 Differential mechanical diagnosis of shoulder pain. In: Proceedings, Fourth Biennial Conference of Manipulative Therapists Association of Australia, Brisbane, pp 284–297

Tulving E, Thomson D M 1973 Encoding specificity and retrieval processes in episodic memory. Psychological Review 80: 352–373

Tuma D T, Reif F 1980 Problem solving and education: issues in teaching and research. Lawrence Erlbaum, Hillsdale

Voytovich A E, Rippey R M, Suffredini A 1985 Premature conclusions in diagnostic reasoning. Journal of Medical Education 60: 302–307

Walton H J, Matthews M B 1989 Essentials of problem-based learning. Medical Education 23: 542–558

Watts N T 1985 Decision analysis: a tool for improving physical therapy practice and education. In: Wolf S L (ed) Clinical decision making in physical therapy. F A Davis, Philadelphia, ch 1

Watts N T 1989 Clinical decision analysis. Physical Therapy 69: 569–576

Weinstein M C, Fineberg H V, Elstein A S, Frazier H S, Neuhauser D, Neutra R R, McNeil B J 1980 Clinical decision analysis. W B Saunders, Philadelphia

Willems J 1981 Problem-based (group) teaching: a cognitive science approach to using available knowledge. Instructional Science 10: 5–21

Wolf S L 1985 Clinical decision making in physical therapy. F A Davis, Philadelphia

Appendix: clinical reasoning form

UNIVERSITY OF SOUTH AUSTRALIA

MASTER OF APPLIED SCIENCE IN MANIPULATIVE PHYSIOTHERAPY

CLINICAL REASONING FORM

NAME ....DATE ....PATIENT'S NAME ....

PERCEPTIONS AND INTERPRETATIONS ON COMPLETION OF THE SUBJECTIVE EXAMINATION

1. MECHANISMS OF SYMPTOMS
   List the supporting evidence for the mechanisms of symptoms:

Peripheral Initiated/maintained	Centrally Initiated/maintained	Autonomic Initiated/maintained	Affective

2. THE SOURCE(S) OF THE SYMPTOMS
2.1 List in order of likelihood all possible structures at fault for each area/component of symptoms.

Area				
Possible structures at fault				

2.2 Highlight with * those structures which must be examined DAY 1

2.3 Do the symptoms appear to fit those commonly associated with a particular syndrome/disorder/pathological factors? ....
....
....

2.4   Are there any contributing factors associated with the patient's symptoms?
      Specify...
      ....
      ....
      ....

3.   THE BEHAVIOUR OF THE SYMPTOMS

3.1   Give your interpretation for each of the following:

● Severity |— — — — — — — |— — — — — — —|
             low   high

● Irritability |— — — — — — — |— — — — — — —|
                 non-irritable   very irritable

Give example: ....
....
....

● Relationship of symptoms — behavioural ....
....
....
                              — historical ....
....
....

● Precautionary questions ....
....
....

3.2   ● Is the disorder predominantly inflammatory or mechanical?
         |— — — — — — —|— — — — — — —|
         inflammatory   mechanical

List those factors that support and those that negate your decision.

Support	Negate

4.   HISTORY OF THE SYMPTOMS

4.1   Give your interpretation of the history (present and past) for each of the following:

- Nature of the onset ....
....
....

- Extent of tissue damage/change ....
....
....

- Progression since onset (including stage & rate of impairment & stability of the disorder) ....
....
....
....

- Does the history fit with the nature of the disorder? ....
Explain ....
....

5.   PRECAUTIONS AND CONTRAINDICATIONS TO PHYSICAL EXAMINATION AND MANAGEMENT

5.1   Does the subjective examination indicate caution? ....
Explain ....
....
....

5.2   Do the symptoms indicate the need for specific testing? ....
Explain ....
....

5.3   At which points under the following headings will you limit your physical examination? Circle the relevant description. Refer to your answers to Q 3.1.

Local symptoms	Referred symptoms	Dysthesia	Dizziness/Other VBI symptoms
	Short of P1	Short of Production	
Point of onset/ increase in resting symptoms	Point of onset/ increase in resting symptoms	Point of onset/ increase in resting symptom	Point of onset/ increase in dizziness
partial reproduction	partial reproduction	partial reproduction	partial reproduction
total reproduction	total reproduction	total reproduction	

5.4   Considering your answers to Q3.1 & 5.1 and in addition to your answer to Q5.3, at which point will you limit the extent of your physical examination? Tick the relevant description.

Active examination	**Passive examination**
Active movement short of limit	• Passive movement short of R1
Active limit	• Passive movement into
Active limit plus overpressure	moderate resistance
Additional tests	• Passive movement to full
	over-pressure

5.5   Is a neurological examination necessary? Why?...
....
....

5.6   Do you expect a comparable sign(s) to be easy/hard to find? ....
Explain ....
....
....

5.7   What are the clues (if any) in the subjective examination to the treatment
techniques that may be used? ....
....
....
....

PERCEPTIONS, INTERPRETATIONS, IMPLICATIONS FOLLOWING THE PHYSICAL EXAMINATION AND FIRST TREATMENT

6.   CONCEPT OF THE PATIENT

6.1   What is your concept of the patient and how he/she is affected by the
problem?..
....
....

6.2   Do you anticipate this affecting your management or the prognosis? ....
....
....
....

7.   THE SOURCES AND/OR PHYSICAL CONTRIBUTING FACTORS TO THE SYMPTOMS

7.1   List the mechanisms and components of symptoms identified in Sections 1.0
and 2.1 and number in order of likelihood the possible structure(s) at fault for
each apparent component. Then identify supporting and negating evidence
from the subjective and physical examination for each structure.

Component	Possible structure(s) at fault	Supporting evidence	Negating evidence

Mechanisms of symptoms	Supporting evidence	Negating evidence

7.2 ● Indicate your principal hypothesis regarding the primary syndrome/disorder.

....

● Briefly note the key features of the underlying pathophysiology for this disorder. ....

....

....

7.3 What are your thoughts regarding prognosis?

Favourable	Unfavourable

IMPLICATIONS OF PERCEPTIONS AND INTERPRETATIONS
ON ONGOING MANAGEMENT

8. **MANAGEMENT**

8.1   Do the signs fit with the symptoms? If not, how might this influence your management and treatment prognosis?...
....
....
....

8.2   Is there anything about your physical examination findings which would indicate the need for caution in your management? ....
Explain ....
....
....
....

8.3   Does your interpretation of the P/E change the emphasis of treatment as outlined?..
....
....

8.4   What was your first treatment technique(s)?...
....
What P/E findings support your choice? (Include in your answer a movement diagram of the most comparable passive sign). ....
....
....
....
....

C ┌─────────────────────────────┐ D
  │   │
  │   │
  │   │
  │   │
A └─────────────────────────────┘ B

MOVEMENT DIAGRAM

8.5   What was the effect of today's treatment (first visit)? ....
....
....
What is your expectation of the patient's response over the next 24 hours?
....
....
....

8.6   What is your plan and justification of management for this patient? (rate of progression; addressing other problems/components; sources/ contributing factors; appreciation of pathophysiology, etc:)...........................
....
....
....
....
....

9.   REFLECTION ON SOURCE(S), CONTRIBUTING FACTOR(S) AND
      PROGNOSIS

AFTER THIRD VISIT

9.1   How has your understanding of the patient's problem changed from your
      interpretations made following the first treatment? ....
      ....
      ....
      ....
      ....

9.2   On reflection, what clues (if any) can you now recognize that you inititally
      missed, misinterpreted, under- or over-weighted? ....
      ....
      ....
      ....
      ....

AFTER SIXTH VISIT

9.3   How has your understanding of the patient's problem changed from your
      interpretations made following the third treatment? ....
      ....
      ....
      ....
      ....

9.4   On reflection, what clues (if any) can you now recognize that you initially
      missed, misinterpreted, under- or over-weighted? ....
      ....
      ....
      ....
      ....

AFTER DISCHARGE

9.5   How has your understanding of the patient's problem changed from your
      interpretations made following the sixth treatment? ....
      ....
      ....
      ....
      ....

9.6   In hindsight, what were the principal source(s) and mechanisms of the
      patient's symptoms?
      ....
      ....

      Identify the key subjective and physical features (i.e. clinical pattern) that
      would help you recognize this disorder in the future.

Subjective	Physical

35. Principles of the physical examination

M. A. Jones   H. M. Jones

INTRODUCTION

The aim of the physical examination at the first consultation is to obtain the physical information required for the most appropriate treatment decision and form hypotheses for the most effective ongoing management. The physical examination continues at subsequent consultations guided by further information from the patient, including the response to initial treatments. Further physical examination may result in confirmation of initial hypotheses about the most effective form of ongoing management or modification of the management plan. This chapter will outline general principles that guide the clinician's clinical reasoning and decisions throughout the physical examination. Discussion will be confined to physical examination of the patient's neuro-musculo-skeletal structures and will not cover other forms of assessment, such as investigative procedures, work-site or functional work capacity assessments.

PHYSICAL EXAMINATION AS AN EXTENSION OF THE SUBJECTIVE EXAMINATION

To make the numerous clinical decisions required for effective management of the patient's disorder, information is required regarding the following categories of hypothesis:

- source of the symptoms and/or dysfunction
- contributing factors
- precautions and contraindications to physical examination and treatment
- management
- prognosis.

This information is obtained throughout the subjective and physical examination as well as during the ongoing management. The evolving clinical picture provides the clinician with both supporting and negating evidence for different hypotheses within each of these categories of hypothesis. Ultimately, an hypothesis is accepted (e.g.

examine this, treat this, take this level of precaution) on the strength of this cumulative evidence.

The subjective examination is not simply a routine set of questions to be asked of all patients with decisions withheld until the examination is completed. While a core of information is sought from all patients, the details pursued are specific to each patient. Thus, information obtained will contribute to evolving hypotheses which, in turn, direct the search for further information. This clinical reasoning process is discussed in Chapter 34, where an example is used to illustrate the evolving nature of the clinician's thoughts.

Similarly, the physical examination is not simply the indiscriminate application of routine tests, but rather should be seen as an extension of the subjective examination. As with the subjective examination, a core set of tests are used for each region of the body; however, these are not only for the purpose of collecting additional information but also for specifically testing hypotheses considered from the subjective examination. For example, if adverse neural tension were hypothesized from the subjective examination as a component source of a patient's symptoms, specific neural tension testing should then be performed as a test of this hypothesis. Information from the subjective examination also assists in guiding variations of standard examination procedures. For example, positions noticed by the patient to aggravate or ease the symptoms may lead to the use of a non-routine test, such as a neural tension test from a combined physiological movement position.

As with 'source of the symptoms', all categories of hypothesis are further tested in the physical examination. A 'contributing factor' is any predisposing or associated factor in the development and/or maintenance of the patient's problem, be it environmental, behavioural, emotional, physical or biomechanical. For example, if the subjective examination implicated a lack of muscle endurance as a potential contributing factor to the development of the patient's symptoms, it would be essential to examine muscle function to support or negate this hypothesis.

491

Hypotheses formed in the subjective examination regarding 'precautions and contraindications to physical examination' are also further tested in the physical examination. For example, a subjective picture of vertebral instability necessitates specific stability, and muscle function tests are performed in the physical examination.

Subjective evidence of the need for caution dictates the extent of physical examination. This includes how far specific movements are performed and how many movements should be tested. Factors which influence these hypotheses include the severity and irritability of the disorder, whether the disorder is progressive, the rate of impairment, the stability (i.e. predictability/variability) of the disorder, general health and the presence of any indicators of more sinister pathology, such as unexplained weight loss or relevant difficulties with bowel or bladder control. For example, a patient's complaint of very little activity eliciting severe symptoms that take hours to settle reflects an 'irritable' disorder requiring caution in the physical examination and treatment.

'Management' hypotheses formulated through the subjective examination are further supported, negated, and new ones entertained as additional information is obtained in the physical examination. For example, a patient presenting with severe and irritable low-back pain may describe a specific position of side-lying in some flexion and rotation as the only means in which his constant symptoms can be eased. If the irritability of the disorder warranted caution, the physical examination would be limited and attention given to identifying a pain-easing treatment position. The physical examination would therefore include assessment of this position, and further examination from this position would endeavour to determine the combination of physiological movements in side-lying that provide maximal relief.

Much of the same information from the subjective examination used for hypotheses of caution/contraindications will also provide an indication of 'prognosis'. Physical examination at the initial consultation adds further information to the assessment of prognosis. For example, a mechanical, non-irritable and stable picture of a disorder gleaned from the subjective examination would support a favourable prognosis. However, if the physical examination revealed passive intervertebral movement signs at appropriate levels with pain elicited before resistance and movement limited by pain, a less favourable prognosis may be expected. The ultimate hypothesis regarding prognosis involves weighing up the evidence of favourable versus less favourable factors gleaned throughout the initial and ongoing examinations.

PLANNING THE PHYSICAL EXAMINATION

By the end of the subjective examination the clinician will have determined which structures to examine, including whether a neurological examination is necessary and whether any special tests, such as vertebro-basilar insufficiency or instability tests, are indicated. Before proceeding with the physical examination the clinician will also need to decide the extent to which the physical examination can be taken without risk to aggravating the patient's disorder. Presentations by patients can be placed into one of two broad categories which relate to the extent to which the physical examination should be taken at the first consultation:

1. Limited examination. Examination procedures can be taken to where symptoms are produced or start to increase. The number of procedures may also need to be limited.

2. Full examination. Examination procedures are taken to their full extent, including the addition of passive overpressure to all active and passive movements.

Limited examination

The decision to limit examination procedures to the point of production or increase of symptoms is made on the basis of any feature of the subjective examination that indicates the need for caution in the physical examination. An irritable disorder and severe symptoms are examples of such features. Similarly, pathology such as rheumatoid arthritis, recent severe trauma or a disorder that is worsening are other features requiring the physical examination to be limited and gentle. It is important to recognize that the clinical decision regarding the degree of caution is not based on any single factor. A non-irritable disorder may still require caution if an underlying pathology such as rheumatoid arthritis were present. Patients who fall into this category will typically have symptoms at rest and pain felt early in the range of movement. Therefore, when examination procedures are limited to the point of production or increase in symptoms, what happens through the remaining movement, including the behaviour of pain, resistance and spasm is not known to the clinician. Despite this, limiting the physical examination in this manner still enables the clinician to obtain information regarding the pattern of movement restriction and the relative involvement of the joint, muscular, neural and vascular systems without aggravating the symptoms. Examination without aggravation of symptoms makes it possible to treat the disorder effectively at the first consultation. This is possible only because the clinical reasoning through the subjective examination has enabled the clinician to prioritize which examination procedures are most important to selection of treatment for this presentation of the patient. The complete clinical picture will gradually be revealed through subsequent consultations as the improving presentation allows further examination.

To illustrate a limited examination consider a patient

presenting with constant and worsening severe low-back pain aggravated by only minimal movement and taking hours to settle. This patient must be examined with great care. All test procedures would be limited to the first point of increased pain, with care taken to ensure that symptoms had settled between movements. Any build-up of symptoms necessitates omitting the examination of remaining movements. While the relative involvement of active physiological movements is important in the examination of all patients, the aim with this patient is not to provoke any further symptoms but rather to ease the constant pain. This requires reasoning where non-aggravating or less-aggravating movement directions become important clues to possible positions of treatment. These non-aggravating movement directions may even be examined further with the use of combined movements from that position to ascertain the least aggravating movement/position (see Ch. 41 on combined movements). If a neurological examination were indicated, and any attempt to flex the legs in supine provoked pain, these tests of muscle power would be foregone with either the use of only distal muscle testing or even a neurological examination limited to sensory and reflex testing. Assessment of soft-tissue palpation and intervertebral mobility would also need to be modified to ensure that the standard position of prone lying itself was not aggravating to the patient's symptoms. Modifications such as pillow(s) under the lower abdomen to flex the lumbar spine, or examination in side-lying with pillows under the waist preventing lateral flexion and pillows between the knees preventing hip adduction, may also be necessary. Examples of the limitations and modifications of examination for this patient could continue with the main point being the extreme care necessary when examining this patient in order to be able to help in the initial acute phase.

Full examination

Taking the examination to the full extent enables the clinician to obtain the complete clinical picture on which to base treatment and management decisions. Examination procedures can be taken to their full extent without risk of aggravation of symptoms if the disorder is non-irritable, not severe, and the nature, history and progression of the disorder do not dictate the need for caution. This situation is ideal for physical methods of treatment. With access to all the available information the clinician can be more confident in weighing up the presenting signs and determining the relative involvement of the different potential sources and contributing factors. This situation is optimal for formulating the most appropriate management plan.

Active and passive movements are examined to their full available range with the addition of passive overpressure. The significance of pain provoked by the passive pressure applied at the limit of range and the degree of stiffness or end-feel, can be determined by comparison with the same movement to the other side. For spinal movement to be classed as 'normal', it must have full physiological and intervertebral range of movement and provoke the same degree of sensation or discomfort with application of overpressure as the movement to the other side, and as one would expect considering the patient's age and somatotype.

There is still need to prioritize examination procedures despite being able to perform a full physical examination. The time available at the first consultation may limit the number of procedures possible. This requires planning of the physical examination where the most probable systems and structures are given priority in examination. However, the complete clinical pattern of presentation should be clear in the first two to three consultations.

To illustrate a full examination consider a patient with chronic minimal low-lumbar aching that is provoked only by driving a truck for longer than 10 hours, and which is then relieved by walking around for half an hour. To reproduce a symptom in the physical examination which, in everyday life, requires considerable mechanical force or activity to aggravate, is non-irritable, and has a history indicating a long-standing and stable disorder, it would be necessary to take the examination to its full extent. As any physical abnormality is likely to be minimal, strong over-pressure needs to be applied to all accessory, physiological and combined movements. Routine physiological and resisted movements are unlikely to provide enough information on which to base treatment even with the use of strong over-pressure. Combined movements, sustained movements and tests specific to that patient's aggravating activity may be necessary to reproduce the symptoms and to detect physical abnormality. Compression through the lumbar spine, repeated and/or combined physiological movements, combined accessory movements and neural tension tests, all in the simulated driving position are likely to provide useful information. It may even be necessary to 'pre-sensitize' the structures at fault and examine the lumbar spine immediately after the patient has been driving the truck, that is, while the symptoms are present.

Naturally, to categorize all patients into two categories is an over-simplification. In reality there is a continuum from that presentation where extreme care is needed to avoid seriously aggravating the patient's symptoms, to the presentation requiring additional test procedures with increased loads or repetitions.

The decision to limit the physical examination or to take it to its full extent does not lead to a singular consequent action but rather a spectrum of possible actions. There is a range of extent to which the physical examination can be limited or taken. The ability to make this complex decision accurately is gained with experience of a variety of clinical presentations, that is, experience in weighing up the various factors in the subjective examination which guide hypotheses regarding the caution necessary in the physical examination.

THE PHYSICAL EXAMINATION

Recognition of clinical patterns

As previously stated, the aim of examining the patient is to obtain the information required for a management decision. This requires recognition of clinical patterns. A clinical pattern of the structure(s) at fault may be given a diagnostic label; however, this alone is insufficient to identify the most effective management. That is, variations of a clinical pattern will exist within the same diagnosis with different treatments indicated for the various presentations. For example, a diagnosis of a lumbar posterior intervertebral joint disorder can have numerous presentations requiring significantly different treatments which may range from gentle oscillatory techniques from a pain-easing position to a localized rotation manipulation. To recognize both the general 'diagnostic' clinical pattern and, more importantly, the particular variation of the presenting patient, considerable detail is needed in the physical examination to guide the clinician in treatment selection.

Which structures to examine

All potential sources (structures) implicated through the subjective examination must eventually be tested in the physical examination. These include:

- all structures which underlie the area of symptoms
- all structures which can refer to the area of symptoms (e.g. spinal somatic referral).

Similarly, all potential contributing factors implicated through the subjective examination must be tested. These include:

- all structures which can chemically and/or nutritionally affect symptom production elsewhere (i.e. chemical effects along a nerve as in the double-crush syndrome and vascular compromise)
- all structures which can mechanically affect other structures contributing to symptom production (e.g. hypomobile thoracic segments predisposing to the development or maintenance of cervical symptoms).

These structures are hypothesized as potential contributing factors because of their ability to alter stress, tension, loads and chemical/fluid flows on the structure(s) which are the actual source of the symptoms. This principle is fundamental to the rationale for examination of seemingly remote areas to the patient's complaint, including pelvic and lower extremity biomechanics, mobility, muscle strength and length which can clearly influence stresses imparted on the spine.

It is important that the clinician examine all potential sources and not only those considered most likely. That is, structures must be examined not only to incriminate their involvement but also to establish their lack of involvement. However, it is obvious from the numerous physical tests described in this book alone, that it is neither practical nor necessary for all tests to be used with every patient at the first consultation. An hypothesis-testing approach through the subjective examination enables the clinician to identify the most likely sources and prioritize those tests to be used in the first consultation and those which can be left to the second or third appointment.

Different clinicians will look at different tests and perform them in different ways. The differences in training and experience creating this variability should serve to broaden our clinical knowledge base. Essential to all clinicians, regardless of their approach, is that the examination be relevant to the individual patient's unique presentation and that all hypotheses regarding the potential structures involved be eventually tested.

Which physical findings implicate a structure's potential involvement?

There are numerous physical signs which will alert the clinician to a structure's potential involvement in the symptom presentation. These include:

- abnormal appearance (e.g. bony asymmetry, muscle contours and trophic changes)
- abnormal movement (e.g. functional, active, passive and resisted)
- abnormal feel on palpation (e.g. temperature, thickening, tightness and swelling).

These signs must be interpreted in the light of the patient's age and somatotype.

The potential involvement of a structure is strengthened if:

- altering the abnormality (e.g. asymmetry, pattern of movement) affects the patient's symptoms
- directly or indirectly stressing a structure reproduces the patient's symptoms
- directly or indirectly stressing a structure capable of directly referring the symptoms reveals abnormality of that structure (e.g. hypomobility and local pain produced on testing the C5/6 posterior intervertebral joint in a patient complaining of lateral shoulder pain)
- directly or indirectly stressing a structure capable of contributing to the predisposition of symptom development reveals abnormality of that structure (e.g. tight hip flexor muscles for a patient complaining of low-back pain).

The relationship between symptoms and movement and posture significantly assists the clinician in identifying the potential source(s) of the symptoms, contributing factor(s) and management. A physical test which provokes symptoms can be said to be stressing the source of the symptoms. Abnormal signs in the absence of comparable symptom production suggests that the structure tested is not the direct source of symptoms, however, these signs may still be significant as contributing factors by their secondary effect on the symptomatic structures.

The patient is the best resource in identifying the source and, knowingly or not, will ultimately guide the attentive clinician to the appropriate management. In order to establish clearly this relationship of symptoms to movement and posture it is essential that the clinician continually clarify the following:

- presence of symptoms at rest
- onset or increase in symptoms with active, passive and resistive tests
- behaviour of symptoms through movement
- provocation of symptoms to palpation.

Interpreting passive movement tests

Passive movement testing provides the added advantage of correlating symptoms with passive feel. The relationship between the soft-tissue resistance to passive movement and the symptoms reported by the patient throughout the range of movement is fundamental information in the physical examination. On one passive movement test, an abnormally high degree of resistance may be perceived well before the report of symptoms. On another, pain may be reported early in the range of movement before resistance is felt.

This important clinical skill of passive movement or soft-tissue 'feel' and its interpretation in relation to symptoms has important implications for both weighing up the significance of an abnormal passive movement and the choice of treatment technique. A passive movement is most likely to be directly stressing the source of the symptoms if pain is the dominant feature through the movement with or without abnormal resistance.

Similarly, the relationship between resistance and pain can assist in guiding selection of treatment technique. For example, a passive movement with abnormal resistance and minimal comparable pain will require treatment with stronger passive stretching, whereas if pain is the dominant feature the passive technique will need to be more gentle, taking into account the patient's symptoms. This concept of assessing the relationship between the resistance to passive movement and symptom production is discussed in detail elsewhere (Maitland 1991).

Components of the physical examination

Each patient's unique presentation will determine the appropriate physical examination. The components of the spinal physical examination which should be considered for all patients include assessment of:

- observation and posture
- the patient's functional aggravating factor
- physiological movements (active and passive)
- passive accessory movements
- soft tissue
- nervous system
- muscle performance
- vascular system
- extremities.

It is not the aim of this chapter to describe all possible findings of a physical examination; rather, it is hoped to point out the principles of this assessment and how it fits into the reasoning of the entire patient examination. All components of the physical examination offer an opportunity to test hypotheses entertained in the subjective examination. The additional information will also contribute to new hypotheses being considered or existing ones being modified.

Observation and posture

The patient's general body posture and willingness to move should be observed during the subjective examination and while he/she is entering the room, undressing, sitting down and so on. Posture should be assessed in the physical examination with observation of the patient in standing and sitting. Posture should be viewed from the front, behind and side-on. To avoid over attendance to the symptomatic area, posture should initially be viewed more globally as though viewing through a 'wide-angle lens'. This enables the recognition of postural faults outside the immediate area of symptoms which may represent contributing factors to the symptomatic structures. Closer 'telescopic' attention can then be given to the symptomatic area. In general, the clinician is looking for asymmetries in regional and local spinal posture in all three planes as well as muscle contours, pelvic asymmetry and both upper and lower limb postures.

Postural deformities. Postural deformities may be protective, non-protective structural and non-protective behavioural. A protective deformity occurs as the patient consciously, or frequently unconsciously, assumes a posture that is relatively pain-easing. Examples of protective deformities include wry necks, lumbar lists and lower extremity postures such as decreased weight-bearing, increased lateral rotation of the hip and knee flexion. Attempts to correct a protective deformity will worsen the patient's symptoms.

The classic example of a non-protective structural deformity is a long-standing structural scoliosis, although any of the above examples may also be non-protective structural if the deformity cannot be corrected and attempts to do so do not elicit pain. However, muscle spasm can also prevent correction of a deformity. When correction of a deformity is painless and the spasm undetected, this may be interpreted as non-protective structural. If the deformity is corrected with treatment, the existence of muscle spasm masking a protective deformity is implicated.

In some cases, a non-protective structural deformity is thought to remain as a mechanical malfunction from a condition in which it was a protective mechanism. In long-standing non-protective structural deformities a compensatory curve will develop. Unlike protective deformities, the non-protective structural deformity will remain after symptoms have been relieved with treatment. While this type of deformity is not the immediate effect of irritation to a painful structure, it may still represent a contributing factor as its presence may have predisposed to the development and/or maintenance of abnormal stress on the symptomatic structures.

A non-protective behavioural deformity is one which is due to the patient's 'personality' or 'emotions' or simply to a lack of body awareness. It can be passively corrected without eliciting pain. Thus, this deformity is not seen as an attempt to move away from the painful structure, although, as alluded to above, it may contribute to the symptoms.

A postural deformity is frequently associated with a predictable pattern of muscle performance and musculoskeletal flexibility. Thus, when the presence of a postural deformity is hypothesized to be related to the patient's symptoms, further physical testing will be indicated to determine the need for incorporating treatment directed at these components of the problem. For example, an increased lower lumbar lordosis which is contributing to the patient's symptoms should prompt the clinician to examine potential causes of the increased lordosis. These may include hypomobile intervertebral segments, weak low abdominals and intersegmental stabilizers, tight lowback extensors, tight hip flexors and any associated lower extremity imbalances (Janda 1983, Kendall & McCreary 1983).

Analysis of the provoking activity

Analysis of the provoking posture or movement as reported in the subjective examination provides useful initial clues to the structures and component movements involved. Once the patient adopts the aggravating posture and symptoms are produced, the therapist can stabilize the relevant body parts and each component movement can be altered individually. With each component movement the effect on the pain is assessed. For example, if buttock pain is provoked at the extreme back swing of a golf drive this action would be analysed. In the position of the drive where pain is being provoked the clinician

stabilizes the pelvis, thereby minimizing any increase in hip rotation. The therapist then increases the lumbar rotation and the pain response is assessed. With the patient back in the initial test position, and with the same degree of buttock pain being provoked, the clinician then stabilizes the trunk and accentuates rotation at the hip. The pain response is compared. If it were established that the trunk movement provoked more pain, the component lumbar movements could be compared in a similar manner, for example, using the same starting position and comparing the effect of over-pressure into rotation versus lateral flexion. Further analysis in this example may include altering hip adduction versus spinal lateral flexion, hip flexion/extension versus spinal flexion/extension and adding/subtracting remote movements (e.g. neck flexion or ankle dorsiflexion) to test for neural tension involvement.

Many provoking activities require dynamic movement to reproduce symptoms, and this movement can be analysed in a similar manner. Using the example of the golf backswing again, the swing is performed in the normal manner and the pain response established. It is then repeated with exaggerated hip rotation, for example, by starting the swing with the hip already in some rotation. The effect on the buttock pain is noted and any influence of hip rotation is confirmed by lessening the rotation through the drive, that is, by starting in the opposite rotation. Accentuating trunk rotation could be achieved by the clinician providing some stabilization of the pelvis while the patient attempts a full backswing.

Analysis of the provoking movement provides a meaningful form of re-assessment for therapist and patient. While a patient may be unimpressed by 10° increase in vertebral rotation, a decrease in pain on a functionally limited activity will be appreciated. It is important to re-emphasize that the analysis of the provoking movement provides only an initial clue to the source of symptoms which will be further supported or negated on continued physical testing.

Active physiological movements

It is insufficient simply to note the gross range of a physiological movement and whether or not symptoms are reproduced. Details such as the quality of the active movement, symptoms at rest and the relationship between change in symptoms and quality of movement provide valuable information. Similarly, symptoms and resistance are assessed with passive over-pressure. For example, a patient reports no symptoms at rest, and on thoracic rotation has equal gross range of movement to the left compared to the right. On closer examination of the quality of thoracic rotation it is noted that while it is easy for the patient to achieve a full range of left rotation, he/she has to push through the last 30° to achieve a full range of right rotation. On passive over-pressure there is increased resistance to right rotation and thoracic symptoms are reproduced. Detailed examination of physiological movement provides a more accurate and clear pattern of clinical presentation.

The patient should be given clear instructions regarding what is required prior to any physical test. The patient must understand that the presence of any symptoms during a movement or test is of interest to the clinician. This is particularly important if tests are to be limited to the point of onset or increase of symptoms, as this requires the cooperation of the patient.

The following is an example of the value of detailed information on the symptoms the patient is experiencing. On gross examination a patient reports back, buttock, posterior thigh and calf pain at the limit of lumbar flexion which is measured by the level of the finger tips to the mid-shin. On physical examination at the next consultation this finding is unchanged and it is concluded that treatment at the initial consultation was not beneficial. However, more detailed information from the patient revealed that, at the initial consultation, lumbar flexion produced back and buttock pain when finger tips were at the level of the mid-thigh, thigh pain when the finger tips were to the patellae, and calf pain at the level of mid-shin along with decreased low-lumbar intervertebral movement. On re-assessment at the next treatment, the back, buttock and thigh pain were produced at the level of finger-tips to upper-shin, and the calf pain at the level of mid-shin with improved intervertebral movement indicating that the previous treatment had affected the symptoms.

The active physiological movements of spinal flexion, extension, lateral flexion and rotation are routine in the examination of spinal dysfunction. General ease of movement, deviation from the expected plane of movement, intervertebral movement and range of movement, as well as the behaviour of symptoms through the movement are noted with each physiological movement.

Observation of the quality of a physiological movement often requires different views of focus. For example, observing cervical flexion from in front enables any deviation from the frontal plane to be noted, whereas intervertebral movement is better observed from a side view. Any asymmetry or deviation with movement must be corrected to assess its relevance to the symptoms. For example, a list to the left on cervical flexion may be a pain-avoiding mechanism or it may be a movement characteristic of that patient irrelevant to the presenting symptoms. If the list is a pain-avoiding mechanism, correction of the list during the active movement should produce symptoms and is also likely to result in further limitation of range of movement.

If the examination is to be taken to its full extent, passive over-pressure at the limit of the movement will estab-

lish the end-feel of the physiological movement and the effect on symptoms, both local and referred. It is important to continually re-establish the status of the symptoms between physiological movements. The clinician needs to be alerted to any build-up of symptoms, especially if the decision has already been made to limit the examination.

If the examination is to be taken to its full extent and routine physiological movements have not reproduced the symptoms, there will usually be clues in the subjective examination as to how the tests can be refined. It may be that sustained positions or repeated movements aggravate the symptoms, or that the injuring movement was a specific combination of physiological movements. On the basis of clues such as these, tests of physiological movements can be refined with the aim of reproducing symptoms and detecting abnormalities in the quality of these movements. For example, lumbar extension and lateral flexion may be full-range and pain-free on routine examination. However, if lumbar extension is performed from a position of full lateral flexion to the right it may be limited and painful. Comparison with the combined movement of extension from a position of left lateral flexion, which is full-range and pain-free, confirms that this is an abnormal finding. Any clues from the subjective examination can be followed up in this manner, and common refinements of physiological movement tests include sustained movements, repeated movements, combined movements, movements under compression or distraction and varying speeds of movement.

Passive physiological intervertebral movements (PPIVMs)

There are a variety of techniques for performing PPIVMs all aiming to assess the available range of physiological movement at each intervertebral level. Intervertebral movement is palpated during passive flexion, extension, lateral flexion and rotation and the available range of movement is compared with the expected range of movement for that intervertebral segment. PPIVMs are used to detect intervertebral hypomobility, hypermobility and structural instability.

In the cervical spine the movement of the motion segment is palpated bilaterally at the posterior intervertebral joints. It is possible to feel the superior facet gliding and translating on the inferior facet during the passive physiological movement. In the thoracic and lumbar spines movement is assessed via the gliding and translation of the spinous processes, the posterior intervertebral joints being inaccessible. As with any passive test, achieving relaxation of the patient by confident and comfortable handling is of paramount importance. For more detailed discussion of PPIVMs the reader is referred to manual therapy texts such as Grieve (1988) and Maitland (1986).

Passive accessory intervertebral movements (PAIVMs) and palpation examination

PAIVMs are performed as part of the spinal palpation examination which includes the following tests:

1. Skin temperature and sweating. An area of increased temperature may indicate an inflammatory process, and a change in temperature and/or sweating may be indicators of autonomic nervous system involvement in the disorder.

2. Soft-tissue changes. Palpation can detect soft-tissue changes such as thickening, swelling, muscle tightness and spasm.

3. Position of vertebrae. The position of one vertebra relative to another can be palpated, as can the symmetry of a single vertebra. The interpretation of this information is difficult as there are little clinical or research data to establish its significance.

4. Movement of vertebrae. Passive accessory intervertebral movements (PAIVMs) can be produced by pressures in an antero-posterior, postero-anterior, and transverse direction or in any combination of these directions. The pressures can be applied through the spinous processes, at any point along the laminae, over the posterior intervertebral joints or at the transverse processes where accessible. In the thoracic spine, pressures can also be applied over the ribs, producing accessory movement at the costovertebral, costotransverse and posterior intervertebral joints of the related vertebra. If applied more anteriorly, accessory movement of the rib can also assess the costochondral and sternochondral joints. At each intervertebral level the available range of movement, the quality of movement through range, including end-feel, and the relationship of any abnormalities detected to symptoms is assessed. Detailed and skilled assessment of PAIVMs ensures the early detection of any movement abnormality and acccuracy of location of an intervertebral source of symptoms.

Palpation and PAIVMs help differentiate between an intervertebral source of symptoms, a contributing factor and 'irrelevant' soft-tissue changes. For example, painless joint stiffness and hard thickened soft tissue indicate chronic abnormality which is not the direct source of the symptoms. If, however, there is swelling on palpation and hypermobility and pain on passive accessory testing at an adjacent vertebral level it is reasonable to hypothesize that while the hypermobile joint is the source of the symptoms, the stiff joint may be a contributing factor. Abnormality detected in more remote segments to the symptomatic area (e.g. thoracic or lumbar spine abnormality in a patient with cervical symptoms) may also prove to be a significant contributing factor. However, this can be determined only in retrospect following treatment to the areas in question and re-assessment of all presenting signs and symptoms.

The changes that are detectable by palpation and by PAIVMs at an intervertebral level are:

1. Soft-tissue changes. Examples include localized taut skin, swelling, muscle thickening or spasm and ligamentous and/or capsular thickening.

2. Altered range of movement—either hypomobility or hypermobility.

3. Abnormal quality of resistance to passive movement—for example, early and increased resistance and the almost unyielding quality of muscle spasm.

4. Provocation of symptoms (local or referred). The pain response felt by the patient during the palpation examination and with PAIVMs is important. The most significant pain response is reproduction of the patient's symptoms. This can be differentiated from local soft-tissue soreness by comparison with other asymptomatic joints. A local pain response, different from the patient's symptoms, is still significant as an indicator of a source of symptoms if it is provoked at an intervertebral level capable of producing the patient's symptoms.

Accessory movements are assessed initially with the spine in a mid-position. The joint may then be placed in a comparable position to one that has been found during testing of physiological and combined movements to reproduce signs and symptoms.

In contrast, when testing accessory movements in an irritable disorder which is easily aggravated, the spine should be placed in a position of maximum comfort. Clues to this position should come from the pain-easing positions offered by the patient in the subjective examination and further by any postures and physiological movements (cardinal and combined) from the physical examination which were either pain-easing or less aggravating. For more detail on spinal palpation and passive accessory intervertebral movement testing see Chapter 37.

Examination of the nervous system

The nervous system is assessed by testing relevant upper and lower motor neurone and peripheral nerve function and by testing the normal mobility of the nervous system. The mobility of the nervous system is assessed by a series of passive movement tests. Any abnormality detected, such as symptom production and/or abnormal resistance, implicates a neural component to the patient's disorder.

Function of lower motor neurones and peripheral nerves is assessed by testing relevant reflexes, muscle power, and sensitivity to pin-prick and light touch. Upper motor neurone assessment includes examination of sensation, muscle tone, muscle reflexes, Babinski reflex and clonus. A neurological examination should be performed whenever the patient presents with symptoms which are neural in character—such as numbness, paresthesia, hyperesthesia and weakness. In addition, a neurological examination is indicated when symptoms are present in the limbs and for any disorder with either a history of trauma or where the progression of symptoms reveals a worsening condition. Details of neurological testing are outlined in Grieve (1988) and Maitland (1986).

Straight leg raise (SLR), passive neck flexion (PNF), prone knee bend (PKB), upper limb tension tests (ULTTs) and the slump test are passive movements used to assess nervous system mobility. Details of these tests and the many variations and combinations used in the examination of the nervous system are discussed in Chapter 44.

Examination of the vascular system

Physiotherapists are limited in their ability to test physically for vascular compromise. Apart from the more obvious physical signs of peripheral cyanosis—decreased skin temperature, swelling, altered pulses and nystagmus (in the case of vertebral artery insufficiency)—spinal vascular deficiencies are difficult to detect by manual therapy physical testing. Medical tests such as doppler studies and arteriography are more definitive.

The strongest evidence for vascular involvement in a patient's symptoms will come from the behaviour of symptoms obtained through the subjective examination. Examples include symptoms of vertebrobasilar insufficiency (VBI) such as dizziness and double vision associated with cervical movements, and symptoms of vascular claudication such as pain or cramping associated with a predictable amount of exercise and immediately eased by rest (independent of spinal posture). Peripheral pulses are the only vascular physical assessment we have at our disposal. These can be tested as resting pulses or in postures known to compromise the vascular system such as thoracic outlet tests (see Ch. 29). Clearly, vascular compromise will often occur in conjunction with other neuromusculo-skeletal disorders. In this case, treatment of the other neuromusculo-skeletal structure(s) will enable the clinician restrospectively to attribute the remaining symptoms to the vascular system.

Vertebrobasilar insufficiency testing. There is a growing international appreciation for the need to perform vertebrobasilar insufficiency testing of the cervical spine for all patients prior to cervical manipulation (Grant & Trott 1991). Subjective clues such as symptoms of dizziness, lightheadedness, strange sensation in the head, dysarthria, diplopia, drop attacks, blackouts, disturbances of vision and tinitis contraindicate cervical manipulation. However, as other forms of physical therapy may be utilized, it is essential that these symptoms be continually monitored through all physical tests and treatments. This will establish a detailed baseline relationship between these symptoms and any provocative physical test enabling the clinician to monitor the effect of treatment and retrospectively incriminate other non-vascular sources. Premanipulative testing is carried out in those patients who respond negatively to specific testing regarding symptoms suggestive of vertebrobasilar insufficiency. Details of specific premanipulative tests are outlined in Chapter 26.

Examination of the muscular system

Muscles can be involved as either a direct 'contractile' source of the symptoms or a contributing factor responsible for the accumulation of excessive stress to other structures.

When pain is elicited on isometric contraction and stretch, a contractile lesion is implicated. Care is needed with interpreting these tests as other non-contractile structures will also be stressed. Palpation examination will assist as a contractile lesion will be tender to palpation locally and may have palpable soft-tissue changes.

Clues of muscular involvement as a contributing factor to the patient's symptoms will come from the subjective examination. For example, a patient who has no difficulty with household activities in the morning yet experiences an accumulation of spinal ache later in the day associated with these same activities may reflect a 'postural' disorder where muscular fatigue predisposes to increasingly poorer posture and excessive stresses on spinal structures. The hypothesis of muscular involvement is further tested in the physical examination.

Resting posture typically provides the first physical evidence of a muscular component. For example, a forward head posture combined with elevated, protracted shoulders and abducted, rotated scapulae will typically be associated with variable involvement of tightness in upper cervical extensors, sternocleidomastoids, levator scapulae, upper trapezius, pectorals and shoulder medial rotators with weakness in the deep neck flexors and lower scapular stabilizers (Janda 1988). This presentation will often have an associated imbalance in the lower body. Thus one should not view any region in isolation, but rather consider its relationship to the whole.

The muscular imbalance hypothesized from the observation of posture requires confirmation through specific tests of muscle length, strength and endurance. Additional functional muscle assessment should be performed with the aim of determining the patient's ability to assume and sustain an improved posture. This can be assessed from a range of developmental, functional work and home-required postures as well as the patient's ability to maintain this control during movement from one posture to another. The patient's performance will be the result of numerous factors including joint, neural and soft-tissue resistance, pain inhibition, muscle strength and endurance, and his/her individual motivation and body awareness. The non-muscular factors will be assessed separately, allowing the clinician to gauge the degree to which each factor contributes. The cognitive factor requires skilled education of the movement or postural correction ensuring that the patient's performance reflects primarily a muscular ability.

Physical testing of muscular performance not only confirms the need for improved muscle function but also enables the clinician to identify functionally and specifically from where treatment should commence. That is, the muscular examination should reveal where the patient has postural control and where that control is lost. For example, a patient may be able to assume the desired posture whilst sitting and standing, but cannot control the posture when movement is required, as in arising from sitting or in walking. This degree of detail, along with measures of endurance, allows the clinician to design a treatment programme working from the patient's strengths (e.g. postures of control), while planning ongoing treatment to incorporate those functional postures and activities relevant to that patient.

Examination of peripheral structures

With more complex spinal neuromusculoskeletal presentations it is necessary to evaluate the relative contribution of spinal and peripheral involvement. Spinal disorders can present with limb symptoms exclusively or, more commonly, with a combination of spinal area and limb symptoms. Spinal and limb abnormalities can also exist as separate and either related or unrelated disorders. Detailed physical examination of both spinal and peripheral structures enables the therapist to hypothesize regarding their relative contribution to the symptoms and direct treatment accordingly.

When limb symptoms are present, the peripheral structures under the area of symptoms and those capable of referring to the area of symptoms or capable of contributing to the predisposition of symptom development must be examined. Consider a patient with anterior, upper-thigh pain whose lumbar spine examination reproduced this pain on lumbar extension with strong pressure over the right mid-lumbar posterior intervertebral joints. There is a limitation of right knee extension in the slump test but without reproduction of anterior thigh pain. While these findings may be relevant to the symptoms and may even be adequate to treat the symptoms, the full pattern of presentation of this disorder will not be revealed, and learning will be limited, if the peripheral structures are not examined. Examination of hip movements reveals limited and painful flexion and extention, abduction greater than adduction and internal rotation. There is a specific point of tenderness over the mid-groin and a positive prone knee-bend test with exact reproduction of the symptom. Tests for other structures hypothesized as likely sources of the symptoms, for example muscles of the groin and anterior thigh region, were negative. Detailed examination of the peripheral structures reveals a more complete pattern of presentation on which to base treatment. The clinician needs to weigh up the significance of the spinal, peripheral and neural movement signs and treat accordingly, reassessing the effect of the treatment on each of these components to the clinical presentation.

ONGOING EVALUATION OF TREATMENT MODALITIES

Continued examination after the first consultation is necessary to complete any tests considered non-essential at the initial examination and to monitor the effect of ongoing treatment. Ongoing evaluation of treatment enables the therapist to test hypotheses formed through the subjective and physical examinations. When treatment fails to produce the desired effect it often reflects an error of reasoning and continued examination is warranted. Certain structures may require re-examination while some tests may need to be taken further, such as a combination of physiological movements and a neural tension position not previously considered.

Assessing the effect of treatment requires attention to both the subjective report of what the patient feels and the physical signs. Only the physical re-assessment will be considered here; however, improvement in physical signs is relevant only when associated with a corresponding improvement in symptoms. For a more detailed discussion of subjective and physical re-assessment the reader is referred to Maitland (1991).

It is not practical or necessary to re-assess every physical sign. Rather, the therapist should identify a key sign to re-assess for each hypothesized spinal and peripheral component. The depth and detail of information obtained in the initial physical examination (e.g. quality of movement through range and precise relationship of symptoms to movement) allows more sensitive detection of change when these key signs are re-assessed.

Re-assessment of the treatment movement itself will assist the therapist's interpretation of the other potential components. That is, if reasonable change has been made to the intervertebral mobility of the segment treated and no change occurs in a peripheral sign, it suggests that peripheral abnormality is not related to the segment treated. While this must be substantiated through repeated and varied attempts at treating the segment in question, this principal of re-assessment is fundamental to guiding one's decision-making.

There are four important times when the patient's key physical signs should be monitored. These are: during the performance of a technique, after the application of the technique, at the end of the treatment session and at the beginning of the next treatment session.

Assessment during performance of a technique should include both the patient's report of what he/she is feeling and any change to the resistance to movement as the technique is delivered. Both will determine whether the technique is achieving the desired aim.

Re-assessment after the application of technique is used to prove the value of the technique. Re-assessment at the end of the treatment session provides a base-line level of improvement for comparison to the start of this treatment session and the beginning of the next. The physical signs at the beginning of the next treatment session should then be compared to the signs at the beginning and end of the last treatment session. This will indicate how much physical improvement was gained and maintained from the last treatment. The subjective and physical responses should correlate. That is, an improvement in physical signs without a corresponding subjective improvement renders that physical improvement less relevant.

SUMMARY

Principals of the physical examination have been reviewed. The physical examination should not be the indiscriminate application of routine tests, but rather should be seen as an extension of the clinical reasoning through the subjective examination. Hypotheses regarding suspected sources and contributing factors to the patient's symptoms are tested, and additional information is obtained assisting further hypothesis formation and refinement.

Consideration of hypotheses regarding precautions and contraindications to physical examination and treatment enables the clinician to conduct an appropriate 'limited' or 'full' examination without worsening the patient's disorder.

Management hypotheses entertained through the subjective examination are further modified as the physical presentation unfolds. This requires recognition of clinical patterns which may receive a diagnostic label, but more importantly contain the necessary detail of presenting signs and symptoms to guide the clinician's choice of treatment.

All potential sources and contributing factors implicated through the subjective examination must eventually be tested in the physical examination. Initial physical clues to a structure's involvement are available on observation of the patient's posture and further implicated through specific active, passive, resistive and palpatory physical tests.

Correlating the patient's symptom production with physical testing is invaluable. It requires meticulous attention to detail, including clarifying symptoms at rest, onset or increase in symptoms with physical testing, and the behaviour of symptoms through movement. This will assist the clinician in identifying different components of the patient's disorder and differentiating between a direct source of the symptoms and potential contributing factors.

The physical examination should include assessment of the patient's posture, physiological movements (active and passive), passive accessory movements, soft-tissue, nervous, muscular and vascular systems. Each of these components of the physical examination have specific criteria which implicated their involvement.

While the physical examination will culminate in a treatment/management decision, continual evaluation of treatment modalities is essential to test hypotheses formed through the subjective and physical examinations and guide ongoing management.

Whether examining a patient in private practice, in a hospital, for a 'specialist' opinion, or in preparation for a legal case, the principles of physical examination outlined here are the same. The clinician must always endeavor to tailor the examination and treatment to the individual patient presentation. This requires skilled clinical reasoning where subjective clues guide physical tests which, in turn, contribute to an evolving understanding of the patient's problem. Physical tests should be conducted to not only test a structures involvement but also to prove a structure's lack of involvement. In this way clinicians can challenge existing clinical patterns and, in the process, broaden the repertoire of clinical patterns which they can recognize.

REFERENCES

Grieve G 1988 Common vertebral joint problems, 2nd edn. Churchill Livingstone, Edinburgh
Grant R, Trott P H 1991 Pre-manipulative testing of the cervical spine —the APA protocol three years on. In: Proceeding of the Seventh Biennial Conference of Manipulative Physiotherapists Association of Australia, Blue Mountains, New South Wales, pp 40–45
Janda V 1983 Muscle function testing. Butterworths, London
Janda V 1988 Muscles and cervicogenic pain syndromes. In: Grant R

(ed) Physical therapy of the cervical and thoracic spine. Churchill Livingstone, New York, ch 5
Kendall F P, McCreary E K 1983 Muscles testing and function, 3rd edn. Williams & Wilkins, Baltimore
Maitland G D 1986 Vertebral manipulation, 5th edn. Butterworths, London
Maitland G D 1991 Peripheral manipulation, 3rd edn. Butterworths, London

36. Influence of circadian variation on spinal examination

L. S. Gifford

Since man's habits are governed largely by regular environmental and social rhythms it is not surprising that many physiological measurements (e.g. temperature) show a more or less regular 24 hour variation. The term 'diurnal' is frequently used for a rhythm whose period is one day. As the word is also used to distinguish night and day, Conroy & Mills (1970) preferred the use of 'circadian' to indicate a period of approximately 24 hours. Both terms are used in current literature.

Recently there has been a significant upsurge in interest in diurnal 'variation' or 'changes', especially as they relate to changes in height, the disc, and, to some extent, to joint ranges and flexibility.

VARIATION IN HEIGHT

In 1777 de Montbeillard described the decrease in height of his son during the course of the day and this variation has since been demonstrated by several workers. In a much-quoted paper, De Puky (1936) showed from a sample of over 1200 people that, on average, a person is 1% shorter by evening compared with the morning. In addition to this he mentioned a corresponding figure of 2% for children and 0.5% for 70–80 year olds.

Tyrell et al (1985) noted that 54% of the total diurnal change was lost in the first hour after rising and 83% in the first 3 hours and 45 minutes. Some 71% was regained in the first half of the night. The mean circadian variation that they recorded was 19.3 mm, or 1.1% of stature. It is generally agreed in the literature that these observed changes in stature are more a result of being horizontal or vertical than of any intrinsic, or endogenous, circadian rhythm. Goode & Theodore (1983) demonstrated this in two subjects who rose at 7 a.m. and immediately returned to bed for 3 hours. When they were measured again their heights had not changed. The substantial effects of gravity on body height is exemplified by astronauts who apparently show increases of up to 10 cm on returning to earth (Kazarian 1974).

The disc has been implicated as a major factor in daily height fluctuation, (De Puky 1936, Markolf & Morris 1974) and it is well established that the disc exhibits viscoelastic properties (Virgin 1951, Markolf 1972). The disc responds elastically to loading and unloading for short periods of time, as in vibrations or shocks. However, if a load is applied for a long time, in addition to the elastic response, creep deformation of the annulus fibrosus occurs as well as fluid loss from the disc generally (Koeller et al 1984). During the recumbency of sleep, the loading on the intervertebral discs is reduced, and their relatively unopposed swelling pressure leads to absorption of fluid and increase in volume (Urban & McMullin 1988).

Average fluid loss from an individual lumbar disc which has lost height in vitro is 12% from the annulus and 5% from the nucleus (Adams & Hutton 1983). Losses from discs of subjects under 35 years were noted as almost twice this amount. Age-related variation in disc hydration and water loss may partly explain the age variations in height loss noted by De Puky (1936).

Traction may mimic or even accelerate the overnight effects of recumbency. Warden & Humphry (1964) have shown 'substantial' increases in body height as a result of traction forces on the spine. Twomey (1985) has demonstrated vertebral separation occurring on lumbar cadaver material with only 9 kg of force.

VARIATION IN FLEXIBILITY

Variation in flexibility over 24 hours is of much concern to those of us who base a large part of our treatment protocol on observed, and measured, changes in ranges of movement. The subject has been reviewed and discussed in detail elsewhere (Gifford, 1985, 1987), but it should be emphasized that this area of research is as yet virtually untouched. Like height variation one would expect flexibility to vary depending on the subjects activity level. Results from preliminary normative studies show that this may not wholly be the case (Gifford 1985).

Variation in flexibility in finger-tip-to-floor distance shows a clear pattern of: maximum 'stiffness' occurring

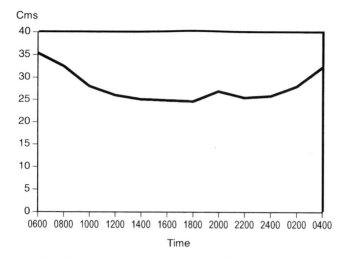

Fig. 36.1 Circadian variation in finger-tip-to-floor (mean values) (Gifford 1985).

early in the morning at, or prior to, rising; maximum flexibility occurring around 6.00 p.m., and, in some subjects, a slight stiffening occurring in the early evening (Fig. 36.1). The mean variation in the 25 subjects investigated was 14.4 cm and ranged from 5.5 cm to as much as 26.2 cm (Gifford 1985, 1987).

Diurnal changes in lumbar flexion have been confirmed recently by Adams et al (1987), but only two measures were made, one in the early morning and one in the afternoon. These authors interestingly found that the early morning result, taken 10 minutes after rising, could also be achieved up to 2 hours after rising on subsequent measures, by getting the subject to lie down before the test for a period of time equal to the time spent between rising and lying down. This suggests that recumbency *is* a strong factor in this measure. Of the 21 subjects they examined, all achieved more range in the afternoon regardless of age, sex, lumbar lordosis in standing or extent of lumbar flexion. The average increase was $5.0° \pm 1.9°$.

Work undertaken by Gifford (Gifford 1985) on 25 subjects measured every 2 hours, showed a mean variation of $13.12°$ (SD = $3.11°$), quite a lot more than the $5.0°$ of Adams and co-workers. Gifford (1987) commented that gradually increasing flexibility occurred from 6 a.m. and peaked during late afternoon or early evening. It seems as if lumbar flexibility starts to improve before rising, continues through the day, and then decreases during the evening before going to bed. It is possible that performing only two measurements in this kind of research will give a false overall picture (Conroy & Mills 1970). Adams et al (1987) found that in vitro 'creep-loading' an individual lumbar segment produced increases in range of between 2 and 3°, which is equivalent to about 12.5° for the whole lumbar spine (Adams et al 1990)—a figure closer in value to the 13.12° given above.

Lumbar extension, also investigated by Gifford (1985), shows an overall 24 hour change similar to lumbar flexion,

although maximum flexibility occurred slightly earlier at around 2 p.m. Two subjects were noted whose pattern was a reversal of this in that they showed a progressive stiffening through the day and an increase in flexibility overnight. A mean variation in extension range over 24 hours of $9.64°$ (SD = $3.51°$) was recorded.

A diurnal pattern of straight leg raising, while showing a rise in range through the day and fall at night did not provide a very dramatic picture (Gifford 1985, 1987). The mean variation over 24 hours was $9.92°$ (SD = $2.74°$). Recent work by Porter & Trailescu (1990) on the analysis of diurnal changes in pathologically limited straight leg raises, sheds interesting light on disc diagnosis and mechanisms of pathology. They looked at 28 patients who had a diagnosis of lumbar disc protrusion. Typical symptoms were of a sciatic distribution below the knee and signs of limited SLR of 50° or less, and either a 'list', or at least two neurological changes. Measurements of the range of SLR were performed in all patients before getting up and then at intervals of ¼ hour, ½ hour, 1 hour, 3 hours and 5 hours. Twenty of the patients had mean increases in SLR range of $16.9°$ (SD = $7.1°$), one showing as much as $38°$. The authors noted that most of the gains occurred in the first hour after rising, and that two hours of recumbency after testing brought the range *back* to near the baseline value recorded on rising. The remaining eight patients showed unimpressive or no diurnal changes. Porter & Trailescu (1990) explained their results in terms of disc hydration and changes in the tension of a disc protrusion. They hypothesized that a weakened disc protrusion acts like a safety valve, bulging further with increasing hydration (as in recumbency), the outer fibres becoming tense at the expense of increasing the disc space (vide supra).

When the patient stands upright, initially there is even more tension in the outer annular fibres as the external load is increased, but gradually the fluid is expressed from the disc with a reduction in its volume, until a new equilibrium is reached. When the patient then lies down for the examination of straight leg raising, a reduction in the external load produces a relatively flaccid protrusion. Straight leg raising if it is related to the tension of the protrusion, will then be improved. This cycle requires a protrusion which has intact outer annular fibres. (Porter & Trailescu 1990)

Porter & Trailescu (1990) acknowledged that changes in disc height will increase tension on a tethered nerve root and that diurnal changes in lumbar lordosis would also affect the root. They laudably suggest that all factors may act in combination. It is interesting to note, and supportive of their hypothesis, that five of the eight patients who showed little diurnal change, or none at all, went to surgery and were found to have complete annular tears or frank protrusions. A trunk list away from the painful side may be an attempt to decrease the symptom provoking annular bulge on the other side. Trunk lists which are worse in the morning and improve through the day may be a result of diminishing disc hydration and hence the size and tension of the bulge. Similar diurnal changes might explain why many patients with a disc protrusion need help with their socks or stockings in the morning, but have little difficulty later in the day (Porter & Trailescu 1990).

Porter & Trailescu (1990) observed that proven L5/S1 disc protrusions showed less diurnal change than those at L4/5 and suggested that this may be due to the relatively reduced proteoglycan content (decreased osmotic pressure) and the low hydration of the lumbosacral disc.

DIURNAL VARIATION IN BIOMECHANICS OF THE SPINE

Diurnal changes in disc volume, responsible for height variations, are likely to have marked effects on vertebral relationships and as a result affect biomechanics and pathological and anatomical relationships. Adams et al (1987) recorded average losses of 1.53 mm per lumbar disc in their creep-loaded specimens. They calculated that the lumbar spine would account for 7.65 mm loss in body height and that the thoracic and cervical spines would represent 10.2 mm and 3.06 mm respectively—this total of 20.9 mm being similar to the physiological height changes of 19.3 mm noted by others.

As disc volume decreases so the vertebrae approximate, the intervertebral foramen diminish in size, the disc bulges radially, the zygapophyseal joints progressively share more of the compressive loads, and all longitudinal ligaments tend to slacken—as do the capsular, supraspinous and interspinous ligaments.

THE INTERVERTEBRAL FORAMEN AND NERVE ROOT

Since the average height of the lumbar intervetebral foramen is about 15 to 20 mm (Panjabi et al 1983) a loss of 1.5 mm could have a significant effect, especially when there is pathological invasion of the space. Radial disc bulging may further complicate matters. Inferences from the work of Brinckmann & Horst (1985) suggest that for a diurnal reduction in disc height of 1.5 mm there should be an increased radial bulge of about 0.5 mm. A bulge of only 0.2 mm was caused by increasing compressive forces from 300 N to 1000 N, the equivalent of going from lying down to light manual work.

The influence upon root canal stenosis of diurnal changes in disc bulging is also likely to have provocative effects on the nerve root.

Segmental nerve roots and, for that matter, the whole length of the spinal canal, neuraxis, brain and meninges, are probably influenced by increased tension in the morning due to the spine's increased length. This may relate clinically to the behaviour of many spine-related symptom pictures, including headache syndromes. Problems in juveniles who have just undergone a growth spurt

of the spine and whose symptoms are worse through the night and ease on rising could relate to changes in tension of an already tight neuraxis and meningial sheath.

ZYGAPOPHYSEAL JOINTS

With loss of height the zygapophyseal joints will be brought more closely together and the facet tips will start to resist compressive forces. Spinous processes also move closer. Adams & Hutton (1983) noted that a loss in height of only 0.9 mm would cause the facets to resist about 16% of the compressive force in the erect posture. Apparently the forces can be as high as 70% (Adams et al 1990). Further insight into the daily stresses suffered by these joints is made if one considers that the lumbar lordosis increases by about 3° during the day (Adams et al 1990). High stress concentrations tend to occur in the lower margins of the joint surfaces (Dunlop et al 1984) and in the adjacent capsule (Yang & King 1984) in more extended postures. As a consequence of this it could be argued that lumbar extension and rotation would diminish as the day progresses. However, Adams et al (1988) demonstrated that simulating height loss by creep loading lumbar spine material reduced the disc's resistance to backward bending by about 40%. They proposed that this increase in disc suppleness balanced the increased resistance from the zygapophyseal joints and spinous processes and that the range of extension would not be altered via this mechanism. Most of the subjects in the study by Gifford (1985) demonstrated moderate increases of extension range, and the range of two subjects actually decreased through the day. Perhaps this highlights the inter-subject variability of biomechanical and anatomical factors involved.

THOUGHTS ON VULNERABILITY AND ADVICE TO PATIENTS

As the spine loses height so its flexion range tends to increase. This may be as much as 2–3° per segment in the lumbar spine. Adams et al (1987) determined that a disc's resistance to bending would be reduced by about 84% and the ligaments by 44%. Thus, any form of bending (or extending, or combinations of) undertaken in the early morning will generate considerably higher stresses than later in the day. Calculations suggest that, in life, bending stresses on the lumbar discs and ligaments can be increased by 334% and 79% respectively in the early morning (Adams et al 1987). It has been found that it is far harder to induce a posterior prolapse in disc material which has been creep-loaded (to simulate height loss) than it is in specimens which have not (Adams & Hutton 1982, Adams et al 1987). This is more than likely to apply in vivo and should make us aware that the disc especially is under greater stress in the first few hours of the day and will be far more susceptible to injury.

From most of the available literature it would appear that the first 3–4 hours after rising are the most critical 'danger' times. The 'key' safety time may be less than this in normal spines. Edwards (1989) and Sullivan & McGill (1990) noted a rapid decrease in height when subjects first stood up in the morning, and Reilly et al (1984) noted a 54% loss in height during the first hour after rising. However loss in stature does seem to relate to the type of activity undertaken and the amount of physical stress one is subject to. Heavy labour will have a greater effect, and in less time, than sedentary activity (Adams et al 1990). Foreman & Troup (1987), investigating stature loss in nurses, noted that this loss was greatest during their 8 hour working shifts than during a 12 hour period on their days off. They may be more susceptible either to the disc accumulating fatigue damage or to sudden injury such as prolapse, firstly, early in their shift, and secondly, during the rest day if they undertake any sudden or heavy physical activity.

Even the type of chair seems to influence the rate of height loss, slight gains in height being shown in easy chairs where plenty of back and arm support is available (Eklund & Corlett 1984).

Older subjects may lose height more quickly after rising (Edwards 1989). Older and more degenerate discs tend to creep at a faster rate than younger less degenerated discs (Keller et al 1987) and are presumably less likely to be susceptible to the type of mechanisms under discussion.

In an attempt to quantify the effects of vibration on loss of height as experienced by workers such as bus drivers, heavy construction and equipment operators and aircraft pilots, Sullivan & McGill (1990) revealed some interesting and rather unexpected results. They found that when their subjects were exposed to a controlled vibration test they demonstrated a rapid loss of height as expected. Height losses soon recovered to their average 'creep response' within 2 hours. However, they found that all subjects exposed to vibration actually were taller later in the day than they were on control days. They hypothesized that the vibration actually caused minor mechanical injury with a consequent inflammatory response causing accumulation of protein-rich exudate within the disc as well as additional fluids. The combination of increased fluid and raised osmotic pressure within the discs resulted in the relative increase in height later in the day. This may in part explain the mechanism of stiffening experienced by these types of workers, and even manual workers, at the end of the day after sitting in easy chairs.

TRACTION

It seems reasonable to assume that one of the major effects of spinal traction is to decrease disc swelling pressure and hence increase its fluid content, thus partially overcoming its natural tendency to lose height with upright activity. It is not uncommon for post traction forward flexibility and SLR range to decrease significantly in patients with presumed 'disc' pathology. This fits nicely with the pathological model outlined by Porter & Trailescu (1990) discussed above. Short periods of traction may mimic the effects of the 2 hour recumbency mentioned in their paper and could be used as a diagnostic aid. These authors suggest that 'if the size of a protrusion changes, then imaging a disc also may be affected by diurnal changes, perhaps explaining some negative radiculograms in patients with surgically proven discs.' The examination of diurnal disc changes by MRI imaging is alluded to in their paper (Porter & Trailescu 1990) and the results will be of great interest. It may be that the use of traction prior to repeat imaging or radiculogram in these 'negative' categories will confirm the gross effects of traction suggested above.

OTHER FACTORS IN FLEXIBILITY VARIATION

So far the disc has been highlighted as a major influence on patterns of changes in flexibility. Small changes in range of movements have been attributed to muscle 'warm up' factors (Baxter 1987). Adams et al (1987) noted variation in hip movements but felt that there was unlikely to be any variation in the mechanical properties of the underlying joints.

Connective tissues

It is well known that collagenous tissues express fluid and progressively elongate when they are repeatedly stretched and released (Hukins 1982). On removal of the stress the fluid driven out is slowly re-absorbed, or recovered, and the tissue slowly creeps back to its original length. The longer the stress is applied the longer the tissue takes to recover (Twomey & Taylor 1982). This could partially account for increasing flexibility when joints are repetitively stressed through the day and their slow recovery during recumbency. It should be realized that connective tissues are stressed during movements in mid-range positions. Johns & Wright (1962) demonstrated that, in the cat wrist joint, the contributions of various tissues to joint stiffness in the mid-range were: capsule 47%; muscle 41%; tendons 10%; and skin 2%. Thus, mid-range joint movements driving out fluid from tissues responsible for limiting movement would aid in increasing that joint's range of movement. Any end-range posture or stretching movement would obviously speed up the process.

Muscle

Collagenous tissues within muscle will be subject to the same effects as those discussed above. Certainly these components of muscle are regarded as the main restrictors to muscle stretch (Banus & Zetlin 1938, Kabo et al 1982). Additional factors highlighted by Gossman et al (1982) may be relevant to diurnal flexibility variation. They believe that length-associated changes can take place from within a few hours of a muscle being immobilized. Typically the number of sarcomeres decrease if the muscle remains in a shortened position. Further, the presence of any neurological hyperactivity, as in pain states or spasticity, leads to the more rapid and greater development of muscle tightness. Williams & Goldspink (1984) have shown that very rapidly increasing concentrations of perimysium occurs in immobilized rabbit muscle.

Muscle tone may be an important consideration. It seems feasible that circadian changes in flexibility, through changes in muscle tone, are a result of fluctuations in central nervous system activity.

Remember that the patient's ability to bend forward involves passive stress on tissues such as joints, ligaments, nerves and meninges as well as active elongation of muscle groups such as the hamstrings (Ortengren & Andersson 1977). Some hamstring muscle activity has been recorded during gentle stretching of the SLR (Moore & Hutton 1980).

Arthritis and inflammation

Morning stiffness accompanied by severe discomfort has long been recognized as part of the symptomatic picture in rheumatoid arthritis and some inflammatory arthropathies such as ankylosing spondylitis (Bennett & Birch 1967). However, it is also a common feature of injury-related disorders as well as the more benign degenerative arthropathies. Inflammation appears to be the common denominator and oedema is believed to be a major factor in causing stiffness (Wright 1959, Scott 1960, Kowanko et al 1981). Variation in oedema may be merely a result of the mechanical effects of movement, or more subtle circadian variations in things such as adrenal corticosteroid production, blood neutrophil counts and immune complexes (Harkness et al 1982).

The duration of symptoms/stiffness is also of diagnostic significance (McKenna & Wright 1990) and is often used as an indicator of the severity of inflammation. Thus administration of steroids or non-steroidal anti-inflammatory drugs significantly diminishes morning stiffness and reduces pain in many 'inflammatory' conditions.

CLINICAL THOUGHTS

The 24 hour variation in symptoms and signs seen in daily clinical evaluation are a result of a combination of physiological and mechanical responses. The following is an example of the type of thinking that knowledge of diurnal changes can give us. It should be emphasized that many other features of examination—such as history, behaviour of symptoms related to movement and the general nature of the disorder—must be considered as well.

Pain progressively worse overnight: mechanisms

Increasing disc fluid pressure

It is likely that an intrinsic focus of damage to a disc will cause pain since the outer fibres of the annulus are innervated via the sinuvertebral nerve. Normal overnight increases in fluid pressure may slowly irritate already sensitive damaged disc tissues. Pain will be provoked markedly on first rising and is quite likely to be relieved by manoeuvres which reduce disc pressure—such as taking weight through the arms, and traction. Beware of short-duration but severe post-traction pain. Increasing disc pressure could place irritative mechanical forces onto damaged or pathological vertebral body end-plates

Increasing spinal canal length

1. Increasing spinal canal length puts a longitudinal tension on meningeal tissues and the neuraxis. It therefore may have irritative mechanical effects on sensitive dura/arachnoid/dural ligaments as well as on major and minor cord lesions such as cord neuopraxia. Longitudinal changes may also influence any pathological tethering of the dura. Diurnal changes in neurological symptoms and signs may be enlightening. Barring other irritative forces, symptoms should decrease on rising and improve through the day. Traction should provoke symptoms.

2. Increased tension will occur on all longitudinal ligaments, supraspinous ligaments, interspinous ligaments, ligamentum flavum and the zygapophyseal capsule.

Increasing tension on nerve root

This can occur (a) within the spinal canal, (b) at the intervertebral foramen, or (c) possibly beyond the intervertebral foramen. Many other factors obviously have to be considered such as limb position which effects the tension on peripheral nerves and their roots. The behaviour of symptoms at these areas will most likely depend on abnormalities such as disc bulging/herniation, spinal stenosis and degenerative changes. Thus, a sensitive dural sleeve in a stenotic lateral recess may be aggravated by the physiological effects of recumbency on the spinal canal length but relieved with upright postures and gentle activity.

Increasing tension on sensitive tissues due to increasing inflammatory exudate/oedema/swelling

It is most likely that the source of symptoms in either injury or degenerative disorders is primarily a physiological response and that mechanical factors are imposed secondarily. The effect of movement and posture on fluid within connective tissues and specialized tissues such as the disc have been discussed. These issues may go part way in explaining diurnal changes in flexibility in normals. It is likely that similar forces brought to bear on inflamed tissues will cause a dispersal of oedema and, if these forces are non-irritative to sensitive tissues, they will bring about a short-term cessation of symptoms and increase in pain-free ranges of movement. The example of a minor sprain of the lateral ankle ligaments, which are stiff and cause limping for the first 10 to 30 minutes after rising, illustrates this simply. Gentle mobilizing techniques easily improve range, but later, rest results in a return of stiffness. The more severe the inflammation the longer it takes to free in the morning and the quicker it returns with rest. This is exemplified by typical rheumatoid arthritis and nasty flare-ups in degenerative disorders such as hip arthrosis and spondylosis.

The last clinical thought is to stress that day-to-day changes in ranges of movement occur even at the same time of day (Gifford 1985, 1987) and that ranges change markedly through the day. If therapists base success of treatment solely on gains in range of movement they are entering a very questionable area. Emphasis must be on symptomatic relief. Consideration of the effects of diurnal variations on symptoms and signs must be considered vital.

Research that involves accurate recording of range of movement has to consider the time at which the measurements were made and knowledge of any day-to-day fluctuations before any reliable conclusions can be drawn.

REFERENCES

Adams M A, Hutton W C 1980 The effect of posture on the role of the apophysial joints in resisting intervertebral compressive forces. Journal of Bone and Joint Surgery 62B: 358–362

Adams M A, Hutton W C 1982 Prolapsed intervertebral disc: a hyperflexion injury. Spine 7: 184–191

Adams M A, Hutton W C 1983 The effect of posture on the fluid content of lumbar intervertebral discs. Spine 8: 665–671

Adams M A, Dolan P, Hutton W C 1987 Diurnal variations in the stresses on the lumbar spine 12: 130–137

Adams M A, Dolan P, Hutton W C 1988 The lumbar spine in backward bending. Spine 13: 1019–1026

Adams M A, Dolan P, Hutton W C, Porter, R W 1990 Diurnal changes in spinal mechanics and their clinical significance. Journal of Bone and Joint Surgery 72B: 266–270

Banus G M, Zetlin A M 1938 The relation of isometric tension to length in skeletal muscle. Journal of Cellular and Comparative Physiology 12: 403–420

Baxter C E 1987 Low back pain and time of day: a study of their effects of psychophysical performance. Thesis submitted for PhD, University of Liverpool (cited in Adams et al 1990)

Bennett P H, Birch T A 1967 Bulletin of Rheumatic Disease 17: 453 (cited by Wright et al 1969)

Brinckmann P, Horst M 1985 The influence of vertebral body fracture, intradiscal injection, and partial discectomy on the radial bulge and height of human lumbar discs. Spine 10: 138–145

Conroy R T W L, Mills J N 1970 Human circadian rhythms. J & A Churchill, London

De Puky P 1936 The physiological oscillation of the length of the body. Acta Orthopaedica Scandinavica 6: 338–347

Dunlop R B, Adams M A, Hutton W C 1984 Disc space narrowing and the lumbar facet joints. Journal of Bone and Joint Surgery 66B: 706–710

Edwards C L 1989 A pilot study of diurnal variation in body height. Proceedings of the Sixth Biennial Conference of the Manipulative Therapists Association of Australia, Adelaide

Eklund J A E, Corlett E N 1984 Shrinkage as a measure of the effect of load on the spine. Spine 9: 189–194

Foreman T K, Troup J D G 1987 Diurnal variations in spinal loading and the effects on stature: a preliminary study of nursing activities. Clinical Biomechanics 2: 48–54

Gifford L S 1985 Circadian variation in human flexibility and grip strength. Unpublished thesis, South Australian Institute of Technology

Gifford L S 1987 Circadian variation in human flexibility and grip strength. Australian Journal of Physiotherapy 33: 3–9

Goode J D, Theodore B M 1983 Voluntary and diurnal variation in height and associated surface contour changes in spinal curves. Engineering in Medicine 12: 99–101

Gossman M R, Sahrmann S A, Rose S J 1982 Review of length associated changes in muscle. Physical Therapy 62: 1799–1808

Grieve G P 1981 Common vertebral joint problems. Churchill Livingstone, Edinburgh

Harkness J A L, Richter M B, Panazi G S, Van de Pette K, Krger A, Pownall R, Geddawi M 1982 Circadian variation in disease activity in rheumatoid arthritis. British Medical Journal 284: 551–554

Hukins D E L 1982 Biomechanical properties of collagen. In: Weiss J B, Jayson M I (eds) Collagen in health and disease. Churchill Livingstone, Edinburgh

Johns R J, Wright V 1962 Relative importance of various tissues in joint stiffness. Journal of Applied Physiology 17 824–828

Kobo J M, Goldsmith W, Nystrom M 1982 Stretch characteristics of whole muscle. Journal of Biomechanical Engineering 104: 253–255

Kazarian L E 1974 NASA (unpublished data) USA. (cited by Grieve 1981)

Keller T S, Spengler D M, Hansson T H 1987 Mechanical behaviour of the human lumbar spine. 1. Creep analysis during static compressive loading. Journal of Orthopaedic Research 5: 467–478

Koeller W, Funke F, Hartmann F 1984 Biomechanical behaviour of human intervertebral discs subjected to long lasting axial loading. Biorheology 21: 675–686

Kowanko I C, Pownall R, Knapp M S, Swannell A J, Mahoney P G C 1981 Circadian variations in the signs and symptoms of rheumatoid arthritis and in the therapeutic effectiveness of flurbiprofen at different times of day. British Journal of Clinical Pharmaceutics 11: 477–484

McKenna F, Wright V 1990 Pain and stiffness in the rheumatic diseases: the relevance of a diurnal variation to diagnosis. British Journal of Rheumatology 29 (suppl 1): 24

Markolf K L 1972 Deformation of the thoracolumbar intervertebral joints in response to external loads: a biomechanical study using autopsy material. Journal of Bone and Joint Surgery 54A: 511–533

Markolf K L, Morris J M 1974 The structural components of the intervertebral disc. Journal of Bone and Joint Surgery 56A: 675–687

Moore M A, Hutton R S 1980 Electromyographic investigation of muscle stretching techniques. Medicine and Science in Sports and Exercise 12: 322–329

Ortengren R, Andersson G B J 1977 Electromyographic studies of trunk muscles, with special reference to the functional anatomy of the lumbar spine. Spine 2: 44–52

Panjabi M M, Takata K, Goel V K 1983 Kinematics of lumbar intervertebral foramen. Spine 8: 348–357

Porter R W, Trailescu I F 1990 Diurnal Changes in Straight leg raising. Spine 15: 103–106

Reilly T, Tyrell A, Troup J D G 1984 Circadian variation in human stature. Chronobiology International 1: 121–126

Scott J T 1960 Morning stiffness in rheumatoid arthritis. Annals of Rheumatic Disease 19: 361–367

Sullivan A, McGill S M 1990 Changes in spine length during and after seated whole-body vibration. Spine 15: 1257–1260

Twomey L T 1985 Sustained lumbar traction an experimental study of long spine segments. Spine 10: 146–149

Twomey L T, Taylor J R 1982 Flexion creep deformation and hysteresis in the lumbar vertebral column. Spine 7: 116–122

Tyrell A R, Reilly T, Troup J D G 1985 Circadian variation in stature and the effects of spinal loading. Spine 10: 161–164

Urban J P G, McMullin J F 1988 Swelling pressure of the lumbar intervertebral discs. influence of age, spinal level, composition and degeneration. Spine 13: 179–187

Virgin S J 1951 Experimental investigation into the physical properties of the intervertebral disc. Journal of Bone and Joint Surgery 330: 607–611

Warden R E, Humphry T L 1964 Effect of spinal traction on the length of the body. Archives of Physical Medicine and Rehabilitation 45: 318–329

Williams P E, Goldspink G 1984 Connective tissue changes in immobilised muscle. Journal of Anatomy 138: 343–350

Wright V 1959 Some observations on diurnal variation of grip. Clinical Science 18: 17–23

Wright V, Dowson D, Longfield M D 1969 Joint stiffness—its characterisation and significance. Bio-Medical Engineering 4: 8–14

Yang K H, King A I 1984 Mechanism of facet load transmission as a hypothesis for low-back pain. Spine 9: 557–565

37. Examination of the articular system

G. A. Jull

Trauma, dysfunction and pathology in the spinal articular system are expressed as painful motion abnormalities. The regional physiological movements may have altered range both in their primary and coupled motions (Fielding 1964, Pope et al 1985, Battie et al 1990, Hindle et al 1990). At the segmental level, some joints exhibit hypomobility or a reduced range of motion while others may display hypermobility. The segment may have an altered pattern, quality or quantity of movement through range being demonstrated in both its rotations and translations. Movement may exceed normal physiological limits and present as marked instability (Stokes et al 1981, Dimnet et al 1982, Farfan & Gracovetsky 1984, Panjabi et al 1984, Seligman et al 1984, Goel et al 1985, Dvorak et al 1987a, 1988b, Friberg 1987).

The primary physical methods used clinically to assess spinal joint dysfunction are examination of active, functional movements and assessment of passive motion at the segmental level by manual examination. The information gained helps to build the picture of the nature, location and extent of the patient's movement dysfunction. As physiotherapists treat with movement, the examination also provides directives for selection of techniques for both the segmental dysfunction and movement dysfunction in the whole kinetic chain.

This chapter overviews the process of the physical examination of spinal joints and considers the possible effects of these mechanical tests on spinal articular tissues, interpretative possibilities and the possible value and limitations of these testing methods.

EXAMINATION OF ACTIVE MOVEMENTS

Movement loads and stresses the spinal tissues. In vitro biomechanical research has documented the segmental compliance and restraints to loads in the different movement directions in the various spinal regions. The mechanical and kinesiological behaviour of segments whose structures have been sectioned (or artificially 'injured') have been investigated, as have the properties of the degenerative segment (Markolf 1972, Ten-Have & Eulderink 1980, Panjabi et al 1983, Goel et al 1985, Pal & Routal 1986, Panjabi et al 1986, Shirazi-Adl et al 1986, Dumas et al 1987, Shirazi-Adl & Drouin 1987, Moroney et al 1988).

The use of this information should assist diagnosis in the clinical setting by incriminating certain structural compromise and pathology when particular movements or combinations of movements are abnormal. In a number of cases, an accurate correlation between the movement abnormality and nature of pathology or structural lesion is present (Dvorak et al 1987a,b).

Unfortunately, in many cases of spinal dysfunction, even in current times, the precise cause of pain and the nature of pathology cannot be nominated with great certainty (Mooney 1987). Despite a wealth of knowledge gained from in vitro experimentation, the in vivo state is very different. As yet no positive relationships have been determined between proposed types of pathology and precise patterns of movement abnormality (Dupius et al 1985, Nachemson 1985, Tibrewal et al 1985, Jackson et al 1988, Hindle et al 1990).

This discordance between in vitro knowledge and the clinical state may occur as the pain-sensitive spinal structures lie in quite close juxtaposition and the complex load-sharing between structures in human function is difficult to replicate in vitro. Very significantly, the activity of the spinal muscles in protection, restraint, control and the effect they have on motion patterns cannot be accounted for in in vitro research.

Spinal pathology or dysfunction and movement abnormalities are interrelated. Despite the difficulties and variables which will be encountered, clinicians and researchers have to persist with attempts to correlate symptomatic complaints, movement abnormalities and structural compromise. This is important to the advancement of the accuracy of clinical diagnosis and the efficiency of management and preventive procedures.

The major aims of the active movement examination are four-fold:

1. To reproduce all or part of the patient's pain
2. To identify and document the pattern, quality, range and pain-response for each direction of movement
3. To identify physical factors in the patient's movement pattern which may have predisposed to or arisen from the disorder
4. To gain objective physical signs on which to assess the effectiveness of treatment.

1. A basic tenet of the physical examination of the spinal pain patient is to prove that the disorder arises from a mechanical disorder of the musculoskeletal system by aggravating and relieving symptoms by mechanical compromise. This is a sound working principle but it is not infallible. Non-mechanical spinal pathology and some systemic pathologies may have pain aggravated by spinal postures and movements (Grieve 1988a, Boissonnault & Bass 1990a, b, c). The clinician correlates the pattern of the subjective complaint with that of the physical findings and refers the patient for medical consultation if discrepancy exists.

A second reason for reproducing the pain or eliciting a comparable physical sign (Maitland 1986) is to identify, at least, the regional source of the disorder. The clinician is well aware of the spinal joint's propensity to cause referred pain which can mimic extremity disorders or, on occasion, visceral symptoms (Lewit 1985, Grieve 1986).

Instances of total hip replacement surgery when the source of pain and pathology was located in the spine can be avoided by thorough and precise examination (Offierski & Macnab 1983).

2. In the examination of active movements, the range in each direction, the quality of motion and the pain response are assessed. Information is sought about the relative amount of movement restriction, the limiting factors to motion and whether any aberrant movement occurs through range.

While pathoanatomical interpretation may be in hypothesis form, the nature of the movement abnormalities contributes unequivocally to the mechanical diagnosis of the physical dysfunction.

Caution is required in interpreting the relevance of absolute range of movement, in isolation, as a criterion for abnormality. There is huge variability in range of movement between individuals of any gender or age group and motion also decreases with advancing years in each spinal region (Taylor & Twomey 1980, Fitzgerald et al 1983, O'Gorman & Jull 1987, Burton 1988, Burton & Tillotson 1988, Lind et al 1989, Battie et al 1990). Persons with a current or past history of back pain often demonstrate restricted motion as compared to controls (Mayer et al 1984, Pope et al 1985, Burton et al 1989, Battie et al 1990) but when large populations are studied, individual variability and the ageing influence virtually masks this difference (Burton et al 1989, Battie et al 1990). The

relevance of the total range is more in its proportional relationship to other movements (for diagnosis) and its use as a control for assessment of improvement.

While many studies have concentrated on the end point of range to investigate abnormality, the dynamic aspects of movement (or the pattern and quality of motion through range) may have greater significance. At the segmental level, altered centrode patterns suggest erratic motion through range (Gertzbein et al 1985). Translatory motion can be excessive even when segmental flexion–extension range is hypomobile or normal (Panjabi et al 1983, Boden & Wiesel 1990, Kalebo et al 1990). External measurement of three-dimensional physiological motions of the lumbar spine normally reveals a fairly regular pattern in primary and associated coupled rotations. In a study of a heterogeneous back pain group, not only were there restrictions in primary directions but altered relationships through range in the movements in the associated planes were identified (Hindle et al 1990).

The evidence of abnormal motion through range, highlights the importance of careful observation of the pattern of motion in the clinical examination. Many signs of abnormal quality and patterns of movement are readily identified. However the level of sensitivity of clinical observation to detect such abnormalities is unknown. The results of initial small studies relating to external measurement of segmental hypomobility and visualization of altered coupled motion are not encouraging (Stokes et al 1987, Hindle et al 1990). Further co-operative research, testing clinical observational skills against quantified motion abnormalities measured externally, need to be undertaken.

3. The active movement examination is essentially divided into two parts. The first is to identify the local signs of movement dysfunction and to locate the joint(s) or other structures immediately causing the patient's symptoms.

The second part of the motion examination is the analysis of the patient's total spinal motion pattern to identify physical factors which may have predisposed to their problem. Postures and movements of spinal regions and adjacent extremities are interdependent, and ideally there is a non-stressful relationship between form and movements of the various regions. A lack of movement in one region may overstress the articular tissue in an adjacent region which then becomes painful. These altered relationships between movement parts may result from previous trauma or joint dysfunction, the patient's inherent motor control and patterning and imbalances in the muscle system (Kendall et al 1952, Janda 1986, 1988, Sahrmann 1988). Careful observation and analysis for joint, muscle and movement dysfunction are critical for the definition of the patient's whole physical dysfunction.

4. Objective measures of movement are commonly used for assessment and monitoring improvement in peripheral joint problems. Similar objectivity is needed for spinal

joint problems but is less commonly employed in the clinical setting. This is perhaps understandable in acute cases when movements are grossly limited by muscle spasm and change is rapid, but objective measurement is desirable for evaluation and valid reassessment in sub-acute and chronic cases (McCombe et al 1989).

External methods of measuring spinal motion have limitations when compared to radiographic methods (Portek et al 1983). Even so, there are now some sophisticated methods for external measurement of three-dimensional spinal motion (Pearcy 1986, Pearcy & Hindle 1989, Alund & Larsson 1990, Hindle et al 1990). While these will probably be reserved for research purposes, there are several simple methods which show good reliability for basic movement measurement and are easily used in the clinical setting. These include spondylometers, inclino-meters and flexicurves (Twomey & Taylor 1979, Mayer et al 1984, Burton 1986, Mellin 1986a).

PROCEDURES OF ACTIVE MOVEMENT EXAMINATION OF THE ARTICULAR SYSTEM

The construction of the active movement examination is such that it progressively moves and loads the articular structures and their related soft tissues in each direction of motion until sufficient information is obtained about the nature of the joint dysfunction and the cause of symptoms. Several progressive steps are taken in the examination. A decision is made before the commencement of the examination regarding the extent of the assessment. This decision is based on the severity and irritability of symptoms and the nature of pathology (Maitland 1986). If necessary, the examination may be initially curtailed and frequently not all stages are necessary.

Posture

Initially, both static and dynamic posture are examined. This can provide a wealth of information about potential stress areas in the articular system, muscle form and motor performance. It is a very comprehensive examination, the details of which are beyond the scope of this chapter.

Pertinent to the evaluation of the articular system, basic body skeletal alignment, the position of the spinal joints and the girdles are viewed in the three body planes. The clinician observes for asymmetry between sides in the frontal plane, any axial rotation of segments or regions of the spine and the shape of the spinal curves in the sagittal plane. The body can withstand some degree of asymmetry without producing symptoms (Dieck et al 1985). Changes in the shape of spinal curvatures also occur as a factor of age (Schmorl & Junghanns 1971, O'Gorman & Jull 1987; Dalton & Coutts in Ch. 25). There is a degree of positional tolerance before joints become symptomatic but associations are beginning to emerge between postural

forms and chronic or recurrent spinal pain. For instance, the forward head posture is more accentuated in cervical headache patients (Watson 1990). A decrease in pelvic inclination associated with flattening of the lumbar curve is more prevalent in back pain sufferers and is apparent in younger and older age groups (Klausen 1986, Takemitsu et al 1988, Sward et al 1990). Conversely, Ohlen et al (1989) in a study of 64 gymnasts (who repeatedly load extension) found that those who suffered back pain had a marked lordosis compared to those without back pain.

Joint dysfunction and pathology can present with acute postural compensations. The clinician is very familiar with the lateral flexion deformity associated with an acute wry neck and the 'cock-robin' deformity of atlanto-axial joint fixation (Ono et al 1985, White & Healy 1987). Lumbar lists associated with back or back and leg pain are not uncommon (Porter & Miller 1986, Khuffash & Porter 1989).

Thorough analysis and documentation of postural deficiencies assist in defining the mechanical dysfunction and in some circumstances contribute positively to structural diagnosis. Furthermore they establish objectives of assessment and treatment both for the current dysfunction and long-term preventative measures.

Primary physiological movements

The primary physiological movements of flexion, extension, lateral flexion and axial rotation are examined initially. Movements are performed to stress specifically the relevant regions of the spine. The clinician assesses the range of movement, eliciting from the patient the onset, location and behaviour of any symptoms produced by the movement, and on recovery. The limiting factors to movement are assessed. When abnormal, these may be pain, protective muscle spasm, lack of extensibility in soft tissues (one or more of articular, muscular or neural tissue) or limitation from adverse compressive loads.

Most importantly, the clinician assesses the rhythm, quality, regional and segmental distribution of the movement. A blockage at two or more levels or an evident 'give' at a segment often has symptomatic and pathological significance (Weitz 1981, Paris 1985).

Abnormal out-of plane motions may occur with the primary motion — for example, excessive lateral deviation (list) during lumbar flexion. When this occurs, the movement is repeated while the clinician counters and prevents the deviation. The relationship of the aberrant motion to the range of the primary movement and the symptom response are determined.

The patient is encouraged to move to the limit of available range — except in cases when the severity or nature of pathology contraindicate it. Overpressure is then applied to detect more accurately the available range and the nature of limiting resistance. The clinician gently and in an exploratory manner passively increases the range until the apparent limit is achieved. This technique is important and informative. Total range of movement is a combination of motion in the joint's neutral zone (or zone of relatively free movement) and elastic zone (where the soft tissue restraints are increasingly stressed to limit movement). In many spinal joints, movement through the elastic zone accounts for the greatest range (Panjabi et al 1988, Yamamoto et al 1989). The application of overpressure to the spinal region or segment helps to ensure that it moves through its true physiological range. The validity of the overpressure procedure was demonstrated by Dvorak et al (1988a) in a radiological study measuring cervical segmental flexion and extension in neck pain patients. Range was compared when movement was performed actively by the patient and passively by the examiner. When overpressure was applied, an increase in segmental movement of up to 2–3° was recorded. Furthermore, the number of segments previously regarded as hypermobile increased and those hypomobile, decreased. These findings suggest that pain, muscle spasm or the patient's voluntary effort may mask the true nature of the movement dysfunction if the active movement alone is assessed.

Functional and combined movements

Human function uses complex movement. The single test movements may not adequately reveal the nature of the joint dysfunction or may fail to reproduce or aggravate the patient's symptoms (Maitland 1986, Grieve 1988b). It is valuable to request the patient to assume the position or move in the way that aggravates the pain. The clinician analyses the components of the movement and the times during which certain structures are compromised. Selective loading of the components at their point of compromise may more accurately locate and define the cause of the dysfunction (Magarey 1986).

The combined nature of spinal movement and the nature of the dysfunction may be more formally assessed by loading the joints through an intended sequence of movements. The principles of this combined movement examination are based on the similarities and relationship between movements and stresses on the articular tissues of the primary physiological movements (Edwards 1979, 1987, 1988, Brown 1988, 1990, Oliver 1989). The rationale and methods of examination of combined movements and the implications for treatment are fully discussed in Chapters 41 and 54.

Movements under different loading modes

In function, the spinal joints are subjected to various modes and rates of loading. The tissues of the spine are viscoelastic and thus the mechanical response and some-

times the tissues resisting the loads are different under different conditions. When the movement examination thus far has failed to reveal adequately the dysfunction, it is appropriate to extend the examination procedures to investigate the effects under these different conditions. The patient's subjective complaints of aggravating factors frequently direct which tests are appropriate. The effects of these different modes of loading apply both to active movement and passive manual examination.

Repeated movements

Viscoelastic tissues expend energy and elongate with repeated movements (hysteretic effect) (White & Panjabi 1978). The articular tissues will stretch further into range. This may expose painful limits to motion more accurately or the stretching effect may ease mechanical compromise and reduce symptoms.

Sustained movements

Sustaining a movement at end of range evokes the property of tissue creep or tissue extension over time (Kazarian 1972). In vitro studies have shown that the segmental tissue deformation through creep, occurs chiefly in the first 15 seconds after loading (Berkson 1977) which gives direction for the timing in clinical tests. Movements may be sustained in any direction or combination, and an adverse pain response may occur either in the position or on recovery to the neutral position.

Movement with speed

The extensibility and stiffness of tissues varies with the rate of loading (Noyes et al 1974). When loaded quickly, they become stiffer and less extensible. This has implications for the nature of injury and the method of application of manual examination procedures. During the active movement examination, movements performed slowly may be painless but they may be painful when tissues are forced to resist movement abruptly.

Movements under compression

Compression is a functional mode of loading which spinal joints should be able to resist painlessly. Dysfunction due to compressive stress can be elicited by applying compression to the spinal segments in their neutral position, in a combined movement position or throughout their range of movement. In this way, compression can embarrass the anterior or posterior elements of the motion segment or compromise the size and contents of the intervertebral foramen (Pal & Routal 1986, Viikari-Juntura et al 1989).

CLINICAL EXAMINATION OF REGIONAL ACTIVE MOVEMENTS

This section will investigate aspects of the methods of clinical examination of active movements of the various spinal regions, highlighting how tests might be adapted to stress specific regions of the spine.

There is reticence to presenting lists of examination techniques as they conjure a routine or recipe-like approach. This is not the method of examination. Even though technical aspects of examination are important to elicit accurately the dysfunction, it is the thought and interpretative processes that are fundamental to successful physical and perhaps pathoanatomical diagnosis.

Before examination techniques are overviewed, the possible interpretative processes will be outlined. Examples are presented from different regions of the spine to highlight the difficulties in this process.

Possible interpretative processes in active movement examination

It is not possible to state unequivocally that a certain deficit in movement means that a particular structure is at fault. A restriction in active movement may be pathognomonic of various and different factors. At a very basic level, movement stresses all mobile tissues — be they articular, muscular or neural tissues. A restriction of upper cervical flexion, for instance, could be due to adhesions or contracture of the C_{0-1} or C_{1-2} joint structures or regional posterior ligaments, tightness in the short sub-occipital extensors or the long extensors attaching to the occiput, or adhesions preventing free movement of the dura or nerve roots in this upper cervical region. Conversely, any one structure — for example, a lumbar zygapophyseal joint — could be symptomatic in any movement direction as different parts of its capsule and joint surfaces are stressed in the various movement planes.

In defiance of a rigid approach to interpretation of patterns of movement abnormality, variation between individuals is marked. This occurs in normal gross physiological movements. Logically, this is the case when segmental movement is measured (Pearcy et al 1984, Lind et al 1989, Mimura et al 1989). As well as the variation in primary motion, coupled motions are not necessarily predictable. This was well illustrated in the studies of Pearcy and Tibrewal (1984) and Pearcy et al (1984) of normal lumbar mobility by biplanar radiography. Likewise, in the cervical spine, where there is a strong ipsilateral relationship reported between lateral flexion and rotation from C_{2-7} (White & Panjabi 1978, Penning & Wilmink 1987, Penning 1988), Mimura et al (1989) found that the coupling at C_{2-3} was contralateral in vivo.

These variations in movement patterns probably reflect factors such as the limitations of in vitro studies and, anatomically, the frequent differences in orientation, shape and size of the articular facets (Overton & Grossman 1952, Mestdagh 1976, Singer et al 1989). Tropism, particularly in the transitional areas of the spine, would exert a significant influence (Farfan 1973, Cyron & Hutton 1980, Malmivaara et al 1987, Burkus 1988, Singer et al 1989). Our once-clear understanding of spinal kinematics is becoming less clear as more precise methods of in vivo measurement evolve.

When examining an active movement, the clinician questions which structures are stressed or relieved of stress, the implications of the quality, range and pain response to movement, and whether a pattern is emerging.

Many studies have investigated the load distribution between the structures of the spinal motion segment in the various directions of movement. The effects on the spinal foramina have also received attention. A few examples of these works are cited (Panjabi et al 1975, Adams et al 1980, Twomey & Taylor 1983, Yang & King 1984, Adams et al 1988, Cusick et al 1988, Liyang et al 1989, Schnebel et al 1989, Parke & Watanabe 1990). Generally, movement will compress the segmental structures on the side to which movement is occurring and place tensile strains on the opposite side. In vivo, the effect of other soft tissues of the trunk need to be considered (Kippers & Parker 1984, Raftopoulos et al 1988).

There are some variations in load distribution in the various areas of the spine relative to their structure and form. (Andriacchi et al 1974, Lang 1986, Dvorak et al 1987a,b, 1988b). However, using lumbar spine flexion as the example, the clinician may consider the following factors in interpretation of examination findings:

Lumbar flexion limited range, pain-provoking

- Anterior disc and ligaments compressed
- Intradiscal pressure increases
- Posterior disc stretched
- Compressive force from a herniated nucleus pulposus increased on nerve root
- Zygapophyseal joint capsules stretched
- Coronally orientated surface of zygapophyseal joint compressed at end of range
- Long and segmental posterior ligaments stretched
- Movement and elongation of neural tissue
- Muscles stretched: segmental and polysegmental paravertebral muscles, hamstrings.

Lumbar flexion, relief of pain

- Widening of central and lateral canal
- Relief of compressive forces from zygapophyseal joints and posterior elements.

While considering the structures under stress during the movement, the clinician also observes the quality and rhythm of the movement to try to localize which structure

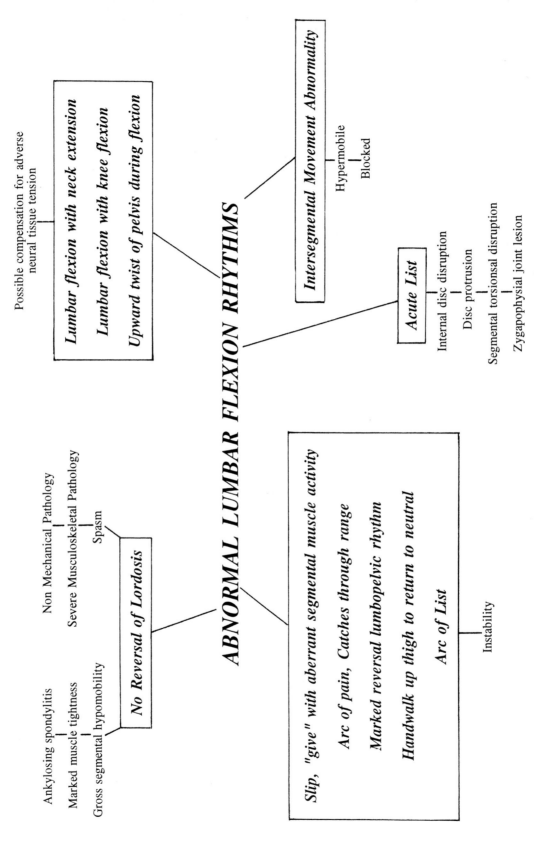

Fig. 37.1 Interpretative possibilities for some movement abnormalities observed during lumbar flexion.

is compromised and the nature of its dysfunction. Figure 37.1 displays possible interpretations of some signs that may be found, using again lumbar flexion as the example. Validation of these observations is important to establish the specificity and sensitivity of clinical examination.

All directions of movement for each spinal region are carefully examined in this way. Information from each is combined to define precisely the patient's movement abnormality. Patterns in physiological movement restriction and pain responses may emerge which may help make a provisional pathoanatomical diagnosis.

Cervical spine

Movements in the cervical segments are coupled (Worth & Selvik 1986, Penning & Wilmink 1987, Mimura et al 1989), but when the whole spine is measured three-dimensionally by external apparatus, the patterns are not strong. In the study of Alund and Larsson (1990), flexion and extension were recorded as virtually single-plane movements. Although some ipsilateral coupling was measured during lateral flexion and rotation, the amount was not as great as recorded for segments in vitro. Alund and Larsson (1990) considered that the contralateral coupling at the craniocervical joints could counteract the appearance of the ipsilateral coupling at the other cervical levels, especially when patients are requested to perform the movements in pure planes. Therefore, clinically, visually evident and quite marked out-of-plane movements accompanying any direction of cervical motion could be abnormal. The response to repeating the movement with correction would bring clarification.

In examination, distinction is made between the craniocervical, cervical and cervicothoracic regions. Even though movements are largely interdependent, full range of craniocervical flexion, for instance, cannot occur concomitantly with mid, lower cervical flexion (Worth 1988).

Flexion

Cervical flexion is initially examined as a spontaneous forward bend of the whole cervical spine. The clinician (as for all movements) observes rhythm, where movement is or is not occurring, eliciting the pain response and measuring range. Manual overpressure is applied over the C_2 level to realize the full potential of mid, low cervical and upper thoracic flexion. This hand position avoids unnecessary stress through the craniocervical joints. If the area or nature of the symptom response suggests that flexion is restricted by adverse mechanical tension of the nervous system in the spinal canal, these tissues can be sensitized by adding trunk flexion to the cervical flexion. Superimposition of knee extension and ankle dorsiflexion will maximize stretch (Troup 1986).

To test the upper cervical joints, the patient nods the head forward 'to make a double chin'. A different response may be elicited by requiring the patient to make a double chin by a retracting action. The position of the posterior arch of the atlas, in relation to the occiput, differs in the two actions, the latter shifting the atlas away from the occiput which may induce a better stretch on posterior soft tissues (Penning 1978, Bogduk 1985).

Extension

The whole cervical spine is fully extended when the head is rolled maximally backward. For regional localization, gentle manual direction or overpressure is applied to the total movement (mid, lower cervical spine), and to the upper cervical and the cervicothoracic joints (Maitland 1986).

Lateral flexion

The lateral curve of the neck is carefully observed during the movement for any regional segmental block or a more general deficit in the whole range. Localized segmental overpressure can be applied by placing the ulnar border of the hand on the occiput (C_{0-1}) and the lamina of each successive cervical vertebra (Fig. 37.2).

A more global deficit in contralateral range of lateral flexion could indicate tightness in the scalene muscles. Tightness in these muscles directs the examiner to consider the position and movement of the first rib. In investigating the thoracic outlet syndrome, Lindgren et al (1990) found an association between an elevated and hypomobile first rib and restriction of contralateral rotation with added lateral flexion.

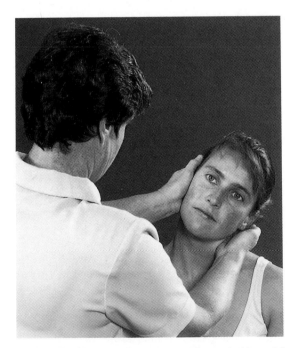

Fig. 37.2 Localized segmental overpressure in cervical lateral flexion.

Alternatively, the general deficit in contralateral lateral flexion may be a preliminary sign of neural tissue tension in the mid, lower cervical nerve roots or spinal nerves.

Axial rotation

The cervical spine is most flexible in axial rotation with more than half of the motion occurring at the atlanto-axial joints (Penning & Wilmink 1987, Panjabi et al 1988, Mimura et al 1989). A marked loss of rotation could in itself suggest dysfunction at this level for motion here generally precedes that of other levels. In the presence of a restriction in rotation, the contribution to the range of the C_{0-1}, C_{1-2} joints can be more selectively viewed if the patient preflexes the whole cervical spine and then rotates the head. Jirout (1979) has further demonstrated that rotation can be more localized to the C_{2-3} segment if the upper cervical spine is preflexed and the head is rotated in this position. As with lateral flexion, overpressure can be applied locally to stress each cervical level in the rotation direction.

As previously discussed, the examination can be extended to assess movements in combination or repeat movements under different loading conditions.

Thoracic spine

The thoracic spine presents a joint complex in the true sense of the word. Movement dysfunction and pain may arise from any of the three joints of the thoracic spinal segment and those of the ribs namely costovertebral, costotransverse and sternocostal joints. The individual components of the rib cage are quite flexible and movement of the ribs accompanies that of intersegmental motion. However, the presence of the ribs — and particularly their attachment to the sternum, as a whole — adds considerable stiffness to the thoracic spine (Andriacchi et al 1974). The joints of the thoracic spine and ribs are subjected to considerable loads during normal function, as is revealed by the frequent presence of degenerative changes and bony hyperostosis (Malmivaara et al 1987, Macones et al 1989).

Movements occur in each plane in the thoracic spine and are of a coupled nature. In the upper thoracic segments, lateral flexion and axial rotation follow the pattern of the cervical spine and are coupled ipsilaterally (Penning & Wilmink 1987). However, the pattern becomes less distinct and variable in the mid- to lower thoracic joints.

The active movements of the upper thoracic joints (T_1–T_4) are examined by leading with cervical movements and superimposing thoracic movement. The mid-thoracic joints (approximately T_4–T_{10}) are assessed in a sitting position, while the lower thoracic segments (approximately T_{10}–L_1) are examined in a standing position in association with lumbar movements. Attention will focus on the examination of the mid-thoracic region.

Flexion

Thoracic flexion is a curling action of the trunk. A flat or almost lordosed group of segments is not uncommonly observed and often indicates segmental hypomobility. The ribs should spread posteriorly, the rib cage almost flaring as it is displaced slightly forward.

The direction of overpressure must carefully increase the thoracic curl (Fig. 37.3). Its angle of application can be adjusted to stress segments more superiorly or inferiorly in the thoracic region. When neural tissue tension is thought to contribute to a painful limitation of movement, this gentle overpressure can be applied to thoracic flexion with the neck preflexed and, if necessary, with the knees also extended.

Extension

Care is taken to instruct the patient in thoracic extension, rather than allow lumbar or even hip extension to occur. Overpressure can be applied segmentally by placing the thumb pad and knuckle of the proximal interphalangeal joint on the laminae of the relevant segment. The limitation to extension should be perceived as a firm end-feel due to contact of adjacent spinous processes and the inferior articular processes with the lamina below.

Lateral flexion

The patient curls his or her shoulder down towards the hip. Any interruption to the arc of the sideways curve may indicate segmental hypomobility and often adjacent segmental hypermobility. The ribs should fan contralaterally

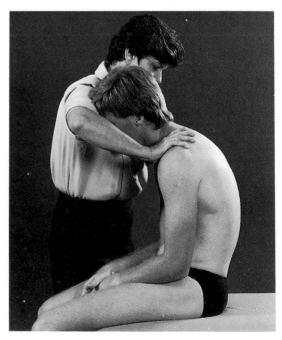

Fig. 37.3 Overpressure to thoracic flexion.

and approximate ipsilaterally. Overpressure can be directed towards a particular segment by placing the ulnar border of the hand on the associated rib, utilizing it as a local lever.

Axial rotation

The thoracic spine is most flexible in axial rotation. Initially the patient rotates to either side in an upright position. Rotation can be accentuated in the mid, lower thoracic levels by preflexing the upper, mid segments before turning to each side. There is some rib slide during rotation, but the attachment of the ribs to the sternum limits this motion. Because the ribs have some elasticity, they distort slightly such that their shape appears slightly more convex on the side to which rotation is occurring and slightly flatter on the opposite side. As for lateral flexion, overpressure can be applied segmentally by manual pressure on the associated rib.

Functional movement

Two more functional tests are valuable adjuncts to the formal assessment of thoracic movements. These are movements of the upper limbs and respiration.

Thoracic spine motion is an integral component of the upper limb movement. The thoracic spine contralaterally laterally flexes and rotates during single arm elevation. The thoracic segments extend with bilateral shoulder flexion (Crawford & Jull 1990). In examining arm movement, the clinician observes for any abnormal segmental motion, any deficits or differences between sides in range of shoulder movement, and seeks any production of thoracic symptoms.

Rib movement and associated thoracic movement are tested routinely in the functional mode of full inspiration and expiration. On full inspiration, the ribs rotate around their respective axes which, in sum, increases the transverse, antero-posterior and vertical diameters of the rib cage. Requiring the patient to cough as part of the assessment strongly loads both the thoracic joints and rib articulations.

Lumbar spine

The assessment of lumbar spine movements takes into account motion of the thoracolumbar, lumbar and lumbo-pelvic-hip complex. The joints and muscles of the lower limb, particularly those of the pelvis and hip, can have a profound influence on the nature of lumbar spine mobility. The pelvic joints have received considerable attention in this text (see Chs 10, 32). Additionally, many aspects of clinical theory on the role of imbalances in muscle length and hip joint mobility in back pain, have been supported by the findings of several studies which indicate that limited hip mobility is often a distinguishing feature between low back pain populations and normal controls (Magora 1975, Fairbank et al 1984, Mayer et al 1984, Mellin 1986a,b). Assessment of the contribution of these structures to the total lumbar motion pattern, as well as individual and specific assessment of the hip and pelvic joints, associated muscles and neural tissue, are mandatory parts of the total examination of lumbar articular dysfunction.

Flexion

Lumbar flexion is initially examined as a spontaneous movement. A measure of range should be made and the relative distribution of the movement occurring in the hip, lumbar and lower thoracic areas also noted.

Flexion normally appears as a single plane movement (Hindle et al 1990). If aberrant trunk lateral flexion or rotation is observed, or if the patient maintains the head and neck towards extension (an antalgic manoeuvre for neural tissue tension), flexion is repeated with these movements corrected. The effects on range of movement and pain response are noted.

Overpressure should reveal a firm but springy, painless resistance of a predominantly collagenous nature. It is often valuable to sustain the overpressure for 15–20 seconds or longer if indicated by the patient's symptomatic complaints. This may provide some indication of the lumbar tissues' ability to recover after some creep deformation.

Extension

An important aspect of the examination of extension is observation of the distribution of motion between segments. A loss of segmental motion is not uncommon. Extension induces compressive forces on the posterior aspect of the disc, the zygapophyseal joints and posterior elements and narrows both the spinal canal and intervertebral foramina. Conversely, pain may be related to tissue stress from sometimes inordinate degrees of hyperextension often maximized at the low lumbar segments. A hypermobile segment may be present, adjacent to ones which are stiff. This occurrence has been clearly demonstrated after spinal fusion (Lee & Langrana 1984).

Overpressure may be applied to extension of the total thoracolumbar region by gently curling the spine backwards through the shoulders or it may be applied at the segmental level.

Lateral flexion

The lumbar spine is quite flexible in lateral flexion, and observation of the lateral curve can reveal segmental blocks or whole blocks to regional movements which could be suggestive of muscle tightness (e.g. quadratus lumborum). The range of lateral flexion can be reasonably reliably monitored by measuring the distance the hand moves down the thigh (Mellin 1986a).

Coupled flexion and contralateral rotation normally accompany lateral flexion (Hindle et al 1990) but excessive degrees of flexion should be corrected. Lateral flexion is a sensitive movement in both acute pathology (Weitz 1981) and in chronic back pain. In comparing range of movement between chronic back pain subjects and controls, Mellin (1986a, 1987) found that deficits in lateral flexion and axial rotation correlated more strongly with back pain than did sagittal movements.

Axial rotation

Examination of rotation is conducted in the standing position. It is often appropriate to allow the patient (with feet facing straight ahead) to perform full trunk, hip and lower limb rotation so that the whole pattern and distribution of rotation can be viewed. By stabilizing the pelvis, rotation can be limited to the trunk. Because the adjacent thoracic region is quite mobile in axial rotation, localization of the movement to the lumbar spine by these methods is difficult, and often this movement provides less information than that gained from other directions.

Functional movements

Assessment of the patient's spontaneous aggravating movement and the more formal assessment of movements in combination are valuable in definining lumbar dysfunction (see Ch. 54).

Formal examination of lumbar spine movement conventionally involves assessment of trunk motion. Movements of the lumbar joints should also be assessed using the pelvis as the primary lever. This not only mimics the movement of our bipedal function but also more directly and primarily stresses the lower lumbar levels. To the conventional examination is added anterior and posterior pelvic tilt, axial rotation of the pelvis and pelvic side shift. These movements as well as other variations of pelvic and lumbar movement should be conducted with care and precision as, when performed correctly, they may more acutely embarrass the low lumbar joints.

MANUAL EXAMINATION OF THE ARTICULAR SYSTEM

The second phase of the articular examination involves the assessment of passive motion at the segmental level by manual examination. By this method, the physiological movements in each plane and many of the associated translatory motions, can be examined at the individual intervertebral segment. The examiner seeks the interrelationship between the active regional and passive segmental motion dysfunction.

The aims of manual examination are:

1. To identify and localize the symptomatic segment(s)
2. To define, in physical terms, the nature of the segmental motion abnormality
3. To identify associated areas of segmental motion abnormality
4. To provide the basis for selection of appropriate treatment techniques.

To practitioners of manipulative physiotherapy, manual examination is a fundamental method of examination and a primary physical diagnostic technique. Historically, manual examination has often been regarded by those not directly in the field as an empirical skill or 'art form' rather than a rationally based physical diagnostic testing method. It is therefore appropriate to review briefly the nature of manual examination to assess its contribution to clinical diagnosis of spinogenic pain.

Manual examination can be described as a very basic in vivo test of spinal segmental mechanics, testing particularly the elastic properties of the viscoelastic spinal tissues. In examination, a manual force is applied rhythmically and repeatedly either directly or indirectly on the motion segment to produce a particular direction of motion. What is measured perceptually is the displacement and the segmental tissue resistance to the applied force. In other words, the clinician is measuring the basic load displacement characteristics for a particular segmental direction of motion. This is a very appropriate measure. Pathology, injury, reactive muscle spasm, the fibrosis of repair or tissue contracture alters tissue compliance when a load is applied which, in turn, alters the displacement characteristics of the segment (Panjabi et al 1983, 1984, Farfan & Gracovetsky 1984, Goel et al 1985, Dvorak et al 1987a).

The measure of manual examination is not a qualitative estimate of absolute range of movement per se, but rather a combined measure of displacement and, more importantly, the nature of tissue resistance both through range and at the limit of range. Manual examination tests the segment well within normal physiological loading limits moving the joint through the neutral zone of unrestrained movement and into the elastic zone where the segmental tissues gradually stiffen to limit motion. The findings can be recorded pictorially (movement diagrams: Maitland 1986) and these can be likened to the load displacement curves calculated in vitro for each movement of the vertebral motion segments (Markolf 1972). Alternatively, the nature of tissue compliance can be recorded on a motion rating scale indicating progressive states of hypomobility or hypermobility (Kaltenborn & Lindahl 1969, Gonnella et al 1982).

There are different tissue restraints to directions of movements in various spinal regions. Therefore, the examiner becomes cognisant with the normal 'feel' of joint movement and restraint to have a basis for decisions of abnormality. For example, segmental lumbar flexion is resisted in its intermediate angles largely by the disc and capsular ligaments, and at the end of range the posterior ligamentous system begins to resist strongly (Adams et al 1980, Panjabi et al 1982). Therefore, in examining a normal segment, the clinician would expect to feel some initial free displacement followed soon by gradual and progressive stiffening of the segment as the collagenous structures resist further displacement. In contrast, axial rotation at the lumbar segment is limited principally by facet compression with some contribution from the disc and opposing capsular ligaments (Schultz et al 1979, Adams & Hutton 1981, Stokes 1988). Consistent with this, the resistance to motion perceived during manual examination is that of an initial, small free phase of motion followed by a short period of progressive stiffening ending in a relatively abrupt and hard resistance to further displacement.

Not only do clinicians familiarize themselves with the manual perception of motion and resistance to motion in normal 'ideal' segments, but any clinical judgement takes into account the factor of age. Spinal motion decreases with advancing age. Two studies have documented upper cervical and lumbar intersegmental motion, as assessed by manual examination, in normal populations of a wide age range (Jull 1986, Jull & Bullock 1987a,b). Results supported those of other studies, but even though incidences of moderate hypomobility were found, the mean loss of segmental motion was not extensive in pain-free individuals and tended towards a slight loss of mobility with advancing age. Of note, some segments exhibited more age-related motion changes than did others. In the lumbar spine, the L_{3-4} and L_{4-5} segments demonstrated most hypomobility, and, in a manual study of thoracic segmental motion (T_{1-8}) in normal subjects ages 17 to 34 years, Minucci (1987) determined that the T_{4-5} segment was the most hypomobile.

Individual variability is also taken into account. Persons have different body types. Even at the level of the intervertebral disc, there is variability in the total amount, relative proportions and topographical distribution of type 1 and type 2 collagen which will influence flexibility (Adams et al 1977). Differences in the orientation of facet planes between individuals, as well as facet asymmetry within a segment, will influence the nature of motion. Even though the clinician is aware of normal, average spinal mobility, judgements of normality or abnormality are always made on an individual basis.

Many texts of manipulative therapy describe physical signs for diagnosing symptomatic motion abnormality at the segmental level (Lewit 1985, Maitland 1986, Bourdillon & Day 1988, Grieve 1988b). A study (Jull et al 1988) confirming the accuracy of manual diagnosis for cervical zygapophyseal joint pain syndromes validated the following criteria as pathognomic of symptomatic joint dysfunction:

- altered displacement
- abnormal quality of physical resistance to joint motion
- provocation of pain (local or referred) by the testing procedure.

These criteria are not necessarily structure-specific or pathology-specific. However, an 'increased thickness' in the perceived resistance to motion could be consistent with segmental tissue fibrosis, an effused zygapophyseal joint, or early signs of capsular fibrosis. Segmental muscle spasm offers an often sudden and firm resistance to manual pressure, but it has a 'giving' quality unlike that of the hard, abrupt unyielding resistance of a markedly arthrotic joint. Conversely, the segment may be felt to have too little resistance through range which may indicate instability (Paris 1985, Schneider 1987). This may or may not be associated with an absolute increase in physiological range.

The contribution of manual examination to diagnosis of spinal dysfunction

It is considered that manual examination is an essential component of the examination of the spinal articular system. The spine is a multisegmental structure. External measurement of active range of movement does not accurately reflect the nature of the segmental motion when comparisons are made with either radiographic or manual methods (Jull & Lane 1983, Portek et al 1983). This is not unexpected when considering the variability in range of movement between individuals, the segmental aberrant movements which may occur, and the influence that external factors such as muscle and neural tissue length may have. Therefore, for an accurate knowledge of spinal motion, examination must include segmental analysis.

There are currently some very sophisticated methods of radiographic examination which can accurately quantify certain pathologies and segmental motion abnormalities. It is therefore reasonable to question the role of manual examination because, to the sceptics, it is a clinical, subjective method of measurement.

To appreciate the place of manual examination in the whole spectrum of spinal diagnostic techniques, the full picture of spinogenic pain and dysfunction needs to be considered. It would not be an exaggeration to state that millions of people world-wide seek diagnosis and treatment of their spinal pain each month. The highly sophisticated, expensive and often invasive radiological methods of segmental examination are used for a small minority of patients — for instance, those who are likely surgical candidates, those where trauma has led to clinical suspicion of loss of structural integrity, or when non-mechanical pathology such as malignancy is suspected. Additionally, there is still the problem that, in many cases of benign spinal pain (as occurs in some other common medical disorders), there are currently no radiological or other laboratory tests that can depict the pathology or the mechanical dysfunction.

Medical investigation of the spinal segment for the vast majority of spinal pain patients consists usually of standard plain X-rays of the spinal region or the qualitative motion analysis of single plane flexion–extension views. It is well appreciated that these methods are basic and often unreliable, both for locating the symptomatic segment and depicting a motion abnormality. Additionally, plain X-rays give negligible indication of the soft-tissue status of the spinal segment, and no information either on the changes in segmental tissue compliance or the presence of pain — all of which are common components of spinal segmental dysfunction.

In contrast, the nature of manual examination is such that it has the capacity to locate the symptomatic segment and, at least, qualitatively define the tissue changes and motion dysfunction. Furthermore, manual examination is a non-invasive, non-destructive, low-cost method of assessment of intersegmental dysfunction which can be used with safety to examine the vast majority of patients with benign spinal disorders.

To be an accepted examination method within the whole medical diagnostic proforma for spinal pain, manual examination has to be reliable in detecting the symptomatic segment. While manipulative physiotherapists would contend that it is, based on their clinical experience, scientific validation is only in its infancy. An initial study has proven the sensitivity and specificity of manual examination for diagnosing the level and side of cervical zygapophyseal joint syndromes (Jull et al 1988). Results of a preliminary pilot study indicate some sensitivity for manual examination for detecting instability associated with a lumbar disc protrusion (Schneider 1987).

The results of these studies are positive, but many more need to be undertaken before the place of manual examination is secure. In the first instance, basic research questions should be posed. For example, does the level of segmental dysfunction determined by manual examination correlate with the segment proven symptomatic by a reliable medical diagnostic technique? Once this basic level of validation has been firmly established, more sophisticated questions — such as those regarding the pathological and structural significance of different tissue compliance patterns — can be posed. It is only through such rigorous research that a true appraisal of the value, place and limitations of manual examination can be established.

PROCEDURES OF MANUAL EXAMINATION OF SEGMENTAL MOTION

Manual examination incorporates soft-tissue palpation, palpation of vertebral alignment and segmental motion

testing to gather a clear understanding of the physical aspects of the segmental dysfunction. The manual techniques of examination for each segment and region of the spine are numerous and it is well outside the scope of this chapter to describe the performance of all techniques in detail. The reader is referred to manipulative therapy texts for this purpose (Maitland 1986, Bourdillon & Day 1988, Grieve 1988b). Rather, each section of the examination will be presented, giving examples from the various spinal regions.

Soft tissue palpation

During any manual palpation procedure it is essential that the examiner's hands are confident, yet relaxed, gently 'sinking' into and moving tissue rather than 'pressing or poking'. False-positive results are readily gained by poor handling.

Segmental dysfunction is manifest in both the joints and soft tissues. The skin of the spinal region is first palpated to detect any temperature changes or changes in skin texture or mobility. The longer muscles of the region are examined for tightness or the presence of painful trigger points (Travell & Simons 1983). The soft tissues between and around the spinous processes, the muscles in the areas of the laminae and transverse processes are gently and deeply palpated. Frequently segmental muscle spasm (most likely in the multifidus muscle) can be felt over a symptomatic joint. In the cervical spine, exostoses may be palpated over the severely degenerative zygapophyseal joint.

Localized soft-tissue thickness and tenderness are often very relevant findings of segmental dysfunction (Helbig & Lee 1988). However, care must be taken with the interpretation of the significance of all findings as paravertebral or interspinous soft-tissue thickening can present in asymptomatic individuals — as revealed in a study of the thoracic region (Minucci 1987). Additionally, such signs can present without a musculoskeletal cause. For instance, via somatovisceral and notably viscerosomatic reflexes, thoracic segmental tenderness can be a symptom and sign of a visceral disorder (Lewit 1985, Grieve 1986). Notably, the converse can be true.

Alignment

The position of bony prominences and the alignment of the vertebrae in each spinal region are carefully palpated and positional anomalies sought. The concept of perfect symmetry of bony prominences, a straight spine in the coronal plane and a smooth regular position of spinous processes in the sagittal curves is an ideal rather than a reality. Minor asymmetries and positional deviations are common. They are usually well within normal physiological limits and are incidental. A general guideline is that a positional abnormality is a significant finding when associated with movement abnormalities.

The bony prominences, namely, the spinous processes, laminae and transverse processes are palpated. In the sagittal plane, spinous processes may be felt to be unduly prominent or depressed. These may be found in any region of the spine and are commonly associated with an extension or flexion motion restriction. In the thoracic spine, two or three neighbouring segments may be involved. Palpation of a true step between adjacent spinous processes is the most overt anomaly in the sagittal plane and may be associated with a spondylolisthesis.

When making decisions on rotation abnormalities, the position of the spinous process, laminae and transverse processes are considered concurrently. Reliance on the position of the spinous process alone is highly unreliable. In the cervical region, one side of the bifid spinous process may be elongated or absent (Maitland 1986, Boquet et al 1989) which can give the erroneous impression of rotation. In the thoracic region, spinous processes commonly and inconsequentially deviate to one side (Minucci 1987). An off-centre position of the low lumbar spinous process may indicate a torsional deformity of the neural arch (Farfan 1984) but this deviation, too, may be of no significance (Van Schaik et al 1989).

True segmental rotational abnormalities are not uncommon and can be quite marked. This is especially so in the craniocervical region in acute or late stage unresolved cases of atlanto-axial fixation (Ono et al 1985, Grieve 1988b). Careful palpation in association with movement analysis (and often radiological findings) can realize the significance of this and other alignment abnormalities.

Segmental motion testing

Manual examination is able to test the physiological movements of flexion, extension, lateral flexion and axial rotation at each segment in every spinal region. In principle, the examiner produces, locally the pertinent direction at the segment and palpates the displacement and tissue resistance to displacement between the two vertebrae of the segment (Fig. 37.4). The bony parts usually palpated are the spinous processes of adjacent vertebrae and in the cervical spine, motion between laminae is assessed when examining lateral flexion and rotation. Due to the unique anatomical configuration of the atlas, the atlanto-occipital joints are assessed by palpating the occipital condyles or mastoid process relative to the arch or transverse process of the atlas (Fig. 37.5).

The translatory (accessory) motions along the Z axis (antero-posterior, postero-anterior glides), Y axis (long axis distraction, compression) and X axis (lateral translation) may be tested, although regional anatomical

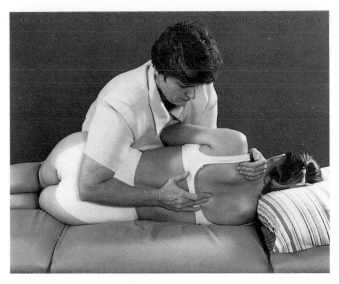

Fig. 37.4 Manual examination of intersegmental thoracic rotation. Motion is produced by rhythmically rotating the thoracic spine through the sternum and anterior shoulder. Segments distal to that being tested are stabilized by the examiner's forearm and hand with the palpating finger pad fixing the lower spinous process of the segment, the tip perceiving the rotary motion of the upper spinous process.

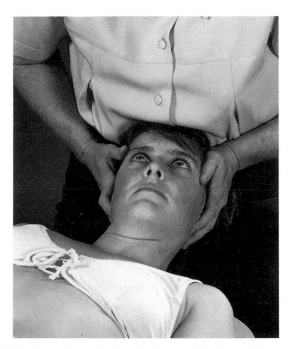

Fig. 37.5 Manual examination of atlanto-occipital lateral flexion. Movement between the transverse process of the atlas and mastoid process is palpated.

configurations govern which directions can be performed effectively. For instance, the presence of the rib cage obviously prevents the direct inducement of antero-posterior glide in the thoracic spine. The conceptualization of testing a pure translation in many cases is incorrect and a proportion of the associated rotation at

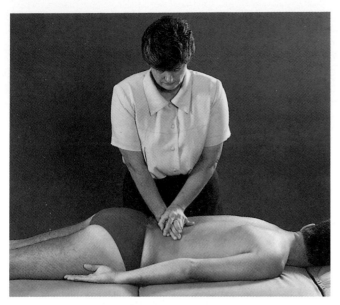

Fig. 37.6 Lumbar segmental postero-anterior translatory (accessory) glide is tested by producing the movement directly through the spinous process.

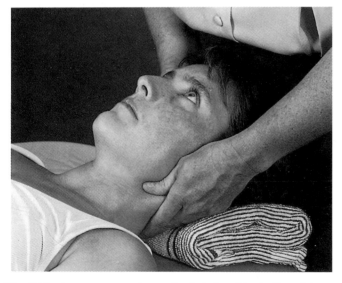

Fig. 37.7 An antero-posterior motion is induced in the line of the facet plane of the C_{2-3} zygapophyseal joint to induce the motion of the C_2 inferior facet which occurs with extension.

the segment will accompany the induced translation. The translatory/accessory motion is usually produced and tested by direct oscillatory, manual pressure through the relevant bony part of the vertebra (Fig. 37.6). The direct application of manual pressure can also test the facet slide which occurs with the physiological movement of the related segment (Fig. 37.7).

Examination of the costotransverse/costovertebral, sterno-costal and rib motion is a routine part of the manual ex-

amination of the thoracic spine. Examination of the upper ribs is included in cervical spine examination. Other special tests may be appropriate for instance, craniovertebral ligament tests (Aspinall 1990) or shear tests for segmental instability (Kaltenborn 1970, Maitland 1986).

The influence of and interrelationship between spinal segments and spinal regions suggests that the examination should include, at least, a basic examination of the whole spine and a detailed regional examination of the symptomatic area. Manual examination seeks to locate the immediate source of symptoms as well as identifying segments and structures which may be adversely influencing or influenced by the symptomatic area.

As for any manual assessment procedure, the higher the level of skill of the clinician, the more accurate will be the information gained. It is necessary for the clinician to become very conversant and competent in the basic procedures of examination. The direction of application, the rate, rhythm and the manual force used to produce motion are all important for consistent responses from the viscoelastic tissues of the spinal segment (Jull & Gibson 1986). Nevertheless, as stressed, there is variability between individuals, and the direction of injurious stresses and resultant dysfunction can have unique effects on joints. For these reasons, as well as conducting standard tests, the clinician must be prepared to 'explore' the spinal joints. Manual pressure can be directed at different angles and different rates. Physiological movements may be tested in various joint positions or translatory motion tested in different positions of the physiological range (see Chs 41, 54). Information gained from the active movement examination guides these extended assessment procedures.

A competent and 'thinking' examination will reveal the nature and extent of the segmental dysfunction and, together with information gained from all aspects of the examination, will guide the approach to appropriate management.

CONCLUSION

The assessment of active movements and manual examination of segmental motion is the foundation for the clinical evaluation of the spinal articular system. It is believed that such tests reveal a wealth of diagnostic information on the nature of spinal joint dysfunction. However, many clinical tests require scientific quantification and validation before their value, sensitivity and specificity are fully realized. It is the physiotherapists who have the high levels of training and expertise in clinical analysis of movement disorders and therefore it is the physiotherapist who should assume a large part of the responsibility for initiating and undertaking such research.

REFERENCES

Adams M A, Hutton W C 1981 The relevance of torsion to the mechanical derangement of the lumbar spine. Spine 6: 241–248

Adams M A, Hutton W C, Stott J R 1980 The resistance to flexion of the lumbar intervertebral joint. Spine 5: 245–253

Adams M A, Dolan P, Hutton W C 1988 The lumbar spine in backward bending. Spine 13: 1019–1026

Adams P, Eyre D R, Muir H 1977 Biochemical aspects of development and ageing of human lumbar intervertebral discs. Rheumatology and Rehabilitation 16: 22–29

Alund M, Larsson S 1990 Three-dimensional analysis of neck motion. A clinical method. Spine 15: 87–91

Andriacchi T, Schultz A, Belytschko T, Galante J 1974 A model for studies of mechanical interaction between the human spine and rib cage. Journal of Biomechanics 7: 497–507

Aspinall W 1990 Clinical testing for the craniovertebral hypermobility syndrome. Journal of Orthopaedic and Sports Physical Therapy 12: 47–54

Battie M C, Bigos S J, Fisher L D, Spengler D M, Hansson T H, Nachemson A L, Wortley M D 1990 The role of spinal flexibility in back pain complaints within industry. A prospective study. Spine 15: 768–773

Berkson M H 1977 Mechanical properties of the human lumbar spine flexibilities, intradiscal pressures and posterior element influences. Proceedings of the Institute of Medicine of Chicago 31: 138–143

Boden S D, Wiesel S W 1990 Lumbosacral segmental motion in normal individuals. Have we been measuring instability properly? Spine 15: 571–576

Bogduk N 1985 The anatomical basis of coupled movements in the cervical spine. Proceedings of the Fourth Biennial Conference, Manipulative Therapists Association of Australia, Brisbane, pp 12–29

Boissonnault W G, Bass C 1990a Pathological origins of trunk and neck pain: Part I — Pelvic and abdominal visceral disorders. Journal of Orthopaedic and Sports Physical Therapy 12: 192–207

Boissonnault W G, Bass C 1990b Pathological origins of trunk and neck pain: Part II — Disorders of cardiovascular and pulmonary systems. Journal of Orthopaedic and Sports Physical Therapy 12: 208–215

Boissonnault W G, Bass C 1990c Pathological origins of trunk and neck pain: Part III — Diseases of the musculoskeletal system. Journal of Orthopaedic and Sports Physical Therapy 12: 216–221

Boquet J, Boismare F, Payenneville G, Leclerc D, Monnier J C, Moore N 1989 Lateralisation of headache: possible role of an upper cervical trigger point. Cephalalgia 9: 15–24

Bourdillon J F, Day E A 1988 Spinal manipulation. 4th edn. Heinemann, Oxford

Brown L R T 1988 Introduction to the treatment and examination of the spine by combined movements. Physiotherapy 74: 347–353

Brown L R T 1990 Treatment and examination of the spine by combined movements — 2. Physiotherapy 76: 66–74

Burkus J K 1988 Cervical facet syndrome simulating facet dislocation. Spine 13: 118–120

Burton A K 1986 Regional lumbar sagittal mobility; measurement by flexicurves. Clinical Biomechanics 1: 20–26

Burton A K 1988 Patterns of lumbar mobility and their predictive value in the natural history of back and sciatic pain. Clinical Biomechanics 3: 190–191

Burton A K, Tillotson K M 1988 Reference values for 'normal' regional lumbar sagittal mobility. Clinical Biomechanics 3: 106–113

Burton A K, Tillotson K M, Troup J D G 1989 Variation in lumbar sagittal mobility with low-back trouble. Spine 14: 584–593

Crawford H J, Jull G A 1990 The influence of thoracic form and movement on range of shoulder flexion. Unpublished data, Department of Physiotherapy, University of Queensland, Australia

Cusick J F, Yoganandan N, Pintar F, Myklebust J, Husasan H 1988 Biomechanics of cervical spine facetectomy and fixation techniques. Spine 13: 808–812

Cyron B M, Hutton W C 1980 Articular tropism and stability of the lumbar spine. Spine 5: 168–172

Dieck G S, Kelsey J L, Goel V K, Panjabi M M, Walters S D, Laprade M H 1985 An epidemiological study of the relationship between postural asymmetry in the teen years and subsequent back and neck pain. Spine 10: 872–877

Dimnet J, Pasquet A, Krag M H, Panjabi M M 1982 Cervical spine motion in the sagittal plane: kinematic and geometric parameters. Journal of Biomechanics 15: 956–969

Dumas G A, Beaudoin L, Drouin G 1987 In situ mechanical behaviour of posterior spinal ligaments in the lumbar region. An in vitro study. Journal of Biomechanics 20: 301–310

Dupius P R, Yong-Hing K, Cassidy J D, Kirkaldy-Willis W H 1985 Radiological diagnosis of degenerative lumbar spinal instability. Spine 10: 262–276

Dvorak J, Hayek J, Zehnder R 1987a CT — functional diagnosis of the rotatory instability of the upper cervical spine — 2. An evaluation on healthy adults and patients with suspected instability. Spine 12: 726–731

Dvorak J, Panjabi M M, Gerber M, Wichmann W 1987b CT — functional diagnostics of the rotatory instability of upper cervical spine. 1. An experimental study on cadavers. Spine 12: 197–205

Dvorak J, Froehlich D, Penning L, Baumgartner H, Panjabi M M 1988a Functional radiographic diagnosis of the cervical spine: flexion/extension. Spine 13: 748–755

Dvorak J, Schneider E, Saldinger P, Rahn B 1988b Biomechanics of the craniocervical region: the alar and transverse ligaments. Journal of Orthopaedic Research 6: 452–461

Edwards B C 1979 Combined movements of the lumbar spine: examination and clinical significance. Australian Journal of Physiotherapy 25: 147–152

Edwards B C 1987 Clinical assessment: the use of combined movements in examination and treatment. In: Twomey L T, Taylor J R (eds) Physical therapy of the low back. Churchill Livingstone, New York, pp 175–198

Edwards B C 1988 Combined movements of the cervical spine in examination and treatment. In: Grant R (ed) Physical therapy of the cervical and thoracic spine. Churchill Livingstone, New York, pp 125–152

Fairbank J C T, Pynsent P B, Van Poortvliet J A, Phillips H 1984 Influence of anthropometric factors and joint laxity in the incidence of adolescent back pain. Spine 9: 461–464

Farfan H 1973 Mechanical disorders of the low back. Lea & Febiger, Philadelphia

Farfan H 1984 The torsional injury of the lumbar spine. Spine 9: 53

Farfan H, Gracovetsky S 1984 The nature of instability. Spine 9: 714–719

Fielding J W 1964 Normal and selected abnormal motion of the cervical spine from the second cervical vertebra to the seventh cervical vertebra: based on cineroentgenography. Journal of Bone and Joint Surgery 46A: 1779

Fitzgerald G K, Wyveen K J, Rheault W, Rothschild B 1983 Objective assessment with establishment of normal values for lumbar spinal range of motion. Physical Therapy 663: 1776–1781

Friberg O 1987 Lumbar instability: a dynamic approach by traction compression radiography. Spine 12: 119–129

Gertzbein S D, Seligman J, Holtby R, Chan K H, Kapasouri A, Tile M, Cruickshank B 1985 Centrode patterns and segmental instability in degenerative disc disease. Spine 10: 257–261

Goel V K, Goyal S, Clark C, Nishiyama K, Nye T 1985 Kinematics of the whole lumbar spine. Effects of discectomy. Spine 10: 543–554

Gonnella C, Paris S V, Kutner M 1982 Reliability in evaluating passive intervertebral motion. Physical Therapy 62: 436–444

Grieve G P 1986 Thoracic joint problems and simulated visceral disease. In: Grieve G P (ed) Modern manual therapy of the vertebral column. Churchill Livingstone, Edinburgh, pp 377–395

Grieve G P 1988a The masqueraders. Proceedings of the International Federation of Orthopaedic Manipulative Therapists Congress, Cambridge, pp 27–28

Grieve G P 1988b Common vertebral joint problems. 2nd edn. Churchill Livingstone, Edinburgh

Helbig T, Lee C K 1988 The lumbar facet syndrome. Spine 13: 61–64

Hindle R J, Pearcy M J, Cross A T, Miller D H T 1990 Three-dimensional kinematics of the human back. Clinical Biomechanics 5: 218–228

Jackson R P, Jacobs R R, Montesano P X 1988 Facet joint injection in low back pain. A prospective statistical study. Spine 13: 966–971

Janda V 1986 Muscle weakness and inhibition (pseudoparesis) in back pain syndromes. In: Grieve G P (ed) Modern manual therapy of the vertebral column. Churchill Livingstone, Edinburgh, pp 197–201

Janda V 1988 Muscles and cervical pain syndromes. In: Grant R (ed) Physical therapy of the cervical and thoracic spine. Churchill Livingstone, New York, pp 153–166

Jirout J 1979 The rotational component in the dynamics of the C_{2-3} spinal segment. Neuroradiology 17: 177–181

Jull G A 1986 Clinical observations of upper cervical mobility. In: Grieve G P (ed) Modern manual therapy of the vertebral column. Churchill Livingstone, Edinburgh, pp 315–321

Jull G A, Bullock M I 1987a A motion profile of the lumbar spine in an ageing population assessed by manual examination. Physiotherapy Practice 3: 70–81

Jull G A, Bullock M I 1987b The influence of segmental level and direction of movement on age changes in lumbar motion as assessed by manual examination. Physiotherapy Practice 3: 107–116

Jull G A, Gibson K 1986 Aspects of therapist reliability in manual examination of lumbar intersegmental motion. Proceedings of the Australian Physiotherapy Association National Conference, Hobart, pp 129–137

Jull G A, Lane M B 1983 Aspects of lumbar spinal mobility in a normal population. In: Bower K (ed) Proceedings of the International Conference on Manipulative Therapy, Perth, pp 65–84

Jull G A, Bogduk N, Marsland A 1988 The accuracy of manual diagnosis for cervical zygapophysial joint pain syndromes. Medical Journal of Australia 148: 233–236

Kalebo P, Kadziolka R, Sward L 1990 Compression-traction radiography of lumbar segmental instability. Spine 15: 351–355

Kaltenborn F 1970 Mobilisation of the spinal column. New Zealand University Press, Wellington

Kaltenborn F, Lindahl O 1969 Reproducerbarheten vid Rorelseundersokning av Enskilda Kotor. Lakartidningen 66: 962–965

Kazarian L 1972 Dynamic response characteristics of the human vertebral column. Acta Orthopaedica Scandinavica 146: 54–117

Kendall H O, Kendall F P, Boyton D A 1952 Posture and pain. Williams & Wilkins, Baltimore

Khuffash B, Porter R W 1989 Cross leg pain and trunk list. Spine 14: 602–603

Kippers V, Parker A W 1984 Posture related to myoelectric silence of erectores spinae during trunk flexion. Spine 9: 740–745

Klausen K 1986 The shape of the spine in young males with and without back pain. Clinical Biomechanics 1: 81–84

Lang J 1986 Craniocervical region. Osteology and articulation. Neuro-Orthopaedics 1: 67–92

Lee C K, Langrana N A 1984 Lumbosacral spinal fusion: a biomechanical study. Spine 9: 574–581

Lewit K 1985 Manipulative therapy in rehabilitation of the locomotor system. Butterworths, London

Lind B, Sihlbom H, Nordwall A, Malchau H 1989 Normal range of motion of the cervical spine. Archives of Physical Medicine and Rehabilitation 70: 692–695

Lindren K-A, Leino E, Hakola M, Hamberg J 1990 Cervical spine rotation and lateral flexion combined motion in the examination of the thoracic outlet. Archives of Physical Medicine and Rehabilitation 71: 343–344

Liyang D, Yinkan X, Wenming Z, Zhihua Z 1989 The effect of flexion–extension motion of the lumbar spine on the capacity of the spinal canal: an experimental study. Spine 14: 523–525

Macones A J, Fisher M S, Locke J L 1989 Stress-related rib and vertebral changes. Radiology 170: 117–119

Magarey M E 1986 Examination and assessment in spinal joint dysfunction. In: Grieve G P (ed) Modern manual therapy of the vertebral column. Churchill Livingstone, Edinburgh, pp 481–497

Magora A 1975 Investigation of the relationship between low back pain and occupation. Scandinavian Journal of Rehabilitation Medicine 7: 146–151

Maitland G D 1986 Vertebral manipulation. 5th edn. Butterworths, London

Malmivaara A, Videman T, Kuosma E, Troup J D G 1987 Facet joint orientation, facet and costovertebral joint osteoarthrosis, disc degeneration, vertebral body osteophytosis and schmorl's nodes in the thoracolumbar junctional region of cadaveric spines. Spine 12: 458–463

Markolf K L 1972 Deformation of the thoracolumbar intervertebral joints in response to external loads: a biomechanical study using autopsy material. Journal of Bone and Joint Surgery 56A: 511–533

Mayer T G, Tencer A F, Kristoferson S, Mooney V 1984 Use of noninvasive techniques for quantification of spinal range-of-motion in normal subjects and chronic low-back dysfunction patients. Spine 9: 588–595

McCombe P F, Fairbank J C T, Cockersole B C, Pynsent P B 1989 Reproducibility of physical signs in low-back pain. Spine 14: 908–918

Mellin G 1986a Accuracy of measuring lateral flexion of the spine with a tape. Clinical Biomechanics 1: 85–89

Mellin G 1986b Chronic low back pain in men 54–63 years of age. Correlations of physical measurement with the degree of trouble and progress after treatment. Spine 11: 421–426

Mellin G 1987 Correlations of spinal mobility with degree of chronic low back pain after corrections for age and anthropometric factors. Spine 12: 464–468

Mestdagh H 1976 Morphological aspects and biomechanical properties of the vertebroaxial joint (C_2–C_3). Acta Morphologica Neerlando-Scandinavica 14: 19–30

Mimura M, Moriya H, Watanabe T, Takahashi K, Yamagata M, Tamaki T 1989 Three-dimensional motion analysis of the cervical spine with special reference to the axial rotation. Spine 14: 1135–1139

Minucci A 1987 Palpation of the thoracic spine T_{1-8} In: Dalziel B A, Snowsill J C (eds) Proceedings of the Fifth Biennial Conference, Manipulative Therapists Association of Australia, Melbourne, pp 367–376

Mooney V 1987 Where is the pain coming from? Spine 12: 754–759

Moroney S P, Schultz A B, Miller J A A, Andersson G B J 1988 Load–displacement properties of lower cervical spine motion segments. Journal of Biomechanics 21: 769–779

Nachemson A 1985 Lumbar spine instability. A critical update and symposium summary. Spine 10: 290–291

Noyes F R, DeLuca J L, Torvik P J 1974 Biomechanics of anterior cruciate ligament failure; an analysis of strain-rate sensitivity and mechanics of failure in primates. Journal of Bone and Joint Surgery 56A: 236–252

Offierski C M, Macnab I 1983 Hip–spine syndrome. Spine 8: 316–321

O'Gorman H, Jull G 1987 Thoracic kyphosis and mobility: the effect of age. Physiotherapy Practice 3: 154–162

Ohlen G, Wredmark T, Spangfort E 1989 Spinal sagittal configuration and mobility related to low-back pain in the female gymnast. Spine 14: 847–850

Oliver M 1989 A biomechanical basis for classification of movement patterns in combined movements examination of the spine. In: Jones H M, Jones M A, Milde M R (eds) Proceedings of the Sixth Biennial Conference of the Manipulative Therapists Association of Australia, pp 138–145

Ono K, Yonenobu K, Fuji T, Okada K 1985 Atlantoaxial rotatory fixation. Radiographic study of its mechanism. Spine 10: 602–608

Overton L M, Grossman J W 1952 Anatomical variations in the articulation between the second and third cervical vertebrae. Journal of Bone and Joint Surgery 34A: 155–161

Pal G P, Routal R V 1986 A study of weight transmission through the cervical and upper thoracic regions of the vertebral column in man. Journal of Anatomy 148: 245–261

Panjabi M M, White A A, Johnson R M 1975 Cervical spine mechanics as a function of transection of components. Journal of Biomechanics 8: 327–336

Panjabi M M, Goel V K, Takata K 1982 Physiologic strains in the lumbar spinal ligaments. Spine 7: 192–203

Panjabi M M, Takata K, Goel V K 1983 Kinematics of lumbar intervertebral foramen. Spine 8: 348–357

Panjabi M M, Krag M H, Chung T Q 1984 Effects of disc injury on mechanical behaviour of the human spine. Spine 9: 707–713

Panjabi M M, Summers D J, Pelker R R, Videman T, Freidlaender G E, Southwick W O 1986 Three-dimensional load–displacement curves due to forces on the cervical spine. Journal of Orthopaedic Research 4: 152–161

Panjabi M M, Dvorak J, Duranceau J, Yamamoto I, Gerber M, Rauschning W, Bueff H U 1988 Three-dimensional movements of the upper cervical spine. Spine 13: 726–730

Paris S 1985 Physical signs of instability. Spine 10: 277–279

Parke W W, Watanabe R 1990 Adhesions of the ventral lumbar dura. An adjunct source of discogenic pain. Spine 15: 300–303

Pearcy M 1986 Measurement of back and spinal mobility. Clinical Biomechanics 1: 44–51

Pearcy M, Hindle R J 1989 New method for the non-invasive three-dimensional measurement of human back movement. Clinical Biomechanics 4: 73–79

Pearcy M J, Tibrewal S B 1984 Axial rotation and lateral bending in the normal lumbar spine measured by three-dimensional radiography. Spine 9: 582–587

Pearcy M, Portek I, Shepherd J 1984 Three-dimensional X-ray analysis of normal movement in the lumbar spine. Spine 9: 294–297

Penning L 1987 Normal movement of the cervical spine. American Journal of Roentgenology 130: 317–326

Penning L 1988 Differences in anatomy, motion, development and aging of the upper and lower cervical disk segments. Clinical Biomechanics 3: 37–47

Penning L, Wilmink J T 1987 Rotation of the cervical spine. A CT study in normal subjects. Spine 12: 732–738

Pope M H, Bevins T, Wilder D G, Frymoyer J W 1985 The relationship between anthropometric, postural, muscular and mobility characteristics of males ages 18–55. Spine 10: 644–648

Portek I, Pearcy M J, Reader G P, Mowat A G 1983 Correlation between radiographic and clinical measurement of lumbar spine movement. British Journal of Rheumatology 22: 197–205

Porter R W, Miller C G 1986 Back pain and trunk list. Spine 11: 596–600

Raftopoulos D D, Rafko M C, Green M, Schultz A B 1988 Relaxation phenomenon in lumbar trunk muscles during lateral bending. Clinical Biomechanics 3: 166–172

Sahrmann S A 1988 Postural applications in the child and adult. Neurodevelopment aspects. In: Kraus S L (ed) TMJ disorders. Management of the craniomandibular complex. Churchill Livingstone, New York, pp 295–309

Schmorl G, Junghanns H 1971 The human spine in health and disease. 2nd edn. Grune & Stratton, New York

Schnebel B E, Watkins R G, Dillin W 1989 The role of spinal flexion and extension in changing nerve root compression in disc herniations. Spine 14: 835–837

Schneider G 1987 Degenerative lumbar instability. In: Dalziel B A, Snowsill J C (eds) Proceedings of the Fifth Biennial Conference of the Manipulative Therapists Association of Australia, Melbourne, pp 91–105

Schultz A B, Warwick D N, Berkson M H, Nachemson A L 1979 Mechanical properties of the human lumbar spine motion segments — Part I: Responses in flexion, extension, lateral bending and torsion. Journal of Biomechanical Engineering 101: 46–52

Seligman J V, Gertzbein S D, Tile M, Kapasouri A 1984 Computer analysis of spinal segmental motion in degenerative disc disease with and without axial loading. Spine 9: 566–573

Shirazi-Adl A, Drouin G 1987 Load bearing role of of facets in a lumbar segment under sagittal plane loadings. Journal of Biomechanics 20: 601–613

Shirazi-Adl A, Ahmed A M, Shrivastava S C 1986 A finite element study of a lumbar motion segment to pure sagittal plane moments. Journal of Biomechanics 19. 331–350

Singer K P, Breidahl P D, Day R E 1989 Posterior element variation at the thoracolumbar transition: a morphometric study using computed tomography. Clinical Biomechanics 4: 80–86

Stokes I A F, Wilder D G, Frymoyer J W, Pope M H 1981 Assessment of patients with low-back pain by biplanar radiographic measurement of intervertebral motion. Spine 6: 233–240

Stokes I A F, Bevins T M, Lunn R A 1987 Back surface curvature and measurement of lumbar spine motion. Spine 12: 355–361

Sward L, Erikssen B, Peterson L 1990 Anthropometric characteristics, passive hip flexion and spinal mobility in relation to back pain in athletes. Spine 15: 376–382

Takemitsu Y, Harada Y, Iwahara T, Miyamoto M, Miyatake Y 1988 Lumbar degenerative kyphosis. Clinical radiological and epidemiological studies. Spine 13: 1317–1326

Taylor J R, Twomey L T 1980 Sagittal and horizontal plane motion of the human lumbar vertebral column in cadavers and in the living. Rheumatology and Rehabilitation 19: 223–232

Ten-Have H A, Eulderink F 1980 Degenerative changes in the cervical spine and their relationship to its mobility. Journal of Pathology 132: 133–159

Tibrewal S B, Pearcy M J, Portek I, Spivy J 1985 A prospective study of lumbar spine movements before and after discectomy using biplanar radiography. Spine 10: 257–263

Travell J G, Simons D G 1983 Myofascial pain and dysfunction. The trigger point manual. Williams & Wilkins, Baltimore

Troup J D G 1986 Biomechanics of the lumbar spinal canal. Clinical Biomechanics 1: 31–43

Twomey L T, Taylor J R 1979 A description of two new instruments for measuring the ranges of sagittal and horizontal plane motions in the lumbar region. Australian Journal of Physiotherapy 25: 201–203

Twomey L T, Taylor J R 1983 Sagittal movement of the lumbar vertebral column: a quantitative study of the role of posterior vertebral elements. Archives of Physical Medicine and Rehabilitation 64: 322–325

Van Schaik J P J, Verbiest H, Van Schaik F D J 1989 Isolated spinous process deviation. A pitfall in the interpretation of AP radiographs of the lumbar spine. Spine 14: 970–976

Viikari-Juntura E, Porras M, Laasonen E M 1989 Validity of clinical tests in the diagnosis of root compression in cervical disc disease. Spine 14: 253–257

Watson D H 1990 Cervical headache: an investigation of natural head posture and upper cervical flexor muscle performance. Thesis, South Australian Institute of Technology, Australia

Weitz E M 1981 The lateral bending sign. Spine 6: 388–397

White G M, Healy W L 1987 Tumor-associated atlanto-axial rotatory fixation. Spine 12: 406–408

White A A, Panjabi M M 1978 Clinical biomechanics of the spine. J B Lippincott, Philadelphia

Worth D 1988 Biomechanics of the cervical spine. In: Grant R (ed) Physical therapy of the cervical and thoracic spine. Churchill Livingstone, New York, pp 15–25

Worth D R, Selvik G 1986 Movements of the cervical spine. In: Grieve G P (ed) Modern manual therapy of the vertebral column. Churchill Livingstone, Edinburgh, pp 86–102

Yamamoto I, Panjabi M M, Crisco T, Oxland T 1989 Three-dimensional movements of the whole lumbar spine and lumbosacral joint. Spine 14: 1256–1260

Yang K H, King A I 1984 Mechanism of facet load transmission as a hypothesis for low back pain. Spine 9: 557–565

38. Stress tests of the craniovertebral joints

E. Pettman

INTRODUCTION

A patient presents complaining of facial pain, occipital headaches, tinnitus, metallic taste in the mouth, numbness of the tongue, dizziness, nausea, retro-occular pain, a feeling of a lump in the throat, possibly even episodes of nightmares or 'stress attacks'.

In isolation, any of these symptoms would lead one to ponder the eventual diagnosis. In combination, they present any medical or paramedical professional a formidable task of diagnosis. Unfortunately, for many patients the provisional, and even eventual, diagnosis will be 'hysteria', 'compensation litigitis' or the universal 'IDK'.

To any clinician involved in the rehabilitation of patients who have sustained injury from high inertial assault (e.g, rear-end motor vehicle accidents), these symptoms, in isolation or various combinations, are probably prosaic.

A knowledge of the sensory innervation of the upper three cervical joints would lend credence to the probability of trauma to the articular or peri-articular structures of one of these joints.

Concurrently, such a patient may complain of (or may have had immediate, initial complaints of), or on further examination may demonstrate signs and/or symptoms of:

1. an overt loss of balance in relation to head movements, usually presented as a history of 'drop attacks'
2. facial lip paraesthesia, reproduced by active or passive movements
3. bilateral or quadrilateral limb paraesthesia, either constantly, or reproduced/aggravated by head or neck movements
4. nystagmus, (usually 'lateral' or 'abduction') produced by active or passive movements of the head or neck.

Such signs and symptoms are considered to be extremely important as they suggest either vertebral/basilar artery insufficiency (1,2 and 4), or cervical cord compression (3).

Because of their significance in inferring overt craniovertebral joint instability, during this chapter, the above four signs and symptoms will be referred to as *cardinal*. If such symptoms can be initiated, reproduced, or aggravated, by passive linear (planar) motions to the craniovertebral joints, then it is reasonable to assume that instability exists within this joint complex.

It is quite possible that any of the symptoms mentioned in the initial paragraph could also be elicited as a linear stress test is performed. However, clinical experience has shown that if at least one of the cardinal signs and symptoms (as listed above, 1–4) is not present as well, then follow-up tests done by the patient's physician (e.g. flexion X-rays) are most likely to be negative. Unfortunately, it is not unknown for a false-negative to be recorded both on visual diagnostics and on active angular motion tests (e.g. Sharp–Perser test) because of the restraining effects of sub-occipital muscle spasm.

It is well to remember, also, that reproduction of pain is of questionable importance when stress testing for instability (as it is e.g. in a knee joint examination), and it should be made quite clear to the patient what information one is looking for during performance of the testing procedure by using phrases such as '*Tell me if you feel anything other than pain . . .* '.

However, when faced with a patient who complains of headaches, dizziness, nausea and a feeling of 'a lump in the throat', all, apparently, reproduced by one or more stress tests, it is difficult not to be concerned.

It must be remembered that the inert tissues being stressed are heavily innervated by the trigeminal nucleus, adjacent to the C2/3 segment, which in turn is joined by a branch of the vagus nerve. If the signs and symptoms of craniovertebral joint dysfunction are as complex as the neurology of this region appears to be, then 'obscure' or 'bizarre' complaints may merely be a reflection of our collective ignorance.

To avoid what is viewed by some as 'craniovertebral hysteria' (on the part of the therapist, not the patient!), it might be as well to reflect on the differences between the signs and symptoms given in the first paragraph, from those enumerated as 'cardinal' signs and symptoms earlier.

It would also be beneficial to realise the different forces in play between an angular motion test and a linear motion test. The disparate effect, of each, on the vertebral artery, for example, is a useful case in point.

Active movements, e.g. extension and rotation, create primarily angular motion at the joints of the cervical spine, creating marked changes in length or tension within the artery itself. Linear stress tests, on the other hand, because of the minimal, or lack of, motion permitted by ligaments or bony opposition, cannot normally affect the length or tension of the arteries, but can produce transectory occlusion of the vessel(s) if excessive intersegmental linear motion is present.

It might well be concluded that if 'cardinal' signs and symptoms are absent during linear stress tests but present during active range of motion testing, then a damaged artery is more likely to be responsible than craniovertebral joint instability. The converse appears to be true, also.

It is clear from the information above that stress tests are necessary to determine whether serious instability exists. However, it has been the author's experience that such pathology is rare, or at least, not frequent enough, in itself, to warrant routine stress tests. This argument has been used by some therapists to justify their conviction for not stress-testing the craniovertebral joint region routinely, if at all. One wonders whether these therapists use the same argument when it comes to assessment of the knee joint.

It needs to be emphasized that linear and/or accessory movements must be stressed to test adequately inert tissue structures, e.g. ligaments and joint capsule, for damage. Surely no one can deny that any examination of the knee joint which does not include ligament stress tests is incomplete. Are the craniovertebral joints different? Indeed they are not. Like other synovial joints, in the periphery, the craniovertebral joints must be subjected to linear and accessory stresses to see whether those structures which limit or prevent such movements have been damaged. In this particular instance, it would be a mistake to consider pain to be the most relevant symptom, since the aggravation of non painful symptoms of trigeminal origin (as decribed earlier) is just as likely.

If symptoms are correlated with end-feel, then not only can the degree of possible inert tissue tearing be determined, but also the nature of any existing instability. For example, using pain as the comparitive symptom, if there appears to be excessive motion, in the absence of pain, with a soft, yielding end-feel, then a complete tear of a ligament is likely. In the following text this will be referred to as a *ligamentous instability*. If, however, this painless excessive motion had a hard, unyieding end-feel, then intra-articular deterioration is suspected. In the text this will be referred to as an *arthrotic instability*. Obviously,

from a prognostic view alone, the differentiation between ligamentous and arthrotic instability is important.

It has been the author's experience that segmental, post-traumatic, arthrotic instability is undoubtedly responsible for many of the chronic symptoms eventually suffered by patients involved in high inertial injuries.

Our nemesis, as a specialized group, are those physiotherapists, physicians and surgeons who, through ignorance, lack of skill, or the lure of financial remuneration, continue to maintain that palpation of segmental spinal motion (of any kind) is not feasible. 'Dare to be different, so many would rather be orthodox than right.' (Fryette).

THE DISTRACTION TESTS

No doubt most of us have experienced the disturbing onset of unexpected signs and symptoms reported by patients, during or following manual, as well as mechanical traction techniques to the cervical spine. Such signs and symptoms may range from simple feelings of dizziness, disorientation and nausea, to the more disquieting onset of distal paraesthesia. Since this conventional modality is in widespread use as a decompressive technique for mid- to lower-cervical spinal dysfunction, without concurrent extensive reports of such adverse reactions, and, since it has been shown that tractional forces do not have a deleterious effect on normal vertebral arteries (if given without other, combined movements), it can be deduced that the onset of such symptoms is an indication of either:

1. an inability of the inert structures of the cervical spine to withstand such a force, or,
2. that the arterial vessels of the neck are, somehow, being abnormally stressed.

With specific regard to the craniovertebral region one can surmise that the fault must lie with:

1. damage to the longitudinally oriented ligaments, or,
2. a traumatized or abnormally stretched (from longitudinal instability) vertebral artery.

From cadaveral investigations, done by the author, it seems that, due to their posterior orientation, the ligaments that resist distraction also restrict flexion of the craniovertebral joint complex. This is especially true of the tectorial membrane, which has been shown to be the the major restraint to distraction of the head from the atlas and axis, and, also in the author's own cadaveral observations, to be maximally stressed with atlanto-axial flexion. The distraction test, therefore, has two components:

1. A general distraction technique performed with the head and neck in neutral, made more comfortable by gently cupping the occiput in between the thenar emminences.

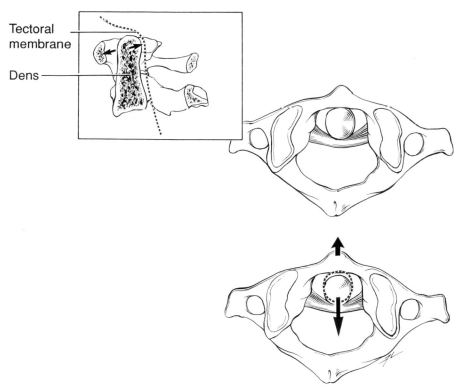

Fig. 38.1 Craniovertebral flexion stressing tectoral membrane.

2. If the response to this test is negative, then the ligaments are further stressed by repeating the distraction stress in craniovertebral flexion.

To make the test more specific to the craniovertebral joints, if the patient can tolerate it, the C2 neural arch is fixated gently in both tests. If the cervicothoracic junction is simultaneously flexed, this will eliminate the stabilizing effect of the ligamentum nuchae (see Fig. 38.1).

LINEAR AND ACCESSORY STRESS TESTS

The commonest accidents causing craniovertebral symptoms appear to be either the rear-end collision or the head-on collision. From the car occupant's point of view, the inertia of impact produces a rapid acceleration, followed by an equally rapid deceleration as either the seat belt restrains the individual or he hits something (or somebody) within the vehicle. So, if the patient's head is facing forward at impact the head and neck will be forced to move through a sagittal plane.

In the case of a rear-end impact the acceleration will be into extension, and a head-on impact into flexion.

It is during this initial phase, before muscle protection can be instigated, that most damage appears to occur.

A review of cervical anatomy will show that most of the muscle power and ligamentous restraint is designed to resist flexion, the same position we are most likely to be forced into as we confront nature's own high inertial force of gravity. There is even a convenient bony block to hyperflexion movement as the chin hits the chest.

A look at structures resisting extension, however, gives one a much bleaker picture. There is a striking paucity of muscular and ligamentous restraints, and if one reflects on how structure is invariably related to function it is easier to see why this is so. It really is hard to imagine any *mundane* cause of a high-velocity, *horizontal* trauma, such as that delivered by a rear-end collision.

So far, this discussion has been limited to what occurs if the head and neck are in a relatively neutral position, and free to move, at the moment of impact. Patients who have reported being struck whilst their head was turned often have a poorer prognosis than those whose heads were in neutral. To understand this better, one only needs to turn one's own head fully, and then try to extend the neck — imagine this movement being forced by a high inertial impact! Such damage in a head-on collision would be almost impossible, as the forward momentum would derotate the neck towards neutral. It might be a good idea to ponder these anatomical and biomechanical facts before making sweeping statements regarding the authenticity of many patients suffering from the now infamous, 'whiplash syndrome'. However, one must remember that head-on collisions also have serious dangers.

The impression one gets, from literature reviews, and discussion with doctors involved in vehicle trauma, is that whilst most chronic disabilities result from rear-end collisions, most fatalities result from head-on collisions. The main factor here is what decelerates the initial impact. In the case of unrestrained drivers (or passengers), it is often their head striking something hard, e.g. steering wheel, windscreen. One of the more serious consequences to the cervical spine is a posterior dislocation of the atlanto-occipital joint, with or without fractures of the atlas or axis.

At least one investigator feels that if there is concomitant head injury associated with a motor vehicle accident, a cervical fracture is not just possible, it is probable.

It is clear from the above that there is a tremendously large spectrum of cervical injuries that can occur in motor vehicle or any high-velocity trauma accidents, ranging from a minor muscle tear . . . to death! Our job as therapists is to deal with those individuals whose injury falls between these two extremes. Which end of the spectrum is your next patient closest to? For those individuals referred for outpatient physiotherapy, linear and accessory stress tests performed in the three spacial planes will help to elucidate matters.

Sagittal stress tests

Posterior stability test of the atlanto-occipital joint (Fig. 38.2)

Fixation. The sides of the cranium are gently compressed with the palms of both hands. The head is kept on a pillow.

Stress. With the pads of the index fingers over the arch of the axis, bilaterally, by using a lumbrical muscle action an attempt is made to translate anteriorly the axis/atlas under a fixed occiput.

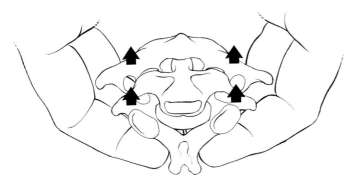

Fig. 38.2 Posterior stability test atlanto-occipital joint.

Anterior stability test of the atlanto-occipital joint (Fig. 38.3)

Fixation. The pads of fingers 2 to 5 gently cradle the occiput. The pads of the thumbs are turned medially to fix *gently* the anterolateral aspect of the transverse masses of the atlas and axis.

Stress. By simultaneously, and bilaterally, producing

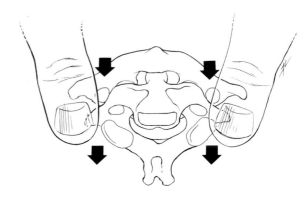

Fig. 38.3 Anterior stability test atlanto-occipital joint.

a lumbrical action at metacarpophalangeal joints 2 to 5, together with flexion at the thenar MCP joint, an anterior translatory force will occur at the atlanto-occipital joint.

Anterior stability of the atlanto-axial joint (Fig. 38.4)

The *'Sharp–Perser' test*, developed by the study of radiographically confirmed instability at the atlanto-axial joint in rheumatoid arthritic patients, analyses the onset of cardinal signs or symptoms (usually distal paraesthesia) following full flexion of the head and neck, and, more importantly, the reduction of such signs and symptoms by a posterior translation of the occiput/atlas.

Fixation. The patient is asked to flex fully the head and neck. The spinous process of the axis is then gently fixed by a 'pinch' grip of thumb and fingertip pads.

Stress. Through palmar pressure on the forehead, the occiput and atlas are translated posteriorly. The unique feature of this test is that the stress component is intended to *relieve* symptoms rather than aggravate them.

Anterior stabilization of the atlas on axis is the responsibility of the transverse ligament. It has sometimes been stated that the transverse ligament restricts flexion of the atlanto-axial joint complex. The author found no sign of this in cadaveral studies; rather, the transverse ligament was found actually to facilitate flexion at this joint by *creating* its coronal axis.

It was also noted (on cadaveral study) that, once the transverse ligament was incompetent (artificially transected), anterior translation of the atlas on axis was possible in flexion, neutral and even extension. At the same time, if the function of the suboccipital muscles could be simulated to prevent flexion of the atlas on axis (? inferior oblique; rectus capitus posterior minor), it seemed that flexion of the cervical spine could be obtained without anterior translation of the atlas on axis.

If these rather crude observations represent what could happen in a living, traumatized individual, then the use of the Sharp–Perser test in the assessment of post-traumatic patients would certainly be questionable. Though it appears to be the most clinically reproducible test for craniovertebral instability, its reliability seems to have been demonstrated on chronic, degenerative joints, where muscle spasm or muscle guarding is probably not a factor.

As mentioned before, anterior translation of the atlas did appear possible, in any position, as long as the transverse ligament was incompetent, and as long as a linear stress — rather than angular stress — was applied to the atlas. Thus, in acute or subacute patients, although tests involving active (angular) movements may be prone to false negatives, it is unlikely that tests involving linear stresses will be. The main disadvantage with the linear stress test about to be described is that it requires a modicum of palpatory skill, which may not be attainable for everybody.

Direct anterior translation stress of atlas on axis (Fig. 38.5)

Fixation. The patient is lying supine, with the head in a neutral position. The pads of the index fingers of the therapist lie over the skin adjacent to the posterior arch of the atlas, and the fingers 3 to 5 gently cup the occiput.

Fixation of the axis (C2) is dependent upon the patient's tenderness to palpation of the anterior part of its transverse processes. Ideally, one should try to fix the axis

(C2) with gentle thumb pressure over these processes, but if this proves impossible, then one must rely on the weight of the body (via the C3) to retard anterior motion of the axis (C2).

Stress. With the axis (C2) fixed (directly through the thumbs, or indirectly, through body weight), the atlas and head are simultaneously lifted away from the bed in a vertical direction. If this stress produces no reaction from the patient, other than pain, then the test can be considered *negative*. If a cardinal sign or symptom is produced, then the test must be considered *positive*.

Unfortunately, mid-cervical instability can also be aggravated by this test, and the signs and symptoms elicited can sometimes be alarming, e.g. distal or facial paraesthesia; a feeling of dizziness or nausea; a distinctly uncomfortable feeling of a 'lump in the throat'.

In an effort to differentiate mid-cervical from craniovertebral instability, the test is repeated with the head in craniovertebral flexion. This time the attempted translation is through a slightly different plane, i.e. in terms of the therapist, upwards and forwards.

By altering the test in this manner, the nuchal ligament is tightened by craniovertebral flexion, thereby somewhat stabilizing the mid-cervical spine whilst, at the same time, increasing the stress on any existing anterior atlanto-axial

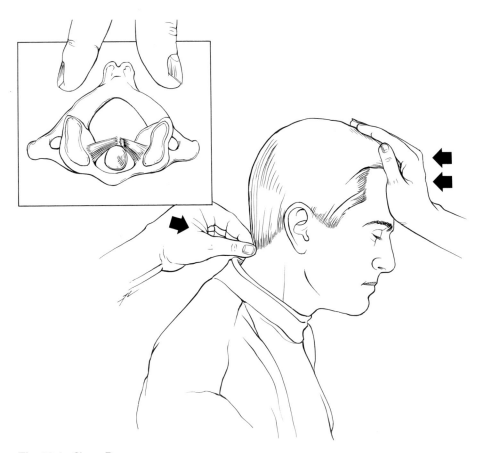

Fig. 38.4 Sharp-Perser test.

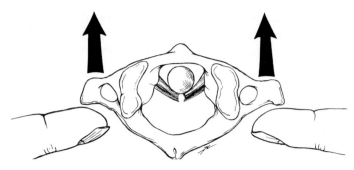

Fig. 38.5   Stress test of transverse ligament.

instability. Thus, if the aforementioned symptoms are increased with this modified test, or, if symptoms are produced earlier, then it would be prudent to assume that the cause might be craniovertebral instability and medical consultation is advised.

Coronal stress tests (Figs 38.6, 38.7)

Lateral stability tests of the atlanto-occipital joints

These, together with rotary stress tests of the atlanto-occipital joints, are in the text describing the 'alar ligament tests'.

Lateral stability of the atlanto-axial joint complex

It should be remembered that the atlanto-axial joint complex consists of three joints. It is the median joint that, although it has no weight-bearing function, is extremely important in maintaining stability, whilst at the same time, facilitating motion within this joint complex. Stability of this joint, in turn, is dependent upon a normal and intact dens. Listed below are some of the reasons why this may not be the case in certain individuals:

1. Anomalies of the dens
   (a) Os odontoidium — a condition where the intervertebral disc between the developing bodies of axis and atlas does not ossify
   (b) Congenital absence of the dens
   (c) Underdeveloped dens whose lack of height renders it unchecked by the transverse ligament
2. Pathologies affecting the dens
   (a) Demineralization or resorption of dens — Grissl's syndrome, rheumatoid arthritis
   (b) Old, undisplaced fractures, which originally escaped diagnosis, and subsequently formed a pseudarthrosis. It must be emphasized that the stress test about to be described is *contra-indicated if a recent dens fracture is suspected.*
3. Developmental considerations. The body of the dens is not of sufficient size to be retained in the osseoligamentous ring of the atlas until a child is approximately 12 years old. One must assume,

therefore, that the atlanto-axial joint of a child under this age is *naturally unstable.* It goes without saying that great care should be taken with any mobilization or manipulative technique performed on a patient within this age group.

Unfortunately, it is not just the young who exhibit deviations from anticipated norms. In a series of sagittal prosections examined at the University of British Columbia, it was evident that the median atlanto-axial joint structure can also vary at the latter end of our spectrum of human development. The anatomical differences (? anomalies) seemed to be most prevalent in cadaveral specimens exhibiting a marked forward head posture. If the observations represent anatomical relationships in life, the abnormal stress of continuous extension at the atlanto-axial joint can not only change the shape of the dens, but also the relationship between the dens and the anterior arch of the atlas.

In one specimen the dens was clearly arcuate, or 'bent' posteriorly. In another, the dens appeared to have migrated inferiorly to the point where its tip was barely in contact with the anterior arch of atlas.

By far the most fascinating, however, was a specimen in which the dens was actually *anterior* to the arch of the atlas, without any obvious evidence of prior structural damage.

Until further evidence suggests that these observations are somehow invalid, the author's impression is that the wisdom of performing high-velocity thrust techniques on elderly patients, especially those who exhibit a marked forward head posture, should be brought into serious consideration.

Lateral stability stress test of the atlanto-axial joint

Fixation. With the patient supine, one of the therapist's hands, e.g. right hand, cradles the occiput with the palm and fingers 3 to 5. The pads of the index finger of this hand lie across the right arch of the atlas. With the other hand, e.g. left hand, the therapist's index finger lies across the left arch of the axis. No other contact is made with this hand.

Stress. This test is probably more often falsely positive than any of the other stress tests. The main reason for this is that the soft-tissue slack is not taken up first. When this is done properly, a more accurate end-feel is perceived. To achieve this initial step, the index fingers of both hands are *gently and slowly* pressed into the neck.

Once the slack appears to have been removed, the left hand becomes a fixed point. A lateral shear of the atlas on axis can now be attempted by *gently and slowly* applying pressure from the right hand, especially the index finger, attempting to push the atlas and occiput to the left.

In the author's experience, one can identify lateral

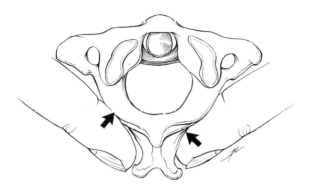

Fig. 38.6 Finger position for lateral stability stress test.

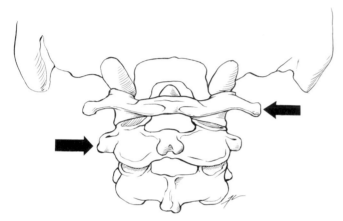

Fig. 38.7 Stress test for lateral stability of atlanto-axial joint.

instability with this test without the reproduction, or aggravation, of any symptoms. In such cases, even where trauma has been involved, one would have to question the clinical relevance of such a finding. However, as a premanipulative safety check, its importance is obvious.

Alar ligament stress tests (see Figs 38.8–38.14)

Of all the stress tests done in the craniovertebral region, alar ligament tests are the most troublesome. It is the author's opinion that these tests have been the least understood, the most poorly performed, and consistently misconstrued.

Current investigation of the alar ligaments shows that they are extremely variable in their anatomical arrangement. However, cadaveral experiments appeared to suggest that an alar ligament would resist contralateral side-bending, regardless of its anatomical orientation. However, the orientation appears to determine the position of the head in which the ligaments would be tightest, i.e. flexion or extension. More sophisticated investigation shows that the alar ligaments are consistently stressed by passive, contralateral side-bending of the occiput, on

axis, and also contralateral rotation of occiput on axis. Use is made of both these findings in alluding the presence of an incompetent alar ligament.

Side-bending stress test for alar ligaments

Side-bending of the occiput is accompanied by an *immediate* ipsilateral rotation of the axis under atlas, e.g. right side-bending is accompanied by right rotation of the axis under atlas (or left rotation at the atlanto-axial joint). It is assumed that the resulting tension in the alar ligaments is responsible for the rotation. This motion can be easily monitored by palpation of the spinous process of C2, which, in the example used here, would be felt to move to the left. Such palpation, for immediate motion of the spinous process, has been taught by some as a test for alar ligament stability. It should be emphasized, however, that this cannot be considered an accurate *stress test* since it does not involve the *fixation* of one bone whilst the other is moved.

Fixation. The key to an accurate test is adequate, but comfortable, fixation of the C2 (axis). The neural arch of the C2 should be fixated in such a way that both rotation and side-bending movements are restricted. Continuing with the example of right side-bending, with the patient in supine, the therapist's left thumb is placed across the patient's left neural arch of C2. This will block right rotation of the C2. The therapist's left index finger is placed across the right neural arch of C2. This will block right side-bending of the C2, thus localizing the stress to the craniovertebral joints.

Stress. The therapist's right hand must somehow be able to move the head into *craniovertebral* right side-bending. To facilitate this it is recommended that, along with the side-bending motion, the therapist introduces some compression, in effect trying to push the patient's right ear towards the left side of his neck. If the C2 is adequately fixed and the alar ligament is intact, there should be *no motion* of the head permissible. This attempted motion will stress the *left alar ligament*.

To take into account the anatomical variations within the alar ligaments, the test is performed in neutral, flexion and extension. A negative in any one position indicates

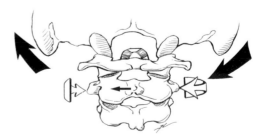

Fig. 38.8 Right side-bending accompanied by immediate right rotation of C2.

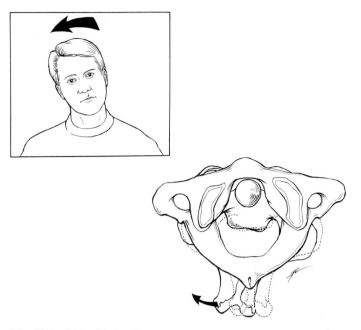

Fig. 38.9 Right side-bending accompanied by <u>immediate</u> right rotation of C2.

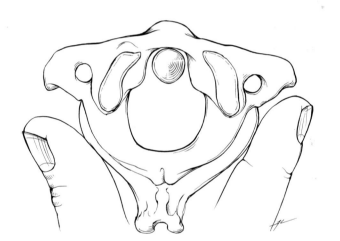

Fig. 38.10 Fixation of C2 for alar ligament stress test.

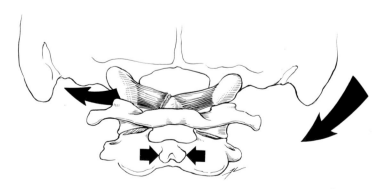

Fig. 38.11 Stress test for left alar ligament.

that the (left) alar ligament is intact. It will be noticed that some 'play' appears in almost everybody in one or other of the positions tested, and this must be considered normal. It is only those patients for whom the test is positive in all three positions that an alar ligament tear, or laxity, is considered a possibility. The ligament must then be stress tested in rotation to confirm such a possibility.

Rotational stress test for the alar ligaments

The 'side-bending' alar ligament test produces a lateral translation force at the atlanto-occipital joint. Therefore, arthrotic instability, as well as ligamentous instability, will show up as positive in the preceding tests. It is obviously important to distinguish these two forms of instability, both for prognosis and treatment.

Since an alar ligament helps to restrict motion in both side-bending and rotation to the opposite side, if side-bending right were felt to be slack, then right rotation should also be excessive if a damaged ligament is the cause of the instability. If, on the other hand, right rotation was not excessive, but left rotation was, then this combination represents an arthrotic instability.

Fixation and stress. The patient is seated. With a 'lumbrical' grip (as opposed to a 'pinch' grip) fixation of C2, again across the lamina instead of just the spinous process, the head is rotated to the right. Under normal circumstances rotation of the head would stop at about 20–30°, due to the effect of the left alar ligament. Rotation could be continued only if the head were side-bent left to slacken the left alar ligament.

If the therapist is able to induce an excessive amount of right rotation, without having to left side-bend the head, then the left alar ligament is *confirmed as incompetent.*

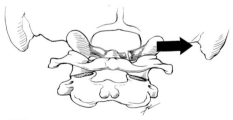

Fig. 38.12 Right translation due to torn alar ligament.

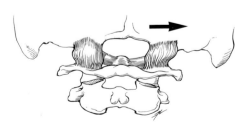

Fig. 38.13 Right translation due to arthrotic changes.

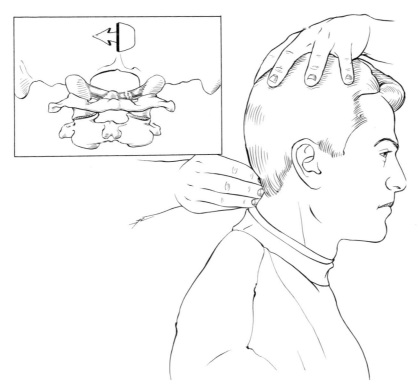

Fig. 38.14   Confirmiratory rotation stress test for torn alar ligament.

If this test proves negative, then the head is passively rotated to the left. If the rotation proves to be excessive (without any right side-bending) then an arthrotic instability might be suspected.

CONCLUSION

Stress tests to the craniovertebral joints have been the basis of abundant clinical and academic dialogue. In support of such tests is the risk of damage which might be caused by the inappropriate use of manual therapy to this area.

While there are those who propagate the belief that primary, traumatic instability of the craniovertebral region is commonplace, in the author's experience, and the adamant assertion of other *clinically oriented* physiotherapists who deal with such problems on a day-to-day basis, the original discovery of life-threatening complications due to high velocity trauma is *rare*.

So why do stress tests?

1. As rare as it is, if there exists even the suspicion of a life-threatening instability, and we believe, as a profession, that we can perform tests that will elucidate this, then the appropriate stress tests should obviously be performed.

2. In the craniovertebral joints, unlike the rest of the spine, the structures restraining angular motion do not necessarily restrain linear or accessory motion. In the spinal column below the craniovertebral joints, the main restraints to both angular and linear motion would appear to be, predominantly, the intervertebral disc and the zygapophyseal joints.

Since the discs are absent from the upper two segments, and their zygapophyseal joints actually facilitate motion, the responsibility for motion restraint is obviously different from the inferior spinal segments. It is more analogous to the peripheral joints, where *muscle* restrains *angular* motion, but *ligaments, bony opposition or intra-articular congruence* restrain *linear and/or angular* motion.

It is quite possible, therefore, that a patient may exhibit angular *hypo*mobility of a craniovertebral motion (through protective muscle guarding), whilst, at the same time, exhibiting linear or accessory *hyper*mobility (because of ligamentous laxity or intra-articular attrition), i.e. *instability*.

If only for consistency of assessment procedures, but knowing there is so much more to be gained, stress tests of the craniovertebral joints should be a routine part of functional cervical evaluation.

39. The reliability of assessment parameters: accuracy and palpation technique

D. H. Evans

INTRODUCTION

Assessment of the quality and amount of intervertebral mobility by palpation and passive movement testing is an integral part of the routine examination of the spine by manipulative therapists. The origins of manipulative therapy are ancient, and the reliability and validity of palpation findings have until recently been accepted untested by successive generations of manipulative physiotherapists.

When an early attempt was made to demonstrate the reliability of passive movement testing (Kaltenborn & Lindahl 1969), strong opposition was voiced, both to that study in particular (Magnusson 1969, Nachemson 1969) and to the general principle that palpation was a sufficiently accurate method of spinal examination (Lysell 1969, Nachemson 1969). Following that controversial exchange there was a lapse of 10 years before publications appeared on the reliability and validity of palpation findings.

This review, which is not exhaustive, of studies relevant to the accuracy and reliability of palpation techniques is divided into three sections.

The first section deals with some of the early attempts to validate palpation as an accurate and reliable means of assessment of spinal movement.

The second section is intended as an introduction to the research described in the third section. It is a brief review of research into tactile acuity in areas relevant to the understanding of the processes involved in assessment by palpation.

The third section deals primarily with research carried out at the South Australian Institute of Technology (now the University of South Australia). This was of a substantially different nature to that described in the first section. In these studies attempts were made to measure palpation skills in a quantitative rather than a comparative manner.

ASSESSMENT OF SPINAL MOBILITY

Practitioners of spinal manipulation place major emphasis on the assessment of gross intersegmental spinal mobility in the examination of patients with spinogenic symptoms. Although some authors (Cyriax 1970) do not rank the assessment of passive intersegmental mobility highly, the majority (Mennell 1952, Maigne 1972, Stoddard 1981, Maitland 1986, Grieve 1988) do value palpation findings highly and describe in detail various techniques for the assessment of passive intervertebral motion.

Until recently little work had been done to measure the accuracy of palpation techniques either directly or indirectly, but some insight into the order of accuracy expected may be deduced from the following exercises recommended to develop sensitivity to various aspects of palpation (Frymann 1963).

a. With eyes closed, gently palpate the surface of a table and find the position of the table legs. There will be less resilience and greater resistance in those areas.
b. Find a small coin under a telephone directory.
c. Find a human hair under several pages of the telephone directory. An elevation of the smooth surface of the page will be noted.

There was no evidence to suggest that performance of those tasks enhanced the ability to assess accurately spinal intervertebral mobility.

The earliest recorded attempt to validate palpation findings (Kaltenborn & Lindahl 1969) was a study in which 10 teachers of manipulative therapy assessed selected spinal levels on four patients. The movements tested were occipito-atlantal lateral flexion in patients 1 and 2, sagittal mobility in the thoracic spine at T6–7, T7–8 and T8–9 in patients 1 and 3, and sagittal mobility of L3–4, L4–5 and L5–S1 in patient 4. The description of the technique of assessment indicated that examination was performed using only palpation of the spine during specific passive movements. The findings were graded from 1 to 4: 1. total stiffness; 2. marked stiffness; 3. normal mobility; 4. hypernormal mobility. Analysis of the results was based on the number of deviations from the reference standard set by the findings of the principal examiner. That choice of reference standard effectively meant that the results were presented in the most favourable light, with some 17 deviations out of a total of 130 readings. One critic (Nachemson 1969) commented that, had examiner 10 been chosen as the reference standard, the number of variations would have been 47, and expressed the opinion that radiographic measurement may be more accurate than palpation. He doubted that it was possible to palpate millimetre displacements of a vertebra with only the aid of one's fingers.

Subsequent palpation studies have consisted of inter-examiner and intra-examiner reliability studies, and have taken various forms. Those which have been published have been tests of physiological movement, either gross, motion testing (Johnston 1982, Johnston et al 1982a, b), intersegmental movement testing (Johnston 1976, Johnston et al 1978), or a combination of both (Gonella et al 1982). The complexity of these studies varied. The simplest (Johnston 1976) recorded findings as positive or negative with an analysis of the discrepancies between examiners. The most complex analysis (Gonella et al 1982) was performed in a study in which five physical therapists evaluated the passive mobility of the vertebral column in five normal subjects. The mobility of six intervertebral levels (from T12–L1 to L5–S1) was assessed and graded on a 7-point scale:

0. Ankylosed
1. Considerable restriction (hypomobility)
2. Slight restriction (hypomobility)
3. Normal
4. Slight increase (hypermobility)
5. Considerable increase (hypermobility)
6. Unstable.

Intra-therapist reliability was found to be dependable, but inter-therapist reliability was not.

Studies evaluating the reliability of palpation assessment of passive accessory intervertebral motion (Jull 1977, Melrose 1979, Scanlon 1979) were each performed as a secondary part of another study, and precise figures were not published. All of these studies were of cervical spine mobility. The techniques for the assessment of passive accessory intervertebral motion were performed by the application of a postero-anterior pressure:

a. centrally over the spinous process, and
b. unilaterally over the apophyseal joints.

In the first instance, the motion produced by a central pressure most nearly approximates a postero-anterior gliding between adjacent vertebrae, whereas the motion produced by a unilateral pressure produces a complex combination of gliding and rotation. The assessment of intersegmental mobility was based on the scale:

1. Hypermobile
2. Normal

3. Slightly stiff
4. Stiff
5. Very stiff.

The inter-examiner reliability varied from 80 to 90% agreement.

More recent comparative studies in the cervical spine (Nansel et al 1989), thoracolumbar spine (Love & Brodeur 1987) and lumbar spine (Keating et al 1990) show similarly variable but generally poor inter- and intra-therapist reliability.

In stark contrast, Jull et al (1988) demonstrated accurate diagnosis of symptomatic apophyseal joint syndromes by testing passive accessory joint motion. To be diagnosed, the joint concerned had to exhibit all of the following: abnormal 'end feel' (i.e. abnormal resistance at the limit of motion); abnormal quality of resistance to motion; and reproduction of either local or referred pain. Confirmation was by radiologically-controlled diagnostic nerve blocks.

RECORDING OF PASSIVE MOVEMENT AND PALPATION FINDINGS

The literature reveals little information on techniques for recording the findings of passive movement tests or mobilizing techniques. Of the various methods of notation available, the Benesh movement notation has been suggested (Papas 1974) as the most appropriate system for the recording of examination findings by physiotherapists. Although application of the system has been described for recording gross trunk or limb movement, no application has yet been described for recording spinal intersegmental motion.

The first reports of notation for the recording of passive peripheral or intervertebral joint movement (Hickling & Maitland 1970, Maitland 1970) were to record the response of the joint to passive movement in the form of a graph or movement diagram. Compilation of the diagram relied heavily on the experience and judgement of the person drawing the diagram, as reference could be made only to adjacent joints, and to memory, for the relationship between the movement characteristics found on testing and 'normal' when determining the joint's range of movement. Similar difficulties exist for magnitude scaling of the variables pain, resistance and muscle spasm.

A comprehensive recording technique, assessment pictography (Stillman 1974, 1979) is a system which allows pictorial representation of any active or passive movement of any joint. All the information contained on a movement diagram may be recorded by that technique. Although the 'star' diagram (Maigne 1972) shows some similarity to the assessment pictograph, only gross active movement was recorded with that method.

No matter which notation system is used, the same

decision problems exist for the location within range and magnitude scaling of the variables to be recorded. In spite of their wide usage, the literature fails to reveal any studies which test the validity of reliability of these notation systems.

CUTANEOUS SENSATION AND TACTILE ACUITY

Assessment of tactile acuity has fallen within the realms of neurology and psychophysics. The following is a summary of research into the accuracy of various touch sensations.

The sensations experienced as result of stimulating normal skin endowed with normal sensory apparatus have been classified into four broad introspective groups (Sinclair 1973).

1. Touch group: touch, pressure vibration, tickle, tingling
2. Pain group: 'metaesthesia', discomfort, itch, pricking pain, burning pain
3. Thermal group: cold, warm
4. Sensory blends: wetness, smoothness, heat, etc.

Although touch and pressure are introspectively different, they are united by a continuous spectrum of intermediate sensations, and as a consequence are generally regarded as forming part of the same modality of sensation.

Touch

The early studies related to touch and accuracy of the touch sensation were aimed at determining absolute threshold, two-point discrimination and point-localization error, and comparing the results for different parts of the body. The following information relating to the early investigations is from review articles (Sinclair 1967, Kenshalo 1978). Most techniques which measure touch threshold involve application of the stimulus by a hair or fine stylus. An alternative method is to deliver a puff of air, but the results show a different order of sensitivity compared with touch by hair or stylus. The most common instrument used was the von Frey 'hair' (von Frey aesthesiometer), which indicated threshold stimuli of 0.9 mg for the pad of the index finger, and 1.0 mg for the pad of the thumb. Measurement of two-point discrimination either by (blunt) compass points, or by edges formed to make a V-shape indicate accuracy of 2.3–3.0 mm as the threshold distance at the index finger pad, and 3.5 mm for the thumb pad.

Scaling (or 'loudness') of touch sensations have proved difficult to measure because of the conditions of measurement. Sites of high or low sensitivity, rate of loading the force increment, increasing as opposed to decreasing the force, and the interval between the application of the force and its increment are some of the factors which influence the perception of increments of the touch sensation. An alternative approach using single skin indentations of various depths (0 to 22.8 mm) rather than incremental changes to indentation, has shown that touch loudness increases linearly with the depth of indentation in glabrous skin (to a depth of 5 mm) but is a power function of the indentation depth of hairy skin.

Active touch

The studies cited above have relied on experimental conditions where stimuli have been applied to a passive receptor field. Under normal conditions, touch is an exploratory sense rather than purely receptive, and it is becoming increasingly evident that tactile acuity is enhanced in active exploration when compared with passive reception. An early indication of the phenomenon may be seen in an examination of the parameters of perception required to read Braille (Meyers et al 1958). The dots are separated by 2.3 mm, which is close to the threshold value for two-point discrimination at the pad of the index finger. Reduction of the inter-dot space to 1.9 mm only moderately reduces the legibility of the Braille text. No attempt was made to reduce further the dot space, so no lower limit of legibility was obtained. The superiority of active versus passive touch has been questioned on the basis of results obtained in a study on surface roughness (Lederman 1981). In this study, however, the movement was of the object being touched (by a stationary finger pad) rather than by movement of the finger pad over the surface. These findings are difficult to reconcile with those of a similar study (Loomis 1979) which demonstrated heightened tactile acuity for spatial interval discrimination, point localization and spatial resolution on a moving surface. In these studies, the kind of perception involved has been related to cutaneous stimuli with a minimum of kinaesthetic input. A difference has been shown in the perception of distance when the arm is moved out to touch an object, compared with when an object touches a stationary partially outstretched arm (Schlater et al 1981). No conclusion could be drawn regarding the respective accuracy of one method of perception over the other, only that the two methods produced different results.

The main aims of current research into tactile sensibility are to relate the psychophysical phenomena of tactile spatial resolution (two-point discrimination, gap detection, grating resolution etc.) with both neural mechanisms and the nature of mechanoreceptive units in glabrous skin. Knibestol and Vallbo (1980) were unable to demonstrate any relationship between the stimulus–response functions of slowly adapting mechanosensitive units with receptive fields in glabrous skin of the hand and psychophysical magnitude estimation. Neural patterns have been recorded and measured in macaque monkeys, and results suggest that the critical dimensions below which spatial neural patterning breaks down is of the order of 1.0 mm, and that the slowly adapting afferent fibres are responsible for that limit in monkeys (Johnson & Lamb 1981, Phillips & Johnson 1981).

Although there has been a recent expansion in the knowledge of both cutaneous mechanoreceptor function and the psychophysical parameters of touch perception, the reconciliation of the two is yet some distance in the future.

Kinaesthetic sensibility

With any movement, the mechanoreceptors in skin, muscle and joints provide a barrage of information to the spinal cord and higher levels of the central nervous system. The extent to which each of the above components contributes to the awareness of body or limb position, and more particularly to the fine control of movement, is not yet fully understood. Although most authors favour control as being principally from the muscle spindle (McCloskey 1978, Boyd 1980, Burke 1980, Abbruzzese et al 1981, McCloskey et al 1983) some authors still favour joint receptors as the principal source (Wyke 1972, Tracey 1980). It has also been suggested that cutaneous afferents may be an important source of kinaesthetic information (Moberg 1983).

The argument in favour of joint receptor activity hinges on the production of arthrokinetic reflexes by the alteration of afferent discharges from the joint receptors. While this effect cannot be ignored, the overwhelming majority of workers favour predominantly muscle-spindle control. Arguments to support this hypothesis are that: (a) the anaesthetization of joints impairs kinaesthetic sensation only when accompanied by anaesthetization of the skin, and (b) that total joint replacement by prosthesis causes only minimal kinaesthetic impairment (McCloskey 1978). Abbruzzese et al (1981) observed the effects of active and passive finger movements on somatosensory evoked potentials (SEP) produced by median nerve stimulation. Both active and passive movements produced a marked change in the amplitude of the primary cerebral response. It was concluded that the activation of peripheral receptors (probably muscle spindle endings) induced a gating effect at both cortical and subcortical (thalamic) levels, giving a potential for selective modulation of different sensory inputs to the cortex.

As can be seen, the finest discrimination was performed with 'active' rather than 'passive' touch, suggesting input from several afferent sources provided the finest discriminatory decisions to be made, although the design of those tests was not directly comparable to the task of assessment by palpation.

The quantitative measurements were not encouraging when the measured accuracy of the various forms of touch were nearly equal to the full range of intervertebral movement.

MEASUREMENT OF PALPATION TECHNIQUES

Two approaches have been taken with measurement of palpation to obtain quantitative information regarding the accuracy with which palpation tasks could be performed.

One approach was to measure forces applied to the body during mobilizing techniques. Indirect measurement, using a force platform (Banting 1982, Mitchell 1983) showed poor inter and intra-therapist reliability, with Matyas and Bach (1985) questioning the reliability of the palpation techniques studied. The studies were criticized (Stoelwinder et al 1986) on a number of grounds, particularly the necessarily indirect methodology of the force platform.

Direct measurement has been made (Jull & Bullock 1987, Jull 1988) using a capacitive pressure transducer placed over the L4 spinous process. Good intra-therapist reliability over three trials was recorded for the one manipulative physiotherapist used.

Both direct (Jull & Gibson 1986) and indirect (Lee et al 1990) methods have been used to assess student performance and training. In both instances, the students 'improved' by more closely approaching the standard performance of the relevant manipulative physiotherapist.

The measurement of force application to human subjects has two major limitations. Firstly, all mobilizing and examination techniques involve movement (usually rhythmical and oscillatory) which cannot be measured. Secondly, the use of living body tissue to provide resistance allowed variation of the task during the course of the study.

The second approach involved the development of an instrument which would fulfil two functions (Evans 1982). Firstly, it had to provide acceptable simulation of a task required during spinal palpation, and secondly, it had to be able to record accurately the performance of the therapist. The task chosen for simulation was that of antero-posterior pressure on a spinous process, applied by the thumbs as for palpation of the cervical spine.

Palpation simulator

For the first study (Evans 1982) the instrument was a prototype and consequently constructed as simply as possible. It consisted of a box-like structure with a flat upper platform through which protruded a vertical plunger. The shape of the upper platform and plunger arrangement permitted a hand position similar to that for palpation of the thoracic or lumbar spinal areas, the fingers being spread wide for support on the platform with the thumbs disposed vertically, pads resting on the plunger. This position was not ideal as the task to be performed more closely

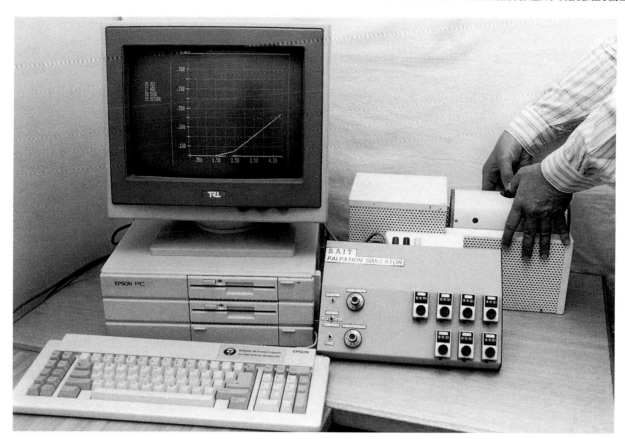

Fig. 39.1 Palpation simulator with control panel and Epson PC. Note hand position on the plunger. The task being performed is displayed on the screen, displacement (0–5 mm) on the X-axis, force (0–1000 gm) on the Y-axis.

related to cervical spine palpation in terms of the amplitude of a plunger movement. For a subsequent study (Christie 1983) the contour was altered, along with several other design modifications.

The amplitude of movement of the plunger was set at 4.0 mm, which was consistent with measurement of postero-anterior movement in the upper cervical spine (Worth 1980), and enabled simple calibration of the recording apparatus.

Measurement of the plunger displacement was detected using two strain gauged beryllium–copper cantilevers. With a standardized power supply and appropriate amplification, the output from the strain gauges enabled measurement of plunger displacement with a repeatability better than could be detected on a dial gauge resolving to 0.01 mm.

The control of the plunger position, and the application of resistance to depression of the plunger was provided by an electromagnetic force transducer. In the prototype this was provided by a piston diaphragm loudspeaker (Evans 1982). The mechanical properties of the loudspeaker produced some hysteresis and non-linearity of resistance to plunger movement, precluding accurate quantitative force measurement. Modifications for a subsequent study allowed the measurements to be made (Christie 1983).

Expansion of interest in the area has led to the development of a second palpation simulator (Watson & Burnett 1990) capable of measuring the amplitude of mobilization techniques with an estimation of forces involved.

Another approach (Harvey & Byfield 1991) was to construct a mechanical model of the spine using universal joints to permit movement, or to immobilize totally the adjacent vertebrae. The subjects (chiropractors and final-year student chiropractors) were able to identify the mobile segments, but had difficulty locating the immobilized segments. The construction of the model did not permit a quantitative analysis of the techniques employed by the subjects.

Palpation tasks

Two palpation tasks were performed in the studies by Evans (1982) and Christie (1983). The tasks consisted of locating the onset of different amounts of resistance which were added electromagnetically to the plunger movement. As there were no parameters for the magnitude of resistance necessary prior to the studies, the increase in resistance was arbitrarily adjusted by the author to provide an 'easy' and a 'difficult' task.

The subjects in the studies (manipulative physiotherapists and untrained subjects) were instructed that, at some point within the range of plunger movement, a force would be applied and should be perceived as resistance to movement of the plunger. The subjects were asked to report at what point in the downward travel of the plunger they first perceived the resistance (R_1), and to hold the plunger still at that point. When the subject reported that R_1 had been located, that position of the plunger was recorded. The subject then returned the plunger to the starting point (zero depression) and repeated the task. In all, 15 recordings were made for each subject for both tasks.

In both studies, the 'easy' task was used as part of the familiarisation procedure, with no significant differences demonstrated between groups. With the 'difficult' task, however, significant differences were obtained (Evans 1982):

a. Manipulative physiotherapists detected resistance earlier in the range than did the untrained subjects ($P <0.01$).
b. Manipulative physiotherapists showed greater precision in the location of onset of resistance as was in evidence by a smaller deviation from the mean value. (Manipulative therapists SD 0.163, untrained subjects SD 0.790, $P <0.01$).

Comparison of the magnitude of force necessary for the location of R_1 (Christie 1983) was again plagued by non-linearities because of the small forces involved. An estimation was possible however, with manipulative physiotherapists perceiving resistance with an applied force* of 5 gm to 7 gm, whereas untrained subjects required 10 gm to 25 gm. In this study, tactile sensibility (light touch threshold and two-point discrimination) were also measured. No relationship could be demonstrated between tactile sensibility and palpation skill.

Subsequent studies have attempted to identify, analyse and quantify the components of a palpation task which allow decisions to be made with regard to identification of the onset and nature of resistance. Trott et al (1988) assessed the ability of 37 experienced manipulative physiotherapists and 9 postgraduate students to detect the onset of resistance in order to determine whether the perception of the onset of resistance was related to:

a. the gradient (g/mm) of the resistance
b. the amount of force (gm) exerted on the plunger
c. the position on R_1 in the range of plunger movement.

They also examined the ability of the manipulative physiotherapists to record the perceived R_1 position on a visual analogue scale (VAS). They found that the accu-

racy of detection was directly related to the gradient of resistance ($P = 0.05$). The amount of force necessary to detect resistance varied both with the position of R_1 and the gradient. Once the gradient reached or exceeded 37 g/mm, there was no significant difference between mean forces (11–12 gm) recorded for the detection of R_1. When the R_1 was at the beginning of plunger movement, or early in the plunger travel (0.5 mm), significantly greater force was necessary (18–20 gm, $P <0.001$) for the perception of R_1.

The ability of the subjects to record their findings showed that there was a significant difference between the perceived position of R_1 and the recorded position on the VAS. These differences varied from 0.1 to 0.55 mm, which represent an error of 2% to 10% when considering the context of the task being assessed.

Trott et al (1989) in an extension of the authors' investigation into the ability of manipulative physiotherapists to palpate resistance to movement, examined the ability of manipulative physiotherapists to perceive changes in the force/displacement curve. Subjects were given three diagrams to illustrate the force/displacement curves they might palpate. The first showed a single linear gradient of resistance (R_1). The second showed the original gradient with an additional linear gradient (R_{1a}), producing a change in gradient. The third showed how the test would be varied, namely, by varying the distance between changes in gradient and by varying the slope of the second gradient.

Their conclusions were that, for a change in gradient to be detectable, the distance between R_1 and R_{1a} had to be greater than 1.00 mm, and that the ratio of the second gradient to the first was 2.0 or greater ($P <0.05$). The results suggested that the accumulated force increment may be the factor responsible for the perception of the gradient change. Whether the relationship is linear or logarithmic was not shown in this study.

The use of the palpation simulator in the assessment of grade III and IV mobilization techniques (Li 1990) showed that both qualified manipulative therapists and third-year physiotherapy students (who had completed and passed the vertebral component of their musculo-skeletal training programme) were able to perform consistent grade III and IV mobilization techniques. The most significant finding was that both groups performed the technique with more than the ideal of defined 50% of available resistance (Magarey 1986) as the end-point of the technique. The techniques were performed to 75% of the resistance, namely, grade IV+ and III+ mobilizations.

The palpation simulator has also been used to examine the effects of feedback on the learning of a palpation skill (Dempsey 1988). The skill studied was that of the location of the onset of resistance (R_1) by third-year physiotherapy students (who had passed the spinal assessment and treatment component of the musculo-skeletal training

---

*Forces are those which would be exerted by a mass equal to the number of grams shown.

programme). Three groups were used. All groups had an initial test on the equipment, a practice period, then were re-tested. The control group had no feedback regarding their performance. The first experimental group was given feedback on the results of their practice session verbally and visually (via the computer visual monitor). The second experimental group received feedback during practice by being permitted to view the cursor movement on the computer visual monitor while depressing the plunger. Both experimental groups showed a learning effect, the most significant result being the improvement in accuracy for the second (knowledge of performance) group.

Discussion

Studies which attempt to measure the performance parameters of palpation are expanding the understanding of the processes involved in assessment by palpation, performance of passive mobilization techniques and the teaching of palpation and mobilizing techniques.

The results of research using the palpation simulator indicate:

a. The instrument (palpation simulator) was able to provide a task which manipulative therapists were able to perform significantly more accurately than untrained subjects. This suggests that the simulated palpation task was sufficiently similar to assessment of the spine by palpation for the experienced subjects to be able to use a learned skill to determine the onset of resistance.

b. The reliability with which the onset of resistance was detected by the manipulative therapists (± 0.16 mm) suggests that palpation is a sufficiently precise technique for the assessment of intervertebral movement.

c. Detection of resistance to plunger movement was more difficult (greater force exerted before 'resistance' being recognized) when the resistance began at or near (within 0.5 mm of) the beginning of the movement.

d. The ability of subjects to record their findings showed that there was a significant difference between the perceived position of R1 (recorded digitally via computer) and the subjects' recording on a visual analogue scale. This undoubtedly highlights one of the hazards of assessing palpation skill solely by the use of scores recorded on a VAS.

e. Perception of a change in resistance (to plunger movement) could be made when the distance between R_1 and R_{1a} was greater than 1 mm and the ratio of the second gradient to the first was 2.0 mm or greater. Where changes were less than the above figures, only one smooth resistance was perceived.

f. Grade III and IV passive mobilization techniques were performed more strongly than expected from accepted definitions.

g. The ability to monitor visually the performance of a palpation task enhanced the learning of that task on the palpation simulator.

It is clear that further investigation into the nature of the perception of resistance is essential to establish whether or not a linear, logarithmic or some other relationship exists. Improved understanding of that relationship may suggest modification of the definition of forces for various strengths (III, III+ etc.) of mobilizing techniques. Use of a palpation simulator may enhance the teaching of palpation and recording skills.

REFERENCES

Abbruzzese G, Ratto S, Favale E, Abbruzzese M 1981 Proprioceptive modulation of somatosensory evoked potentials during active or passive finger movements in man. Journal of Neurology Neurosurgery and Psychiatry 44: 942–949

Banting J 1982 Inter-therapist reliability in the performance of a grade II mobilisation movement. Unpublished postgraduate diploma dissertation, Department of Physiotherapy, Lincoln School of Health Sciences, La Trobe University, Melbourne

Boyd I A 1980 The isolated mammalian muscle spindle. Trends in Neurosciences 3: 258–265

Burke D 1980 Muscle spindle function during movement. Trends in Neurosciences 3: 251–253

Christie A D 1983 Hand sensibility — a comparative study of light touch and two-point discrimination thresholds, and palpation skill in naive and experienced subjects. Thesis, South Australian Institute of Technology

Cyriax J 1970 A textbook of orthopaedic medicine. vol 1, 5th edn. Bailliere Tindall and Cassell, London, ch 6, p 101

Dempsey D P 1988 The motor learning of palpation. Thesis, South Australian Institute of Technology

Evans D H 1982 Accuracy of palpation skills. Thesis, South Australian Institute of Technology

Frymann V M 1963 Palpation part 1. Its study in the workshop. Academy of Applied Osteopathy Year Book, pp 16–20

Gonella C, Paris S V, Kutner M 1982 Reliability in evaluating passive intervertebral motion. Physical Therapy 62: 436–444

Grieve G P 1988 Common vertebral joint problems. Churchill Livingstone, Edinburgh, ch 9, pp 473–475

Harvey D, Byfield D 1991 Preliminary studies with a mechanical model for the evaluation of spinal motion palpation. Clinical Biomechanics 6: 79–82

Hickling J, Maitland G D 1970 Abnormalities in passive movement and diagrammatic representation. Physiotherapy 56: 105–114

Johnson K O, Lamb G D 1981 Neural mechanisms of spatial tactile discrimination: neural patterns evoked by braille-like dot patterns in the monkey. Journal of Physiology 310: 117–144

Johnston W L 1976 Interexaminer reliability in palpation. Journal of the American Osteopathic Association 76: 286–287

Johnston W L 1982 Passive gross motion testing part 1. Its role in physical examination. Journal of the American Osteopathic Association 81: 298–330

Johnston W L, Hill J L, Elkiss M L, Marino R J 1978 A statistical model for evaluating stability of palpatory cues. Journal of the American Osteopathic Association 77: 473–474

Johnston W L, Beal M C, Blum G A, Henra J L, Neff D R, Rosen M E 1982a Passive gross motion testing part III. Examiner agreement on selected subject. Journal of the American Osteopathic Association 81: 309–313

Johnston W L, Elkiss M L, Marino R J, Blum G A 1982b Passive gross motion testing part II. A study of interexaminer agreement. Journal of the American Osteopathic Association 81: 304–308

Jull G A 1977 The upper cervical spine. Thesis, South Australian Institute of Technology

Jull G A 1988 Monitoring aspects of the development of undergraduate student skills in manual techniques. International Federation of Orthopaedic Manipulative Therapists, Congress, pp 31–32

Jull G A, Bullock M 1987 A motion profile of the lumbar spine in an ageing population assessed by manual examination. Physiotherapy Practice 3: 70–81

Jull G A, Gibson K 1986 Aspects of therapist reliability in manual examination of lumbar intersegmental motion. Proceedings of the Australian Physiotherapy Association, National Conference, Hobart, 129–137

Jull G, Bogduk N, Marsland A 1988 The accuracy of manual diagnosis for cervical zygapophysial joint pain syndromes. Medical Journal of Australia 148: 233-236

Kaltenborn F, Lindahl O 1969 Reproducerbarheten vid rorelsundersckning av enskilda kotor. Lakartidningen 66: 962–965

Keating J C, Bergmann T F, Jacobs G F, Finer B A, Larson K 1990 Interexaminer reliability of eight evaluative dimensions of lumbar segmental abnormality. Journal of Manipulative and Physiological Therapeutics 13: 463–470

Kenshalo D R 1978 Biophysics and psychophysics of feelings. In: Carterette E C, Friedmann M P (eds) Handbook of perception. vol VIb. Academic Press, New York, ch 2, pp 30–63

Knibestol M, Vallbo A B 1980 Intensity of sensation related to activity of the slowly adapting mechanoreceptive units in the human hand. Journal of Physiology 300: 251–267

Lederman S J 1981 The perception of surface roughness by active and passive touch. Bulletin of the Psychonomic Society 18: 253–256

Lee M, Moseley A, Refshauge K 1990 Effect of feedback on learning a vertebral joint mobilisation skill. Physical Therapy 70: 97–104

Li L 1990 Aspects of mobilisation: a quantitative measurement. Thesis, School of Physiotherapy, South Australian Institute of Technology

Loomis J M 1979 An investigation of tactile hyperacuity. Sensory Processes 3: 289–302

Love R M, Brodeur R R 1987 Inter- and intra-examiner reliability of motion palpation for the thoracolumbar spine. Journal of Manipulative and Physiological Therapeutics 10: 1–4

Lysell E 1969 Motion in the cervical spine. Acta Orthopaedica Scandinavica (suppl 123)

Magarey M E 1986 Examination and assessment in spinal joint dysfunction. In: Grieve G P (ed) Modern manual therapy of the vertebral column. Churchill Livingstone, Edinburgh, pp 481–497

Magnusson R 1969 Manipulation med vetenskap (1). Lakartidningen 66: 1726–1727

Maigne R 1972 Orthopaedic medicine. A new approach to vertebral manipulation. Charles Thomas, Springfield, ch 4, pp 52–62

Maitland G D 1970 Vertebral manipulation. Butterworths, London

Maitland G D 1986 Vertebral manipulation. 5th edn. Butterworths, London, ch 4, p 71

Matyas T A, Bach T M 1985 The reliability of selected techniques in clinical arthrometrics, a response to letter. Australian Journal of Physiotherapy 32: 195–199

McCloskey D I 1978 Kinesthetic sensibility. Physiological Reviews 58: 763–820

McCloskey D I 1980 Knowledge about muscular contractions. Trends in Neurosciences 3: 311–314

McCloskey D I, Cross M J, Hommer R, Potter E K 1983 Sensory effects of pulling or vibrating exposed tendons in man. Brain 106: 21–37

Melrose G R 1979 Cervical rotation. Thesis, South Australian Institute of Technology

Mennell J 1952 The science and art of joint manipulation. vol 2. Churchill, London, ch 5, p 50

Meyers E, Ethington D, Ashcroft S, 1958 Readability of Braille as a function of three spacing variables. Journal of Applied Psychology 42: 163–165

Mitchell W 1983 Reliability in the performance of grade II and grade III mobilisation movements. Unpublished postgraduate diploma dissertation, Department of Physiotherapy, Lincoln School of Health Sciences, La Trobe University, Melbourne

Moberg E 1983 The role of cutaneous afferents in position sense, kinaesthesia and motor function of the hand. Brain 106: 1–19

Nachemson A 1969 Manipulation med veteskap (2). Lakartidningen 66: 1727–1729

Nansel D D, Peneff A L, Jansen R D, Cooperstein R 1989 Interexaminer concordance in detecting joint play asymmetries in the cervical spines of otherwise asymptomatic subjects. Journal of Manipulative and Physiological Therapeutics 12: 428–433

Papas M E 1974 An introduction to Benesh movement notation and its relevance to physiotherapy. Australian Journal of Physiotherapy 20: 70–74

Phillips J R, Johnson K O 1981 Tactile spatial resolution II. Neural representation of bars, edges and gratings in monkey primary afferents. Journal of Neurophysiology 46: 1193–1203

Pubols P H, Pubols L M 1982 Magnitude scaling of displacement and velocity of tactile stimuli applied to the human hand. Brain Research 223: 409–423

Scanlon E 1979 Facilitated segment C5–6. Thesis, South Australian Institute of Technology

Schlater J A, Baker A H, Wapner S 1981 Apparent arm length with active versus passive touch. Bulletin of the Psychonomic Society 18: 151–154

Sinclair D 1967 Cutaneous sensation. Oxford University Press, London, ch 2, pp 19–31

Sinclair D 1973 Psychophysiology of cutaneous sensation. In: Jarrett A (ed) The physiology and pathophysiology of the skin. vol 2. Academic Press, London, ch 30, pp 430–439

Stillman B C 1974 Assessment pictography. Australian Journal of Physiotherapy 20: 75–81

Stillman B C 1979 Assessment pictography: a method for recording passive movement treatment techniques and related assessment findings. Proceedings of a Multidisciplinary International Conference on Manipulative Therapy, Melbourne, pp 156–159

Stoddard A 1981 Manual of osteopathic technique. 3rd edn. Hutchinson Medical, London

Stoelwinder E, Henderson G, Zito G, McCahey P, Jull G, Johnston P, Trott P H, McCormick G 1986 The reliability of selected techniques in clinical arthrometrics. Letter to the editor. Australian Journal of Physiotherapy 32: 194–195

Tracey D J 1980 Joint receptors and the control of movement. Trends in Neurosciences 3: 253–255

Trott P H, Evans D H, Baghurst P, Pugatschew A 1988 Manual palpation of resistance to movement — Part II, a study of the skills of manipulative physiotherapists. Proceedings of the International Federation of Orthopaedic Manipulative Therapists, Congress, Cambridge, p 22

Trott P H, Evans D H, Frick R 1989 Accuracy of manual palpation skills: the ability of manipulative physiotherapists to detect changes in force and displacement on a palpation simulation. Proceedings of Sixth Biennial Conference, Manipulative Therapists Association of Australia, Adelaide, pp 207–214

Watson M J, Burnett M 1990 Equipment to evaluate the ability of physiotherapists to perform graded postero-anterior central vertebral pressure type passive movements of the spine by thumb pressure. Physiotherapy 76: 611–614

Worth D R 1980 The kinematics of the craniovertebral joints. Master's thesis, Victorian Institute of Colleges

Wyke B 1972 Articular neurology — a review. Physiotherapy 58: 94–99

40. Temperature testing by manipulative physiotherapists in spinal examinations

A. Lando

INTRODUCTION

Physiotherapists specializing in manipulation for musculo-skeletal problems rely heavily on an extensive initial examination in arriving at a clinical diagnosis. Apart from questioning regarding the extent and the behaviour of the symptoms, and testing of range, ease and strength of movement, manipulative physiotherapists put great store on their palpatory findings. The first step in the palpation procedure is to feel for abnormally high or low skin temperature (Maitland 1986). The reason for this is the fact that increased temperature has long been considered one of four cardinal signs of inflammation and, as such, gives an immediate indication of where the patient's symptoms may stem from. Furthermore, evidence has been provided (Uematsu & Long 1976) that decreases in skin temperature commonly occur over areas of chronic pain. Therefore, temperature determination can be an important first step in the localization of the culprit structures, whether the symptoms are of recent onset or long-standing.

Thermal patterns in patients suffering from low-back pain (LBP) have been measured, recorded and mapped in the past by the use of thermography (Raskin et al 1976, Wexler 1980, Pochaczevsky & Feldman 1982) and have been found to be as accurate a diagnostic test as myelography. Thermistor couples used on the skin overlying the temperomandibular joint have been used in establishing thermal patterns in patients suffering from rheumatoid arthritis (Tegelberg & Kopp 1988).

In the field of inter- and intra-examiner reliability, the literature is generally agreed on the greater accuracy being achieved in intra-examiner trials, be it in relation to the use of goniometers (Low 1976, Gonnella et al 1982) or other measuring devices.

As far as low-back pain and temperature testing is concerned, there are two main areas of interest to the manipulative physiotherapist. First, does the skin temperature of the low back vary significantly between patients with low-back problems and normal subjects? Secondly, can manipulative physiotherapists palpate skin temperature accurately and reproducibly? These questions were addressed by six experiments described below.

MATERIALS

Normal subjects

One group of 20 normal subjects was used. It consisted of 3 men and 17 women; their ages ranged from 22 to 45. They were fit and had never sought medical or other help for low-back pain.

Patients

Two groups of patients were used. Both were taken from a larger group of patients referred to the physiotherapy department complaining of LBP and/or buttock and leg pain. The groups consisted of (i) 5 men and 16 women, and (ii) 7 men and 13 women; their ages ranged from 23 to 70, and from 20 to 70, respectively. Only patients who were able to lie in the prone position for 30 minutes were selected.

Examiners

The two examining physiotherapists, both of whom are members of the Manipulation Association of Chartered Physiotherapists, had had extensive post-registration training in manipulative physiotherapy.

Infra-red thermometer

An infra-red thermometer (Linear Laboratories C-600M, Biotherm infra-red thermometer) was used as an objective measure of the skin temperature of the low back (Fig. 40.1). This instrument has a cone-shaped, non-contact probe suitable for use with patients. The thermometer has an accuracy of 0.1°C at a distance of 1.5–2 cm from the surface being measured. For these studies the thermometer was mains-operated with a voltage-stabilizing device incorporated in the circuit.

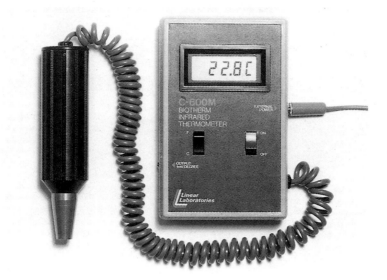

Fig. 40.1 Infra-red thermometer used for the measurement of low-back temperature.

Perspex grid

The infra-red thermometer was used in conjunction with a perspex grid (Fig. 40.2) in order to ensure that the location of the area of skin measured in each subject was the same. The grid had 36 holes large enough to hold the temperature probe, 18 on each side of the mid-line, making it possible to take six readings of each lumbar and thoracic paraspinal area. The grid had two perspex rods attached to its underside which were 4 cm high and which rested lightly on the back. The lower rod was placed on the spinous process of L5 and the other, centrally, in the lower thoracic spine.

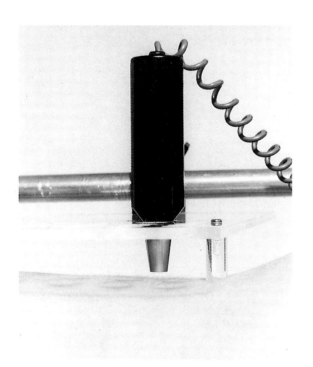

Fig. 40.2 Infra-red thermometer in situ in perspex grid.

Thermal testing apparatus

The testing apparatus consisted of a metal disc (oblong) with a lead attached to a transducer unit which was operated by a computer program. Sensitivity to cooling and to heating was tested for the dorsum of the fingers using a 15 cm² metal disc. The apparatus was operated in the following manner. The disc was held in firm contact with the area being tested by the subject. The computer was then switched on to either a heating or a cooling programme. The subject was told which programme was being used and then informed that they would hear a bleep following which there would be an increase in the temperature of the metal disc (if the heating programme were being used), or alternatively nothing would happen. They were asked to indicate these sensations with 'yes' for increase and 'no' for no change. Their response was recorded on the computer and this procedure was then repeated 10–15 times. The temperature increases were stepped, and the order in which an increase was induced or not was randomized.

The apparatus was developed by Dr C. Fowler of the Middlesex Hospital for similar work by Lele et al (1954) and kindly loaned to the author.

METHODS

The area of the low back which was being palpated and measured for temperature variations was demarcated with a biro on the spinous processes of L1, L3 and L5 (Fig. 40.3), so creating four lumbar quadrants with L3 forming the horizontal mid-line. The area extended 10 cm lateral to the spinous processes as this is the average width of the four fingers being used for the palpation. The lower thoracic paraspinal region, i.e., 10 cm above L1 and 10 cm away from the mid-line, was chosen as the area of reference.

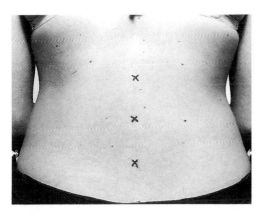

Fig. 40.3 Demarcation of the lumbar spine into four quadrants.

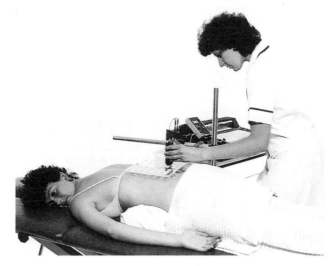

Fig. 40.4 Measurement and recording of skin temperatures of the low back.

The examiners were asked to use the dorsum of their fingers for the temperature palpation as was their usual practice. No other instructions were given in relation to the palpation.

The recording of the palpation findings was done on forms on which four quadrants were drawn representing the lumbar upper and lower quadrants (right and left).

The scale used for temperature estimations had four points of change by reference to the arbitrary zero of the reference area:

++ much increase
+ some increase
0 no change
− some decrease
− − much decrease

This scale was printed on the recording forms as a reminder to the examiners. Once the form had been completed it was given to the author but not made available to the other examiner.

EXPERIMENTS 1 AND 2. DETERMINATION OF LOCAL VARIATIONS IN BACK TEMPERATURE IN NORMAL SUBJECTS, AND PATIENTS REFERRED WITH LOW-BACK PAIN

Each subject was asked to undress and lie prone on the plinth. The subject's back was then lightly marked with a pen at the spinous processes of L1, L3 and L5, and the perspex grid lightly placed on the back as described above. Thirty-six measurements were taken and recorded for each subject (Fig. 40.4).

EXPERIMENT 3. DETERMINATION OF THERMAL SENSITIVITY OF THE DORSUM OF THE FINGERS OF THE HUMAN HAND USING A PHYSICAL MODEL

The thermal sensitivity thresholds of 20 physiotherapists

were tested using the thermal testing apparatus as detailed above.

EXPERIMENT 4. PALPATION FOR SKIN TEMPERATURE VARIATIONS IN THE LOW BACK OF 21 PATIENTS REFERRED WITH LOW-BACK PAIN BY TWO EXAMINERS OPERATING SEPARATELY

Each patient was asked to undress to their underwear and lie on the examination plinth in the prone position. The patient's back was marked with a biro at the levels of L1, L3 and L5. The examiner would then enter, do the temperature palpation, leave the cubicle and record the findings on the form using the scale described.

EXPERIMENT 5. PALPATION FOR SKIN TEMPERATURE VARIATIONS IN THE LOW BACK OF 20 NORMAL SUBJECTS BEFORE AND AFTER INDUCED HEATING OF ONE AREA OF THE LUMBAR SPINE

In this experiment the examiners knew they were palpating healthy subjects but were blindfolded before entering the cubicle to avoid any complications due to visual indications of temperature change. The subjects were asked to undress and lie down in the prone position. The skin temperatures of the lower thoracic and the lumbar paraspinal areas were then measured using the infra-red thermometer and the grid (Fig. 40.4). The examiners were then blindfolded, one at a time, and led into the cubicle by the author, who guided their hands into position (Fig. 40.5). This time, the order in which the examiners palpated was randomized. They were then led out of the cubicle, the blindfold removed, and the form filled in. One of the lumbar quadrants was then selected at random, and this

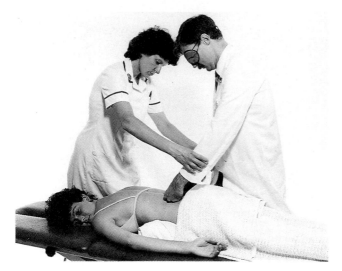

Fig. 40.5 Palpation of the low back by blind-folded examiner.

was then heated with a 40 watt spotlight at a distance of 5–7 cm from the skin surface for 2 minutes. The surrounding areas were screened, using towels. After the heating the towels were removed, the skin temperature measured and the palpations performed blind as before. The temperature of the untreated areas was measured and was unaffected by these procedures.

The subject was then left lying with the back exposed for 10 minutes. The skin temperature was then again measured and the palpations performed.

EXPERIMENT 6. PALPATION FOR SKIN TEMPERATURE VARIATIONS IN THE LOW BACK OF 30 SUBJECTS (PATIENTS AND NORMALS) WHERE THE TEMPERATURE WAS MEASURED AND RECORDED

The skin temperature was measured and palpated for in the same way as described in experiment 5.

RESULTS

Experiments 1 and 2. Determination of local variations in back temperature in normal subjects, and in patients referred with low-back pain

The overall mean temperatures and standard deviations for 20 normals and 20 patients were calculated and tabulated. Using different parts of the grid as reference points, Student's t-tests (Swinscow 1976) were performed on both sets of results (not all given).

Significant differences were found to exist between the mid-line and more peripheral areas in both groups ($P < 0.001$). In the patient group there was a significant difference ($P < 0.01 – P < 0.001$) between the thoracic/upper lumbar regions by comparison with the (cooler) lower lumbar regions (Tables 40.1 and 40.2). This differential was not present in the normal population and clearly demonstrates a difference in thermal pattern between the normal and symptomatic populations.

Experiment 3. Determination of thermal sensitivity of the dorsum of the fingers of the human hand using a physical model

The thermal sensitivities of the hands of the physiotherapists to heated and cooled metal can be seen in Table 40.3. The mean result was that temperature differences of 0.2°C could be detected.

Experiment 4. Palpation for skin temperature variations in the low back of 21 patients referred with low-back pain by two examiners operating separately

There are two main points of interest in these results:

1. Complete agreement on estimation of the skin temperature in all four quadrants occurred in 3 out of 21 cases.
2. Agreement on individual quadrants occurred in 36/84

Table 40.1 Student t-test performed comparing the uppermost of the thoracic readings with the lower readings

	NORMALS							PATIENTS					
L.T.	†††	†††	R	R	††	†††		†††	††	R	R	NS	††
	†††	††	R	R	†	†††		†††	†††	R	R	††	†††
U.L.	†††	†††	R	R	†††	†††		†††	†††	R	R	††	†††
	†††	†††	R	R	†††	†††		†††	†††	R	R	††	†††
L.L.	†††	†††	R	R	†††	†††		NS	†	R	R	†	†††
	†††	††	R	R	††	†††		††	NS	R	R	NS	†††

† = P < 0.05
†† = P < 0.01
††† = P < 0.001
NS = Not Significant
R = Reference point

Table 40.2 Student t test performed comparing the uppermost of the lumbar readings with the rest

	NORMALS							PATIENTS							Legend
L.T.	†	NS	NS	NS	NS	NS		NS	NS	NS	NS	NS	NS	† = P < 0.05
	NS	NS	NS	NS	NS	NS		NS	NS	NS	NS	NS	NS	†† = P < 0.01
U.L.	R	R	R	R	R	R		R	R	R	R	R	R	††† = P < 0.001
	NS	NS	NS	NS	NS	NS		NS	NS	NS	NS	NS	NS	NS = Not Significant
L.L.	NS	†	NS	†	NS	NS		NS	NS	NS	NS	NS	NS	R = Reference point
	†	NS	NS	NS	NS	NS		††	†††	†††	†††	††	†	

instances. A one-step difference occurred in 36/84 instances. A two-step difference occurred in 10/84 instances. A three-step difference occurred in 2/84 instances.

Experiment 5. Palpation for skin temperature variations in the low back of 20 normal subjects before and after induced heating of one area of the lumbar spine

The following points should be made:

1. In palpations 1 and 2 there was complete agreement in all four quadrants in one subject, and in palpation 3 there was no complete agreement.

2. The agreement in individual quadrants was as follows:

	Agreement	1-Step	2-Step	3-Step difference
Palpation 1	31/80	47/80	2/80	–
Palpation 2	36/80	41/80	3/80	–
Palpation 3	30/80	48/80	1/80	–

Table 40.3 Results of the heat and cooling test (in °C) performed on the hands of 20 physiotherapists

	Heat test (digits 15 cm)*	Cool test (digits 15 cm)*
1	0.1	0.3
2	0.3	0.3
3	0.3	0.2
4	0.1	0.2
5	0.4	0.6
6	0.1	0.1
7	0.3	0.2
8	0.2	0.1
9	0.1	0.1
10	0.4	0.1
11	0.1	0.4
12	0.1	0.2
13	0.2	0.1
14	0.4	0.2
15	0.1	0.1
16	0.1	0.1
17	0.3	0.1
18	0.3	0.2
19	0.1	0.3
20	0.3	0.1

* Mean values: heat test digits: 0.2, 0.13; cool test digits: 0.2, 0.13.

3. In palpation 2, i.e. directly after the induced heating, examiner B indicated the heated quadrant in 17/17 subjects (due to random selection of quadrants only 17/20 subjects were heated), and examiner A in 16/17 subjects with a minimum of a one-step difference between the heated and the non-heated quadrants. At the time of this palpation the mean temperature increase in the heated quadrant was 1.3°C ± 0.5°C.

4. In palpation 3, i.e. after the 'cooling' of the back for 10 minutes, the quadrant originally heated was still identified with a one-step difference in 10/17 subjects by both examiners. At the time of this palpation the heated quadrant still had an increase of 0.5°C ± 0.4°C.

5. The temperature variation boundaries of each examiner were very consistent in the second and third palpation, although these boundaries were not the same for both examiners.

Experiment 6. Palpation for skin temperature variations in the low back of 30 subjects (patients and normals) where the temperature was measured and recorded

The results of this experiment are given in Table 40.4. Of note were:

1. Complete agreement in the estimation of the skin temperature in all four quadrants occurred in 14/30 cases.

2. The agreement for the individual quadrants was: agreement 17/120, one-step difference 46/120.

3. The temperature variation boundaries for the 0 rating was 0.16°C for both examiners, although examiner A used the 0 rating 81/120 times, and examiner B used it in 54/120 instances.

DISCUSSION

The purpose of the two initial experiments reported in this chapter was to ascertain whether temperature changes in the backs of patients with low-back pain exist in the way which manipulative physiotherapists 'feel' and say they do.

Table 40.4 Palpation of the low back of 30 subjects (random mix of patients and normals)*

	1	2	3	4	Examiner A				Examiner B			
					1	2	3	4	1	2	3	4
1	0.01	0.16	0.00	−0.03	0	+	0	0	+	+	−	−
2	0.03	0.00	0.01	0.04	0	0	0	0	0	0	0	0
3	−0.01	−0.03	−0.08	−0.08	0	0	0	0	0	0	0	0
4	−0.07	0.52	−0.17	−0.23	0	0	0	0	+	0	+	0
5	−0.22	−0.20	−0.12	−0.34	+	0	0	+	+	+	0	0
6	−0.05	0.30	0.15	0.47	0	−	0	−	0	−	0	−
7	0.52	0.88	0.58	0.68	−	−	− −	− −	−	−	−	−
8	0.36	0.63	0.39	0.87	0	0	0	0	0	0	0	0
9	0.32	0.60	0.19	0.65	0	0	0	0	0	−	0	−
10	0.45	1.02	0.38	0.70	0	−	0	−	0	−	0	−
11	0.07	−0.10	−0.13	−0.20	0	0	0	+	+	0	+	0
12	0.11	0.06	0.17	−0.02	0	0	0	0	0	0	0	0
13	−0.25	−0.08	0.26	0.41	0	0	0	0	0	0	0	0
14	0.25	0.50	0.15	0.62	0	0	0	0	−	−	−	−
15	−0.70	−1.10	−0.67	−1.35	+	++	+	++	+	++	+	++
16	−0.03	−0.58	0.27	−0.46	0	0	0	0	−	+	−	+
17	0.09	1.24	−0.92	0.18	+	0	+	0	+	0	+	0
18	−0.61	−1.63	−0.19	−1.24	0	+	0	+	+	++	+	++
19	0.00	1.04	0.29	1.32	−	− −	−	− −	−	−	−	−
20	0.32	0.65	0.20	0.35	0	−	0	−	−	−	0	0
21	0.27	1.32	0.28	1.08	0	−	0	−	0	−	0	−
22	0.29	0.75	0.37	0.77	0	0	0	0	0	−	0	−
23	−0.26	−0.10	−0.68	−0.56	+	+	+	+	++	++	++	++
24	0.23	0.03	−0.02	−0.04	0	0	0	0	0	0	0	0
25	0.27	− 0.38	0.56	0.95	−	0	−	− −	−	−	−	−
26	0.12	0.34	−0.11	−0.10	0	0	0	0	0	0	0	0
27	0.32	0.47	0.11	0.10	0	0	0	0	0	0	0	0
28	−0.07	0.60	0.24	0.84	0	−	0	−	−	− −	−	− −
29	0.55	0.60	0.30	0.06	0	0	0	0	−	−	−	−
30	0.18	0.83	0.14	0.02	0	−	0	−	0	−	0	−

* The values in the first four columns relate to the mean temperature in each of the lumbar quadrants, each of which has been deducted from the mean temperature of the two thoracic quadrants.
1 and 3 represent the upper lumbar quadrants, left and right;
2 and 4 represent the lower lumbar quadrants, left and right.

These studies looked at the thermal patterns of the lower backs of normal and low-back pain patients rather than for absolute temperature variations, as this has been advocated as being more relevant by previous workers (Salisbury et al 1983).

On mapping the thermal patterns for the normal group, the author achieved the same thermal picture as previous workers (Raskin et al 1976, Uematsu & Long 1976, Pochaczevsky et al 1982) in relation to central readings compared with more peripheral readings. It is perhaps of some interest to note the similarities in results between this study and other similar studies mentioned as the methods used varied considerably. These studies were carried out in a physiotherapy department where badly fitted windows provided continuous variation in room temperature and humidity. The subjects were not requested not to have a hot drink or a cigarette, or not to run up the stairs, and were not put through a 20-minute 'stabilizing' period, all of which are common procedures when using thermography.

The result of greatest interest in the mapping of thermal patterns was the one of reduced temperature in the lower lumbar regions in the symptomatic population. This

warrants a closer look. It has been shown (Salisbury et al 1983) that in the case of acute inflammation there is a noticeable change in the thermal pattern of the skin overlying the affected area. Uematsu and Long (1976), when performing thermographic studies on 101 patients with chronic pain, observed that the skin overlying the painful area was consistently cooler than asymptomatic areas. Gunn and Milbrant (1978) make the observation that longstanding partial nerve disturbance that develops concurrently with degenerative joint changes causes a cooling of the related dermatome. Pochaczevsky and Feldman (1982) looked at two groups of patients, one group suffering from nerve root compression syndromes in cervical or lumbar regions and one group with musculoligamentous injuries. The following observations were made: the lumbar patients demonstrated thermographic changes both centrally (increased temperature) and peripherally (decreased temperature). Group two showed thermographic changes (increased temperature) which were localized to the paraspinal areas of the affected levels. The duration of these symptoms was not stated.

The mean length of time for which low-back symptoms had been present in this study's patient group was 6.4 years (range 2 weeks to 20 years). These symptoms were not constant but appeared in a varying number of bouts and with varying intensity. In other words the patients were in the category of chronic pain sufferers.

This study then went on to look at the ability of physiotherapists to detect temperature variations and found that they had a high degree of sensitivity ±0.2°C. Clearly, it is possible to detect absolute differences, but in the clinical situation physiotherapists are palpating large skin areas across which a temperature gradient exists. Therefore, how reproducible are the findings? Two manipulative physiotherapists were used. Despite extensive postgraduate experience they both independently changed their methods of temperature palpation at an early stage of the first experiment. Using one hand for each side of the areas they palpated by using the reference point (lower thorax) initially and then feeling the upper lumbar area, returning to their reference point and then feeling the lower lumbar area. This was then repeated for the other side. They both adopted this procedure at the same time and so this cannot be the reason for their apparent lack of agreement. Incidentally, this finding has consequences for the teaching of palpation procedure.

A closer look at the results shows the apparent lack of inter-examiner agreement not to be a 'true' one. There is a high level of accuracy in the detection of significant temperature variations by both examiners (almost to 100%) but they have not chosen to describe these variations in the same way. The use of an arbitrary grading system does not, in these experiments, demonstrate this finding. From this it follows that inter-examiner studies performed in order to validate the subjectively estimated examination findings need a grading system in conjunction with objective measurements.

The results of the sixth experiment show a great increase in inter-examiner agreement and also a convergence in the way in which both examiners used the grading system. The probable reason for this was that a learning effect

had taken place. By the time the last trial had been carried out the examiners had palpated a great number of backs in the manner described not only as part of this study but on a daily basis with their own patients. It should be stressed at this point that, throughout these experiments, the examiners were asked not to discuss their findings with one another neither were they told the results of the trial—thus ruling out discussion as a possible source of convergence in the results.

CONCLUSIONS

1. Statistically significant variations exist in the thermal patterns of the low back in patients suffering from long-standing low-back pain.

2. Manipulative physiotherapists were able to detect pathologically significant (>1.0°C) temperature increases with virtually 100% accuracy, and increases of 0.5°C with 50% accuracy.

3. The use of an arbitrary scale in the validation of palpation findings may not fully and correctly demonstrate the inter-examiner agreement.

4. Repeated skin temperature palpations on patients and healthy subjects induced a convergence between the two examiners and also narrowed the temperature boundaries in the use of the four-point scale. This could indicate a learning effect despite the fact that the examiners were experienced manipulative physiotherapists, and suggests that sustained practice is an important element in the accuracy of temperature estimation.

Acknowledgements

I wish to extend my thanks to the Colt Foundation for the financial support for this project. I also thank Mr P. E. Wells and my other colleagues for their collaboration, and Mr S. Brown for the illustrations.

REFERENCES

Gonnella C, Paris S V, Kutner M 1982 Reliability in evaluating passive intervertebral motion. Physical Therapy 62: 436–444

Gunn C C, Milbrant W E 1978 Early and subtle signs in low back sprain. Spine 3: 267–281

Lele P P, Weddell G, Williams C M 1954 The relationship between heat transfer, skin temperature and cutaneous sensibility. Journal of Physiology 126: 206–234

Low J L 1976 The reliability of joint measurement. Physiotherapy 62: 227–229

Maitland G D 1986 Vertebral manipulation, 5th edn. Butterworth, London

Pochaczevsky R, Feldman F 1982 Contact thermography of spinal root compression syndromes. American Journal of Neuroradiology 3: 243–250

Pochaczevsky R, Wexler C E, Meyers P H, Epstein J A, Marc J A 1982 Liquid crystal thermography of the spine and extremities. Its value in

the diagnosis of spinal root syndromes. Journal of Neurosurgery 56: 386–395

Raskin M M, Martinez-Lopez M, Sheldon J J 1976 Lumbar thermography in discogenic disease. Radiology 119: 149–152

Salisbury R S, Parr G, De Silva M, Hazelman B L, Page-Thomas D P 1983 Heat distribution over normal and abnormal joints: thermal patterns and quantification. Annals of the Rheumatic Diseases 42: 494–499

Swinscow T D V 1976 Statistics at square one. British Medical Journal

Tegelberg A, Kopp S 1988 Skin surface temperature over the masseter muscle in individuals with rheumatoid arthritis. Acta Odontologica Scandinavica 46: 151–158

Uematsu S, Long D M 1976 Thermography in chronic pain. Medical thermograph theory and clinical application. Brentwood Publishing, pp 52–58

Wexler C E 1980 Thermographic evaluation of trauma (spine). Acta Thermographica 5: 3–11

41. Examination of the high cervical spine (Occiput–C2) using combined movements

B. C. Edwards

INTRODUCTION

The high cervical spine (Occiput–C2) is an area of the vertebral column which does not lend itself easily to physical examination. It is however subject to a wide variety of mechanical disorders. The so-called cervical headache (see also Chs 22 and 23) has its origin, in many cases, at these levels, as do a number of associated mechanically caused symptoms. Stoddard (1962, 1969) discusses common mechanical headaches, as does Jackson (1967). The common areas of pain from these high cervical mechanical disorders are:

1. sub-occipital and occipital
2. frontal
3. frontal and occipital
4. unilateral from high cervical to over and in the eye
5. parietal and/or occipital
6. band around the head
7. occipital and crown
8. orbit (with accompanying watering of the eye)
9. nasal.

Pain is often accompanied by:

- nausea
- blurring of vision
- vertigo
- enforced rest
- duffed concentration.

Some of the above symptoms can, of course, be related to conditions other than a cervical headache and are not suitable for manual therapy techniques; such conditions include, for example, migraine, vertebral artery syndromes and cranial or cervical tumours. However, mechanical disorders of the cervical spine can often mimic these more serious conditions. In cases where true migrainous symptoms are present, manipulation has no part to play. However, many migraine sufferers have a cervical component in the genesis of their symptoms and often the severity of migrainous attacks can be lessened after the cervical component has been corrected. Unfortunately, signs and symptoms in the high cervical spine are often overlooked, due to inadequate examination.

The anatomy of the high cervical spine is unique and to some degree more complicated than the rest of the vertebral column. The shapes of the bones and their articulations are distinctly different between the occiput and atlas, atlas and axis and C3. Such a marked change in anatomy does not occur in such close proximity anywhere else in the vertebral column.

The atlas has no body, but rather an anterior and posterior arch, which joins the lateral masses. The superior articular facets are concave and face upwards and medially. The inferior articular surfaces are slightly convex and face downwards and medially. The transverse processes are long.

The axis is quite a different shape. The superior articular facets are slightly convex and laterally inclined. The inferior articular facets are set more posteriorly and are directed downwards and anteriorly to articulate with the third cervical vertebra.

Between the superior articular surfaces of the axis, the stout odontoid process projects upwards. At its base posteriorly is a facet for the transverse ligament of the atlas.

Anteriorly, there is a smooth oval facet for articulation with the posterior surface of the anterior arch of the atlas. The transverse ligament passes between the medial tubercles on the lateral masses of the atlas and continues superiorly as the superior longitudinal band to attach to the foramen magnum. Inferiorly, it continues as the inferior band and attaches to the posterior aspect of the body of C2.

From the tip of the odontoid process the apical ligament passes up to be attached to the foramen magnum, anteriorly to the superior longitudinal band of the cruciate ligament. The alar ligaments diverge upwards from the sides of the odontoid process to the medial aspects of the occipital condyles.

It is interesting to note that the articulations of the

occipito-atlantal and atlanto-axial joints are situated approximately 1 cm anterior to the articulations of second and third cervical vertebra.

Although the articular surfaces of the atlanto-occipital and atlanto-axial joints vary somewhat, it is generally agreed that those between the occiput and atlas are concavo-convex, and between the atlas and axis slightly biconvex (excluding the articulation between the odontoid peg and the anterior arch of the atlas). The main movements which occur between the occiput and atlas are flexion and extension. Because the joint surfaces are concavo-convex, the condyles of the occiput and the articulating surface of the atlas follow the simple concavo-convex rule of relative movement.

Although there is some dispute as to whether any rotation occurs between occiput and atlas, passive testing between mastoid process and transverse process of C1 reveals that a small amount of passive rotation is possible.

PHYSIOLOGICAL MOVEMENTS

On flexion of the head, the condyles of the occiput move dorsally on the superior articulating surfaces of the atlas, tightening the posterior part of the capsule as well as tightening the posterior atlanto-occipital membrane (Fig. 41.1). On extension, the condyles of the occiput move ventrally on the superior articular surface of the atlas and in doing so tighten the anterior atlanto-occipital membrane and the apical ligament (Fig. 41.2).

Lateral flexion of the occiput on the atlas causes the condyles of the occiput to move in the opposite direction to which the head is laterally flexed. There is also some

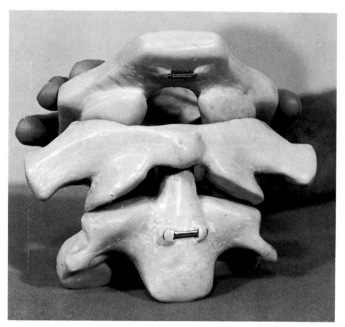

Fig. 41.2 Extension occipito-atlantal joint.

evidence to suggest that lateral flexion is combined with rotation to the opposite side (see Ch. 4). However, when examining the occipito-atlantal complex with combined movements, the movement of lateral flexion is not as useful as flexion or extension primarily, as it is difficult to increase or decrease the stretch or compression effects of combining lateral flexion with either flexion or extension.

Due to the shape of the articulating surfaces between atlas and axis, the movements which occur are quite different to those occurring between occiput and atlas. Braakman and Penning (1971) suggest that the occiput and axis should be considered as a segment, rather than the atlas and the axis. This is because of the attachment of the apical superior longitudinal band of the cruciate, the apical ligament from the odontoid tip to the occiput and the alar ligaments from the occiput to the axis. However, while this is a useful concept, any examination of the high cervical spine is not complete without endeavouring to test the individual movements between the occiput and atlas, and atlas and axis. On extension, there is an approximation of the posterior arch of the atlas and the spinous process of the axis and a gapping of the articular surfaces anteriorly (Fig. 41.3). On flexion, the distance between the posterior arch of the atlas and the spinous process of the axis increases and there is a gapping of the articular surfaces posteriorly (Fig. 41.4). On rotation, say to the right, of the atlas on the axis, the left inferior articular surface of the atlas moves forward on the left superior articular surface of the axis and the right inferior articular surface of the atlas moves backwards on the right superior articular surface of the axis (Fig. 41.5).

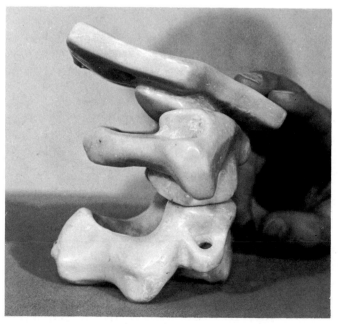

Fig. 41.1 Flexion occipito-atlantal joint.

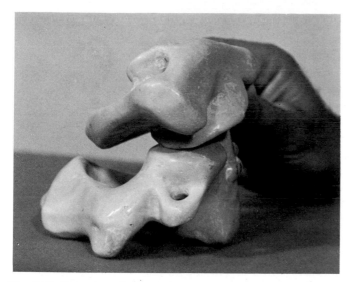

Fig. 41.3   Extension atlanto-axial joint.

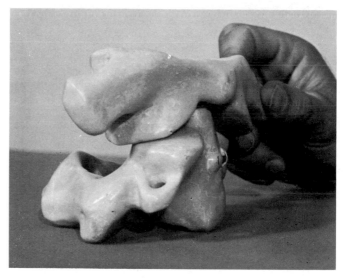

Fig. 41.5   Right rotation atlanto-axial joint.

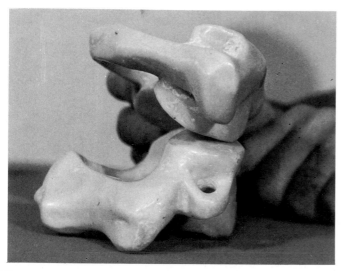

Fig. 41.4   Flexion atlanto-axial joint.

stretch is placed on the right-hand posterior part of the capsule of the occipito-atlantal joint (Fig. 41.6).

Method of testing

The therapist supinates his left forearm and extends the left wrist. The web between the left index finger and left thumb is placed over the symphysis menti. The right hand is placed over the crown of the head with the finger tips extending down to grasp the skull below the external occipital protuberance. The head is flexed on the cervical spine. Right rotation is added in such a manner as to

EXAMINATION OF THE OCCIPITO-ATLANTAL COMPLEX USING COMBINED MOVEMENTS

The combining of movements when examining the cervical and lumbar spine has already been described (Edwards 1979, 1980, 1992). The principles when combining movements in the high cervical spine are the same as with the rest of the vertebral column, i.e. movements are combined which tend to stretch or compress the joints and surrounding structures.

Testing in flexion and right rotation

On flexion, the condyles of the occiput move backwards in relation to the articular surface of the atlas. If this is combined with rotation, say to the right, an increased

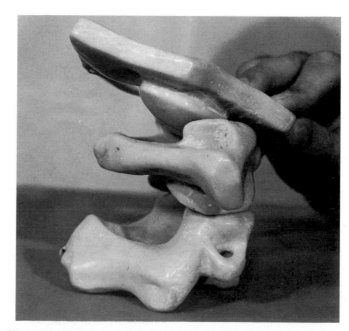

Fig. 41.6   Flexion and right rotation.

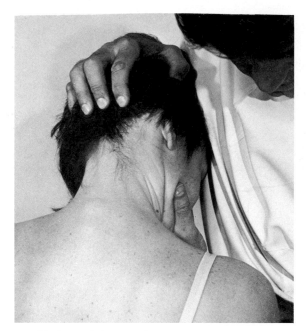

Fig. 41.7   Flexion and right rotation.

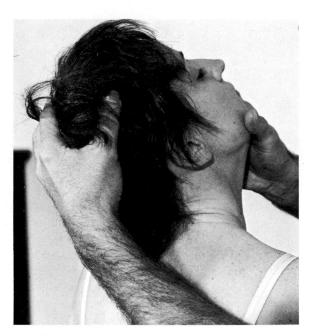

Fig. 41.9   Extension and right rotation.

increase the stretch on the right posterior atlanto-occipital membrane (Fig. 41.7).

Testing in extension and right rotation

On extension, the condyles of the occiput move forwards in relation to the articular surface of the atlas. If this is combined with rotation to the right, an increase in the stretch on the anterior capsule of left occipito-atlantal joint is obtained (Fig. 41.8).

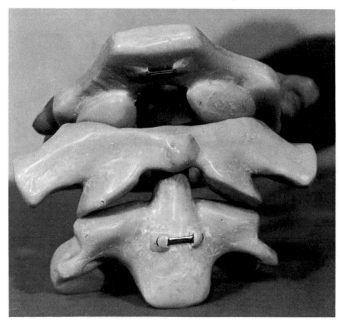

Fig. 41.8   Extension and right rotation.

Method of testing

The left hand is placed over the crown of the head and the right hand under the chin. The head is then extended on the neck and rotation to the right of the head is added, so as to increase the stretch of the anterior part of the capsule of the left occipito-atlantal joint (Fig. 41.9).

EXAMINATION OF THE ATLAS–AXIS COMPLEX USING COMBINED MOVEMENTS

Right rotation and flexion

On rotation to the right of the atlas on the axis, the left inferior articular surface of the atlas moves forward on the left superior articular surface of the axis. The opposite occurs on the right hand side. If flexion is then added, an increase of the stretch of the left and right posterior aspect of the atlanto-axial joint is obtained (Fig. 41.10).

Method of testing

The left hand is placed over the posterior aspect of C2 so that the left middle finger is over the anterior aspect of the left transverse process of C2. The left index finger is placed on the left hand side of the spine of C2 and the left thumb is placed over the posterior aspect of the superior articulation of C2. The right hand and arm hold the patient's head so that the right little finger comes around the arch of C1. The head is then rotated to the right, just until C2 moves. Flexion of the occiput and C1 is then added so that an increase of the stretch on the left and right posterior aspect of the atlanto-axial joint is obtained (Fig. 41.11).

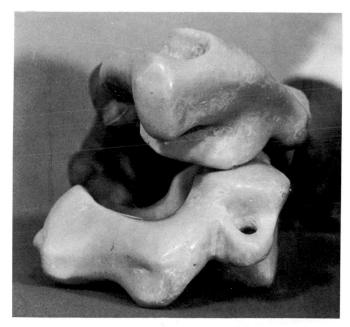

Fig. 41.10 Right rotation and flexion.

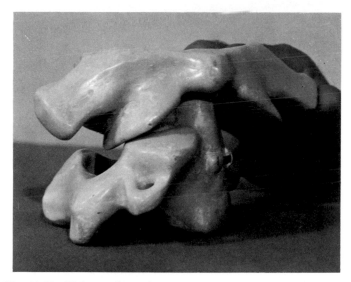

Fig. 41.12 Right rotation and extension.

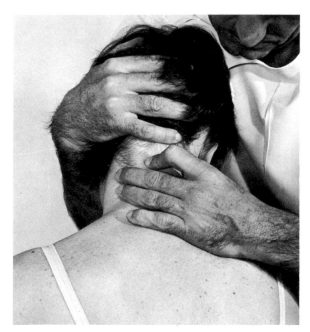

Fig. 41.11 Right rotation and flexion.

Testing in right rotation and extension

On rotation to the right of the atlas on axis, the left inferior articular surface of the atlas moves forwards on the left superior articular surface of the axis and the opposite occurs on the right hand side. If extension is added, there is an increase in the stretch on the right and left anterior part of the capsule of the atlanto-axial joint (Fig. 41.12).

Method of testing

The same hand positions are adopted as above, with extension now added so that there is an increase of stretch on the right and left anterior part of the capsule of the atlanto-axial joint (Fig. 41.13).

The passive testing procedures described above will elicit signs which are more often related to restriction of movement rather than reproduction of specific areas of pain. For that reason, confirmation by palpation is essential. Very often, specific signs and symptoms are more easily isolated by palpation than by passive physiological testing.

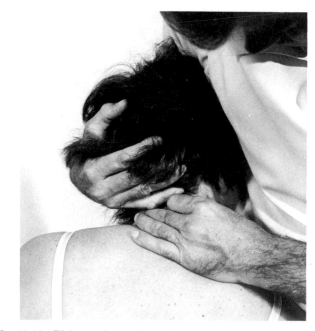

Fig. 41.13 Right rotation and extension.

CONFIRMATION BY PALPATION

Occipito-atlantal articulation

The patient lies prone with the therapist standing at her head. The patient's head is flexed and rotated to the right. The tips of both thumbs are placed over the right side of the posterior arch of C1 and the fingers of both hands are allowed to rest comfortably over the sides of the patient's head. Palpatory oscillating pressure is then applied so as to increase the stretch of the right occipito-atlantal articulation (Fig. 41.14). Palpation over the anterior aspect of the transverse process of C1 will decrease the stretch on the right (Fig. 41.15). With the head in extension and right rotation, palpation over the posterior arch of C1 on the left will decrease the stretch on the anterior aspect of the left atlanto-axial joint (Fig. 41.16). Palpation over the anterior aspect of the left of C1 will increase the stretch on the left anterior occipito-atlantal joint (Fig. 41.17).

Atlas-axis articulation

With C1/2 in right rotation and flexion, palpation over the anterior aspect of the left transverse process of C1 will decrease rotation between the atlas and the axis and therefore decrease the stretch on the posterior aspect of the left and right atlanto-axial articulation (Fig. 41.18).

With the patient in the same position as above, palpation over the left anterior aspect of C2 transverse process will increase the stretch on the posterior aspect of left and right atlanto-axial articulations (Fig. 41.19).

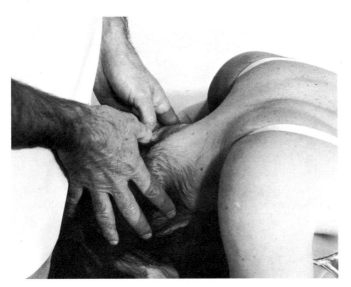

Fig. 41.14 Posterior palpation of C1 in right rotation and flexion.

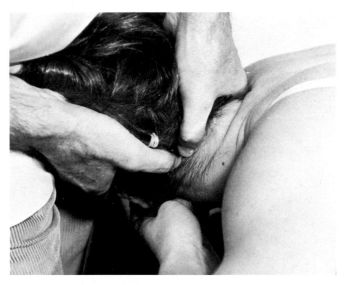

Fig. 41.16 Posterior palpation on the left of C1 in extension and right rotation.

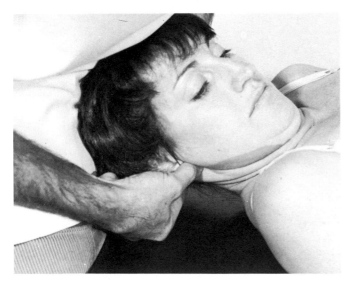

Fig. 41.15 Anterior palpation on the right of C1 in right rotation and flexion.

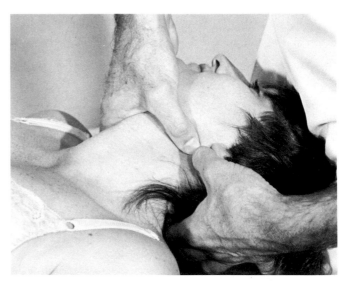

Fig. 41.17 Anterior palpation on the left of C1 in extension and right rotation.

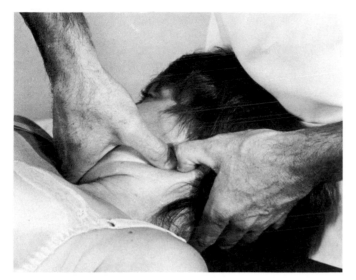

Fig. 41.18 Anterior palpation on the left of C1 in right rotation and flexion.

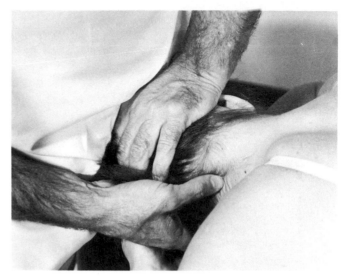

Fig. 41.20 Posterior palpation over left posterior aspect of C1 in right rotation and flexion.

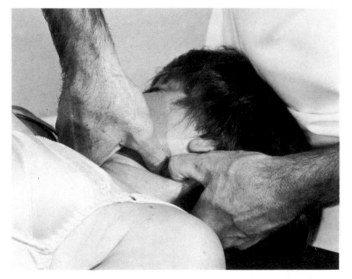

Fig. 41.19 Anterior palpation on the left transverse process of C2 in right rotation and flexion.

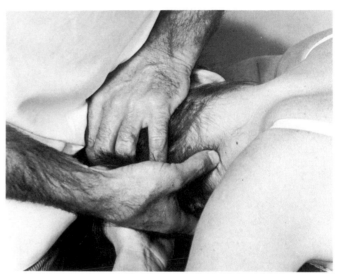

Fig. 41.21 Palpation over the posterior aspect of the left of C2 will decrease the rotation and therefore decrease the stretch on the posterior aspect of the atlanto-axial articulations.

With the patient in the same head/neck relationship as described above, palpation over the left posterior aspect of C1 will increase the stretch on the posterior aspect of the atlanto-axial articulations (Fig. 41.20).

With the patient in the same position as above, palpation over the posterior aspect of the left of C2 will decrease the rotation and therefore decrease the stretch on the posterior aspect of the atlanto-axial articulations (Fig. 41.21).

In the position of right rotation and extension, palpation over the right anterior aspect of the transverse process of C1 will increase the rotation of C1 on C2 and increase the stretch on the anterior aspect of the right and left atlanto-axial joints (Fig. 41.22).

Palpation over the right anterior aspect of C2 will de-

crease the rotation and stretch on the anterior aspect of the right and left atlanto-axial joints (Fig. 41.23).

Palpation over the posterior aspect of the right of C1 in rotation extension will decrease the rotation of C1 on C2 and decrease the stretch on the anterior aspect of the right and left atlanto-axial joints (Fig. 41.24).

Palpation over the posterior aspect of the right of C2 in right rotation and extension will increase the rotation and increase the stretch on the anterior aspect of the right and left atlanto-axial joints (Fig. 41.25).

TREATMENT

Accessory movements have been found to be the most useful type of technique when treating headaches arising

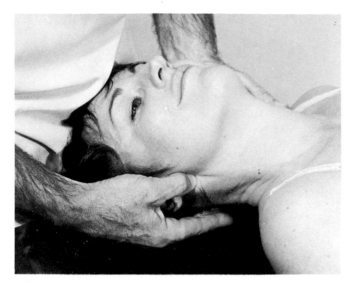

Fig. 41.22   Anterior palpation over C1 in right rotation and extension.

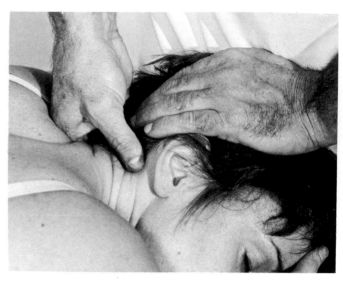

Fig. 41.24   Posterior palpation over the right C1 in right rotation and extension.

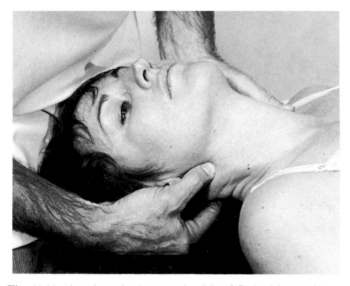

Fig. 41.23   Anterior palpation over the right of C2 in right rotation and extension.

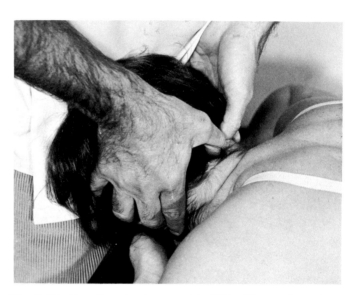

Fig. 41.25   Posterior palpation over right C2 in right rotation and extension.

from the joints and soft tissue of the upper cervical spine (Edwards 1992). Choice of technique is made using the mechanical principles outlined above. Examination of the physiological combinations of movement will often reveal a significant movement combination, but such positioning usually demonstrates a restriction of movement or produces local pain rather than referred symptoms. Once the most significant position is found, confirmation of the particular joint at fault can be made using palpation. For example, if the primary combination is flexion and right rotation with symptoms on the right of 0/1 origin, then the following accessory technique could be used to attempt to reproduce the headache or detect significant movement restriction.

Thus the movement at 0/1 may be enhanced.

If, for example, 0/1 is to be treated, the following sequence is a way of progressively increasing the stretch being applied to the joint.

Right-sided headache of 0/1 origin, primary combination flexion and right rotation.

  (i)   ⤵   C1 in neutral
 (ii)   ⤴   C1 in flexion and right rotation
(iii)   ⤵   C1 in flexion and right rotation

For right-sided headache of 1/2 origin with right rotation and flexion as the primary combination, the following sequence may be used.

  (i)   ⤴   C2 in neutral
 (ii)   ⤵   C1 in neutral

(iii) ⌐↘ C2 in neutral
(iv) ↗ C1 in neutral
(v) ↗ C2 in right rotation and flexion
(vi) ⌐↘ C1 in right rotation and flexion
(vii) ⌐↘ C2 in right rotation and flexion
(viii) ↗ C1 in right rotation and flexion

Greater detail on the subject of treatment is presented in Chapter 54.

SUMMARY

Because of the unique shapes of the articulations between the occiput, atlas and atlas on axis, the examination of this area requires different techniques to those used for the rest of the vertebral column. Many signs associated with the common cervical headache may be more easily highlighted if specific movement procedures are carried out. These movement procedures need to be related to the shapes of the articular surfaces between occiput and atlas, and atlas and axis. Passive physiological procedures, when combined, can help in highlighting specific signs. However, these findings should be confirmed by palpation and these procedures should be carried out in similar combined positions. In using these procedures, it is not unusual to find that what initially appear to be minor local signs are in fact substantial signs, often exactly underlying the headache and other symptoms for which the patient is seeking treatment. After establishing the exact locality and nature of these signs, a more accurate selection of technique can be made, therefore increasing the efficiency of the application of manual therapy procedures.

CONCLUSIONS

The physical examination of the high cervical spine requires a high degree of skill. Signs and symptoms arising from this area are often difficult to isolate by usual movement procedures. The combining of various movement may assist in increasing or decreasing the stretch or compression forces on particular joints and therefore highlighting signs which may not be obvious with the standard examination procedures. These combined movements, including a method of confirmation by palpation, have been described. Treatment has also been briefly described.

Acknowledgement

I would like to thank Mr D. Watkins, Photographer, Department of Physiotherapy, Western Australian Institute of Technology, for his assistance with photographs.

REFERENCES

Braakman R, Penning L 1971 Injuries of the cervical spine. Excerpta Medica, Amsterdam, ch 1, p 3–30
Edwards B C 1979 Combined movements of the lumbar spine: examination and clinical significance. Australian Journal of Physiotherapy 25: 141–152
Edwards B C 1980 Combined movements in the cervical spine (C2–C7): their value in examination and technique choice. Australian Journal of Physiotherapy 26: 165–171

Edwards B C 1992 Manual of combined movements. Churchill Livingstone, Edinburgh
Jackson R 1967 Headaches associated with disorders of the cervical spine. Headache 6: 175–179
Stoddard A 1962 Manual of osteopathic technique. Hutchinson, London
Stoddard A 1969 Manual of osteopathic practice. Hutchinson, London, pp 229–232

42. The use of repeated movements in the McKenzie method of spinal examination

P. M. Van Wijmen

INTRODUCTION

Traditionally, in the assessment of patients with spinal pain, examination of movement is performed in order to establish whether there is a movement loss and, if so, whether the restriction is painful or not. To this end, movements are performed once, or possibly a few times, until the necessary information about the range of motion has been obtained.

Frequently, significant differences are observed when comparing the effects of single movement performance with repeated movements. In the McKenzie approach to mechanical disorders both diagnosis and treatment are based on the symptom behaviour observed during and after repeated movement testing.

This chapter deals with the rationale for and method of dynamic mechanical evaluation (repeated movement testing) as introduced by McKenzie (1981, 1990); it provides an analysis of the effects of repeated movements, and includes a brief discussion of the rationale for static mechanical evaluation.

RATIONALE FOR DYNAMIC MECHANICAL EVALUATION

The aims of repeated movement testing are diagnostic (1, 2, 4, 5), prognostic (2, 3), therapeutic (4, 5, 6, 7) and prophylactic (7); specifically, the aims are to:

1. Identify the syndrome(s) responsible for the patient's present symptoms
2. Identify conditions for which mechanical therapy is unsuitable or contraindicated
3. Predict treatment outcome
4. Identify the correct direction of movement to be utilized in treatment
5. Determine the stability of healing following trauma and derangement
6. Provide a comprehensive premanipulative testing protocol prior to applying therapist technique
7. Provide guidelines for safe exercising (home

programmes) and identify warning signs that may lead to exacerbations or recurrence of symptoms.

Diagnosis of syndromes

In the majority of patients with spinal problems it is difficult, if not impossible, to identify precisely the actual structures causing the symptoms (Nachemson 1980, Dixon 1980, Spitzer et al 1987) and to arrive at a diagnosis based on existing pathologies. Therefore McKenzie, in 1981, proposed a different method of classification based on the way symptoms are produced and influenced by patients' own normal spinal movements and positions. The categorization of patients into the postural, dysfunction and derangement syndrome, and the further classification of the derangement syndrome into subgroups, depend mainly on accurate evaluation of the effects of repeated end-range movements and sustained end-range positions on the symptoms. The determination of the intensity and location of symptoms while at rest, and the subsequent changes in these symptoms caused by movement repetition or sustained positioning, play an important part in this method of patient evaluation.

In 1987, Spitzer et al recommended in the Quebec Task Force (QTF) report a classification of activity-related spinal disorders. The first four categories (11 in total) are based on the location of the symptoms and the presence or absence of neurological deficit. These groups contain the vast majority of patients seen in clinical practice. There is a remarkable resemblance between the three syndromes of McKenzie and the first four QTF classifications (see Ch. 28).

In order to stress the spine and related joints adequately during the examination without causing exacerbation of symptoms, mechanical forces in the form of a series of test movements and, if necessary, test positions are applied in a controlled manner. The aim of repeated movement testing is to influence the patient's symptoms. This may be achieved in three ways: (i) the symptom status is altered during movement testing, i.e. symptoms are reproduced,

565

increased, decreased, or abolished; (ii) a lasting change results after movement testing; (iii) both (i) and (ii) may take place. With sufficient knowledge and understanding of the three syndromes and their specific pain behaviours in response to the predetermined test movements and positions, patterns characteristic for each syndrome can be identified. It as also possible to recognize disorders which do not respond typically to the application of mechanical force, thereby exposing non-mechanical pathologies. In conclusion, the information obtained by deliberately stressing the structures involved will lead to classification of patients into one or more of the McKenzie syndromes. Additionally, pathological categories outside this framework, including serious or sinister pathologies, may be identified. In this way patients with pathologies unsuited to mechanical therapy will be eliminated early in the process of conservative care.

The McKenzie syndromes are dealt with in detail in Chapter 28 and elsewhere (McKenzie 1981, 1990, Van Wijmen 1986a, b). For the purpose of this chapter it will suffice to state how pain is produced in each of the syndromes and relate this to the testing procedures. In McKenzie's conceptual model postural pain is produced by end-range stress of normal structures, i.e. by static loading in end-range positions. Pain caused by dysfunction is produced by end-range stress of shortened structures, i.e. by static or dynamic loading in end-range positions and movements. The pain of derangement is produced by mid- or end-range stress of intervertebral joints, the contents of which are internally or externally displaced, i.e. by static or dynamic loading in mid- or end-range positions and movements.

It must be emphasized that, in patients with the pure postural syndrome, symptoms are not reproduced by movements but only by prolonged positioning. Therefore, the postural syndrome may be exposed when no symptoms are present prior to testing and repeated movements do not provoke pain. When symptoms are reproduced during movement testing, in essence the purpose of evaluating the effects of repeated movements on these symptoms and, consequently, the range of movement, is to be able to identify the type of pain behaviour and movement loss typical for derangement and dysfunction.

McKenzie (1981) described a clinical phenomenon whereby, as a result of movement repetition, the patient's most distal symptoms are relocated in a more proximal or central position. Known as the centralization phenomenon, this is described in detail in Chapter 55 and elsewhere (McKenzie 1981, 1990, Donelson et al 1990). The exact mechanisms underlying the centralization phenomenon are not yet fully understood. However, there is ample scientific evidence that, in a disc with an intact hydrostatic mechanism, annular/nuclear displacement results from offset loading of the intervertebral segments involved (Park 1976, Shah et al 1978, Hickey & Hukins 1980, Adams & Hutton 1982, 1985, Krag et al 1987, Wilder et al 1988, Shepperd et al 1990, Kramer 1990). Following removal of the loading, replacement of displaced disc material will occur (Kramer 1990).

Centralization and peripheralization of symptoms, and the simultaneous changes in symptom intensity, occur only and predictably in patients suffering from the derangement syndrome. The explanation for these phenomena may lie in the conceptional model of displacement (peripheralization) and replacement (centralization) of the annular/nuclear complex occurring under defined circumstances as a result of movements and positions of the vertebral column.

Changes in pain location and intensity are not likely to result from a single movement but can readily be observed during or after one to five sequences of 5- to 15-movement repetitions. In certain conditions it may be necessary to repeat one or more movements many times, possibly over a 24 hour period, before centralization or peripheralization becomes apparent. It is only through the systematic performance of repeated movement testing and careful analysis of the effects on the symptoms, that it is possible to verify the presence or absence of the centralization phenomenon and arrive at a mechanical diagnosis.

In general terms the typical response of the three McKenzie syndromes to repetitive end-range motion can be summarized as outlined in Table 42.1.

Table 42.1 Effects of repeated movements on the McKenzie syndromes

Syndrome	Effects of repeated movements
Postural syndrome	Pain is not reproduced Pain present when stationary is not present during testing
Dysfunction syndrome	Pain is produced at end-range of movement only Stops shortly on release of end-range stress Fixed pain pattern during testing (same end-range pain) Will radiate slightly during testing of nerve root adherence Condition unchanged after testing (no better or worse) No rapid and lasting changes as a result of testing
Derangement syndrome	Symptoms are produced or altered within movement range Painful arc may exist Variable pain pattern during testing Progressive decrease or increase during testing Centralization or peripheralization during testing Condition remains better or worse after testing Rapid and lasting changes as a result of testing

Identification of unsuitable conditions and contraindications

Examination by repeated movement testing will, early in the process of conservative care, eliminate those patients whose pathology is unsuitable for mechanical treatment. If, during examination, no position or movement can be found to reduce, centralize or abolish the symptoms, mechanical therapy may be of no value, at least not at this stage (McKenzie 1981). If symptoms are only increased or peripheralized it is likely that more advanced pathology exists, such as an extruded disc fragment, fracture or other condition, and mechanical therapy is contraindicated. If symptoms are not affected at all by mechanical measures (e.g. movements or positions, rest or activity, loading or unloading of the spine) or respond atypically to their application, the underlying cause may not be mechanical, and further investigation is indicated.

Although dynamic mechanical evaluation on the first examination may identify patients with pathologies unsuitable for mechanical therapy, the exact nature of the pathology may not as yet have been determined (McKenzie 1987).

Prediction of the outcome of treatment

Kopp et al (1986) proposed that, in patients admitted to hospital with herniated nucleus pulposus (HNP) and radiculopathy, the presence of a positive extension sign, i.e. the inability to achieve extension as a result of repetitive passive extension exercises, is an early predictor of the need for surgical intervention. Patients who, in this study, had a negative extension sign were subsequently treated conservatively. At long-term follow-up, Alexander et al (1990) reported that the extension sign was able to predict, in 91% of cases, those patients who will respond well to non-operative treatment of HNP. An extension sign that changed within 5 days from positive to negative was a strong predictor that surgery may not be required.

Donelson et al (1990) reported that patients who could not achieve centralization of symptoms as a result of repeated movements, did not respond well to conservative therapy and generally had a poor treatment outcome. All patients who subsequently had proven surgical disc pathology were non-centralizers. Donelson recommended that non-centralization be regarded as an early predictor of the need for surgical intervention.

From these two studies the following conclusions may be drawn. Patients are likely to have a more complex pathology if they are unable to achieve at least some extension or centralization of symptoms during repeated movement testing at examination or during the first few days of treatment. The condition of such patients is often not rapidly reversible and they may have a less favourable prognosis with regard to conservative management.

Identification of the correct direction of movement in treatment

While repeated movement testing is essential to arrive at a diagnosis, it is equally important to determine the positions and movements that are to be employed in treatment. In the treatment of derangement, the test movements that reduce, centralize or abolish the symptoms must be used. Conversely, movements that, at examination, peripheralize the symptoms should be avoided. In the treatment of dysfunction, test movements that reproduce and enhance the symptoms must be used. From this it can be seen that, for treatment to become successful, it is essential to have established the correct diagnosis. It has been found elsewhere (Stevens & McKenzie 1988, Kilby et al 1990) that failure to diagnose correctly leads to slower and less effective treatment.

In a recent two-part prospective randomized study, Donelson (1991a, b) documented the response of pain location and intensity to single and repeated spinal end-range movement testing in both the sagittal and frontal planes. In the first study the effects of lumbar flexion and extension on low-back and referred pain were evaluated. Movement testing was performed with the spine loaded while standing and unloaded while lying. Of the patients in this study, 40% improved with extension and 7% with flexion, and no subject experienced a decrease in pain during both movements. Donelson concluded that repeated extension significantly decreased central and distal pain intensity and centralized referred pain, while flexion had the opposite effect.

Only 47% of subjects in this study experienced centralization with testing procedures limited to motion in the sagittal plane. One of the characteristics of the remaining patients is that their symptoms had been present for longer than in those who responded to sagittal motion. According to McKenzie (1981) patients who do not respond to sagittal movements may experience centralization as a result of lateral or rotational movements. Therefore, patients who did not benefit from sagittal motion were subsequently evaluated for their response to lateral spinal end-range movements, first unloaded and then loaded. Of those who improved as a result of lateral movements, 69% improved by side-gliding towards the side of symptoms (or moving the hips away from the pain), 12% by side-gliding away from the symptomatic side (or moving the hips towards the pain), and 19% by side-gliding in both directions.

Donelson concluded that dynamic mechanical evaluation utilizing repeated movement testing and monitoring the pain response, enables the clinician to establish a mechanical profile and identify the beneficial exercises for patients with spinal pain.

Determination of the stability of healing

Repeated movement testing is essential to determine the stability of repair following tissue damage by derangement or trauma. This applies not only to spinal structures but also to soft tissue elsewhere in the body. During the healing process natural tension applied to the repair is necessary to prevent the development of a painful and weak scar resulting from cross-linkage of collagen (Evans 1980). However, this tension must not be of such a degree that healing is disrupted. The traffic-light guide as introduced by Rath (1989) provides an excellent assessment tool for therapists and patients alike (see Ch. 55).

To establish whether stressing the repair can safely be commenced after derangement or trauma, the following criteria should be adhered to:

1. If, on repetition, a movement becomes *progressively more painful and symptoms peripheralize*, stressing the repair using this movement should not be initiated. Testing indicates that continuation of the same stress will most likely cause recurrence of derangement or disrupt the still weak repair following trauma.

2. If, on repetition, a movement causes *pain of the same intensity to be felt in the same location at the end of the movement range*, it is safe and necessary to commence the application of stress. Testing indicates that the repair process following trauma and derangement has been completed and reduction of derangement appears stable.

3. If, on repetition, a movement becomes *progressively less painful*, the application of stress may commence. Testing indicates that the repair following derangement and soft-tissue injury is not yet dense or contracted but strong enough to adapt to forces of stress without being damaged. Some caution is indicated as recently repaired structures may be fragile, and overstretching may lead to recurrence of the problem.

Performance of premanipulative testing

McKenzie (1989) stated: 'Dynamic testing by repetitive motion should always precede the application of hands-on procedures and is a vital part of any mechanical assessment programme'. By applying patient-generated forces in the form of repeated movements, the stability of healing and reduction of derangement is tested and potentially unstable pathologies are exposed. The progressive increase of the applied stress from patient-generated to therapist-generated forces is a built-in safeguard of the McKenzie approach. Once improvement ceases or slows, or centralization remains incomplete, the next progression utilizing an increase of applied stress is indicated. In this way repeated movement testing serves as premanipulative testing prior to the use of therapist technique.

Provision of guidelines for safe exercising and identification of warning signs as prophylactic measures

Testing by repeated movements must be incorporated in the self-treatment programme of all patients, in particular when performing stretching exercises or potentially harmful movements. This serves as a safeguard against over-exercising which could lead to microtraumata in dysfunction or recurring episodes in derangement. For patients with a long-term preventative home exercise programme, self-testing will enable them to recognize warning signs and predisposing circumstances that may lead to recurrence of symptoms.

The same criteria used to determine whether stressing the repair following injury can be commenced safely can be applied to identify warning signs. Again, the traffic-light guide (Rath 1989, see Ch. 55) is very useful when self-testing by repeated movements. Patients should be taught to compare symptoms felt during the first movement in a series of exercises with symptoms felt during movement repetition. They must learn to differentiate between good pains (centralizing pain, or end-range pain of the same intensity and in the same location on movement repetition) and bad pains (pain progressively increasing and/or peripheralizing on movement repetition). The onset of bad pains during self testing or exercising must be recognized as a warning sign, and patients should be taught how to respond purposefully and effectively to avoid exacerbation.

The criteria to identify warning signs should be part of the guidelines for safe exercising that must be given to all patients with home exercise programmes.

METHOD OF REPEATED MOVEMENT TESTING

In repeated movement testing a series of normal movements are performed with the aim of causing a change in the symptoms. To achieve this the structures involved must be stressed sufficiently. It is essential, therefore, that patients be encouraged to move to the limit of range each time movement is performed (Stevens & McKenzie 1988). Active and passive end-range movements, the application of overpressure, and loading or unloading of the spine are evaluated for their effects on the symptoms.

Nearly all patients with mechanical spinal pain can be subjected to an assessment process that involves dynamic or static mechanical evaluation. Exceptions are patients with very severe pain for whom movement testing would be intolerable, or those derangement patients who exhibit acute deformities with major movement and posture obstructions that do not allow normal resting postures. A number of patients may have co-existing medical or other problems which may preclude or severely limit the extent of the examination procedures or require considerable modifications.

In patients with very severe and constant symptoms, repeated movements may cause only little change, if any, in pain intensity and location. In such cases, in particular, if distal symptoms are consistently being worsened it is necessary to abandon the testing procedures at this time. These patients should be re-evaluated after a few days of rest to determine whether mechanical therapy can be instituted at that stage.

The significance of the presence of distal paresthesiae, numbness and neurological motor deficit must not be underestimated. Such symptoms indicate interference with nerve root conduction. Frequently during repeated movement testing, low-back pain is greatly reduced as peripheral symptoms become more prominent. If attention is paid only to proximal symptoms in the low back, it may appear that improvement is occurring when in fact the condition is worsening. Patients must be encouraged to focus on their most distal symptoms during the examination. Naturally this will assist in determining whether centralization or peripheralization is taking place. During repeated movement testing patients should frequently be asked: 'What is happening to your most peripheral symptoms whilst performing these movements?' or 'Have your most distal symptoms changed as a result of performing these movements?'.

When symptoms in the extremity extend below the elbow or knee, especially when they are constant, it is important to examine reflexes and strength of key muscles representing certain nerve roots (motor conduction) as well as sensation prior to performing the test movements and closely monitor any changes during testing.

The entire sequence of test movements does not necessarily have to be completed at the initial examination. If a patient is in severe pain or has an acute deformity or unstable derangement that is easily disturbed, examination procedures will be very limited and may include only those movements that are most likely to lead to improvement of the symptoms.

In patients who do not present with an acute deformity (i.e. an acute obstruction to curve reversal), sagittal movements should be explored first, even when the symptoms are unilateral or bilateral but much more on one side than the other. Many of these patients respond well to sagittal procedures (McKenzie 1990, Donelson 1991a). If no significant alteration in the symptoms results, the effects of unilateral procedures, such as sidegliding, side-bending or rotation need to be explored (Donelson 1991b, see Ch. 55).

If following the test movements no conclusion can be drawn, it is possible that the affected structures have not been stressed adequately. A common problem is that patients often stop a test movement at the first sign of pain rather than continuing to move, despite the pain, to the end of the possible range. To facilitate the diagnostic process the following may be required: (i) ensure that movements are performed to the limit of the range; (ii) apply mechanical force more vigorously; (iii) sustain postures; (iv) increase the number of repetitions; (v) increase the frequency of repetitions; (vi) use alternative starting positions; (vii) stress the joints in one direction and check the effects on pain and movement range for motion in the opposite direction. In patients with a minor derangement, flexion or extension may have to be repeated many times or over a longer period of time (e.g. 24 hours) before the symptoms are reproduced.

If symptoms are not provoked with repeated movements, it could be that the pain is of pure postural origin. In patients with the postural syndrome, static end-range loading in the painful position is required for pain to be reproduced. It may also be possible that the symptoms originate in a different part of the spine than where they are actually felt. A good example is the reference of pain to the mid-thoracic and scapular region by discs lesions in the cervical spine (Cloward 1959). Alternatively, it could be that the cause of the problem does not lie in the spine or its surrounding tissues. In such cases it may be necessary to investigate possible involvement of joints in adjacent areas (sacro-iliac, hip, shoulder or acromioclavicular joints). Finally, the pain may not be mechanical in origin. Mechanical pain is always affected to some extent by mechanical factors such as movements and positions, rest and activity, loading and unloading of the spine.

The assessment by repeated movements must be methodical. Only if many patients are evaluated in the same logical way can patterns be seen to emerge that are typical for each of the syndromes. In addition, atypical pathologies will be identified very quickly.

The physiotherapist must control the mechanics of the assessment. Movements must be performed from the correct starting position to the limit of the range, in a rhythmic manner and not too quickly, applying intermittent pressure ('pressure on—pressure off'), relaxing between repetitions, and avoiding trick movements.

In order to be able to determine adequately the effects of movements on the symptoms, it is important to evaluate carefully the intensity and location of the symptoms, in particular the most distal symptoms, at three different stages:

1. The status of pain and other symptoms at rest prior to the commencement of repeated movement testing
2. The behaviour of pain and other symptoms during movements while repeated movement testing is performed
3. The status of pain and other symptoms at rest after repeated movement testing is completed.

Recording of the assessment findings must be accurate, clear and concise. In addition to noting alterations in intensity and location of symptoms, it is necessary to watch for changes in range of movement. There should be a correlation between reported changes in symptoms and observable changes in obstruction to movement. For example, if a patient reports a rapid decrease and centralization of symptoms with repeated lumbar extension, one would expect to see a corresponding increase in the range of lumbar extension.

In the latest version of the assessment forms (McKenzie Institute International 1993) changes have been made to the section dealing with repeated movement testing (Fig. 42.1). The typical McKenzie conventions, used when recording the effects of movement on the symptoms, are outlined. Allowance is made for description of pretest symptoms before test movements are performed in loaded and unloaded positions. The test movements that usually are examined first, are listed first. Under 'If required' follow the movements that do not always need to be examined. Finally, there is a new section that allows recording of the effects of standard static tests.

At times testing procedures other than the regular ones need to be explored. These may include alternative starting positions, the application of overpressure or manual overcorrection, or a variety of resting positions. It may be useful for the examiner to document any alterations or additions to the usual testing procedures on a separate sheet.

Commonly, 8 to 15 movement repetitions will sufficiently affect the symptoms to expose the presenting syndrome. When a fewer or a greater number of repetitions are required, it is useful to note this on the assessment form. This will give an indication of the fragility of the condition and the stability of the repair following trauma or derangement. For example: 'Repeated Flexion in Lying × 4 (RFIL × 4) – Peripheralizes' indicates that only four repetitions were required to worsen the condition; and 'RFIL × 50 – No Effect' indicates that even after 50 repetitions the symptoms were not affected.

Sequence of testing procedures

Evaluation of movement status prior to testing

Prior to repeated movement testing the quality of movement must be evaluated. Firstly, the available range of motion should be established for each of the test movements. This is usually done with the patient in the standing position for the lumbar spine and in sitting for the cervical and thoracic spine. It is necessary to grade any movement loss subjectively (major, moderate, minor or nil), and to determine whether or not the loss of movement is associated with pain. Painful movements are identified and noted, but behaviour of pain in response to movement is not assessed at this stage. Factors to be

TEST MOVEMENTS   Describe effects on present pain — produces, abolishes, increases, decreases, centralizes, peripheralizes, better, worse, no better, no worse, no effect

TEST MOVEMENTS		PDM	ERP
Describe pretest pain standing: (1)		(3)	(3)
FIS (2)			
Rep FIS (2)			
EIS (2)			
Rep EIS (2)			
Describe pretest pain lying: (1)			
FIL (2)			
Rep FIL (2)			
EIL (2)			
Rep EIL (2)			
If required SGIS (R)			
Rep SGIS (R)			
SGIS (L)			
Rep SGIS (L)			

(1) Record pre-test symptoms:
1. Presence/absence of symptoms
2. Location of symptoms
3. Nature of symptoms (pain, numbness, pins and needles)

(2) Record effects of testing:
1. Production or alteration of symptoms (use McKenzie conventions)
2. No effect

(3) Record where in movement range symptoms are affected:
1. Tick under PDM if pain during movement
2. Tick under ERP if end-range pain

Fig. 42.1   Lumbar assessment form — repeated movement section

observed in addition to the range of movement are: (i) the quality of curve reversal; (ii) the type of movement loss; (iii) the presence of deviation from the mid-sagittal movement pathway during flexion and extension; and (iv) the patient's ability and willingness to move.

In order to determine the type of movement loss it is important to establish the relationship between the loss of motion and pain. Not only will this information provide essential clues about the syndrome causing the problems, it will also act as a guide regarding the possible vigour and extent of the repeated movement testing that is to follow. Dysfunction is characterized by a *restriction of movement* which may cause only minor to moderate discomfort at the end of the possible range. In some instances there is a pain-free loss of motion. In derangement, there is frequently an *obstruction to movement* and acute pain may appear in the early part of the range with attempts to force the blocked movement.

Examination of the quality of movement will provide essential baseline information against which any change achieved with repeated movement testing and treatment will be compared. It is imperative to have a clear picture of this information in order to make a judgement of improvement or deterioration in the patient's condition. One or more of the painful, restricted or obstructed movements can be used as a measure for re-assessment. By establishing the relationship between movement loss and pain, and evaluating the changes in movement range that may develop later on in the examination or over the next few days with treatment, it will be possible to determine the effectiveness of the treatment and predict the treatment outcome.

Evaluation of symptom status prior to testing

Before commencing the loaded or unloaded test movements it is necessary to establish the symptoms present at rest. With the patient in the appropriate starting position, the location, nature (i.e. pain, numbness, pins and needles) and, in some instances, intensity of pain and other symptoms—in particular, the most peripheral symptoms—are defined. The presence or absence of symptoms is recorded in the appropriate section on the assessment form (see Fig. 42.1). This will provide a baseline to determine whether repeated movement testing produces new symptoms or leads to a change in existing symptoms, and whether these developments have a lasting effect. Evaluation of pain intensity may be facilitated by the use of a numeric pain rating scale (0 = no pain, 10 = the worst pain you could experience) or a visual analogue scale to which subsequent changes in the pain intensity can be related.

Evaluation of the effects of testing

First, the patient is asked to perform a test movement once only and report any effects during that movement. Depending on the symptom status prior to testing, symptoms may be produced or altered (increased, decreased, centralized, peripheralized, abolished), and this may occur during the movement itself or at the end of the existing range. Alternatively, movement may not alter the symptom status prior to testing.

Production or alteration of symptoms, or the fact that movement does not influence the symptoms, is recorded in the appropriate section on the assessment form (see Fig. 42.1). To indicate whether pain occurred during or at the end of the movement range the appropriate column on the assessment form is marked (see Fig. 42.1).

Secondly, the patient is asked to repeat the same movement a certain number of times and to compare the behaviour of symptoms during movement repetition to what happened during the first movement. Similar effects can be observed as described above and there will be concomitant changes in movement range. The most peripheral symptoms must be watched closely for possible changes in location and intensity. The number of repeti-

tions required depends on the fragility of the condition and the clarity of response to repeated movements. For example, in an acute patient a clear picture of increasing pain may emerge after only five repetitions. In this case there is no need to pursue the matter further. However, in a patient with a long-standing minor problem, two or more sets of 10 repetitions may be required to show changes in the pain pattern.

The effects of repeated movements are again recorded in the appropriate section on the assessment form and symptom changes occurring during or at the end of the movement range are indicated by marking the appropriate column (see Fig. 42.1). Table 42.2 explains the symbols and terms that are used in recording.

Table 42.2 Glossary of symbols and terms used in recording of symptoms during testing

Symbols	Word/phrase	Explanation
P	Produces	There are no symptoms at rest and the applied mechanical force* (AMF) produces symptoms
I or ↑	Increases	There are symptoms at rest and AMF increases the intensity
Periph	Peripheralizes	There are symptoms at rest and AMF relocates the symptoms further away from the spine
D or ↓	Decreases	There are symptoms at rest and AMF decreases the intensity
Centr	Centralizes	There are symptoms at rest and AMF relocates the symptoms closer to the spine
A	Abolishes	There are symptoms at rest and AMF eliminates symptoms in some or all areas
NE	No effect	1. There are no symptoms at rest and AMF does not produce symptoms 2. There are symptoms at rest and AMF does not alter the symptoms
PDM	Pain during movement or mid-range pain	Pain is produced or increased in the mid-range of movement or in a mid-range position
ERP	Pain at the limit of movement or end-range pain	Pain is produced or increased at the limit of movement or in an end-range position

* The applied mechanical force can be: (i) dynamic loading by repeated movements, or (ii) static loading by sustained positions.

Evaluation of symptom and movement status following testing

This part of evaluation establishes whether or not there are any lasting changes as a result of repeated movement testing. After a few minutes of rest or walking around, the patient is asked whether the original symptom status is unchanged or has altered. If, during testing, symptoms were produced or increased, the patient is asked whether he/she remains worse as a result. If, during testing, symptoms were reduced or abolished, the patient is asked whether he/she remains better as a result. Frequently, symptoms are produced or altered during repeated movements, but once movement has stopped the symptoms return to what they had been prior to movement testing. Occasionally, symptoms do not appear to be influenced during movement testing, but once movement has stopped the patient reports a lasting change. Table 42.3 explains the symbols and terms used when recording the after-effect of movement testing.

Table 42.3 Glossary of symbols and terms used in recording of symptoms after testing

Symbols	Word/phrase	Explanation
W	Worse as a result of testing	Symptoms produced or increased during application of a mechanical force* (AMF), remain worse after testing
NW	Not worse as a result of testing	Symptoms produced or increased during AMF, do not remain worse after testing
B	Better as a result of testing	Symptoms decreased or abolished during AMF, remain better after testing
NB	Not better as a result of testing	Symptoms decreased or abolished during AMF, do not remain better after testing

* The applied mechanical force can be: (i) dynamic loading by repeated movements, or (ii) static loading by sustained positions.

Summary of sequence of testing procedures

1. Establish movement status prior to testing, i.e. the presence or absence of restriction or obstruction to movement.
2. Establish symptom status prior to testing.
3. Perform test movement once, evaluate and record the effects on symptoms, and determine whether symptoms are affected at mid-range or at end-range.
4. Repeat test movement as required, evaluate and record the effects on symptoms, and determine whether symptoms are affected at mid-range or at end-range.
5. Compare the effects of repeated movements with the effects of the first movement.
6. Establish symptom status after testing, compare with symptom status prior to testing, and determine whether or not there are lasting changes.
7. Establish movement status after testing, compare with movement status prior to testing, and determine whether or not there are lasting changes. This is not routinely done in all patients. For example, in acute derangement patients provocative movements will be avoided, whereas potentially reductive movements can be checked safely.

Analysis of the effects of repeated movements

Typically, the derangement syndrome has a variable pain pattern: as a result of repeated movements, symptoms may change in intensity (increase, decrease), location (centralization, peripheralization) and constancy (constant, intermittent). Furthermore, the point in the range where the pain is felt may alter and, after testing, there may be a lasting change in the baseline symptoms. *The dysfunction syndrome is characterized by a fixed pain pattern:* on movement repetition the same end-range pain is felt in the same location and, after testing, the patient is no better and no worse.

The following criteria are essential when relating the effects of repeated movements to the three McKenzie syndromes:

1. The effect on the production of symptoms. If there are no symptoms prior to testing and repeated movements produce symptoms, the presenting problem is likely to be dysfunction or derangement. When no symptoms are produced with movements, the testing procedures provide insufficient force to reproduce the symptoms and end-range positioning will be required instead. Commonly, patients with this type of response will subsequently be classified in the postural syndrome category or they may have a minor displacement problem.

2. The point in the movement pathway where symptoms or symptom changes are first perceived. Pain produced or increased *within the movement range* is a strong indication of the presence of derangement. In minor derangements, or in the early stages of the development of derangement, only end-range pain may be felt rather than pain during motion. However, as a result of sufficient movement repetition or static loading of movements at end-range, the derangement syndrome will eventually emerge.

Pain produced *at the limit of movement only*, usually indicates dysfunction. This is particularly so when, on repetition of movement, the fixed pain pattern characteristic for dysfunction becomes apparent in addition to the end-range pain.

3. The effect on the location of symptoms. A change in location of the symptoms during repeated movement testing indicates the variable pain pattern of the derangement syndrome. Symptoms may disappear in one area but appear elsewhere. For example, low-back pain may disappear as thigh pain appears, or left-sided low-back pain may be abolished as right-sided low-back pain develops. It is also possible that, in addition to symptoms felt in one area, symptoms appear in a new area. Production and abolition of symptoms occurring during movement, may indicate that centralization or peripheralization is taking place.

Symptoms that are always felt in the same location, especially if they arise at the limit of movement, may be part of the fixed pain pattern of dysfunction. In nerve root adherence, which is a form of dysfunction, symptoms will radiate when the adherent structure is stressed. Provided the same mechanical force is applied on repeated movement testing, the same radiation will occur in the fixed pain pattern of dysfunction.

4. The effect on the intensity of symptoms. With the application of the same mechanical force during repeated movements, rapid and progressive changes in pain intensity (progressive increase, decrease or abolition) may be felt in derangement. This is part of the variable pain pattern of derangement. In dysfunction, the pain will have the same intensity with application of the same mechanical force during repeated movements. This is part of the fixed pain pattern of dysfunction.

5. The effect on the constancy of symptoms. Constant symptoms may be chemical or mechanical in origin. Of the three McKenzie syndromes, constant pain occurs only in the derangement syndrome. In addition to the mechanical causes of pain in derangement, changes in the intradiscal chemistry may well be responsible for at least part of this constant pain (Mooney 1987, McCarron et al 1987). Intermittent pain must be mechanical in origin and can be caused by each one of the three McKenzie syndromes.

Whether the mechanical pain of derangement is constant or intermittent depends merely on the size and location of the displacement within the disc. A change in symptoms from constant to intermittent, and vice versa, during or as a result of repeated movement testing, reflects the variable pain pattern of derangement.

6. The effect on the symptom status prior to testing. Rapid and lasting changes in the original symptoms following the test movements indicate the variable pain pattern of the derangement syndrome. After testing, the patient may have symptoms which originally were not present, symptoms may have peripheralized, centralized or completely disappeared. The truly lasting nature of these changes will only become apparent over a longer time period (e.g. 24 hours) and it may not be possible to evaluate this adequately during the assessment. Patients must be instructed to note carefully how long it takes for symptoms, brought on by the examination, to subside.

In dysfunction there are no rapid and lasting changes following the test movements and, unless the amount of applied mechanical force has been excessive, the patient feels about the same as prior to testing. Adaptive shortening, contracture or scaring of soft tissues takes place over a long period of time. It will require stretching over a similar duration before changes in symptom will be noticeable. This is consistent with the fixed pain pattern of dysfunction.

Chronic patients with long-standing severe dysfunction and nerve root involvement may experience an increase in symptoms for a day or longer following testing, especially if lately they have been quite inactive and have been avoiding painful movements and activities. On re-assessment there is usually no appreciable change in movement restriction. The increase in symptoms may merely indicate that shortened structures have finally been mobilized. Naturally, the history of such patients will assist to clarify the diagnosis.

7. The effect on the movement status prior to testing. When dealing with a rapidly reversible condition, as frequently occurs in the derangement syndrome, rapid changes in some or all of the affected movements are often seen to accompany symptom changes. In such conditions the range of the affected movements may increase or decrease in a matter of minutes as pain, caused by movement obstruction, decreases or increases. This can often be observed during the first assessment.

When dealing with a condition that is not rapidly reversible, as occurs in the dysfunction syndrome, rapid changes will not be observed in the affected movements. The movement range will gradually increase over days or even weeks as the shortened structures are being stretched and the movement restriction gradually decreases.

The McKenzie syndromes are described as separate entities but frequently they co-exist. In such cases the pictures emerging from repeated movement testing may be less clear. This commonly leads to difficulty with interpretation of repeated movement findings. In patients with a confusing clinical picture, the diagnosis will often be clarified by relating the objective to the subjective findings. The following key questions may assist in decision making. Is there a variable pain pattern with symptoms changing in location and intensity? What is the number of repetitions required to affect the symptoms? Is it necessary to sustain positions rather than perform movements?

Common errors with repeated movement testing are: (i) failure to take movements to end-range; (ii) failure to repeat movements enough times; (iii) skipping portions of the examination; (iv) avoiding provocative movements out of fear of exacerbation; (v) inadequate recording of repeated movement findings; (vi) inadequate evaluation of the effects of repeated movements on the symptoms; (vii) failure to relate the objective findings to the subjective findings.

RATIONALE FOR STATIC MECHANICAL EVALUATION

If dynamic testing procedures with or without overpressure do not provoke or alter the symptoms, the problem may be purely postural, or a minor displacement may exist which remains unaffected by repeated movements. In these cases symptoms will be reproduced only by replacing the repetitive motion (dynamic loading) by sustained positioning (static loading). The time factor introduced by static loading will stress the structures involved for a longer period. This will provide the additional mechanical deformation required to reproduce the symptoms and arrive at a diagnosis. The same three stages of symptom evaluation as used in repeated movement testing should be explored in testing by sustained positioning. The same symbols and terms are used in recording (see Tables 42.2 and 42.3).

In the evaluation of patients with the postural syndrome, static end-range loading is applied by maintaining the painful postures. The length of time a posture needs to be maintained to become painful varies for each patient. Generally this ranges from 10 to 60 minutes, but in some patients more time may be required to reproduce the symptoms.

When aiming to expose a minor derangement, static loading is applied by sustaining potentially provocative movements at end-range. Again the time period varies with each patient. Usually up to 3 minutes is sufficient but in some cases more time may be required and 2 to 3 hours is not unknown.

Williams et al (1991) demonstrated that sitting with the lumbar spine supported in lordosis resulted in a significant reduction of low-back and leg pain and centralized distal symptoms. In patients with an acute derangement who are unable to tolerate assessment by repeated movements, comparing the behaviour of the symptoms in different mid- and end-range positions may assist in identifying the correct position and direction of movement to be used in treatment.

CONCLUSIONS

Nelson et al (1979) recommended that the reliability of examination procedures increases when the information to be gained is kept to a minimum. The McKenzie assessment aims at obtaining the essential information required to arrive at a mechanical diagnosis. For a variety of reasons (insufficient time, lack of understanding, lack of confidence, fear of exacerbation), short cuts are frequently made when assessing spinal patients. Unfortunately, it is usually the repeated movement section that is left out. This part of the examination provides the most relevant and reliable information regarding the nature, severity and prognosis of the patient's problem. Skipping this section may interfere significantly with the process of clinical decision-making which should evolve from the assessment of all patients.

Kilby et al (1990) noted that the use of repeated movements to evaluate pain behaviour is one of the mainstays of the McKenzie assessment. In examining the reliability of back pain assessment by physiotherapists using a McKenzie algorithm, these workers reported good levels of agreement on the interpretation of pain patterns resulting from movement. It has been stated elsewhere (Matyas & Bach 1985, McCombe et al 1989, Spratt et al 1990) that the determination of pain behaviour in response to active physiological spinal movements provides reliable signs in low-back pain assessment.

An assessment that evaluates the performance of one single movement, or a few movements in each direction, to note the available range of movement and the presence or absence of pain, does not provide adequate information about the underlying pathology and the state of the structures involved (McKenzie 1990). This type of testing merely identifies a problem movement. It does not provide any clues about the nature of the problem, its underlying cause, suitable mechanical therapy that may resolve it, or the stability of the structures involved. In fact, if clinical decision-making is based on the effects of one movement or a few movements only, the patient's problems may not be solved. For example, when one movement significantly increases peripheral symptoms, frequently all further testing is abandoned. However, repetition of the problem movement could well indicate a potential to centralize and abolish the symptoms. Without movement repetitions this information would not be gained. In this way the most reliable indicator for a possible successful treatment outcome, the presence of the centralization phenomenon would not be exposed.

Dynamic mechanical evaluation forms the basis of the McKenzie method of spinal examination. Under certain circumstances dynamic movement testing must be substituted by static mechanical evaluation. However valuable other assessment findings, such as subjective examination, examination of posture and range of movement, radiological and laboratory investigations, may appear to be, it is the behaviour of the pain in response to repeated movements and sustained positioning that ultimately determines the mechanical diagnosis. The presence or absence of centralization and peripheralization are the key factors in arriving at this diagnosis.

REFERENCES

Adams M A, Hutton W C 1982 Prolapsed intervertebral disc: a hyperflexion injury. Spine 7: 184–191

Adams M A, Hutton W C 1985 Gradual disc prolapse. Spine 10: 524–531

Alexander A H, Jones A M, Rosenbaum D M 1990 Non-operative management of herniated nucleus pulposus: patient selection by the extension sign—long-term follow-up. Proceedings North American Spine Society Annual Meeting, Monterey, California, August 1990

Cloward R B 1959 Cervical diskography. A contribution to the etiology and mechanism of neck, shoulder and arm pain. Annals of Surgery 150: 1052–1064

Dixon A St J 1980 Diagnosis of low back pain—sorting the complainers. In: Jayson M I V (ed) The lumbar spine and back pain, 2nd edn. Pitman Medical, Tunbridge Wells, ch 6

Donelson R, Silva G, Murphy K 1990 Centralization phenomenon. Its usefulness in evaluating and treating referred pain. Spine 15: 211–213

Donelson R, Grant W, Kamps C, Medcalf R 1991a Pain response to sagittal end-range spinal motion: a prospective, randomised multicentered trial. Spine 16: S206–S212

Donelson R, Grant W, Kamps C, Medcalf R 1991b Low back and referred pain response to mechanical lumbar movements in the frontal plane: a prospective, multi-centered study. Presented at the International Society for the Study of the Lumbar Spine annual meeting, Heidelberg, Germany, May 1991

Evans P 1980 The healing process at cellular level: a review. Physiotherapy 66: 256–259

Hickey D S, Hukins D W L 1980 Relation between the structure of the annulus fibrosus and the function and failure of the intervertebral disc. Spine 5: 106–116

Kilby J, Stignant M, Roberts A 1990 The reliability of back pain assessment by physiotherapists using a 'McKenzie Algorithm'. Physiotherapy 76: 579–583

Kopp J R, Alexander A M, Turocy R M, Levrini M G, Lichtman D M 1986 The use of lumbar extension in the evaluation and treatment of patients with acute herniated nucleus pulposus. A preliminary report. Clinical Orthopedics and Related Research 202: 211–218

Krag M H, Seroussi R E, Wilder D G, Pope M M 1987 Internal displacement distribution from in vitro loading of human thoracic and lumbar spinal motion segments: experimental results and finite theoretical predictions. Spine 12: 1001–1007

Kramer J 1990 Intervertebral disc diseases. Causes, diagnosis, treatment and prophylaxis. Georg Thieme Verlag, Stuttgart

McCarron R F, Wimpee M W, Hudkins P G, Laros G S 1987 The inflammatory effect of the nucleus pulposus: a possible element in the pathogenesis of low back pain. Spine 12: 760–764

McCombe P F et al 1989 Reproducibility of physical signs in low-back pain. Spine 14: 908–918

McKenzie R A 1980 Treat your own back. Spinal Publications, Waikanae, New Zealand

McKenzie R A 1981 The lumbar spine. Mechanical diagnosis and therapy. Spinal Publications, Waikanae, New Zealand

McKenzie R A 1987 Mechanical diagnosis and therapy for low back pain: toward a better understanding. In: Twomey L T, Taylor J R (eds) Physical therapy of the low back. Churchill Livingstone, New York, ch 6, pp 157–173

McKenzie R 1989 A perspective on manipulative therapy. Physiotherapy 75: 440–444

McKenzie R A 1990 The cervical and thoracic spine. Mechanical diagnosis and therapy. Spinal Publications, Waikanae, New Zealand

McKenzie Institute International 1993 Lumbar and cervical assessment form. Spinal Publications, Waikanae, New Zealand

Matyas T A, Bach T M 1985 The reliability of selected techniques in clinical arthrometrics. Australian Journal of Physiotherapy 31: 175–195

Mooney V 1987 Where is the pain coming from? Presidential address, International Society for the Study of the Lumbar Spine, Dallas, 1986: Spine 12: 754–759

Nachemson A 1980 A critical look at the conservative treatment for low back pain. In: Jayson M I V (ed) The lumbar spine and back pain, 2nd edn. Pitman Medical, Tunbridge Wells, ch 16

Nelson M A, Allen P, Clamp S E, De Dombal F T 1979 Reliability and reproducibility of clinical findings in low-back pain. Spine 4: 97–101

Park W M 1976 Radiological investigation of the intervertebral disc. In: Jayson M I V (ed) The lumbar spine and back pain. Pitman Medical, Tunbridge Wells

Rath W 1989 Personal communication

Rath W 1991 Personal communication

Shah J S, Hampson W G H, Jayson M I V 1978 The distribution of surface strain in the cadaveric lumbar spine. Journal of Bone and Joint Surgery 60B: 246–251

Shepperd J, Rand C, Knight G, Wetheral G 1990 Patterns of internal disc dynamics, cadaveric motion studies. Presented at the International Society for the Study of the Lumbar Spine annual meeting, Boston, June 1990

Spitzer W O, LeBlanc F E, Dupuis M 1987 Scientific approach to the assessment and management of activity-related spinal disorders. A monograph for clinicians. Report of the Quebec Task Force on Spinal Disorders. Spine 12: 7s

Spratt K F, Lehmann T R, Weinstein J N, Sayre H A 1990 A new approach to the low-back physical examination. Behavioral assessment of mechanical signs. Spine 15: 96–102

Stevens B J, McKenzie R A 1988 Mechanical diagnosis and self treatment of the cervical spine. In: Grant R (ed) Physical therapy of the cervical and thoracic spine. Churchill Livingstone, New York, ch 14, pp 271–289

Van Wijmen P M 1986a Lumbar pain syndromes. In: Grieve G P (ed) Modern manual therapy of the vertebral column. Churchill Livingstone, Edinburgh, ch 41, pp 442–462

Van Wijmen P M 1986b The management of recurrent low back pain. In: Grieve G P (ed) Modern manual therapy of the vertebral column. Churchill Livingstone, Edinburgh, ch. 73, pp 756–776

Wilder D G, Pope M H, Frymoyer J W 1988 The biomechanics of lumbar disc herniation and the effect of overload and instability. Journal of Spinal Disorders 1: 16–32

Williams M M, Hawley J A, McKenzie R A, van Wijmen P M 1991 A comparison of the effects of two sitting postures on back and referred pain. Spine 16: 1185–1191

43. The investigation of arm pain: signs of adverse responses to the physical examination of the brachial plexus and related neural tissues

R. L. Elvey

INTRODUCTION

Elvey (1979) conceptualized the physical examination of the neural tissues of the upper quarter in the investigation of arm pain and regional pain syndromes of the upper quarter. At the time the thought behind this conceptualization was predominantly related to a better understanding and a differential diagnosis of difficult shoulder conditions (Elvey 1984) which were reticent to manual therapy and physiotherapy treatments. In addition, the thoughts behind the physical examination processes which were outlined at the time were to gain a better understanding of conditions such as whiplash syndrome, where there had been an apparent progressive pathological state over a period of months and years following what appeared at times to be relatively minor trauma (Elvey 1979). In these conditions, neck pain had progressed to arm pain and painful limitation of shoulder mobility.

Since the original description of the brachial plexus tension test (Elvey 1979), the author has expanded the entire concept of the testing techniques to indicate that, when physically testing the role which neural tissues may play in regional pain syndromes, it is in fact muscle responses to the tension imparted to sensitized and possibly inflamed neural tissues that are being examined. As a result, the original name of brachial plexus tension test, which has also been referred to as upper limb tension test, tends to convey an incorrect impression of the whole thought process behind assessment of conditions when using physical examination tests of neural tissues.

The author prefers now to describe the whole concept of testing manoeuvres as the responses to the physical examination of neural tissues, when those neural tissues are related to regional pain syndromes or symptomatic disorders.

With the original description of the brachial plexus tension test (Elvey 1979), it was demonstrated that tension could be imparted to the cervical nerve roots comprising the brachial plexus via the median nerve. This description was outlined at the time to simplify the testing procedures to gain early and more ready acceptance of their use on a clinical basis. Since the testing techniques were first demonstrated (Elvey 1979, 1988) it has been shown, in the concept of testing, that there is a very definite requirement for the involvement of all peripheral nerve trunks of the upper limb in various manoeuvres in order to obtain an overall clinical assessment of pain or syndromes involving the upper quarter. More latterly this has been documented by Butler (1991) (see Chs 2, 44 and 50).

With an increased popularity of the topic of neural tissue and the investigation of arm pain it has been found, on teaching assignments, that the use of descriptions of lower-limb techniques in the physical examination of neural tissues enables course participants to gain a more ready appreciation of the overall role of neural tissues in the neuromusculoskeletal system and the need to test neural tissues in the physical examination.

Although there appears to be general acceptance of the requirement to examine neural tissues on a physical basis, there still remains some criticism in the interpretations of responses. This criticism relates mostly to ranges of motion and responses of tissues with the thought that range and response of muscles may be misinterpreted for neural tissue. Generally this is simply due to a lack of understanding and appreciation of the ability that the clinician has to change the anatomical relationships of the different structures in the limbs in order to impart more tension to neural tissue than overlying muscle tissue, or vice versa. In particular, this applies to straight leg raising techniques to examine the sciatic nerve and lumbosacral plexus in leg pain syndromes. Critics of straight leg raising as a clinical test for conditions such as sciatica state that the range of straight leg raising and responses obtained cannot be distinguished between neural tissue or muscles such as the hamstring muscle group. In addition, it is said that straight leg raising may also be limited by hamstring muscle spasm as a result of facet joint arthrosis (Mooney & Robertson 1976). However, various positions and manoeuvres of the lower limb can be used so that greater tension is imparted to the sciatic nerve rather than the hamstring and other muscle groups. It is stressed that it is not simply a matter of demonstrating a range of straight leg raising as an angle from the horizontal together with the onset of pain. However, the important requirement is to examine the feel-through range of the straight leg raising manoeuvre and the end-feel.

It has been demonstrated by Smythe and Wright (1958) that inflamed nerve roots are hypersensitive to any manual stimulation and that uninflamed nerve roots are not sensitive and do not produce the same responses of radiating leg pain. Smythe and Wright (1958) also demonstrated how the range of straight leg raising from the horizontal was markedly reduced when inflamed nerve roots were stimulated post-surgery with nylon sutures whereas, when non-inflamed nerve roots were stimulated, straight leg raising was unaffected and was reported as being of normal range.

Xavier et al (1990) have demonstrated the capacity for a nerve root lesion to cause sensitization of peripheral nociceptors which causes pain to be perceived in the buttock, leg and foot. The means of distal pain perception is caused by antidromic discharge along the course of the sciatic nerve and subsequent afferent impulses to the central nervous system as a result of peripheral nociceptor discharge.

It therefore becomes very apparent that it is possible for neural tissues to be directly implicated in peripheral or regional pain syndromes and that the neural tissues which involve the nerve root and the peripheral nerve trunks need to be throughly examined in the physical examination of these syndromes.

With respect to the adverse responses that are assessed when physically examining sensitive or inflamed neural tissue, Nordin et al (1984) have demonstrated that there is a sensory discharge in conditions of sciatica when straight leg raising of the affected limb is performed. The sensory discharges appear to be very pertinent to the physical examination of sensitive neural tissues when the clinician can feel a gradual muscular contraction of muscles which overlie or protect the neural tissue being implicated in the test manoeuvres.

The author feels that muscles have a very definite role of protection of neural tissues when they are sensitive to movement or tension or when they are inflammed. In a straight leg raising test in the presence of sciatica, a point will be reached where neural tissue nociceptors (sensitized by pathology) will discharge. This will result in central nervous system mechanisms causing increased muscular tone in muscle groups related to the sciatic nerve, in particular the hamstring group. The skilled clinician is capable of feeling this increased tone as a gradually increasing muscle contraction up to the point where the muscles attempt to prevent further movement. This feel-through range and muscular contraction end-feel is quite different to that during straight leg raising of a normal limb or the non-involved leg. In the latter case, the feel-through range is one of physiological lengthening of the hamstring group (in particular) with an end range feel of anatomical end length which is a hard end-feel and which precedes significant rotation of the pelvis. Experience is required in order to appreciate these fine aspects, and very careful and precise clinical testing techniques are necessary.

In addition to this basic approach to straight leg raising, examination of many different manoeuvres can be included. These form a means of retesting any hypothesis that is formed on initial testing and provide a means of a test and retest approach where the hypothesis can be tested in a number of different ways. This type of approach, where there is test and retest, also tends to implicate strongly the neural tissue rather than, for instance, arthrosis or pathology of zygapophyseal joints (facet joints) or other structures that may be causing referred pain into the limb. For example, if the initial hypothesis implicates the neural tissue as a dominant factor, in adverse responses produced with a straight leg raising test, there must be a predictable increase in responses when dorsiflexion of the ankle is added or, importantly, when adduction of the hip is carried out in a position of 70–90° of hip flexion and full-range medial rotation. This latter manoeuvre selectively changes the anatomical relationships of the sciatic nerve and the hamstring group to the axis of motion at the hip joint. The result is greater tension of the sciatic nerve than the hamstrings.

In the examination of the upper quarter, similar principles apply. The upper limb, the shoulder girdle, the head and neck are placed in many different positions, and many different manoeuvres are made which involve the various peripheral nerve trunks, brachial plexus and cervical nerve roots, in combinations or singularly, in order to assess fully on a test and retest basis. With respect to this method of examination, the testing techniques do not have a positive or negative outcome. The test techniques serve to help the clinician form an hypothesis which, in turn, must have collaborative support from the entire physical examination, subjective complaint and history. Only then can neural tissues be said to be a dominant factor in a condition and a diagnosis be made.

BIOMECHANICS

When the shoulder girdle is depressed the neurovascular bundle at the level of the shoulder becomes taut. This can be readily seen on cadaveric experimentation at autopsy and has been documented previously by Frykholm (1955). As the neurovascular bundle becomes taut, movement is seen to occur in the cervical nerve roots from C4 to C8 and the first thoracic nerve root. The 4th cervical nerve root is involved in these dynamics due to its relationship within the shoulder girdle as it courses from its exit at C3/4 to the shoulder as the supraclavicular nerve. The roots from C5 to T1 are involved due to their relationship to the brachial plexus. As the 'slack' is taken up in the neural tissue during movement, tension is imparted throughout its length from the cervical spine to the shoulder.

Movement and tension also occur in the subclavian artery and vein on shoulder girdle depression. This can also readily be demonstrated in cadaveric experimentation.

When the shoulder girdle is fixed and the cervical spine is laterally flexed to the contralateral side, movement and tension are seen to occur in the cervical nerve roots from C4 to C8 and the first thoracic nerve root. Most movement is observed in the roots from C4 to C7, and little movement is observed at C8 and T1. Because of a lack of any direct anatomical attachment to the cervical spine, no movement is observed in either the subclavian artery or vein.

When the arm is abducted at the glenohumeral joint with the shoulder girdle fixed so that it cannot elevate, movement and tension is observed in the neurovascular bundle, in the cervical nerve roots from C5 to C8, and in the first thoracic nerve root. Most movement occurs at C5, C6 and C7, with little movement occurring at C8 and T1, and little movement occurring in either the subclavian artery or vein.

With arm abduction the amount of movement in a pin placed in the median nerve at the level of the shoulder was measured in one adult cadaver to be 1 cm. This demonstrates a considerable amount of movement and tension of the peripheral nerve trunk which is transferred to the lateral cord of the brachial plexus and thence to the C5, C6 and C7 nerve roots. A pin placed in the C5 nerve root in the same cadaver moved 4 mm at the level of the intervertebral foramen of C4/5 on arm abduction with the shoulder girdle fixed. Again, this amount of movement is considerable and is an indication of the tension which is imparted to the nerve root by the same manoeuvre.

In order to gain an understanding of the biomechanics related to these neural tissue dynamics, an X-ray of the author's shoulder girdle was taken with the arm by the side. A further X-ray where the arm had been abducted at the glenohumeral joint but without incurring movement of the shoulder girdle was superimposed on the first. A marker placed mid-way along the shaft of the humerus allowed a measurement to be made from the coracoid process with the arm by the side and again in the abducted position. There was a relative increase of 2.4 cm in length from the arm by the side position to the abducted position. This appears to occur due to the geometry of the humeral head. As a result of this relative increase in distance, the neurovascular tissue—as it traverses across and inferior to the glenohumeral joint—has to accommodate to the abduction position. If the shoulder girdle elevates with the abduction movement the neurovascular tissue maintains its relaxed undulated appearance. However, if the shoulder girdle is fixed—in order to prevent it elevat-

ing—then the neurovascular tissue moves relative to the abduction movement and tension occurs in it. This tension is transferred to the nerve roots.

If the arm is fixed in abduction at the glenohumeral joint with the shoulder girdle also fixed and the elbow is then extended, the neurovascular bundle continues to behave in the same manner. That is, further tension is imparted to the related cervical nerve roots. If the wrist is extended along with extension of the elbow, even greater tension is imparted to the neurovascular bundle and the cervical nerve roots.

The mechanics of this tension are a result of the peripheral nerve trunk dynamics in the arm. Wrist and elbow extension, as can be observed, cause tension in the median nerve. This tension is then transferred along the length of the median nerve to the brachial plexus. Similarly, the other peripheral nerve trunks will cause tension. However, it should be noted that different physiological positions of the glenohumeral, elbow and wrist joints need to be considered when implicating the radial or ulnar nerves.

It becomes clear on observing the biomechanics of neural tissue that it takes part in the dynamics of the musculoskeletal system and that it is a relatively mobile tissue to all its fascial and anatomical surrounds in normal function. In other words, neural tissue—whether it be nerve root or peripheral nerve trunk—has to comply with, and accommodate to, musculoskeletal function. This fact makes it possible to use manual orthopaedic tests to stress the neural tissue of the brachial plexus in such a way whereby it can be objectively assessed in order to examine a condition affecting the upper quarter. This assessment involves differentiating the neural tissue from the articular tissue and the muscle tissue so that it can be selectively examined within the musculoskeleton of the upper quarter.

TEST CONCEPTS (see Figs 43.1–43.5)

As a result of the cadaveric observations of the biomechanics of the brachial plexus, and by careful assessment of patients presenting with radiculopathies associated with cervical spine pathologies demonstrated radiologically, it is evident that various tests can be carried out which place tension on the cervical spinal nerve roots from C5 to T1 as a means of clinical assessment of the upper quarter. This clinical assessment can thus be likened to the straight leg raise or slump tests used in the assessment of low-back and leg conditions.

Because of the multiple variations of positions the upper quarter can be placed in, tension can be varied and there can be variations applied to each test procedure. This allows for careful differentiation between neural tissue, articular tissues and muscles as having a role in the condition or if there may be a combination of structures involved. In other words, there is not a standard brachial

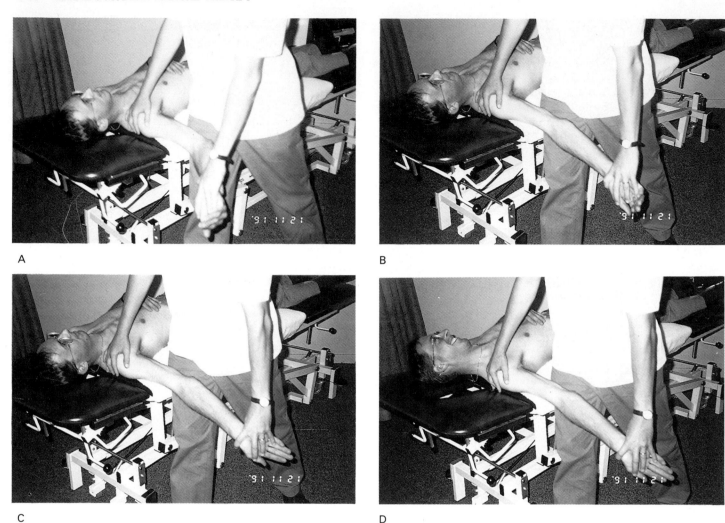

Fig. 43.1 The basic test concept. **A.** Patient lies supine. The arm is abducted and externally rotated at the glenohumeral joint, and the upper arm is then supported against the therapist's thigh. The shoulder girdle is gently and lightly fixed in a position which would be equivalent to the upright position where the 'slack' of the supporting muscle tissues is taken up. **B.** The elbow is extended carefully so that the 'feel' of the movement can be assessed. It is the 'feel' of the movement as well as the range of elbow extension which are the important aspects to an objective assessment. For this purpose it is essential for the therapist to have the hand lightly applied to the patient's shoulder girdle and wrist/hand region as shown. In this manner, as tension is applied to the neural tissue the therapist can 'sense with the hands' any involuntary rising of the shoulder girdle and flexion of the elbow. This is similar in many respects to a flexion withdrawal reflex and similar to pelvic rotation and knee flexion during the examination of SLR in a sciatic condition. **C.** In further assessing a condition and, depending upon the acuteness, sensitivity and irritability of the condition, wrist extension can be added. This component may be used as a ready differential indicator as to whether or not the glenohumeral joint is involved in a condition, or whether or not shoulder girdle muscle imbalance may be related to the condition. Many other examples can be given to differentiate conditions by varying the components of the procedure. **D.** In some conditions it may be necessary to impart maximum tension to the neural tissue. This may well be so in chronic, non-irritable or non-sensitive conditions. This involves the same previous manoeuvres together with shoulder girdle depression and lateral flexion of the cervical spine to the contralateral side. This position may be likened to the slump position when maximum tension is required through the vertebral canal and sciatic complex. In this position, as can be done in all other positions, the different components of the test can be varied to gain differential information. This is performed in a manner similar to the slump technique, when different components of the slump position are changed to give varying responses.

plexus tension test for the upper quarter but a concept of testing which involves many techniques. This is important to realize at the outset for it answers the questions concerning which tissues are being stressed and it can separate, in a differential manner, anatomical structures. For example, on abduction of the arm with the shoulder girdle fixed, stress will be imparted to the cervical nerve roots and the subclavian artery and vein. If this position is maintained and the cervical spine is laterally flexed to the contralateral side, further stress is imparted to the cervical nerve roots but not to the subclavian artery or vein. The response to this manoeuvre can then be assessed in order to differentiate neural tissue from vascular tissue. However, the lateral flexion component causes tension within the scalene muscle groups, in particular, and other muscle groups of the shoulder girdle. Further differentiation

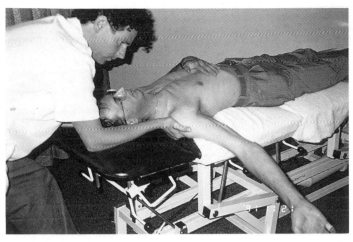
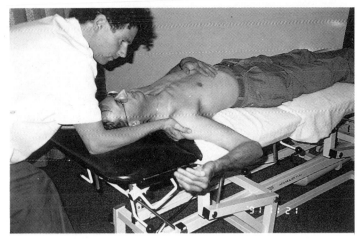

A

B

Fig. 43.2 Further test concept. **A.** A similar effect to the basic test techniques on the neural tissues of the upper quarter can be gained by the position illustrated. Here, the peripheral nerve trunks are placed under tension due to the shoulder girdle fixation with the arm in abduction and external rotation in the glenohumeral joint. As a result of tension being imparted to the brachial plexus peripherally from the peripheral trunks, the cervical spine is limited in lateral flexion to the contralateral side. As before, the therapist's grip with both hands must be light and must enable a careful objective assessment of 'feel' through the movement of lateral flexion and 'end feel' of the movement together with range of movement. This objective assessment is again correlated with the subjective response. **B.** The position of this basic technique can also be varied in many ways so that further objective and subjective information can be gained in order to make differential judgements and a differential diagnosis. By flexing the elbow, as shown, the peripheral nerve tension is released somewhat—but not the tension which may be imparted to shoulder girdle muscles such as the scalene group. Hence, the response—whether changed or unchanged—gives more information. Further information may be gained by varying other components. In all test techniques it is important to compare left side to right side, to compare against what has been established for 'normal neural tissue tension response' for the upper limb (Kenneally, 1986) and to correlate the responses to all other findings of the complete examination. The test techniques are not 'positive' or 'negative' but are complementary to a complete examination. In this context they may be said to be positive for a particular diagnosis providing the rest of the examination process indicates a diagnosis supported by the neural tissue tension techniques. The techniques indicate the presence or otherwise of adverse responses to neural tissue tension. They do not indicate a pathology or the site of pathology which may be the cause of the adverse tension. For example, carpal tunnel syndrome or a radicular syndrome may have the same effect on the same neural tissue. Only by a complete examination can a diagnosis and determination of the anatomical site of pathology causing adverse neural tissue responses be made. This process of complete examination is of the utmost importance to the clinician when using these techniques.

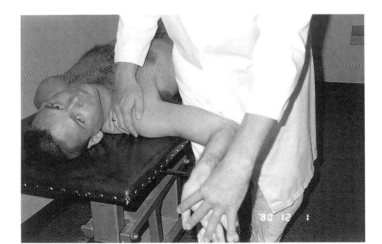
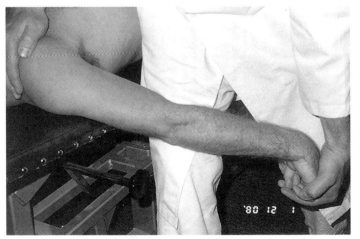

Fig. 43.3 Ulnar nerve test concept. In order to reproduce symptoms related to the lower trunk of the brachial plexus or along the distribution of the ulnar nerve, a position of strong shoulder girdle depression, shoulder abduction/external rotation, elbow flexion and wrist extension is adopted. Contralateral lateral flexion of the cervical spine will increase the response. The therapist can retest from proximal to distal by adopting the position of Figure 43.2A but with the arm in the position of tension for the ulnar nerve described above.

Fig. 43.4 Radial nerve test concept. In order to reproduce symptoms in the region of the radial nerve and, in particular, in the region of the lateral aspect of the elbow/forearm, a position of shoulder girdle depression, shoulder abduction/internal rotation, elbow extension, wrist/finger flexion is adopted. Contralateral lateral flexion of the cervical spine will increase the response. The therapist can retest from proximal to distal by adopting the position of Figure 43.2A but with the arm in the position of tension for the radial nerve described above.

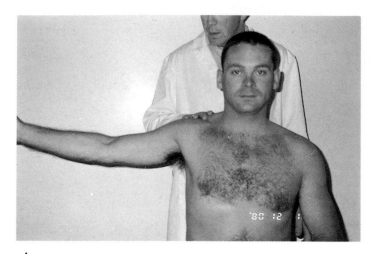

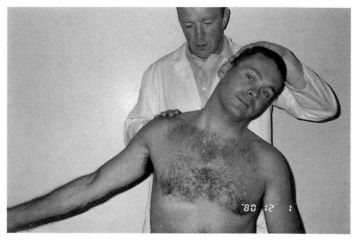

A   B

Fig. 43.5   Central peripheral relationships. **A.** In assessing the relationship between limited glenohumeral joint mobility and possible cervical nerve root pathology, the patient abducts the arm, as shown, and range and symptoms are assessed with the shoulder girdle lightly fixed so as it does not elevate as fully as it normally would. **B.** The cervical spine is laterally flexed to the contralateral side, thus fixing the cervical nerve roots and imparting tension to the brachial plexus. The arm is again abducted and the therapist lightly fixes the shoulder girdle in the position as shown in (A). The range of abduction and the response is assessed. If there is nerve root pathology the range of abduction will be decreased.

between muscles and neural tissue can then be made by flexing and extending the elbow, by flexing or extending the wrist or by varying the amount of abduction of the arm. These manoeuvres change the tension in the nerve roots but not in the muscles, and hence the response can once again be assessed and a judgement made. These are just two simple examples of differential tests. The clinician with anatomical knowledge can work the patient through a variety of screening tests similar to these examples.

Kenneally et al (1988) demonstrated in 100 asymptomatic individuals that, in the position of shoulder girdle fixation and arm abduction, the elbow can be fully extended. Kenneally's study has therefore given a base-line for extensibility of the neural tissue associated with the brachial plexus and upper limb.

Hence, in the objective assessment during the test technique, when the elbow is extended in a normal individual, the therapist should be able to move the elbow into extension freely with a 'hard end-feel' and without a feeling of an attempt to elevate the shoulder girdle. In the symptomatic individual, the therapist may well feel an increasing 'elastic type feel' to the extension movement and, at a certain point towards the end of available range, a sensation of attempted elevation of the shoulder girdle and an attempted flexion of the elbow. The final range would be without the normal 'hard end-feel'.

The 'feel' of the elbow extension movement through range when examining neural tissue extensibility and the end-range 'feel' gives a very good objective clinical assessment of a condition. This objective assessment is then correlated with the subjective response to the test such as reproduction of symptoms in terms of area where they may be perceived by the patient and type of symptoms.

DISCUSSION

A number of studies on topics concerned with adverse responses to brachial plexus tension tests have been completed and the conclusions of these studies have been favourable both to the validation of the testing procedures and to the use of such tests in the clinical examination. Some of these studies and their conclusions are listed below:

1. The study of Kenneally et al (1988)—'The upper limb tension test—the SLR of the arm'—showed that brachial plexus tension tests were clinically effective and that there was a 'normal' extensibility or range of neural tissue from the cervical spine to the hand accompanied by 'normal' responses.

2. The results of the study of Selvaratnam (1987)—'the discriminative validity of the brachial plexus tension test'—indicated that the test was a discriminatively valid test and had a moderate to high intra-examiner reliability.

3. The results of the study by Rubenach (1985), 'The upper limb tension test—the effect of the position and movement of the contralateral arm', indicated that in young, right-hand dominant, asymptomatic subjects, tension in pain-sensitive neural structures was transmitted across the cervical spinal canal.

4. Reid's (1987) study, 'The measurement of tension changes in the brachial plexus', showed that the buckle force transducer (a device to measure longitudinal tension) can be used effectively to measure tension changes in neural tissues during the brachial plexus tension test. In other words it demonstrated tension within the neural tissue.

5. Bell's (1985) study, 'An investigation of responses to the brachial plexus tension test with leg position', a

change in the response was noted —thus indicating that neural tissue tension is transmitted through the vertebral canal when using the test techniques.

One study (Zuluaga 1986) on the inter-therapist reliability of the test technique showed a poor result. However, it becomes plainly obvious to the practising clinician that, in testing for adverse responses to brachial plexus tension, the various articulations and components of the tests are such that it is quite a difficult task to position the upper quarter in the same posture each time. The response to the techniques can be changed dramatically with just the slightest change in postural position and so constancy of position is a critical obstacle to overcome otherwise results will be predictably poor.

Yaxley and Jull (1991), in an inter-examiner reliability trial of a 'Modified upper limb tension test', indicated that there was no significant variation of results between two testers. Furthermore, in an intra-examiner repeatability trial there was no significant difference in measurement between the trials—thus indicating that the examiner could reproduce measurements repeatedly.

Sunderland (1974) has stated that '. . . the 5th, 6th, and 7th cervical nerve roots are firmly tethered to the gutters of their respective transverse processes'. He stated that this is a protective measure and that it prevents neural tissue mobility from occurring in the intervertebral foramen. This statement insinuates that tension tests for nerve root pathology may be unlikely to have the same acceptance in the cervical region as they do in the lumbosacral region. However, experiments on cadavers, as indicated earlier, do not support this. It appears that movement of the nerve root on movement of the arm in certain directions (provided that the shoulder girdle is not elevated) is carried on beyond the intervertebral foramen and into the vertebral canal where the dura is clearly seen to be involved. The author has documented such events on film taken during cadaveric experiments. Studies listed above also demonstrate this occurrence where a response in one upper limb during the testing technique can be varied by involving the contralateral limb or the lower limbs, thus implying that the tension is transmitted across or through the vertebral canal.

It should also be considered that the tests can be used in a differential screening manner not only with regard to nerve root, neural tissue, articular tissue or muscle tissue but to peripheral nerve trunks. For instance, the basic techniques described place much greater tension on the median nerve than does extension of the wrist when the elbow is flexed with the arm by the side. This fact makes it appear that carpal tunnel syndrome may be examined more thoroughly using the techniques described which place the median nerve on full tension. Similarly, ulna nerve entrapment at the elbow may be examined much more thoroughly using the tests described here, but with the elbow flexed, thus placing the ulna nerve on full tension and assessing and correlating the response of the technique to the patient's symptoms. The same applied to all the other peripheral nerves, and, importantly, to the suprascapular nerve which appears to have a common clinical implication. The examination process in each case involves full tension to the particular peripheral nerve via the cervical nerve roots and brachial plexus with the peripheral nerve being placed under tension by positioning it in a physiological posture according to its anatomical placement in the limb or shoulder girdle.

In addition to peripheral nerve entrapments, it has been the experience of the author that thoracic inlet syndromes can be assessed in a differential manner using the techniques. The possibility of extraneural tissue adhesions causing loss of shoulder mobility following trauma or surgery, for example radical mastectomy, can be assessed in a differential manner very efficiently using tests for adverse neural tissue tension. Stiff painful shoulder and pseudo-frozen shoulder are common conditions which require a very careful assessment which should include consideration of neural tissue. It follows that if neural tissue has relative mobility in the dynamics of the musculoskeletal system then sensitivity of the neural tissue may well cause an impairment of articular mobility.

This would appear quite feasible as far as the glenohumeral joint is concerned (Elvey 1984). A sensitive cervical nerve root could possibly alter the mobility of the glenohumeral joint and shoulder as a whole, thus mimicking a true glenohumeral condition. Tests such as those for the determination of adverse responses to brachial plexus tension are therefore required in the differential examination to make a clear distinction. Although this subject is beyond the scope of this chapter it should be mentioned that limited active glenohumeral abduction can be assessed quickly as far as neural tissue involvement is concerned by adding in lateral flexion of the cervical spine to the contralateral side. Similarly, the shoulder quadrant position as described by Maitland (1985) can be assessed with the shoulder girdle in elevation or in depression with or without contralateral lateral flexion of the cervical spine, thus relaxing and tensioning the neural tissue. The different objective and subjective responses, if any, are then assessed, and differential judgement may be made as a complementary addition to the complete examination.

In addition, signs of adverse responses to brachial plexus tension may give the clinician a ready guide as to the dominant tissue causing active mobility limitation of the cervical spine.

In manual therapy examination, the signs which relate to the symptoms usually indicate a dysfunction of the musculoskeletal system. The same signs will then guide the clinician in the choice of treatment technique to regain normal musculoskeletal function. This also applies to signs of adverse responses to brachial plexus tension.

A number of techniques of treatment have been documented for use in the treatment of conditions accompanied by signs of adverse responses to brachial plexus tension (Elvey 1986, Butler 1991). In additon to the treatment techniques, postulations can be given for the development of adverse responses to tension in neural tissue (Elvey 1986, 1987) and, importantly, why the onset of neural tissue symptoms may take some time following trauma and why the symptoms may take a long time to settle relative to joint symptoms (Elvey 1987).

SUMMARY

Many difficulties are encountered by the clinician in making a differential diagnosis of upper-quarter symptoms. One such difficulty is the ability to apply tension selectively to neural tissue, which may, if sensitive as a result of a condition, give the response and reproduction of symptoms which are being sought.

By considering the biomechanics of the neural tissues of the upper quarter, and by considering the anatomical relationships of these tissues with various physiological posture changes of the upper quarter, tension tests can be applied in a differential diagnostic manner. These tests, referred to as brachial plexus tension tests, can be varied according to the response. The tests form a concept of testing for signs of adverse or abnormal responses to neural tissue tension. These signs, when placed in the overall examination, become very valuable to the clinician, particularly on an objective basis.

Alone, signs of adverse neural tissue tension do not mean anything other than the fact that the neural tissue examined does not have normal extensibility because it is sensitive to stretch or tension. Signs of adverse neural tissue tension, when present, must be complementary to some condition determined by the overall examination before their meaning can be discerned. With regard to this, signs of adverse response to brachial plexus tension may be due to a condition of the peripheral nerve trunks, the brachial plexus, the cervical nerve roots or anatomically related tissues in these regions. However, the most value gained in using techniques to examine for these signs is in the examination for cervical nerve root conditions and for the differential judgement of glenohumeral joint signs from cervical spine signs as a cause of dysfunction in the region of the shoulder.

In this chapter, only the basic techniques are given, and it is hoped that this will encourage assessment in greater depth using the outline given as a basis for clinical study. For example, movement of the 4th cervical nerve root was mentioned under biomechanics, and with this knowledge it is possible to develop tests to differentiate between C4 radiculopathy and other conditions. Many other examples are also possible.

In using the concepts of testing for signs of adverse responses to brachial plexus tension, the clinician requires a careful and detailed objective approach, an open mind, and the time to repeat the same examination in a number of ways. Above all, consideration by the clinician must be given to the fact that the neural tissue being examined may be in a highly sensitive state which will cause an aggravated response to stretch or tension imparted to it.

Gentleness of technique is therefore a key element in the successful examination for signs of adverse responses to brachial plexus tension in conditions of the upper quarter.

REFERENCES

Bell A 1985 An investigation of responses to the right upper limb tension test and the effect on them of leg positon in young asymptomatic right hand dominant subjects. Unpublished thesis, Adelaide SAIT

Butler D 1991 Mobilisation of the nervous system. Churchill Livingstone, Edinburgh

Elvey R L 1979 Brachial plexus tension tests and the pathoanatomical origin of arm pain. In: Glasgow E F, Twomey I (eds) Aspects of manipulative therapy. Lincoln Institute of Health Sciences, Melbourne, pp 105–110

Elvey R L 1980–1991 Teaching assignments. Curtin University of Technology. Courses conducted internationally

Elvey R L 1984 Abnormal brachial plexus tension and shoulder joint limitation. Proceedings, of the IFOMT Vancouver, pp 132–139

Elvey R L 1986 Treatment of arm pain associated with abnormal brachial plexus tension. Australian Journal of Physiotherapy 32: 225–230

Elvey R L 1987 Pathophysiology of radiculopathy. Proceedings of the MTAA 5th Biennial Conference, Melbourne

Elvey R L 1988 The clinical relevance of signs of adverse brachial plexus tension. Proceedings of the IFOMT Congress, Cambridge

Frykholm R 1955 Cervical nerve root compression resulting from disc degeneration and root sleeve fibrosis. A clinical investigation. Acta Chirurgica Scandinavica (suppl) 160

Grieve G P 1981 Common vertebral joint problems. Churchill Livingstone, Edinburgh

Kenneally M, Rubenach H, Elvey R L 1988 The upper limb tension test — the SLR of the arm. In: Grant R (ed) Clinics in physical therapy. The cervical and thoracic spine. Churchill Livingstone, New York

Maitland G D 1985 Peripheral manipulation, 3rd edn. Butterworths, London

Mooney V, Robertson J 1976 The facet syndrome. Clinical Orthopaedics & Related Research 115: 149–156

Nordin M, Nystrom B, Wallin V, Hagbarth K E 1984 Ectopic sensory discharges and paraesthesiae in patients with disorders of peripheral nerves, dorsal roots and dorsal columns. Pain 20: 231–245

Reid S 1987 The measurement of tension changes in the brachial plexus. Proceedings of the MTAA 5th Biennial Conference, Melbourne, pp 79–90

Rubenach H 1985 The upper limb tension test. The effect of the position and movement of the contralateral arm. Proceedings of the MTAA 4th Biennial Conference, Brisbane

Selvaratnam P 1987 The discriminative validity and reliability of the brachial plexus tension test. Proceedings of the MTAA 5th Biennial Conference, Melbourne, pp 325–350

Smyth M J, Wright V 1958 Sciatica and the intervertebral disc. Journal of Bone and Joint Surgery 40A: 1401

Sunderland S 1974 Mechanisms of cervical nerve root avulsion injuries of the neck and shoulder. Journal of Neurosurgery 41: 705–714

Xavier A V, Farrell C E, McDanal J, Kissin I 1990 Does antidromic

activation of nociceptors play a role in sciatic radicular pain? Pain 40: 77–79

Yaxley G A, Jull G A 1991 A modified upper limb tension test: an investigation of responses in normal subjects. Australian Journal of Physiotherapy 37: 143–151

Zuluaga M 1986 Intertherapist reliability study of the brachial plexus tension test (research notes). Australian Journal of Physiotherapy 34: 57

44. The dynamic central nervous system: examination and assessment using tension tests

H. Slater   D. S. Butler   M. O. Shacklock

INTRODUCTION

The concept of altered nervous system mechanics is not new to manual therapy, and clinically the link with some neuro-orthopaedic syndromes such as discogenic low-back pain is well recognized. However, there are other disorders, including the T4 syndrome, headache and whiplash, where a neurogenic component has previously gone unrecognized, or has been underestimated. By examining neural mechanics, tension testing offers the clinician a method of inferring that symptoms have a neurogenic component. Although tension testing still requires validation, it nonetheless provides a simple, effective and repeatable method of clinical examination. With the emergence of more refined tension testing, based on anatomical and biomechanical knowledge combined with enquiry strategies and clinical reasoning processes, new opportunities are emerging to examine and treat neuro-orthopaedic disorders.

Integral to the concept of tension testing in relation to vertebral disorders is an appreciation of the continuity of the nervous system. The separation into peripheral and central systems is purely artificial, as is the division into somatic and autonomic. There is physiological and mechanical continuity of the nervous system. This is important because a vertebral disorder may well involve altered nervous system function in the periphery. Similarly, few clinicians would contend that peripheral disorders do not commonly have a vertebral component. Tension tests such as the slump test, the straight leg raise and the upper limb tension test offer the clinician a means of detecting and determining the nature and extent of neural pathomechanics.

While this text is concerned with vertebral disorders, the present chapter emphasizes the interplay, via the nervous system, between vertebral and peripheral symptoms. It emphasizes the need for the clinician to take a multistructural and multilevel approach to the examination of all neuro-orthopaedic disorders. The use of structural differentiation in examination to support a neurogenic component is introduced. Pathological processes which underlie the abnormal responses to tension testing are briefly described. Examination and assessment via tension tests are detailed along with documented normal responses. This chapter should be read in conjunction with Chapters 2 and 50.

PATHOLOGICAL PROCESSES

There is a growing body of support for Breig's (1978) long-held contention that altered nervous system function forms part of many syndromes. Mackinnon and Dellon (1988) have pointed out that involvement of the radial sensory nerve in de Quervain's syndrome is quite common, and yet it often goes unrecognized. It is known that the symptoms of multiple sclerosis can be evoked by mechanical stress on the neuraxis. Quintner (1989) found a high incidence of positive upper limb tension tests in whiplash sufferers. Clinically, the authors have found a link between signs of altered nervous system function and many common syndromes, including sympathetic maintained pain syndromes, whiplash, dural headache, tennis elbow and plantar fasciitis. Associated anatomical and neurobiomechanical considerations of altered nervous system function are clearly documented in Chapter 2.

It is contended that many common orthopaedic syndromes that have previously gone unrecognized as having a neurogenic component may represent a group of minor neuropathies. Butler (1991) suggests that what clinicians are often assessing and treating could well be a precategory 1 nerve injury as classified in Sunderland (1978). Significantly, these more minor neuropathies may have no measurable conduction changes. The diagnosis of neuropathy is made by information obtained from enquiry strategies and physical examination, in conjunction with structural differentiation. While the logic of structural differentiation implies that symptoms may have a neurogenic component, this contention has not been experimentally validated. The relationship between the pathological processes in these minor neuropathies and the mechanical loading that is placed by tension tests requires investigation.

There are some pathological processes that the clinician needs to be familiar with to enable interpretation of subjective and physical findings, in order to treat the condition appropriately, and on which to base a prognosis.

Altered microcirculation and axonal transport

The majority of experimental work has been performed on the peripheral nervous system. Common physiological features exist between the peripheral and central nervous systems, and it is logical that similar pathophysiological processes operate.

At low compression forces there is temporary compromise of intraneural microcirculation (Lundborg 1988). This means impaired oxygenation and slowed axonal transport. If this loading is sustained, the cell body/axon/target tissue relationship deteriorates and the neurone becomes 'sick'. The neurone in its entirety becomes more susceptible to compressive forces (Dahlin et al 1986b). As well as mechanical factors, physiological instability of the sympathetic nervous system may contribute to altered intraneural microcirculation (Selander et al 1985).

Pressure gradients

Pressure gradients exist within the fluids and tissues of the nervous system and surrounding structures. As Sunderland (1976) stated, the arterial pressure in the vasa nervorum must be greater than the capillary and venous pressures for optimal neuronal nutrition. Even slight alterations in these pressure gradients can be sufficient to effect changes in blood flow and axonal transport. Sunderland (1976) has documented a model for altered pressure gradients in the carpal tunnel in relation to the carpal tunnel syndrome. It is believed that this model is equally applicable elsewhere in and around the nervous system, especially at common sites of neural compromise (Ch. 2).

Recent literature has pointed out that both blood and axoplasmic flow is readily slowed by mechanical compression of pressures less than those around the median nerve in mild carpal tunnel syndrome (Rydevik et al 1980, Dahlin & McLean 1986a). Altered axoplasmic flow is regarded as the basis of the double crush syndrome where there is serial impingement along the nervous system. This may explain why a local injury is sometimes followed by a spread of symptoms elsewhere. For example, patients with carpal tunnel syndrome are more likely to get compression of the ulnar nerve in Guyon's canal (Cassvan et al 1986), and those suffering carpal tunnel syndrome frequently have the symptoms bilaterally (Hurst et al 1985). There may be patients with multiple crush where the spread of symptoms involves multiple sites and structures. This concept should be applied universally so that the coexist-ence of lumbar and cervical symptoms can be interpreted as a central manifestation of the double crush syndrome.

Pathomechanics

Pathology that affects the mechanics of the nervous system either from within (intraneural), or from outside (extraneural), can alter the nervous system/mechanical interface relationship with the potential for symptoms. Intraneural pathology affects the elasticity of the nervous system. Sunderland (1976) referred to a fibrosed nerve setting up a friction fibrosis elsewhere along the nerve. Taking up tension at one point in the nervous system means that less slack is available further along the system. Osteophytic impingement on an emerging nerve root may change neural mechanics, again with the possibility of symptom production. The likelihood of small changes in physiology and mechanics producing symptoms is magnified by anomalies. Common examples are split emerging nerve roots, congenital spinal canal stenosis, and spinal dysraphisms. The clinician needs to appreciate the significance of pathological processes, including disease and anomalies, in regard to the variation in recovery rates of some patients.

COMPONENT CONCEPT

Introduction

Signs and symptoms may originate from local and remote neural and non-neural sources. Component thinking involves considering all possible sources of signs and symptoms. It also provides a valid reason for the clinician to examine areas remote from the site of symptoms. The nervous system, being continuous and supplying structures throughout the body, is inevitably implicated either directly or indirectly in symptomatology. It is emphasized that the clinician must take a multistructural and multilevel (both vertebral and peripheral) approach in order effectively to examine vertebral disorders involving altered nervous system function.

Structural differentiation provides a means of supporting the supposition that symptoms have a neurogenic component. By moving a component remote from the site of the symptoms a change in the symptom response infers that symptoms are, at least in part, neurogenic. For example, a patient may complain of low-back pain at 30° of straight leg raise (SLR) and the addition of cervical extension decreases the pain. The inference is that the symptoms are neurogenic as the most direct structural connection between the pain and where the movement was applied is the nervous system.

Guidelines for component thinking

- Identify all possible sources of the symptoms. The

concept of thinking along the length of the nervous system will lead to the inclusion of more sources than previously considered. An example of the possible sources of inter-scapular symptoms is shown in Table 44.1.

- Establish whether these sources present any physical signs.
- Demonstrate physical signs that are relevant to the patient's disorder, and that can be retested following treatment of a specific component. For example, if the cervical component is treated, does this change the inter-scapular symptoms and signs?

Table 44.1 Possible sources of interscapular symptoms

Source	Local	Remote
Joint	Mid-thoracic intervertebral, costovertebral, costotransverse; scapulothoracic	Low cervical: zygapophyseal/ intervertebral disc; sternocostal
Muscle	Middle/low trapezius, rhomboids, iliocostalis	
Nerve	Spinal cord, meninges, sympathetic trunk, intercostal nerves	Spinal cord (cervical and lumbar), meninges, brain
Other	Blood vessels, bone, fascia, skin	Viscera

Analysis of the neural components

Both local and remote components need consideration. Local components may involve intraneural or extraneural pathology, similarly remote components which lie proximal or distal to the site of symptoms. Combinations of local and remote components are common; for instance, a local intraneural component such as thoracic dural scarring may be compounded by a remote extraneural problem such as spinal canal stenosis in the lumbar region.

Structures that must be considered include:

- the nervous system as a whole and its interfacing tissues—for example muscle, bone, and ligamentous structures
- the neurones as the conducting elements of the nervous system, including autonomic neurones
- the connective tissue components of the central nervous system (meninges) and the nerve supply (sinuvertebral nerve), and the connective tissue components of the peripheral nervous system (epineurium, perineurium, endoneurium) and their intrinsic nerve supply (nervi nervorum)
- neural blood vessels.

IDENTIFICATION OF ABNORMAL NERVOUS SYSTEM FUNCTION

Early identification of abnormal nervous system function will help the clinician to form priorities in the physical examination. There will be some subjective clues to support such an hypothesis.

Definitions

Mechanical interface. This may be defined as 'that tissue or material adjacent to the nervous system that can move independently of the system'.

Activity-specific mechanosensitivity refers to 'a common movement pattern associated with repetitive movements . . . or overuse of a limited part of the nervous system's range'. In these cases there seems to be a specific nervous system/mechanical interface relationship that may become symptom-provocative.

Subjective examination

Area and nature of symptoms

Common patterns of presentation are proposed for verte-bral conditions where abnormal nervous system function is implicated in the symptomatology.

Patients may complain of clumps of pain which typi-cally (co)exist at anatomic sites where the nervous system is vulnerable to mechanical compromise. Common exam-ples are the C5/6, T5/6/7 and L3/4/5 vertebral levels (Butler 1991). There may be a spread of symptoms, being a possible example of the central manifestation of the double/multiple crush syndrome.

Bizarre descriptive terms such as crawling, ant-like, pulling like a tight string, dry, woody, and dragging may be used. Patients may report sensations or areas of swelling, for instance at the cervicothoracic and lumbosacral junctions. Altered sweating patterns are not uncommon. Dilation of superficial blood vessels may be evident and commonly appear in a cluster at the cervicothoracic junc-tion, the mid-thoracic region sometimes extending around the rib cage and in the mid-lumbar spine area. It is proposed that some of these symptoms may relate to autonomic nervous system dysfunction, specifically the sympathetic nervous system.

Behaviour of symptoms

Symptoms may be aggravated by recognized positions that load the nervous system. Examples include slump whilst driving or taking a bath, SLR when kicking a foot-ball, or the upper limb tension test (ULTT) when reach-ing for a seat-belt. Specific and repetitious movement combinations at particular speeds may provoke symp-toms. Some examples are keyboard operating and playing the violin.

Symptoms frequently vary at night, possibly in relation to decreased blood pressure, altered tissue pressure gradients—for instance, the dorsal root ganglion compartment syndrome as described by Rydevik et al (1988) and pathomechanics. Pathophysiological processes such as inflammatory reactions, compromised microcirculation and slowed axonal transport develop over time, and symptoms may exhibit latency in relation to these processes.

The patient may be caused to adopt antalgic postures. Common examples include a lumbar disc protrusion causing an ipsilateral or contralateral list, and a chronic cervicothoracic complaint resulting in a forward head posture and/or a dowager's hump.

History

Either directly or indirectly, injury must inevitably involve the nervous system. There are certain histories that are suggestive of nervous system dysfunction.

A history of trauma, in particular high-velocity trauma such as a motor vehicle accident, implicates the nervous system. This may have occurred some years previously, and may not be considered by the patient as significant to the current complaint. However, it is proposed that the aftermath of trauma and the effect of even slight changes to nervous system mechanics is often underestimated. An old crush fracture in the low thoracic spine can alter nervous system mechanics, and this may predispose to symptoms locally or elsewhere. The concept of 'prespondylosis', that is, insidious attrition of other functions of the nervous system, especially the trophic aspect, is discussed in detail by Gunn (1980) and Gunn and Milbrandt (1978). This may also help to explain why some patients are slower to respond to treatment and their symptoms are often more severe than would be antipicated from the history of injury.

Chronicity of symptoms is common in vertebral disorders. This is particularly so when there has been no treatment in the acute stage, or all the possible structures and levels implicated in the symptomatology (that is non-neural and neural, peripheral and vertebral) have not been thoroughly examined, or adequately treated.

The patient may have had surgical intervention, for instance laminectomy or spinal fusion. The outcome of surgery may offer only temporary or partial relief of symptoms. If there is persistent neural pathomechanics elsewhere in the body there may be no change at all.

A progressive spread of symptoms may be reported. These are typically proximal and distal to the original complaint, often to sites of nervous system compromise such as C6, T6, and L4.

There may be a rapid growth spurt in adolescence when the lengthening of the nervous system lags behind the growth rate of bone. It is interesting to consider the possibility of a link between neural pathomechanics and the high incidence of conditions such as osteochrondritis that occur during adolescence.

General health considerations that are known to affect nervous system function and connective tissue structure should be considered. Examples include diabetes, systemic lupus erythematosus, multiple sclerosis, peripheral vascular disease and acquired immune deficiency syndrome.

Physical examination

Examination of vertebral disorders with altered neural function will include:

- tension testing
- examination of conduction, the nature of which is guided by subjective enquiry strategies and physical tests
- palpation of the vertebral column
- palpation of the peripheral nervous system when appropriate.

If the symptoms involve the nervous system, an indication of the area of compromise can be gained from:

- awareness of vulnerable anatomic sites (Ch. 2)
- area of symptoms, including the number of sites involved and whether referred symptoms are dermatomal in distribution
- palpation of peripheral nerves along their anatomical courses
- selective loss of muscle power and altered reflexes
- examination of surrounding structures, particularly the interfacing structures
- knowledge of the possible role of the sympathetic nervous system in maintained pain syndromes
- knowledge of anomalies of both the nervous system and the musculoskeletal system.

PRINCIPLES OF TENSION TESTING

Tension tests are not specific to the nervous system alone as they inevitably affect non-neural structures. However, it is possible to infer a neural component by using structural differentiation to alter component movements remote from the site of symptoms. These movements are known as sensitizing tests. For example, when the SLR test reproduces low-back pain and the addition of passive neck flexion (PNF) alters the symptoms, there has been minimal effect on non-neural structures while the position of the neuraxis and meninges has changed in relation to the spinal canal. The addition of PNF will cause neuromechanical changes and this may result in a change in symptoms.

Often it is only in retrospect and by treating one of the affected tissues or structures that a clear diagnosis can be made. Clinically, it is common to find disorders that involve a number of structures, both neural and non-neural, at a number of both vertebral and peripheral levels and with combinations of intraneural and extraneural pathology.

Guidelines to effective tension testing

To examine effectively using tension testing the clinician should consider the following points.

Certain precautions and contraindications apply to the use of all tension tests. The author strongly recommend that clinicians are familiar with these. A detailed list appears in Butler (1991).

The patient should be relaxed during the testing procedures, and the patient's response to tension testing should be established on the asymptomatic side first. The clinician needs to be familiar with the documented normal responses to tension testing.

The same starting position should be used each time the tension tests are repeated. The behaviour of symptoms at rest and during testing should be recorded. It may be necessary to experiment with possible combinations and refinements of tension tests in order to provoke a patient's symptoms.

When performing tension tests, careful handling will allow repeatable and accurate results. The addition of sensitizing tests to enable structural differentiation also relies on finesse in handling. It is often small or subtle changes in remote movement components that effect a symptomatic change. Gross handling may sacrifice this information.

Classification of responses to tension tests

For a tension test to be of diagnostic value it must reproduce the patient's symptoms, or symptoms relevant to the disorder. It is not always possible to reproduce the same symptoms; however, a response that is different from normal, or different from the contralateral limb response, may still be relevant. Butler (1991) has introduced a classification of responses that is clinically useful:

- *Physiological.* This refers to the normal responses to tension testing where symptoms may come from neural and non-neural sources. Possible neural sources are the innervated supporting connective tissues, or hypoxic axons from temporary vascular compromise (Sunderland 1976).
- *Clinical physiological.* The patient may report symptoms that are similar to, but not quite, the symptoms of which they are complaining. The symptoms can be in a different but related area; they can occur in a different sequence during testing from the other side or from normals. This is similar to Maitland's (1986) concept of 'comparable' signs on physical examination. An example of a clinical physiological response is a patient complaining of right buttock pain, with a 20° limitation of right knee extension in the slump position, and pulling in the right calf. With left knee extension there is a 10° limitation in the slump position with a pulling sensation in the posterior thigh and knee. While the slump test has not reproduced the symptoms complained of, it is likely to be relevant that there is greater limitation of knee extension on the right, and a different area of response from the left leg.
- *Neurogenic.* Classically this term applies to symptoms arising from the peripheral nervous system. Butler (1991) uses 'neurogenic' when referring to symptoms arising from either the central or peripheral nervous system. The neurogenic response is supported by careful structural differentiation. For example, the upper limb tension test (ULTT) reproduces a headache, and adding an SLR alters the response. It can be inferred that the symptoms are at least in part neurogenic.

Interpretation of tension tests

The clinician should consider the following points when interpreting tension tests:

- The response on the contralateral limb(s) where appropriate.
- The range of the tension test, and, where relevant, any changes in range, or symptom response with the addition of sensitizing tests. Even small changes in range or response can be relevant.
- The behaviour of the symptoms through range.
- The sequence of area response. For example, with a left SLR the response may be initially in the calf then the hamstring. Conversely, the right SLR produces hamstring symptoms initially and then calf pulling. In conjunction with other physical signs this may indicate altered neural mechanics.
- The area of response. For instance, a right ULTT may reproduce shoulder pain extending along the length of the arm, while the left ULTT causes a slight pulling sensation in the cubital fossa. There is a significant difference in the area of response, and in this case it will be relevant to right arm symptoms.
- The effect of sensitizing manoeuvres on tension test responses (area, range, symptoms). For example, in a slump position right knee extension is limited by 20° and reproduces a headache and this is aggravated by the addition of ankle dorsiflexion. There is no limitation of left knee extension and there is no symptom response. A symptom reproduced by a remote sensitizing test is a clue to examine the whole nervous system, including interfacing structures.
- There may be no obvious pathomechanics; however, a tension test may reproduce an abnormal response. For instance, an SLR test causes dizziness which can be altered by changing the range of the SLR.
- An activity-specific mechanosensitivity disorder may require a combination of tension tests of varying speeds, or in conjunction with varying joint or muscle positions. There should be subjective clues to guide the clinician to appropriate tension testing.

• Clinical experience has shown that, in many cases, if symptoms are predominantly distal and non-irritable, taking up the distal component first makes the tension test more sensitive. For example, if a patient is complaining of suprascapular pain, performing the ULTT with shoulder depression first will often reproduce symptoms more effectively than adding the distal components first.

TENSION TESTS

Tension tests such as the SLR, the prone knee bend (PKB) and PNF have long been used as part of the routine examination of neuro-orthopaedic disorders. What is more recent is the concept of movement and tension alterations of the nervous system, and the link between this and disorders such as neural headache, sympathetic maintained pain syndromes, plantar fasciitis and tennis elbow that have traditionally been considered as predominantly musculoskeletal in origin.

The slump test and the ULTT have been developed from the recognition that altered neural mechanics form part of many common neuro-orthopaedic disorders. In combination with the SLR, PKB and PNF, the slump test and ULTT collectively form the basis for examination of neural mechanics. These tests are simple, repeatable, and have documented normal responses.

The complexity of the nervous system, its interconnections and anomalies, mean that while these tension tests may have a particular peripheral nerve trunk bias, they cannot be thought of as moving or tensioning only one nerve trunk and its central extensions. The effects are transmitted to varying degrees along the peripheral nervous system to the neuraxis and meninges. The skilled clinician with a knowledge of neuroanatomy, neurophysiology, neurobiomechanics and the effect of pathology on nervous system function will be able to refine and adapt tension tests most effectively to reproduce variations in patient symptomatology.

The base tests

• Straight leg raise (SLR)
• Passive neck flexion (PNF)
• Prone knee bend (PKB)
• Slump
• Upper limb tension test (ULTT)

Terminology and recording

The base tests will be described for a non-irritable disorder. Each test will be discussed under the following headings:

• Historical perspective

• Biomechanics
• Method
• Normal responses
• Sensitizing tests
• Indications.

Notation of tension tests should include the test performed, the sequence of component movements, any symptomatic responses, the ranges of movement and resistance to movement. For a detailed discussion of notation refer to Butler (1991).

THE STRAIGHT LEG RAISE

Historical perspective

According to Dyck (1984), a Serbian named Lazar Lazarevic in 1880 was the first person to notice that pain produced with the SLR test had, as its origin, the sciatic nerve. It is more widely documented that Lasègue in 1864 described the SLR, with his pupil Forst bringing Lasègue's test into prominence. The test was described as the extended knee being lifted to the point of pain. The knee was then flexed and the diagnosis of sciatica confirmed if the pain ceased.

Biomechanics

It is clear that the SLR test affects not just the sciatic nerve but other structures including soft tissues such as hamstrings, and vertebral, hip and sacro-iliac joints. This chapter concentrates on the effect of the SLR test on neural structures, in particular the sciatic nerve and its branches.

The SLR moves and tensions the nervous system from its terminal extensions in the foot, via the sciatic nerve, to and along the neuraxis and meninges. There is considerable caudad movement of lumbosacral roots in relation to the intervertebral foramen (Goddard & Reid 1965). Breig (1978) demonstrated that an SLR also moves the sympathetic trunk in the lumbar spine in relation to interfacing tissues.

The nervous system does not move in just one plane, and is composed of many structures possessing differing properties. With certainty there will be some movement in the anteroposterior and lateral directions too. The axis of joint movement may well influence neural mechanics. For instance, there will probably be a different nervous system/mechanical interface relationship if the SLR is performed with the hip joint as the axis of movement, compared with that when the knee joint is the axis of movement.

The addition of dorsiflexion of the foot and ankle to the SLR increases tension along the tibial branch of the sciatic nerve (Macnab 1971, Breig & Troup 1979). The sequence of addition of dorsiflexion can influence the available range of SLR. This probably relates to variations in neural mechanics. For example, in a patient with lumbar symptoms, dorsiflexing the foot and ankle before the SLR may elicit symptoms at 60° SLR. In comparison, the addition of dorsiflexion after an SLR may not elicit symptoms until 90°.

The response to an SLR is clinically different from that of a bilateral SLR (BSLR). The combination of more lumbar spine flexion and the lack of neural fixation by the contralateral leg cause different mechanical events. It is reasonable to suggest that locally there will be less neural tension but perhaps more neural movement with a BSLR compared with a unilateral SLR. This is supported clinically, where it is common to find a limitation of unilateral SLR, and frequently BSLR is either unlimited or limited later in the range.

Method

The method will describe a right SLR.

The patient lies supine, relaxed and comfortable on the side of the examination bed. The trunk, shoulders and hips should be in a neutral position. The head should be flat where possible. If a pillow is used it must be used on retesting for consistency.

The examiner fixes the knee into extension by placing the left hand above the knee. The right hand supports the patient's foot and ankle under the heel allowing it to assume a neutral position. The right leg is elevated in a sagittal plane, moving at a fixed point about the hip joint. It may be necessary to fix the left leg by placing the examiner's right thigh above the patient's left knee. The leg is elevated to the symptomatic point, the examiner noting the onset of symptoms, their behaviour through range, and the available range of SLR. A comparison is made with the left SLR, and with what the examiner expects to be normal for that patient.

Normal responses

The range of the SLR varies widely and is by itself of little clinical value. More importantly, it must be interpreted in combination with the range of the asymptomatic SLR, the area and intensity of response, the sequence of area response and physical findings. Other tension tests should be performed to support the supposition that the symptoms have a neurogenic component.

Miller (1987) and Slater (1989) examined the SLR in 100 and 49 normal individuals respectively. Findings were similar with the areas of symptoms falling into three main regions, namely, the posterior thigh, the posterior knee, and the posterior calf extending to the foot. The response to the SLR was described as a deep, moderate stretch

sensation in the posterior thigh and posterior knee, extending to the calf region and plantar aspect of the foot.

Sensitizing tests

The most commonly used sensitizing tests for the SLR are:

- Ankle dorsiflexion
- Ankle plantarflexion/inversion
- Hip adduction
- Hip medial rotation
- Cervical flexion/extension
- Combinations of sensitizing tests. Examples include dorsiflexion and inversion, or hip adduction, medial rotation, dorsiflexion and eversion. A sensitizing test can be added either after a tension test, for example SLR/DF, or it can be performed first with the addition of the tension test after. The test would then be recorded as DF/SLR. The sequence of adding components to tension tests is discussed in more detail by Shacklock (1989).

Ankle dorsiflexion (SLR/DF)

Ankle dorsiflexion will increase tension in the tibial branch of the sciatic nerve and the sural branch. When dorsiflexion is added after the SLR (SLR/DF) the patient's heel rests on the examiner's shoulder, and the examiner then uses the hand to dorsiflex the patient's ankle. It is proposed that the addition of dorsiflexion/inversion of the foot and ankle to the SLR (SLR/DFInv) increases tension, particularly on the sural branch of the sciatic nerve.

These sensitizing tests are useful when examining patients with symptoms indicative of an S1 nerve root problem. The SLR/DFInv test is also valuable when examining lateral calf, heel or foot symptoms.

Ankle plantarflexion/inversion (SLR/PFI)

The addition of PFI to the SLR will increase tension along the common peroneal branch of the sciatic nerve (Nobel 1966, Sunderland 1978, Luk & Pun 1987, Styf 1988, Slater 1989). The sequence of addition of PFI can be varied as described for DF, i.e.: SLR/PFI or PFI/SLR.

To test SLR/PFI, the SLR is performed and the patient's heel is then placed on the examiner's shoulder. The examiner maintains the knee extension with the hand above the knee, while using the other hand to move the patient's ankle and foot into PFI. It is suggested that the toes are also flexed to maximize the response to this test (Slater 1989).

The PFI/SLR test is most easily performed by the examiner standing to the side of the patient, slightly facing the patient's feet. The foot is then placed into PFI using the examiner's two hands. The examiner's forearm lies along the shaft of the tibia, a downward pressure maintaining the knee extension (Fig. 44.1).

It is suggested that, in some patients with lumbar symptoms, it is possible to relate PFI of the ankle to pathology/pathomechanics of the L5 nerve root. This test is also valuable in the diagnosis of lower limb disorders such as chronic ankle sprains, anterior compartment syndrome, shin splints, and when there is a neurogenic component involving the common peroneal nerve.

Hip adduction (SLR/HAd)

Breig and Troup (1979) and Sutton (1979) reported the powerful sensitizing effect of hip adduction on the response to the SLR. This test increases neural tension as the position of the sciatic nerve is lateral to the ischial tuberosity. It is important to maintain the same range of SLR when applying hip adduction to clarify the effect of the sensitizing test. If a small amount of adduction is required, the test is easily performed from the position for the SLR described. When a greater degree of adduction is necessary, it may be more practical for the examiner to stand on the patient's left side.

Hip medial rotation (SLR/HMR)

This test also increases tension in the sciatic nerve (Breig & Troup 1979). It possibly increases tension in the common peroneal branch more than the tibial branch, as this branch lies most laterally. The SLR/HMR test may be sensitive for lower limb and lumbar symptoms. The examiner can perform SLR/HMR in the same position as the SLR test. The rotation is achieved by synchronous rotation of both the examiner's hands, so that the rotation is from combined femoral and tibial movement.

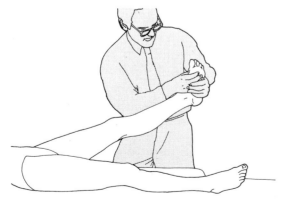

Fig. 44.1 Plantarflexion/inversion of the foot and ankle, in addition to the SLR, biases tension toward the common peroneal tract. (Reproduced from Butler 1991 with kind permission.)

Cervical flexion/extension (SLR/CF, SLR/CE)

This is a useful remote examination technique. It was initially suggested by Cyriax (1978), and studied later by Lew (1979) and Lew and Puentedura (1985). These studies found that cervical flexion added to an SLR would alter the symptom response and the range of the SLR test. Clinically, the authors have found that cervical extension and lateral flexion can also be valuable sensitizing additions in some patients. The sequence of performing the test will influence the symptom response. The most reliable method of effecting changes in cervical positions is with an assistant.

Other alternatives include positioning the cervical spine in flexion or extension using the movable section of an examination couch, using pillows either under the head and neck for flexion, or under the thoracic spine for extension. The patient may be able to assist by actively moving the cervical spine into flexion, or lowering it into extension.

Variations of the SLR test

Well-straight-leg-raise test

The well-leg-raising test describes the reproduction of ipsilateral leg symptoms with a contralateral asymptomatic SLR. The test is diagnostically valuable in patients with prolapsed discs, possibly because the irritated or adhered dural theca is brought into contact with the prolapsed or extruded disc material.

Bilateral straight-leg test (BSLR)

From the BSLR position either leg can be taken further into SLR, adducted, medially rotated or alterations in cervical positions performed.

Side-lying straight-leg-raise

It may be relevant or necessary to perform the SLR in a side-lying position. This does alter the range of and the response to the SLR as shown by Miller (1987). The alteration is thought to relate to an increase in tension of the neuraxis and meninges on the downmost side, and a decrease in tension on the uppermost side (Breig 1978).

Prone straight-leg raise

It is possible to perform an SLR in the prone position. The patient lies close to the edge of the examination couch, the examiner easing the leg to the floor. It is easy to sensitize the SLR by asking the patient to place the dorsiflexed foot to the floor. In this position the examiner can palpate the tensioned sciatic nerve in the buttock region.

Hip flexion/knee extension (HF/KE)

The examiner flexes the patient's hip and knee. The patient's thigh is supported by the examiner's thorax. The examiner's other hand is placed under the patient's heel to extend the leg. When symptoms are of an irritable nature this test will be less likely than the SLR test to aggravate the symptoms.

Indications

The SLR is a diagnostic test that has traditionally been used to help in the diagnosis of lumbar spine disorders and lower limb symptoms. Its application is now recognized as far wider, and the authors suggest it as a routine test in all neuro-orthopaedic disorders. This should be qualified by stating that unstable/progressive lumbar disorders and symptoms of an irritable nature may contraindicate the use of the SLR test. (Specific contraindications are listed in Butler 1991). As the disorder stabilizes it may become appropriate to examine the SLR.

The SLR test and its derivatives may be relevant to other vertebral disorders including neural headache, sympathetic maintained pain syndromes, the T4 syndrome and, peripherally, upper limb overuse syndromes, recurrent ankle sprains, plantar fasciitis and achilles tendonitis. The SLR test can also be valuable in remote and irritable disorders where local tension testing is likely to exacerbate the symptoms. An example is examining the SLR of a patient with irritable cervical symptoms.

PASSIVE NECK FLEXION

Historical perspective

According to O'Connell (1946), as early as 1909 Brudzinski was using PNF as a clinical sign of meningitis. Breig (1978) has presented a detailed analysis of the effects of cervical flexion and extension on the biomechanics of the neuraxis and meninges. This work is described more fully in Chapter 2. Lew and Puentedura (1985) have supported Breig's findings with a normative study that showed an altered response to the SLR with the addition of PNF.

Biomechanics

Breig and Marions (1963), Breig (1978) and Tencer et al (1985) have shown in cadaveric studies that passively flexing the head and neck moves and tensions the neuraxis and meninges in the lumbar spine and to a lesser extent the sciatic nerve. This provides support for both in vivo studies (Troup 1981), and clinical findings (Lew 1979, Lew & Puentedura 1985) that PNF can alter lumbar and lower limb symptoms.

As a remote tension test PNF is useful as there is little movement of lumbar spine structures including muscles,

the sacro-iliac joints, the posterior intervertebral joints, and the intervertebral discs. This offers the clinician a simple and effective test using structural differentiation.

Method

The patient lies supine, the head preferably unsupported. If a pillow is used the examiner must use this on repeat testing for consistency. The patient's arms rest at the side of the thorax, and the legs are together and in line with the body.

The examiner slides one hand under the patient's occiput, and gently raises the head a little. The examiner's other hand is then placed along the cervical spine to the cervicothoracic junction. This allows good support of the patient's head and neck. If the patient is small, the examiner may find one hand can support the head and neck along the examiner's forearm. The thorax can then be stabilized by the examiner's other hand. The head and neck are then taken into flexion in a 'chin on chest' direction (Fig. 44.2). The examiner notes the available range of PNF, the onset of symptoms, and their behaviour through range.

Normal responses

In a normal state other than a pulling sensation in the cervicothoracic region, the result of strain on both neural and non-neural structures, PNF should be asymptomatic. Any other response may be differentiated as neurogenic by the addition of remote tension tests such as the SLR.

Sensitizing tests

Upper and lower cervical flexion (PNF/U, PNF/L)

It may be possible to differentiate the upper or lower cervical spine as the predominant source of neural mechanics. For instance, in patients suffering neural headache

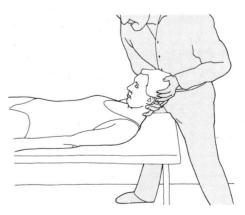

Fig. 44.2 Passive neck flexion performed as a 'chin on chest' movement. (Reproduced from Butler 1991 with kind permission.)

PNF in combination with SLR may reproduce a hint of the headache. The addition of upper cervical flexion may further aggravate the headache. Cervical retraction (PNF/RE) is often a useful addition to PNF in combination with other tension tests, especially the SLR, PKB and the ULTT.

Cervical lateral flexion or rotation (PNF/LF, PNF/RO)

Any neck movement will influence neural mechanics. When the clinician wants to provoke the symptoms it may be appropriate to combine PNF with cervical lateral flexion or rotation. These combinations are commonly sensitive in nervous system disorders that involve positive ULTTs.

Thoracic flexion or extension (THF/THE)

Positioning the thoracic spine into extension, or adding thoracic flexion to PNF, is often an effective means of altering the symptomatic response to PNF. This is usually done in combination with other tension tests such as PKB, ULTT, SLR.

Indications

Any neuro-orthopaedic disorder in the vertebral region may be sensitive to PNF. Examples include lumbar spine symptoms, headaches, and the T4 syndrome. Upper limb and lower limb symptoms may also be altered by PNF. It is recommended that PNF be performed as a routine tension test where symptoms are suspected to have a neurogenic component. It may be useful as a remote tension test where symptoms are too irritable to allow for more local tension testing.

PRONE KNEE BEND

Historical perspective

According to Estridge et al (1982), Wasserman (1919) first documented PKB as a physical sign used to reproduce anterior thigh and shin pain in soldiers. The PKB moves and tensions the nervous system via the L2/3/4 nerve roots, in particular the femoral nerve and its branches. O'Connell (1946) suggested that hip extension (HE) in addition to the PKB, would further increase tension via the femoral nerve and lumbar nerve roots. However, in a normative study Davidson (1987) found a more significant response to PKB without the addition of hip extension. In symptomatic patients, for instance patients with 'meralgia parasthetica', it is clinically evident that PKB/HE frequently reproduces symptoms more effectively than does the PKB alone. The different neural anatomy and mechanics may be the key to the differences

in response to PKB between symptomatic and asymptomatic subjects. In symptomatic cases it may be a movement-related pathology rather than a problem of altered neural tension.

Biomechanics

Tension is transmitted via the femoral nerve and its soft-tissue attachments to the L2/3/4 nerve roots and to the neuraxis and meninges (Estridge et al 1982). As the saphenous nerve lies behind the axis of knee flexion and extension it is unlikely to be effectively tensioned by the PKB alone. In comparison, the lateral femoral cutaneous nerve which lies anterior to the axis of hip flexion and extension is under more tension with PKB/HE, provided that the lumbar spine does not extend.

As with any of the tension tests, interpretation of pathomechanics of the PKB must not be limited to symptoms that relate only to increases in tension. The symptomatic response may relate to altered movement of the neural structures in relation to the surrounding interfaces. While this is a simplistic view of complex neural mechanics, based on current patho-anatomical knowledge and clinical reasoning processes, it is a logical explanation of the differing responses to tension tests.

Method

The patient lies prone near the side of the examination couch with the head rotated towards the examiner, so that for a right PKB the patient's head is rotated to the right side. The examiner stands at the patient's side, and with the hand grasps the patient's shin just proximal to the ankle. The knee is then flexed, the examiner noting the range of PKB, any symptoms reproduced and the behaviour of these symptoms through range. The contralateral leg is tested to allow a comparison of symptom response.

Normal responses

The normal responses to the PKB in a large group of asymptomatic subjects have not been documented. From clinical observations it has been noted that, in the majority of subjects, it is possible to flex the knee so that the heel approximates the buttock. Subjects usually report a pulling sensation in the anterior thigh. This response should he compared to the other side and to what the clinician has found to be a normal response.

The diagnostic value of the test is confused by movement and stretch of non-neural structures. For instance, the rectus femoris muscle is placed on stretch and the pelvis tilted anteriorly, thereby extending the lumbar spine and presumably lessening the tension on the femoral nerve roots. Structural differentiation enables the clinician to clarify the extent of neurogenic involvement. An example is with the patient in a side-lying position, adding PNF to the PKB.

Sensitizing tests

Hip extension (PKB/HE)

As mentioned, adding hip extension may increase the response to the PKB. In combination with PKB, variations of hip adduction/abduction, and medial/lateral rotation may be relevant in some vertebral presentations. As these movements are unlikely to cause more than slight increases in neural tension, it is probably the different neural and mechanical relationships that cause changes in the symptom response. The examiner can support the hip in extension either by using the thigh under the patient's anterior thigh or by using folded towels.

Slump (PKB/slump)

A useful means of structural differentiation between symptoms of predominantly neural origin or musculoskeletal origin, and those reproduced by the PKB, is provided by the addition of slump to the PKB. Davidson (1987) described this test and suggested performing it in a side-lying position, preferably with the help of an assistant.

The patient lies on the examination couch slightly to one side, with the PKB/slump to be examined uppermost. The patient is instructed to curl up, the examiner ensuring that the cervical and thoracic spines are fully flexed. The assistant stabilizes the cervical and thoracic spines in this position. The patient grasps the underneath knee, and takes the hip into flexion. The examiner stands behind the patient using one hand to stabilize the hip and trunk through the buttock, the other hand holding the patient's shin and performing the PKB to achieve the desired symptomatic response (Fig. 44.3) The assistant can then release the cervical flexion component of the slump, and any alteration in symptoms is noted. Cervical flexion can then be added again to confirm the response.

Davidson (1987) reported that the addition of cervical flexion to the PKB/slump increased the response in 62.5% of asymptomatic subjects, and decreased it in 12.5%. Cervical extension was found to decrease the response in 20% of subjects and increase the response in 30% of subjects.

Hip abduction

The saphenous branch of the femoral nerve terminates with a cutaneous supply at the instep of the foot. Butler (1991) proposes that it is possible to tension the saphenous nerve if, in hip extension and knee extension, the leg is abducted and laterally rotated and the ankle everted.

This can be useful as both a diagnostic test and a treatment technique where vertebral and lower limb symptoms are neurogenic, and related to pathology particularly of the L2/3/4 neural structures.

Bilateral PKB (BPKB)

If indicated, a BPKB can be performed and any difference in range is easily identifiable in this position. Different neurobiomechanics from that of the PKB will mean that the symptom response will also be different.

Indications

It is suggested that the PKB be indicated as a routine tension test for all non-irritable vertebral neuro-orthopaedic conditions. It should also be examined where there is a suspicion that peripheral symptoms involve a neurogenic component, particularly from the L2/3/4 neural structures. Examples include anterior thigh and medial knee symptoms. There may be subjective indicators that the PKB should be examined—for instance, in a patient who experiences pain in both the anterior thigh of the behind leg and the lumbar spine when hurdling.

It is not uncommon to find that patients with a limitation of SLR also exhibit a symptomatic PKB. This may be contralateral or ipsilateral depending on the pathology. It is important to recognize the close anatomical relationship of the femoral and sciatic nerve roots, and the implications of pathomechanics of one neural complex on the other.

THE SLUMP TEST

Historical perspective

According to Woodhall and Hayes (1950), Petren, as early as 1909, used knee extension in sitting as a tension test. Cyriax (1942) used combinations of knee extension

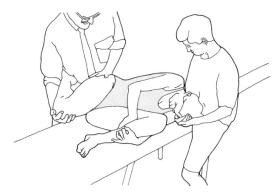

Fig. 44.3 Prone knee bend in a sidelying 'slump' enables the clinician to perform structural differentiation via cervical movements. (Reproduced from Butler 1991 with kind permission.)

in sitting combined with cervical flexion to diagnose 'sciatic perineuritis'. Inman and Saunders (1942) described combinations of trunk flexion and SLR to attempt to localize the origin of lumbar symptoms. Where lumbar symptoms increased with an increase in SLR range, lower lumbar pathology was indicated. Conversely, an increase in symptoms when the trunk was flexed suggested upper lumbar pathology. Clinically, the authors have found that this differentiation is not always correct. There is a diversity of symptomatic responses that presumably relate to variations in anatomy and pathomechanics.

Maitland (1979) performed a normative study using the combination of trunk flexion, cervical flexion and SLR to assess movement of the spinal neural structures. He named this the 'slump test'. This tension test is one of the most important as it moves and tensions both the neural and connective tissue components of the nervous system from both ends, that is, from the brain to the terminal branches of the sciatic nerve in the foot. It combines the PNF and the SLR tension tests and effects unique neural and mechanical interface relationships. It also provides a valuable base test for assessment of neural mechanics from which a number of more refined additions offer the clinician a wide range of sensitive neural examination techniques.

Biomechanics

The biomechanics of the slump test have not been extensively studied. The authors' interpretation of the mechanics of the slump test relies on information from several studies. These include investigations by Smith (1956), Reid (1960), Adams and Logue (1971), cadaveric studies by Louis (1981), dissections by Penning and Wilmink (1981), a few in vivo studies and extrapolation from clinical studies of the PNF and SLR tests.

According to Louis (1981), the C6, T6 and L4 intervertebral levels are areas where the neural and mechanical interface relationship remains relatively constant during movement of the spinal canal. Butler (1991) stresses the importance of examining these areas and adjacent vertebral levels for early signs of altered neural mechanics.

Penning and Wilmink (1981) found in their dissections that there was anteroposterior movement of the dural sac in the lumbar spinal canal during flexion and extension. This emphasizes that neural mechanics are not limited to cephalad and caudad movement but occur in many directions and combinations of directions.

Maitland' s (1979) study found that, in the complete slump test position, releasing cervical flexion allowed an increased range of knee extension and ankle dorsiflexion and associated changes in the symptom response. These changes cannot be explained by local factors alone. The most direct structural connection is the nervous system.

While the slump test places tension over a greater length of the nervous system than any other tension test it may not necessarily reproduce a patient's symptoms. If the primary pathology affects extraneural movement rather than neural tension, the slump test may not simulate the symptomatic relationship. The SLR or PNF tests might prove more sensitive in some presentations as they allow more movement to occur at the unfixed end (that is, cephalad and caudad, respectively). It is important that this is considered when interpreting an asymptomatic slump test, especially when no other tension test has been examined. The danger of forming a diagnosis based on the slump test alone, as a test which places 'maximal' uniform tension on the nervous system, is evident. Tension tests such as the SLR, PKB and ULTT may produce greater localised neural tension than does the slump test.

Method

It must be impressed that the following method of performing the slump test is described for a non-severe, non-irritable disorder. Modifications and limitations to slump testing are often indicated and will be discussed following a description of the test. For contraindications and precautions refer to Butler (1991).

The patient sits on the examination couch with the knee creases approximating the edge. The thighs are fully supported and the knees together. The patient's hands are linked loosely behind the back. The examiner stands close to the patient's side. The examiner notes any resting symptoms, and the behaviour of these are observed throughout each stage of testing. The range of movement of each component is visually estimated.

The patient is asked to 'slump' or 'sag' the trunk. The cervical spine is kept in a neutral position. The examiner applies overpressure to thoracolumbar flexion, aiming to 'bow' the spine rather than to increase hip flexion (Fig. 44.4A). The sacrum must remain upright. Butler (1991) suggests stabilizing the patient's cervicothoracic region with the examiner's axilla. This allows the examiner to use the thorax and forearm to bow the spine and still maintain an even downward pressure on the patient's trunk. Symptom responses and ranges of movement are noted.

Maintaining this position, the patient is asked to sag the head down onto the chest. The examiner applies gentle overpressure to the cervical flexion. Symptom responses and ranges are noted.

The patient is asked to straighten actively the left knee, the examiner noting the response (Fig. 44.4B). While it is suggested, that, for consistency, the sequence of knee extension is left and then right, if the patient has a symptomatic side testing should commence on the asymptomatic side first.

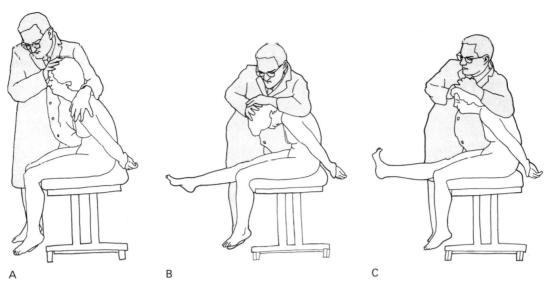

Fig. 44.4   The slump test in sequence (refer to test detail): **A.** The patient 'slumps' the trunk, the examiner maintaining the cervical spine in neutral. **B.** The examiner maintains the trunk flexion and cervical flexion, while the patient extends the knee. **C.** The patient actively dorsiflexes the ankle, the examiner assessing the response. Any change in response is noted as the cervical flexion component is released. (Reproduced from Butler 1991 with kind permission.)

The patient is then asked to 'pull your left foot up', that is, to dorsiflex the left ankle. The examiner releases the cervical flexion, and monitors any changes in response (Fig.44.4C). It may be essential to take the cervical spine into some extension before any change in response occurs. In some patients there will be no alteration of symptoms, while others may experience an increase or a decrease of symptoms.

The same method is repeated for the other leg. The examiner can then compare any differences in ranges or symptom response. Finally, in the slump position, the patient is asked to extend both knees together. Any difference in ranges of knee extension is clearly visible. The symptom response is noted.

The slump test stresses many neural and non-neural structures. Skilled handling and consistent method are essential prerequisites for clear interpretation of responses. It must be emphasized that the slump test may be contraindicated when the disorder is irritable or unstable—for instance, a disc prolapse with impending nerve root compression, or when underlying pathology such as the tethered cord syndrome is recognized.

A patient's symptoms may be reproduced in the early stages of the slump test. An example is trunk flexion and cervical flexion components reproducing lower limb symptoms. There is no need for completing the full slump test if the symptoms are adequately reproduced with certain components only. As the symptoms improve with treatment the test can then be progressed to the full slump test as the clinician examines for residual signs of pathomechanics.

Normal responses

Maitland (1979) has pointed out that even in normal subjects it is common to experience some pain or discomfort in response to the slump test. The following responses are suggested as normal descriptions from studies of approximately 250 asymptomatic subjects (Maitland 1979, Grant 1983, Leung 1983, Butler 1985).

Normally, there is no discomfort on assuming the trunk flexion position. With the addition of cervical flexion, a stretch pain is commonly reported in the T8/9 region. When knee extension is added pain is often felt in the posterior region of the extended knee and the posterior thigh, and there is commonly some limitation of knee extension. This limitation should be symmetrical. Ankle dorsiflexion in addition to this position is frequently limited and may increase the lower limb symptoms.

Finally, on release of cervical flexion there is a decrease in all symptoms, in all areas, and an increase in the ranges of both knee extension and ankle dorsiflexion.

Sensitizing tests and other variations

While the standard slump test is useful as a base tension test, the clinician may need to alter the sequence of component movements or experiment with combinations of sensitizing movements to reproduce the symptoms. It may be appropriate to combine the slump test with joint motion testing. For example, unilateral postero-anterior pressures on the costotransverse joints in the slump position. Butler (1991) suggests that in the slump position abduction of the extended leg can reproduce groin symptoms of neurogenic origin. Structural differentiation can be used to assist in this diagnosis. Similarly, in vertebral disorders resulting in upper limb symptoms combinations of the slump test and the ULTT may be diagnostically valuable.

The essence of diagnosis using the slump test is examination and interpretation of responses based on normative data and clinical reasoning processes. Good handling skills will allow the clinician effectively to experiment with combinations of neural and mechanical interface relationships that are the most likely to reproduce relevant signs and symptoms.

The slump test in long sitting (slump LS)

The slump test can also be performed by loading the neural structures from caudad to cephalad. It is an easily performed test that is diagnostically valuable and useful for treatment both in the clinic and for the patient at home. Asymmetrical restriction of ranges such as knee extension are immediately visible. Antalgic postures are often exaggerated. Confirmation of a neurogenic component can quickly and easily be made by using a remote sensitizing test. For instance, in a patient with a pronounced forward head posture the examiner can slightly flex the knees and note any change in the head position.

It is hypothesized that slump LS may be a particularly effective tension test for pathomechanics of the sympathetic trunk. The idea that the sympathetic trunk (and the sympathetic nervous system) responds mechanically and physiologically to movement has received little attention in the literature. We propose that altered tension and movement of the sympathetic trunk can occur, and that this may be a potent and underestimated part of certain pain syndromes. Via its widespread connections to target tissues and its interconnections with the somatic nervous system, it is inevitable that body movements affect sympathetic nervous system movement and function. It follows that tension tests must also affect sympathetic neurobiomechanics. This includes the SLR, PNF, PKB and ULTT tension tests. The anatomy of the sympathetic trunk suggests that it will be loaded by the slump LS test. The load is perhaps increased on the sympathetic trunk by contralateral lateral flexion of the body.

Common disorders that exhibit symptoms suggestive of sympathetic involvement are the 'T4' syndrome, chest and upper limb symptoms simulating cardiac disease, the shoulder/hand syndrome, neural headaches, thoracic outlet syndrome and Raynaud's syndrome. Structural differentiation again forms the basis of confirming that symptoms have a neurogenic component.

Slump LS method

The patient assumes a long sitting position on the examination couch. The knees are extended and held together. When appropriate, ankle dorsiflexion can be added by the patient placing the feet against a wall. The patient sags into a position of trunk flexion. The examiner either kneels on the couch behind the patient, or stands beside the examination couch where they effectively can guide the component movements whilst maintaining trunk flexion. Cervical flexion is then added by the examiner (Fig. 44.5). In this position combinations of cervical/thoracic/hip/knee and ankle movements can be added to reproduce symptoms of a complex nature. The ULTT can also be added in the slump LS position.

Indications for slump and slump LS tests

Slump

The authors suggest that the slump test should be a routine part of examination in all non-irritable neuro-orthopaedic disorders with the exception of those vertebral conditions that are unstable or progressive as mentioned earlier, or listed as contraindications by Butler (1991).

The slump test can he a particularly useful examination technique in disorders where:

- There are vertebral symptoms.
- There are subjective indicators that the slump test may be relevant. For example, exacerbation of symptoms when a patient flexes the head to get into/out of a vehicle.
- Treatment via the nervous system involves using other tension tests such as the ULTT and PKB. The slump test is then useful for re-assessment purposes.
- Symptoms indicate neural pathomechanics and these symptoms have not been reproduced by other tension tests.
- Normal neurobiomechanics are required prior to discharge.

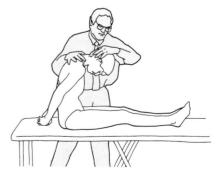

Fig. 44.5 Slump longsitting test with cervical flexion. (Reproduced from Butler 1991 with kind permission.)

Slump LS

The same contraindications as those listed for the slump test apply to the slump LS test. The slump LS test should be particularly examined in neuro-orthopaedic disorders where:

- This position is reported as symptom-provocative—for instance sitting in a reclining chair.
- The history of injury indicates that a force occurred in the slump LS position. An example is an injury that occurs in the final stage of long jumping.
- The symptoms cannot be adequately reproduced by the slump test.
- The slump test is used as a treatment technique; then, slump LS is an effective re-assessment tool.
- The sympathetic trunk is suspected of contributing to the symptomatology.
- The patient needs an easy self-mobilization home exercise that involves the slump test. It is easy to perform on the floor and, if done carefully, is safe.

More details of home exercises specifically for the nervous system are discussed in Chapter 50.

THE UPPER LIMB TENSION TEST

Historical perspective

The ULTT has been described as the upper limb analogue to the SLR. This is a useful analogy as it intimates movement and tension of neural tissue in the upper limb and spinal canal. While both the neuro-anatomy and neurobiomechanics of the upper limb are much more complex than those of the lower limb, there is no doubt that the nervous system develops tension and moves in relation to surrounding structures with movements of the fingers, wrist, elbow, shoulder, and body (Pechan & Julius 1975, McLellan & Swash 1976). These adaptive mechanisms to movement are not limited to the upper limb: they also affect the neuraxis and meninges.

In 1978, Elvey documented in cadavers that certain movements of the arm selectively moved and tensioned the cervical nerve roots, their investing sheaths and dura. Elvey's (1979) work has formed the basis of the standard ULTT. Other observations on cadavers (Rubenach 1987, Ginn 1989, Selvaratnam et al 1989) support the supposition that the neural structures can be mechanically tested with little associated movement of interfacing structures. Over the past decade, tension testing of the upper limb has progressed considerably with established patterns of responses to the ULTT in approximately 1000 upper limbs, through normative studies at the University of South Australia (Fardy 1985, Kenneally 1985, Rubenach 1985, Bell 1987, Landers 1987).

Clinical validation of the ULTT, linking some syndromes with abnormal responses to the ULTT is developing. Elvey et al (1986) reported a symptomatic ULTT in 98% of patients diagnosed with repetitive strain injury. Quintner (1989) documented a high incidence of symptomatic ULTTs in patients suffering from whiplash. Young (1989) also found a high rate of abnormal responses to the ULTT in post-Colles' fracture patients. More clinical research is needed to explore the relationship between vertebral disorders such as neural headache, T4 syndrome, thoracic outlet syndrome, some sympathetic maintained pain syndromes and altered responses to the ULTT. There is also a need for wider medical support of the ULTT, by surgical correlates and other medical investigations.

Biomechanics

The complexity of the neuro-anatomy of the upper limb is coupled by the complexity of its neurobiomechanics. To a large extent the mechanics of the standard ULTT (ULTT1) is based on extrapolation from cadaver studies (Elvey 1978, Rubenach 1987, Ginn 1989, Selvaratnam et al 1989) and a few in vivo studies. The ULTT1 affects predominantly the median nerve via the C5/6 nerve roots, and to a lesser extent the C7 nerve root (Elvey 1979, Rubenach 1987, Kenneally et al 1988). Based on these findings, Butler (1991) has described the ULTT1 as a median nerve bias test.

Butler also describes radial nerve bias (ULTT2), and ulnar nerve bias (ULTT3) tension tests. In some patient presentations these base tests can be useful for localizing symptoms to particular vertebral levels and peripheral nerve trunks. The way in which each base ULTT affects neural mechanics will be different, and this may explain the variations in symptom response between the tests.

Method

The ULTT1 consists of three basic movements, as described by Elvey (1979) and outlined by Kenneally et al (1988). The clinician should be aware of the symptom response and range for each component movement.

With the patient supine, lying to the side of the examination couch, the head unsupported, the shoulder is slightly depressed with the examiner's fist. The shoulder is taken to 110° abduction in the coronal plane, and then lateral rotation of the glenohumeral joint is added.

The arm is held in this position and the forearm is supinated and the elbow extended. Maintaining this position the wrist and fingers are extended (Fig. 44.6).

The ULTT1 can be performed in a different sequence, with the last addition being elbow extension. This sequence is preferred because the radial and median nerves are stronger at the elbow than the wrist. Also any loss of

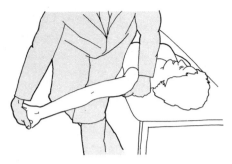

Fig. 44.6 Upper limb tension test 1, end position. (Reproduced from Butler 1991 with kind permission.)

range is easily visible. Shoulder depression is omitted, keeping the ULTT1 as a simple base tension test.

If the upper limb symptoms are distal, taking up the distal components first will usually be the most sensitive ULTT1. Conversely, if the problem lies proximal it is usually most effective to perform shoulder and elbow movements before adding the distal components.

Normal responses

Kenneally et al (1988) documented the responses to the ULTT in 400 normal volunteers. Volunteers reported a deep stretch or ache in the cubital fossa (99% of volunteers) extending down the anterior and radial aspect of the forearm and into the radial side of the hand (80%). Some subjects experienced a definite tingling sensation in the thumb and first three fingers. A small percentage of subjects felt a stretch in the anterior shoulder area. Contralateral cervical lateral flexion increased the response in approximately 90% of normals. Cervical lateral flexion towards the tested side decreased the response in 70% of normals.

Sensitizing tests and other variations

The most commonly used sensitizing tests are placing the opposite upper limb in the ULTT1 position (Rubenach 1987), cervical lateral flexion (Kenneally et al 1988) and the SLR test (Bell 1987). There are many other variations of body and limb movements that are valuable when wanting to provoke symptoms of a specific nature. Some examples are cervical flexion and lateral flexion; cervical lateral flexion with trunk lateral flexion; and combinations of wrist positions.

Indications

Although the ULTT1 may have a median nerve bias, it must also move and tension the nervous system from the finger tips along the arm to the neuraxis and meninges and the sympathetic trunk, to the contralateral arm. It may provoke symptoms anywhere along the nervous sys-

tem, and the authors have noted that patients report symptoms in areas as remote as the lumbar spine and lower limbs.

It is therefore recommended that the ULTT is examined for neuro-orthopaedic disorders in the upper quadrant, including the thoracic spine. However, contraindications apply to all the ULTTs and it is strongly advised that clinicians review these (Butler 1991).

There are two specific precautions for the ULTT. The first is that it is far easier to aggravate upper-limb symptoms than lower-limb symptoms. Neural structures are weaker and have a more complex configuration in the upper limb. It is therefore more likely that the clinician will aggravate the irritated nervous system.

The second precaution relates to the test. The ULTT involves many component movements and affects many non-neural as well as neural structures. It is easy to overlook a particularly sensitive structure and thereby exacerbate the symptoms. These precautions should be observed especially if the clinician is not familiar with tension testing.

THE UPPER LIMB TENSION TEST 2

The ULTT2 has been developed as a functional refinement of the ULTT1. The ULTT2 emphasizes the powerful sensitizing effect of shoulder depression and protraction on tension of the neural structures in the cervical spine and upper limb. It combines these components with the work posture typical of many patients with upper quadrant symptoms. In some disorders, the ULTT2 may be provocative and the response to the ULTT1 normal. The reverse may also be true. This illustrates the clinical value of examining all the base ULTTs when indicated.

Butler (1991) has described a median nerve bias ULTT2 (Mb) and a radial nerve bias ULTT2 (Rb) Peripherally, the ULTT2 (Mb) is proposed to move and tension predominantly the median nerve. The use of shoulder girdle depression means that the ULTT2 (Rb) affects the same nerve roots (C5/6/7) but may move and tension predominantly the radial nerve. This does not infer that the neurobiomechanics of these ULTTs are the same. It is quite likely that they move and tension neural structures in a different way. This is probably especially so in pathological conditions. A good example is C6 nerve root compression, where the ULTT2 (Rb) can be expected to produce a different and often more provocative symptomatic response than either ULTT2 (Mb) or ULTT1.

Method ULTT2 (median bias)

The examiner notes any symptom response and the available ranges of movement.

The patient lies to the side of the examination couch

with the scapula free of the couch. The legs and trunk are angled to the other side of the bed so that the patient feels supported. The examiner's thigh rests against the patient's shoulder, supporting the patient's arm at the elbow and wrist. The shoulder will need to be in approximately 10° of abduction so that the arm is free from the couch. The examiner's thigh is used to depress the patient's shoulder girdle. Protraction may be examined independently or in combination with depression, by the examiner slightly squatting and picking up the shoulder girdle with the thigh (Fig. 44.7A). The shoulder girdle can also be retracted using the same method.

The shoulder girdle position is held, and for a median nerve bias the patient's elbow is extended, the shoulder externally rotated and the forearm supinated. This position is maintained and the examiner's hand slides down into the patient's hand, the examiner's thumb lying between the patient's thumb, and index finger (Fig. 44.7B). This means the examiner has good control of the patient's thumb, fingers and wrist and can alter the degree of radial/ulnar deviation and pronation/supination.

In this position the shoulder can be abducted or extended, and the wrist components, or cervical positions,

altered. These changes will help to support a neurogenic component in the disorder. Note that if the symptoms are neurogenic even a slight release of shoulder depression will usually ease the symptoms.

Method ULTT2 (radial bias)

The anatomical course of the radial nerve suggests that it may be tensioned by shoulder girdle depression/protraction/retraction/medial rotation/elbow extension/forearm pronation/wrist/finger/thumb flexion and ulnar deviation.

The method for the ULTT2 (Rb) is the same as for the ULTT2 (Mb) to the point of shoulder girdle depression/protraction. The patient's shoulder is then internally rotated and the elbow extended. The examiner can maintain the patient's elbow extension by blocking it with the elbow. Wrist and finger movements can then be added using the other hand (Fig. 44.8).

Variations

Sometimes it is appropriate to perform the ULTT2s with the patient lying prone. The examiner again uses the thigh to control retraction of the shoulder girdle, and gravity assists the protraction as well as displacing the neuraxis and meninges forward. This position also offers the clinician an opportunity of mobilizing the cervical and thoracic spines in combinations of ULTT2.

Similar combinations of sensitizing tests can be added to the ULTT2 as those described for ULTT1. For example, chin retraction with cervical extension/lateral flexion is often a sensitive combination, particularly where symptoms are non-irritable in nature and proximal in distribution. In prone ULTT2, it is possible to add a bilateral PKB or trunk contralateral lateral flexion.

Normal responses

Yaxley & Jull (1991) documented the normal sensory re-

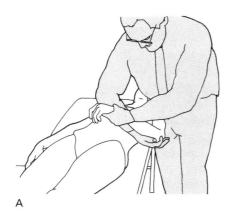

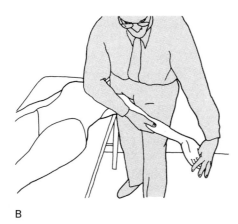

Fig. 44.7 Upper limb tension test 2 (median bias): **A.** Protraction/depression of the patient's shoulder girdle, is the essence of the ULTT2. **B.** End position ULTT2 (median bias). (Reproduced from Butler 1991 with kind permission.)

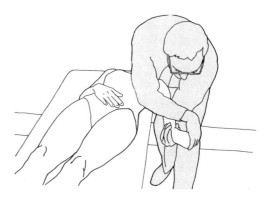

Fig. 44.8 Upper limb tension test 2 (radial bias). Note the internal rotation of the shoulder, wrist pronation and flexion. (Reproduced from Butler 1991 with kind permission.)

sponses to the ULTT2 (Rb) in 50 subjects. The test produced a strong painful stretch over the radial aspect of the proximal forearm and elbow. This was often accompanied by a stretch pain in the dorsum of the hand, lateral upper arm and biceps brachii. Approximately 40° of glenohumeral abduction was available in the final position. These areas of sensory response were different from the ULTT1. This suggests that the ULTT2 (Rb) does have different neural mechanics.

Indications

Similar indications and contraindications apply for ULTT2 as those described for ULTT1. Where symptoms have a clear postural relationship that involves shoulder depression and protraction/retraction, and the disorder is non-irritable, the ULTT2 should be examined. Symptoms that follow a median nerve or radial nerve distribution can often be reproduced with ULTT2. Both ULTT1 and ULTT2 are base tests and often it will be combinations of these, other tension tests and sensitizing movements that reproduce symptoms.

THE UPPER LIMB TENSION TEST 3

Pechan (1973) described a manoeuvre to test mechanics of the ulnar nerve in the cubital tunnel. Butler (1991) has proposed an extension of this test—the ulnar nerve tension test (ULTT3). The ULTT3 emphasizes shoulder girdle depression and abduction in combination with pronation of the forearm, wrist extension, elbow flexion and shoulder lateral rotation. The ULTT3 should be considered as a base test, and when appropriate, examined in conjunction with the ULTT1 and ULTT2.

Method

The examiner should note any symptom response and the available ranges of movement. The suggested sequence offers the most convenient handling especially for the examiner who may not be familiar with ULTT3.

The patient lies supine and to the side of the examination couch. The patient's elbow lies supported on the examiner's thigh. The examiner usually fans out the hand to lie palm against the volar aspect of the patient's fingers. The examiner's thumb rests against the dorsum of the patient's index and ring fingers at the metacarpal joints. This allows good control of wrist and finger extension and means that the amount of pronation/supination and radial/ulnar deviation can be varied.

The patient's wrist and fingers are held in extension, the forearm is pronated and the elbow fully flexed. The examiner rests the patient's flexed elbow in the groin. Using a clenched fist, the examiner depresses the patient's shoulder girdle before adding shoulder lateral rotation. With this position maintained the shoulder is then ab-

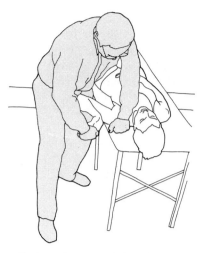

Fig. 44.9 Upper limb tension test 3 (ulnar bias). Note wrist supination; clinically, pronation is more sensitive. (Reproduced from Butler 1991 with kind permission.)

ducted (Fig. 44.9). At this stage the patient's hand should lie flat against the side of the head, the fingertips pointing caudad.

Variations

The ULTT3 can also be examined with the patient in a prone position. This is a useful position as it allows the clinician to examine/mobilize both the thoracic spine and the cervical spine with the nervous system in tension. Combinations of shoulder girdle protraction and retraction, or cervical positions, can be added to the ULTT3 in either the prone or supine position. Similarly, trunk side-flexion, a PKB or a contralateral ULTT, can be examined with the ULTT3 maintained. In some cases, the ULTT3 will elicit vertebral symptoms more effectively with the cervical spine or thoracic spine prepositioned in lateral flexion or the symptomatic position. Handling techniques will need to be modified according to the combination of component movements.

Normal responses

There have been no normative studies to document responses to ULTT3. As with the ULTT2 tests, the clinician must become familiar with responses and ranges of movement to ULTT3 in normals, and compare symptomatic and asymptomatic responses within individual patients. It is worth remembering that even small changes in range, or a different sequence of area responses, may constitute a relevant finding.

Indications

The authors have found that the ULTT3 can be an effective examination and treatment technique in upper quadrant conditions. It has proved to be particularly effective in the assessment and treatment of chronic and stable nerve root disorders at the C8/TI intervertebral level. The ULTT3 is also valuable when examining disorders that have symptomatic ULTT1 and ULTT2.

OTHER UPPER LIMB TENSION TESTS

It is not only possible to examine the mechanics of neural structures in the upper quadrant using these base ULTTs: by following the anatomy of other upper limb peripheral nerve courses, and combining this with a knowledge of neurobiomechanics, it is possible to develop tension tests for the long thoracic nerve, the musculocutaneous nerve, the axillary nerve and the suprascapular nerve. Butler (1991) details the component movements that bias tension testing towards these nerves and their central continuations.

SUMMARY

The approach of manual therapy to examination and treatment of neuro-orthopaedic disorders needs to include consideration of the potential of the nervous system to contribute to symptoms. Our thinking must be flexible and questioning in terms of our knowledge of the anatomy, biomechanics and pathology of the nervous system, and what we discover with enquiry strategies, clinical reasoning processes and on physical examination. We need to appreciate the interplay between nervous system dysfunction and musculoskeletal disorders.

Tension testing provides the clinician with a simple and reliable examination procedure that explores the relationship between altered neural mechanics and symptomatology. Tension testing emphasizes the mechanical and physiological continuity of the nervous system, an often forgotten fact of significance to the correct diagnosis and treatment of many common vertebral and peripheral disorders. In combination with other routine joint, soft-tissue and neurological examination techniques, tension testing offers a comprehensive means of assessment of neuro-orthopaedic disorders.

REFERENCES

Adams C B T, Logue V 1971 Studies in cervical spondylitic myelopathy. Brain 94: 557–568

Bell A 1987 The upper limb tension test-bilateral straight leg raising—a validating manoeuvre for the upper limb tension test. Proceedings of the Fifth Biennial Conference of the Manipulative Therapists' Association of Australia, Melbourne

Breig A 1978 Adverse mechanical tension in the central nervous system. Almqvist & Wiksell, Stockholm

Breig A, Marions O 1963 Biomechanics of the lumbosacral nerve roots. Acta Radiologica 1 Diagnosis 1141–1160

Breig A, Troup J D G 1979 Biomechanical considerations in the straight-leg-raising test. Spine 4: 242–250

Butler D S 1985 The effects of age and gender on the slump test. Unpublished thesis, South Australian Institute of Technology, Adelaide

Butler D S 1991 Mobilisation of the nervous system. Churchill Livingstone, Edinburgh

Cassvan A, Rosenberg A, Rivers L F 1986 Ulnar nerve involvement in carpal tunnel syndrome. Archives of Physical Medicine and Rehabilitation 67: 290–292

Cyriax J 1942 Perineuritis. British Medical Journal 578–580

Cyriax J 1978 Textbook of orthopaedic medicine, 7th edn. Baillière Tindall, London, vol 1

Dahlin L B, McLean W G 1986a Effects of graded experimental compression on slow and fast axonal transport in rabbit vagus nerve. Journal of the Neurological Sciences 72: 19–30

Dahlin L B, Sjostrand J, McLean W G 1986b Graded inhibition of retrograde axonal transport by compression of rabbit vagus nerve. Journal of the Neurological Sciences 76: 221–230

Davidson S 1987 Prone knee bend: an investigation into the effect of cervical flexion and extension. In: Dalziel B A, Snowsill J C (eds) Proceedings of the Manipulative Therapists' Association of Australia, Fifth Biennial Conference, Melbourne

Dyck P 1984 Lumbar nerve root: the enigmatic eponyms. Spine 9: 3–6

Elvey R L 1979 Painful restriction of shoulder movement: a clinical observational study. In: Proceedings, Disorders of the knee, ankle and shoulder. Western Australian Institute of Technology, Perth

Elvey R L, Quintner J L, Thomas A N 1966 A clinical study of RSI. Australian Family Physician 15: 1314–1322

Estridge M N, Rouhe S A, Johnson N G 1982 The femoral nerve stretching test. Journal of Neurosurgery 57: 813–817

Fardy E 1985 The upper limb tension test and the effect of passive movement of the head in sagittal and coronal planes in young asymptomatic subjects. Unpublished thesis, South Australian Institute of Technology, Adelaide

Ginn K 1989 An investigation of tension development in upper limb soft tissues during the upper limb tension test. In: Proceedings of the International Federation of Orthopaedic Manipulative Therapists' Congress, Cambridge

Goddard M D, Reid J D 1965 Movements induced by straight leg raising in the lumbosacral roots, nerves and plexuses and in the intra-pelvic section of the sciatic nerve. Journal of Neurology, Neurosurgery and Psychiatry 28: 12–18

Grant A 1983 The slump test. Unpublished thesis, South Australian Institute of Technology, Adelaide

Gunn C C 1980 Prespondylosis and some pain syndromes following denervation supersensitivity. Spine 5: 185–192

Gunn C C, Milbrandt W E 1978 Early and subtle signs in 'low back sprain'. Spine 3: 267–281

Hurst L C, Weissberg D, Carroll R E 1985 The relationship of the double crush to carpal tunnel syndrome (an analysis of 1000 cases of carpal tunnel syndrome). Journal of Hand Surgery 10B: 202–204

Inman V T, Saunders J B 1942 The clinico-anatomical aspects of the lumbosacral region. Radiology 38: 669–678

Kenneally M 1985 The upper limb tension test: In: Proceedings of the Manipulative Therapists' Association of Australia, Fourth Biennial Conference, Brisbane pp 259–273

Kenneally M, Rubenach H, Elvey R 1988 The upper limb tension test: the SLR test of the arm. In: Grant R (ed) Physical therapy of the cervical and thoracic spine. Clinics in physical therapy 17. Churchill Livingstone, Edinburgh

Landers J 1987 The upper limb tension test. In: Dalziel B A, Snowsill J C (eds), Proceedings of the Fifth Biennial Conference of the Manipulative Therapists' Association Australia, Melbourne

Leung A L 1983 Effects of cervical lateral flexion on the slump test in normal young subjects. Unpublished thesis, South Australian Institute of Technology, Adelaide

Lew P C 1979 The straight leg raise and lumbar stiffness. Unpublished thesis, South Australian Institute of Technology, Adelaide

Lew P C, Puentedura E J 1985 The straight-leg-raise test and spinal posture. In: Proceedings of the Fourth Biennial Conference of the Manipulative Therapists' Association of Australia, Brisbane, pp 259–273

Louis R 1981 Vertebroradicular and vertebromedullar dynamics. Anatomia Clinica 3: 1–11

Luk K D K, Pun W K 1987 Unrecognized compartment syndrome in a patient with a tourniquet palsy. Journal of Bone and Joint Surgery 69B 1: 97–99

Lundborg G 1988 Nerve injury and repair. Churchill Livingstone, Edinburgh

Mackinnon S E, Dellon A L 1988 Surgery of the peripheral nerve. Thieme, New York

McLellan D C, Swash M 1976 Longitudinal sliding of the median nerve during movements of the upper limb. Journal of Neurology, Neurosurgery and Psychiatry 39: 556–570

Macnab I 1971 The whiplash syndrome. Orthopaedic Clinics of North America 2: 389–403

Maitland G D M 1979 Negative disc exploration: positive canal signs. Australian Journal of Physiotherapy 25: 129–134

Maitland G D M 1986 Vertebral manipulation, 5th edn. Butterworths, London

Miller A M 1987 Neuro-meningeal limitation of straight leg raising. In: Dalziel B A, Snowsill J C (eds) Proceeding of the Fifth Biennial Conference of the Manipulative Therapists' Association of Australia, Melbourne

Nobel W 1966 Peroneal palsy due to haematoma in the common peroneal nerve sheath after distal torsional fractures and inversion ankle sprains. Journal of Bone and Joint Surgery 48A: 1484–1495

O'Connell J E A 1946 The clinical signs of meningeal irritation. Brain LXIX: 9–21

Pechan J 1973 Ulnar nerve manoevre as a diagnostic aid in its pressure lesions in the cubital region. Ceskoslovenska Neurologie 36: 13–19

Pechan J, Julius F 1975 The pressure measurement in the ulnar nerve: a contribution to the pathophysiology of cubital tunnel syndrome. Journal of Biomechanics 8: 75–79

Penning L, Wilmink J 1981 Biomechanics of the lumbosacral dural sac. Spine 6: 398–408

Quintner J L 1989 A study of upper limb pain and parathesiae following neck injury in motor vehicle accidents: assessment of the brachial plexus tension test of Elvey. British Journal of Rheumatology 28: 528–533

Reid J D 1960 Effects of flexion-extension movements of the head and spine upon the spinal cord and nerve roots. Journal of Neurology, Neurosurgery and Psychiatry 23: 214–221

Rubenach H 1985 The upper limb tension test: the effect of the position and movement of the contralateral arm. In: Proceedings of the Manipulative Therapists' Association of Australia, Fourth Biennial Conference, Brisbane

Rubenach H 1987 The upper limb tension test. In: Proceedings of the World Congress of Physical Therapy, Sydney

Rydevik B, McLean W G, Sjostrand J, Lundborg G 1980 Blockage of axonal transport induced by acute graded compression of the rabbit vagus nerve. Journal of Neurology, Neurosurgery and Psychiatry 43: 690–698

Rydevik B L, Myers R R, Powell H C 1988 Tissue fluid pressure in the dorsal root ganglion. An experimental study on the effects of compression. Proceedings of the 34th Annual Meeting of the Orthopaedic Research Society, Atlanta Georgia, p 135

Selander D, Mansson L G, Karlsson L et al 1985 Adrenergic vasoconstriction in peripheral nerves in the rabbit. Anesthesiology 62: 6–10

Selvaratnam P J, Glasgow E F, Matyas T 1989 Differential strain produced by the brachial plexus tension test on C5 to T1 nerve roots. In: Jones H M, Jones M A, Milde M (eds) Proceeding of the Manipulative Therapists' Association of Australia, Sixth Biennial Conference, Adelaide

Shacklock M O 1989 The plantarflexion/inversion SLR. Unpublished thesis, South Australian Institute of Technology, Adelaide

Slater H 1989 The effect of foot and ankle position on the SLR responses. In: Jones H, Jones M A, Milde M (eds) Proceedings of the Sixth Biennial Conference of the Manipulative Therapists' Association of Australia, Adelaide

Smith C G 1956 Changes in length and posture of the segments of the spinal cord with changes in posture in the monkey. Radiology 66: 259–265

Styf J R 1988 Diagnosis of exercise induced pain in the anterior aspect of the lower leg. American Journal of Sports Medicine 16: 165-169

Sunderland S 1976 The nerve lesion in carpal tunnel syndrome. Journal of Neurology, Neurosurgery and Psychiatry 39: 615–626

Sunderland S 1978 Nerve and nerve injuries, 2nd edn. Churchill Livingstone, Edinburgh

Sutton J L 1979 The straight leg raising test. Unpublished thesis, South Australian Institute of Technology, Adelaide

Tencer A N, Allen B L, Ferguson R L 1985 A biomechanical study of thoracolumbar spine fractures with bone in the canal. Part III. Mechanical properties of the dura and its tethering ligaments. Spine 10: 741–747

Troup J D G 1981 Straight-leg-raising (SLR) and the qualifying tests for increased root tension. Spine 6: 526–527

Troup J D G 1986 Biomechanics of the lumbar spinal canal. Clinical Biomechanics 1: 31–43

Wilgis E F S, Murphy R 1986 The significance of longitudinal excursion in peripheral nerves. Hand Clinics 2: 761–766

Woodhall B, Hayes G J 1950 The well leg raising test of Fajersztajn in the diagnosis of ruptured intervertebral disc. Journal of Bone and Joint Surgery 32A: 786–792

Yaxley G A, Jull G A 1991 A modified upper limb tension test: an investigation of responses in normal subjects. Australian Journal of Physiotherapy 37: 143–152

Young L 1989 The upper limb tension test response in a group of post Colle's fracture patients. Unpublished thesis, South Australian Institute of Technology, Adelaide

45. Modern imaging of the spine: the use of computed tomography and magnetic resonance

M. J. Warren

During the last two decades exciting advances in imaging have revolutionized the investigation of spinal disorders. X-ray technology has reached its zenith in the form of computed tomography (CT), and magnetic resonance imaging (MRI) is the most significant development since the discovery of X-rays by Roentgen in 1895. The first human in vivo images were obtained using CT in 1973 (Ambrose & Hounsfield 1973), and four years later using MRI (Damadian 1971, Hinshaw et al 1977, Mansfield & Maudsley 1977). CT is now widely available but the dispersion of MRI has been slower because of its expense and the technical limitations of early machines.

In the first section of this chapter the imaging methods applicable to the spine will be briefly reviewed, and the second section will concentrate on pathology as demonstrated by CT and MRI.

IMAGING TECHNIQUES

Investigation for each patient must be planned individually with knowledge of their symptoms, signs and provisional clinical diagnosis. It behoves those who request investigations, which may be unpleasant or potentially hazardous, to consider how the result will affect patient management. CT and MRI are both sensitive techniques which may detect abnormalities unrelated to the current clinical condition. This factor must be considered before abandoning further investigation or advising surgical intervention.

Plain radiographs

Low-back pain has an annual prevalence of between 2 and 5% with an incidence of 80% (Nachemson 1985) resulting in numerous requests for radiographs the value of which must be critically assessed. Many of these radiographs will show signs of degenerative disc disease but similar changes may be found in asymptomatic patients (Magora & Schwartz 1976, McNab 1977, Biering-Sorensen et al 1985, Frymoyer et al 1986). Similarly, in the cervical spine McRae (1960) found that more than 50% of patients over 40 years had degenerative spondyloarthropathy which correlated poorly with symptoms.

The main purpose of lumbar spine radiography is that it may detect other pathology such as spondylolisthesis, ankylosing spondylitis, vertebral collapse, metastasis and Scheuermann's disease (McNab 1977, Nachemson 1985). However, radiographs have poor sensitivity and provide limited information mostly about bony structures; thus they are a poor method of excluding pathology.

The medical use of ionizing radiation has significant carcinogenic and genetic risks (NRPB 1990). Patient dosage may be reduced by avoiding unnecessary repeat radiographs and limiting projections. In the lumbar spine for instance a single lateral projection has been advocated (Eisenberg et al 1979) and if CT is planned plain radiographs may be omitted since equivalent information is provided by the scout or topogram. Digital imaging requires considerable financial outlay but delivers a lower radiation dose than conventional radiography and has been advocated for the follow up of scoliosis (Kushner et al 1986, Kling et al 1990).

Ultrasound

In adults the bony elements of the vertebral column provide a poor acoustic window to the spinal canal. Attempts have been made to measure spinal canal dimensions (Porter et al 1978) and assess spinal stenosis (Engel et al 1985) but ultrasound is of little use in the individual patient (Nachemson 1985).

Ultrasound (US) has poor sensitivity compared with other methods in the detection of lumbar disc herniation (Merx et al 1989a).

Intra-operative US is useful for monitoring manoeuvres during surgical treatment of spinal fractures (Quencer et al 1985), cervical cord trauma (Mirvis & Geisler 1990), lumbar disc herniation and spinal stenosis (Montalvo et al 1990), extradural abscess (Donovan Post et al 1988) and tumours of the spinal cord (Quencer et al 1984).

The incompletely ossified posterior spinal elements of normal infants and those with spina bifida enable US examination of the spinal canal. Meningocoele, myelomeningocoele and intraspinal lipomas may be identified and postoperative assessment of residual lipoma is possible (Naidich et al 1983a, Scheible et al 1983, Rubin et al 1988). However, despite its simplicity and safety, ultrasound cannot be used as the sole imaging method in dysraphism but rather as an adjunct to CT and MRI.

Nuclear medicine

Bone scintigraphy may be used to confirm abnormality suspected on other investigations or as a screening technique in patients with back pain of obscure origin. Metastases, infection and arthritides are examples of pathology which are well displayed, although the appearances may be non-specific (Fogelmann 1989, Holder 1990).

Myelography

Myelography entails the injection of water-soluble iodinated contrast media into the subarachnoid space either by lumbar puncture or lateral puncture in the cervical spine at C1/C2. It is unpleasant for the patient and made more difficult if they are immobile due to paraplegia, rheumatoid disease, ankylosing spondylitis or scoliosis. Infants and some children may require general anaesthesia or sedation. Traditionally a short in-patient stay has been advised post-myelography because of side-effects such as nausea, vomiting and dizziness and headache reported in 20–30% of patients (Grainger 1983). More recent data indicate a lower incidence of side-effects, and outpatient myelography has been demonstrated to be safe (Tate et al 1985, Vezina et al 1989, Boulos & Free 1991). If neurological examination fails to localize the spinal segmental level of abnormality myelography is a quick method of examining the whole spinal cord.

Myelography shows the normal nerve roots and spinal cord indirectly as filling defects surrounded by radiopaque contrast (Fig. 45.13a). Pathology is also detected indirectly because of distortion or displacement of these structures. Myelography followed by CT (MYELO-CT, Fig. 45.13a,b) may provide additional information, although Dublin et al (1983) found it useful in only 40% of cases. In the lumbar spine MYELO-CT must be delayed for several hours to allow dilution of intrathecal contrast and thus reduce artefact.

Computed tomography

CT produces cross-sectional grey scale images of the body based on the X-ray attenuation produced by its constituent tissues. Attenuation values are expressed in Hounsfield Units (HU) on a scale of −1000 to +1000 relative to water—which has a value of zero at the centre of the scale. The other conventional radiographic densities of air, fat and calcium have a characteristic range of HU by which they may be identified. Since the human eye can distinguish only about 20 grey tones the video image must be manipulated to display different tissues to best advantage. The *window width* selects the width of the band of HU that is displayed in grey scale form, thus altering the image contrast. The *window level* specifies the central value of this band and affects which type of tissue is optimally displayed.

CT has far superior contrast resolution compared to conventional radiography and it is this factor coupled with the cross-sectional imaging capability which accounts for the impact of CT despite its spatial resolution being inferior to conventional radiography (Anderson & Berland 1989). Scan planes are limited by the positions in which the body can be placed in the gantry aperture and by the range of gantry angulation (usually ± 25°).

A digital radiograph (*topogram* or *scout*) is first produced to facilitate selection of section thickness and interval, examination area and gantry angulation. Decreasing the section thickness increases the spatial resolution at the expense of increased noise, producing a 'grainy' image. Section interval is closely related to the section thickness and the site and type of pathology being sought. Scan time for each section varies according to machine specification but may be as short as one second. A longer scan time increases image quality at the expense of increased radiation dose and a greater risk of encountering movement artefact. Unco-operative adults and children may require sedation or general anaesthesia.

The major hazard of CT is its high radiation dose (Katz 1987) which varies according to examination technique and machine type (Nishizawa et al 1991). Recent British data indicate that CT (all body parts) and lumbar spine radiography contribute 17% and 15% respectively of the total collective radiation dose to the population from all medical X-ray examinations (NRPB 1990). While the image quality of modern machines is superior to that of earlier generation machines this improvement has been achieved at the expense of higher radiation doses.

The data obtained during an axial scan can be reformatted in other planes or used to produce three-dimensional images (3D CT). The spatial and contrast resolution of reformatted images is inferior to that of axial images, and for best results thin contiguous sections are required—thus increasing the radiation dose. 3D CT is not in routine use because it consumes much computer time (Wojick et al 1987), although improvements in computing may change this situation.

Most spinal CT examinations are non-invasive but they may be augmented by the use of intravenous or intrathecal water-soluble iodinated contrast. The newer low osmolarity contrast media produce fewer adverse reactions when injected intravenously than do high osmolarity media (Grainger 1984), but they still carry a small risk of a fatal anaphylactic reaction (Grainger & Dawson 1990). In the lumbar spine the theca and nerve roots can usually be identified because of the presence of abundant extrathecal fat; elsewhere, intrathecal contrast is required for reliable identification of these structures.

A limitation of the CT cross-sectional plane is that the suspected level of abnormality must be well localized since it is not practical to examine long segments of spine. A routine lumbar spine examination for disc prolapse extends from L3/4 to L5/S1 and will miss a conus medullaris lesion which would require MYELO-CT of the thoracolumbar junction for detection. However, Love (1944) found that only 5% of patients with spinal cord tumours presented with clinical features of disc protrusion. Additional features of a more proximal lesion are often present and Heitoff (1990) considered that in practice this disadvantage of CT is not a major problem.

CT may be used to guide a biopsy needle to a site of pathology by measuring the depth and angle of safe approach from the CT image. Cervical vertebral (Kattapuram & Rosenthal 1987) and lumbar intradural extramedullary lesions (Castillo & Quencer 1988) have been biopsied under CT guidance. However, for vertebral lesions fluroscopic guidance of a large-bore cutting needle is often simpler and obtains a larger sample for histology or microbiological examination (Stoker & Kissin 1985, Cotty et al 1988).

Table 45.1 shows the advantages and disadvantages of CT and contraindications to its use.

Magnetic resonance imaging

The physical basis has been well described (Balter 1987, Fullerton 1987, Merritt 1987, Pavlicek 1987, Porter et al 1987, Lufkin 1990a) and only a brief outline follows.

MRI is based on the magnetic spin properties of hydrogen atoms and their recovery after excitation by radiofrequency electromagnetic radiation while in a powerful uniform magnetic field. Hydrogen with a single proton in its nucleus has a strong magnetic moment, and because of its abundance in the body (mostly in the form of water or fat) it is utilized for MRI.

The strength of the magnetic resonance signal emitted from a particular tissue depends on many factors including proton density, molecular composition and flow effects such as occur in blood vessels or cerebrospinal fluid (CSF). Brief radio frequency pulses are applied in complex sequences which exploit the differences in these factors so that various tissues can be distinguished by the strength of the emitted signal.

The spin–echo sequence is commonly used and the recovery (or relaxation) of protons after excitation can be measured by the time constants T1 and T2. These are determined by the rate at which protons lose energy by two distinct mechanisms:

1. T1 Dissipation of the energy into the overall molecular environment also known as *spin–lattice* or *longitudinal* relaxation
2. T2 Energy exchange between protons also known as *spin–spin* or *transverse* relaxation.

Pulse sequence parameters are varied to produce images based on signal strength and which are predominantly dependent on either the T1 or T2 values of the body tissues and these are referred to as T1- or T2-weighted images (T1 W or T2 W).

Acquisition time for T2 W images is longer than for T1 W images but the use of gradient echo (GE) techniques shortens acquisition time whilst providing similar information to T2 W images.

In recent years there has been a remarkable improvement in MRI image quality along with a shortening of examination time due to advances in equipment, pulse sequences and artefact suppression. MRI was once considered lengthy and prohibitively expensive, but since it may replace other, invasive investigations, and high patient throughput is possible with modern systems, these objections are now no longer valid.

Unlike CT, the grey scale ordering of the tissues on MRI is not constant and depends on the conditions of measurement. However, tissues with a low proton density such as cortical bone (or calcium), fibrous tissue, tendons and air have a low signal whatever pulse sequence is used; thus, they appear as dark areas. Tissues with high proton density such as fats and fluids have a variable appearance. As a broad approximation, T1 W images are sensitive to fat and show excellent anatomical detail. T2 W or GE images are more influenced by water and demonstrate pathology which generally alters the water content of tissues. Sagittal T2 W or GE images of the spine have a superficial resemblance to a myelogram since the high signal intensity CSF appears white and surrounds a darker (lower signal intensity) cord or cauda equina and this

Table 45.1 Advantages and disadvantages of, and contraindications to, CT

Advantages of CT
Good tissue contrast
Good bony detail
Guided biopsy quick

Disadvantages of CT
Ionizing radiation
Limited scan planes
Artefact from metallic implants and prostheses
Intrathecal contrast often needed in thoracic and cervical region

Contraindications to CT
Pregnancy unless maternal health jeopardized

is sometimes referred to as the 'myelographic effect' (Figs 45.7, 45.9).

The main advantages of MRI over CT are its superior soft tissue contrast and multiplanar capability achieved non-invasively without the use of ionizing radiation. Sagittal plane MRI is ideal when the segmental level of abnormality is uncertain and, for example, the whole lumbar spine and the conus can be included in one examination. Phased array surface coils are now available (Kricun et al 1990) which allow simultaneous sagittal imaging of all spinal segments without moving the patient. However, at present most MRI units require separate consecutive examinations of cervical, thoracic and lumbar regions to cover an entire adult spine. Volume acquisition MRI allows rapid reformation of data in any plane after the examination (Kricun et al 1990). MRI-guided biopsy is possible (Duckwiler et al 1989, Gronemeyer et al 1990) but at present CT guidance is simpler and quicker.

Successful MRI examination requires a co-operative patient who will remain still for several minutes (e.g. 2–10 minutes depending on imaging sequence and MRI unit design). Sedation may be required and sometimes enables examination of claustrophobic patients.

Intravenous gadolinium has been shown to be a safe MRI contrast agent with minimal side-effects (Goldstein et al 1990), and there has been only a single reported case of severe anaphylactic reaction (Lufkin 1990b). Gadolinium alters the local magnetic field within body tissues and accelerates both T1 and T2 relaxation (Gibby 1988) but its practical use is for T1 W imaging. Abnormal contrast enhancement with gadolinium (i.e. tissue appears brighter on the grey scale T1 W image obtained after gadolinium compared to the T1 W image before gadolinium) either reflects increased tissue vascularity or breakdown of the blood/central nervous system barrier (Figs 45.11, 45.14).

The operation of an MRI unit poses potential hazards to both patients and staff because of the powerful magnetic field. The most dramatic of these is the projectile effect by which ferromagnetic objects may be attracted to the magnet at high velocity. Cardiac pacemakers malfunction in a magnetic field and are an absolute contraindication to MRI (Shellock 1988, Kanal et al 1990). Certain ferromagnetic prostheses, implants and foreign bodies also contraindicate MRI. With adequate safety precautions MRI has no known adverse effects and is the preferred method of spinal imaging in pregnancy. Although there is no definite evidence of teratogenic effects at the magnetic field strengths used in clinical imaging, MRI is generally avoided during the first trimester provided that maternal health is not jeopardized. However, continued vigilance is required regarding possible adverse effects (NRPB 1991).

Table 45.2 shows the advantages and disadvantages of MRI and contraindications to its use.

Table 45.2 Advantages and disadvantages of, and contraindications to, MRI

Advantages of MRI
Excellent tissue contrast
Multiplanar capability
No known adverse effects
Safe in pregnancy

Disadvantages of MRI
Expense/lack of availability
Artefact—patient movement, cardiac, respiratory and CSF motion, metallic implants
Cortical bone and calcium poorly seen
Potential claustrophobia

Contraindications to MRI
Cardiac pacemakers
Cardiac valve prostheses*
Intravascular coils*
Intracranial surgical clips*
Cochlear implants*
Foreign bodies
    Metallic intra-ocular
    Bullets near vital structures**
† Obesity
    weight limit, e.g. 135 kg
    excessive girth, e.g. magnet bore diameter 55 cm
Artificial ventilation, special apparatus required

---

* Shellock 1988—depending on degree of ferromagnetism.
** Teitelbaum et al 1990.
† These limits vary with MRI unit design.

PATHOLOGY

Vertebral body and ligaments

Trauma

Plain radiographs should be performed initially since the whole spine may be rapidly surveyed, and in severe trauma multiple contiguous or distant levels are involved in up to 20% of cases (Calenoff et al 1978, Korres et al 1981). In adults, fractures most commonly occur in the following segments: C1 to C2, C5 to C7 and T12 to L1 (Jefferson 1928, Calenoff et al 1978) which may be difficult to demonstrate on plain radiographs, especially in an immobile patient. Further information may be obtained using conventional tomography (TOMO) or CT, and these techniques may be complimentary. Movement of a patient with an unstable spinal injury may produce or worsen neurological deficit, and CT involves less disturbance to the patient than TOMO. TOMO allows several vertebral levels to be surveyed simultaneously and both fractures of C2 and cervical vertebral facets may be more easily appreciated on TOMO than on CT (Fagan & Rogers 1990). Sagittal reformatting and 3-D CT may aid understanding of some complex cervical injuries (Wojick et al 1987).

CT is the best method of demonstrating the full extent of vertebral fractures (Angtuaco & Binet 1984, Acheson et al 1987), especially those involving the posterior elements, and it allows assessment of bony encroachment on the spinal canal (Fig. 45.1). Vertically orientated fractures are

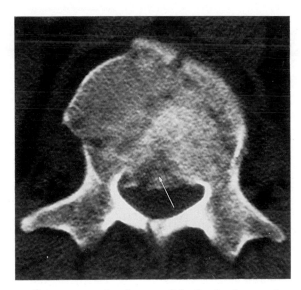

Fig. 45.1 Burst compression fracture of the first lumbar vertebra: axial CT. Arrow = retropulsed bone fragments narrowing spinal canal. There is also a fracture through the neural arch on the right.

well demonstrated by CT but those in the axial plane may be missed or difficult to appreciate.

Once a level of injury has been located its stability must be assessed. Whitesides (1977) defined stable injuries as those able to withstand stress without progressive deformity or further neurological damage. In the three-column model of thoracolumbar fractures (Denis 1984) the middle column consists of the posterior longitudinal ligament, posterior annulus fibrosus and posterior part of the vertebral body. If the middle column is intact the injury is, in general, a stable one.

In 17% of cases with neurological signs of traumatic cord injury no obvious fracture or dislocation can be seen radiologically (Riggins & Kraus 1977). Many such cases are caused by hyperextension injury of the cervical spine (Scher 1976, Schneider et al 1954, Selecki 1970), and elderly patients with pre-existing narrowing of the spinal canal due to degenerative disease are particularly susceptible. When signs of spinal cord dysfunction are present further investigation is required to detect remediable conditions such as intervertebral disc herniation or extradural haematoma.

Many pieces of life-support apparatus will not function in a strong magnetic field, and patients with unstable injuries may need transportation to an MRI unit. In addition, some traction devices and braces are ferromagnetic and produce artefacts (Clayman et al 1990). As a result, MYELO-CT has often seemed more practical, although this situation is changing due to the development of MRI compatible equipment.

MRI is superior to CT myelography in the detection of cervical disc herniation but inferior to CT in the detection of fractures—especially those of the posterior elements (Mirvis et al 1988). On sagittal MRI vertebral mal-

alignment is more easily appreciated than it is on axial CT, although sagittal reformatting provides similar information.

MRI directly demonstrates injuries to the spinal cord, intervertebral discs and ligaments which would be undetected by other methods (Davis et al 1991). T1 W images are required to demonstrate the anatomy of the cord and ligamentous structures, and T2 W images are most sensitive for the detection of parenchymal lesions. Abnormalities detected in the traumatized cord range from signal changes thought to represent oedema, haemorrhage, infarction or necrosis through to complete cord transection (Gebarski et al 1985, Beers et al 1988, Goldberg et al 1988, Mirvis et al 1988). The acute appearances may give clues regarding prognosis (Bondurant et al 1990, Yamashita et al 1990). Late complications which may cause clinical deterioration such as syrinx formation (Fig. 45.2) and cord atrophy may be assessed with MRI (Yamashita et al 1990).

Brachial plexus injuries often result from road traffic accidents and produce persistent disability. MYELO-CT

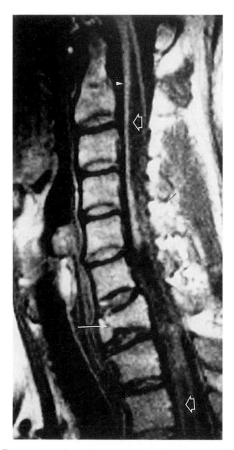

Fig. 45.2 Post-traumatic syrinx, cervical cord: sagittal MRI T1 W. The cord has been severely disrupted at the level of the fracture and the patient was paraplegic. Arrow = flexion compression tear-drop fracture of the seventh cervical vertebra with displacement of bone fragments into the spinal canal; arrowhead = CSF; open arrow = syrinx in cervical and thoracic cord (both CSF and syrinx are fluid and are of low signal intensity so that they appear black).

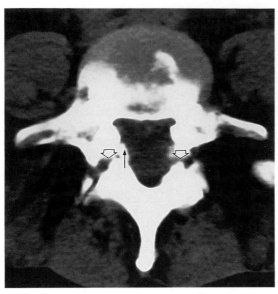

Fig. 45.3 Spondylolisthesis of the fifth lumbar vertebra: axial CT. Open arrows = pars interarticularis defects; arrow = bone fragments and callus.

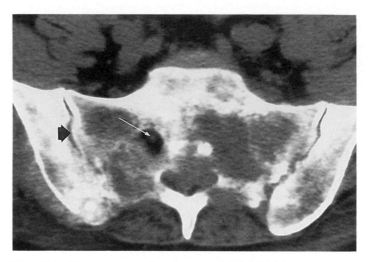

Fig. 45.4 Bone metastases in sacrum: axial CT. Multiple lytic metastases with soft-tissue masses involving the left S1 root and the sacral canal. White arrow = normal right S1 nerve root in bony canal; black arrow = right sacro-iliac joint.

is useful for detecting only intradural nerve root lesions (Roger et al 1988) and is limited by the axial plane and artefact from shoulders (Gebarski et al 1982). MRI displays distal brachial plexus anatomy and pathology including fibrosis, neuroma and meningocoele (Gupta et al 1989). MRI may become the investigation of choice for surgical planning, but it needs further evaluation.

The aetiology of spondylosis and spondylolisthesis is a source of controversy but is probably the result of repetitive trauma (Newman & Stone 1963). CT is the best method of demonstrating the bony defect of the pars interarticularis (Fig. 45.3) and any adjacent bone fragments (Rothman & Glenn 1984). While MRI will also demonstrate the pars interarticularis defect, the adjacent bone fragments, which may produce nerve root impingement, are poorly delineated (Grenier et al 1989a). Complications of spondylolisthesis such as spinal stenosis and degenerative disease of the facet joints and intervertebral discs may be demonstrated using CT or MRI. The multiplanar capability and superior soft tissue contrast of MRI may prove to be advantageous, but further research is required.

Neoplasia

Plain radiographs are an insensitive method of detecting vertebral metastasis (Edelsyn et al 1967) and are unreliable for distinguishing between benign and malignant vertebral compression deformities. Bone destruction by metastases can be demonstrated on CT and is useful in areas such as the sacrum (Fig. 45.4) which are difficult to assess on radiographs.

Bone scintigraphy may be equivocal, and MRI

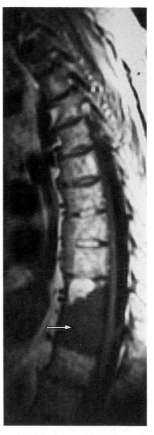

Fig. 45.5 Bone metastases (carcinoma of the prostate), thoracic spine: sagittal MRI T1 W. Arrow = metastases (low signal intensity dark grey) involving part of D9 and the whole of D10. Normal vertebrae have higher signal intensity (light grey) because of fat in marrow.

(Fig. 45.5) is the most reliable technique for detecting metastases (Avrahami et al 1989, Baker et al 1990, Algra et al 1991).

Primary vertebral tumours are much rarer, but Beltran

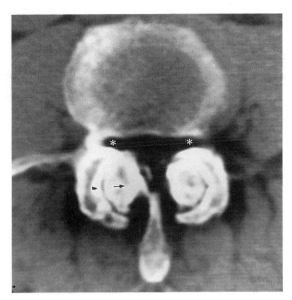

Fig. 45.6 Facet joint hypertrophy, lumbar spine L3/4: axial CT. The central canal has become trefoil in shape and both lateral recesses are narrow. Arrow = right inferior articular process of L3; arrowhead = right superior articular process of L4; asterisks = narrow lateral recesses.

et al (1987) found MRI to be superior to CT and equivalent to MYELO-CT for assessment of the extent of disease, although CT provided better demonstration of critical bone destruction.

Arthropathy

Facet joint osteoarthritis (Fig. 45.6), which is well demonstrated by CT (Carrera et al 1980), may cause low-back pain, and facet joint injection with local anaesthetic has been advocated as a diagnostic test (Lewinnek & Warfield 1986).

The cervical spine is frequently affected in rheumatoid disease and cord compression may occur. Methods of investigation prior to surgery have included plain radiographs, myelography and CT myelography (Stevens et al 1986).

MRI demonstrates the relationship of the odontoid peg to the skull base and narrowing of the spinal canal due to vertebral subluxation. In addition, distortion of ligaments, fat pads and bursae due to either bony displacement or extradural soft-tissue masses (pannus) is uniquely displayed by MRI. The degree of compression of the medulla and cord along with signal changes in the cord probably due to oedema may be directly demonstrated with MRI (Aisen et al 1987, Bundschuh et al 1988, Pettersson et al 1988, Larsson et al 1989a). After flexion and extension radiographs have been performed in order to assess stability, MRI is the preferred method for further evaluation of rheumatoid myelopathy.

The cauda equina syndrome is a rare complication of ankylosing spondylitis but may be more common than has been previously believed. MYELO-CT demonstrates the characteristic bony erosions and arachnoid diverticula (Mitchell et al 1990) but the diagnosis may also be made using CT and MRI without the need for intrathecal contrast (Abello et al 1988, Rubenstein et al 1989).

Atlanto-axial subluxation is another rare complication of ankylosing spondylitis which has been demonstrated by CT when conventional radiographs were not diagnostic (Leventhal et al 1990).

Spinal stenosis

The spinal canal may be congenitally narrow, as an isolated feature, or may occur in skeletal dysplasias such as achondroplasia. More often stenosis is acquired due to a combination of factors which are especially significant when superimposed on a congenitally narrow canal. Degenerative spondylosis, buckling of the ligamentum flavum and hypertrophic arthropathy of the facet joints may narrow the central canal or lateral recess (Fig. 45.6). After leaving the thecal sac the nerve roots pass through the lateral recess to exit via foramina beneath the pedicles. The nerve roots are immobile and may be compressed by hypertrophic superior articular facets (Helbig & Casey 1988, Schellinger et al 1987). Other acquired causes of spinal stenosis include Paget's disease, trauma and malignant disease of the vertebrae.

On T1 W MRI ostephytes may have either high signal intensity, if they contain fatty marrow, or a low signal intensity if there is bony sclerosis (Grenier et al 1989b). The latter type may be confused with other capsulo-ligamentous structures or degenerate intervertebral disc. At present, MRI is not as sensitive as MYELO-CT for the detection of lateral recess stenosis (Epstein et al 1990) but further research is required.

Intervertebral disc pathology

Degenerative

On plain radiographs degenerative disc disease can be inferred from loss of disc space height and vertebral end-plate osteophytosis, but osteophytes alone are not a reliable indicator (Quinnell & Stockdale 1982). In severe degeneration, gas (vacuum phenomenon, Knutsson 1942, Resnick 1985), or calcification, may be seen within the disc space on plain radiographs or CT. Disc degeneration results in facet joint arthrosis, ligamentous and capsular hypertrophy, spinal instability and eventually spinal stenosis (Harris & McNab 1954, Schellinger et al 1987).

Discography was once the best method of detecting abnormality of the intervertebral disc; it involves passing a needle into the disc under fluroscopic control and injecting iodinated contrast. Conventional radiography (Lindbloom 1951, Brodsky et al 1979) or CT (Schneiderman et al 1987, Bernard 1990) is then performed. Important functional information may be obtained by careful monitoring of symptom reproduction during the procedure (provocative discography, Simmons & Segil 1975, Colhoun et al 1975).

MRI provides a unique anatomical display of the intervertebral disc (Yu & Haughton 1990) and allows detection of the subtle and early changes of disc degeneration. The normal nucleus of the intervertebral disc contains 85–90% water, and the annulus contains 80% water, (Lipson & Muir 1981a, b). On T2 W or GE images the normal disc has a high signal intensity and appears white. In degenerate discs the amount of water in both components of the disc is reduced to about 70% and there are complex biochemical changes. As a result there is loss of signal so that the disc appears darker on T2 W or GE images (Fig. 45.7). Further study of the signal changes may enable characterization of the biochemical changes (Modic et al 1984, 1988). Gas or calcium within the disc produce a signal void on MRI (Grenier et al 1987) but these features are more reliably demonstrated by CT or plain radiographs. Disc degeneration also results in signal changes in the adjacent vertebral body marrow (Aoki et al 1987, de Roos et al 1987, Modic et al 1988).

MRI has been shown to be as accurate as discography in detecting disc degeneration (Gibson et al 1986, Schneiderman et al 1987). Discography requires multiple injections whereas the preferred technique of sagittal MRI demonstrates several levels non-invasively (Modic et al 1988). Abnormal discographic morphology with normal MRI has been reported (Zucherman et al 1988) although such discs may be asymptomatic (Collins et al 1990). If MRI identifies several degenerate discs and surgery is planned then provocative discography is required to identify those responsible for symptoms as this cannot be predicted from the MRI appearance (Collins et al 1990). However, MRI generally reduces the number of levels at which discography is required.

An intact annulus fibrosus is important for maintenance of disc integrity and annular tears may lead to disc degeneration (Friberg 1948, Hirsch & Schajowicz 1952).

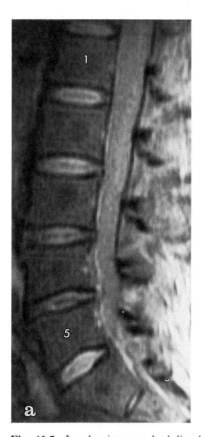 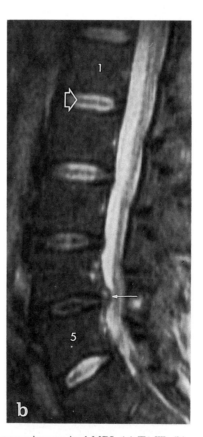

Fig. 45.7 Lumbar intervertebral disc degeneration: sagittal MRI. (**a**) T1 W, (**b**) gradient echo demonstrating the lower signal (dark grey) from desiccated L3/4 and L4/5 discs compared to normal discs at levels above and below. There is mild loss of height at the L4/5 disc space with a small disc bulge indenting the theca. Axial images showed no evidence of root compression. Note 'myelographic' effect (CSF of high signal intensity appears white). Arrow = posterior longitudinal ligament/outer annulus complex and L4/5 disc bulge; open arrow = normal intervertebral disc with central low signal intensity band (internuclear cleft).

Annular tears may cause back pain (Vanharanta et al 1988); however, Yu et al (1988) found a high prevalence of annular tears in cadavers suggesting that they are not always symptomatic. There is also controversy regarding the relative sensitivities of discography and MRI in the detection of annular tears, but in a cadaver study (Yu et al 1989) MRI demonstrated only two-thirds of the tears seen on discography. Further research on the significance and imaging of annular tears is required.

Myelography has been used for over 50 years in the diagnosis of lumbar disc herniation (Hampton & Robinson 1936). CT allows direct demonstration of a herniated disc as effectively as myelography (Haughton et al 1982, Schipper et al 1987). However, there has been considerable controversy regarding the relative merits of the techniques (Bell et al 1984, Aprill 1985, Heitoff 1985, Raskin 1985, Rothman & Glenn 1985, Rothman et al 1986, Weitz 1985, Wiesel 1985, Kardaun et al 1989).

There are two well recognized sources of myelographic error in diagnosis of lumbar disc herniation. Myelography has poor sensitivity for far lateral disc herniation which compresses the exiting nerve root after it has lost its thecal covering, and, at the L5/S1 level, disc prolapse may occur without indentation of the theca because of the large extradural space (Haughton et al 1982, Schipper et al 1987). In view of these drawbacks, and its non-invasive nature, CT (Fig. 45.8) is preferable to myelography as a first-line investigation in suspected disc prolapse (Schipper et al 1987). Sources of error on CT include conjoined nerve roots (Peyster et al 1985) misinterpreted as herniated disc, and large central disc herniation may be difficult to appreciate (Buirski 1989). In the majority of cases CT provides equivalent information to MYELO-CT but the latter may be useful if there is discrepancy between CT findings and the patient's symptoms (Fagerlund 1988).

MRI is as accurate as CT for the detection of lumbar disc herniation (Fig. 45.9) and lumbar canal stenosis (Modic et al 1986a). MRI demonstrates the outer annulus/posterior longitudinal ligaments complex as a very low signal thin line in contrast to the inner annulus/nucleus pulposus (Figs 45.7, 45.9). Disruption of the posterior longitudinal ligament may be reliably identified on MRI (Grenier et al 1989b) enabling classification of disc herniation which is important for therapeutic decisions and determining prognosis (Masaryk et al 1988). A disc herniation through a defect in the posterior longitudinal ligament into the spinal canal may become completely detached from its parent nucleus. This is referred to as a *sequestered* disc and surgical treatment is preferred as chemonucleolysis (Gentry et al 1985) or percutaneous discectomy (Onik et al 1985, Kahanovitz et al 1990) may be ineffective.

Most disc herniations occur posteriorly or posterolaterally, but 1–11% of lumbosacral disc herniations are lateral or extraforaminal. While they are poorly detected by myelography they may also be overlooked on CT (Fig. 45.10) or MRI if the entity is not fully appreciated (Osborn et al 1988). Epstein et al (1990) found that myelography and MYELO-CT was superior to CT and MRI in identification of lateral recess stenosis coexisting with lateral disc herniation. However, in the young patient who is unlikely to have lateral recess stenosis MRI is the investigation of choice for suspected lumbar disc herniation.

Before the advent of MRI, myelography followed by CT was the usual method of investigation for suspected thoracic disc herniation. Symptomatic thoracic disc herniation may be demonstrated with similar accuracy using MRI (Ross et al 1987) although the distinction between osteophyte, low signal degenerate disc or meningioma may not be possible. Gadolinium may be helpful in diagnosis since meningioma shows enhancement while disc material itself does not, although epidural veins adjacent to herniated disc may be enhanced (Parizel et al 1989a).

Thoracic disc herniation is regarded as rare but Williams et al (1989a) have reported a 14.5% prevalence of asymptomatic thoracic disc herniation in oncology patients undergoing MRI.

CT without intrathecal contrast is of little use in the diagnosis of nerve root or cervical cord compression due to spondylosis. MYELO-CT is an accurate method of assessing these structures (Scotti et al 1983, Modic et al 1986b, Penning et al 1986) because it is able to distinguish bone from disc and demonstrate bony encroachment on the neuroforamina.

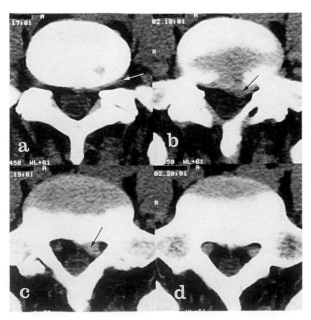

Fig. 45.8 Lumbar intervertebral disc herniation L5/S1: CT. **a-d.** Cranial to caudal sections at 5 mm intervals. White arrow = normal left L5 nerve root; black arrow = herniated disc material compressing the left S1 nerve root.

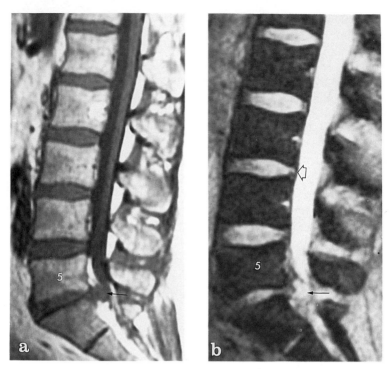

Fig. 45.9 Lumbar intervertebral disc herniation L5/S1: sagittal MRI.
(**a**) T1 W, (**b**) gradient echo (note 'myelographic' effect). Open arrow =
posterior longitudinal ligament/outer annulus complex; arrow = large disc
herniation which, on axial images, was seen to compress the left S1 nerve root.

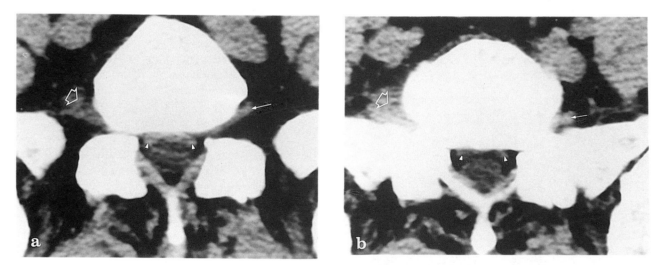

Fig. 45.10 Far lateral lumbar intervertebral disc herniation L5/S1: axial CT; (**b**) is 5 mm caudal to (**a**) Arrow = normal left L5 nerve
root; open arrow = herniated disc material compressing the right L5 nerve root lateral to exit foramen; arrowheads = normal S1 nerve
roots.

The role of MRI in cervical radiculopathy is still under investigation. MRI has inferior spatial resolution compared to CT using the same field of view and is unable reliably to distinguish between osteophyte and disc material. Modic et al (1986b) found MRI as sensitive as CT myelography for the identification of disease, but less specific—particularly so for lateral disc herniations (Karnaze et al 1987). Hedberg et al (1988), using GE imaging, found good correlation with CT myelography and surgery in cervical radiculopathy and proposed MRI as the initial procedure of choice for this condition. Further improvements in MRI sequences, such as 3-D gradient echo (Tsuruda et al 1990, Yousem et al 1991), show promise but need further evaluation.

Central cervical disc herniation is probably better demonstrated by MRI than CT myelography (Modic et al 1986b, Nakstad et al 1989). However, the clinical relevance of any abnormality must always be considered as MRI evidence of cervical disc degeneration and herniation may be found in asymptomatic individuals (Teresi et al 1987).

MRI demonstrates cord deformity, compression and atrophy secondary to cervical spondylosis (Nagata et al 1990). High signal intensity on T2 W images has been demonstrated; this is believed to correspond to gliosis, myelomalacia or demyelination. In other cases areas of low signal intensity on T1 W images are thought to represent cystic necrosis or secondary syrinx formation. It has been proposed that the high signal intensity on T2 W images is an early manifestation of myelopathy which is followed by cystic degeneration and finally syrinx formation and cord atrophy (Takahashi et al 1987, Al-Mefty et al 1988).

Postoperative spine

Persistent or recurrent symptoms following spinal surgery occur in 25–40% of patients (Djukic et al 1990). Important causes of the failed back surgery syndrome are failure to recognize or adequately treat lateral recess stenosis, recurrent or persistent disc herniation and arachnoiditis (Burton et al 1981). The distinction between postoperative fibrosis and recurrent disc herniation on CT may be difficult, and reoperation on scar tissue without associated disc material gives poor results (Finnegan et al 1979). The use of CT with intravenous iodinated contrast has been advocated (Teplick & Haskin 1983, Braun et al 1985) since, in general, fibrous tissue shows enhancement (i.e. increase in HU value so that tissue appears lighter on grey scale) but disc material does not. However, the degree of enhancement depends on the age of the scar, and disc material involved with granulation tissue may show enhancement (Bundschuh et al 1990). On the contrary, McKinstry & Bell (1991) concluded that non-contrast CT was sufficient for diagnosis of true recurrent disc prolapse in the majority of cases.

MRI enables the distinction between scar and disc material to be made on the basis of configuration and margination (Hochhauser et al 1988) and is more effective than enhanced CT (Sotiropoulos et al 1989). Ross et al (1990), using MRI pre- and postgadolinium, reported an accuracy of 96% in distinguishing scar tissue from disc material as the former shows enhancement while the latter does not (Fig. 45.11). The degree of enhancement of fibrous tissue is variable and images must be obtained immediately after injection of gadolinium since disc material may also enhance if there is a delay. The postoperative spine still presents a diagnostic challenge, but MRI using gadolinium as appropriate is the investigation of choice.

Infection

Radiographic abnormalities, which may be subtle, often occur late in the clinical course of spinal infection. Bone scintigraphy is sensitive early in the disease but is often

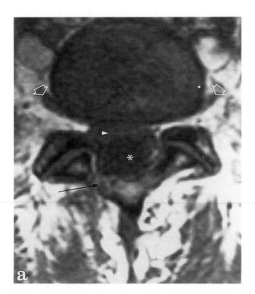
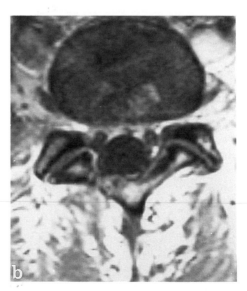

Fig. 45.11 Postoperative fibrosis, lumbar spine L4/5: axial MRI. T1 W (**a**) before gadolinium and (**b**) after gadolinium. Arrow = site of previous laminectomy for removal of herniated disc; open arrow = normal L5 nerve roots; asterisk = thecal sac; arrowhead = low-signal-intensity material surrounding both S1 nerve roots. This enhances (signal intensity increases and appears brighter) after gadolinium (b).

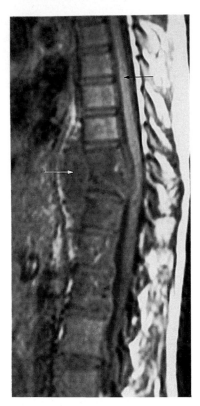

Fig. 45.12 Tuberculous osteomyelitis, thoracic spine: sagittal MRI T1 W. Five contiguous vertebrae are involved and have abnormally low signal (dark grey) compared to the marrow of normal vertebrae (light grey). There are large paravertebral and epidural abscesses, the latter producing distortion of the lower thoracic cord. (Black arrow = normal thoracic cord; white arrow = paravertebral mass. There is partial collapse of the vertebra just below the level of the white arrow.

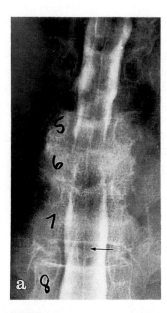

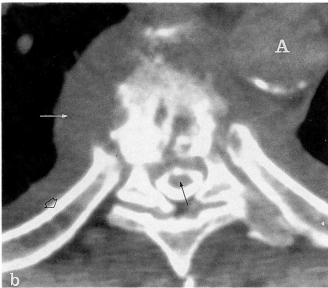

Fig. 45.13 Infective discitis and osteomyelitis, thoracic spine: (**a**) myelogram AP, (**b**) axial CT at D5/6 postmyelogram. (a) Black arrow = normal thoracic cord seen as filling defect outlined by contrast in subarachnoid space. More superiorly from D5–D7 the subarachnoid space appears incompletely filled. (b) White arrow = paravertebral mass with bone lysis in body of D5; black arrow = thoracic cord surrounded by contrast in subarachnoid space. The thecal sac is distorted anteriorly by an epidural abscess due to *Staphylococcus aureus*. A = descending thoracic aorta; open black arrow = right 5th rib.

non-specific and may be negative in early aggressive disease (Thrush & Enzmann 1990). Infection and neoplasm may be indistinguishable on radiographs but CT may clarify and more accurately defines the extent of disease (van Lom et al 1988). MRI demonstrates characteristic changes in discitis and osteomyelitis and is very sensitive (Fig. 45.12). Tuberculosis may mimic metastatic disease on MRI (Smith et al 1989), and although there may be certain distinguishing features (Thrush & Enzmann 1990) further experience is required. The presence of an epidural abscess increases morbidity and mortality and alters management. Detection of epidural abscess by MRI is not reliable (Modic et al 1985, Donovan-Post et al 1988) although the use of fat suppression techniques (Bertino et al 1988) or gadolinium (Donovan-Post et al 1990) may improve visualisation. If there is clinical suspicion of epidural abscess MYELO-CT (Fig. 45.13) is required for exclusion. However, MRI can be recommended as the primary investigation in suspected spinal infection as it is probably the most sensitive modality in the early stages of disease and best demonstrates its full extent. Biopsy is often required to obtain a histological or microbiological diagnosis and thus plan treatment.

Spinal cord and meningeal pathology

Extradural lesions

In cases of acute spinal cord compression emergency myelography, followed by CT of abnormal areas, was a standard method of investigation before the availability of MRI. Myelography may be technically difficult, and if there is a CSF block a second puncture may be required to demonstrate the upper and lower limits of a tumour and exclude a second level of involvement. MRI is a preferable technique in suspected spinal cord compression assuming that it can be performed without delay. Extradural cord compression due to metastatic disease is diagnosed by MRI with a degree of accuracy similar to that of myelography. MRI also demonstrates multiple levels of involvement more simply than myelography and is superior for the detection of metastatic disease involving bone marrow (Carmody et al 1989, Williams et al 1989b).

Intradural extramedullary lesions

Masses such as meningiomas and neurofibromas which displace and compress the spinal cord generally give a signal intensity similar to that of cord on T1 W and T2 W MRI. Both enhance with gadolinium and were easier to visualize (Parizel et al 1989b).

Chronic adhesive arachnoiditis has a variety of causes, including agents injected into the subarachnoid space (contrast media, anaesthetics, intradural steroids), infection, trauma, surgery and intrathecal haemorrhage (Quiles et al 1978). Among contrast agents, iophendylate (Myodil or Pantopaque), in particular, has been implicated and is no longer used (Occleshaw 1987). The correlation between CT myelography and MRI in moderate and severe cases of arachnoiditis is good (Delmarter et al 1990, Johnson & Sze 1990). Variable enhancement of affected nerve roots occurs with gadolinium but plays little role in diagnosis (Johnson & Sze 1990). In mild arachnoiditis the abnormality may be confined to one nerve root sheath, and MYELO-CT must be relied upon for diagnosis of these cases but further research is required.

A variety of primary malignancies metastasize to the leptomeninges, including those of breast, lung, gastrointestinal tract, skin (melanoma), haemopoietic system and paediatric brain (Wasserstrom et al 1982, Sorensen & Scott 1984). The presence of leptomeningeal metastasis will alter management, which may ameliorate symptoms and improve survival. Unenhanced MRI compares unfavourably with CT myelography in the detection of leptomeningeal metastases partly because of their small size (Barloon et al 1987, Davis et al 1988, Krol et al 1988). Preliminary experience suggests that the use of gadolinium (Sze et al 1988, 1989) improves the rate of detection of leptomeningeal metastases and may even demonstrate pial metastases (Lim et al 1990). Gadolinium enhanced MRI and MYELO-CT are probably equally sensitive (Blews et al 1990), but further experience is required to determine the rate of false-negatives with gadolinium enhanced MRI, and CSF cytology will continue to be necessary.

Intradural intramedullary lesions

Acute multiple sclerosis (MS) may produce cord swelling due to oedema and in chronic disease cord atrophy develops. Both of these features are well demonstrated on T1 W MRI. T2 W images may show MS plaques as elongated areas of high signal intensity which enhance after gadolinium when disease is clinically active (Larsson et al 1989b). However, MRI of the brain is usually performed to diagnose MS more reliably, even when there are clinical features suggesting spinal cord involvement.

Intramedullary neoplasms of the cord, such as astrocytoma and ependymoma, may be well defined by MRI but if they give a signal intensity similar to that of normal cord their limits are indistinct and cord expansion may be the major feature. After administration of gadolinium these tumours enhance (Fig. 45.14), enabling the limits of their margins to be defined, and solid components may be distinguished from cystic areas and syrinx (Slasky et al 1987, Valk 1988, Sze et al 1989, Dillon et al 1989, Parizel et al 1989b, Sze et al 1990). These distinctions aid planning of surgery or radiotherapy.

Intramedullary and perimedullary arteriovenous malformations with intramedullary extension may be demonstrated on MRI. The central nidus may show a flow void on T2 W images, and T1 W images may show haemorrhage above and below the nidus (Dormont et al 1988, Minami et al 1988, Dillon et al 1989). Gadolinium enhancement of vessels and the spinal cord in patients with myelopathy due to dural arteriovenous malformations has been observed (Terwey et al 1989). However, at present myelography is still indicated in all MRI negative

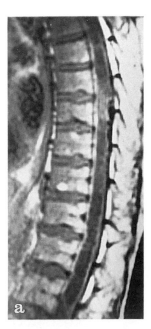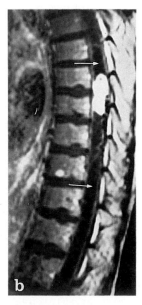

Fig. 45.14 Intramedullary primary neoplasm of thoracic cord: sagittal MRI T1 W (**a**) before and (**b**) after gadolinium. Intense enhancement of the tumour occurs after gadolinium, enabling its margins to be defined. White arrows = extensive syrinx throughout the thoracic cord.

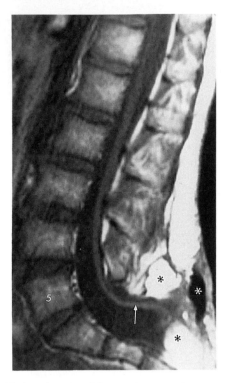

Fig. 45.15 Tethered cord and lipoma, lumbar spine; sagittal MRI T1 W. Arrow = tethered cord or filum terminale lying posteriorly. It was not possible to identify reliably the level of the conus in this case; black asterisks = associated lipoma; white asterisk = meningocoele.

cases, and spinal angiography remains the definitive investigation.

Congenital malformations

The term 'spinal dysraphism' refers to a heterogeneous collection of intrauterine developmental anomalies resulting from imperfect differentiation and fusion of midline dorsal structures. The best known form is meningomyelocoele, which is clinically apparent and involves cutaneous, mesodermal and neural elements. Occult spinal dysraphism includes abnormalities such as diastematomyelia, intra- and paraspinal masses including lipomas, dermoids and teratomas (Figs 45.15, 45.16).

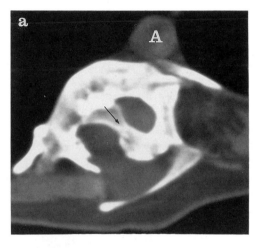

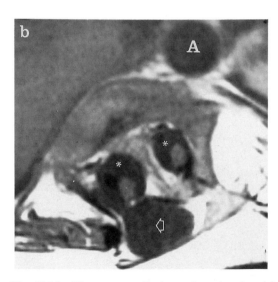

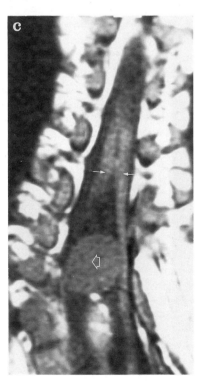

Fig. 45.16 Diastematomyelia, lower thoracic spine: (**a**) axial CT, (**b**) axial MRI, (**c**) coronal MRI. Black arrow = bony spur seen best on CT, but in this patient it is also well demonstrated on MRI; white arrows = two hemicords; open white arrow = intradural mass, probably a teratoma; asterisks = the two separate thecal sacs surrounding each hemicord; A = descending thoracic aorta.

In one series of patients with congenital scoliosis 18% had occult intraspinal anomalies (McMaster 1984). Patients may be asymptomatic or there may be an insidious and slowly progressive onset of complex neurological abnormalities. Before surgical correction of scoliosis occult dysraphism must be excluded as it is generally believed that neurological deficit may be induced unless intraspinal anomalies are also dealt with.

One major purpose of investigation is to detect a tethered cord (Fig. 45.15) since surgery is based on the thesis that freeing a tethered cord will halt neurological deterioration. According to conventional teaching the normal lower level of the conus medullaris is L3 at birth and it ascends throughout childhood to reach L1 by adulthood (Harwood-Nash & Fitz 1976). On the contrary, MRI (Wilson & Prince 1989) has shown that the conus medullaris does not ascend throughout childhood and attains the adult level during the first few months of life. A conus level of L2/3 or above is normal at any age, but with a conus level of L3 the cord may be normal or tethered.

Until recently the standard method of investigation in dysraphism was myelography with or without CT. Myelography has a good correlation with surgical findings, and MYELO-CT improves the demonstration of neural tissue–CSF relationships and bony anomalies including diastematomyelia spurs (Naidich & Harwood-Nash 1983, Naidich et al 1983b, Rothwell et al 1987, Scatcliff et al 1989, Merx et al 1989b).

MRI correlates well with surgical findings in dysraphism (Altman & Altman 1987) and is the investigation of choice (Doyon et al 1987, Davis et al 1988, Raghavan et al 1989, Tortori-Donati et al 1990). Dysraphism is also associated with anomalies of the cerebella tonsils and medulla oblongata (Arnold-Chiari malformation) and MRI is the definitive investigation for this condition. In complex scoliosis multiple imaging planes may be required but further development of volume acquisition may simplify examination. Certain intradural mass lesions, such as lipomas (Fig. 45.15), have characteristic appearances. MYELO-CT may still be necessary if more detailed information about the disposition of neural tissue is required. The spur of diastematomyelia (Fig. 45.16) may be fibrous, cartilaginous or bony, and difficult to detect on MRI, and the use of CT will resolve equivocal cases.

Acknowledgements

I would like to acknowledge my colleagues Dr S Barker, Dr R Bodley, Dr A J Molyneux and Dr N R Moore for their assistance in collecting the illustrations.

REFERENCES

Abello R, Rovira M, Sanz M P et al 1988 MRI and CT of ankylosing spondylitis with vertebral scalloping. Neuroradiology 30: 272–275

Acheson M B, Livingston R R, Richardson M L et al 1987 High resolution CT scanning in the evaluation of cervical spine fractures: comparison with plain film examinations. American Journal of Roentgenology 148: 1179–1185

Aisen A M, Martel W, Ellis J H et al 1987 Cervical spine involvement in rheumatoid arthritis: MR imaging. Radiology 165: 159–163

Algra P R, Bloem J L, Tissing H et al 1991 Detection of vertebral metastases: comparison between MR imaging and bone scintigraphy. Radiographics 11: 219–232

Al-Mefty O, Harkey L H, Middleton T H et al 1988 Myelopathic cervical spondylitic lesions demonstrated by magnetic resonance imaging. Journal of Neurosurgery 68: 217–222

Altman N R, Altman D H 1987 MR imaging of spinal dysraphism. American Journal of Neuroradiology 8: 533–538

Ambrose J, Hounsfield H 1973 Computerized transverse axial tomography. British Journal of Radiology 46: 148–149

Anderson D J, Berland L 1989 CT techniques. In: Lee J K T, Sagel S S, Stanley R J (eds) Computed body tomography with MRI correlation, 2nd edn. Raven Press, New York, ch 3, p 35

Angtuaco J C, Binet E F 1984 Radiology of thoracic and lumbar fractures. Clinical Orthopaedics and Related Research 189: 43-57

Aoki J, Yamamoto I, Kitamura N et al 1987 End plate of the discovertebral joint: degenerative change in the elderly adult. Radiology 164: 411–414

Aprill C 1985 Editorial: on CT scanning and metrizamide myelography. Spine 10: 691–692

Avrahami E, Tadmor R, Daily O et al 1989 Early MR demonstration of spinal metastases in patients with normal radiographs and CT and radionuclide bone scans. Journal of Computer Assisted Tomography 13: 598–602

Baker L L, Goodman S B, Perkash I et al 1990 Benign versus pathological compression fractures of vertebral bodies: assessment with conventional spin-echo, chemical shift, and STIR MR imaging.

Radiology 174: 495–502

Balter S 1987 An introduction to the physics of magnetic resonance imaging. Radiographics 7: 371–383

Barloon T J, Yuh W T C, Yang C J C et al 1987 Spinal subarachnoid tumour seeding from intracranial metastasis: MR findings. Journal of Computer Assisted Tomography 11: 242–244

Beers G J, Raque G H, Wagner G G et al 1988 MR imaging in acute cervical spine trauma. Journal of Computer Assisted Tomography 12: 755–761

Bell G R, Rothman R H, Booth R E et al 1984 A study of computer-assisted tomography II. Comparison of metrizamide myelography and computed tomography in the diagnosis of herniated lumbar disc and spinal stenosis. Spine 9: 552–556

Beltran J, Noto A M, Chakeres D W et al 1987 Tumours of the osseous spine: staging with MR imaging versus CT. Radiology 162: 565–569

Bernard T N 1990 Lumbar discography followed by computed tomography refining the diagnosis of low back pain. Spine 15: 690–707

Bertino R E, Porter B A, Stimac G K et al 1988 Imaging of spinal osteomyelitis and epidural abscess with short T1 inversion recovery (STIR). American Journal of Neuroradiology 9: 563–564

Biering-Sorenson F, Rolstead Hansen F, Schroll M et al 1985 The relation of spinal X-ray to low back pain and physical activity among 60-year-old men and women. Spine 10: 445–451

Blews D E, Wang H, Kumar A J et al 1990 Intradural spinal metastases in pediatric patients with primary intracranial neoplasms: Gd-DTPA enhanced MR vs CT myelography. Journal of Computer Assisted Tomography 14: 730-735

Bodurant F J, Cotler H B, Kulkarni M V et al 1990 Acute spinal cord injury: a study using physical examination and magnetic resonance imaging. Spine 15: 161–168

Boulos R S, Free T W 1991 Outpatient iohexol lumbar, cervical and total column myelography in 883 patients. Neuroradiology 33 (suppl): 89–91

Braun I F, Hoffman J C, Davis P C et al 1985 Contrast enhancement in CT between recurrent disk herniation and post operative scar: prospective study. American Journal of Neuroradiology 6: 607–612

Brodsky A E, Binder W F 1979 Lumbar discography its value in diagnosis and treatment of lumbar disc lesions. Spine 412: 110–120

Buirski G 1989 Giant central disc prolapse: a pitfall in computed tomographic diagnosis. British Journal of Radiology 62: 274–276

Bundschuh C, Modic M T, Kearney F et al 1988 Rheumatoid arthritis of the cervical spine: surface coil MR imaging. American Journal of Neuroradiology 9: 565–571

Bundschuh C V, Stein L, Slusser J H et al 1990 Distinguishing between scar and recurrent herniated disc in postoperative patients: value of contrast-enhanced CT and MR imaging. American Journal of Neuroradiology 11: 949–958

Burton C V, Kirkaldy-Willis W H, Yong-Hing K et al 1981 Causes of failure of surgery on the lumbar spine. Clinical Orthopaedics and Related Research 157: 191–199

Calenoff L, Chessare J W, Rogers L F et al 1978 Multiple level spinal injuries: importance of early recognition. American Journal of Roentgenology 130: 665–699

Carmody R F, Yang P J, Seely G W et al 1989 Spinal cord compression due to metastatic disease: diagnosis with MR imaging versus myelography. Radiology 173: 225–229

Carrera G F, Haughton V M, Syvertsen A et al 1980 Computed tomography of the lumbar facet joints. Radiology 134: 145–148

Castillo M, Quencer R M 1988 Percutaneous needle evaluation of intradural extramedullary lesions of the lumbar spine. Neuroradiology 30: 551–555

Clayman D A, Murakami M E, Vines F S 1990 Compatibility of cervical spine braces with MR imaging: a study of nine nonferrous devices. American Journal of Neuroradiology 11: 385–390

Colhoun E, McCall I W, Williams L et al 1975 Provocative discography as a guide to planning operations on the spine. Journal of Bone and Joint Surgery 70B: 267–271

Collins C D, Stack J P, O'Connell D J et al 1990 The role of discography in lumbar disc disease: a comparative study of magnetic resonance imaging and discography. Clinical Radiology 42: 252–257

Cotty Ph, Fouquet B, Pleskoff L et al 1988 Vertebral osteomyelitis: value of percutaneous biopsy. Journal of Neuroradiology 15: 3–21

Damadian R 1971 Tumour detection by nuclear magnetic resonance. Science 171: 1151–1153

Davis P C, Hoffman J C, Ball T I et al 1988 Spinal abnormalities in paediatric patients: MR imaging findings compared with clinical, myelographic and surgical findings. Radiology 166: 679–685

Davis S J, Teresi L M, Bradley W C et al 1991 Cervical spine hyperextension injuries: MR findings. Radiology 180: 245–251

Delmarter R B, Ross J S, Masaryk T J et al 1990 Diagnosis of lumbar arachnoiditis by magnetic resonance imaging. Spine 15: 304–310

Denis F 1984 Spinal instability as defined by the three column spine concept in acute spinal trauma. Clinical Orthopaedics and Related Research 189: 65–76

de Roos A, Kressel H, Spritzer C et al 1987 MR imaging of marrow changes adjacent to end plates in degenerative lumbar disc disease. American Journal of Roentgenology 149: 531–534

Dillon W P, Norman D, Newton T H et al 1989 Intradural spinal cord lesions: Gd-DTPA-enhanced MR imaging. Radiology 170: 229–237

Djukic S, Genant H K, Helms C A et al 1990 Magnetic resonance imaging of the postoperative spinal cord. Radiologic Clinics of North America 28: 341–360

Donovan Post M J, Quencer R M, Montalvo B M et al 1988 Spinal infection: evaluation with MR imaging and intraoperative US. Radiology 169: 765–771

Donovan-Post M J, Sze G, Quencer R M et al 1990 Gadolinium-enhanced MR in spinal infection. Journal of Computer Assisted Tomography 14: 721–729

Dormont D, Gelbert F, Assouline E et al 1988 MR imaging of spinal cord arteriovenous malformations at 0.5 T study of 34 cases. American Journal of Neuroradiology 9: 833–838

Doyon D, Sigal R, Poylecot G et al 1987 MRI of spinal cord congenital malformations. Journal of Neuroradiology 14: 185–201

Dublin A B, McGahan J P, Reid M H 1983 The value of computed tomography metrizamide myelography in the neuroradiological

evaluation of the spine. Radiology 146: 79–86

Duckwiler G, Lufkin R B, Teresi L et al 1989 Head and neck lesions: MR guided aspiration biopsy. Radiology 170: 519–522

Edelsyn G A, Gillespie P J, Grebell F S 1967 The radiological demonstration of osseous metastases. Experimental observations. Clinical Radiology 18: 158–165

Eisenberg R L, Akin J R, Hedgecock M W 1979 Single, well centered lateral view of lumbosacral spine: is coned view necessary? American Journal of Roentgenology 133: 711–713

Engel J M, Engel E, Gunn D R 1985 Ultrasound of the spine in focal stenosis and disc disease. Spine 10: 928–933

Epstein N E, Epstein J A, Carras R et al 1990 Far lateral lumbar disc herniations and associated structural abnormalities an evaluation in 60 patients of the comparative value of CT, MRI, and myelo-CT in diagnosis and management. Spine 15: 534–539

Fagan J, Rogers F 1990 Spinal trauma. Current Imaging 2: 31–41

Fagerlund M K J 1988 Computed tomography in low back pain before and after myelography. Acta Radiologica 29: 353–356

Finnegan W J, Fenlin J M, Marvel J P et al 1979 Results of surgical intervention in the symptomatic multiply-operated back patient. Journal of Bone and Joint Surgery 61-A: 1077–1082

Fogelmann I 1989 Radionuclide imaging in the assessment of bone disease. Current Imaging 1: 119–127

Friberg S 1948 Anatomical studies on lumbar disc degeneration. Acta Orthopaedica Scandinavica 17: 224–230

Frymoyer J W, Phillips R B, Newberg A H et al 1986 A comparative analysis of the interpretations of lumbar spinal radiographs by chiropractors and medical doctors. Spine 11: 1020–1023

Fullerton G D 1987 Magnetic resonance imaging signal concepts. Radiographics 7: 579–596

Gebarski K S, Glazer G M, Gebaski S S 1982 Brachial plexus: anatomic, radiologic and pathologic correlation using computed tomography. Journal of Computer Assisted Tomography 6: 1058–1063

Gebarski S S, Maynard F W, Gabrielsen T O et al 1985 Post-traumatic progressive myelopathy. Radiology 157: 379–385

Gentry L R, Strother C M, Turski P A et al 1985 Chymopapain chemonucleolysis: correlation of diagnostic radiographic factors and clinical outcome. American Journal of Neuroradiology 6: 311–320

Gibby W A 1988 MR contrast agents: an overview. Radiologic Clinics of North America 26: 1047–1058

Gibson M J, Buckley J, Mawhinney R et al 1986 Magnetic resonance imaging and discography in the diagnosis of disc degeneration. Journal of Bone and Joint Surgery 68-B: 369–373

Goldberg A L, Rothfus W E, Deeb Z L et al 1988 The impact of magnetic resonance on the diagnostic evaluation of acute cervicothoracic spinal trauma. Skeletal Radiology 17: 89–95

Goldstein H A, Kashanian F K, Blumetti R F et al 1990 Safety assessment of gadopentetate dimeglumine in US clinical trials. Radiology 174: 17–23

Grainger, R G 1983 The spinal canal. In: Whitehouse G H, Worthington B S (eds) Techniques in diagnostic radiology. Blackwell Scientific Publications, Oxford, ch 18, p 280

Grainger, R G 1984 The clinical and financial implications of the low-osmolar radiological contrast media. Clinical Radiology 35: 251–252

Grainger R G, Dawson P 1990 Editorial: Low osmolar contrast media: an appraisal. Clinical Radiology 42: 1–5

Grenier N, Grossman R I, Schiebler M L et al 1987 Degenerative lumbar disc disease: pitfalls and usefulness of MR imaging in the detection of vacuum phenomenon. Radiology 164: 861–865

Grenier N, Kressel H Y, Schiebler M L et al 1989a Isthmic spondylolysis of the lumbar spine: MR imaging at 1.5 T. Radiology 170: 489–493

Grenier N, Greselle J-F, Vital J-M et al 1989b Normal and disrupted lumbar longitudinal ligaments: correlative MR and anatomic study. Radiology 171: 197–205

Gronemeyer D H W, Seibel R M M, Kaufman L 1990 Interventional MRI cracks device and design barriers. Diagnostic Imaging International 6: 32–36

Gupta R K, Mehta V S, Banerji A K et al 1989 MR evaluation of brachial plexus injuries. Neuroradiology 31: 377–381

Hampton A O, Robinson J M 1936 The roentgenographic demonstration of rupture of the intervertebral disc into the spinal canal after injection of lipiodol. American Journal of Roentgenology 36: 782–803

Harris R I, McNab I 1954 Structural changes in the lumbar intervertebral discs their relationship to low back pain and sciatica. Journal of Bone and Joint Surgery 36-B: 304–322

Harwood-Nash D C, Fitz C R 1976 Myelography. In: Neuroradiology in infants and children. C V Mosby, St Louis, p 1133

Haughton V M, Eldevik O P, Magnaes B et al 1982 A prospective comparison of computed tomography and myelography in the diagnosis of herniated lumbar discs. Radiology 142: 103–110

Hedberg M C, Drayer B P, Flom R A et al 1988 Gradient echo (GRASS) MR imaging in cervical radiculopathy. American Journal of Neuroradiology 9: 145–151

Heitoff K B 1985 Editorial: On CT scanning and metrizamide myelography. Spine 10: 692–693

Heitoff K B 1990 Computed tomography and plain film diagnosis of the lumbar spine. In: Weinstein J N, Weisel S W (eds) The Lumbar Spine. W B Saunders, Philadelphia, p 315

Helbig T, Casey C K 1988 The lumbar facet syndrome. Spine 13: 61–64

Hinshaw W S, Bottomley P A, Holland G N 1977 Radiographic thin section of the human wrist by nuclear magnetic resonance. Nature 270: 722 –723

Hirsch C, Schajowicz F 1952 Studies on structural changes in the lumbar annulus fibrosus. Acta Orthopaedica Scandinavica 22: 184–231

Hochhauser L, Kieffer S A, Cacayorin E D et al 1988 Recurrent postdiskectomy low back pain: MR-surgical correlation. American Journal of Neuroradiology 9: 769–774

Holder L E 1990 Clinical radionuclide bone imaging. Radiology 176: 607–614

Jefferson G 1928 Discussion on spinal injuries. Proceedings of the Royal Society of Medicine 21: 21–44

Johnson C E, Sze G 1990 Benign lumbar arachnoiditis: MR imaging with gadopentelate dimeglumine. American Journal of Neuroradiology 11: 763–770

Kahanovitz N, Viola K, Goldstein T et al 1990 A multicenter analysis of percutaneous discectomy. Spine 15: 713–715

Kanal E, Shellock F G, Talagala L 1990 Safety considerations in MR imaging. Radiology 176: 593–606

Kardaun J W P F, Schipper J, Braakman R 1989 CT, myelography, and phlebography in the detection of lumbar disc herniation: an analysis of the literature. American Journal of Neuroradiology 10: 1111–1112

Karnaze M G, Gado M H, Sartor K J 1987 Comparison of MR and CT in imaging the cervical and thoracic spine. American Journal of Neuroradiology 8: 983–989

Kattapuram S V, Rosenthal D I 1987 Percutaneous biopsy of the cervical spine using CT guidance. American Journal of Roentgenology 149: 539–541

Katz D 1987 Computed tomography. In: Ansell G, Wilkins R A (eds) Complications in diagnostic imaging, 2nd edn. Blackwell Scientific Publications, Oxford, ch 25, pp 362–363

Kling T F, Cohen M J, Lindseth R E et al 1990 Digital radiography can reduce scoliosis X-ray exposure. Spine 15: 880–885

Knutsson F 1942 The vacuum phenomenon in the intervertebral discs. Acta Radiologica 23: 173–179

Korres D S, Katasara A, Pontazopoulous T et al 1981 Double or multiple level fractures of the spine. Injury 13: 147–152

Kricun R, Kricun M E, Dalinka M K 1990 Advances in spinal imaging. Radiologic Clinics of North America 28: 321–339

Krol G, Sze G, Malkin M et al 1988 MR of cranial and spinal meningeal carcinomatosis: comparison with CT and myelography. American Journal of Neuroradiology 9: 709–714

Kushner D C, Cleveland R H, Herman T E et al 1986 Radiation dose reduction in the evaluation of scoliosis: an application of digital radiography. Radiology 161: 175–181

Larsson E M, Holtas S, Zygmunt S 1989a Pre- and postoperative MR imaging of the craniocervical junction in rheumatoid arthritis. American Journal of Neuroradiology 10: 89–94

Larsson E M, Holtas S, Nilsson O 1989b Gd-DTPA-enhanced MR of suspected spinal multiple sclerosis. American Journal of Neuroradiology 10: 1071–1076

Leventhal M R, Maguire J K, Christian C A 1990 Atlantoaxial rotatory subluxation in ankylosing spondylitis. Spine 15: 1374–1376

Lewinnek G E, Warfield C A 1986 Facet joint degeneration as a cause of low back pain. Clinical Orthopaedics and Related Research 213: 216–222

Lim V, Sobel D, Zyroff J 1990 Spinal cord plial metastases: MR imaging with gadopentetate dimeglumine. American Journal of Neuroradiology 11: 975–982

Lindbloom K 1951 Backache and its relation to ruptures of the intervertebral disks. Radiology 57: 710–719

Lipson S J, Muir H 1981a Experimental intervertebral disc degeneration morphologic and protoglycan changes over time. Arthritis and Rheumatism 24: 12–21

Lipson S J, Muir H 1981b Proteoglycans in experimental intervertebral disc degeneration. Spine 6: 194–210

Love J G 1944 The differential diagnosis of intraspinal tumours and protruded intervertebral disks and their surgical treatment. Journal of Neurosurgery 1: 275–290

Lufkin R B 1990a The MRI manual. Year Book Medical Publishing Inc, Chicago

Lufkin R B 1990b Severe anaphylactoid reaction to Gd-DTPA. Radiology 176: 879

McKinstry C S, Bell K E 1991 CT of the postoperative lumbar spine: is contrast enhancement necessary? Neuroradiology 33 (suppl): 95–96

McMaster M J 1984 Occult intraspinal anomalies and congenital scoliosis. Journal of Bone and Joint Surgery 66-A: 588–601

McNab I 1977 Backache. Williams & Wilkins, Baltimore, Maryland, ch 8, pp 131–132

McRae D L 1960 The significance of abnormalities of the cervical spine. American Journal of Roentgenology 84: 3–25

Magora A, Schwartz A 1976 Relation between the low back pain syndrome and X-ray findings. Scandinavian Journal of Rehabilitation Medicine 8: 115–125

Mansfield P, Maudsley A A 1977 Medical imaging by NMR. British Journal of Radiology 50: 188–194

Masaryk T J, Ross J S, Modic M T et al 1988 High-resolution MR imaging of sequestered lumbar intervertebral discs. American Journal of Neuroradiology 9: 351–358

Merritt C R B 1987 Magnetic resonance imaging—a clinical perspective: image quality, safety and risk management. Radiographics 7: 1001–1016

Merx J L, Thijssen H O M, Meyer R et al 1989a Accuracy of ultrasonic evaluation of lumbar intervertebral discs by an anterior approach. Neuroradiology 31: 386–390

Merx J L, Bakker-Niezen S H, Thijssen H O M et al 1989b The tethered spinal cord syndrome: a correlation of radiological features and peroperative findings in 30 patients. Neuroradiology 31: 63–70

Minami S, Sagoh T, Nishimura K et al 1988 Spinal arteriovenous malformation: MR imaging. Radiology 169: 109–115

Mirvis S E, Geisler F H 1990 Intraoperative sonography of cervical spinal cord injury: results in 30 patients. American Journal of Neuroradiology 11: 755–761

Mirvis S E, Geisler F H, Jelinek J J et al 1988 Acute cervical spine trauma evaluation with 1.5-T MR imaging. Radiology 166: 807–816

Mitchell M J, Sartoris D J, Moody D et al 1990 Cauda equina syndrome complicating ankylosing spondylitis. Radiology 175: 521–525

Modic M T, Pavlicek W, Weinstein M A et al 1984 Magnetic resonance imaging of intervertebral disc disease clinical and pulse sequence considerations. Radiology 152: 103–111

Modic M T, Feiglin D H, Piraino D W et al 1985 Vertebral osteomyelitis: assessment using MR. Radiology 157: 157–166

Modic M T, Masaryk T, Boumphrey F et al 1986a Lumbar herniated disc disease and canal stenosis: prospective evaluation by surface coil MR, CT and myelography. American Journal of Neuroradiology 7: 709–717

Modic M T, Masaryk T J, Mulopulos G P et al 1986b Cervical radiculopathy: prospective evaluation with surface coil MR imaging, CT with metrizamide, and metrizamide myelography. Radiology 161: 753–759

Modic M T, Masaryk T J, Ross J S et al 1988 Imaging of degenerative disc disease. Radiology 168: 177–186

Montalvo B M, Quencer R M, Brown M D et al 1990 Lumbar disc herniation and canal stenosis: value of intraoperative sonography in diagnosis and surgical management. American Journal of Neuroradiology 11: 31–40

Nachemson A 1985 Advances in low back pain. Clinical Orthopaedics and Related Research 200: 266–278

Nagata K, Kiyonaga K, Ohashi T et al 1990 Clinical value of magnetic resonance imaging for cervical myelopathy. Spine 15: 1088–1096

Naidich T P, Harwood-Nash D C 1983 Diastematomyelia: hemicord and meningeal sheaths; single and double arachnoid and dural tubes. American Journal of Neuroradiology 4: 633–636

Naidich T P, McLone D G, Shkolnik A et al 1983a Sonographic evaluation of caudal spinal anomalies in children. American Journal of Neuroradiology 4: 661–664

Naidich T P, McLone D G, Mutluer S 1983b A new understanding of dorsal dysraphism with lipoma (lipomyeloschsis): radiologic evaluation and surgical correction. American Journal of Roentgenology 140: 1065–1078

Nakstad P H, Hald J K, Bakke S J et al 1989 MRI in cervical disc herniation. Neuroradiology 31: 382–385

Newman P H, Stone K H 1963 The aetiology of spondylolisthesis. Journal of Bone and Joint Surgery 45-B: 39–59

Nishizawa K, Maruyama T, Takayama M et al 1991 Determinations of organ doses and effective dose equivalents from computed tomographic examination. British Journal of Radiology 64: 20–28

NRPB 1990 Patient dose reduction in diagnostic radiology. Documents of the National Radiological Protection Board 1(3)

NRPB 1991 Board statement on clinical magnetic resonance diagnostic procedures. Documents of the National Radiological Protection Board 2(1)

Occleshaw J V 1987 Myelography and cisternography. In: Ansell G, Wilkins R A (eds) Complications in diagnostic imaging, 2nd edn. Blackwell Scientific Publications, Oxford, ch 21, pp 313–314

Onik G, Helms C A, Ginsburg L et al 1985 Percutaneous lumbar disectomy using a new aspiration probe. American Journal of Roentgenology 144: 1137–1140

Osborn A G, Hood R S, Sherry R G et al 1988 CT/MR spectrum of far lateral and anterior lumbosacral disc herniations. American Journal of Neuroradiology 9: 775–778

Parizel P M, Baleriaux D, Zegers de Beyl D et al 1989a Gd-DTPA-enhanced MR in thoracic disc herniations. Neuroradiology 31: 75–79

Parizel P M, Baleriaux D, Rodesch G et al 1989b Gd-DTPA-enhanced MR imaging of spinal tumours. American Journal of Neuroradiology 10: 249–258

Pavlicek W 1987 MR instrumentation and image formation. Radiographics 7: 809–814

Penning L, Wilmink J T, van Woerden H H et al 1986 CT myelographic findings in degenerative disorders of the cervical spine: clinical significance. American Journal of Neuroradiology 7: 119–127

Pettersson H, Larson E M, Holtas et al 1988 MR imaging of the cervical spine in rheumatoid arthritis. American Journal of Neuroradiology 9: 573–577

Peyster R G, Teplick J G, Haskin M E 1985 Computed tomography of lumbosacral conjoined nerve root anomalies potential cause of false-positive reading for herniated nucleus pulposus. Spine 10: 331–337

Porter B A, Hastrup W, Richardson M L et al 1987 Classification and investigation of artifacts in magnetic resonance imaging. Radiographics 7: 271–287

Porter R W, Wicks M, Ottewell D 1978 Measurement of the spinal canal by diagnostic ultrasound. Journal of Bone and Joint Surgery 60-B: 481–484

Quencer R M, Montalvo B M, Green B A et al 1984 Intraoperative spinal sonography of soft tissue masses of the spinal cord and spinal canal. American Journal of Neuroradiology 5: 507–515

Quencer R M, Montalvo B M, Eismont F J et al 1985 Intraoperative spinal sonography in thoracic and lumbar fractures: evaluation of Harrington rod instrumentation. American Journal of Neuroradiology 6: 353–359

Quiles M, Marschisello P J, Tsairis P 1978 Lumbar adhesive arachnoiditis. Etiologic and pathologic aspects. Spine 3: 45–50

Quinnell R C, Stockdale H R 1982 The significance of osteophytes on lumbar vertebral bodies in relation to discographic findings. Clinical Radiology 33: 197–203

Raghavan N, Barkovich A J, Edwards M et al 1989 MR imaging in the tethered spinal cord syndrome. American Journal of Neuroradiology 10: 27–36

Raskin S P 1985 Editorial: on CT scanning and metrizamide myelography Spine 10: 694

Resnick D 1985 Degenerative diseases of the vertebral column. Radiology 156: 3–14

Riggins R S, Kraus J F 1977 The risk of neurologic damage with fractures of the vertebrae. Journal of Trauma 17: 126–133

Roger B, Travers V, Hentz V R 1988 Imaging of post traumatic brachial plexus injury. Clinical Orthopaedics and Related Research 137: 57–61

Ross J S, Perez-Reyes N, Masaryk T J et al 1987 Thoracic disc herniation: MR imaging. Radiology 165: 511–515

Ross J S, Masaryk T J et al 1990 MR imaging of the post operative lumbar spine: assessment with gadopentetate dimeglumine. American Journal of Neuroradiology 11: 771–776

Rothman R H, Wiesel S W, Bell G R 1986 Editorial: on CT scanning and metrizamide myelography. Response from the authors to letters received. Spine 11: 1

Rothman S L G, Glenn W V 1984 CT multiplanar reconstruction in 253 cases of lumbar spondylolysis. American Journal of Neuroradiology 5: 81–90

Rothman S L G, Glenn W V 1985 Editorial: on CT scanning and metrizamide myelography. Spine 10: 693–694

Rothwell C I, St C. Forbes W, Gupta S C 1987 Computed tomographic myelography in the investigation of childhood scoliosis and spinal dysraphism. British Journal of Radiology 60: 1197–1204

Rubenstein D J, Alvarez O, Ghelman B et al 1989 Cauda equina syndrome complicating ankylosing spondylitis: MR features. Journal of Computer Assisted Tomography 13: 511–513

Rubin J M, DiPietro M A, Chandler W F 1988 et al Spinal ultrasonography intraoperative and pediatric applications. Radiologic Clinics of North America 26: 1–27

Scatcliff J H, Kendall B E, Kingsley D P E et al 1989 Closed spinal dysraphism: analysis of clinical, radiological, and surgical findings in 104 consecutive patients. American Journal of Neuroradiology 10: 269–277

Scheible W, James H E, Leopold G R et al 1983 Occult spinal dysraphism in infants: screening with high resolution real-time ultrasound. Radiology 146: 743–746

Schellinger D, Wener L, Ragsdale B D et al 1987 Facet joint disorders and their role in the production of back pain and sciatica. Radiographics 7: 923–944

Scher A T 1976 Cervical spinal cord injury without evidence of fracture or dislocation. South African Medical Journal 50: 962–965

Schipper J, Kardaun J W P F, Braakmann R et al 1987 Lumbar disc herniation: diagnosis with CT or myelography. Radiology 165: 227–231

Schneider R C, Cherry G, Pantek H 1954 The syndrome of acute central cervical spinal cord injury. Journal of Neurosurgery 11: 546–577

Schneiderman G, Flannigan B, Kingston S et al 1987 Magnetic resonance imaging in the diagnosis of disc degeneration: correlation with discography. Spine 12: 276–281

Scotti G, Scialfa G, Pieralli S et al 1983 Myelopathy and radiculopathy due to cervical spondylosis: myelographic-CT correlations. American Journal of Neuroradiology 4: 601–605

Selecki B R 1970 Cervical spine and cord injuries mechanisms and surgical implications. Medical Journal of Australia 1: 838–840

Shellock F G 1988 MR imaging of metallic implants and materials: a compilation of the literature. American Journal of Roentgenology 151: 811–814

Simmons E H, Segil C M 1975 An evaluation of discography in the localisation of symptomatic levels in discogenic disease of the spine. Clinical Orthopaedics and Related Research 108: 57–69

Slasky S S, Bydder G M, Niendorf P et al 1987 MR imaging with Gadolinium-DTPA in the differentiation of tumour, syrinx, and cyst of the spinal cord. Journal of Computer Assisted Tomography 11: 845–850

Smith A, Weinstein M A, Mizushima A et al 1989 MR imaging characteristics of tuberculous spondylitis vs vertebral osteomyelitis. American Journal of Neuroradiology 10: 619–625

Sorensen S C, Scott M 1984 Meningeal carcinomatosis in patients with primary breast or lung cancer. Mayo Clinic Proceedings 59: 91–94

Sotiropoulos S, Chafetz N I, Lang P et al 1989 Differentiation between postoperative scar and recurrent disk herniation: prospective comparison of MR, CT, and contrast enhanced CT. American Journal of Neuroradiology 10: 639–643

Stevens J M, Kendall B E, Crockard H A 1986 The spinal cord in rheumatoid arthritis with clinical myelopathy: a computed myelographic study. Journal of Neurology, Neurosurgery and Psychiatry 49:140–151

Stoker D, Kissin C 1985 Percutaneous vertebral biopsy: a review of 135 cases. Clinical Radiology 36: 569–577

Sze G, Abrahamson A, Krol G et al 1988 Gadolinium-DTPA in the evaluation of intradural extramedullary spinal disease. American Journal of Neuroradiology 9: 153–156

Sze G, Bravo S, Krol G 1989 Spinal lesions: quantitative and qualitative temporal evolution of gadopentetate dimeglumine enhancement in MR imaging. Radiology 170: 849–856

Sze G, Stimac G K, Bartlett C et al 1990 Multicenter study of gadopentetate dimeglumine as an MR contrast agent: evaluation in patients with spinal tumours. American Journal of Neuroradiology 11: 967–974

Takahashi M, Sakamoto Y, Miyawaki M et al 1987 Increased signal intensity secondary to chronic cervical cord compression. Neuroradiology 29: 550–556

Tate C F, Wilkov H R, Lestrange N R et al 1985 Outpatient lumbar myelography. Radiology 157: 391–393

Teitelbaum G P, Yee C A, Van Horn D D et al 1990 Metallic ballistic fragments: MR imaging safety and artifacts. Radiology 175: 855–859

Teplick J G, Haskin M E 1983 Computed tomography of the post operative spine. American Journal of Roentgenology 141: 865–884

Teresi L M, Lufkin R B, Reicher M A et al 1987 Asymptomatic degenerative disk disease and spondylosis of the cervical spine: MR imaging. Radiology 164: 83–88

Terwey B, Becker H, Thron A K et al 1989 Gadolinium-DTPA enhanced MR imaging of spinal dural arteriovenous fistulas. Journal of Computer Assisted Tomography 13: 30–37

Thrush A, Enzmann D 1990 MR imaging of infectious spondylitis. American Journal of Neuroradiology 11: 1171–1180

Tortori-Donati P, Cama A, Rosa M L et al 1990 Occult spinal dysraphism: neuroradiological study. Neuroradiology 31: 512–522

Tsuruda J S, Norman D, Dillon W et al 1990 Three-dimensional gradient recalled MR imaging as a screening tool for the diagnosis of cervical radiculopathy. American Journal of Neuroradiology 10: 1263–1271

Valk J 1988 Gd-DTPA in MR of spinal lesions. American Journal of Neuroradiology 9: 345–350

Vanharanta H, Guyer R D, Ohnmeiss D D 1988 Disc deterioration in low-back syndromes a prospective, multi-center CT/discography study. Spine 13: 1349–1351

van Lom K J, Kellerhouse L E, Pathria M N et al 1988 Infection versus tumour in the spine criteria for distinction with CT. Radiology 166: 851–855

Vezina J L, Fontaine S, Laperriere J 1989 Outpatient myelography with fine-needle technique: an appraisal. American Journal of Neuroradiology 10: 615–617

Wasserstrom W R, Glass J P, Posner J B 1982 Diagnosis and treatment of leptomeningeal metastases from solid tumours: experience with 90 patients. Cancer 49: 759–772

Weitz E M 1985 Editorial: On CT scanning and metrizamide myelography. Spine 10: 694

Whitesides T E 1977 Traumatic kyphosis of the thoracolumbar spine. Clinical Orthopaedics and Related Research 128: 78–92

Wiesel S W 1985 Editorial: On CT scanning and metrizamide myelography. Spine 10: 695

Williams M P, Cherryman G R, Husband J E 1989a Significance of thoracic disc herniation demonstrated by MR imaging. Journal of Computer Assisted Tomography 13: 211–214

Williams M P, Cherryman G R, Husband J E 1989b Magnetic resonance imaging in suspected metastatic spinal cord compression. Clinical Radiology 40: 286–290

Wilson D A, Prince J R 1989 MR imaging determination of the normal conus medullaris throughout childhood. American Journal of Neuroradiology 10: 259–262

Wojick W G, Edeiken B S, Harris J H 1987 Three dimensional computed tomography in acute cervical spine trauma: a preliminary report. Skeletal Radiology 16: 261–269

Yamashita Y, Takahashi M, Matsuno Y et al 1990 Chronic injuries of the spinal cord assessment with MR imaging. Radiology 175: 849–854

Yousem D M, Atlas S W, Goldberg H I et al 1991 Degenerative narrowing of the cervical spine neural foramina: evaluation with high-resolution 3DFT gradient-echo MR imaging. American Journal of Neuroradiology 12: 229–236

Yu S, Haughton V M 1990 Anatomic-radiographic correlations in the spine. Current Imaging 2: 105–116

Yu S, Haughton V M, Sether L A et al 1988 Annulus fibrosus in bulging intervertebral discs. Radiology 169: 761–763

Yu S, Haughton V M, Sether L A 1989 Comparison of MR and discography in detecting radial tears of the annulus: a postmortem study. American Journal of Neuroradiology 10: 1077–1081

Zucherman J, Derby R, Hsu K et al 1988 Normal magnetic resonance imaging with abnormal discography. Spine 13: 1355–1399

A review of clinical procedures and rationale

46. A review of manual therapy for spinal pain

D. W. Lamb

INTRODUCTION

Manual therapy is a specialization within physical therapy. The training, now increasingly incorporating higher standards at the undergraduate level, is further developed in postgraduate courses. This training considerably amplifies the theoretical basis and the technical skill received during the diploma or degree necessary for certification as a physical therapist. This basic training originally included a diploma training of 3 years. This is being replaced by degrees either at the baccalaureate or master's level, depending on the different educational focus in countries.

Consideration is being given by some training institutions in the USA to extending postgraduate training to attain professional doctoral degrees, e.g. PT.D. This would address the questionable desirability of having the research degree, e.g. Ph.D., as the only pathway available to manual therapists of gaining a doctorate and the status which goes along with this. Chiropractors have long recognized the professional status gained in the public eye from the use of the title 'doctor'.

The manual therapy training may be provided on a continuous part-time basis where a sequential course of study is followed. This includes theoretical, practical and clinical practise recognized or sponsored by the national association. It may also be more formalized into longer full-time courses provided by universities or institutes of tertiary education.

A further development is the recognized specialist in manual therapy. This has been implemented in Australia to provide patients already receiving manual or physical therapy access to further expertise so that their treatment may be modified if necessary. This service is recognized by paying agencies as an expert service, so that a higher service fee is paid. A proposal along similar professional lines is at the final stages of acceptance in Canada (Contact 1990). A number of criteria will be required:

1. Expertise in manual therapy, competency proven in examination

2. Graduate-level courses in research design and statistics
3. Publishing of research and clinical articles in peer-reviewed journals or published textbooks.

The manual therapist provides comprehensive conservative management for spinal and peripheral joint pain of musculoskeletal dysfunction. Manual therapists work within the medical team, providing a specialized service following referral.

Easy access to treatment is essential; long waits tend to promote chronicity as well as emphasize the severity of the problem. A very active treatment regime seems to promote rapid independence from formalized treatment (Mitchell & Carmen 1990). In the UK (Ellman et al 1982) open access to hospital physiotherapy services, for family practitioners, is successfully being provided. In Canada, family practitioners have full hospital privileges and thus open access has existed for a long time. Additionally, in many Canadian provinces, and in other countries, registered independent practices are included in the government-funded medicare system and are funded on a fee-for-service basis. Independent insurance companies also include the provision of physical therapy services. The increasing costs of medical services of all kinds are placing the various systems under great pressure to analyse the cost effectiveness of the different treatment regimens.

It is important to compare the different regimes in similar circumstances. A recent review (Meade et al 1990) which compared chiropractic care to treatment received in hospital physiotherapy outpatients showed the superiority of the former. However, it failed to analyse the effect on patients of immediate access to a practitioner of their choice, the effect of paying for treatment, and the difference in atmosphere of a private office compared to the more harassed environment of the hospital outpatient department. Perhaps the effect of the 'total chiropractic experience' could have been duplicated in the private offices of manual therapists and osteopaths. As the superiority of chiropractic shown in this study related to chronic or severe pain perhaps the more personalized approach is necessary in the former and the immediacy of availability of treatment in the latter.

One interesting aside is that chiropractors are relative newcomers in the UK, as compared with osteopaths. It says much for the political acumen of chiropractors that they should be chosen as the group performing the manipulation which was a fundamental part of the protocol.

The variety of practice allows physical therapists the choice of career structure, provides the public and the physician with a variety of treatment choices and treatment delivery, and facilitates speedy referral and treatment.

In many developed countries physiotherapists in private practice are effectively operating as 'first-contact' therapists, providing ethical and responsible specialist service in this field of minor orthopaedics. Occasionally, legislation exists requiring the therapist to contact the physician following initial assessment and to maintain contact throughout the course of treatment (Manitoba 1981). In jurisdictions where this is not a requirement reports have not become prevalent of inappropriate treatment performed on inappropriate patients because of the lack of skill in differential diagnosis in manual therapists. This is often cited as a reason for restricting first-contact privileges. One Canadian province has recently allowed this new development in an effort to reduce the costs of treatment. The policy will be reviewed after one year to assess the feasibility of expansion. Where 'first contact' exists it is probably wise to exclude certain groups of patients — for example, where external factors have caused trauma, such as a fall or a motor vehicle accident where radiographs would be advisable, or where the family history of inflammatory arthritis suggests the desirability of blood tests. However, many sophisticated tests have been developed by manual therapists to test the integrity of segments to absorb stress revealing hypermobility and instability at the cranioverterbral and all spinal levels. The role of manual therapists in the diagnostic process should be expanded.

Probably the most efficient team in treating spinal dysfunction comprises the orthopaedic physician and manual therapist working in close contact.

In relation to the common vertebral syndromes, physiotherapy practice has undergone very considerable changes in the last 30 years. In a climate of dissatisfaction, both of the therapist and the patient, critical evaluation of treatment results has shown the inadequacy of the uncritical application of thermal and electrical agencies, back extension exercises, lumbar flexion routines, various traction protocols and external splinting of various kinds. Patients may have recovered in spite of, rather than because of, the treatment applied. More recent advances have demonstrated the poor therapeutic value of illogically selected thrust techniques or bilateral (generalized) rotation manipulation.

Under the guidance of Cyriax (1983), Grieve (1988a), Kaltenborn (1970, 1974), Evjenth (1986), Maitland (1986), Mennell (1960), Paris (1965) and others, manual therapists have developed a systematic assessment and treatment approach. This approach has remained non-doctrinal, based on a careful analysis of establishing dysfunction in the vertebral segment with consequential changes on neuromusculoskeletal structures. Appropriate physiotherapy techniques are used to normalize function, such as massage, proprioceptive neuromuscular facilitation (PNF), rhythmic and sustained traction, passive maintenance movements, various thermo-hydro-electro agencies, ergonomic analysis, specific exercise techniques for strengthening, flexibility and stabilization, group teaching in the 'Back School' — to name some — as well as specialized manual techniques.

The graduate therapist has had experience in treating a wide variety of disease processes in all body systems under the scientific medical model. This wide clinical exposure to patients is essential in developing handling skills, both physical and psychological, and enables the manual therapist to treat the whole person, observe precautions and recognize contraindications. This thorough training, with its clinical basis, compares more than favourably with the training of other health professionals, such as chiropractors for example. The observation of manual therapists (Schmidt 1991) who have done the chiropractic training is the emphasis on high velocity thrust (HVT) and paucity of training in mobilization with specific localization and muscle-based techniques.

THE CONTEXT OF MANUAL THERAPY

Consideration will be given to the multifactorial causation of spinal dysfunction and especially its multistructural effects. To look for one cause of mechanical spinal dysfunction or one universal treatment would be foolish. The concept of a single cause of dysfunction is attractive but simplistic and unrealistic. Bogduk (1990) reviewed the anatomical multi-causal basis of lumbar spinal pain. This analysis, with slight changes for spinal regional variations, is appropriate for all regions of the spine.

Often there is a particular position or strain which produces immediate pain, frequently accompanied by a 'giving' sensation or sound. Thus, distortion produces a particular mechanical problem in the moving parts — the assumption being that some structure has been moved or trapped. Superficially it would seem rational that a carefully contrived force, applied in the opposite direction to the deforming stress, would correct the problem. Some suggestions that studying regular radiographs would indicate the direction in which the thrust should be applied is difficult to accept as most structures producing pain in the spinal segment are radiotranslucent. Unfortunately, this is infrequently the case, and the results of treatment are unpredictable. The damage which has occurred is usually part of an ongoing process of degenerative change in the neuromusculoskeletal system, with wide ranging consequences other than that of a simple mechanical block. Often the treatment has to be comprehensive, directed towards immediate management, restoration of function, and future prevention.

Simple biomechanical principles

The functional unit of the spine is the mobile vertebral segment (Schmorl & Junghanns 1971). This consists of two contiguous vertebrae, the intervening disc, the zygapophyseal joints, interconnecting ligaments and intrinsic muscles. In the cervical spine the neurocentral joints are a factor, and in the thoracic spine consideration must be given to the rib joints. However, the segment is functionally much more complex, having axial components both mechanical and physiological but also embryologically related peripheral components.

Dysfunction is much more complex than simple alteration in the position of the mechanical components. The osteopathic definition of somatic dysfunction succinctly expresses it thus: 'an area of impaired function of the related components of the musculoskeletal system (muscle fasciae ligament) and its associated or related parts of the vascular, lymphatic and nervous system' (Rumney 1975).

The healthy joint is well constructed to absorb mechanical stresses. In the lumbar spine torsion stresses are absorbed partially by the zygapophyseal joints which are positioned as outriggers, set at a distance from the instantaneous centre of rotation. For example, the factor of facet apposition on the side opposite to the direction of rotation is more efficient in absorbing torsion than the capsular tension produced by facet gapping on the side to which rotation is directed (Adams & Hutton 1981). The zygapophyseal joints work in concert with the lamellae of the annulus fibrosus, particularly the outer fibres, in absorbing torsional loading.

Compression is absorbed by the nucleus with the force dissipated vertically via the end plates and laterally by the annular fibres. The efficiency of the vertebral body in resisting crush is increased by the engorgement of venous blood prevented from exiting the vertebral body by the valve effect of the posterior longitudinal ligament on the nutrient foramen. This mechanism is facilitated by segmental flexion (Farfan 1977a).

Resistance to flexion is also provided by the posterior ligamentous structures which exert their combined effect several centimetres behind the instantaneous centre of rotation. This mechanism is more efficient than that provided by the intrinsic extensor muscles in keeping the increase in compression to a minimum (Farfan 1977, Gracovetsky & Farfan 1986). In addition, this mechanism is enhanced by the abdominal oblique muscles which increase intra-abdominal pressure. Probably more important for continuous support is the attachment of the abdominal oblique muscles to the thoracolumbar fascia, which, acting on the spinous processes posteriorly, controls the tendency to vertebral shear (Farfan 1975). Forward shear is also resisted efficiently by the orientation and configuration of the zygapophyseal joints (Adams & Hutton 1983). The mechanisms comprise the balanced vertebral segment resisting movement, reducing compression and shear (Gracovetsky et al 1977).

The muscular control of the cervical spine is a major consideration in the absorption of forces generated in motor vehicle accidents. In rear-end collisions with the head facing directly forward, the zygapophyseal joints do not impact efficiently to prevent extension, thus placing a greater requirement on the deep cervical muscles to prevent excessive extension. Slight rotation of the head more efficiently engages the facets on the ipsilateral side, and while the anterior muscles are less damaged impaction damage occurs in the zygapophyseal joints. The slight rotational positioning in slight flexion renders the alar ligaments much more vulnerable to damage in the absence of damage to the transverse ligaments (Dvorak 1987).

Penning (1988) described the difference in motion in the cervical spine in the sagittal plane as gliding in C3–5 and tilting in C6–7. The gliding motion is more profound, and the uncovertebral joints are much better developed in segments which have gliding, presumably as this requires more control. The tendency for well developed transverse splits to occur parallel to the vertebral bodies starting at the uncovertebral joints in these gliding segments seems to protect these from frank disc prolapse. This phenomenon is much better seen at C6–7 where uncovertebral joint development is negligible. The completeness of uncovertebral joint development increases the relationship of side flexion rotation coupling.

The mechanisms of degenerative change

The lumbar vertebral segment is subjected to considerable loading throughout life. It has been calculated that a 77 kg man lifting 91 kg weight may develop 940 kg reaction at the lumbosacral disc (Morris et al 1961).

The repetitive absorption of stress, particularly torsion, causes gradual attrition of the segment, slowly exhausting the adaptive potential. It seems likely that compression loading causes fractures in the end plate, with subchondral bone compression and radial tears of the annulus fibrosus. Torsion produces circumferential tears between the outer layers of the annulus, providing potentially weak areas which precede subsequent bulging of the disc (Farfan 1973).

The efficiency of absorption of the deforming forces is determined by the anatomical factors described, including the shape and the surface area of the vertebral body and the efficiency of the muscular support.

Structural anomalies such as facet tropism (asymmetry of facet plane orientation) seriously compromise the efficiency of the facets in absorbing torsion; with coronal facets, damage is seen earlier in the outer annulus of the disc, diagonally opposite the coronal facet.

Fahrni (1976) has described compression of the posterior annulus, as seen in lordosis, as a major factor in attrition of the disc prior to the classical posterolateral disc bulging, particularly if this is aggravated by the prone lying positions for sleep which impede corrective healing.

All spinal segments are influenced by their functional and mechanical relationship to the whole column. An increase in the lumbosacral angle accentuates the primary and secondary curves, increasing the posterior lamellae compression and increasing the shear effect.

Alteration in the head–neck relationship, typically the forward head carriage of the slumped or fatigue posture, increases the extension of the occipito-atlantal region. Mechanoreceptor-driven reflexes of the cervical spine increase muscle activity in the antigravity muscles, generally increasing fatigue and producing aching through persistent stress on the ligaments and the accumulation of metabolites (Lewit 1985).

The excessively straight spine is also prone to injury. Excessive compression forces generate in the discs not being dissipated by increases in the spinal curves. Also, rotation produces torsion strains in the segments, whereas in the normally curved spine rotation often produces some degree of flexion which is more easily handled by the spine.

It is interesting to note how easily vertebral joint damage occurs in the recumbent position. This probably occurs because unloading reduces the approximation of the facets allowing a greater excursion of motion in the presence of reduced muscular tone.

In the cervical spine falling asleep on a couch with the head in an awkward position allows slow deformation (creep) to occur. Sudden movement, e.g. on being wakened suddenly by a telephone, can produce acute joint symptoms such as those caused by the incarcerated meniscoids seen in one kind of acute wry neck.

Contiguous regions are coupled functionally, e.g. the H-P-L complex (hip–pelvis–lumbar spine). Changes in one component of the complex, such as a stiff hip or a short leg, will be compensated for in other parts of the complex. This, however, imposes sustained abnormal stress, gradually exhausting the adaptive potential and leading to secondary joint dysfunction, often involving laxity. Unilateral ilial rotation will directly influence the lumbosacral joint by producing rotation which produces compensatory rotoscoliosis at higher levels.

The gradual attrition within the disc creates resorption resulting in loss of disc height. There is a loss of stiffness (firmness) of the disc. Thus, changes occur in the relationship of the two vertebrae involved in the segment. The bodies move closer together causing the superior facet of the inferior vertebrae to move upwards and anteriorly encroaching on the intervertebral segment. This gives rise to retrolisthesis, as seen on radiographs. This effect is increased if the segment is subject to torsion. Thus, the A/P diameter of the foramen is compromised, creating intermittent lateral entrapment (Kirkaldy-Willis et al 1978).

The biomechanical inadequacies of the segment result in anomalies of motion. The normal arthrokinematics will be modified, with an increase in the forward and lateral shear. The arthrotic destruction of the medial curvature of the anterior margin of the facet also allows more anterior shear, creating the potential for degenerative spondylolisthesis.

It seems reasonable to postulate that a state of mild hypermobility — and thus insufficiency — exists in the early stages of arthrosis, followed by gradual fibrosis of the disc and thickening of the joint capsule which reduces movement in the segment whence it becomes less painful (Kirkaldy-Willis 1978).

A comparative functional interdependence with comprehensive dysfunction occurs in stiffness in flexion of the cervicothoracic junction. This results in:

1. Forward head carriage with chronic extension of the occipito-atlantal joint
2. Reduced movement in the cervical spine
3. Altered positional set of the scapula altering the force couple of the supraspinatus leading to chronic tendinitis
4. Reduced movements of the glenohumeral joint in elevation and lateral rotation
5. Increased tightness in the pectoral muscles with weakening of the interscapular muscles
6. Reduction in the inspiratory excursion of breathing.

Successful treatment is predicated upon influencing the primary dysfunction, particularly the mobility of the C–T junction by rhythmical mobilization and reducing the extension of the O–A segment with muscle-based techniques. The secondary events then fall within the scope of orthodox physical therapy with which the manual therapist is thoroughly familiar.

Thus it is possible to trace pathological wear through various structures. It is less easy to predict the consequences of such change on all structures within the segment, or the behaviour of these structures during movement.

The wider implications

Being able to ascertain, with any accuracy, a fault in a single component is usually not possible. Various workers have stated a preference for naming specific structures or functions responsible:

Cyriax (1983)   The disc
Mennell (1960)   Loss of accessory joint
                         motion
Travell & Simons (1983) Presence of myofascial
                         trigger points
Gunn (1989)   Neuropathic pain origins
Chiropractors (States 1968) Changes in vertebral
                         alignment
Osteopaths (Johnston 1975) Abnormalities of segmental
                         motion.

These do not address the pathological consequences. Thus, for the most part, the exact nature of segmental dysfunction remains speculative, and even in cases of the classical disc protrusion with neurological signs changes throughout the segment must be considered.

The approach by MacNab (1977) as:

disc degeneration without root irritation
disc degeneration with root irritation

may, in its generality, be more accurate.

Gitelman (1975) expresses it thus: 'Subluxation is a process and not a static condition. A state of living tissue undergoing constant change. These changes include hyperaemia, congestion, oedema, minute haemorrhages, fibrosis, local ischaemia, atrophy and eventually rigidity and adhesions which form not only in the joint capsules but also in the ligaments, tendons and muscles themselves'. Thus, Gitelman has moved from the classical chiropractic theory of segmental positional fault, although the terminology still implies displacement and altered bony relationship (States 1968).

Pain

Pain on movement and/or attaining or maintaining certain positions is the key presenting symptom in most cases encountered in manual therapy practice.

It is often accompanied by limited movement, the existence of terminal deflection or dynamic deviation, or the presence of painful arcs. Indeed, it is expected that the inculpated neuromusculoskeletal tissue should produce a painful reaction when subjected to damaging stresses. In general, tissues related to the moving parts are stressed in the spine as well as in all regions of the body by testing: active and passive movement and isometric contraction of muscle. Pain derived from visceral tissues referred to the body wall in general are exculpated by these procedures, although, as Grieve (1988b) described in 'Masqueraders', this is by no means foolproof.

Segmental dysfunction will be detected by the nociceptive system which has a ubiquitous distribution in the intervertebral segment. A complete account is provided by Bogduk et al (1981), Bogduk and Twomey (1987), Wyke (1975, 1980) and Yoshizawa et al (1980).

In a brief summary, Lamb (1979) described a rich distribution to the facet joint and sacro-iliac joint capsules. There are fibres to the ligamentous structures of the intervertebral segment, with a dense distribution to the fibro-areolar fat pad between the posterior longitudinal ligament and the posterior aspect of the disc. The periosteum of the vertebrae, connective tissue aspects of the bone, the vascular system of the segment, the anterior dura mater, the dural root sleeves and epidural areolar adipose tissue within the intervertebral foramen are all innervated by the nociceptive system. Additionally, all the intrinsic muscles are well supplied.

Recent studies (Yoshizawa et al 1980, Bogduk et al 1985) provide strong supporting evidence indicating that the full circumference of the outer annulus is well supplied with free nerve endings. The inner annulus and the nucleus of the disc are noteworthy by the absence of innervation.

Specific treatment requires specific mechanical diagnosis. As many of the spinal structures are translucent to ionizing radiation, and the use of modern techniques such as MRI is not foolproof, is expensive and is not universally available, much of the conclusions on the origin of musculoskeletal pain is based on clinical impressions. The creation of pain and patterns of referral from different musculoskeletal structures has been well documented: facet joint (Mooney & Robertson 1976, Bogduk & Jull 1985), dural tissue (Cyriax 1945), ligaments (Feinstein 1977), myofascial trigger points (Simons & Travell 1983) and nerve root irritability (Smythe & Wright 1958).

The characteristics of the pain (burning, aching, lancinating, numbness etc.) have been listed in exhaustive detail (Melzack 1973). The dermatomal fields and skin distribution affected by the individual structures was drawn in the studies cited above.

Some generalizations may be drawn:

1. The greater the irritation produced, the greater the pain and the more extensive the spread into the dermatomes.
2. If the pain did not extend into the distal parts of the dermatome, the less accurate could be conclusions on the segmental origins of the pain.
3. Often the pain extended beyond the dermatomal field — inexplicable when related to the segmental anatomy of relationships of myotomes dermatomes and sclerotomes.

This latter point may be explained in part by extrasegmental spread of pain by irritation of structures such as dural sleeves. Additionally the segmental dysfunction may affect several structures simultaneously at the same segment and may extend over several segments. The concept of segmental innervation is also erroneous as the individual segment is supplied from at least two or three contiguous levels (Paris 1988) in the lumbar spine and up to five levels in the cervical spine (Wyke 1979). This makes essential the process of obtaining objective information to define the tissue responsible such as:

1. Presence or absence of signs of nerve root compromise
2. Evidence of signs of altered motion such as hypermobility or hypomobility
3. Tissue texture abnormalities (Greenman 1989).

Damage produces tissue reaction, the more obvious signs of acute inflammation, or the milder but no less significant milder persistent irritation (repetitive strain injuries) producing fibroblastic reaction with collagen proliferation typical of chronic inflammation (Lee 1989).

Abnormality in the tissues is created by dysfunction. This is detected by depolarization of the free nerve endings of the nociceptive system. Depolarization can be triggered by marked deformation caused by excessive mechanical force (which also affects the Ad system) and production of the inflammatory cascade which includes chemical substances resulting from tissue damage, e.g. polypeptide kinins, 5-hydroxytryptamine, histamine, and metabolic derivatives such as lactic acid and potassium ions. The early changes produce alteration in the normal tissue fluid exchange and add to the general stasis which allows a lingering effect of the damage derivatives.

Activation of the nociceptive system can give rise to pain, but not invariably so, and certainly the degree of irritability and pain produced is not a direct relationship. Activation in the pain-conducting system may be modulated by ongoing activity in the other receptor systems, especially the type I and II mechanoreceptors situated in the synovial joint capsules, by central inhibitory control systems and by endogenous neuropeptide opiates (Watson 1986).

Complicating the matter further is the finding that tissues are not consistently reactive throughout the day; Porter and Trailescu (1990) found a difference in the diurnal behaviour of SLR, and Adams (1990) described the infinitely greater stresses on the lumbar segment early in the day when presumably the disc has imbibed fluid during the night. Flexion in the morning can increase the stress on the ligaments of the neural arch by as much as 80%. This presents a challenge in that exercises not only have to be carefully chosen but some consideration should be given to the time of day when they are performed.

Within the segment the facet joints have a rich distribution of nociceptors, and it is reasonable to assume they are a common cause of pain. Mooney and Robertson, previously cited, have shown these to be capable of mimicking mild discogenic features such as limited SLR (not under 45°) weakness in the myotomes and reduced reflex response. These improved immediately after an arthrographically confirmed injection of local anaesthetic into the facet joint cavity.

The disc can be the source of pain by activating the nociceptive system of the connective tissue anterior to the posterior longitudinal ligament and the outer circumference of the annulus. Perhaps the annular innervation could be stimulated by chemical changes in the disc, particularly when coalescing of radial tears and circumferential tears allow exposure of the intra-annular layers with the nuclear material. Within the foramen, the nerve root can cause pain when exposed to the chemical products of inflammation or by pressure once the inflammatory process has affected the nerve root. The microcirculation of the nerve root is very vulnerable to distortion or pressure, which can create occlusion producing ischaemia and oedema. Rydevik (1984) has graphically illustrated these events. The changes are ubiquitous in that the events in the nerve root show great similarities to the events described by Lankford (1983) for the production of reflex sympathetic dystrophy.

Muscle splinting (discrete guarding spasm) is a significant reaction in segmental dysfunction (Gunn et al 1989). He coined the term 'neuropathic pain', listing the following characteristics:

1. Pain in the absence of an ongoing tissue-damaging process
2. Delay in onset after a precipitating injury
3. Abnormal or unpleasant sensations such as 'burning or searing pain' (dysesthesia) or 'deep, aching pain' which is more common in musculoskeletal pain syndromes
4. Pain felt in the region of sensory deficit
5. Paroxysmal brief 'shooting or stabbing' pain
6. Painful mild stimuli (allodynia)
7. Pronounced summation and after reaction with repetitive stimuli.

The pain is accompanied by:

1. Muscle shortening from spasm and/or contractions
2. Tender myofascial trigger points
3. Autonomic and trophic effects of neuropathy
4. Degrading of related collagenous structures.

These changes may be found in the spinal segmental area supplied by the appropriate posterior primary ramus and the peripheral segmental areas supplied by the anterior primary ramus.

A similar reaction has been illustrated by Paris (1989), the muscle reaction being caused by, and then perpetuating, the joint dysfunction.

The segment is a neuromusculoskeletal unit with axial and peripheral components, in the sense that peripheral musculoskeletal tissues and somatic nerves retain the parenthood of their embryological source, segment by segment, corresponding approximately with the dermatomes.

The appreciation of pain in the dermatome may be

remote from the origin of pain, which may arise in any of the axial or peripheral components of the segment.

It is essential therefore that the assessment procedure for mechanical dysfunction includes a systematic examination of all the components, focusing on those requiring detailed study and clearing others.

Examination

The contribution of Cyriax (1983) in analysing segmental joint dysfunction is incalculable. He devised a scheme of systematically reviewing function in the total segment in a sequential way. By careful review of the symptoms, the inculpated area is determined. The reactivity and abnormal behaviour of the dysfunctional joint are ascertained. The history includes pertinent information such as medication, intercurrent diseases, history of past episodes and the results of treatment. Then, by following a sequence of tests for objective signs, a profile of joint dysfunction is obtained. For example, in the lumbar spine, testing key muscles, reflexes, skin sensation and straight leg raising and prone knee bend indicates the conductivity and mobility of the nerve roots respectively.

The following summary, related to the lumbar spine, indicates the completeness of the Cyriax scanning examination:

Patient's profile
  Subjective: Site of pain or paraesthesia (especially S4 symptoms)
  Type of pain
  Behaviour of pain
  Bladder or bowel involvement
  Aggravating factors
  Previous history
  Previous or concurrent treatment
  Previous or concurrent illness
  Previous or concurrent medication

  Objective: Gait analysis
  Postural profile
  Gross movement profile
  Muscular profile
  Neurological profile
  Vascular profile
  Localizing techniques
  Exclusion

Summary of the objective analysis:
Gait analysis
Postural profile
  The existence of developmental or acquired deformity such as lateral deviation to obtain the antalgic position; position of the pelvis for leg length discrepancies

Movement profile
  Indicates the degree of involvement; produces suggestive patterns, e.g. arthrotic pattern, discogenic patterns; non-correlating patterns: comparison later with other signs; provides salient signs for evaluating the efficacy of the treatment procedures
Neurological profile
  CNS and cauda equina
  Dural signs
  Reflexes
  Plantar response
  Peripheral nervous system
  Key muscle strength
  Reflex response
  Areas of anaesthesia
  SLR and PKB — root tension and movement
Muscular profile
  This is probably the only weak link; isometric muscle activity of the trunk muscles is tested; this is discussed later as a much more detailed analysis is required
Vascular profile
  Testing the peripheral pulses to differentiate between the symptoms of spinal stenosis and intermittent claudication of peripheral vascular origin
Localizing techniques
  These comprise palpation and direct vertebral pressures to confirm or establish level of involvement
Exclusion
  Inculpation of, or clearing peripheral components
Radiographs
  To exclude serious pathology.

All manual therapy assessments use the elegant Cyriax scanning examination to form a framework on which additional information can be built. It is relevant to all spinal areas, although specific questions may be more relevant to one area than to another. For example, in the cervical spine a number of questions should be asked (Kleynhans & Terrett 1985). Grieve (1980) has listed these:

1. X-rays, particularly when trauma has occurred in the upper cervical spine
2. Presence of inflammatory arthritides, the most important of which are rheumatoid arthritis and ankylosing spondylitis
3. Anticoagulant therapy, including aspirin
4. Dizziness, where it is essential to differentiate between vertebrobasilar occlusion, craniovertebral ligament laxity, labyrinthine involvement and cervical vertigo derived from segmental dysfunction; special manual therapy tests have been developed
5. Corticosteroid medication, because of the possibility of bone absorption in the vicinity of the transverse ligament of the dens

6. Upper respiratory tract involvement in children —
Grisel's syndrome
7. Symptoms in the lower trunk and legs created by
neck movements
8. Unremitting night pain not relieved by recumbency
9. Bowel and bladder problems
10. Down's syndrome, because a significant proportion
of these patients have craniovertebral anomalies.

The system is concise and convenient, and short cuts
should not be countenanced.

To summarize the results and precisely record the
salient findings, a compact but comprehensive recording
system was developed by Grieve (1984). An attempt was
made by Lamb (1980, 1991) to put the subjective section
of the record into a questionnaire form to increase the
patient's participation at the first visit (Figs 46.1–46.4).

Figure 46.5 contains a diagram developed by Maigne
and modified by Fowler and Lamb (1970). This allows a
set of kinetic events to be depicted on a static diagram. As
the movement profile frequently provides the salient signs,
an accurate record of range and behaviour of movement
is vital.

The movement diagram illustrated in Figure 46.6 is
a composite to illustrate usage; the profile indicated is
unlikely. In normal use, patterns possibly indicating
arthrosis, discogenic pathology and minor facet pathology
can be recognized.

The Cyriax system is relevant in reviewing dysfunction
of discogenic origin with neurological signs. In clinical
situations, where the signs and symptoms are less marked,
further detailed analysis of the involved segment is
necessary.

Several methods of analysis are employed:

1. Testing passive intervertebral joint motion (IVJM).
The vertebral segment is passively moved through a range
of movement around each major axis if appropriate. The
movement at the various segments is compared and the
end feel of the joint in various ranges is ascertained.

Passive movement is rated on a 0–6 scale, ranging from
0 = ankylosis and 3 = normal to 6 = unstable. This is
useful in providing a numerical recording but can also be
used in treatment planning, for example:

0 = Ankylosis	No treatment appropriate
1 = Markedly hypomobile	Use mobilization only; if spasm present mobilize away from pain
2 = Slightly hypomobile	Mobilize or manipulate into the stiff hypomobile range
3 = Normal	Maintain by lifestyle and exercise
4 = Slightly hypermobile	Low-grade mobilization for vascular hypermobile and mechanoreceptor effect
5 = Markedly hypermobile	Stabilization exercises, external support such as a back brace, a cervical collar
6 = Unstable	May require surgical stabilization

This analysis is mandatory if manipulation (HVT) is
contemplated because hypermobile joints are often the
source of pain and should never be subjected to high-
velocity thrusts.

Other accessory motions are also tested, in particular
distraction and compression. If the pain is produced by
discrete separation of the vertebral segment it is an important indicator that passive or active movement is likely
to cause a reaction, and other techniques such as rest,
external support, transcutaneous electrical nerve stimulator
(TENS), ultrasound or thermal agencies should be used
initially. This is particularly important in planning the
treatment protocol of acceleration/deceleration injuries
of the cervical spine.

Certain local passive rotary stress procedures, demonstrated by Farfan have proved useful in establishing rotary
instability in the lumbar spine.

2. Application of specific pressures on bony vertebral
processes. This method, refined by Maitland, uses discrete pressures of controlled depths on spinous and transverse processes to ascertain the irritability of the segment.

Maitland has emphasized the importance of the pain-
range–spasm relationship. This is a sophisticated analysis
of the end feel of joint range (Jull et al 1988), and can be
quantified on a diagram which is reliably reproducible
for interpretation by different examiners (Maitland 1970,
Grieve 1984). As well as expressing joint irritability, this
relationship also determines the approach to treatment,
the grade of movement being predicated upon the pain
and spasm elicited by the testing movements. As these are
objectively reduced, more positive grades of mobilization
movements are applied.

3. Joint position. Irritability within the segment produces local guarding muscle spasm. The braking effect of
muscle when the segments are explored passively may be
the physiological explanation for so-called joint bind
(Korr 1975, Stoddard 1983, Greenman 1989).

However, positional faults are also described in neutral
and the extremes of flexion and extension (Mitchell et al
1979). The latter are classified as type II lesions, usually
of a single segment and traumatic in origin, i.e. ERS, FRS
(e.g. extended rotated side flexed) implying fixation at
the extremes of extension (ERS) or flexion (FRS) with
simultaneous spasm in the rotators and side flexor
muscles. Although these are called positional faults they
denote the inability of the segment to move symmetrically
over its full range, and movement restriction, as well as
position, is an integral part of this concept. Often a com-

PARKLAND PHYSIOTHERAPY CLINIC

Please fill in the following information: TODAY'S DATE:

YOUR NAME: YOUR AGE:

YOUR MEDICAL DOCTOR: YOUR WORK:

Please shade in the areas of pain or
abnormal sensation where appropriate,
using the following code (signs).   CIRCLE underlined words
ACHING: // //   BURNING: X X X   or numbers which are
                               X X X   most appropriate.
NUMBNESS: O O O O   SHOOTING ↓ ↓ ↓
          O O O O   OR   Since the onset of
                     STABBING ↓ ↓ ↓   this problem have you
                                              had:

                                            1.) Difficulty in
                                                control of bowel or
                                                bladder function.
                                                    YES   NO

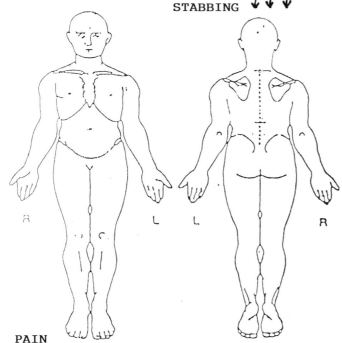

                                            2.) Any numbness in the
                                                genital or anal area.
                                                    YES   NO

                                            3.) Any dizziness or
                                                drop (fainting) attacks.
                                                    YES   NO

PAIN
DEGREE: (mild) 1 2 3 4 5 (severe)

NATURE: Sharp Dull Throbbing
          Constant Periodic Occasional
          Increasing Static Decreasing.

It is AGGRAVATED by: Sitting Rising from sitting
                      Coughing Sneezing Straining
                      Taking a deep breath   Sustained bending

Is the pain made worse or eased by activity?

Is it made worse or eased by rest?

Fig. 46.1 Patient questionnaire. Subjective analysis.

Do you have pain at night?   <u>YES</u   <u>NO</u>

If <u>YES</u>:   Is it present only while lying still?   <u>YES</u>   <u>NO</u>

Is it present only when changing position?   <u>YES</u>   <u>NO</u>

Are you very stiff getting out of bed in the morning?   <u>YES</u>   <u>NO</u>

What are the effects of normal movement on stiffness?   <u>EASE</u>   <u>NO EFFECT</u>

During the day overall does the pain   <u>DECREASE</u>   <u>INCREASE</u>   <u>NO CHANGE</u>
towards the evening?

Any additional things which ease the pain? Specify:_____

_____

Do you lie on your stomach for any length of time?   <u>YES</u>   <u>NO</u>

What kind of mattress do you use? Specify?_____

How many pillows do you use?_____   TYPE: <u>Feather</u>
                                                         <u>Foam - Solid</u>
                                                                    <u>Chip</u>
                                                         <u>Fibre</u>
                                                         <u>Contoured</u>

Have you any history of: <u>DIABETES</u>
                           <u>HEART DISEASE</u>
                           <u>PACE MAKER</u>
                           <u>INFLAMMATORY ARTHRITIS</u>
                           <u>CANCER</u>
                           <u>STRESS RELATED TENSION</u>
                           <u>METAL IMPLANTS</u>

If appropriate, is there any chance you may be pregnant at this time?
                                                         <u>YES</u>   <u>NO</u>

Have you had any <u>RECENT SURGERY</u>?   _____

                                         _____

<u>MEDICATIONS</u>:   Are you currently, or have recently taken any:
                       <u>STEROIDS</u> (e.g.: Cortisone)
                       <u>MUSCLE RELAXANTS</u>
                       <u>ANTI INFLAMMATORIES</u>
                       <u>BLOOD THINNERS</u> (incl. aspirin)
                       <u>PAIN KILLERS</u>
                       <u>OTHERS</u>

Fig. 46.2   Subjective analysis.

GIVE A BRIEF ACCOUNT OF THE PRESENT ATTACK: INJURY   NO INJURY

_____

_____

Have you had any previous history of similar problems?   YES   NO

What helped the most to relieve the previous attacks?   _____

_____

LIFE STYLE CHARACTERISTICS

Are you currently involved in:

    1.) Regularly walking any distance.   YES   NO

    2.) Physical activity programme.   YES   NO
            Specify.

    3.) Stress management, relaxation,   YES   NO
        meditation, etc.
            Specify.

LOW BACK PATIENTS: PLEASE MARK WITH A CROSS (X) WHICH ACTIVITIES CAUSE
YOU PAIN.
    DATE

Lying still in bed
Turning over in bed
Standing up for short periods
Walking across a room
Putting on shoes, socks, stockings
Coughing or sneezing
Sitting in a straight-back (dining) chair
Sitting in a low (easy) chair
Getting out of an easy chair
Stepping forward over a wash basin
Standing for more than fifteen minutes
Walking for more than one quarter mile

THANK YOU FOR COMPLETING THIS QUESTIONNAIRE.

NOTE: THE LAST SHEET IS FOR THE THERAPIST'S ASSESSMENT.

Fig. 46.3   Lifestyle and activities of daily living (ADL).

PALPATION FINDINGS

O Tender   ✕ Stiff Segment   ⋔ Hypermobile
● Sore   ‖‖ Thickened (deep)   Segment
            Ƶ Elicited Spasm   ⊗ Prominent

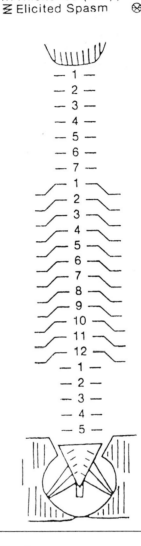

MOVEMENT PROFILE:

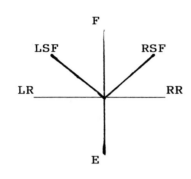

OTHER TESTS

S.I.   T/M

                    A/C

S.L.R.   S/C

                    Shoulder

Hip

PKB   Elbow

Knee   Wrist

Foot   Hand

ISOMETRIC TESTING (MUSCLES AND ATTACHMENTS)

VERT. A.

C.V. LIGS.   TRANS.
                ALAR.

NEUROLOGICAL EXAMINATION

Neck F.

Weakness   POSTURE/ANTALGIC SPASM

Wasting

Reflexes

Sensation

Fig. 46.4 Objective examination — includes movement diagram.

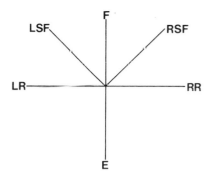

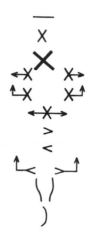

——	Limitation of range.
X	Central pain.
	Will denote the severity of symptoms.
	Central pain with radiation to L or R.
	Central pain with radiation into L or R leg.
	Central pain with bilateral radiation.
>	Pain on the R.
<	Pain on the L.
	Pain on L or R with radiation into limb
	Deviation to L or R.
	Arc of pain.

Fig. 46.5 Movement diagram (including symbols).

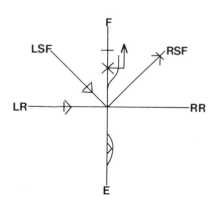

Flexion.	Movement limited to two thirds normal range.
	Central pain with radiation into the right leg at half of normal range.
	Deviation to the R. as movement is attempted.
Extension.	Full range movement with an arc of pain R. at half range.
Side Flexion L.	One third of normal movement with pain on the R.
Side Flexion R.	Almost full range with some pain on the R. at the end of range.
Rotation L.	Movement restricted at half the normal range with pain on the R.

Fig. 46.6 Movement diagram showing use of symbols.

pensatory scoliosis, or antalgic deviation develops above or at the site of the primary lesion. The segment with the type II lesion is often at the junction areas and at the caudal end of the compensatory curve, whilst with type I or neutral lesions the vertebra showing the greatest rotation is at the apex of the curve.

This system forms the basis of a more precise positional analysis and treatment by muscle energy techniques being increasingly used by manual therapists (see Ch. 57). It can also form the basis for correction by HVT.

Prognosis

From the basic scanning examination plus the individual segment assessment an accurate profile can be obtained of the dysfunctional segment.

Certain key features or salient signs should be noted. These are used to plan treatment and to chart the progress of the case and the efficiency of the treatment.

Other factors are useful in predicting the speed of response, i.e. prognosis. Maitland (1986) refers to these as guiding factors; Cyriax (1983) includes some under the criteria for reducibility.

In lumbar spine dysfunction, indicators of poor prognosis are:

Symptoms	Constant unremitting pain affecting sleep
	Pain more peripheral than proximal
	Previous manipulation has failed
Signs	Movement causes peripheralization of pain
	All movements including flexion are painful
	No movement affects pain
	Side flexion causes pain on the ipsilateral side (compression pain)
	Presence of lateral deviation especially if towards the side of pain
	SLR less than 30°, especially if contralateral pain is provoked
	Presence of neurological signs
	Existence of fasciculation in peripheral myotomes

Gunn and Millbrandt (1976) have shown that if painful motor areas exist in the myotomes of the affected segments in the absence of neurological signs, progress is only marginally better than where neurological signs exist.

Some symptoms have a favourable prognostication. Donelson et al (1990) described as favourable the centralizing phenomena of pain. In lumbar spine derangement, movement of pain out of the lower limb and buttock by repetition of a favourable movement, often correction of the lateral deviation or passive back extension, was very suggestive of a favourable outcome. This is done by the patient either from standing or, often, from the prone lying position.

Factors such as drug dependency, low self-esteem, job

dissatisfaction or an outstanding claim for compensation can all materially influence the speed of recovery (Bigos 1990, Magnusson et al 1990).

Thus, the examination performed by the manual therapist establishes certain characteristics of dysfunction, of lifestyle and of the patient's personality and weighs these in order of prognostic significance.

For example, the planning and application of treatment in the case of lumbar segment dysfunction with antalgic lateral deviation would be as follows, in order of preference:

1. Lateral deviation with neurological signs.
a. Rest in bed for a short period with anti-inflammatory medication.
b. Manual: specific distraction accommodating the deviation. The use of 3-D tables greatly enhances this technique. Single leg pulls, maintaining the distraction and allowing only a very slow recoil. The pull should use the leg which does not straighten the deviation.
c. Traction sustained, pulling along the line of the deviation; three-dimensional auto traction.
2. Lateral deviation without neurological signs.
a. McKenzie (1981) protocol. This involves manual correction of the use of lateral shift of the pelvis, observing the centralization phenomenon, followed usually by passive correction to obtain the normal lordosis.
b. Three-dimensional traction using the mobilization table (see Fig. 46.7).
c. Muscle energy techniques.
d. Distractive manipulation along the line of the deviation, taking care to avoid all rotation at the affected segment. A further technique which shows some promise has been developed by Evjenth (1990). A side flexion thrust in a position of the appropriate coupled rotation (to ensure that rotation is not produced by the technique) simulates the X-ray finding of antalgic deviation demonstrating side-flexion without rotation.

Fortunately, the McKenzie protocol is so successful that other alternatives are often not necessary.

MODERN MANUAL THERAPY

The manual therapy philosophy of basing treatment on the clinical profile of dysfunction is well founded. Nachemson (1975) stated that, in the majority of patients, the true cause of back pain is unknown. Haldeman (1977) favours a definition of subluxation which may make no reference to a particular symptomatology and gives no particular significance to the subluxation which may be considered a clinical finding rather than a pathological entity.

A review of the favoured pathologies indicates how much is purely speculative. The approach taken by the manual therapist is scientifically honest and non-doctrinal.

This brings into discussion the role of the manual therapist in providing care in neuromusculoskeletal dysfunction of the spine.

In the workshop on the Research Status of Spinal Manipulative Therapy in 1975, manual therapists were not invited to participate — although Wardwell (1975) suggested that they should have contributed, particularly as the outcome of such a meeting could affect their right to practise. Wardwell also postulated that physiotherapists are the physicians' traditional assistants in physical medicine, and to train them as manipulators is as inefficient as a surgeon standing by whilst an assistant performs the surgery. He felt that they would have to duplicate the role of chiropractors and thus have their training. This conclusion was also stated by the Royal Commission on Chiropractic in New Zealand in 1978. Wardwell indicates that professionalism requires the ability to evaluate a patient's suitability, to make a differential diagnosis, to know when to modify the treatment, when to refer, and to recognise the contraindications for treatment.

The manual therapist works in the medical team on a referral basis. In those cases where 'first contact' policy exists, early medical consultation and progress reports are in the best interests of the patients and, of course, are professionally necessary.

Differential diagnosis is the responsibility of the medical doctor. Once the neuromusculoskeletal system has been implicated, and the possibility of mechanical cause established, the detailed examination is taken over by the manual therapist who establishes the clinical findings.

Wardwell's discussion illustrates profound misunderstanding of the present state of the training of manual therapists who form a distinct professional group. It illustrates a lack of understanding of the complexities of spinal joint dysfunction. Spinal manipulative therapy provides the total therapeutic answer for only a small percentage of cases. The rest require a much more comprehensive management.

In a much more enlightened vein, Haldeman (1991), in a tri-journal editorial, accepts the fact that manipulation is provided by practitioners of different schools of manual therapy. He states 'the rivalry still exists, though it has changed to a healthy competition to gain excellence'.

A review of the treatment agencies in which a manual therapist is competent is given by Grieve (1988a) and Kaltenborn (1974). It is reasonable to ask whether any other professional group can come close to providing such a comprehensive approach.

It appears that the simpler the concepts of subluxation, the more the preoccupation with the complexity of specific spinal manipulation. Manual therapists are highly competent in the use of specific manipulations not only of the spine but also of the peripheral joints. It is a small but important part of the comprehensive treatment and management programme. A review of the work of Evjenth (1984) Kaltenborn and Evjenth (1988) using spinal movements with specific and semi-specific techniques using locking of the caudal and cranial segments exemplifies this. The exploration of movement using arthrokinematic principles with a selection of the most appropriate procedures predicated on end-feel from muscle-based to HVT is seen at the highest technical level in the cranioverteral region.

These techniques and principles should be celebrated by manual therapists as the highest level of excellence and should be used to counter any suggestion that SMT should be the monopoly of any one group.

Training

The postgraduate training of the physical therapist in manual therapy can be made by reviewing the work of some of the major contributors in the field. This is particularly appropriate now as some of the most distinguished members have now retired from active clinical practice and this marks the necessity of the new generation to continue the work.

Kaltenborn (1974, 1988) has a distinguished record of developing a treatment and educational system for manual therapists. His influence has been great both technically and politically. He derived much of his background from English osteopathic thought. He has had a particularly fruitful association with Evjenth, and the K E system of musculoskeletal management has been very influential all over the world. In this system, after the scanning examination, great emphasis is placed on testing intervertebral joint motion to establish hypermobility and hypomobility with any possible instability. Particular emphasis is placed on the effect of discrete distraction, the latter being the primary therapeutic manoeuvre.

Soft tissues are examined, particularly for tightness, which could subsequently interfere with recovery.

Kaltenborn has developed therapeutic techniques which closely relate to the arthrokinematics of joint motion. Briefly, with the active component — which has a concave or female surface — the accessory joint motion is induced in the same direction as the angular motion. When the active component has a convex or male surface the joint motion is induced in the opposite direction to the angular motion. This latter is exemplified in the motion of the occipito-atlantal joint, where the occipital condyles are convex. Passive motion to restore flexion at this joint requires that the condyles be coaxed in a posterior direction. In regaining side flexion at this joint the condyles must be glided opposite to the angular movement ensuring that the coupled movement of opposite rotation is in no way impeded.

Specificity is emphasized, with very accurate stabilization in this very comprehensive system.

The educational system which Kaltenborn devised, and which has been further developed in Norway as their current system, involves a controlled training sequence with a number of consecutive courses, involving both peripheral and vertebral joint content of increasing complexity: E1V1-E3V3-V4 etc. (E = extremity; V = vertebral). This policy is also followed by Mennell in his teaching courses. He feels that competency in handling peripheral joints should be gained before spinal manipulation is taught.

First-level examination tests competence in assessment, mobilization and total management. Manipulation (i.e. thrust techniques) is taught only in a clinical setting once the Part 1 examination has been passed and competence has been shown in the manipulation of peripheral joints.

Kaltenborn was responsible for convening an International Seminar in 1973. This was repeated in 1990. This brought together manual therapists from all over the world to study under his team which included European physicians skilled in manual medicine. The 1990 meeting heard the last public lecture of Dr Alan Stoddard, and shortly after this meeting the death of Dr W. Hinsen was announced. Both these physicians have had illustrious careers in manual medicine and have been very influential in the development of manual therapists' training.

The 1973 meeting allowed manual therapists to take examinations conducted by physicians of impeccable credentials in manual medicine in an attempt to establish an international standard. This worthy aim has not proven internationally workable in practice, although some countries, e.g. Canada, used the opportunity to give credibility to their own examiners who took the examination.

However, as an extension of this worthwhile enterprise a rigorous code of educational standards was produced for the International Federation of Orthopaedic Manipulative Therapists — which countries must adopt in order to obtain membership of the organization.

Maitland has done much in the English-speaking world to increase the acceptability of controlled passive movement treatment by the orthodox medical establishment. His text, *Vertebral Manipulation* (1986), gives a detailed description of the rationale and application of passive movement to spinal joints. It emphasizes the importance of the pain–range–spasm relationship referred to earlier in this chapter.

Maitland's approach is the basis of training in Australia, the United Kingdom, South Africa and Switzerland. The earlier training in Australia involved one full year of postgraduate education, with rigorous control of clinical training. Participants were required to undertake a comprehensive and arduous survey of world literature related to this subject. This training has now been incorporated into the tertiary institutes of education and further developed. A further extension of this system is the specialist manual therapy qualification which allows manual therapists access to a group of government-recognized manual therapy specialists in the field for advice, and for patients to obtain very specific help should their condition warrant.

Clinically, there is a strict protocol of approach, determined by the presence or absence of neurological signs, and then by symptoms. A set sequence of techniques is performed, determined eclectically over the years by careful clinical observation. In general, unilateral pain is treated by techniques which affect the segment asymmetrically, whereas central or bilateral pain is treated by moving the segment symmetrically.

The initial grade of movement is determined by the end-feel. Failure to effect a change in the salient signs results in the selection of the next technique in the sequence.

A very happy spin-off of the Australian system has been the development of many innovations by manual therapists (Edwards et al 1986).

Comparison

It is helpful to compare the approaches of three leaders within orthodox manual medicine, reviewing only the application of passive movement. Cyriax (1974) used a set sequence of techniques. The safety was engendered by meticulous analysis of the scanning examination and weighing the factors indicating likely success.

The techniques are manipulation manoeuvres, for the most part performed under strong traction. The more reactive the segment the less the articular motion induced, with traction being optimally maintained. Key signs are tested after each technique to test the efficacy of the procedure in improving the clinical picture.

Kaltenborn (1970) uses techniques predicated on arthrokinematic principles. Once again, the scanning examination is the basis of planning treatment. Discrete distraction of the affected segment is used as the 'trial treatment'. If this proves beneficial the provisional diagnosis of mechanical dysfunction is now confirmed. Other techniques may now be added to restore the abnormally affected motion. Unless the trial treatment has proven beneficial, high-velocity techniques would not be used. In manipulation, great emphasis is placed on distraction and gliding while minimizing rotation.

Maitland (1986) uses a set sequence determined by the site of pain and the behaviour of the joint to the testing movement. These considerations are secondary to the information gained from the scanning examination.

The safety is enhanced by the use of graded movements performed as a 'trial treatment'. Greater depth or motion is not permitted unless there is a change in the end-feel of the segmental movement and a beneficial alteration in the salient signs. Aggravation of symptoms will be determined rapidly, and undue exacerbation can be prevented.

Manipulation, i.e. grade V techniques, would be done only if the advanced grades of mobilization suggest the desirability of this.

Reviewing these approaches, which use different movements on a different conceptual basis, common ground is plain:

1. All strictly observe the scanning examination.
2. All use carefully controlled movements, the effects of which are determined immediately by subsequent analysis of the salient signs.
3. All strictly adhere to the rules regarding precautions and absolute contraindications.

Thus mobilization or manipulation as performed by manual therapists is not a hit-or-miss affair, but planned, logical, safe and effective.

Historically, the whole subject of manual treatment has always been contentious, and at times acrimonious, with much factional, internecine and interprofessional rivalry. All groups providing these treatments are the extension of a long line of bone setters going back to the earliest days of healing (Schiotz & Cyriax 1975). Each group developed to meet a need and to fill a niche. Any group claiming a monopoly is cultist, and such claims should be resisted vigorously.

Other major contributors

It is fitting in this overview to mention briefly the unique contribution made to manual therapy by Grieve (1988a, b), McKenzie (1971), Paris (1965) and Rocabardo (1977). Others have contributed greatly but these manual therapists have given manual therapy an exposure far beyond our own group. The brevity of the description in no way reflects their major contributions.

Grieve has made significant contributions as a clinician, teacher and author. The publication of his textbook, *Common Vertebral Joint Problems* (1988a) has been a major event for manual therapists. It is a book of utmost scholarship. Its publication has enhanced the prestige of manual therapists everywhere. Further, as a research volume, and as a learning resource for manual therapists in the field, it is unsurpassed and rates with the first volume of Cyriax' *Textbook of Orthopaedic Medicine* (1983) in its significance. Grieve also edited *Modern Manual Therapy* (1986) which enabled manual therapists from different parts of the world to elaborate on recent developments in the field.

McKenzie has developed a total system of classifying and treating mechanical disorders of the lumbar and cervical spines. He has classified problems as postural, dysfunction and derangement. Of singular significance is his contribution in the treatment of acute derangement which exhibits lateral spinal deviation, often with loss of lordosis. His approach has revolutionized the treatment of this difficult problem. It is a genuinely original method, developed eclectically after making sound clinical observations. It is a safe, highly effective method requiring patient involvement. This prepares the way for continuing prophylaxis, and future self-treatment if this should prove necessary. This method has received more analysis and has greater orthopaedic participation than other manual therapy-derived procedures.

To Paris must go much of the credit for the present standards of manual therapy in the USA. He has developed a structured training system containing all the necessary elements of comprehensive manual therapy training. He has initiated a postgraduate degree programme in manual therapy. In possessing a doctoral research degree he carried the message of manual therapists to many prestigious spine societies and has always been an outspoken proponent of the place the modern manual therapist should take in the treatment of musculoskeletal disorders.

Rocabardo has taught that the temporomandibular joint dysfunction involves much more than a clicking or locking joint, or one with limited opening. He has contributed to the concept that stomatagnathic dysfunction produces effects on the cervical spine with consequences affecting total spinal and bodily functions. In holding a full professorial appointment at the University of Chile in Santiago he has helped to develop the association between manual therapists, orthodontists, oral surgeons and dentists involved in occlusal therapy. Further consideration of the effects of tempromandibular joint (TMJ) dysfunction can be obtained from Gelb (1977) and Royder (1981).

The role of muscles

Mention has been made on the role of muscles in controlling the vertebral segment. No consideration of this could be made without reviewing the work of Janda (1978, 1983) and Lewit (1985).

The scanning examination does not adequately test the total function of the trunk muscles, although assessment of the key muscles selected from the peripheral myotomes is of course undertaken.

The Cyriax concept of isometric contraction specifically testing the contractile elements, uncritically accepted in the past, is faulty. Visible joint movement may not occur, but static muscle contraction produces considerable compression and joint shearing, with consequent rise in interdiscal pressure. Nachemson (1970) demonstrated considerable rise in pressure in performing simple exercises and straining for example.

The analysis of trunk muscle function in the scanning examination may produce false results. Any evidence of insufficiency or lack of extensibility, such as found in marked postural lordosis with tightness in the iliopsoas,

requires a full examination of muscle function to be performed and a muscle profile established.

In treating dysfunction of the segment, possibly too much emphasis has been given to restoring normal joint motion by passive movement, often neglecting other components of the segment such as muscle. Inadequacy of strength, endurance, reaction time and flexibility while not being immediately apparent, will certainly slow recovery and contribute to reactivation of the problem.

Janda suggests that dysfunctional responses of muscle follow definite rules comprising recognisable patterns of muscle groupings. In response to segmentally mediated pain, muscles with phasic function tend to become inhibited, becoming weak and atrophic, whereas postural muscles tend to tighten and lose extensibility. After Janda, Lewit (1985) has described total patterns of dysfunction such as the lower and upper crossed syndrome and the stratification syndrome.

This antalgic relationship will lead to a state of imbalance, the tightness of the antagonistic group impeding contraction and accentuating weakness of the agonist. The back extensors tend to shorten, while the abdominal muscles tend to weaken. Additionally, altered recruitment occurs. Even in the basic 'sit-up' exercise there was marked EMG activity in the erector spinae group as well as rectus abdominis (Janda 1978). A similar situation exists in the cervical spine. The preponderance of muscle distribution is reminiscent of quadruped origins, with the posterior muscles far exceeding the strength, bulk and individual segmentalization of the lateral and anterior muscles. Tight suboccipital muscles are very dysfunctional in perpetuating the forward head posture. A further example of abnormal muscle patterns in the cervical spine shows the trapezius, scaleni, levator scapulae and pectoralis minor and major tighten while the rhomboids and deep neck flexors weaken. Thus it may be more effective to stretch the shortened muscles primarily and to strengthen their antagonists secondarily.

DISCUSSION

Earlier manipulators emphasized the 'mechanical' basis of joint dysfunction. Therapy was aimed at restoring normal movement to the segment. The widespread consequences of somatic dysfunction were recognized but not stressed.

In this review the more comprehensive approach has been discussed but greater emphasis has been placed on the various aspects of passive movement — this because greater professional acrimony exists concerning these techniques, and the manual therapists' raison d'etre had to be unequivocally established.

Comparison of mobilization and manipulation

Manipulation and mobilization are quite distinct groupings of passive movement. Manipulation involves a high-velocity thrust of small amplitude performed at the limit of available movement. As mentioned earlier only grade 2 limitation should be present which represents only a few degrees loss of movement. On the whole, little irritability should be encountered when testing end-feel. In general, manipulation is used to restore joint range by:

1. Releasing minor adhesions
2. Altering the position of an intra-articular loose body
3. Reducing a displaced articular meniscoid
4. Reducing discrete muscle spasm by affecting the input through the gamma loop system (Rahlmann 1987).

Mobilization involves repetitive passive movement of varying amplitudes of low velocity applied at different parts of the range depending on the effects desired. On the whole they constitute a more powerful group of techniques because of the variety of joint reactions over which they can be applied. They are used extensively by osteopaths as well as by manual therapists.

As has been discussed previously, two important manual therapy contributions have been the arthrokinematic basis of movement and the development of technique, grading and end-feel.

Mobilization produces several distinct physiological effects. It is reasonable to postulate that repetitive rhythmical movement will:

1. Affect the hydrostatics of the disc and the vertebral bodies
2. Activate the type I and II mechanoreceptors in the capsule of the facet joint influencing the spinal gating mechanism (Melzack & Wall 1965, Wall 1978)
3. Alter the activity of the neuromuscular spindle in the intrinsic muscles of the segment subsequently affecting bias in the grey matter cells
4. Assist the pumping effect on the venous plexus of the vertebral segment.

A vast array of mobilization techniques exist. In spite of the variety of names they are linked by similarities. For example, in functional technique (Bowles 1981) and combined movements Brown (1988) the most pain-free starting position, using a combination of movements, is sought, and superimposed on this starting position is one movement done as gentle repetitive motion. In the strain and counterstrain position Jones (1964, 1983) places the patient in the most antalgic position and maintains this for a period. The active relaxation techniques and totally non-painful movements, which are actively performed in a repetitive fashion, play a fundamental role in the management of chronic pain in the 'Pain Clinic' approach.

The common physiological theme in all these approaches is obtaining an antalgic starting position with subsequent reduction in the input from the depolarized

nociceptors. This is replaced by a more normal input which is non-painful in character.

Although the mechanical effect can be described, brought about by segmental motion, probably far more important is the neurophysiological effect derived from depolarization of the proprioceptors and exteroceptors, which, in the absence of nociceptor stimulation, will do much to normalize activity in the neural segment with consequent reduction in the abnormal activity in the segmentally innervated structures.

Application of the mobilizing techniques has been greatly assisted by the research and development of new equipment which complements the skills of manual

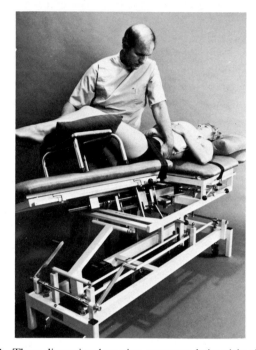

Fig. 46.7 Three-dimensional traction, accommodating right-side flexion, left rotation deviation.

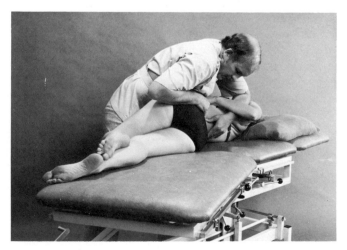

Fig. 46.8 Distraction in extension.

therapists. For example (Figs 46.7–46.11) the Canadian Mobilization Table has been developed and thoroughly tested in the clinical situation to allow mobilization techniques to be done rhythmically with precision, and with proper control of the mobilizing forces regardless of the size, or gender of the therapist or the patient.

Wider applications

Somatic dysfunction has been defined previously as an area of impaired dysfunction of the interdependent components of the musculoskeletal system (bone, muscle, fasciae, ligament) and its associated parts of the vascular, lymphatic and nervous systems.

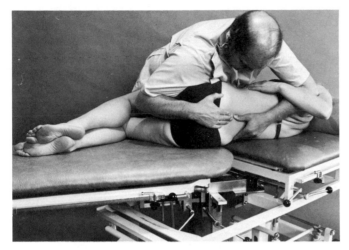

Fig. 46.9 Specific flexion at L4/5.

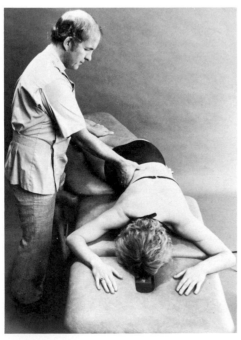

Fig. 46.10 Specific right-side flexion.

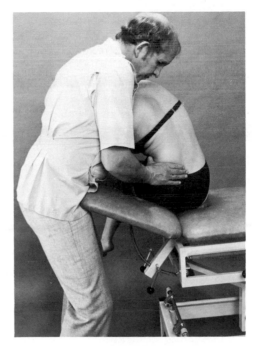

Fig. 46.11 Muscle energy technique for ERSR L4/5.

The question exists as to whether the influence of the somatically mediated dysfunction deleteriously influences other bodily systems; if so, can manual therapy play a role in treatment beyond the strict boundaries of joint problems?

Korr (1948) postulated:

1. The body is a unit: all parts function in the context of the entire organism.

2. Disease is a reaction of the body as a whole. Abnormal stress on one part exerts abnormal stress on the entire organism.

3. The organism has an inherent capacity to defend itself, repair itself and resist serious upsets in its equilibrium.

4. The nervous system plays a dominant role in this repair process.

5. There is a somatic component to every disease. It is a manifestation of that disease but also a contributory factor.

6. The somatic component, when appropriately treated, also leads to an improvement in the other components, to a varying degree.

Thus there is a concept of 'wellness', with the somatic system (neuromusculoskeletal) playing an important role — much more so than merely restoring joint motion would imply.

The classical changes associated with joint dysfunction are: added asymmetry, loss of joint motion and tissue texture abnormality. The first two have been considered previously but it is important to note that symmetry is very rare in the human organism, if it exists at all.

Tissue texture abnormality includes changes in the tissues to a variety of stimuli. Alterations are found in the sensitivity, consistency, temperature and dampness of the skin. So, within the parameter of somatic dysfunction is an integrated dysfunction involving many systems. One highly important common denominator is the sympathetic component of the autonomic nervous system.

To summarize briefly, in the thoracic spinal segments, because of preganglionic connections of the white rami communicantes of the thoracolumbar outflow, dysfunction can have widespread and bizarre effects. In dysfunction of the other segments there will be a sympathetic involvement but the effects will be more restricted to the segment. This may be an explanation for repetitive strain injuries and degradation of collagen tissue proposed by Gunn (1989) in his hypothesis of neuropathic pain, findings being found in both the anterior and posterior primary rami distribution.

Persistent segmental bombardment from the depolarized nociceptors will create a hyperactive vertebral segment, depolarizing the anterior horn cells. This is the basis of the 'facilitated segment'.

Korr states:

1. Long-term hyperactivity of a particular sympathetic pathway is deleterious to the target tissues and may indeed have a rather generalized clinical significance.

2. Abnormally high-density impulse traffic in selected sympathetic pathways may be related to neuromusculoskeletal dysfunction, especially in the spinal and paraspinal areas.

The increase in sympathetico-tonia is part of the stress adaption of the body — the flight or fight response; and is not conducive to healing. In effect, a self-perpetuating devitalized area exists, created in part by the sympathetically induced increased tone of the arterioles, causing a persistent low-grade ischaemia.

Physiotherapists have long been concerned with total rehabilitation following orthopaedic, neurological, circulatory and respiratory disorders to itemize a few. It is a natural extension of this training that manual therapists should be concerned with the restoration of total bodily function, using comprehensive analysis of somatic dysfunction, selection and application of appropriate techniques, and advice on management and prophylaxis, thus helping to attain total body harmony and wellness.

REFERENCES

Adams M A 1983 Mechanics of the lumbar spine. Newsletter of the Manipulative Association of Chartered Physiotherapists 14: 1–5

Adams M A 1990 Spinal mechanics. Journal of Bone and Joint Surgery, March

Adams M A, Hutton W C 1981 The relevance of torsion to the mechanical derangement of the lumbar spine. Spine 6: 241–248

Adams M A, Hutton W C 1983 Mechanical function of the lumbar apophysial joints. Spine 8: 327–330

Bigos S 1990 Symposium on sports medicine for working people

Bogduk N, Jull G 1985 The theoretical pathology of the acute locked back: a basis for manipulative therapy. Manual Medicine 1: 78

Bogduk N, Twomey L T 1987 Clinical anatomy of the lumbar spine. Churchill Livingstone, Melbourne, pp 92–102

Bogduk N, Tynan W, Wilson A S 1981 The nerve supply of the human intervertebral disc. Journal of Anatomy 132: 39–56

Bowles C H 1981 Functional technique: a modern perspective. Journal of the American Osteopathic Association 80: 326–331

Brown L 1988 An introduction to the treatment and examination of the spine by combined movements. Physiotherapy 74: 347–353

Contact 1990 Canadian Physiotherapy Association Sept:1

Cyriax J 1945 Lumbago: the mechanics of dural pain. Lancet: 427

Cyriax J 1974 Textbook of orthopaedic medicine. 8th edn. Bailliere Tindall, London, vol 2

Cyriax J 1983 Textbook of orthopaedic medicine. 8th edn. Bailliere Tindall, Eastbourne, vol. 1

Donelson R, Silva G, Murphy K 1990 Centralization phenomenon: its usefulness in evaluating and treating referred pain. Spine 15: 211

Edwards B 1979 Combined movements of the lumbar spine: examination and significance. Australian Journal of Physiotherapy 25: 147–152

Edwards B, Elvey R, Jull G, Worth D 1986 Contributing writers. In: Grieve G P (ed) Modern manual therapy. Churchill Livingstone, London, 561, 530, 547, 77

Ellman R, Adams S M, Reardon J A, Curwen I H M 1982 Making physiotherapy more accessible: open access for general practitioners to a physiotherapy department. British Medical Journal 284: 1173–1175

Evjenth O 1990 Personal communication

Fahrni H W 1976 Backache, assessment and treatment. Musqueam, Vancouver, ch 2

Farfan H F 1973 Mechanical disorders of the low back. Lea & Febiger, Philadelphia, ch 4

Farfan H F 1975 Muscular mechanism of the lumbar spine and the position of power and efficiency. Orthopaedic Clinics of North America 6: 135–144

Farfan H F 1977a Techniques demonstrated at the 3rd seminar. International Federation of Orthopaedic Manipulative Therapists, Vail

Farfan H F 1977b Pathological basis for manipulative therapy. In: Kent B (ed) Proceedings of the 3rd Seminar of the International Federation of Manipulative Therapists. Haywood, California, pp 135–143

Feinstein B 1977 Referred pain from paravertebral structures. In: Buerger A A, Tobis J F (eds) Approaches to the validation of manipulation therapy. Thomas, Springfield, p 139

Gitelman R 1975 Treatment of pain by spinal manipulation. In: Goldstein M (ed) Research status of spinal manipulative therapy. US Department of HEW publication 76–998, Bethesda, pp 277–285

Gracovetsky S, Farfan H F 1986 The optimum spine. Spine 11: 543

Gracovetsky S, Farfan H F, Lamy C 1977 A mathematical model of the lumbar spine using an optimised system to control muscles and ligaments. Orthopaedic Clinics of North America 8: 135–153

Greenman P E 1977 Manipulative therapy in relation to total health care. In: Korr I M (ed) Neurobiological mechanisms in manipulative therapy. Plenum Press, New York, pp 43–52

Greenman P E 1989 Principles of manual medicine. Williams & Wilkins, Baltimore, ch 2

Grieve G P 1984 Mobilization of the spine. 4th edn. Churchill Livingstone, Edinburgh

Grieve G P 1988a Common vertebral joint problems. Churchill Livingstone, Edinburgh

Grieve G P 1988b Masqueraders. Lecture given to International Federation of Manipulative Therapy Congress, Cambridge

Gunn C C 1989 Treating myofascial pain. University of Washington, Seattle

Gunn C C, Milbrandt W E 1976 Tenderness in motor points: a diagnostic and prognostic aid for low back injury. Journal of Bone and Joint Surgery 58A 815–825

Haldeman S 1977 Why one cause of back pain? In: Buerger A A, Tobis J S (eds) Approaches to the validation of manipulation therapy. Thomas Springfield, Illinois, pp 187–197

Janda V 1978 Muscles, central nervous regulation and back problems. In: Korr I M (ed) The neurobiological mechanisms of manipulative therapy. Plenum Press, New York, pp 27–41

Janda V 1983 Muscle function testing. Butterworth, London

Johnston W L 1975 Role of static and motion palpation in structural diagnosis. In: Goldstein M (ed) Research status of spinal manipulative therapy. US Department of HEW publication 76–998, Bethesda, pp 249–253

Jones L H 1964 Spontaneous release by positioning. Doctor of Osteopathy 4: 109

Jones L H 1983 Strain and counterstrain. American Academy of Osteopathy, Colorado Springs, Colorado

Jull G, Bogduk N, Marsland A 1988 The accuracy of manual diagnosis for cervical zygapophyseal joint pain syndromes. Medical Journal of Australia 148: 17–20

Kaltenborn F 1970 Mobilization of the spinal column. New Zealand University Press, Wellington

Kaltenborn F 1974 Manual therapy for extremity joints. Bokhandel, Oslo

Kaltenborn F, Evjenth O 1988 Manuelle mobilisation der wirbelsaule. ISOMT publication. Scheidegg, Germany

Kirkaldy-Willis W H, Wedge J H, Yong-Hing K, Reilly J 1978 Pathology and pathogenesis of lumbar spondylosis and stenosis. Spine 3: 319–328

Kleynhans A M, Terrett A G J 1985 The prevention of complications from spinal manipulative therapy. In: Glasgow et al (eds) Aspects of manipulative therapy. Churchill Livingstone, Melbourne, pp 161–175

Korr I M 1948 The emerging concept of the osteopathic lesion. Journal of the American Osteopathic Association 48: 127–138

Korr I M 1975 Proprioceptor and somatic dysfunction. Journal of the American Osteopathic Association 74: 123–135

Korr I M 1977 Sustained sympathetico-tonia as a factor in disease. In: Neurobiological mechanisms of manipulative therapy. Plenum Press, New York, pp 229–268

Lamb D W 1979 Neurology of spinal pain. Physical Therapy 59: 971–973

Lamb D W 1983 Canadian mobilization table. Cardon Rehab. Mississauga, Ontario

Lamb D W 1991 Unpublished, for personal clinical use

Lankford L L 1983 Reflex sympathetic dystrophy. In: Evarts C M (ed) Surgery of the musculoskeletal system. Churchill Livingstone, Edinburgh, vol 1, p 145

Lee D 1989 The pelvic girdle. Churchill Livingstone, Edinburgh, p 63

Lewit K 1985 Manipulative therapy in the rehabilitation of the motor system. Butterworth, London, p 172

Lomax E 1975 Manipulative therapy: an historical perspective. In: Buerger A A, Tobis J S (eds) Approaches to the validation of manipulative therapy. Springfield, Illinois, ch 12

McKenzie R A 1981 The lumbar spine. Spinal Publications, Waikanae, NZ, ch 11, p 12

MacNab I 1977 Backache. Williams & Wilkins, Baltimore, ch 9, p 10

Magnusson M, Granqvist M, Jonson R, Lindell V, Lunberg U, Wallin L, Hansson T 1990 The loads on the lumbar spine during work at the assembly line. Spine 8: 774

Maigne R 1965 The concept of painless and opposite spinal motion in spinal manipulations. American Journal of Physical Medicine 44: 55–69

Maitland G D 1970 Peripheral manipulation. 2nd edn. Butterworths, London

Maitland G D 1986 Vertebral manipulation. 5th edn. Butterworths, London

Manitoba 1981 Province of Canada Physiotherapists' Act

Meade T W, Dyer S, Browne W, Townsend J, Frank A O 1990 Low back pain of mechanical origin: randomized comparison of chiropractic and hospital outpatient treatment. British Medical Journal 300: 1431–1437

Melzack R 1975 The McGill pain questionnaire. Pain 1: 277

Melzack R, Wall P D 1965 Pain mechanisms: a new theory. Science 150: 971–979

Mennell J M 1960 Back pain. Little Brown, Boston

Mitchell R I, Carmen G M 1990 Results of a multicenter trial using an intensive active exercise program for the treatment of acute soft tissue and back injuries. Spine 15: 514–521

Mitchell F L, Moran P S, Pruzzo N A 1979 An evaluation and treatment manual of osteopathic muscle energy procedures. Published by the authors: PO Box 371, Valley Park, MO 63088, USA, part 111

Mooney V, Robertson J 1976 The facet syndrome. Clinical Orthopaedics and Related Research 115: 149–156

Morris J M, Lucas D B, Bresler B 1961 The role of the trunk in the stability of the spine. Journal of Bone and Joint Surgery 43A: 327–351

Nachemson A 1970 Intravital dynamic pressure measurements in lumbar discs. Scandinavian Journal of Rehabilitation Medicine suppl 3–40

Nachemson A 1975 A critical look at the treatment for low back pain. In: Goldstein M (ed) The research status of spinal manipulative therapy. US Department of HEW publication 76–998, Bethesda, pp 287–293

Paris S V 1965 The spinal lesion. Pegasus, Christchurch

Paris S P 1988 In: Kirkaldy-Willis W (ed) Managing low back pain. Churchill Livingstone, New York

Penning L 1988 Differences in anatomy, motion, development and aging of the upper and lower cervical disk segments. Clinical Biomechanics 3: 37–47

Porter R W, Trailescu I F 1990 Diurnal changes in straight leg raising. Spine 15: 103

Rahlmann J F 1987 Mechanisms of intervertebral joint fixation: a literature review. Journal of Manipulative and Physiological Therapeutics 10: 177–187

Rocabado M 1977 Relationship of the temporomandibular joint to cervical dysfunction. In: Kent B (ed) Proceedings of the 3rd Seminar of the International Federation of Manipulative Therapists, Hayward, California, pp 103–111

Royal Commission on chiropractic 1978 Government of New Zealand

Royder J O 1981 Structural influence in temporomandibular joint pain and dysfunction. Journal of the American Osteopathic Association 80: 460

Rumney I 1975 The relevance of somatic dysfunction. Journal of the American Osteopathic Association 74: 723–725

Rydevik B 1984 Pathoanatomy and pathophysiology of nerve root compression. Spine 9: 7

Schmidt D 1991 Personal communication

Schmorl G, Junghanns H 1971 The human spine in health and disease. 2nd American edn. Grune & Stratton, New York

Shiotz E H, Cyriax J 1975 Manipulation past and present. Heinemann, London

Simons D G, Travell J G 1983 Myofascial origins of low back pain. Postgraduate Medicine, February 73

Sjostrand J, Rydevik B, Lunborg G, McLean W G 1977 Impairment in intraneural microcirculation, blood barrier and axonal transportation in experimental nerve ischaemia and compression. In: Korr I (ed) Neurobiological mechanisms of manipulative therapy. Plenum, New York, pp 337–355

Smythe M J, Wright V 1958 Sciatica and the intervertebral disc. Journal of Bone and Joint Surgery 40A: 1401

States A Z 1968 Spinal and pelvic technic. National College of Chiropractic, Lombard

Stoddard A 1981 Manual of osteopathic technique. 3rd edn. Hutchinson, London

Stoddard A 1983 Manual of osteopathic practice. 2nd edn. Hutchinson, London, ch 1

Travell J G, Simons D G 1983 Myofascial pain and dysfunction: the trigger point manual. Williams and Wilkins, Baltimore

Wall P D 1978 The gate control of pain mechanisms, a re-examination and re-statement. Brain 101: 1–18

Wardwell W 1975 Discussion. The impact of spinal manipulative therapy on the health care system. In: Goldstein M (ed) The research status of spinal manipulative therapy. US Department of HEW, publication 76–998, Bethesda, pp 53–58

Watson J 1986 Pain and nociception — mechanisms and modulation.

In: Grieve G P (ed) Modern manual therapy. Churchill Livingstone, Edinburgh

Wyke B D 1975 Morphological and functional features of the innervation of costovertebral joints. Golia Morph 23: 296

Wyke B D 1979 Neurology of the cervical spinal joints. Physiotherapy 65: 72–76

Wyke B D 1980 The neurology of low back pain. In: Jayson M (ed) Lumbar spine and back pain. Pitman Medical, Tunbridge Wells, ch 11

Yoshizawa H, O'Brien J P, Smith W T, Trumper M 1980 The neuropathology of intervertebral discs removed for low-back pain. Journal of Pathology 132: 95–104

47. What does manipulation do? The need for basic research

M. Zusman

INTRODUCTION

Despite the remarkable growth in the use and popularity of therapeutic methods of manually delivered passive joint movements (MPM) over the past 100 years, there is unfortunately no conclusive answer to the question 'What does manipulation do?'. The specific in vivo effects of MPM are still not known. Extensive basic anatomical and physiological research using suitable animal and, where possible, human models and material needs to be carried out. Clinical trials comparing MPM with some other or no treatment are obviously of limited value in this regard.

The prevalence and cost of spinal pain, particularly chronic disabling spinal pain, continue to escalate (Frymoyer & Gordon 1989). The future of unproven treatments founded on what are viewed by some to be simplistic and confusing explanations for the cause and treatment of this symptom, is being threatened (Editorial 1989). Evidence exists, and has to be recognized, that some of the explanations advanced for MPM may indeed be inadequate. Certain of the evidence cited is often not readily reconcilable with clinical experience and may be challenged on this and possibly other grounds. The impact such evidence might have on the wider scientific medical community is less easy to dismiss. Available evidence needs to be considered in an objective and unselective manner when advancing proposals and formulating research hypotheses for the clinical observations and effects of MPM. Some hypotheses warrant further investigation; others would seem at this time to be less sound and should be revised or discarded.

Selected clinical presentations and observations together with evidence from related and specific research relevant to these will be discussed. It is hoped that, in doing so, the urgent need for specific basic research will be reinforced and directions which this research might take will emerge. Important elements intrinsic to the patient–practitioner encounter, such as reassurance, expectations, confidence, enthusiasm, beliefs, perceptions and the so-called placebo effect are not considered here.

'LOCKED JOINT'

One of the most dramatic effects obtainable with MPM is the relatively rapid restoration of range(s) of joint movement combined with the decrease in severe pain experienced by patients with an acute locked spinal joint. The speed and (to the uninitiated) apparent ease with which this effect may be achieved have done much to promote the cause of various sects and systems of MPM.

There is not yet complete agreement as to the precise basis for this acute onset presentation. Some impediment to normal joint function — loose body, disc material, synovial fringe or meniscoid entrapment — are among causes that have been proposed (Kos & Wolf 1972, Cyriax 1974, Bogduk & Engel 1984, Bogduk & Jull 1985, Taylor & Twomey 1986, Jones et at 1989). The assumption is that MPM moves or frees the impediment, permitting movement and halting nociceptive input and associated reflex muscle spasm. It has still to be demonstrated that both these proposed causes and mechanisms occur in the clinical situation. Magnetic resonance imaging is one method which might be suitable for this purpose (Jones et al 1989), as well as for other areas of MPM.

RECENT SOFT-TISSUE DAMAGE

There is now general agreement that, with most types of soft-tissue damage, prolonged total immobilization results in a number of undesirable effects (Enneking & Horowitz 1972, Donatelli & Owens-Burkhart 1981, Akeson et al 1987). It is acknowledged that most of these undesirable effects may be avoidable or minimized by earlier resumption of appropriate activity (Videman 1987).

Soft-tissue injury and repair involve a series of reasonably well researched and documented events (van der Meulen 1982). Depending on the nature and extent of the damage, there remains a somewhat variable period before essential adequate, but still fragile, vascularization is present (Lehto et al 1985). Collagen fibrils, precursors of the subsequent collagen bundles which constitute the

651

fibrous tissue of most repair, begin to be laid down by fibrocytes somewhat later (Evans 1980, Kellett 1986). Movement, including MPM, of damaged tissues prior to this time would appear to be of negligible value in directly facilitating the laying down and subsequent optimal formation of collagen, and the prevention of contracture (which, if unregulated, occurs from about the third week to the sixth month of repair (Evans 1980). Intermittent movement after this time could be of benefit in these respects. Responsible practitioners of MPM can also make an important contribution to minimizing the risk of subsequent chronicity in these situations by the informed prescription and supervision of appropriate activity (stretch/exercise routines), and encouraging the early safe resumption of a normal lifestyle (Waddell 1987).

Exercise training

Activity which transmits gradually increasing forces to ligamentous tissue and tendons (and bone) will at least maintain, and mostly increase, the strength and functional capacity of these structures (Tipton et al 1975, Woo et al 1982). However, the precise mechanism(s) by which exercise facilitates repair of these tissues is still not clear. For example, Tipton et al (1986) propose that exercise training enhances repair via an exercise-induced hormone (luteinizing, testosterone) release, and by increasing the blood supply and vascularization of the repairing tissue. That is, restoration of strength, extensibility and endurance in repairing soft tissues with exercise training may be in part due to the creation of a hypermetabolic state. Hence, though, strictly speaking, MPM involves passive and not active movement, it would be valuable if some such vascular/metabolic effect were shown to occur during the early as well as subsequent period of management of recent soft-tissue damage.

Passive motion

There is now also considerable evidence for the use and value of continued passive movement in the early stage of soft-tissue repair (Frank et al 1984). However, it is premature to conclude that the effects of MPM might, for example, be comparable with (and therefore its early use endorsed by) those which have been extensively researched and documented for the mechanical device, CPM (Salter 1989).

Many of the recommended and clinically practised movement parameters for the two treatments are usually different. Furthermore, with candidates for CPM repair is generally initiated surgically. Clinically, integrity of the method and materials of restoration (sutures/grafts) is tested through a full range of joint movement at surgery (Noyes et al 1987). Surgical repair was also used in experimental studies where, over a 12-week period, only 5

minutes of passive movement were performed daily through gradually increasing ranges (e.g. Gelbermann et al 1982). Fronek et al (1983) obtained good results with experimentally damaged, but non-surgically repaired, ligament. However, passive motion was delivered mechanically for 40 hours per week over a 6-week period.

Before the effects of MPM can be compared with, and its use for these reasons considered a possible viable alternative to, other methods and types of active and passive movements, adequate exclusive investigations of MPM need to be carried out using appropriate animal and human models. With one such study the results were inconclusive (D James, personal communication). It should not be difficult to conduct further controlled studies of the influence particular and uncontaminated MPM manoeuvres has on many of the dependent variables investigated in the experiments mentioned above.

Chemically mediated pain

Recent soft-tissue damage is accompanied by chemically mediated (inflammatory) pain. Most patients seek and many report an albeit often temporary and varying decrease in pain after, or even during, a session of expert treatment. It is necessary to acknowledge that decrease in pain can be a specific and worthwhile effect of MPM and not simply a secondary and fortuitous consequence of some other proposed effect. Wall (1987) has recently drawn attention to the growing recognition of the clinical significance of pain per se, and therefore its relief. This is nowhere more so than for spinal pain with its often cryptic cause and highly costly propensity for becoming chronic. Any sound and safe approach to the management of different types of spinal pain which might facilitate recovery of function and diminish the likelihood of their becoming protracted would obviously be of considerable value. The current consensus is that an active rather than purely passive approach is likely to be more effective in this regard (Waddell 1987, Mooney 1989). Some measure of pain relief will enhance patient compliance with supplementary stretch/exercise routines and realistic advice.

Mechanisms

The precise mechanism(s) whereby MPM decreases any sort of pain has been the subject of much speculation but remains unknown. This is partly because with some presentations the actual cause of the pain is not always clear. Another limiting factor is that the neurological effects of this treatment have not been specifically investigated. Knowledge of these effects is a necessary prerequisite to the resolution of this debate. Other more or less accepted treatments such as TENS and acupuncture have been and continue to be extensively basically researched (MacDonald 1989, Woolf 1989). It is now time to do likewise with MPM. Until specific neurological research is carried out the only evidence available for consideration is from related studies. It is emphasized that the parameters for mechanical stimulation in the studies cited are not exactly the same as those which prevail with MPM. Hence, for this and other reasons, the effects may be different. However, any differences and additional effects which might exist will become apparent only when similarly investigated.

Passive movement of experimentally inflamed joints. In order better to understand chemically mediated (inflammatory) pain, numerous experiments have been carried out utilizing different means of creating inflamed joints in a range of animal models. With many of these experiments various directions and intensities of passive joint movements are preferred stimuli for producing responses in nerves supplying the joints (e.g. Coggeshall et al 1983). The effects of such stimuli have also been examined centrally in certain areas of the spinal cord, thalamus and cerebral cortex (Gautron & Guilbaud 1982, Menetrey & Besson 1982, Lamour et al 1983). The intention is to mimic as far as possible neurophysiological events which may occur at rest and during movement in patients with chemically mediated pain. In this regard there appears to be a good relationship between observed behavioural responses of the conscious animal and the electrophysiological responses recorded experimentally, to the same sorts of mechanical stimulation (Levine et al 1984, Kanaka et al 1985, Steranka et al 1988). In general, the results show that, both when the joint is at rest and when moved passively, there are significant differences in neural discharge characteristics between inflamed and normal joint preparations in the areas recorded from throughout the neuraxis.

It appears that under normal circumstances a substantial proportion of mainly small-diameter joint and other somatic afferents are relatively or completely inactive (McMahon & Koltzenburg 1990). The majority of those normally silent small-diameter fibres are able to be activated, and sensitized to mechanical stimuli, by various chemicals intrinsic to the inflammatory response (Neugebauer et al 1989, Handwerker 1990).

Schmidt (1990) recorded a five-fold increase in resting discharges and a seven-fold increase in passive-movement-evoked discharges in nerves supplying the inflamed, compared with the normal, knee joint of the cat. Such an unaccustomed barrage of nociceptive (C fibre) input from deep structures has been shown to produce profound changes in the response properties of spinal cord (and supraspinal) neurones (Woolf 1983a, Woolf & Wall 1986). In addition to other changes, this is reflected in central neurones being rendered responsive to intensities and directions of passive movement which were ineffective in the normal animal (Schaible & Schmidt 1988a, b). Naturally tissue-specific neurones become convergent,

responding as well to input from muscle and skin both adjacent to and distant from the joint (Schaible et al 1987a, b). Some neurones which normally did not do so, now responded to contralaterally provoked input. Responses evoked in spinal cord neurones ipsilateral to the mono-articular inflammation were enhanced in normally bilaterally receptive neurones by contralateral mechanical stimuli (Schaible et al 1987b).

Biochemical analyses demonstrated an innocuous passive movement-evoked release of substance P in dorsal and ventral laminae of the spinal cord ipsilateral to the inflamed joint (Oku et al 1987, Schaible et al 1990). Another putative nociceptive peptide, neurokinin A, was released bilaterally (Hope et al 1990). This finding could help account for the spontaneous (or passive/active-movement-provoked) development of contralateral mirror-image presentations sometimes seen clinically. Interestingly some large-diameter joint nerve afferents with corpuscular endings also showed increased activity following inflammation of the joint. It was speculated that discharges from these large-diameter fibres might sum with those of small-diameter fibres on potentially nociceptive neurones in the dorsal horn of the spinal cord and enhance the activity of these central neurones (Schaible & Schmidt 1988b).

Together, this evidence suggests that MPM in the presence of chemically mediated pain would have undesirable consequences. The fact that, when expertly delivered, this is rarely the case clinically, indicates that either MPM does not produce the same effects for passive movements described above and/or has some inhibitory effect which decreases activity (pain) that is already present.

Inhibition. Certain recommended MPM parameters seem to be designed to have the least possible stimulatory potential (Maitland 1985). Also, the considerable attention practitioners give to positioning of patients ('easing') probably has the effect of reducing any naturally occurring postural contribution to pain and spasm. This appears to be a large component of the so-called 'functional technique' and similar manoeuvres (Buerger 1983, Tehan 1985). Hence, some degree of temporary subjective relief is likely to ensue. Any other effect these manoeuvres are designed to, or actually might, achieve is less obvious. Neurologically, there appears to be some variation in chemically mediated sensitization to mechanical stimuli in different classes of fibres in different nerves conveying input from joint and other surrounding tissue (Grigg et al 1986). Focal concentration of the inflammatory reaction in particular clinical presentations could therefore be a reason why some positions and directions/intensities of movement are more comfortable and less aggravating than others.

The mechanisms whereby MPM causes distinct inhibition with chemically mediated and other 'irritable' conditions (e.g. neuropathic pain) are still to be determined. Electrical stimulation of normal skin has been shown experimentally to produce large-diameter mechanoreceptive and small-diameter nociceptive mediated inhibition in the spinal cord (Woolf & Wall 1982, Woolf 1983b). It firstly needs to be shown that electrical stimulation of equivalent afferents supplying joints produces the same sorts of central inhibition. Then experiments could be carried out with normal and chemically inflamed joints, employing various parameters of MPM as the stimulus, although this is likely to be less specific.

Cherished claims for abundant and uncontaminated large-diameter joint afferent mediated inhibition with MPM (Wyke 1972, Paris 1979) are probably not clinically realistic. On the other hand, the cause of MPM is not necessarily helped by the proposal that inhibition is effectively obtained by recruitment of neural input from adjacent skin and muscle. Clinically, such inhibition can be independently produced with appropriate electrical stimulation, vibration and probably massage (Melzack & Wall 1988, Woolf 1989). The important issue to establish is that the peripheral and central inhibitory effects of MPM are at least equivalent to those which have been demonstrated for other types of peripheral nerve stimulation. Animal models such as those used in the experiments mentioned above would appear to be most suitable for conducting these sorts of investigations of MPM.

Indirect investigation of endogenous inhibitory systems using pharmacological manipulations and analyses has so far been inconclusive in any mechanistically and therapeutically meaningful sense with MPM (Payson & Holloway 1984, Vernon et al 1986, Christian et al 1988, Zusman et al 1989). Further investigations employing these approaches are certainly warranted. Though more difficult to perform, consideration could be given to investigation of any effect MPM might have on chemical mediators themselves. Experimentally, prostaglandin synthesis inhibitors (aspirin, indomethacin) suppress increased resting and passive movement-evoked discharges in peripheral joint afferents and neurones in the thalamus (Guilbaud et al 1982, 1986, Heppelmann et al 1986). These findings correlate indirectly with the clinical relief experienced by patients (Heppelmann et al 1986). Were MPM able in some way to attenuate concentrations of these and other mediators of the inflammatory response, this would be of significant benefit to at least those patients for whom medication was ineffective or contraindicated.

Also experimentally, the response characteristics of chemically sensitized articular afferents appear to decline with repeated mechanical stimulation (Guilbaud et al 1985, Schaible & Schmidt 1985). Whether this occurs clinically, and, if so, has any therapeutic significance, is not known and obviously is very difficult to investigate in the conscious living organism. Use of restrained conscious animals for this purpose is complicated by the observation that they become apparently analgesic for several proposed reasons (Basbaum & Fields 1984, Fanselow 1984,

Porro & Carli 1988). Nevertheless, it could be of importance clinically to test specific MPM manoeuvres in the anaesthetized animal if only to determine whether this effect can be produced and their relative potency in this regard (Zusman 1987).

Sympathetic nervous system. There is considerable evidence for at least a contribution by the sympathetic nervous system, directly or indirectly, to most if not all clinical pain states (Melzack & Wall, 1988). Sato et al (1986) and others investigated the effects of various passive movements of normal and inflamed joints on sympathetic nerve activity and resultant consequences. Significant increases in efferent sympathetic nerve activity, adrenal catecholamine secretion, blood pressure and heart rate were observed following non-noxious (through the normal working range) rhythmical or static passive movements of inflamed — compared with normal — knee joints of intact anaesthetized cats. These responses were diminished or abolished in the pathological preparation by section of various hind-limb afferent nerves, complete denervation of the joint, adrenal sympathetic nerve section or transection of the spinal cord at C2. The authors concluded that chemically sensitized joint and other somatic afferents constituted the afferent arm for these reflexly induced effects.

Intense end-of-range sustained passive movement (rotation) of the normal joint also reflexly increased adrenal sympathetic nerve activity and adrenal catecholamine release. Rhythmical or static passive movement through the normal joint's working range had no statistically significant effect on these variables (Sato et al 1986). At this stage there is no sound evidence either way for any autonomic nervous system effects MPM might produce when administered to either painful or normal joints. Somewhat dubious claims for wider beneficial effects aside (Greenman 1978), it is firstly necessary to show experimentally that MPM does not produce the same sorts of undesirable consequences found in these experiments.

Oedema. Persistent oedema retards the metabolic processes necessary for normal repair and is therefore undesirable (Fowler 1989). Moreover, pressure such as might occur with oedema during the inflammatory response has been recognized as having a somewhat selective influence on the terminals of sensory neurones (Melzack & Wall 1988). Mechanical stimulation (pressure, passive movement) of experimentally inflamed joints was found to produce a temporary reduction of resting discharges in nerves supplying the joint (Guilbaud et al 1985, Schaible & Schmidt 1985). This may have been due to movement-induced pressure changes in the local environment. However, early and significant suppression of these resting discharges was afforded by prostaglandin synthesis inhibitors. This observation led Schaible and Schmidt (1985) to conclude that increases in small-diameter afferent resting discharges were mainly chemically mediated. These authors further proposed that the therapeutic effect of such drugs is via a direct action on nerve terminals rather than by producing significant mechanical pressure or thermal changes in the local environment. It was speculated that the pressure-induced increase in responses observed in these experiments may be more attributable to large-diameter low-threshold mechanoreceptors rather than the small-diameter nociceptors. Even so, any beneficial influence MPM might have on oedema and its consequences would be valuable. This needs to be carefully investigated with soundly designed controlled research.

DEFICIENCIES OF JOINT MOVEMENT

The most obvious and recognized means by which MPM might help regain normal movement in certain joints which present with restricted ranges of motion is by stretching, or rupturing, scar tissue. This in turn would help to relieve any pain which was the direct result of such 'stiffness' (Zusman 1986). However, other factors that impede normal joint movement on which MPM might have an influence have been proposed. Some of these will be considered under the headings extra-articular, peri-articular and intra-articular. Clearly, varying proportions of combinations of these categories could co-exist clinically.

Extra-articular

The function, and consequences of nociceptor-initiated reflex muscle spasm are well known and will not be discussed here. If unduly prolonged for any reason, this extra-articular restraint on joint movement could also lead to inappropriate repair and contracture of articular and neural connective tissue, as well as adaptive length changes in normal undamaged tissue. Despite past controversy, many acute and chronic back pain patients probably do have higher than normal EMG responses (spasm) (Arena et al 1989) as well as abnormal muscle movement patterns (Frymoyer & Gordon 1989).

Several ways have been proposed whereby appropriate MPM might at least temporarily reduce EMG levels and permit more normal muscle-movement patterns, reflecting in rapidly observable improvement in ranges of joint movement clinically (Buerger 1983, Terrett & Vernon 1984). Muscle stretch receptor input acting segmentally or via some supraspinal influence on descending motor pathways could result in inhibition of particular muscle groups. This is likely to be expanded by specific golgi tendon organ input. Certain classes of joint and skin afferents, if selectively or predominantly activated, also appear to be capable of effectively inhibiting muscle contraction (Baxendale & Ferrell 1981, Moore 1984).

Simply decreasing excitatory input onto ventral horn motor neurones is another attractive proposal. However,

here again it is necessary to consider any contribution central changes might make to some clinical examination and treatment observations. Experimentally, even a relatively brief barrage of nociceptive input has been shown to cause long-term changes in muscle activity. Thresholds for muscle contraction were substantially lowered, hence excitability raised both ipsilaterally and contralaterally for up to six weeks following such input (Woolf 1984). These changes, together with prolonged response times, are considered to be manifested with clinical pain in the recognized muscle mediated joint signs 'splinting' (decrease in ranges of movement) and distortions of posture ('listing') (Woolf 1984, Woolf & Wall, 1986). Such manifestations of alpha-motorneurone excitability (postural asymmetries) were found to persist after abolition of peripheral nociceptive input with local anaesthetic (Steinmetz et al 1983).

The production, persistence and therapeutic reduction of a reflex muscular basis for deficiencies of joint movement are clearly not simple. It needs to be shown experimentally that in the presence of pathologically produced muscle spasm, MPM manoeuvres actually depress activity in ventral horn motorneurones resulting in measured decreases in specific spinal muscle group EMG levels. The work of Thabe (1986) is an important preliminary investigation in this regard.

Periarticular

As stated earlier, precise graduated, or abrupt, alteration in the length or location of undesirable and restrictive scar tissue emerges as the most logical means by which ranges of joint movement might be improved with MPM. The indication would appear to be best for longer duration ('stiffness') presentations (Hadler et al 1987, MacDonald & Bell 1990). However, appreciation of the effects movement is likely to have on pain accompanying certain chronic presentations, together with accurate identification of the optimal parameters of MPM, are what separate harmless and effective from ineffective and even detrimental treatment (Maitland 1986). For instance, patients with chronic spinal nerve root or trunk pathology may have adaptive limitations and/or develop reparative limitations of (joint) movement. Following demyelination or damage, axons become highly mechanosensitive (and chemosensitive) (Woolf 1987). The naturally responsive nociceptive endings of the nervi nervori may also become sensitized (Ashbury & Fields 1984). These changes contribute to at least the acute (nociceptive) pain of nerve compression syndromes (Vecht 1989). Later, however, pain appears to have a large central component which again might be provoked and exacerbated by mechanically produced input from surrounding normal low-threshold large-diameter mechanoreceptors (Roberts et al 1990). Stimulation-evoked activity in different classes of normal and sensitized peripheral afferents has also been implicated in the production of both neuropathic sympathetically maintained signs and symptoms as well as neurogenic inflammation (Woolf 1987, 1989). The means by which particular parameters of MPM, expertly delivered, improve ranges of movement without exacerbation — indeed, often with pain relief — in these situations are not known and need to be investigated. Animal models with different sorts of soft tissue, including nerve injury, could be considered for this purpose.

Disc-implicated syndromes

Despite continued claims (e.g. Cox 1990) and their superficial appeal, there is not yet conclusive evidence that MPM will, even temporarily, reduce the size (or shape) of a symptomatic bulging annulus of an intervertebral disc. There is no evidence whatsoever that any externally applied manoeuvre will restore herniated nuclear and other material to its former location within the annulus. Neither is there any logical reason to suppose that even were these effects to occur, they would persist for any worthwhile period of time beyond the duration of the treatment.

Symptoms and signs of nerve compromise. Initially, spinal nerve root and/or dorsal root ganglion compromise are likely to cause neural nociceptive pain (sciatica), and motor signs can be present (Arner & Meyerson 1989, Vecht 1989). Later, with fibre and/or cell damage, this changes to a neuropathy with its recognized peripheral and central components.

However, the precise cause and relief of signs and symptoms in either of these situations are not necessarily straightforward (Urban 1981, Kirkaldy-Willis 1984, Loeser 1985). For instance, Tessari et al (1984) treated a sample of 15 patients who had radiologically (CAT, myelogram) documented evidence of L5 and S1 disc herniations, sciatic pain and positive tension signs (Laseques manoeuvre), by infusing guanethedine (effectively, an alpha-adrenagic inhibitor) into the affected leg. All 15 patients obtained substantial or complete pain relief and negative tension signs for hours up to days following the treatment. The authors postulate that the signs and symptoms seen with this sample were initiated proximally by the presumed compromise, and manifested distally by sensitization of nociceptive endings of the nerve fibres to noradrenaline. A vicious circle involving sympathetic efferent outflow, modified afferent input and further sympathetic efferent outflow (Woolf 1987, 1989), may have been largely responsible for the reported observations, and effects of guanethedine in this study.

Involvement of the sympathetic nervous system in a number of spinal syndromes has long been proposed, as has inhibition of the central neurones of this system with MPM (Grieve 1986). It is worth noting that damage, mechanical compromise or even hyperactivity of the sympathetic nervous system itself may not be essential for its involvement (Campbell et al 1990). However, if the experimental findings for chemically mediated joint pain are any indication, proposed passive-movement-produced inhibition with these no less 'irritable' conditions needs to be carefully investigated. Generally, presentations with nerve root involvement have not done well in clinical trials of MPM (Haldeman 1983). Here again, correlation of measures of heart rate, blood pressure, galvanic skin response, perhaps thermography and pain levels would provide preliminary indirect evidence of any effect MPM might have by way of the sympathetic nervous system in these cases. Experimental models of acute and chronic peripheral and spinal root neuropathies could be employed to extend these investigations of MPM (Casey & Dubner 1989).

Nutrition. It has been claimed that, due to the enhancement of fluid exchange, the human intervertebral disc lives because of movement (Kraemer et al 1985).

Thirty minutes of moderate exercise has been shown to improve exchange of nutrients in the disc by about 10% (Holm & Nachemson 1983). However, as is also the case with studies of the effects of prolonged immobilization and active mobilization on joint cartilage (Lowther 1985, Houlbrooke et al 1990), it is unclear as to the extent to which such evidence can be extrapolated to MPM. The variables in question have to be investigated in relation to the specific MPM parameters usually employed in the treatment of particular disc (or facet joint) implicated syndromes. Then it needs to be shown that MPM produces a direct observable therapeutic effect for these reasons.

In a somewhat different vein, the proposal that regular extension movements of the spine help to relieve disc-implicated signs and symptoms by repositioning nuclear material is not supported by work such as that of Gill et al (1987). With repeated extension, increased leakage of intradiscal dye and bulging of the annulus were observed in all three categories of cadaveric spine examined — with normal/slight, moderate and severe disc degeneration. These authors cite the work of McCarron et al (1987) which demonstrated an inflammatory effect for nuclear material on surrounding tissue. It would be of value to show that MPM has some therapeutically beneficial extenuating influence on either such leaking material or the chemical reaction it appears to initiate (Saal et al 1990).

Intra-articular

Both disc and facet joints could be sources of some mechanical impediment to normal movement of spinal motion complexes. Examination findings and responses to particular MPM manoeuvres often create the clinical impression that the impediment emanates from changes within one or other of these articulations.

Static symptomatic as well as non-symptomatic pathological alterations in the position of disc material certainly occur. Transient non-symptomatic alterations in shape and position of this material also occur during the course of normal everyday movement. However, lack of certainty at the present time regarding the capacity of MPM to afford therapeutically relevant changes in disc material confuses any clear understanding of the proposed restrictive role of these changes, and the mechanisms for restoration of normal movement following treatment.

Traumatized or degenerative facet joints are subject to the same internal changes as other synovial joints. Natural movement could be impeded in some presentations by disrupted or free fragments of cartilage which might be non-restrictively repositioned or relocated with MPM (Editorial 1978, Taylor & Twomey 1986).

This entire area is a potential source for extensive in vitro and in vivo research. Are changes in intra-articular and intraosseous pressures involved? If so, what specific and lasting movement facilitation, as distinct from a temporary pain decreasing effect, might MPM have on these pathological changes (inflammatory effusion, vascular engorgement). Does restoration of movement perceived to be deficient in contiguous segments actually reduce abnormal movement at a pathologically hypermobile (unstable) segment? What is the functional relationship between this aim of MPM and the proposed protective role of strong highly trained trunk muscles in 'bracing' sections of the spine at rest and during movement? Mathematical biomechanical models need to be developed to provide some insight into such clinical concepts.

Assuming that these and other proposals have been seriously advanced in relation to MPM, their contribution to movement restriction and susceptibility to treatment require clarification. Suitable cadaver material could be used initially to simulate the in vivo situation. Should this prove encouraging the investigations could be extended in vivo — perhaps through the use of radiological and imaging techniques. It may be that during the course of such investigations other causes of deficiencies of joint movement will emerge which help to explain clinically observed joint 'blocking' and its 'release' with MPM (e g Good 1985, Rahlmann 1987).

CONCLUSION

Failure to treat successfully and halt the rising cost and disruption to lifestyle wrought by benign spinal pain syndromes is currently the cause of considerable concern the world over. However, this failure, and the fact that no single treatment seems to be more successful than any other — or more successful than natural history and the placebo effect (Waddell 1987) — are not reasons for complacency. The ready availability of not inexpensive single treatments, for which there is to date no demonstrable or acceptable basis or prospectively proven longer term benefit, is being questioned (Nachemson 1990). At the present time MPM is seen by some to be one of these treatments which appear to qualify on both accounts.

This attempt to address the question 'What does manipulation do?' was made in relation to some clinical presentations involving the vertebral column seen by practitioners of MPM. Evidence, mainly from related research, was introduced with the major purpose of highlighting areas for future specific research. The constraints on such research are well known: formulation of plausible hypotheses; sound design; availability of expertise and facilities; conformation with internationally approved ethical guidelines (Zimmerman 1983, Casey & Dubner 1989); objective reporting and interpretation of results; adequate finance.

With the exception of the last, these constraints would probably be best satisfied by engaging in collaborative studies with recognized experts and laboratories. Worthwhile collaborative or independent research requires realistic financial backing.

REFERENCES

Akeson W H, Amiel D, Abel M F et al 1987 Effects of immobilisation on joints. Clinical Orthopaedics and Related Research 219: 28–37

Arena J G, Sherman R A, Bruno G M et al 1989 Electromyographic recordings of 5 types of low back pain subjects and non-pain controls in different positions. Pain 37: 57–65

Arner S, Meyerson B 1989 Reply to Dr Vecht's comments. Pain 39: 245–246

Ashbury A K, Fields H L 1984 Pain due to peripheral nerve damage: an hypothesis. Neurology 34: 1587–1590

Basbaum A I, Fields H L 1984 Endogenous pain control systems: brainstem spinal pathways and endorphin circuitry. Annual Review of Neuroscience 7: 309–338

Baxendale R H, Ferrell W R 1981 The effect of knee joint afferent discharge on transmission in flexion reflex pathways in decerebrate cats. Journal of Physiology 315: 231–242

Bogduk N, Engel R 1984. The menisci of the lumbar zygapophyseal joints. A review of their clinical significance. Spine 9: 454–460

Bogduk N, Jull G 1985 The theoretical pathology of acute locked back: a basis for manipulative therapy. Manual Medicine 1: 78–82

Buerger A A 1983 Experimental neuromuscular models of spinal manual techniques. Manual Medicine 1: 10–17

Campbell J N, Ochoa J, Raja S 1990 Sympathetically maintained pain. Pain (suppl 5) S471 (abstract 916)

Casey K L, Dubner R 1989 Animal models of chronic pain: scientific and ethical issues. Pain 38: 249–252

Christian G F, Stanton G J, Sissons D et al 1988 Immuno-reactive ACTH, B-endorphin and cortisol levels in plasma following spinal manipulative therapy. Spine 13: 1411–1417

Coggeshall R E, Hong K A P, Langford L A et al 1983 Discharge characteristics of fine articular afferents at rest and during passive movements of inflamed knee joints. Brain Research 272: 185–188

Cox J M 1990 Low back pain. Mechanisms, diagnosis and treatments. 5th edn. Williams & Wilkins, Baltimore

Cyriax J 1974 Textbook of orthopaedic medicine. vol 2, 9th edn. Bailliere Tindall, London

Donatelli R, Owens-Burkhart H 1981 Effects of immobilisation on the extensibility of periarticular connective tissue. Journal of Orthopaedic and Sports Physical Therapy 3: 67–72

Editorial 1978 Apophyseal joints and back pain. Lancet 247

Editorial 1989 The back pain epidemic. Acta Orthopaedica Scandinavica 60: 633–634

Enneking W F, Horowitz M 1972 The intra-articular effects of immobilisation on the human knee. Journal of Bone and Joint Surgery 54A: 973–985

Evans P 1980 The healing process at cellular level: a review. Physiotherapy 66: 256–259

Fanselow M S 1984 What is conditioned fear? Trends in Neurosciences 7: 460–462

Fowler J D 1989 Wound healing: an overview. Seminars in Veterinary Medicine and Surgery 4: 256–262

Frank C, Akeson W H, Woo S L-Y et al 1984 Physiology and therapeutic value of passive joint motion. Clinical Orthopaedics and Related Research 185: 113–125

Fronek J, Frank C, Amiel D et al 1983 The effect of intermittent passive motion (IPM) in the healing of the medial collateral ligament (ab). Proceedings of the Orthopaedic Research Society 8: 31

Frymoyer J W, Gordon S L 1989 Research perspectives in low back pain. Spine 14: 1384–1390

Gautron M, Guilbaud G 1982 Somatic responses of ventrobasal thalamic neurones in polyarthritic rats. Brain Research 237: 459–471

Gelbermann R H, Woo S L-Y, Lothringer K et al 1982 Effects of early intermittent passive mobilisation on healing canine flexor tendons. Journal of Hand Surgery 7: 170–175

Gill R, Videman T, Shimizu T et al 1987 The effect of repeated extensions on the discographic dye patterns in cadaveric lumbar motion segments. Clinical Biomechanics 2: 205–210

Good A B 1985 Spinal joint blocking. Journal of Manipulative and Physiological Therapeutics 8: 1–8

Greenman P E 1978 Manipulative therapy in total health care. In: Korr I M (ed) The neurobiologic mechanisms in manipulative therapy. Plenum Press, London, pp 43–52

Grieve G P 1986 The autonomic nervous system in vertebral pain syndromes. In: Grieve G P (ed) Modern manual therapy of the vertebral column. Churchill Livingstone, Edinburgh, ch 24, p 259

Grigg P, Shaible H-G, Schmidt R F 1986 Mechanical sensitivity of groups III and IV afferents from posterior articular nerve in normal and inflamed cat knee. Journal of Neurophysiology 55: 635–643

Guilbaud G, Benoist J M, Gautron M et al 1982 Aspirin clearly depresses responses of ventrobasal thalamus neurons to joint stimulation in arthritic rats. Pain 13: 153–168

Guilbaud G, Iggo A, Tegner R 1985 Sensory receptors in ankle joint capsules of normal and arthritic rats. Experimental Brain Research 58: 29–40

Guilbaud G, Kayser V, Benoist J M et al 1986 Modifications in the responsiveness of rat ventrobasal thalamic neurones at different stages of carrageenin-produced inflammation. Brain Research 385: 86–98

Hadler N M, Curtis P, Gillings D B et al 1987 A benefit of spinal manipulation as adjunctive therapy for acute low back pain. Spine 12: 403–406

Haldeman S 1983 Spinal manipulative therapy. A status report. Clinical Orthopaedics and Related Research 179: 62–70

Handwerker H P 1990 Pain and inflammation. Pain (suppl 5) S217 (abstract 428)

Heppelmann B, Pfeffer A, Schaible H-G et al 1986 Effects of acetysalicylic acid and indomethacin on single groups III and IV sensory units from acutely inflamed joints. Pain 26: 337–351

Holm S, Nachemson A 1983 Variations in the nutrition of canine intervertebral disc induced by motion. Spine 8: 866–874

Hope P J, Schaible H-G, Jarrott B et al 1990 Release and persistence of immunoreactive neurokinin A in the spinal cord is associated with chemical arthritis. Pain (suppl 5) S230 (abstract 448)

Houlbrooke K, Vause K, Merrilees M J 1990 Effects of movement and weight bearing on the glycosaminoglycan content of sheep articular cartilage. Australian Journal of Physiotherapy 36: 88–91

James D 1990 Personal communication

Jones T R, James J E, Adams J W et al 1989 Lumbar zygapophyseal joint meniscoids. Evidence of their role in chronic intersegmental hypomobility. Journal of Manipulative and Physiological Therapeutics 12: 374–385

Kanaka R, Schaible H-G, Schmidt R F 1985 Activation of fine articular afferent units by bradykinin. Brain Research 327: 81–90

Kellett J 1986 Acute soft tissue injuries — a review of the literature. Medicine and Science in Sports and Exercise 18: 489–500

Kirkaldy-Willis W H 1984 The relationship of structural pathology to the nerve root. Spine 9: 49–52

Kos J, Wolf J 1972 The intervertebral meniscus and its possible role in intervertebral joint blockage. Journal of Orthopaedic and Sports Physical Therapy 1: 8–9

Kraemer J, Kolditz D, Gowin R 1985 Water and electrolyte content of human intervertebral discs under variable load. Spine 10: 69–71

Lamour Y, Guilbaud G, Willer C 1983 Altered properties and laminar distribution of neuronal responses to peripheral stimulation in the Sm I cortex of the arthritic rat. Brain Research 273: 183–187

Lehto M, Duance V C, Restall D 1985 Collagen and fibronectin in a healing skeletal muscle injury. An immunohistological study of the effects of physical activity on the repair of injured gastrocnemius muscle in the rat. Journal of Bone and Joint Surgery 67B: 820–828

Levine J D, Lau W, Kwiat G 1984 Leukotriene B4 produces hyperalgesia that is dependent on polymorphonuclear leukocytes. Science 225: 743–745

Loeser J D 1985 Pain due to nerve injury. Spine 10: 232–235

Lowther D A 1985 The effects of compression and tension on the behaviour of connective tissues. In: Glasgow E F et al (eds) Aspects of manipulative therapy. 2nd edn. Churchill Livingstone, Melbourne, ch 2, p 16

McCarron R F, Wimpee M W, Hudkins P G et al 1987 The inflammatory effect of nucleus pulposus. A possible element in the pathogenesis of low-back pain. Spine 2: 760–763

MacDonald A J R 1989 Acupuncture analgesia and therapy. In: Wall P D, Melzack R (eds) Textbook of pain. 2nd edn. Churchill Livingstone, Edinburgh, ch 65, p 906

MacDonald R S, Bell C M J 1990 An open controlled assessment of osteopathic manipulation in non specific low-back pain. Spine 15: 364–370

McMahon S B, Koltzenburg M 1990 Novel classes of nociceptors: beyond Sherrington. Trends in Neurosciences 13: 199–201

Maitland G D 1985 Passive movement techniques for intra-articular and periarticular disorders. Australian Journal of Physiotherapy 31: 3–8

Maitland G D 1986 Vertebral manipulation. 5th edn. Butterworths, London

Melzack R Wall P D 1988 The challenge of pain. 2nd edn. Penguin, London

Menetrey D, Besson J M 1982 Electrophysiological characteristics of dorsal horn cells in rats with cutaneous inflammation resulting from chronic arthritis. Pain 13: 343–364

Mooney V 1989 Where is the lumbar pain coming from? Annals of Medicine 21: 373–379

Moore J L 1984 The golgi tendon organ: a review and update. American Journal of Occupational Therapy 38: 227–236

Nachemson A 1990 Management of the back pain patient. Possible solutions to the problem. Refresher courses on pain management. International Association for the Study of Pain VIth World Congress on Pain, Adelaide, Australia

Neugebauer V, Schaible H-G, Schmidt R F 1989 Sensitization of articular afferents to mechanical stimuli by bradykinin. Pflugers Archiv European Journal of Physiology 415: 330–335

Noyes F R, Mangine R E, Barber S 1987 Early knee motion after open and arthroscopic anterior cruciate ligament reconstruction. American Journal of Sports Medicine 15: 149–160

Oku R, Satoh M, Takagi H 1987 Release of substance P from the spinal dorsal horn is enhanced in polyarthritic rats. Neuroscience Letters 74: 315–319

Paris S V 1979 Mobilization of the spine. Physical Therapy 59: 988–994

Payson S M, Holloway H S 1984 Possible complications of using naloxone as an internal opiate antagonist in the investigation of the role of endorphins on osteopathic manipulative treatment. Journal of the American Osteopathic Association 84: 152–156

Porro C A, Carli G 1988 Immobilization and restraint effects on pain reactions in animals. Pain 32: 289–307

Rahlmann J F 1987 Mechanisms of intervertebal joint fixation: a literature review. Journal of Manipulative and Physiological Therapeutics 10: 177–187

Roberts W J, Lynch S A, Lindblom U 1990 Pain from myelinated afferents. Pain (suppl 5) S256 (abstract 489)

Saal J S, Franson R C, Dobrow R et al 1990 High levels of inflammatory phospholipase A2 activity in lumbar disc herniation. Spine 15: 674–678

Salter R B 1989 The biologic concept of continuous passive motion of synovial joints. Clinical Orthopaedics and Related Research 242: 12–25

Sato A, Sato Y, Schmidt R F 1986 Catecholamine secretion and adrenal nerve activity in response to movements of normal and inflamed knee joints of cats. Journal of Physiology 375: 611–624

Schaible H-G, Schmidt R F 1985 Effects of an experimental arthritis on the sensory properties of fine articular afferent units. Journal of Neurophysiology 54: 1109–1122

Schaible H-G, Schmidt R F 1988a Excitation and sensitization of fine articular afferents from cat's knee joint by prostaglandin E2. Journal of Physiology 403: 91–104

Schaible H-G, Schmidt R F 1988b Time course of mechanosensitivity changes in articular afferents during a developing experimental arthritis. Journal of Neurophysiology 69: 2180–2195

Schaible H-G, Schmidt R F, Willis W D 1987a Convergent inputs from articular, cutaneous and muscle receptors onto ascending tract cells in the cat spinal cord. Experimental Brain Research 66: 479–488

Schaible H-G, Schmidt R F, Willis W D 1987b Enhancement of responses of ascending tract cells in the cat spinal cord by acute inflammation of the knee joint. Experimental Brain Research 66: 489–499

Schaible H-G, Jarrott B, Hope P J et al 1990 Acute arthritis in cat's knee joint leads to release of immunoreactive substance P (ir SP) in the spinal cord. Pain (suppl 5) S230 (abstract 447)

Schmidt R F 1990 Experimental arthritis. Pain (suppl 5) S215 (abstract 425)

Steinmetz J E, Beggs A L, Lupica C R et al 1983 Effects of local anaesthesia on persistence of peripherally induced postural asymmetries in rats. Behavioural Neuroscience 97: 921–927

Steranka L R, Manning D C, De Haas C J et al 1988 Bradykinin is a pain mediator: receptors are localised to sensory neurones, and antagonists have analgesic action. Proceedings of the National Academy of Sciences of the USA 85: 3245–3249

Taylor J R, Twomey L T 1986 Age changes in lumbar zygapophyseal joints: observations on structure and function. Spine 11: 739–745

Tehan P J 1985 Functional technique: a different perspective in manipulative therapy In: Glasgow E F et al (eds) Aspects of manipulative therapy. 2nd edn. Churchill Livingstone, Melbourne, ch 14, p 94

Terrett A C J, Vernon H 1984 Manipulation and pain tolerance. American Journal of Physical Medicine 63: 217–225

Tessari L, Fassina A, Corbellini L et al 1984 A regional intravenous guanethidine sympathetic block in the painful leg relieves sciatic pain. Pain (suppl 2) S393 (abstract 580)

Thabe H 1986 Electromyography as a tool to document diagnostic findings and therapeutic results associated with somatic dysfunctions in the upper cervical spinal joints and sacroiliac joints. Manual Medicine 2: 53–58

Tipton C M, Mathes R D, Maynard J A et al 1975 The influence of

physical activity on ligaments and tendons. Medicine and Science in Sports 7: 165–175

Tipton C M, Vailas A C, Mathes R D 1986 Experimental studies on the influences of physical activity on ligaments, tendons and joints: a brief review. Acta Medica Scandinavica (suppl) 711: 157–168

Urban L M 1981 The straight-leg-raising test: a review. Journal of Orthopaedic and Sports Physical Therapy 2: 117–133

van der Meulen J C H 1982 Present state of knowledge on processes of healing in collagen structures. International Journal of Sports Medicine 3: 4–8

Vecht Ch J 1989 Nociceptive nerve pain and neuropathic pain. Pain 39: 243–244

Vernon H T, Dhami M S I, Howley T P et al 1986 Spinal manipulation and beta-endorphin: a controlled study of the effect of a spinal manipulation on plasma beta-endorphin levels in normal males. Journal of Manipulative and Physiological Therapeutics 9: 225–123

Videman T 1987 Connective tissue and immobilisation. Key factors in musculoskeletal degeneration? Clinical Orthopaedics and Related Research 221: 26–32

Waddell G 1987 A new clinical model for the treatment of low-back pain. Spine 12: 632–644

Wall P D 1987 Recent advances in the knowledge of mechanisms of intractable pain. International Disability Studies 9: 22–23

Woo S L-Y, Gomez M A, Woo Y-K et al 1982 Mechanical properties of tendons and ligaments. II. The relationship of immobilization and exercise on tissue remodelling. Biorheology 19: 378–408

Woolf C J 1983a Evidence for a central component of post-injury pain hypersensitivity. Nature 306: 686–688

Woolf C J 1983b C-primary afferent mediated inhibitions in the dorsal horn of the decerebrate-spinal rat. Experimental Brain Research 51: 283–290

Woolf C J 1984 Long term alterations in the excitability of the flexion reflex produced by peripheral tissue injury in the chronic decerebrate rat. Pain 18: 325–343

Woolf C J 1987 Physiological, inflammatory and neuropathic pain. Advances and Technical Standards in Neurosurgery 15: 39–62

Woolf C J 1988 Segmental afferent fibre-induced analgesia: transcutaneous electrical nerve stimulation (TENS) and vibration. In: Wall P D, Melzack R (eds) Textbook of pain. 2nd edn. Churchill Livingstone, Edinburgh, ch 63, p 884

Woolf C J 1989 Recent advances in the pathophysiology of acute pain. British Journal of Anaesthesia 63: 139–146

Woolf C J, Wall P D 1982 Chronic peripheral nerve section diminishes the primary afferent A-fibre mediated inhibition of rat dorsal horn neurones. Brain Research 242: 77–85

Woolf C J, Wall P D 1986 The relative effectiveness of C primary afferent fibres of different origins in evoking a prolonged facilitation on the flexor reflex in the rat. Journal of Neuroscience 6: 1433–1442

Wyke B D 1972 Articular neurology — a review. Physiotherapy 58: 94–99

Zimmermann M 1983 Ethical guidelines for investigations of experimental pain in conscious animals. Pain 16: 109–110

Zusman M 1986 Spinal manipulative therapy: review of some proposed mechanisma and a new hypothesis. Australian Journal of Physiotherapy 32: 89–99

Zusman M 1987 A theoretical basis for the short-term relief of some types of spinal pain with manipulative therapy. Manual Medicine 3: 54–56

Zusman M, Edwards B C, Donaghy A 1989 Investigation of a proposed mechanism for the relief of spinal pain with passive joint movement. Manual Medicine 4: 58–61

48. Manipulation trials

C. E. O'Donoghue

When I took the first survey of my undertaking, I found our speech copious without order, and energetic without rules; wherever I turned my view, there was perplexity to be disentangled, and confusion to be regulated; choice was to be made out of boundless variety, without any established principle of selection; adulterations were to be detected, without a settled test of purity; and modes of expression to be rejected or received, without the suffrages of any writers of classical reputation or acknowledged authority.

Samuel Johnson
A Dictionary of the English Language

INTRODUCTION

The earliest record of treatment for low-back pain can be found in the Edwin-Smith papyrus, a medical text dating from the 16th century BC; it recommends a treatment of bed rest together with a diet of fresh meat and honey. Unfortunately the papyrus is incomplete, and though there is a description of the positioning of a patient prior to manipulation, any description of a thrust is missing. A more complete description of manipulation and treatment dates from the time of Hippocrates (5th century BC), who advocated treatment for posterior curvature of the spine due to either a fall, habit, pain, or advancing years. The patient was tractioned from ankle and axillae, then the surgeon, or 'some person who is strong and not uninstructed, should apply the palm of one hand to the hump and then, having laid the other hand upon the former, he should make pressure, gauging whether this force should be applied directly downwards, or towards the head, or the hips' (Withington 1959).

Ligeros (1937) advocated that the ancient Greeks did not merely attempt a forceful repositioning of the vertebrae, but actually used manipulation to treat slightly luxated vertebrae for a wide variety of dysfunctions. This opinion is not in keeping with most authorities and reads rather more into Hippocrates' writings than is generally accepted. Although Hippocrates' method may seem somewhat dangerous today, similar methods have been reported by anthropologists and historians collecting material from all over the world. If such methods have been found effective in countries as far apart as Norway, Mexico, the Pacific Islands and Greece over many centuries, then the technique must surely have some validity, and is worthy of scientific consideration.

TRIAL DESIGN

Although manipulation has been used as a therapeutic approach to the management of spinal problems for centuries, it is only in the latter half of this century that its value has been subject to critical appraisal. Trials of manipulation are expected to be randomized controlled studies as suggested by the Working Party on Back Pain (Cochrane 1979) which was set up by the Secretary of State for Social Services. This document states: 'The only acceptable way of resolving uncertainty about any particular remedy or management policy is by the conduct of a controlled trial, with random allocation of study subjects to alternative therapy groups between which the only controllable difference is in the therapy to which the groups is exposed.', and this remains the 'bench mark' for all good research.

Bloch (1987), in reviewing the methodology of a number of clinical back-pain trials, suggested that the study architecture should include: (i) careful selection of representative subjects, (ii) clear definition of interventions, (iii) complete follow-up, and (iv) blind outcome assessment.

MANIPULATION TRIALS

Manipulative therapy, involving a thrust technique, is the most controversial of the non-invasive treatments used for the management of spinal problems. Haldeman (1983), in reviewing its status, rates it as the most widely used therapy, with the largest number of adherents among both patients and therapists. He goes on to suggest that manipulation has no acceptable logical basis and no proven role; the only effect is a short-term benefit when used in chronic back pain.

661

For the purpose of this review the studies have been arranged in representative groups, as described below.

Studies based on industrial population

Study 1

Glover et al (1974) conducted the first randomized controlled trial on an industrial population.

Admission criteria. Eighty-four patients with back pain and associated tenderness and hyperaesthesia were randomly allocated to two treatment groups. The hyperaesthesia and tenderness were mapped out at each assessment. Straight-leg-raising and forward flexion were also measured.

Treatment groups. Patients were randomly allocated to: (i) manipulation, or (ii) de-tuned short-wave diathermy; the latter acted as a control group. The manipulation was a non-specific rotational manipulation, carried out by a doctor on one occasion, followed by four 15-minute daily sessions of de-tuned short-wave diathermy. The control group were given five, 15-minute sessions of de-tuned short-wave.

Results. Improvement was monitored by the patients own subjective assessment of relief of pain on a pain scale of 0% (no relief) to 100% (complete relief). Assessments were made at 15 minutes, 3 days and 7 days after treatment. Both groups showed marked and progressive improvement on the pain relief scale during the first 7-day period. There was no demonstrable difference between the two groups, except at the 15-minute stage when the manipulated group showed greater relief of pain than did the control group.

Study 2

Bergquist-Ullman and Larsson (1977) conducted another study in an industrial group of patients.

Admission criteria. Two hundred and seventeen patients with acute or subacute low-back pain, with or without radiation into the thigh and a history in the current episode of no longer than three months, were randomly allocated to three treatment groups.

Treatment groups. The treatment groups were as follows. (i) Back school; patients were given four 45-minute sessions during a two-week period, under the supervision of a physiotherapist. (ii) Combined physical therapy; patients were treated by registered physiotherapists specially trained in manual therapy using techniques developed by Cyriax (1974), Kaltenborn (1975), Lewit (1977) and Janda (1975). (iii) Control; these patients were treated with short-wave diathermy at the lowest possible setting.

Results. Patients made an assessment of their pain on an 11-point scale, ranging from 'terrible' pain (1) to 'insignificant' pain (11). An assessment of the patients' ability to conduct 10 functional activities was also made.

Measurements were made of certain ranges of motion: flexion, lateral flexion, extension and rotation. Two functional dynamic tests were also conducted: the sit-up and the arch-up. After the initial examination, patients were re-assessed after 10 days, 3 weeks, 6 weeks, 3 months, 6 months and 1 year.

This investigation showed that 70% of the patients recovered from the initial episode within 2 months and 86% within three months, regardless of the treatment given. A significantly shorter duration of symptoms was reported by patients receiving either back school therapy or combined physiotherapy (manual therapy) in relation to the control treatment. The back school group showed a further benefit in that they had a shorter absence from work. No statistically significant findings were made in relation to pain, range of motion and functional dynamic tests.

Studies based on hospital populations and general practice

Study 1

Chrisman et al (1964) looked at the use of rotatory manipulation. They studied its use on 39 patients.

Admission criteria. The age range was 19–62 years. All the patients selected for myelography and manipulation had low-back pain with sciatic radiation, pain on one of the sciatic nerve stretch tests, and at least one unequivocal objective neurological sign from the following list: (i) a diminished/absent ankle/knee jerk; (ii) difference in leg circumference of more than ¼ of an inch (64 mm); (iii) diminished tone or strength in the extensor muscles of the hip, ankle or toes by palpation or hand test; (iv) sensory impairment to light touch or pin prick in a dermatomal distribution. The average history of back pain in this group was 6 years. For their last attack, all the patients in the study received conservative treatment ranging from 4 days to 1 year. The treatment ranged from heat and analgesics to traction and corset.

Results. Twenty patients (51%) with an unequivocal clinical picture of ruptured intervertebral disc, unrelieved by conservative care, had good or excellent results after rotational manipulation of the spine under anaesthesia. Of the 10 patients with a list prior to manipulation, eight were upright within 2 days of manipulation. Straight-leg-raising had returned to normal by the second day in 16 patients, had increased by 50% in 14, and was unchanged in the remaining nine. Neurological signs improved more slowly. There were no changes in the appearances of these patients' myelograms before or after manipulation, whether positive or negative; 10 of the patients with positive myelograms had good to excellent results 3 years or more after manipulation. Patients without a demonstrable defect did consistently better than those with a defect.

Study 2

Doran & Newell (1975) reported a large multicentre trial conducted in the London area.

Admission criteria. Four hundred and fifty-six patients with low back pain were randomly allocated to four treatment groups. Patients had to be between 20 and 50 years of age, have painful limitation of movement in the lumbar spine and be suitable for any of the four treatments. Patients were excluded if they had significant root pain in one or both legs, if straight-leg-raising was reduced to less than 30% on either side, or if abnormal reflexes, sensory loss or significant weakness or wasting existed due to this episode.

Treatment groups. The four treatment groups were as follows. (i) Manipulation; techniques used were at the discretion of the manipulator. (ii) Definitive physiotherapy; this included any treatment within the usual practice of the department, except manipulation. (iii) Corset; any corset supplied on admission to the study was acceptable. (iv) Analgesics; this was effectively a control group.

Results. The following objective assessments were made: (i) measurements of lumbar flexion, and (ii) measurements of straight-leg-raising. Further assessments were made of the limitation of spinal mobility by pain, the results of the femoral nerve stretch test, decrease in muscle power, knee and ankle reflexes and impaired sensation. Finally, the doctor assessed the clinical severity as mild, moderate or severe.

Patients were assessed on entry to the study and again at 3 weeks, 6 weeks, 3 months and 1 year. A few patients in this study responded well and quickly to manipulation but there was no way of identifying these patients in advance. The response to a corset was slow, but the long-term effect was at least as good as any other treatment in the study, and the authors concluded that it was certainly less expensive than manipulation or physiotherapy, and safer than drugs.

Study 3

Evans et al (1978) conducted a trial of manipulation on patients with low-back pain in which a double blind, cross-over design was used.

Admission criteria. Patients with pain arising from the inferior angles of the scapulae to the lower sacrum and present for at least 3 weeks, were admitted to the study. Femoral or sciatic radiation was not an exclusion but patients with femoral or sciatic nerve compression signs were excluded. Patients who had previously been treated with traction or any other form of physiotherapy were also excluded. A full clinical examination was conducted, including routine haematological and biochemical profiles. Standard radiographs were taken to exclude any condition other than degenerative changes in the lumbar spine.

Treatment groups. Patients were randomly allocated to two treatment groups: A and B. Group A had three manipulations at weekly intervals, followed by 3 weeks of codeine phosphate taken as necessary; group B had the first 3 weeks on codeine phosphate followed by three manipulations at weekly intervals. The manipulations were given by an experienced medically qualified manipulator using a rotational thrust with distraction both to the right and to the left.

Results. The following parameters were used to assess progress. (i) Measurement of anterior flexion of the lumbar spine. (ii) Daily pain scores on a four-point scale ranging from 0 (= no pain) to 3 (= severe pain). (iii) The number of codeine phosphate tablets taken. (iv) Patient's assessment of progress at the end of each 3-week period using the scale: ineffective, equivocal, effective, highly effective. (v) Patient's preference at the end of the trial as to the best 3-week period. (vi) Patient's overall assessment at the end of the trial comparing their condition at the commencement of the study using the scale: deteriorated, no change, slight improvement, marked improvement.

There was a significant increase in spinal flexion during the 3-week period of manipulation followed by a significant decrease in the period after manipulation. The first week of manipulative treatment was more painful than the corresponding week in the group taking codeine phosphate, which acted as the control group, but in the second and third weeks patients in the manipulated group were less painful. Pain scores were significantly lower at the end of 1 month, but only in the group receiving manipulation as the first treatment. Patients benefiting subjectively from manipulation were more likely to be older than those who derived no benefit. The age of onset of symptoms were significantly later in those who responded.

The radiographic analysis (Roberts & Evans 1978) conducted on this group of patients was of no benefit in predicting or assessing the response of these patients to manipulation. The authors suggest that although it is a commonly requested investigation, it contributes very little to the management of patients with back pain except to exclude serious pathology before any form of physical treatment is carried out.

Study 4

Sims-Williams et al (1978, 1979) conducted a two-part study of mobilization and manipulation for patients with low-back pain. The first study (1978) looked at a group of patients in general practice, while the second study (1979) dealt with a group of patients referred for hospital consultation.

Admission criteria. Patients, aged 20–65 years presenting with low-back pain sufficient for their general practitioner to request radiographs, were admitted to the study. Patients with gross radiological abnormalities of the spine were eliminated, as were patients with bladder or bowel disturbances, muscle wasting and previous spinal surgery. These same criteria applied to both studies.

Treatment groups. Patients were randomly allocated to either active or placebo (control) physiotherapy. The active treatment consisted of mobilization and manipulation of the spine as described by Maitland (1977). Placebo physiotherapy consisted of microwave radiation at the lowest possible setting, given to the lumbar spine for 15 minutes. The same physiotherapists treated all the patients in both studies with comparable degrees of enthusiasm. Treatments were given daily for 1 week and then three times weekly for 3 weeks. However, treatment could be stopped earlier if symptoms were relieved.

Results. Assessments were made by a physician without knowledge of the treatment given. Objective measurements were made of flexion, extension and lateral flexion of the lumbar spine and straight-leg-raising, using a goniometer (Loebl 1967, Reynolds 1975). Lumbar radiographs were scored for changes in the intervertebral disc spaces and vertebral end-plates, the development of osteophytes and apophyseal joint changes. Assessments were made at the end of 4 weeks treatment, 2 months later, and by postal questionnaire after 1 year. Subjective assessments were made on the following: (i) assessment of pain, (ii) return to normal activities, (iii) opinions on the value of treatment, and (iv) the need for further treatment.

Immediately after treatment many patients showed improvements on the various features studied. However, in the treated group of the general practice study, there was a significant increase in ability to do at least light work. This same group also showed a significant increase in the range of straight-leg-raising, compared with the controls. The only differences between the two populations was that the hospital group were significantly: (i) older, (ii) more restricted in activity, (iii) had a longer history of pain, (iv) had more night pain, (v) had greater restriction of movement, and (vi) radiologically showed more osteophytes at L4–5 and L5–S1 levels and more apophyseal arthrosis at L5–S1. No prognostic factors could be found on age, sex, physical activity, mode of onset, precipitating cause, root pain, radiation of pain, straight-leg-raising and radiological changes.

Study 5

Fisk (1979a) studied 10 patients selected from a general practice and compared them with 10 normal subjects with no history of back pain.

Admission criteria. Patients were selected with low-back pain favouring one side of the back. The duration of symptoms ranged from 2 to 35 days; age ranged from 25 to 55 years.

Treatment groups. The author employed a single manipulation using a modified 'million dollar roll' (lumbar rotation technique) resulting in gapping, or cavitation of the apophyseal joint on the side manipulated. The non-painful side was manipulated first, followed by the painful side.

Results. Assessment was made of alterations in the measurement of passive hamstring stretch, a factor which the author has observed to be commonly limited in this type of patient. The measurements (Fisk 1979b) were made by an independent assessor. Tension measurements in both legs were taken at five-degree increments as the legs were passively raised, with the knees extended, both before and after manipulation. When compared with a control group, who were also manipulated and measured, there was a statistically significant alteration in tension measurements after manipulation of the painful side in the back pain group as compared with the controls.

Study 6

Rasmussen (1979) reported a randomized trial on a small group of hospital patients.

Admission criteria. Patients between the ages of 20 and 50 years were admitted to the study. Any patient exhibiting signs of root pressure and having symptoms for longer than 3 weeks was excluded from the trial. The only treatment acceptable prior to entry was analgesics.

Treatment groups. Patients were randomly allocated to two treatment groups: (i) short-wave diathermy, three times a week for 14 days (control), and (ii) manipulation, three times a week for 14 days. The treatment was given either by a physician or a physiotherapist using the same rotational manipulation, in the pain-free direction.

Results. Before starting therapy all 24 patients in the study were subject to a routine clinical examination and X-ray of the lumbar spine. Subsequently, they were re-examined at the end of each week's treatment. The following outcome measures were used: (i) fitness for work, (ii) pain/painlessness, (iii) spinal flexion (using a modified Schober test), (iv) routine rheumatological examination, (v) routine neurological examination.

Patients were considered better if they fulfilled the following criteria: (i) no pain at all, (ii) normal function, (iii) no objective signs of disease, (iv) were fit for work.

Of the patients treated with manipulation, 92% were free of symptoms within the 14-day period. Only 25% of the short-wave diathermy group were symptom-free. The mobility of all patients receiving manipulation improved, whereas only half the control group improved.

Study 7

Coxhead et al (1981) conducted a randomized controlled trial that looked at manipulation as well as a range of other treatments commonly used by physiotherapists.

This study compared the use of manipulation, alone and in combination with other treatments, in a multicentre study which took part in eight hospitals in the London area. A factorial design was adopted in order to study each of the treatments at two levels—given and not given.

Admission criteria. Patients complaining of back pain and/or paraesthesiae of sciatic distribution in the lower limb, radiating at least as far as the buttock crease, between the ages of 20 and 65 years, were admitted to the study. Patients with any obvious preference or dislike for one particular type of treatment were excluded. Further exclusions were: (i) malignant disease, (ii) pregnancy, (iii) surgery to spine, (iv) sacro-iliac and vertebral disease, (v) vertebral collapse and gross structural abnormalities.

Treatment groups. The treatments studied were: (i) exercises, (ii) traction, using 'tru-trac' apparatus, (iii) corsets, (iv) manipulation—based on the work of Maitland (1977).

Because the techniques were carefully graded, they allowed quantification of treatments given and standardization of treatments used in each centre. These were compared with the *control treatment*: one having a minimal mechanical effect on the patient and consisting of short-wave diathermy and a 'back lecture' containing advice on posture and lifting in relation to the patients' work and daily living activities. In order to standardize any beneficial effect this may have had, it was given to all the patients in the study. In addition, a control situation was achieved in the statistical analysis by comparing all those patients who had any one treatment, with those who did not have it.

Allocation to the treatment groups was entirely random. The duration of any given treatment was at the discretion of the physiotherapists and was initially on a daily basis, reducing as the patient's symptoms settled. All the physiotherapists taking part in the study were experienced and had received special training in the use of the manipulative techniques.

Results. All the 334 patients in the study underwent the same procedures, which were: (i) initial examination by a physician in rheumatology or orthopaedic outpatient departments; (ii) initial examination by physiotherapists; (iii) allocation to treatment groups; (iv) standardized X-ray examination; (v) therapy programme for 1 month; (vi) assessment 1 month after commencing treatment, by physiotherapist and also by physician; (vii) further assessment 4 months after entry to the trial; (viii) postal questionnaire 16 months after entry.

Assessment of improvement was made on the following measures. (i) Pain analogue on a three-point scale: better, no change, worse. A further assessment was made during the physician's follow-up examination, the patient being asked to rate improvement or deterioration on a percentage scale of −100% to +100%. (ii) Return to physical activities and work. (iii) Mobility tests. Measurements were made of sagittal and lateral mobility using a spirit goniometer. Hip range and straight-leg-raising were also measured. (iv) Dynamic strength tests—the arch-up and sit-up. (v) Changes in clinical signs such as extent of pain and alterations in ankle and knee jerks. (vi) Radiographic measurements of the lower three levels of the lumbar spine.

There were two significant results from this study:

1. Patients receiving manipulation had significantly less pain than those receiving other treatments, at the 1-month assessment. This result was significant only on the pain assessment.

2. There was a significant increase in symptomatic improvement with increasing numbers of treatments, irrespective of the actual treatments used. This was complemented by a clear tendency for those who received fewer types of treatment during the trial to have further treatment in the ensuing 3 months.

Measurements of mobility did not show any significant changes during the study of the follow-up period. None of the clinical characteristics of the patients in the trial was associated with a tendency to do well or badly with a particular treatment.

A significant number of patients originally receiving manipulation still remained in the same jobs at the 1-year follow-up, compared with those receiving other treatments. There is now supporting evidence of the importance of this finding on the long-term management of back pain: the study of Meade et al (1990).

Study 8

Farrell and Twomey (1982) compared two conservative treatment approaches in the management of acute low-back pain.

Admission criteria. Patients eligible for admission to the study had to fulfil the following criteria: (i) aged 20–65 years; (ii) experience pain on lumbar movements or straight-leg-raising; (iii) complain of pain centrally or paravertebrally between T12 and the gluteal folds; (iv) have symptoms of 3-week duration, or less; (v) have had a pain-free period of 6 months before the onset of the current episode.

Exclusions: (i) previous treatment in the current episode; (ii) pregnancy; (iii) signs of cauda equina pressure, or altered sensation, reflexes or muscle weakness in the lower extremity; (iv) surgery of the lumbar spine; (v) history of fracture in the lower thoracic/lumbar region; (vi) systemic disease (e.g. rheumatoid arthritis, ankylosing spondylitis or carcinoma).

Forty-eight patients completed the study; subsequently, eight were withdrawn as they did not pass the criteria for entry. The remaining subjects were randomly placed into two groups.

Treatment groups. The treatment given to each group was as follows. (i) Passive mobilization and manipulation techniques localized to one motion segment, as described in the literature (Stoddard 1981, Maitland 1977). (ii) Microwave diathermy, isometric abdominal exercises and ergonomic instruction.

All personnel involved in the assessment and treatment of the patients were registered physiotherapists.

Results. Identical procedures were used in each centre. Before treatment commenced, and at intervals thereafter, an independent observer carefully examined each subject. The following assessments were made: (i) patients completed a functional limitation questionnaire as described by Bergquist-Ullman and Larsson (1977); (ii) back pain was assessed on a 0–10 rating; (iii) lumbar movements and straight-leg-raising were measured.

Assessments were made before and after the first treatment, after the third treatment, after the final treatment, and 3 weeks from the date of the initial treatment. There was a significant difference between the two treatments with regard to the number of days taken to become symptom-free. The manipulated group required 3.5 treatments compared with 5.8 treatments from the heat and exercise group.

After 3 weeks treatment there was no significant difference between the subjective pain ratings of the two treatment groups, although there was a trend favouring manipulation. Passive mobilization and manipulation allowed the patients to achieve a greater range of lumbar extension by the final day of treatment. However, this result must be interpreted with caution because of the large number of tests completed for the various lumbar movements over the duration of the study.

A similar uncontrolled study was conducted by Edwards (1969) in which patients with acute low-back pain were treated with either: (i) heat, massage and exercise, or (ii) passive movement techniques of mobilization and manipulation.

The lengths of time taken to obtain an acceptable result were compared. The results did not reach significant levels, although the number of treatments needed to obtain an acceptable result by mobilization and manipulation was approximately half the number required by heat, massage and exercise. It was found that because of the gentleness of the techniques, good results could be obtained with mobilization even if some neurological symptoms were present.

Study 9

Hadler et al (1987) conducted a trial looking at the benefit of spinal manipulation as an adjunctive therapy for low-back pain.

Admission criteria. Forty-five subjects between the ages of 18 and 40 years took part in a controlled trial. All the subjects suffered from low-back pain of less than 1 month's duration and denied any prior episode of back pain within the previous 6 months.

Treatment groups. There were two treatment groups: (i) spinal manipulation consisting of a thrust technique sufficient to move the facet joints, and (ii) spinal mobilization, without the rotational forces and leverages required to move facet joints; the latter group also acted as the control group.

Results. Patients were randomly allocated to one of the two groups. This randomization was also stratified, at the outset, into those whose symptoms had been present for less than 2 weeks and those whose pain had persisted for 2–4 weeks.

Assessment was by means of a functional impairment questionnaire which showed a positive treatment effect of manipulation in the group with more prolonged symptoms. In the first week following manipulation these patients improved to a greater degree and more rapidly than the group with symptoms under 2 weeks.

STUDIES BASED ON THE CERVICAL SPINE

Study 1

A study of manipulation for chronic neck pain was reported by Sloop et al (1982). A controlled, double-blind approach to manipulation of the cervical spine was undertaken in order to demonstrate any benefit manipulation may have in the relief of pain and other symptoms. An attempt was also made to identify any characteristics of the patients which may have prognostic value in the management of chronic neck pain.

Admission criteria. Thirty-nine patients with a diagnosis of either cervical spondylosis or non-specific neck pain were admitted to the study. The criteria for admission to the study were: (i) pain of at least 1 month's duration; (ii) absence of major systemic disease; (iii) no presence of neurological signs; (iv) no extraneous local cause of symptoms.

Eighteen patients were randomly assigned to the control groups and 21 to the treatment group.

Treatment groups. Patients in the treatment group were given an amnesic dose of diazepam followed by manipulation of the cervical spine carried out by a rheumatologist experienced in manipulative techniques. The control group received diazepam only.

A follow-up assessment was conducted after 3 weeks by an independent physician. Patients who had not improved at this point returned for a second, cross-over treatment. Further assessments were made 3 weeks after the second treatment. All patients were re-assessed at 12 weeks.

Results. A baseline examination was performed on all patients together with a minimal radiographic examination. Patients completed the Middlesex Hospital questionnaire and a social re-adjustment rating scale dealing with life changes during the preceding 12 months.

No difference between the two groups were found on age, sex, range of movement, radiological changes, examination for tenderness, tablet count, history of trauma, location of pain and graphic self-assessments of symptoms and disability. Statements of outcome by the patients and mean visual analogue scales for pain and activity showed no significant differences between manipulation and control groups, though tests favoured manipulation. Those patients from this control group who were subsequently treated with manipulation showed no consistent favourable response. The authors therefore concluded that the value of a single manipulation of the cervical spine had not been established.

Study 2

A trial of manipulation for migraine was conducted by Parker et al (1978) over a period of 6 months.

Admission criteria. Eighty-five volunteers under the age of 55 years, suffering from migraine, were selected by a psychiatrist and also by a neurologist. Only those patients who were considered by both assessors to have migraine were admitted to the study after a 2-month observation phase. Patients who reported less than four migraine attacks in the 2-month period were excluded from the study.

Treatment groups. There were three treatment groups, as follows:

1. Chiropractic manipulation. Manipulation was defined as 'movement of joints beyond normal limitations'. The chiropractors were free to manipulate other parts of the spine of patients in this group.

2. Manipulation. Two medical practitioners and four physiotherapists acted as therapists for this group. The definition of manipulation was the same for this group as in the chiropractic group. Therapists were also free to manipulate other regions as well as the cervical spine.

3. Control. One medical practitioner and six physiotherapists were therapists for this group and were required to perform cervical mobilization described as 'movement of joints within normal limitations'.

Patients were randomly allocated to one of three treatment groups. Patients were not treated more than twice a week during the 2-month treatment phase. The medical practitioners and physiotherapists were selected on the basis of their training and practice in spinal manipulation.

Results. All the patients had cervical spine radiographs before entering the trial. They also completed the Eysenck personality inventory (EPI), in order to obtain a score on neuroticism and extroversion, and a 30-item general health questionnaire. Medical details of the headaches and drugs taken were recorded. During the trial patients were requested to complete a 'migraine form' at the end of each attack; this recorded: (i) duration of attack, in hours; (ii) pain, measured on a visual analogue scale; (iii) disability, measured on a five-point scale ranging from 1 (= usual activities not interrupted) to 5 (= had to remain in bed in a darkened room).

For the whole group, migraine attacks were significantly reduced following therapy. Analysis also showed that reduction in frequency of attacks was similar for those with X-ray evidence of a degenerative cervical spine and those with no radiological evidence of degeneration. No differences in outcome were found between those patients who were manipulated either by orthodox therapists or chiropractors and those who received 'control' mobilization. Chiropractic manipulation was no more effective than the other treatments in reducing the frequency, duration or associated disability of the attack; however, the patients did report a greater reduction of pain associated with their attacks.

STUDIES BASED ON OSTEOPATHIC/ CHIROPRACTIC MANIPULATION

Study 1

A retrospective study of 5310 patients was undertaken in a study of back pain in osteopathic practice (Burton 1981). Almost half the patients in this study had their symptoms for over 4 months. Low-back pain was recorded mainly between the L4 and S2 level; 50% of the low-back cases had associated symptoms in the lower limbs, whilst 75% of cervical problems had associated symptoms in the upper limbs.

The most frequently used examination procedures were palpation, observation combined with standard orthopaedic and neurological testing procedures. The following treatments were used:

Deep soft-tissue techniques	69.9%
Passive joint movement	51.9%
High-velocity thrust	48.0%
Manual traction	16.0%
Mechanical traction	2.8%

There was no evidence to show that objective measures of outcome were used, but a satisfactory result was claimed in over 80% of cases.

Because of the design of this study, standardization of both admission criteria and treatment was impossible and records were often incomplete. The results of this type of study must therefore be interpreted with caution but they may be of some value in collecting historical data.

Study 2

Hoehler et al (1981) reported on a randomized clinical trial of 95 patients with low-back pain.

Admission criteria. The main criteria for admission to the study was low-back pain presenting with palpatory cues indicating hyperalgesia or a restricted or painful range of vertebral movement. This decision was made by the examining physician. Patients were excluded for the following reasons: (i) pregnancy, (ii) disorders of the spinal cord or cord equina, (iii) advanced occlusive vertebral artery disease, (iv) spinal disease, (v) recent trauma, (vi) malignancy, (vii) drug abuse, (viii) asymmetric weight-bearing syndrome or marked obesity, (ix) previous back surgery, (x) disability income or pending litigation, (xi) previous experience of manipulation.

Treatment groups. Patients were randomly allocated to two groups: (i) rotational manipulation of the lumbosacral spine using a short, high-velocity thrust applied to the pelvis; (ii) control group—soft-tissue massage of the lumbosacral area.

The number of treatments was variable at the discretion of the treating physician, who was an experienced, qualified osteopath.

Results. Examination and assessment of the patients was carried out by an examining physician who was not told which treatment the patient had received.

Patients completed a number of questionnaires; a shortened version of the MMPI was used—'Mini-Mult'. Assessment of pain was made on a five-point scale ranging from 1 (much better) to 5 (much worse).

Patients were asked to appraise the effects of treatment immediately and after 1 hour, 4 hours, 1 day and 4–5 days. A functional assessment was made on the patients' ability to walk, bend or twist, sit in a chair and in a bed, reach and dress. The origin of pain, rapidity of onset, extent of pain on lateral bending, straight-leg-raising, and forward flexion were recorded.

The only outcome measure that produced statistically significant results was the pain scale assessment. Manipulated patients felt better than the massaged patients during the first few hours after treatment. They also reported longer overall relief of pain.

Study 3

McDonald and Bell (1990) reported on an open controlled trial for patients' non-specific low-back pain.

Admission criteria. One-hundred patients were admitted to the study from a group general practice in an outer London suburb. Patients were between 16 and 70 years of age and presented to their general practitioner with pain between the scapulas and the buttock folds. The duration of symptoms ranged from less than 3 weeks to more than 1 year. There were a number of exclusions including patients suffering from certain specific pathologies, neurological deficit and pregnancy. The general practitioners decided whether patients were eligible for the study and obtained the patients' consent to attend a specialist back clinic set up at the practice. Patients were given an information pack which contained: (i) an instruction booklet on back care, (ii) an explanatory letter about the trial, (iii) a questionnaire on duration and nature of symptoms, and (iv) a self-rating disability assessment.

A twice-weekly back-pain clinic was set up in the group practice; at the first attendance patients were examined by both orthodox and osteopathic methods.

Treatment groups. Patients were allocated to either: (i) control, or (ii) osteopathic manipulation. Both groups received advice on posture, exercise and avoidance of occupational stresses as appropriate to their situation, but the treatment group also received a high-velocity, low-amplitude manipulative thrust. Treatment continued twice weekly until the patients deemed themselves to be recovered or the manipulator decided that no further benefit was likely.

The control patients were told that there was no treatment that had been shown to be superior to the programme of rest and graded resumption of activities on which they had embarked.

Results. Progress was assessed by means of the self-rating disability questionnaire. The form also allowed patients to report their return to either partial or full work and whether they felt fully recovered. Post-entry questionnaires were completed twice-weekly for 3 weeks after the trial and then weekly until the patient reported recovery, or for 3 months if they had not reported recovery. Any recurrence of symptoms within the 3-month observation periods was reported.

After losses to the trial and exclusions due to development of neurological deficit, 49 subjects were in the manipulated group and 46 in the control group. The two groups were well matched in terms of previous history and disability scores at the commencement of the study. The duration of symptoms ranged from 3 weeks to more than 1 year.

The results showed that patients presenting with low-back pain of 14–28 days' duration had a statistically significant response to treatment, which was maximal between the first and second week.

This study had a strict protocol which is well reported; however, a considerable number of assessments had incomplete data on a number of occasions (8.2%). As the results are supported by other workers, it does not appear to have prejudiced the study.

Study 4

The most recent study of mechanical low-back pain compared chiropractic and hospital outpatient treatments (Meade et al 1990).

Admission criteria. Eleven centres were selected where hospitals and chiropractic clinics were within reasonable distance of each other. Patients admitted to the study were between 18 and 65 years of age and had not been treated within the last month. The main criteria for eligibility was that the patients should have no contraindications to manipulation. Of the patients presenting at hospital, 30% were eligible to enter the trial, against 28% who presented to chiropractors. All the patients had radiographic investigations of their lumbar spines. Patients also completed recruitment questionnaires, including psychological and Oswestry questionnaires. Measurements of straight-leg-raising and lumbar flexion were made.

Treatment groups. Provided that the patient was eligible, the general practitioner agreed, and the patient consented to take part, then the patient was randomly allocated to either hospital or chiropractic treatment, described below.

1. Chiropractic treatment was given up to a total of 10 sessions which were intended to be concentrated within the first 3 months but could be spread over a year if considered necessary. Nearly all the patients received chiropractic manipulation (99%) consisting of a high-velocity low-amplitude thrust; a few also received traction (2%) and exercise (9%).

2. Hospital outpatient treatment. Of this group, 72% received Maitland mobilization/manipulation, 12% Cyriax manipulation, 25% traction, 4% corsets, and 30% exercises. Hydrotherapy and short-wave diathermy were used in an unrecorded number. Many patients, especially those treated in hospital, received more than one type of treatment.

Results. In all, 741 patients were recruited from 11 centres and were eligible for treatment; of these, 384 were randomly allocated to the chiropractic group and 357 to the hospital group. At 6 weeks, 29% had completed treatment in the chiropractic group, whereas 79% had completed therapy in the hospital group. Almost all the patients in the hospital group had completed treatment by 12 weeks, whereas it took about 30 weeks for the chiropractic group to complete their treatment—notwithstanding the fact that the hospital therapists treated patients with much longer episodes of back pain. Altogether, 608 patients completed the trial up to 6 weeks without missing any treatment or follow-up. At 2 years the patients treated by chiropractic had improved by 7% more than those treated in hospital ($P = 0.01$). Among patients who had originally attended hospital, there was no difference between chiropractic and hospital outpatient treatment until 2 years after entry. For patients who originally attended a chiropractor, treatment was more effective throughout the follow-up period. There was no difference between the two treatments in those with no history of back pain. Changes in straight-leg-raising and lumbar flexion showed a trend in favour of chiropractic treatment.

In one centre, hospital treatment was more effective than chiropractic. Two centres showed no difference between chiropractic and hospital treatment. The authors concluded that chiropractic was more effective than hospital management mainly for patients with chronic or severe back pain, a benefit that became more evident throughout the follow-up period.

DISCUSSION

Very few manipulation trials have been conducted in relation to the cervical spine, and although all the cervical spine trials reported here failed to show any significant findings, the subject of manipulative therapy in relation to the cervical spine has been inadequately investigated. This may be due, in part, to the increased reporting of incidents and accidents associated with manipulating the cervical spine.

Criticism can always be levelled at clinical trials; some of those reported here had shortcomings associated mostly with outcome measures, but some had shortcomings related to the size or design of the trial.

Outcome measures

Neurological deficit

This is usually considered to be a contraindication to manipulation, but several studies have shown this assumption to be incorrect (Sims-Williams et al 1978, Coxhead et al 1981). Both the studies that confirmed this fact used manipulative techniques that ranged from very gentle (mobilizations/articulations) to forceful (thrust) techniques. This may account for the fact that patients with neurological deficit fared no worse on treatment than patients with no deficit.

Mobility

Nearly all the early studies reported here used changes in mobility as an outcome measure: only three (Evans et al 1978, Sims-Williams et al 1979, Rasmussen 1979) showed any significant increase in mobility due to manipulation. There were no significant changes of mobility in the other studies.

Return to work.

This is obviously a valid outcome measure to use in a population whose problem occurs during their working life; one study has shown significant results on this outcome measure in the short term (Bergquist-Ullman & Larsson 1977). Two have shown long-term benefit on this parameter, with lower frequency and shorter duration of absence from work (Coxhead et al 1981, Meade et al 1990).

Trial design

Definition of manipulation. The problem of conducting good manipulation research is compounded by a lack of clear definition as to what is meant by the word 'manipulation'. Frequently even those conducting the research do not interpret the word correctly. Korr (1978) described manipulative therapy as the 'application of an accurately determined and specifically directed manual force to the body, in order to improve mobility in areas that are restricted; in joints, in connective tissues or in skeletal muscles'. This includes treatments ranging from the reduction of a fracture or dislocation, to massage, connective tissue massage, stretching, passive movements, mobilizations and articulations. Perhaps the most accurate description of the word is given by the Oxford dictionary—'to work with the hands; to handle or manage'.

Control groups. With the meaning of the word manipulation in mind, the trials conducted by Hoehler et al (1981) and Buerger (1980) failed to fulfil the criteria of a randomized controlled trial as the control group was given soft-tissue massage—also a manipulation technique. This may account for the lack of significant results from the study. The control group used by Farrell and Twomey (1982) also fell short of a 'control' in the strict sense of the word. A group having isometric exercises cannot really be accepted as 'no treatment'. The failure to fulfil adequate scientific criteria may have lead to a failure to obtain clinical results in both these trials. There is a risk that patients will be lost to a trial where a control group obviously has no therapy. However, it is scientifically essential that a 'control' situation be included. One of the trials reported here has overcome this problem by using a research design that had a built in 'control' (Coxhead et al 1981).

Numbers. One study (Rasmussen 1979) had very small numbers which must cast doubt on the reliability of the results. The subjects in this study had symptoms of 2–3 weeks' duration and this has subsequently been shown to be the group which responded best to manipulation. This may account for the exceptionally good results reported in this study, together with the fact that the control group showed very little natural history of remission.

Even smaller numbers (10) were used by Fisk (1979a) in his experimental group. Such small numbers cannot adequately evaluate the use of manipulation in increasing straight-leg-raising. This study would have been more reliable had the control group been patients with similar symptoms who were not manipulated, rather than a normal population.

Blindness. A number of studies are described as being 'blind' or 'double blind'. It is impossible for the patient or therapist to be truly 'blind' when manual techniques are being used in the same way as can be established in a drug trial. The trial of Doran and Newall (1975) showed that an attempt to make the examiner 'blind' also failed in 10% of the cases.

Most of the studies discussed, have attempted to make the assessments following treatment, blind.

General factors. Standardization of assessment and treatment is essential in any well conducted investigation and needs particular attention when a multicentre trial is being considered. The study of Coxhead et al (1981) was carefully standardized between the eight centres used. Meade et al (1990) allowed their therapists discretion to select treatment and did not report any attempt to standardize assessments and recording of data.

The study of Doran and Newall (1975) has been widely criticized for lack of standardization, particularly in the use of manipulation. Their non-significant results do not further the question of whether manipulation is an effective treatment.

The results of Meade et al (1990) are at odds with most of the clinical trials in that they showed that manipulation has a more beneficial effect in the later stages of assessments. In discussing the benefit of chiropractic and suggesting it should be introduced into the National Health Service, they appear not to take into account the fact that chiropractic patients received 44% more treatment than those in the hospital group and the profound financial effect this might have on the NHS. The study reported that, in one centre, hospital treatment was more effective than chiropractic, and at two further centres there was no difference between the two. One hospital that performed well had a therapist specially trained as a manipulator and supports the criticism of this trial on the basis of comparing skilled manipulators with skilled but generalist physiotherapists. Further bias may have been introduced by reason of comparing a patient management study (i.e. hospital outpatient treatment) with a treatment (i.e. chiropractic).

Ottenbacher and Dijabio (1985) undertook a quantitative review of 57 studies using manipulation/mobilization, of which only 9 met their strict criteria for inclusion. Their analysis indicates that improvements shown by these studies are short term. A number of studies used combinations of treatments which included manipulation/mobilization, posture and exercises. When such combinations were used, the effect of manipulation was enhanced. Their findings summarized the results of manipulation trial findings to date.

Korr (1978) stated in the preface of his book: 'manipulative procedures, even in the hands of the same practitioner, vary according to the findings and their changes in every visit; they vary from patient to patient and from visit to visit. Manipulative therapy is no more a uniform therapeutic entity than is surgery, psychiatry or pharmacotherapeutics'.

Research is difficult, and clinical research is one of the most difficult types of research to conduct. Manipulation research is a veritable minefield. Wood (1980) pointed out just a few of the pitfalls in discussing the clinical problem of back pain .

Manipulation research has not yet established what structures actually move and how—i.e. the biomechanics of manipulation. Clearing up this problem would make manipulation more specific and leave only the difficulties concerned with the multifactorial nature of back pain. It may also clear up the question of therapeutic skill; a criticism frequently levelled at manipulation trials is that they only measure the skill of the individual manipulator. This is a contentious issue that could be overcome if it were possible to measure what actually happens to the structures manipulated.

Haldeman (1978), in reviewing the clinical basis for discussing the neurobiological mechanisms of manipulative therapy, sounded a note of caution: that research in the neurosciences should not be used to justify a therapeutic approach without adequate clinical research.

CONCLUSION

Seven of the studies reported here have shown an accept-able result in favour of manipulation (Glover et al 1974, Sims-Williams et al 1978, Hoehler et al 1981, Coxhead et al 1981, Hadler et al 1987, Meade et al 1990, McDonald & Bell 1990). This positive finding was seen in the more chronic group of patients, and the effect was short-lived. Only two studies indicated a long-term result on the basis of absence from work (Coxhead et al 1981, Meade et al 1990).

New ways of looking at studies of low back pain, such as those used by (Hadler et al 1987, Sikorski 1985) may clarify which patients are likely to benefit from manipulation.

On reviewing the randomized clinical trials to date, all fall short of the ideal scientific criteria necessary for the perfect study; there is still plenty of room for vigorous scientific work on the subject of manipulation. As Nachemson (1969) says, those who advocate manipulation must demonstrate whether the clinical effect of treatment is superior to other forms of treatment and also for which particular patients. However, in the final analysis it is not the technique that is important but the patient and his management.

REFERENCES

Bergquist-Ullman M, Larsson U 1977 Acute low back pain in industry. Acta Orthopaedic Scandinavia Supplement 170: 1–117

Bloch R 1987 Methodology in clinical back pain trials. Spine 12 (5): 430–432

Buerger A A 1980 A controlled trial of rotational manipulation in low back pain. Manuelle Medizin 18: 17–26

Burton A K 1981 Back pain in osteopathic practice. Rheumatology and Rehabilitation 20: 239–246

Chrisman O D, Mittnach T, Snook G A 1964 A study of the results following rotary manipulation in the intervertebral disc syndrome. Journal of Bone and Joint Surgery 46A: 517–524

Cochrane A L (Chairman) 1979 Working group on back pain. Her Majesty's Stationery Office, London

Coxhead C E, Inskip H, Meade T W, North W R S, Troup J D G 1981 Multicentre trial of physiotherapy in the management of sciatic symptoms. Lancet 1(8229): 1065–1068

Cyriax J 1974 Textbook of orthopaedic medicine, 8th edn. Bailliere Tindall, London, Vol 2: 254–278

Doran D M L, Newell I D J 1975 Manipulation in the treatment of low back pain: a multicentre study. British Medical Journal 2: 161–164

Edwards B C 1969 Low back pain resulting from lumbar spine conditions: a comparison of treatment results. Australian Journal of Physiotherapy 15: 104–110

Evans D P, Burke M S, Lloyd K N, Roberts E E, Roberts G M 1978 Lumbar spine manipulation on trial: Part 1. Rheumatology and Rehabilitation 17: 46–53

Farrell J P, Twomey L T 1982 Acute low back pain. Comparison of two conservative treatment approaches. Medical Journal of Australia 1: 160–164

Fisk J W 1979a A controlled trial of manipulation in a selected group of patients with low back pain favouring one side. New Zealand Medical Journal 90: 288–291

Fisk J W 1979b The passive hamstring test: a comparison of clinical estimates with tension gauge measurements. New Zealand Medical Journal 89: 346–348

Glover J R, Morris J G, Khosla T 1974 Back pain: a randomized clinical trial of rotational manipulation of the trunk. British Journal of Industrial Medicine 31: 59–64

Hadler N M, Curtis P, Gillings D B, Stinnett S 1987 A benefit of spinal manipulation as adjunctive therapy for acute low back pain: a stratified controlled trial. Spine 12(7): 702–706

Haldeman S 1978 The clinical basis for discussion of mechanisms of manipulative therapy. In: Korr I (ed) The neurobiologic mechanisms in manipulative therapy. Plenum Press, New York, pp 53–75

Haldeman D C 1983 Spinal manipulation therapy: a status report. Clinical Orthopaedics and Related Research. 179: 62–70

Hoehler F K, Tobis J S, Buerger A A 1981 Spinal manipulation for low back pain. Journal of the American Medical Association 245: 1835–1839

Janda V 1975 Muskelfunktionsdiagnostik studentlitterature. Lund 8: 13–23, 266–275, 278

Kaltenborn F M 1975 Mobilization 1. Segmenti mobilus columna vertebralis. Olaf Norlis Bokhandel, Oslo

Korr I 1978 Preface: What is manipulation? In: Korr I (ed) The neurobiologic mechanisms in manipulative therapy. Plenum Press, New York

Lewit K 1977 Manuelle medizin in rahmen der medizinischen. Rehabilitation: Vol 2

Ligeros K A 1937 How ancient healing governs modern therapeutics. Putman, New York

Loebl W Y 1967 Measurements of spinal posture and range of movements. Annals of Physical Medicine 9: 103–110

McDonald R S, Bell C M J 1990 An open controlled assessment of osteopathic manipulation in nonspecific low back pain. Spine 15(5): 364–370

Maitland G D 1977 Vertebral manipulation, 4th edn. Butterworths, London

Meade T W, Dyer S, Browne W, Townsend J, Frank A O 1990 Low back pain of mechanical origin: randomized comparison of chiropractic and hospital outpatient treatment. British Medical Journal 300(6737): 1431–1437

Nachemson A 1969 Physiotherapy for low back pain patients. Scandinavian Journal of Rehabilitation Medicine 1: 85–90

Ottenbacher K, Dijabio R P 1985 Efficacy of spinal manipulation/ mobilization therapy. A meta-analysis. Spine 10(9): 833–837

Parker G B, Tupling H, Pryor D S 1978 A controlled trial of cervical manipulation for migraine. Australia and New Zealand Journal of Medicine 8: 589–593

Rasmussen G G 1979 Manipulation in treatment of low back pain (randomized clinical trial). Manuelle Medizin 17: 8–10

Reynolds P M G 1975 Measurements of spinal mobility: a comparison of three methods. Rheumatology and Rehabilitation 14: 180–185

Roberts G M, Evans D P 1978 Lumbar spinal manipulation on trial: Part 2. Rheumatology and Rehabilitation 17: 54–59

Sikorski J M 1985 A randomized approach to physiotherapy for low back pain. Spine 10(6): 571–579

Sims-Williams H L, Jayson M I V, Young S M S, Baddeley H, Collins E 1978 Controlled trial of mobilization & manipulation for patients with low back pain in general practice. British Medical Journal 2: 1338–1340

Sims-Williams H L, Jayson M I V, Young S M S, Baddeley H, Collins E 1979 Controlled trial of mobilization and manipulation for patients with low back pain: hospital patients. British Medical Journal 2: 1318–1320

Sloop P R, Smith D S, Goldberg E, Dore C 1982 Manipulation for chronic neck pain: a double blind study. Spine 7: 532–535

Stoddard A 1981 A manual of osteopathic technique, 3rd edn. Hutchinson, London

Withington E T 1959 Hippocrates with an English translation. Harvard University Press, Cambridge, MA, Vol 3: 8

Wood P H N 1980 Understanding back pain. Lumbar spine and back pain, 2nd edn. Pitman Medical, Tunbridge Wells, pp 1–27

49. Incidents and accidents of manipulation and allied techniques

G. P. Grieve

History teaches that men and women behave wisely only after they have exhausted all other options (Abba Eban)

INTRODUCTION

Spinal musculoskeletal pain, at one time or another, is our almost universal inheritance and, in sum, is probably responsible for more restriction of free physical activity than any other medical or surgical condition. The features of benign spinal joint problems frequently mimic clinical presentation of a wide variety of more serious conditions.

There is a reason for everything — it is no accident that, of all lay practitioners, the overwhelming majority are largely concerned with treating, by one method or another, common aches and pains and other referred symptoms from the spinal locomotor apparatus. Thus the massive extent of the market dictates the extent of the service, however variegated the service may be (Grieve 1988).

Every activity entails a proportion of mischance, of accidents; mechanical/electrical failure, unsafe buildings, poor visibility at sea, treacherous road surfaces, unsuitable equipment, wrongly labelled substances, vagaries of wind when crop-spraying and so on. By contrast, whether working with a technically-sophisticated plinth or a kitchen table and two pillows, the manipulative setting when treating vertebral problems involves only the therapist's concepts, clinical wits, skill and the patient.

Provided the clinical history is *prima facie* trustworthy, and X-rays, when indicated, have excluded significant mechanical defect, significant bony anomaly and bone disease (so far as is possible) the therapist enjoys as much control of the variables as can reasonably be achieved, i.e. need consider only clinical purpose, the patient's temperament and physique, indications, contraindications, conditions requiring extra care, localization of effect, choice of technique, method of application, grading of energy applied and likely after-effects.

INCIDENCE

Writers (Lescure 1954, Brewerton 1964, Schiötz & Cyriax 1975, Dvorak & Orelli 1982, Gutmann 1983) stress the infrequency of accidents reported in the medical journals, compared to the number (here follows this or that astronomical figure) of manipulations performed throughout the world on a single day. Debate may hinge on the word 'reported'. Those experienced in the manipulative field may not wholly subscribe to the implications of these observations. A rough comparison to the frequency of road traffic accidents is probably more realistic, in the sense that while a certain number of serious accident reports feature in national daily newspapers, scores of moderately serious accidents occur each day in any one country without being nationally featured. Very many relatively minor incidents, nevertheless involving a degree of avoidable injury and distress may occur in those 24 hours.

Accidents continue to occur; reports appearing during the eighties are those by Robertson (1981, 1982), Horn (1983), Braun et al (1983), Rosenwasser et al (1983), Fritz et al (1984), Austin (1985), Davis (1985), Katirji et al (1985), Brownson et al (1986), Grayson (1987), Terrett (1987a, b, Fast et al (1987) and Villar et al (1989). Some reports which did not appear in the first edition of this text are those by Kuhlendahl and Hansell (1953), Tomlinson (1955), Shepard (1959), Lindemann and Rossak (1959), Knudsen (1965), Serre and Simon (1968), Cyriax (1971) and LaBan and Meerschaert (1975). There was also a report (Hanus et al 1977) of vertebral artery occlusion as a complication of performing yoga exercises.

Extending the comparison with road traffic accidents, the case-notes of Accident and Emergency Departments and the files of motor insurance companies may more accurately reflect the frequency of road traffic accidents than medical literature reflects the number of manipulation incidents and accidents — or mischance of other treatments, too.

In Great Britain, at least, there is a legal obligation to report vehicular accidents in which persons are injured.

It is not mandatory to likewise report manipulation accidents in the medical journals or to anybody at all, other than within the clinical locality concerned. Were this so, unrealistic as it may be, the literature would very probably feature a much higher proportion of incidents, not all of them necessarily serious. For this reason alone, those which are formally described probably do not accurately reflect the incidence.

While Martienssen and Nilsson (1989) mention that they have reviewed cases of accidents following cervical manipulation, published in the English and German languages, there are also the papers in French (see bibliography) and other languages, too, and few experienced workers would agree with a passage under 'Discussion' in their paper: 'As is the case with all research into rare diseases we are faced with the problem that we have a limited number of cases on which to draw our conclusions'.

Apley (1990) remarked upon 'The tyranny of numbers' and asks '. . . are we sometimes fooled by pseudosciences?'. He also suggests 'We should not substitute bad accounting for good judgement'. Fast et al (1987) observed that an *undetermined* (my italics) number of patients suffer from serious neurological disturbances due to manipulations, and a recent editorial in the journal *Stroke* (Robertson 1981) states that neurological complications following cervical manipulation may be unusual but not rare. Robertson asserted that they are 'far more common than the literature would reflect'.

Perhaps most of those who have spent many decades in this clinical field would agree with the proposal that published examples of manipulation accidents are akin to only the tip of a somewhat larger iceberg. While this does not negate the conclusions of Martienssen and Nilsson — so far as they go — the incidents of their attention are certainly not 'very rare' (their phrase).

The estimation of Hosek et al (1981), that one in a million cervical manipulations will result in a serious vertebrobasilar accident, is possibly based upon incomplete information, i.e. the dearth of fully *reported* cases. As Grant (1988) has suggested, complications may be unusual but they are far from rare.

At a Joint Meeting on Stroke and Cerebral Circulation (Editorial, 1980) in the USA, a Missourian neurologist, D. G. Sherman, reported five cases of vertebrobasilar system infarct, and warned the medical audience that manipulative techniques of rotation, or simply turning the head sharply to look behind, can cause a stroke. A Mayo Clinic neurologist, B. R. Krueger, reported ten more apparently manipulation-induced infarcts, and discussed mechanical trespass upon the atlanto-axial portion of the vertebral artery which cervical rotation and extension combined can produce. His comment, that the number of cases was small compared to the large number of manipulations performed, prompted the Chairman, neurosurgeon J. T. Robertson, to object. He suggested that the numbers were unrepresentative and far too small.

When the Chairman called for a show of hands among the 300 physicians present, approximately a third of them indicated that they had seen at least one case.

In a rebuttal, to correspondents' suggestions following his earlier short paper (Robertson 1981) that complications due to cervical manipulation are rare, Robertson (1982) mentioned that a recent survey, conducted by the Stroke Council of the American Heart Association, uncovered 360 hitherto unreported cases of extracranial arterial injury; two-thirds of the injuries involved the vertebral artery and one-third the carotid artery. These cases were additional to the reports in medical publications. He points out that (i) the data would tend to emphasize that this type of injury is not rare, and (ii) it is alarming that many of the arterial injuries occur in relatively young patients. In his own words (Roberston 1981) '. . . Physicians should suspect the diagnosis in patients with brainstem or cerebral vascular ischaemic symptoms who have had, for various reasons, neck manipulative therapy. This complication can be induced in patients undergoing repetitive rotatory neck activities (e.g. exercises); however, the odds are that most of the injuries are induced by manipulative therapy'.

Livingston (1971) asserted that injury associated with spinal manipulation appears more frequently than North American medical literature may suggest. He remarked that injury may result from manipulations by lay, medical and paramedical workers.

The majority of negative results are of a transient nature and, while temporarily unpleasant for the patient, are soon recovered from and have not merited wide reporting. Nevertheless, with rising standards of care it is these mostly avoidable incidents which should now receive a greater proportion of our concern.

A hoary and now wearisomely familiar list of some 25 cases selected from the literature has been discussed in fair and reasonable terms (Kleynhans 1980), but more important in terms of incidence are those cases which may not feature in the literature. For example: (i) Hanraets (1959) reported patients admitted to his neurological clinic suffering serious neural loss following chiropractic manipulative attentions to the back.

In passing, he remarks on the puzzling regularity, the frequent *repetitions* of manipulative treatment. 'One cannot help but be struck by the following contradiction: Success is claimed to attend one manipulation, or at most once repeated. If, therefore, it happens not to be successful, what useful purpose can be served by undergoing these manipulations regularly for months on end, as the patients coming to us with persistent symptoms have done over and over again?' (Grieve 1991). One of Livingston's (1971) patients had received over 200 'adjustments' in 2 years. (ii) Blaine (1925) described the clinical and X-ray findings in three cases of forward dislocation of the atlas, and mentioned another two cases. All had received manipulative treatment to the spine. During the ensuing discussion, eight further cases were reported by physicians present. (iii) Following formal presentations on the subject (Louyot et al 1967), it is common that ensuing discussion between physicians elicits many further examples of manipulation accidents, in this case more than 20, which may not appear as full clinical reports in the literature. Frequent among these examples (Coste et al 1953, Lievre 1953a, b, De Sèze & Mieg 1955, Attali 1957, Benassy & Wolinetz 1957, Boudin & Barbizet 1958, Maigne 1960, Deshayes & Geoffroy 1962, Lapresle 1965, De Sèze et al 1966) were converting a low back pain into a painful sciatica with neurological involvement requiring surgery. Yet more serious complications are also mentioned, e.g. vertebral fractures in an elderly patient with osteoporosis, paraplegia after a cervical manipulation for torticollis, unduly prolonged medical treatment being necessitated after cervical manipulations, fracture of the sternum in a patient with Kahler's disease (lymphomatosis of bone, or multiple myeloma).

A selection of other reports and views of continental authors (Lievre 1955, Maigne 1955, Boudin 1957, Illoux 1962, Oger 1964, Depoorter 1966, Grossoirs 1966, Rageot 1966, Rieunau 1966, Simon 1966, Thierry-Mieg 1967, Le Corre et al 1971, Maigne 1972) in the middle '50s, '60s and early '70s is of interest.

INCIDENTS AND ACCIDENTS

A distinction can be made between (i) undue consequences in patients who were otherwise normal and healthy and (ii) those patients in whom passive movement techniques should have been used either with extreme care or not at all. Examples are frank lower thoracic disc lesions, osteoporosis, rheumatoid arthritis, spinal tuberculosis, neoplasm, absent odontoid process, gross segmental instability and upper respiratory tract infections, and operations, in children. The full catalogue is familiar enough.

Gutmann (1983) mentions those patients with symptoms of vertebrobasilar insufficiency, recent whiplash or other vertebrocranial injuries, young hypermobile women with autonomic instability and those in whom arteritis is suspected, when symptoms are similar to the aortic arch syndrome. Anticoagulant medication is a contraindication (vide infra) to other than gentle passive movements of moderate range. If 'accident' is defined as some deterioration of the patient's previously healthy condition, as a consequence of the treatment, the degree and duration might possibly be categorized as follows:

A. Unnecessarily hurting the patient. Adding an increase of distress and inconvenience for some 2–3 or more weeks, without ultimate improvement in the presenting condition. This is quite different to briefly transient soreness. Some treatment soreness, following the indicated and successful use of passive movement techniques for vertebral joint restriction, may occur and commonly settle

within a day or two. On occasions it may last 4 days. These are normally expected short-lived reactions and seldom inconvenience the patient to any appreciable degree. It is responsible practice to warn patients about soreness, also that they must promptly report undue or prolonged after effects.

B. Examples could be converting localized neck or low back pain to so-called root pain in the associated limb, respectively brachialgia or sciatica (Lescure 1954, Livingston 1971, Louyot et al 1967, Jung & Kehr 1972). The patient is sharply distressed, inconvenienced and temporarily disabled to a greater or lesser degree. Neurological deficit appears. Hospitalization, with surgical decompression on occasions, may be necessary. Complete recovery is measured in weeks or months. Sequelae are restricted to those involving the vertebral segment and its associated nerve root. Uncomplicated rib fracture, while acutely painful, may be included here.

C. Production of symptoms and signs of cauda equina (Eyre-Brook 1952, Jennett 1956, Jackson 1971, Hooper 1973) and/or central nervous system involvement (Miller & Burton 1947, Kunkle et al 1952, Green & Joynt 1959, Pribeck 1963, Parkin et al 1978, Kewalramani et al 1980) either (i) by trespass upon important vessels with transient ischaemia, or vascular stretching, thrombosis and infarct and/or (ii) direct cauda equina or spinal cord impingement. The patient requires prompt hospitalization and invariably suffers a degree of residual neurological disablement, which may include paraplegia, (Lievre 1953a, b) tetraplegia (Dvorak & Orelli 1982), sphincter disturbance, bouts of dizziness and restriction of locomotor function. Surgery is often necessary. There may or may not be complete recovery, which in any case is prolonged.

D. Death ensues as a consequence, within hours, days or weeks (Pratt-Thomas & Berger 1947, Ford & Clark 1956, Smith & Estridge 1962 Krueger & Okazaki 1980).

Most published reports concern categories C and D because of their serious nature.

Incidents and accidents in category B probably occur much more frequently than appears in the literature, being more often discussed among medical and para-medical colleagues, in clinical teaching and during professional meetings than is reported in journals. Group A are probably never mentioned at all in the literature, despite anxious preoccupation, transient added symptoms such as digital paraesthesiae and a widened pain distribution.

CAUSES

Force is dangerous. Like the sped arrow and the spoken word, errors are not easily retrieved. As silence is golden, so we should stay our hand until indications for thrust techniques are quite unequivocal. This is prevention — well-informed prudence.

Kleynhans and Terrett (1985) remarked that little

appears in the literature on the prevention of complications from the use of manipulative thrust techniques. Whose literature are they talking about? This is a large statement. Also a puzzling one, since it accompanies a reasonably comprehensive bibliography on that topic. Instruction in prevention springs naturally from knowledge of causes, and likelihoods of incident. In a variety of forms there is much in the literature on this aspect (Mennell 1952, Lescure 1954, Maigne 1955, De Sèze et al 1966, Depoorter 1966, Rieunau 1966, Louyot et al 1967, Thierry-Mieg 1967, Jeanblanc 1970, Le Corre et al 1971, Livingston 1971, Maigne 1972, Schiötz & Cyriax 1975, Schmitt & Wolff 1979, Editorial 1980, Gutmann 1983, Maitland 1986, Bourdillon & Day 1987, Grieve 1988, 1989, 1991).

The therapist is responsible — not the patient, the radiographer, the X-rays, the plinth or the floor covering, etc., since it is the therapist's duty to see to these factors.

The causes of incidents and accidents may be marshalled in various ways.

The therapist

Examination

Insufficient awareness, or observance, of contraindications, dangers and those conditions requiring extra care and gentleness.

Not perceiving inappropriate referrals from medical and surgical colleagues.

Poor appraisal of the patient as a reliable witness.

Poor judgement of the patient's temperament, mentality and ideation, i.e. expectations.

Incomplete history-taking.

Inadequate information about co-existing disease and medication, e.g. anticoagulants and systemic steroid drugs.

Poor and insufficiently detailed examination technique, resulting in erroneous assessment of indications, both generally and segmentally.

Palpation technique which is other than comprehensive and meticulous.

Insufficient information from ancillary procedures — X-rays, blood tests, CAT scans, ultrasonography, scintigraphy, magnetic resonance imaging, etc. when history-taking indicates the desirability of these before treatment.

Being in a hurry, or feeling tired at the end of a long day.

Taking short-cuts; this is a potent cause of incidents/accidents.

The wrong type of patient (Grieve 1988).

Technique

Exceeding the bounds of competence. Livingston's (1971) observation '. . . either study spinal manipulation thoroughly or avoid it' applies equally to medical, paramedical and lay practitioners, of course, and is no more than common sense.

Poor technique, excessive force, poor localization of effect, using techniques known to be hazardous, energetically attempting to overcome reflex muscle guarding.

Excessive rotation, with or without extension, of the cervical spine.

Excessive traction of the cervical spine, combined with sudden movement.

Repetition at one session of a somewhat energetic technique, which either does not initially succeed or has already had a negative effect.

Further 'slight' manipulative treatment, or 'tests' in attempting to rectify wrong 'adjustment' just performed, which has manifestly resulted in negative or ominous effects (Gutmann 1983).

Repeated sessions, at regular intervals, of manipulative thrust techniques. This is nonsensical, irresponsible and dangerous.

A mesmeric preoccupation with eliciting the obligatory 'click', or with the importance of manipulation as such.

Simple human stupidity and carelessness.

Unsuitable equipment — wrong height of a couch, unsuitable floor surface.

Technique undertaken on a false or ludicrous clinical premise.

The patient

The poor or inarticulate witness.

Excessive lability, emotional and/or autonomic.

Deliberate concealment of salient information. The writer recalls a patient who, despite careful questioning, withheld the fact of urinary sphincter incompetence associated with her back pain episode. On suspicion of this, she was more directly questioned, and at once referred for neurological consultation. At operation the next day, the cauda equina was decompressed.

The confirmed stoic: 'If it's not hurting me it cannot be doing any good.'

The masochist who secretly welcomes painful distress — 'punishment' — as assuaging a deep sense of guilt for social transgressions, real or imagined. The important factor here is *handling* — pain at the *hands* of another. The occasional patient will actively encourage further manipulative thrust techniques by fulsome accounts of symptomatic improvement.

A fixation with having 'discs put back', and dissatisfaction with other than abrupt, forceful manual techniques. These patients can be very persuasive, and may overcome the clinical self-discipline of weak and obliging therapists.

The concept

Analysis (Kleynhans 1980, Kleynhans & Terrett 1985) of incidents and accidents reported in the literature does not wholly reveal the nature of the problem, only its substrate. The problem is larger than the simple sum of its parts. The old suggestion that bad results of manipulation are due to bad manipulators might include considerations other than technique, e.g. concept. What do we believe we are doing?

What is manipulation FOR?

This is not a frivolous question; the more manipulations are carried out, the greater is the potential for untoward incidents and accidents.

A proportion of manipulators tend to alienate more realistic clinicians by their persistent and 'catch-all' claims that the field of manipulative therapy is much wider than that of musculoskeletal conditions alone. Hanraets (1959) mentions chiropractic theory, and agrees that manipulative treatment is of assistance in mechanical lesions of the musculoskeletal system, but 'as soon as it is claimed that a number of internal diseases can be cured by manual "repositions" of the spine, this therapeutic venture becomes shrouded in mystery'. Hanraets quotes the manipulator Zukschwerdt who, over 30 years ago, wrote 'Hitherto no statistical, anatomical or experimental proof has been adduced of the existence of a disposition to diseases brought about by compression of vegetative (autonomic nerve) fibres in the intervertebral foramen. And that leaves the major part of chiropractic unproven.'. Crelin (1973), who subjected the theory to scientific test, was unable to demonstrate its validity. While Hoyland et al (1989) suggest that venous obstruction in the intervertebral foramen may be a factor in the pathogenesis of perineural and intraneural fibrosis, direct nerve compression was observed in only eight (5%) of the 160 lumbar foraminal specimens examined; the age range was 35–91 years. Despite the increasing volume of chiropractic literature — as witnessed in this chapter's bibliography — there are no studies known to the writer which scientifically support the notion that the genesis of visceral disease lies in nerve root compression and that 'adjustment' of vertebral 'malalignment' will cure it.

Chiropractic is at times presented as almost a sovereign remedy for all ills, virtually an alternative system of total health care. The prestigious *New England Journal of Medicine* reports that a medical committee carried out an experiment in Philadelphia (Barrett 1976). They sent a healthy four-year-old girl for a check-up to five different chiropractors. The first found 'pinched nerves to her stomach and gallbladder', the second noted a 'twisted pelvis', the third worried about future 'headaches, nervousness, equilibrium and digestive problems due to spinal misalignment' which he had detected, the fourth pre-dicted 'bad periods and rough childbirth', if the 'short leg' was not lengthened, and the fifth diagnosed hip and neck misalignment which required instant treatment.

Skrabanek and McCormick (1989) mention that a leaflet published by the recently founded Chiropractic Association of Ireland encourages whole families to come for a check-up 'to ensure early detection of potential nerve interference'. The promised benefits include 'improved digestion, better circulation, improved mental clarity, normalization of reproductive–hormonal imbalances, and easier breathing'.

Among conditions recently mentioned by manipulators as suitable for 'craniosacral' manipulative technique, for example, is brain dysfunction, whether evidenced as dyslexia, hyperkinesis or spastic cerebral palsy (Grieve 1988). Among very many other examples are discussions of the effect of chiropractic 'adjustment' on the behaviour of autistic children (Sandetur & Adams 1987), the chiropractic treatment of mental illness (Goff 1988), the possible role of chiropractic therapy in influencing the body's immune system in the acquired immunodeficiency syndrome (AIDS) (Lucido 1988), and the detection of mild essential hypertension and its chiropractic 'management' (Jamison 1987).

While the writer is certainly no stranger to the importance of the autonomic nervous system (see Chs 20 and 29), and notwithstanding questions of the clinical validity of these notions, the potential for manipulation accidents is much increased if simple manipulative capability prompts an energetic and possible inappropriate search for ever-widening clinical opportunities.

Taken to its logical conclusion, it could be said that if SMT (spinal manipulative therapy) becomes the treatment for anything and therefore everything, then by the simple law of averages the frequency of manipulation accidents would rise proportionately.

Fallacies are not confined to manipulators, of course; even Sir Arthur Conan Doyle, a medical graduate of Edinburgh University, believed in fairies.

Ashley (1987) makes the point that 'acupuncture, osteopathy, homeopathy and similar art forms offer poor substitutes for haemodialysis if your kidneys have stopped working, or for intravenous diuretics if you have acute heart failure, or antibiotics for septicaemia, or surgery for acute appendicitis. Nor have they led to dramatic improvements to the general health comparable to immunisation against poliomyelitis, and they are unlikely to do so until they achieve a solid scientific foundation.'.

Chiropractic theosophy

Despite the fact that modern chiropractic training is long, and of degree standard, that modern chiropractors are skilled manipulators (in their own idiom) and that some ludicrous basic assumptions and dogma are at last being scientifically questioned (Bryner 1987, Charlton 1987, Dulhunty 1987, Keating 1988a), a proportion of chiropractors' writing still has an unreal quality, which begins to induce light-headedness after much reading of it. The maudlin, almost quasi-religious adulation of a late 19th century grocer and 'magnetic healer' (one D. D. Palmer) — who claimed to have discovered chiropractic — has a musty, unrealistic air about it. An example of his writing (Palmer 1910) follows: '. . . knowing that our physical health and the intellectual progress of Innate (the personified portion of Universal Intelligence) depend upon *the proper alignment of the skeletal frame, we feel it our bounden duty to replace any displaced bones* [my italics] so that physical and spiritual health, happiness and the full fruition of earthly life may be enjoyed'. Even allowing for the year of writing, this unbuttoned rhetoric hardly merits serious clinical attention. Yet to this day, these remarks are earnestly discussed and debated in all seriousness by grown men and women who have successfully undergone the rigours of what purports to be a scientific training. Palmer's phrase 'innate . . . intelligence' is a case in point (Donahue 1988a, b, Keating 1988b), where precious space in expensive, glossy chiropractic journals is given to exchanges about the meaning, for modern workers, of this flatulent prose; although Donahue (1988b) does refer to 'shabby philosophising'.

Nevertheless, how are orthodox clinicians, unversed in the doubtful theosophical concepts of chiropractic, expected to try and grasp whether it is scientific logic or chiropractic philosophy which governs the spinal locality, the direction, the degree of vigour and the clinical purpose of a chiropractic manipulation? What is it they believe they are doing?

It is salutory for *all* manipulators — orthopaedic surgeons, physiotherapists, osteopaths, chiropractors and bonesetters — to be able to articulate to other clinicians in simple terms what they believe they are doing, to what tissue, with what predetermined amount of force and why, since each of the disciplines just mentioned have used manipulations which, on occasion, went wrong, and which have been reported in these pages (Eyre-Brook 1952, Jennett 1956, Jackson 1971, Austin 1985, Davis 1985, Villar et al 1989).

In an anecdotal report, Cyriax (1971) remarked: 'I have seen cases of secondary vertebral deposits, chordoma, myeloma and intraspinal neuroma in which lay manipulation had done no harm, but Strohmeyer in Germany reported that, of 40 cases of paraplegia admitted to his neurological unit in 6 months, 28 followed attention by lay manipulators'.

Subluxation theories

As Keating (1988a) remarked: 'Subluxation has become a holy word in chiropractic . . . too many chiropractors have come to equate commitment to chiropractic with belief in subluxation . . . theories have become so overburdened with philosophical and political meaning, and significance to chiropractors, that any criticism of their validity is automatically rejected. This intolerance to critical questions . . . dogmatic belief in subluxations must be tempered . . .'. He goes on to state that the existence of subluxation, as a clinically useful and objectively detectable clinical phenomenon, is *not* well-established in current scientific literature. Dulhunty (1987) now postulates that what chiropractors have called vertebral subluxations do not exist, and a Norwegian radiologist (Dalseth 1976) long ago remarked that the chiropractic X-ray diagnosis of positional faults ('subluxations') is illusory, this probably sums up the view of most realistic clinicians, orthodox or lay.

Brentingham (1988) addressed the question of whether proof exists that manipulation reduces subluxation (in the chiropractic sense) and since such proof as might exist is flimsy, scientific grounds for continuing to use that ridiculous word 'adjustment' (vide infra) become nonexistent.

Keating's (1988a) bibliography includes the work of a colleague (Watkins) who offers an alternative to dogma as a basis for chiropractic. In his view 'the future of the chiropractic profession depends more on the manner by which we choose our methods of patient care than upon any other consideration'. Timely, wise and welcome words indeed.

The disc

Notwithstanding clear evidence (Hitselburger & Witten 1968) that, of 300 patients without symptoms of degenerative disc disease, myelographic abnormalities of the intervertebral disc space were found in 110 (37%), manipulators continue to speak of relieving spinal pain by putting discs back. While the profile of an intervertebral disc may be altered by manipulative techniques (Mathews & Yates 1969) and by traction (Mathews 1968) there are no studies known to the writer which demonstrate permanence of the altered profile, which changes with trunk postural changes anyway. It is maintained that '. . . herniated discs can be *reduced* [my italics] by manipulatory methods . . . torsional force would tend to exert centripetal force, *reducing* the prolapsed or bulging disc material.' (Kleynhans & Terrett 1985).

There appears no evidence to suggest this (Bourdillon & Day 1987). Enthusiastic torsional force is probably often responsible for incidents and accidents in the 'B' group.

Farfan (1977) has readily produced annular failure, as a separation of laminae, when applying torsion, and remarks: 'The relatively small twisting force required to injure the intervertebral joint probably occurs in everyday life; for example, using the flexed thigh as a lever to manipulate the lumbar spine, a manipulator would easily attain a 1000 inch-pounds (113 Nm) of torque by applying a 50 lb (23 kg) force to a femur 20 inches (51 cm) long. In this way, he could easily damage the intervertebral joint.'.

Alignment

The concept that vertebral, muscular, autonomic and sometimes visceral dysfunction may be consequent upon abnormal relationships of vertebrae, one to another, could bear inspection, as could the concept of subluxation. Grice (1980) described one of the mechanical goals of thrust techniques as the 'correction of static misalignment'. The subluxated vertebra requires therapeutic 'adjustment'. 'The adjustive thrust is characterized by a transmission of force using a combination of muscular power and the body weight of the practitioner. The force is delivered with controlled speed, depth and magnitude through a specific contact on a particular structure such as the transverse or spinous process of a vertebra.'

Drum (1975) mentioned the delicacy of some manipulative procedures, which even in the hands of experienced clinicians are not without risk. Further, '... many congenital, traumatic, degenerative or adaptive positional disc-relationships of vertebral motor units may well be irreversible ... there are permanent intervertebral subluxations that cannot be manipulated back into "proper alignment". Markedly abnormal motor units are distorted as a result of advanced breakdown of their stabilizing elements. A manipulation would have to instantaneously restore these degenerated tissues to "hold" '.

Fast et al (1987) observed: '... the manipulable lesion — a term frequently used by manipulators — may indicate local segmental malalignment. This malalignment cannot be identified by roentgenograms and thus is not accepted by most physicians. It is claimed that restoration of full range of motion, up to the "anatomical barrier" of the joint, is responsible somehow for the pain relief obtained immediately following manipulation therapy'.

Asymmetry of contour and attitude need not be of any significance in the context of symptoms reported by the patient. The sometimes unwitting tendency to assume that 'symmetry is all', and that asymmetry must always be 'normalized' for symptoms to be relieved, is an insufficient basis for planning treatment (Grieve 1988).

A more rational concept of relieving pain and restoring normal segmental movement, by persuasive techniques to the patient's tolerance, may be more appropriate than repetitive, abrupt attempts to 'normalize mal-alignment'. In the hurly-burly of clinical practice, the prisoner of concept makes a poor clinician.

The X-ray

The radiographic image of a vertebral body is the *sum* of the shadows cast by the cortex and trabeculae. The lumbar spine, for example: '... is particularly challenging to the radiologist because the shadows cast by the bones form only a proportion of the structures under scrutiny ... a standard examination only portrays one limited modality of a spinal disorder.' Park (1980). Park suggests that routine radiographic investigation of the lumbar spine should be avoided, because of the radiation hazard but also because inappropriate X-ray examination contributes little to the solution of a particular clinical problem and may even obscure it. Many medical and paramedical clinicians, very experienced in the manipulative field, concur with the consensus of current radiological opinion that many patients with musculoskeletal pain do not need to be X-rayed. In the writer's ample orthopaedic experience, after bone disease and significant mechanical defect have been excluded, seeking precise manual treatment indications in X-ray appearances is like attempting to recognize one's friends by the shadows they cast in the street.

The concept of 'mal-alignment' may be stretched beyond the limits of elasticity, to include 'significant mechanical defect'. An inverted pyramid of extrapolation, on this or that often quite innocuous and blameless radiographic appearance, may underlie a proportion of unnecessary treatment by manipulative thrust techniques, when mobilization may be adequate.

The beguiling charm of 'X-rays before and after' may have something to answer for, in impressing the gullible and fostering a life-long concept, in some, that 'misalignment' must needs be corrected or adjusted by manipulative thrust techniques.

When accompanied by symptomatic improvement, before and after X-rays which demonstrate restoration of normal *movement* at a previously hypomobile segment, clinically and accurately determined to be the genesis of symptoms, the films have admissible teaching value. Where *alignment* has been modified (Schmorl & Junghanns 1971), the radiographic distinction between 'malalignment' and simple fixation or block at some point on the normal range of movement (Coutts 1934) is not an exact science, and the face value of these films may require careful qualification. Fielding et al (1978) discuss atlanto-axial rotary deformities, for example, and mention the obscure aetiology of these lesions. *Bone disease* is not immediately revealed by X-rays; as is common knowledge, some 35–40% of bone salts must be lost before osteoporosis becomes radiographically evident. As with osteoporosis, so with *neoplasms*, in that it is unwise to rely completely on the innocence of X-ray appearances.

In cadaver studies (Macnab & McCullough 1990), radiographic changes were shown in only 15% of vertebral

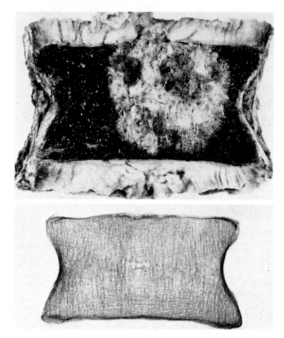

Fig. 49.1 The top photograph is of the cut surface of the vertebral body, showing a large circular metastasis. Below is a radiograph of a 2 mm slice from this surface. The trabeculae are intact. For a time the trabeculae maintain their strength, but with the loss of normal cellular associations they become weak, and the entire body may suddenly collapse. (Reproduced from Carstairs 1959 with permission.)

bodies with gross secondary neoplastic disease (see Fig. 49.1), and it is wise to bear in mind the predilection of metastases for vertebral bodies, ribs and ilium (Grieve 1988).

THE CERVICAL SPINE

Lyness and Simeone (1978) remarked that:

'. . . the upper cervical region is a delicate sanctuary of anatomic features the disruption of which can be accomplished with surprisingly minor trauma. Thus, chiropractic manipulations, yoga exercises, the collision of athletes in contact sports, and voluntary head movement have provided settings in which seemingly trivial neck injuries have resulted in neurologic sequelae ranging from mild transient dizziness to permanent disturbing paralysis or even fatal brain stem syndrome.'

In most cases, it is impossible to modify advanced neurological deficits once they have occurred.

De Kleyn and Nieuwenhuyse (1927) studied the mechanics possibly involved, by perfusion techniques on autopsy specimens, when right rotation and extension markedly restricted flow in the left vertebral artery. Further studies, by De Kleyn and Versteegh (1933), suggested that vertigo and nystagmus tended to occur when circulation was restricted in one vertebral artery (Figs 49.2 and 49.3) and its opposite fellow was either diseased or absent.

Tissington-Tatlow and Bammer (1957) also described

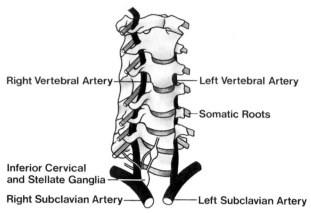

Fig. 49.2 The vertebral arteries. Anterior aspect. (Reproduced from Grieve 1988.)

and illustrated the effect on the contralateral vertebral artery when the head is rotated to one side. Their angiographic cadaver studies demonstrated narrowing of the contralateral vessel, which appears to be the mechanics underlying untoward effects, on occasions, of treatment by passive movement of the cervical spine (Medico-legal abstracts 1937, Bureau of Legal Medicine and Legislation 1952, Ford 1952, Boshes 1959, Nick et al 1967, Lorenz & Vogelsang 1972, Kanshepolsky et al 1972, Mehalic & Farhat 1974, Lyness & Wagman 1974, Davidson et al 1975, Rinsky et al 1976, Mueller & Sahs 1976, Easton & Sherman 1977 Beatty 1977, Nyberg-Hanson et al 1978, Gorman 1978, Schellhas et al 1980, Jaskoviak 1980, Simmons 1982, Cameron & Browning 1982).

During recent years, many have drawn attention to the hazards of manipulation of the neck (Jackson 1966,

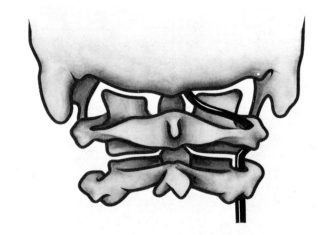

Fig. 49.3 Posterior aspect of the craniovertebral region. After emerging through the foramen transversarium of the atlas, the vertebral artery winds around the articular pillar and, together with the first cervical nerve and veins, pierces the posterior atlanto-occipital membrane, to unite with its fellow on the front of the brain stem to form the basilar artery. On rotation of the head and the atlas to the left, the right vertebral artery is stretched at the level of C1–C2. (Reproduced from Grieve 1988.)

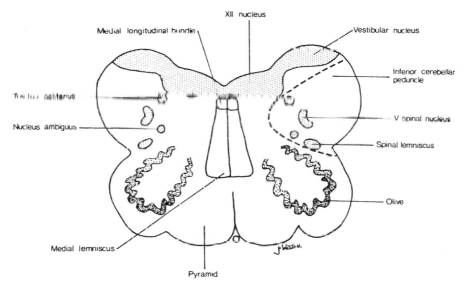

XII nucleus

Medial longitudinal bundle

Vestibular nucleus

Inferior cerebellar peduncle

Tractus solitarius

Nucleus ambiguus

V spinal nucleus

Spinal lemniscus

Olive

Medial lemniscus

Pyramid

Fig. 49.4 Transverse section of medulla. The dotted line encloses the area infarcted by posterior inferior cerebellar artery obstruction. (Reproduced from Jeffreys 1980 with permission.)

Sandifer 1967, Brain & Wilkinson 1967, Wilkinson 1971, Jeffreys 1980) (Fig. 49.4).

It is apparent that disease need not be present for incidents to occur (Schwartz et al 1956, Editorial 1980, Daneshmend et al 1984), although the presence of spondylosis and arthrosis with consequent osteophytosis increase the hazard (Masson & Cambier 1962).

One neurologist's 28 patients (Editorial 1980), six of them fatal, showed the following striking points:

1. The average age was 37.7 — which is unusually low for stroke victims.

2. Only three patients had had any previous neurological symptoms.

3. For all but four, symptoms began during or immediately after chiropractic manipulation.

4. Of the 21 patients whose chiropractic treatment was reported in detail, all had been subjected to neck rotation.

5. Nine patients went back for more manipulation even though they had clearly had ischaemic symptoms during the first treatment.

Lescure (1959) discussed the pros and cons of traction and manipulation to the cervical spine, stressing that they can be as efficacious as they can occasionally be harmful. He mentions that these treatments can put into effect complex phenomena beyond the physiological phenomena of normal movement. Some necks are not normal to begin with (Ch. 17). Wadia (1967) describes a total of 34 cases of myelopathy complicating congenital atlanto-axial dislocation. In all except two, symptoms were precipitated by a sudden, often exaggerated, movement of the neck.

Grinker and Guy (1927) also reported the fatal outcome of a normally innocuous movement, yet the movement need not be gross. Fielding and Reddy (1969)

reported the case of a 65-year-old woman who woke, yawned and twisted her neck, with immediate sharp pain. She could not correct her 'cock-robin' deformity. After 10 days of cervical traction, she turned to the left, increasing the deformity, and died. Ford and Clark (1956) described a similar case of innocuous movement precipitating a catastrophic event. Nagler (1973) described four examples of spinal cord or cerebellar damage after forceful hyperextension of the neck during calisthenic exercises. Okawara and Nibbelink (1974) reported vertebral artery occlusion in a decorator who painted a ceiling with his head in extension and left rotation. His consequent right lateral medullary syndrome appeared secondary to marked narrowing of the right vertebral artery at C1–C2 level.

Neck rotation (Barton & Margolis 1975, Bladin & Merory 1975) or quick voluntary movement of the head (Sherman et al 1981), may induce vertigo, a common consequence of whiplash injury, too, of course (Braaf & Rosner 1962).

Horner's syndrome (Kommerell & Hoyt 1973, Johnson & Spalding 1974), and dysmetria (Zimmerman et al 1978), are among the clinical features in 46 cases tabulated by Jaskoviak (1980). Grundy and McSweeney (1984) mention that cranial nerve lesions (Brodal 1957, 1981) may be due to several causes, including manipulation.

Williams and Wilson (1962) discuss the vascular basis of these lesions. For a comprehensive review by a neurologist who is familiar with the preoccupations of manual therapists, see Chapter 22. A diverse number of lesions may present simply with neck pain, when manual therapy would be ill-advised (Fleischli 1967, Thambyrajah 1972).

It is a fallacy that rotatory manipulations are safe so long as accompanied by traction (Jackson 1966, Parkin et al 1978, Gutmann 1983, Bourdillon & Day 1987) (see Ch. 5).

Cervical vertigo and manual treatment

Since confluence of the vertebral arteries form the basilar artery, and these vessels and their branches supply the brainstem and hindbrain while contributing to the cerebral circulation, freedom of flow in the vertebral arteries is vital. Frequently the vertebral arteries are of markedly unequal calibre, and in only 8% of individuals are the arteries of equal size (Stopford 1916).

It is the combination of developmental narrowness of one or more vessels, cervical spondylosis, arthrosis, atheroma of vertebral arteries and the great variability of central nervous system arterial supply between individuals, which is so productive of symptoms believed due to ischaemia — these may include listing, a brief attack of 'giddiness', a feeling of impending syncope, diplopia or even a drop attack, when the patient suddenly falls to the ground without losing consciousness (Grieve 1988).

Reflex vertigo

Attributing responses to effects produced by certain movements of the neck, and combined movements, is not an exact science and dizziness need not have anything to do with disturbed vascularity. Another factor is that of listing, dysequilibrium, giddiness or 'vertigo' being induced alone by extremes of stress, or abnormal relationships, of the craniovertebral complex of joints and soft tissues and the presence of this may compound findings suspicious of vertebrobasilar insufficiency (Terrett 1983).

Reflex vertigo differs from ischaemic vertigo in that it is not accompanied by the features of vascular disturbance. Together with the eyes and labyrinths, the cervical musculoskeletal structures contribute an important share of the proprioceptive information governing balance.

Whether the origin of tonic neck reflexes lies in the joints and/or the cervical musculature, it is well established that disturbing them can initiate a variety of subjective and motor abnormalities. The location of the disturbance remains unresolved. Some inculpate the cervical joints, others suggest muscular hypertonicity due to sympathetic overactivity. A further view is that strain of the ligaments and intervertebral discs recruits a diverse autonomic response.

Causes of vascular compromise

In a series of patients with atheromatous arterial changes, Biemond (1951) observed that cervical rotation with extension produced nystagmus, dysarthria and transient abnormality of plantar response. He also stressed the long-established finding that, of all cerebral vessels, the basilar artery is most frequently affected by atherosclerosis. Nevertheless, vascular compromise following cervical manipulations can and does occur in young adults with normal arteries (Editorial 1980). Experimental angiographic studies of atlanto-axial occlusion of the vertebral artery have all involved passive physiological rotation of the head. *The circumstances are different in manipulation since, depending on the technique, two additional factors are force and suddenness.* Reports of stroke after manipulation frequently refer to the speed and violence of the manoeuvre suffered by the patient. It appears that these additional factors would increase the likelihood of intimal tearing and its consequences. Trauma to the atlanto-axial segment of the vertebral artery is the most likely explanation for the occurrence of stroke after cervical manipulation (Krueger & Okazaki 1980).

Recognition of potential hazard

When patients present with apparent vertebral artery involvement, manifest as dizziness, cervical vertigo or dysequilibrium — call it what we will — and there is reason to believe that the genesis of symptoms may be musculoskeletal changes of trespass in the neck, it has been standard pre-treatment practice to identify carefully those postures of cervical rotation and/or extension which provoke the symptoms reported. Wisely, these postures were then avoided, of course, and the treatment techniques were modified accordingly.

Tests of vertebrobasilar arterial sufficiency are not really diagnostic tests, as is sometimes asserted, since a positive result does not necessarily provide a diagnosis, only the important information that certain postures and movements are likely to be either reducing flow somewhere in the vertebrobasilar system, initiating aberrant reflex responses, or both, and therefore these postures should be avoided during treatment. Precisely where, when and how the circulation might be restricted by these tests in any one individual, whether these are reflex responses, whether this is a normal effect and has been so for that patient throughout life, *and exactly what relationship a positive result has to the presenting symptoms, are not revealed by these tests alone.*

Grant (1988) quotes findings which corroborate this view, i.e. that a definitive patho-anatomical diagnosis of cervical vertigo is rarely possible; particularly so by simple postural tests alone.

Terrett (1987a) reviewed 107 reported cases of vascular accidents from cervical spine manipulations, and mentioned in a later paper (Terrett 1987b) that vascular accidents have occasioned the major criticism of spinal manipulative therapy. He suggested that the frequency of such accidents would be minimized if all manipulators understood the mechanism of injury, and modified their examination and treatment procedures accordingly.

Pretreatment protocol

An appreciation of the real incidence of manipulation accidents (vide supra) and of the need for rigorous exclusion of possible hazard, has suggested a fully documented protocol of premanipulation testing procedures, should the use of full range mobilizations and/or manipulative thrust techniques be contemplated (Grant 1988). It is recommended that the protocol should include (i) an adequately detailed history of the presence and behaviour of dizziness and associated symptoms, (ii) a comprehensive series of sustained cervical postures which will simulate the controlled stress applied during a higher than grade II rotational mobilization and/or a grade V manipulation, (iii) a full explanation to the patient of the risk, however minor, of manipulative thrust techniques applied to the cervical spine, when clinically appropriate, (iv) the *informed* written consent of the patient and (v) adequate documentation of (a) the patient's consent and (b) the relevant clinical findings at the initial and all subsequent attendances. It is important from the medico-legal standpoint that the documented protocol should be such as could withstand critical analysis in a court of law.

Therapists should be aware that even after receiving the patient's informed and written consent, they remain legally liable if it can be shown that the reasonable screening measures commonly known and available to the profession were not employed.

Uneventful premanipulative tests do not guarantee that the succeeding thrust or rotational manipulation will also be uneventful (Terrett 1983, Lindy 1984, Bolton et al 1989).

The whole time-consuming procedure is itself not without risk, and, plainly, the tail is beginning to wag the dog.

WARNING. Because several full-range rotations, alone and combined with extension, form the basis of these testing procedures, *the tests may induce the very conditions one is seeking to avoid*. They are no longer advocated by the writer (Grieve 1991).

Of those cervical movements which compromise flow in the vertebral artery, the single most effective one is rotation (Toole & Tucker 1960). Wyke (1990) mentions that the combination of hyperextension and full rotation during testing has been known to cause major neurological accident, hence the tests are neither described nor illustrated in new editions of this writer's work.

Since most manipulation accidents involving the neck appear to have occurred following the imposition of full cervical rotation, this technique should be avoided. The addition of traction does not make it any safer (see p. 681).

By now, many readers have concluded that ardent pursuit of the one-shot, dramatic relief of upper cervical problems, by full-range rotational mobilization or a single grade V manipulation, may make more trouble than the possibility of success might merit. Not often, but often enough.

In common with other workers (Paterson & Burn 1985, Bourdillon & Day 1987, Terrett 1987b, Martienssen & Nilsson 1989) who have suggested restricting the field of cervical testing and/or manipulation, the writer abandoned extremes of cervical rotation and extension, both in testing and in treatment, some years ago and also abandoned *all* grade V manipulation thrust techniques above the level of T3. Clinical efficacy and economy of attendances have not been adversely affected.

The attraction of common or garden localized mobilizations, under the patient's control and skilfully used with the patient in neutral or carefully combined positions, becomes understandable (Edwards 1988, Mulligan 1989). These techniques are safe and effective, and there are many from which to choose (Grieve 1991).

Fast et al (1987) have suggested: 'More research is necessary in order to elucidate the exact mechanisms leading to vertebral artery damage during manipulations. Excessive forces, wrong techniques, ignoring contraindications for manipulation (e.g. unstable spine) and fragile bones due to pathological processes, may be but a few of the causes of these complications. Means to document the amount of force used during manipulation should be developed. Adequately controlled studies to evaluate the effects of manipulation are necessary. Only then will the role of manipulative therapy be determined.'

Traction, manual or mechanical, is not without its potential for an unfortunate outcome, particularly if unwisely applied without careful and cautious assessment when treating severe road traffic injuries of the cervical and upper thoracic spine (Grieve 1989). LaBan and Meerschaert (1975) report two cases of paraplegia, following cervical traction in patients with occult epidural prostatic metastasis. (i) A 77-year-old man presented with severe paravertebral neck, bilateral shoulder and precordial pain. Comprehensive examination, which included radiography and electromyography, did not reveal the cause of his complaint. His initial treatment comprised intermittent cervical traction, of 5.5 kg (12 lb), from an overhead suspension point. In two days he developed paraplegia. (ii) A 69-year-old man with a clinical and radiographic diagnosis of cervical spondylosis was started on cervical traction as the treatment. Twelve days later, after the sixth traction treatment, the patient began developing the symptoms of a cerebral vascular accident, with the sudden onset of left-sided arm and leg weakness. Repeated radiography then demonstrated widespread prostatic metastases.

Comment. The authors observe that prostatic cancer is now the fourth most common cause of death from cancer in the American male; and metastatic spread can occur surreptitiously through multiple pathways, including the pelvic venous channels and their connections with the major venous systems (see Ch. 1).

Schaberg and Gainor (1985) reported that, in their

series of 179 patients with metastic bone disease of the vertebral column, prostate tumours were the most frequent neoplasm causing epidural spinal cord impingement (see Fig. 49.1, p. 680).

Pain remains the single most constant early symptom of epidural metastasis, often for five to six months before X-ray identification of the cause. A history of past primary malignancy, even with 'normal' radiographic appearances, is the salient factor. With the benefit of hindsight, of course, the onset of these pains, in patients of this maturity, should suggest caution.

Clark et al (1986) reported the case of a 16-year-old girl admitted for neck pain. She had landed on her head when falling from a horse eight months previously, and presented with a 'cock-robin' deformity, with the head tilted to the right and rotated to the left. She could turn her head 45° to the left but only 10° to the right. Lateral and a–p radiographs revealed atlanto-axial rotatory fixation, and computerized tomography disclosed compensatory occipito-atlantal counter subluxation. On the 13th and 16th day after injury she had visited a chiropractor because of persistent neck pain and stiffness. Cervical 'adjustment', by brisk head rotations to the right were attempted, but did not resolve the condition. The authors make the point that traction for the fixed atlanto-axial deformity could have increased the compensatory occipito-atlantal subluxation, with potentially disastrous results. Because the condition was considered too dangerous for surgical manipulation, the treatment adopted was fusion from posterior occiput to C2, with an iliac crest bone graft. Following immobilization for 3 months, solid fusion was achieved and at 6 months' follow-up the patient was pain-free and neurologically normal. The original X-rays following injury were obtained, revealing that the C0–C1 articulation was properly aligned and appeared to be intact; hence the patient's attempts at 'stretching exercise', to correct her torticollis, may have provoked the compensatory subluxation.

Traction combined with manipulation. As has been mentioned (p. 681), the addition of traction does not make manipulations any safer, despite the widespread belief that it may do so; neither does it even assist the aims of treatment. Martienssen and Nilsson (1989) analysed a small series of reported cerebrovascular accidents following upper cervical manipulation, and among the group were two cases, one in which traction was added to rotation and extension of the cervical spine and one in which traction alone was employed. The latter treatment resulted in the onset of paraesthesiae, and after the former treatment the patient died.

When Brown and Tissington-Tatlow (1963) added traction to rotation of the neck in cadavers, the incidence of total occlusion of the contralateral vertebral artery was more than tripled, i.e. from 5 to 17 instances.

Several clinicians have testified to the possible hazards of employing traction in manipulative techniques (Lescure 1959, Jackson 1966, Parkin et al 1978, Robertson 1981, Gutmann 1983, Bourdillon & Day 1987).

THE THORACIC SPINE

Important considerations when formulating treatment for thoracic joint problems are:

Neoplastic disease

Primary spinal bone tumours are unusual, but metastases are common in the thoracic bony structures (see Ch. 63). Macnab and McCullough (1990) mention that the lumbar vertebrae are the most frequent site of metatastic spread, but over 80% of tumours producing neurological defects occur at thoracic cord level. Radiography reveals bone depletion later rather than earlier.

Manipulators should perhaps bear in mind four useful clinical propositions:

1. A high index of suspicion, that one is confronting the presentation of neoplastic disease rather than evidence of simple degenerative change, becomes more necessary as the average age of our patients goes up.

2. Apparently 'normal' X-rays of mature patients may already present the features of neoplastic disease, which become evident on a closer look and/or repeated films.

3. Thoracic and lumbar neoplasms (primaries and metastases) may be well-established in the presence of normal spinal movements, normal straight-leg-raising (SLR) tests and with no evidence of neurological deficit (Grieve 1991).

4. A single episode of stress or trauma may not always herald an episode of simple musculoskeletal pain but can well be the factor uncovering hitherto covert and silent neoplastic disease. A common example of (1) is that of the onset of backache in a mature adult who has never had backache worth complaining about before. Examples of (2) are the second of the two patients with epidural metastases who were initially treated by cervical traction (p. 683) and those occasions described by Grimer and Sneath (1990) (Ch. 63 p. 850) in discussing the diagnosis of malignant bone tumours. In that instance an initial radiograph, passed as normal in 13 out of 70 cases, was observed on retrospective review to reveal evidence of neoplastic disease.

Examples of (3) are evident in Table 63.5 (p. 845), mentioning 20 cases of primary neoplasms of bone who had no restriction of SLR. On the same page is described a young man, with two disparate thoracic neoplasms, whose spinal motion, SLR test and neurological findings were normal.

Examples of (4) are given on the first page of Chapter

63. This preamble is meant to highlight all four clinical propositions which in the instance to be discussed might have suggested caution. Austin (1985) presented a case of a 53-year-old man, with a 6-month history of thoracic pain which began while he was mending a window. After 3 months the pain worsened; radiographs then were reported as showing only degenerative change. Haemoglobin concentration and a full blood count were normal — the specimen tube for plasma viscosity was lost. Three weeks before presenting himself he had undergone three sessions of manipulation by a physiotherapist. After this his thoracic spine felt unstable; he could only remain upright by levering himself upwards with his thumbs tucked into the waistband of his trousers. Examination revealed a 'knuckle' kyphosis at T9, which was tender. SLR was 90° bilaterally and there was no neurological deficit nor other signs or symptoms of spinal cord compression. Radiographs then showed a pathological crush fracture of the T9 vertebral body, with circumscribed radiolucent areas suggestive of multiple myeloma of ribs and pelvis. A review of the previous films revealed that these deposits were present in those X-rays. Myelomatosis was confirmed on examination of the bone marrow. Pain from the fracture resolved with local radiotherapy and medication with melphalan and prednisone.

It is easy to make these points in hindsight, of course, but the lessons are there, and of the four factors mentioned perhaps the most important is the first, i.e. a high level of suspicion.

Osteoporosis

This can have many causes, not necessarily ageing, and it is wise to enquire about medication because treatment by systemic steroids, or heparin anticoagulant therapy, may induce loss of bone minerals (Dimond 1964, Peters 1983). The ribs are particularly vulnerable, as they are in rheumatoid disease (Grieve 1988).

Anticoagulants

Continuing this theme, manual attentions of any vigour and overpressure to full range movements are unwise in patients on anticoagulants. Stewart-Wynne (1976) reported a patient, receiving warfarin sodium after a myocardial infarct, who attended an osteopath three times for spinal manipulation. The last of these was followed by an ilio-femoral psoas haematoma with femoral neuropathy. Nobel et al (1980) described the anatomical basis for the neuropathy. Pear (1972) discussed the catastrophe of spinal epidural haematoma, mentioning those described by Dabbert (1970). Rajashekhar and Herbison (1974) report cases of retroperitoneal haemorrhage in patients receiving anticoagulants.

Thoracic cord vascularity

It is curious that a particular anatomical circumstance (Ch. 17) does not receive wider attention in the manipulative literature, lay or orthodox. The neural canal between T4 and T9 is a critical vascular zone, where the canal is narrowest and the blood supply poorest. The implications are obvious.

Thoracic disc lesions

Many relatively innocuous spondylotic and/or arthrotic changes in the thoracic region are called 'disc lesions'. This may tend to obscure the real importance of frank localized disc protrusions, usually in the lower half of the region, which can be catastrophic and have not, until recently, enjoyed a good surgical prognosis. It is important to be aware of the implications of unpleasant bilateral lower limb paraesthesiae in patients with body wall pain (Grieve 1988). Thoracic disc trespass in the lower half of the region is a lesion of potential hazard (Simeone 1971, Shaw 1975, Benson & Byrnes 1975).

Livingston (1978) reported a patient with a tuberculous dorsal vertebra who was subjected to spinal 'adjustment' by a chiropractor. She had previously been 'adjusted' for low-back pain by a physiotherapist, who are not blameless in the matter of multiple treatments for which no possible rationale could exist. He described 100 physiotherapy treatments for one patient and 300 chiropractic adjustments for another, and mentioned a rheumatoid patient who received 40 treatments of pressure techniques to the dorsal spine (Livingston 1971).

A further example was that of a 70-year-old patient with multiple myeloma, whose third visit to a chiropractor precipitated paraplegia. The patient developed bronchopneumonia some 3 weeks later and died.

O'Neill and Crawford (1922) described a manipulative treatment, now mainly of historical interest, of quite extraordinary ferocity. It produced intra-abdominal haemorrhage, requiring surgical control.

THE LUMBAR SPINE

Farfan (1973) remarked on the main difficulty with manipulation — the results are unpredictable.

This unpredictability is reduced by comprehensive examination and a clinical method in which no thrust techniques are employed until the assessment of response, to exploratory mobilization, clearly indicates the need. Even then, heavy artillery should not be deployed when good marksmanship with a rifle may suffice.

Schmorl and Junghanns (1971) observed that in certain cases manual therapy may be successful, but it may also displace a disc sequestrum and produce extensive compression on nerve roots. Of those reported, accidents are usually either (i) converting a low-back pain into a painful sciatica with neurological signs; (ii) precipitating a massive cauda equina compression with bilateral muscle weakness and sensibility changes, reflex loss and sphincter paralysis — respectively the 'B' and 'C' groups previously mentioned.

While accidental production of a cauda equina syndrome is serious, it is uncommon (Laderman 1981). The 'B' group of accidents occurs more frequently, and these need not have a direct cause-and-effect relationship between disc trespass, low-back pain and sciatica.

Over-preoccupation with the lumbar intervertebral disc, as the prime cause of low-back pain and sciatica, continues unabated. Disc protrusions, though important, are not always of clinical significance (Farfan 1973).

Examination

However informed and comprehensive examination may be, it remains wise to interpret findings with caution. There are no copper-bottomed guarantees that thrust techniques will be safe. Lower-limb pain and a positive straight-leg-raising test may have nothing to do with disc trespass. The symptoms of the lumbar dorsal ramus syndrome (Ch. 30) and sacroiliac syndromes (Ch. 57) may also be provoked by peremptory attempts to restore symmetry or 'alignment'.

Urban (1986) discussed the clinical significance of the straight-leg-raise (SLR) test. The well-leg SLR, or crossed SLR, test is probably of most value in identifying those patients with large disc herniations in whom manipulation is most unwise. A positive ipsilateral SLR test is of doubtful value in diagnosing disc herniation in young people under 30. Conversely, the more mature the patient, the less does a negative SLR response exclude disc herniation. Positive findings, when employing the prone-knee flexion test to enhance reflex suppression and muscle weakness, are not necessarily pathognomonic of disc lesions. They are equivocal (Grieve 1991). Carefully localized injections of local anaesthetic into facet-joint cavities can normalize reduced SLR and depressed tendon jerks within a few minutes (Mooney & Robertson 1976).

Spinal stenosis

Extension postures are known to bulge the annulus posteriorly into the neural canal (Grieve 1988); also, the ligamentum flavum bulges anteriorly. When the canal is developmentally narrow, and a degree of degenerative trespass already exists, vertical thrust techniques on the prone patient are hazardous. When history-taking suggests aggravation by extension and relief by flexed postures, and physical examination confirms this (Weinstein & Ehni 1977), ordinary a–p and lateral lumbar X-rays (Jones & Thomson 1968), and diagnostic ultrasound if

necessary (Porter 1980), will identify developmental stenosis, supposing manipulative thrusts are being envisaged. The wisest course is not to use these techniques in the presence of stenosis, nor rotatory thrust techniques using the thigh as a lever since considerable extra torque is applied this way. Goldthwait's (1911) absorbing account of manipulative techniques employed for 'sacroiliac' lesions appears to be such a case of stenosis.

The 'C' group

Hooper (1973) described two cases where complications might possibly have been avoided by appreciation of contra-indications. Jackson (1971) described a further two cases, where operations were done as emergency procedures to relieve bladder paralysis after manipulative treatment of prolapsed disc lesions — presumably in an orthopaedic environment. Eyre-Brook (1952) and Jennett (1956) each report such a case, which suggests the need for caution during manipulation under anaesthesia. Other reports in this group are by Fisher (1943), Ravault et al (1954), Kuhlendahl and Hansell (1958), Oger et al (1966), Richard (1967) and Dan and Saccasan (1983), who report seven cases including one of vertebral pedicle fracture.

Livingston (1971) described five examples of what appeared to be unnecessarily athletic treatment. '*Manipulation is not manhandling a joint into submission, or acceptable radiographic symmetry, by firm and sometimes unnecessarily vigorous treatment.*'

The importance of suspicion

Weinstein and McLain (1987) have observed that 'Although primary tumours of the spine are uncommon lesions, a wide variety of primary tumours may arise in the bone and soft tissues of the vertebral column. Simply identifying the presence of a tumour may require a high index of suspicion, since the most common early symptom is back pain, an almost universal complaint'. At the other end of the scale, the manual treatment of *assumed spinal musculoskeletal lesions in children* goes hand in hand with heightened awareness of the greater potential for untoward consequences. Apart from the folly of employing any degree of vigour, it is worthwhile improving one's knowledge of dysraphism, anomalies, tumours and juvenile infections (Raimondi 1989). Turner et al (1989) reported the incidence of back pain in childhood, and of the 61 children mentioned, 50% had serious spinal disease. The authors suggest that clinical findings alone can be unreliable in distinguishing such patients. (See also 'The adolescent acute back' in Grieve (1988), p. 410.)

There is nothing in the least morbid about consistently being suspicious of the genesis of seemingly 'musculoskeletal' pain. On the contrary, it is a positive approach amounting to no more than ordinary common sense. Things (especially clinical features) are not always what they seem and it is wise to be wise (McCauley et al 1981).

The variety of effective manual mobilizing techniques, under the patient's control rather than the clinician's, exceeds by far the single, stark choice of *insisting* on segmental movement by peremptory thrust manipulations or abrupt so-called 'adjustments'. While rationale governing use of thrust techniques may differ between manipulators, it is thrust manipulations which most often make the occasions when undesirable consequences are irretrievable — no going back or erasure is possible, and the dismal sequelae must follow as night follows day.

Conclusion

Manipulative treatment belongs to no man exclusively, nor to any one discipline — nor ever will.

All manual therapists, orthodox or lay, will continue to use mobilization and manipulation techniques and to improve their knowledge, skills and efficacy.

Claims to be the only true repository of manual skills, and internecine strife about these claims, are pointless. They are also unwise because they enhance an undesirable aspect of manipulative thrust techniques — that of the 'manipulation dynamic', for want of a better phrase.

As a consequence of its existence, the potent weapon generates its own dynamic — the tail begins to wag the dog. The national possession of a military machine more capable than neighbouring countries tends to generate a restlessness to use it. Manipulative capability may likewise invite rationalization by way of an earnest search for further clinical opportunities, and this tends to occur if the student is not soundly trained first as a *clinician*. The good clinician is more likely to recognize when a particular therapy is, or might well be, inappropriate. The dedicated and zealous manipulator of whatever discipline, orthodox or lay, may not always recognize this. Some of those who expressly train to be manipulators may fall prey to the self-generated dynamic.

A proportion of keen manipulators, having devoted years of study and practice to gaining the necessary skills, seem prone to a euphoric preoccupation with manipulation as such. The manipulative *ethos* begins to be something acquiring virility in itself, psychologically almost resembling a concern with powdered rhino horn. Most of our patients do not *need* to be manipulated. On the other hand, for the smaller proportion who do, we should responsibly use the effective techniques at our disposal.

There is a valuable and considerable place for manual/ mechanical passive movement techniques, when founded on authentic concepts of pathology and used with care, economy and clinical discretion. This view enjoys the manifest support of orthopaedic colleagues (Grieve 1988). Schiötz and Cyriax (1975) observed that contingencies

cannot be wholly guarded against and their occasional occurrence provides no argument against the use of manipulation. The writer's more recent opinion is that, in certain cases, an argument against manipulation *is* provided, i.e. by a more accurate and realistic appraisal of the possible consequences of enthusiastic pre-manipulative testing of cervical structures, and grade V thrust and/ or rotatory techniques to the cervical and cervicothoracic regions.

A positive development is the self-generated improvement in physiotherapy services for musculoskeletal conditions. Umbrella prescriptions for 'heat and exercises' or 'SWD three times weekly' have long since been replaced by 'Physiotherapy please', in the confident knowledge that the patient's need will be accurately assessed and the condition treated according to that need, frequently by manual therapy. A corollary of this is the increasing use of direct General Practitioner referral to physiotherapy departments of National Health Service hospitals in Great Britain, and physiotherapists in private practice responsibly acting as 'first contact' professionals. We owe much to those therapists (Kaltenborn 1970, Evjenth & Hamberg 1980, McKenzie 1983, Maitland 1986) who, over the last three decades, have steadily evolved a more rational and less energetic approach to manual treatment. This is based on scientific evaluation with clear graphic expression of movement abnormalities, and careful grading of treatment procedures. The importance of continuing assessment has been enhanced. A welcome addition to our skills has been recognition of a very common group of low back conditions which do not require manual treatment at all; under therapist instruction these patients do better exercising responsibility for their own wellbeing (McKenzie 1983). When manipulation is not indicated, nor used, accidents cannot occur. The widespread and understandable tendency to view manipulation as a possibly energetic form of treatment does impose upon manipulatively-minded therapists (of whatever persuasion) the obligation to make themselves not only intelligible but also credible to their peers and colleagues (Crelin 1973). These interests are not served by presenting manipulation almost as an alternative system of total health care, by the regular employment of somewhat athletic thrust techniques, by continued repetition of manifestly unsuitable procedures nor by encouraging patients to continue attending for months on end of 'treatment'.

Dedicated manipulators make much of skill, as if skill alone is sufficient (Lewit 1972). This is not so.

Taking up our road traffic analogy, however skilled, careful and experienced the manipulator may be, he is, like the car driver, in charge of a potentially lethal instrument. As in car driving, informed prudence reduces incidents and accidents. There are road conditions, weather and the unpredictability of others to consider.

This unpredictability is illustrated by Lindy's (1984) case in which a 43-year-old male, with a 3-year history of recurrent headache, collapsed within 30 seconds of a direct manipulative thrust technique to the left occipito-atlantal joint in traction. The patient became progressively disoriented and nauseous, complained of feeling cold, became inco-ordinated, inarticulate and began to vomit. Verging on unconsciousness, he was immediately hospitalized but recovered in 24 hours. Brisk head movements provoked slight disorientation for a further 2 weeks, after which he recovered completely.

Previous unspecified manipulative treatment had been successful, for some months at least.

While the mechanisms underlying the sequelae, particularly their short duration, are of interest, the outstanding factor is that of unpredictability, despite premanipulative tests.

Clinical concern is to achieve treatment objectives with the least energetic of procedures available. When preoccupation with manipulative thrust techniques (Grice 1980, Hartman 1985, Latey 1984) becomes quasi-religious, the tail is wagging the dog and thrust manipulations may be used on occasions when they need not. Gainsbury (1985) introduced overdue realism to this tendency for ecclesiastical reverence. Remarking on its limited effectiveness, he adds 'High velocity thrust is frequently a placebo which keeps the patient — and the practitioner — happy while the body's own reparative processes are at work'.

A sound maxim is that when patients do not *need* to be manipulated — DO NOT.

REFERENCES

Apley A G 1990 An assessment of assessment. Journal of Bone and Joint Surgery 72B: 957–958

Ashley J 1987 Anatomy of a hospital. University Press, Oxford, p 25

Attali P 1957 Accidents graves après manipulation intempestive par un chiropractor Revue du Rhumatisme 24: 652

Austin R T 1985 Pathological vertebral fracture after spinal manipulation. British Medical Journal 291: 1114–1115

Barrett S 1976 Chiropractic. New England Journal of Medicine 294: 346

Barton J W, Margolis M T 1975 Rotational obstruction of the vertebral artery at the atlanto-axial joint. Neuroradiology 9: 117–120

Beatty R A 1977 Dissecting haematoma of the internal carotid artery following chiropractic cervical manipulation. Journal of Trauma 17: 248–250

Benassy J, Wolinetz E 1957 Quadriplégie après manoeuvre chiropractique. Revue du Rhumatisme 24: 555–556

Benson M K D, Byrnes D P 1975 The clinical syndromes and surgical treatment of thoracic intervertebral disc prolapse. Journal of Bone and Joint Surgery 57B: 471–477

Biemond A 1951 Thrombosis of the basilar artery and vascularisation of the brain stem. Brain 74: 300–317

Bladin P F, Merory J 1975 Mechanisms in cerebral lesions in trauma to high cervical portion of the vertebral artery — rotational injury. Proceedings of the Australian Association of Neurology 12: 35–41

Blaine E S 1925 Manipulative (chiropractic) dislocations of the atlas. Journal of the American Medical Association 85: 1356–1359

Bolton P S, Stick P E, Lord R S A 1989 Failure of clinical tests to predict cerebral ischaemia before neck manipulation. Journal of Manipulative and Physiological Therapeutics 12: 304–307

Boshes L D 1959 Vascular accidents associated with neck manipulation. Journal of the American Medical Association 171: 1652

Boudin G 1957 Syndrom grave du trone cérébral après manipulations cervicales. Bulletins et mémoires de la Société médicale des hôpitaux de Paris 73: 562–566

Boudin G, Barbizet J 1958 Les accidents nerveux des manipulations du rachis cervical. Revue Practicien 8: 2235-2243

Bourdillon J F, Day E A 1987 Spinal manipulation. 4th edn. Heinemann, London

Braaf M M, Rosner S 1962 Menière-like syndrome following whip-lash injury of the neck. Journal of Trauma 2: 494–501

Brain Lord, Wilkinson M 1967 Cervical spondylosis and other disorders of the cervical spine. Heinemann, London, ch 3, p 120

Braun I F, Pinto R S, De Filipp G J 1983 Brain stem infarction due to chiropractic manipulation of the cervical spine. Southern Medical Journal 76: 1199–1204

Brentingham J W 1988 Commentary: a critical look at the subluxation hypothesis. Journal of Manipulative and Physiological Therapeutics 11: 130–132

Brewerton D A 1964 Conservative treatment of the painful neck. Proceedings of the Royal Society of Medicine 57: 163–165

Brodal A 1957 The cranial nerves: anatomy and anatomico-clinical correlations. Blackwell Scientific, Oxford, p 127

Brodal A 1981 Neurological anatomy in relation to clinical medicine. 3rd edn. University Press, Oxford, p 469, p 532

Brown S T J, Tissington-Tatlow W F 1963 Radiographic studies of the vertebral arteries in cadavers: effect of position and traction of the head. Radiology 81: 80–88

Brownson R J, Zollinger W K, Madeira T 1986 Sudden sensorial hearing loss following manipulation of the cervical spine. Laryngoscope 96: 166–169

Bryner P 1987 Commentary: isn't it time to abandon anachronistic terminology? Journal of the Australian Chiropractors' Association 17: 53–59

Bureau of Legal Medicine and Legislation 1952 Chiropractors: rupture of brain tumour following adjustment. Journal of the American Medical Association 148: 669

Cameron I, Browning S 1982 The vertebral artery. British Osteopathic Journal 14: 11–18

Carstairs L S 1959 Radiology. In: Modern trends in diseases of the vertebral column. Butterworth, London

Charlton K H 1987 Data and Dogma: the use and abuse of information. Journal of the Australian Chiropractors' Association 17: 46–48

Clarke C R, Kathol M H, Walsh T, Elkoury G Y 1986 Atlantoaxial rotatory fixation with compensatory counter occipitoatlantal subluxation. Spine 11: 1048–1050

Coste F, Galmiche P, Brion S, Chabot J, Chaouat Y, Illoux G 1953 Deux cas de mal de Pott révélés par traction ou manipulations. Revue du Rhumatisme 20: 710–711

Coutts M B 1934 Atlanto-epistropheal subluxations. Archives of Surgery 29: 297–311

Crelin E S 1973 A scientific test of the chiropractic theory. American Scientist 61: 574–580

Cyriax J 1971 Manipulation: by laymen or physiotherapists? Journal of the Canadian Physiotherapy Association 23: 236–238

Dabbert O, Freeman D G, Weis A J 1970 Spinal meningeal haematoma, warfarin therapy and chiropractic adjustment. Journal of the American Medical Association 214: 2058

Dalseth I 1976 Chiropractic and radiological diagnosis. Tidsskrift for Den norske laegeforening 11: 642-644

Dan N G, Saccasan P A 1983 Serious complications of lumbar spinal manipulation. Medical Journal of Australia 2: 672–673

Daneshmend T K, Hewer R L, Bradshaw J R 1984 Acute brain stem stroke during neck manipulation. British Medical Journal 288: 189

Davidson K C, Welford E C, Dixon G D 1975 Traumatic vertebral artery pseudoaneurysm following chiropractic manipulation. Neuroradiology 115: 651–652

Davis C 1985 Osteopathic manipulation resulting in damage to the spinal cord. British Medical Journal 291: 1540–1541

De Kleyn A, Nieuwenhuyse P 1927 Schwindclanfallcund Nystagmus bei einer bestimmten Stellung des Koppes. Acta Otolaryngolica 11: 155–157

De Kleyn A, Versteegh C 1933 Uber verchiedeni Foramen von Menière's Syndrome. Deustche Zischr Nerventh 132: 57

Depoorter A F 1966 Indications et contreindications des manipulations vertébrales. In: Proceedings 4th International Congress of Physical Medicine. Excerpta Medica, Amsterdam, pp 150 155

De Sèze, Mieg T 1955 Les munipulations vertébrales. Revue du Rhumatisme 22: 635–650

De Sèze S, Kahn J J, Mieg T, Renoult C L 1966 Les accidents des manipulations vertébrales. In: L'actualité Rhumatologie — Presentee au Practicien. L'Expansion Scientifique, Paris

Deshayes P, Geoffroy Y 1962 Un cas de paralysie plexique supérieure, accident d'une manipulation vertébrale. Revue du Rhumatisme 29: 137–139

Dimond E G 1964 Panel discussion: the clinical uses of heparin. American Journal of Cardiology 14: 49–54

Donahue J H 1988a Dis-ease in our principles: the case against innate intelligence. American Journal of Chiropractic Medicine 1: 86–88

Donahue J H 1988b Letter. American Journal of Chiropractic Medicine 1: 203

Drum D C 1975 The vertebral motor unit and intervertebral foramen. In: Goldstein M (ed) The research status of spinal manipulative therapy. NINCDS Monograph No 15 US Department of Health, Bethesda, ch 3, p 64

Dulhunty J 1987 Basic mechanics of the vertebral subluxation. Journal of the Australian Chiropractors' Association 17: 49–52

Dvorak J, Orelli F V 1982 Wie gefahrlich ist de Manipulation der Halswirbelsäule? Manuelle Medezin 20: 44–48

Easton D J, Sherman D G 1977 Cervical manipulation and stroke. Stroke 8: 594–597

Editorial 1980 Chiropractors urged to consider stroke risk. Medical World News. March 17: 23

Edwards B C 1988 Combined movements of the cervical spine in examination and treatment. In: Grant R (ed) Physical therapy of the cervical and thoracic spine. Churchill Livingstone, New York, p 125

Evjenth O, Hamberg J 1980 Töjning av muskler Del 11 Ryggraden. Alfta Rehab Forlag, Malmo

Eyre-Brook A L 1952 A study of late results from disc operations: present employment and residual results. British Journal of Surgery 39: 289–296

Farfan H F 1973 Mechanical disorders of the low back. Lea and Febiger, Philadelphia, ch 7, p 138; ch 10, p 220

Farfan H F 1977 Pathological basis for manipulative therapy. In: Proceedings of the 3rd Conference International Federation of Orthopaedic Manipulative Therapists, Vail, Colorado, p 135

Fast A, Zinicola D F, Marin E L 1987 Vertebral artery damage complicating cervical manipulation. Spine 12: 840–842

Fielding J W, Reddy K 1969 Atlanto-axial rotatory deformity. Journal of Bone and Joint Surgery 51A: 1672–1673

Fielding J W, Hawkins R J, Hensinger R N, Francis W R 1978 Atlantoaxial rotary deformities. Orthopaedic Clinics of North America 9: 955–967

Fisher E D 1943 Report of a case of ruptured intervertebral disc following chiropractic manipulation. Kentucky Medical Journal 41: 14

Fleischli D J 1967 Lytic lesion in a cervical vertebra. Journal of the American Medical Association 201: 110

Ford F R 1952 Syncope, vertigo and disturbances of vision resulting from intermittent obstruction of the vertebral arteries due to defect in the odontoid process and excessive mobility of the second cervical vertebra. Bulletin of Johns Hopkins Hospital 91: 168–173

Ford F R, Clark D 1956 Thrombosis of the basilar artery with softening in the cerebellum and brain stem due to manipulation of the neck. Bulletin of Johns Hopkins Hospital 98: 37–42

Fritz V U, Maloon A, Tuch P 1984 Neck manipulation causing stroke. South African Medical Journal 66: 844–846

Gainsbury J M 1985 High-velocity thrust and pathophysiology of segmental dysfunction. In: Glasgow E F, Twomey L T, Scull E R, Kleynhans A M, Idczak R M (eds) Aspects of manipulative therapy.

2nd edn. Churchill Livingstone, Edinburgh, ch 13, p 92

Goff P J 1988 Chiropractic treatment of mental illness: a review of theory and practice. Research Forum 4: 4–10

Goldthwait J E 1911 The lumbo-sacral articulation. An explanation of many cases of lumbago and sciatica. Boston Medical and Surgical Journal 164: 365–372

Gorman R F 1978 Cardiac arrest after cervical spine mobilization. Medical Journal of Australia 2: 169–170

Grant R 1988 Dizziness testing and manipulation of the cervical spine. In: Grant R (ed) Physical therapy of the cervical and thoracic spine. Churchill Livingstone, New York, p 111

Grayson M F 1987 Case report: Horner's syndrome after manipulation of the neck. British Medical Journal 295: 1381–1382

Green D, Joynt R J 1959 Vascular accidents to the brain stem associated with neck manipulation. Journal of the American Medical Association 170: 522–524

Grice A S 1980 A biomechanical approach to cervical and dorsal adjusting. In: Haldeman S (ed) Modern developments in the principles and practice of chiropractic. Appleton-Century Crofts, New York, ch 15, pp 332–333

Grieve G P 1986 Psychological aspects of vertebral pain and dysfunction. In: Grieve G P (ed) Modern manual therapy. Churchill Livingstone, Edinburgh, ch 25, pp 270–279

Grieve G P 1988 Common vertebral joint problems. 2nd edn. Churchill Livingstone, Edinburgh, pp 243, 356, 429, 532

Grieve G P 1989 Contraindications to spinal manipulation and allied treatments. Physiotherapy 75: 445–453

Grieve G P 1991 Mobilization of the spine. 5th edn. Preface. Churchill Livingstone, Edinburgh

Grimer R J, Sneath R S 1990 Editorial: diagnosing malignant bone tumours. Journal of Bone and Joint Surgery 72B: 754–756

Grinker R R, Guy C C 1927 Sprain of cervical spine causing thrombosis of anterior spinal artery. Journal of the American Medical Association 88: 1140

Grossiors A 1966 Les accidents neurologiques des manipulations. Annales de Médecine Physique 9: 283–299

Grundy D J, McSweeney T, Jones H W F 1984 Cranial nerve palsies in cervical injuries. Spine 9: 339–343

Gutmann G 1983 Injuries to the vertebral artery caused by manual therapy. Manuelle Medizin 21: 2–14

Hanraets P R M J 1959 The degenerative back and its differential diagnosis. Elsevier, Amsterdam, ch 9, p 579

Hanus S H, Homere Td, Harter D H 1977 Vertebral artery occlusion complicating Yoga exercises. Archives of Neurology 34: 574–575

Hartman L 1985 Classification and application of osteopathic manipulative techniques. In: Glasgow E F, Twomey L T, Scull E R, Kleynhans A M, Idczak R M (eds) Aspects of manipulative therapy. 2nd edn. Churchill Livingstone, Edinburgh, ch 12, pp 81–86

Held J P 1966 Pièges et dangers des manipulations cervicales en neurologie. Annales de Médecine Physique 9: 251–260

Hitselburger W E, Witten R M 1968 Abnormal myelograms in asymptomatic patients. Journal of Neurosurgery 28: 204–206

Hooper J 1973 Low back pain and manipulation. Paraparesis after treatment of low back pain by physical methods. Medical Journal of Australia 1: 549–551

Horn S W 1983 The 'locked-in' syndrome following chiropractic manipulation of the cervical spine. Annals of Emergency Medicine 12: 648–650

Hosek R S, Schram S B, Silverman H 1980 Cervical manipulation. Journal of the American Medical Association 245: 922–927

Hoyland J A, Freemont A J, Jayson M I V 1989 Intervertebral foramen venous obstruction: a cause of periradicular fibrosis? Spine 14: 558–568

Illoux G 1962 Du danger des manipulations vertébrales, Vie Médicale 43: 226–229

Jackson R 1966 The cervical syndrome. 3rd edn. Thomas, Springfield, USA, p 284

Jackson R K 1971 The long term effects of wide laminectomy for lumbar disc excision. Journal of Bone and Joint Surgery 53B: 609–616

Jamison J 1987 Hypertension case finding and management in chiropractic clinics. European Journal of Chiropractic 35: 151–155

Jaskoviak P A 1980 Complications arising from manipulation of the cervical spine. Journal of Manipulative and Physiological Therapeutics 3: 213–219

Jeanblanc J 1970 Indications et limites des manipulations vertébrales. Annales Medicales de Nancy 9: 117–121

Jeffreys E 1980 Disorders of the cervical spine. Butterworth, London, ch 6, p 101

Jennett W B 1956 A study of 25 cases of compression of the cauda equina by prolapsed intervertebral discs. Journal of Neurology, Neurosurgery and Psychiatry 19: 109–116

Johnson R H, Spalding J M K 1974 Diseases of the autonomic nervous system. Blackwell Scientific, Oxford, ch 11, p 208

Jones R A C, Thomson J L G 1968 The narrow lumbar canal: a clinical and radiological review. Journal of Bone and Joint Surgery 50B: 595–605

Jung A, Kehr P 1972 Das Zerviko-enzephale syndrom bei Arthrosen und nach Traumen der Halswirbelsáule. Manuelle Medizin 10: 127–133

Kaltenborn F 1970 Mobilization of the spinal column. University Press, Wellington

Kanshepolsky J, Danielson H, Flynn R E 1972 Vertebral artery insufficiency and cerebellar infarct due to manipulation of the neck. Bulletin of the Los Angeles Neurological Society 37: 62

Katirji M B, Reinmuth O M, Latchaw R E 1985 Stroke due to vertebral artery injury. Archives of Neurology 42: 242–246

Keating J C 1988a Science and politics and the subluxation. American Journal of Chiropractic Medicine 1: 107–110

Keating J C 1988b Dis-ease in our principles (letter). American Journal of Chiropractic Medicine 1: 202–203

Kewalramani L S, Kewalramani D L, Krebs M, Saleen A 1980 Myelopathy following chiropractic cervical spine manipulation. Abstract and Comment: British Association of Manipulative Medicine Newsletter November: 15–16

Kleynhans A M 1980 Complications and contraindications to spinal manipulative therapy. In: Haldeman S (ed) Modern developments in the principles and practice of chiropractic. Appleton-Century Crofts, New York, ch 16, pp 359–384

Kleynhans A M, Terrett A G J 1985 The prevention of complications from spinal manipulative therapy. In: Glasgow E F, Twomey L T, Scull E R, Kleynhans A M, Idczak R M (eds) Aspects of manipulative therapy. 2nd edn. Churchill Livingstone, Edinburgh, ch 24

Knudsen V 1965 Cauda equina syndrom ved lumbal discuprolaps. Nordisk Medicin 74: 898–904

Kommerell G, Hoyt W J 1973 Lateropulsion of saccadic eye movement. Archives of Neurology 28: 313–318

Krueger B R, Okazaki H 1980 Vertebral-basilar distribution infarction following chiropractic cervical manipulation. Mayo Clinic Proceedings 55: 322–332

Kuhlendahl H, Hansell V 1953 Der mediane Massenprolaps der lendenwirbelsaüle mit Kaudakompression. Deutsch Medizinsche Wochenschrift 78: 332–337

Kuhlendahl H, Hansell V 1958 Nil nocere. Munchener Medizinische Wochenschrift 100: 1738

Kunkle C E, Muller C J, Odom G L 1952 Traumatic brain-stem thrombosis: report of a case and analysis of the mechanism of injury. Annals of Internal Medicine 36: 1329–1335

LaBan M M, Meerschaert J R 1975 Quadriplegia following cervical traction in patients with occult epidural prostatic metastasis. Archives of Physical Medicine and Rehabilitation 56: 455–458

Laderman J P 1981 Accidents of spinal manipulation. Annals of the Swiss Chiropracters Association 7: 161–280

Lapresle J 1965 Les myélopathies des cervicarthroses. Seminar des Hôpitaux de Paris 31: 3254–3260

Latey P 1984 An expansion of modern osteopathic theory of technique. British Osteopathic Journal 16: 51–56

Le Corre F, Rageot E, Orsini A, Maigne R 1971 Prévention des accidents des manipulations vertébrales. In: Proceedings 3rd International Congress of Manual Medicine, Monaco

Lescure R J 1954 Incidents, accidents, contreindications des manipulations de la colonne vertebrale. Médecine et Hygiène 12: 546

Lescure R J 1959 Réponses à quelques questions concernant les tractions et manipulations des syndromes cervicaux. Médecine et Hygiène 17: 761–762

Lewit K 1972 Complications following chiropractic manipulations.

Deustche Medizinische Wochenschrift 97: 784

Lievre J A 1953a Paraplégie due aux manoeuvres d'un osteopathe. Revue du Rhumatisme 20: 707

Lievre J A 1953b Paraplegie due aux manoeuvres d'un chiropracteur. Revue du Rhumatisme 20: 708–709

Lievre J A 1955 A propos du traitment des lombalgies et des sciatiques par manipulations vertébrales. Revue du Rhumatisme 26: 651

Lindemann K, Rossak K 1959 Anzeige und gegenanz der Reposition bei Lumbago-Ischias-Syndrom und ihre Komplikationen. Zeitschrift Orthopädie 91: 335–340

Lindy D R 1984 Patient collapse following cervical manipulation: a case report. British Osteopathic Journal 16: 84–85

Livingston M C P 1971 Spinal manipulation causing injury: a three year study. Clinical Orthopaedics 81: 82–86

Livingston M C P 1978 Paramedics, chiropractors and health planners. Canadian Medical Association Journal 119: 1391–1392

Lorenz R, Vogelsang H G 1972 Basilar artery thrombosis after chiropractic manipulation of the cervical spine. Deutsche Medizinische Wochenschrift 97: 36–43

Louyot P, Gaucher A, Jeanblanc J 1967 Indications, Contreindications et accidents des manipulations vertébrales. Annales Medicales de Nancy 6: 1327–1342

Lucido V P 1988 Aids: why it should concern us. Journal of the American Chiropractic Association 25: 5, 8, 9

Lyness S S, Simeone F A 1978 Vascular complications of upper cervical injuries. Orthopaedic Clinics of North America 9: 1029–1038

Lyness S S, Wagman A D 1974 Neurological deficit following cervical manipulation. Surgical Neurology 2: 121–124

McCauley R G K, Goldberg M J, Schwartz A M 1981 Referred pain in the lower leg — a cause of delayed diagnosis. Skeletal Radiology 6: 39–41

McKenzie R 1983 The lumbar spine: mechanical diagnosis and therapy. 4th edn. Spinal Publications, Waikanae

Macnab I, McCullough J A 1990 Backache. Williams and Wilkins, Baltimore

Maigne R 1955 Les manipulations vertébrales: indications, contreindications techniques et résultats. Journal Médicale de Paris 11: 405–418

Maigne R 1960 Les manipulations vertébrales. L'Expansion Scientifique, Paris

Maigne R 1972 Accidents, incidents et abus des manipulations. In: Douleurs d'origine vertébrale et traitments par manipulations, 2nd edn. Expansion Scientifique. Paris, ch 10, pp 130–137

Maitland G D 1986 Vertebral manipulation. 5th edn. Butterworth, London

Martienssen J, Nilsson N 1989 Cerebrovascular accidents following upper cervical manipulation: the importance of age, gender and technique. American Journal of Chiropractic Medicine 2: 160–163

Masson M, Cambier J 1962 Vertebro-basilar circulatory insufficiency. Presse Médicale 70: 1990

Mathews J A 1968 Dynamic discography: a study of lumbar traction. Annals of Physical Medicine 9: 275–279

Mathews J A, Yates D A H 1969 Reduction of lumbar disc prolapse by manipulation. British Medical Journal 3: 696–697

Medico-legal abstracts 1937 Malpractice: death resulting from chiropractic treatment for headache. Journal of the American Medical Association 109: 233–234

Mehalic T, Farhat S M 1974 Vertebral artery injury from chiropractic manipulation of the neck. Surgical Neurology 2: 125–129

Mennell J B 1952 The science and art of joint manipulation. Churchill, London, ch 10, p 193

Miller R G, Burton R 1947 Stroke following chiropractic manipulation of the spine. Journal of the American Medical Association 229: 189–190

Mooney V, Robertson J 1976 The facet syndrome. Clinical Orthopaedics and Related Research 115: 149–156

Mueller S, Sahs A L 1976 Brainstem dysfunction related to cervical manipulation: report of three cases. Neurology (Minneapolis) 26: 547–550

Mulligan B 1989 Manual therapy. Plane Services, Wellington, New Zealand

Nagler W 1973 Mechanical obstruction of the vertebral arteries during hyperextension of the neck. British Journal of Sports Medicine 7: 92–97

Nick J, Contamin F, Nicholls M H 1967 Neurological accidents and accidents due to cervical manipulation. Societé Médicale des Hôpitaux de Paris 118: 435–444

Nobel W, Marks S C, Kubik S 1980 The anatomical basis for femoral nerve palsy following iliacus haematoma. Journal of Neurosurgery 52: 533–540

Nyberg-Hanson R, Loken A C, Tenstad O 1970 Brainstem lesion with coma for five years following manipulation of the cervical spine. Journal of Neurology 218: 97–105

Oger J 1964 Les accidents des manipulations vertébrales. Journal Belge de Médecine Physique et Rhumatisme 19: 2

Oger J, Brumaigne J, Margaux J 1966 Lés dangers et accidents des manipulations vertébrales Revue du Rhumatisme 33: 93–104

Okawara S, Nibbelink D 1974 Vertebral artery occlusion following hyperextension and rotation of the head Stroke 5: 640–642

O'Neill B J, Crawford W W 1922 Intra-abdominal haemorrhage from stomach due to osteopathic treatment: a report of a case. Journal of the American Medical Association 79: 1607

Palmer D D 1910 Textbook of the science, art and philosophy of chiropractic for students and practitioners. Portland Printing House Company, Portland

Park W M 1980 Radiological investigation of the intervertebral disc. In: Jayson M I V (ed) The lumbar spine and back pain. 2nd edn. Pitman Medical, Tunbridge Wells, ch 8, pp 186–187

Parkin P J, Wallis W E, Wilson J L 1978 Vertebral artery occlusion following manipulation of the neck. New Zealand Medical Journal 88: 441–443

Paterson J K, Burn L 1985 An introduction to medical manipulation. MTP Press, Lancaster

Pear B L 1972 Spinal epidural haematoma. American Journal of Roentgenology, Radium Therapy and Nuclear Medicine 115: 155–164

Peters R E 1983 Heparin therapy — contraindication to manipulation. Charter House Publishing, Wagga Wagga, New South Wales

Porter R W 1980 Measurement of the spinal canal by diagnostic ultrasound. In: Jayson M I V (ed) The lumbar spine and back pain. 2nd edn. Pitman Medical, Tunbridge Wells, ch 9, pp 231–245

Pratt-Thomas H R, Berger K E 1947 Cerebellar and spinal injuries after chiropractic manipulation. Journal of the American Medical Association 133: 600–603

Pribeck R A 1963 Brain stem vascular accident following neck manipulation. Wisconsin Medical Journal 62: 141–143

Rageot E 1966 Les accidents et incidents des manipulations vertébrales. In: Proceedings 4th International Congress of Physical Medicine Excerpta Medica, Amsterdam, pp 170–172

Rajashekhar T P, Herbison G J 1974 Lumbosacral plexopathy caused by retroperitoneal haemorrhage: report of two cases. Archives of Physical Medicine and Rehabilitation 55: 91–93

Raimondi A J 1989 The paediatric spine. vol I. Development and the dysraphic state. vol II. Developmental anomalies. vol III. Cysts, tumours and infections. Springer Verlag, London

Ravault P P, Vignon G, Deslous P 1954 La sciatique paralysante. Revue du Rhumatisme 21: 217–224

Richard J 1967 Disc rupture with cauda equina syndrome after chiropractic adjustment. New York State Journal of Medicine 67: 2496–2498

Rieunau G 1966 Pieges et dangers des manipulations vertébrales en orthopédie. Annales de Médecine Physique 9: 260–272

Rinsky L A, Reynolds G G, Jameson R M, Hamilton R D 1976 Spinal cord injury following chiropractic manipulation. Paraplegia 13: 323–327

Robertson J T 1981 Neck manipulation as a cause of stroke. Stroke 12: 1

Robertson J T 1982 Neck manipulation as a cause of stroke. Stroke 13: 260–261

Rosenwasser R, Delgado T, Buchheit W 1983 Cerebrovascular complications of closed neck and head trauma: injuries to the carotid artery. Surgical Rounds 6: 56–65

Sandetur R, Adams E 1987 The effect of chiropractic adjustments in the behaviour of autistic children. American Chiropractic Association Journal of Chiropractic 24: 21–25

Sandifer P H 1967 Neurology in orthopaedics. Butterworth, London, p 52

Schaberg J, Gainor B J 1985 A profile of metastatic carcinoma of the spine. Spine 10: 19–20

Schellhas K P, Latchaw R E, Wendling L R, Gold L H A 1980 Vertebrobasilar injuries following cervical manipulation. Journal of the American Medical Association 244: 1450–1453

Schiötz E H, Cyriax J 1975 Manipulation — past and present. Heinemann, London, ch 10, p 124

Schmitt A P, Wolff H D 1979 Memorandum on the prevention of accidents arising from manipulative therapy of the cervical spine. Manuelle Medizin 17: 53–59

Schmorl G, Junghanns H 1971 The human spine in health and disease, 2nd American edn. Grune and Stratton, London, ch 8 p 222, p 237

Schwarz G A, Geiger J K, Spano A V 1956 Posterior inferior cerebellar artery syndrome of Wallenberg after chiropractic manipulation. Archives of Internal Medicine 97: 352–354

Serre H, Simon L 1968 Dangers des manipulations vertébrales. Revue du Rhumatisme 35: 445–452

Shaw N E 1975 The syndrome of the prolapsed thoracic intervertebral disc. Journal of Bone and Joint Surgery 57B: 412

Shepard R H 1959 Diagnosis and prognosis of cauda equina syndrome produced by protrusion of lumbar disc. British Medical Journal II: 1434–1439

Sherman D G, Hart R G, Easton J D 1981 Abrupt change in head position and cerebral infarction. Stroke 12: 2–6

Simeone F A 1971 The modern treatment of thoracic disc disease. Orthopaedic Clinics of North America 2: 453–462

Simmons K C 1982 Trauma to the vertebral artery related to neck manipulation. Medical Journal of Australia 1: 187–188

Simon L 1966 Pièges et dangers des manipulations cervicales en rhumatologie. Annales de Médecine Physique 9: 272–283

Skrabanek P, McCormick J 1989 Follies and fallacies in medicine. Tarragon Press, Glasgow, p 124

Smith R A, Estridge M N 1962 Neurologic complications of head and neck manipulation. Journal of the American Medical Association 182: 528–531

Stewart-Wynne E G 1976 Iatrogenic femoral neuropathy. British Medical Journal 1: 263

Stopford J S B 1916 The arteries of the pons and medulla oblongata. Journal of Anatomy and Physiology 50: 131–164

Terrett A G J 1983 Importance and interpretation of tests designed to predict susceptibility to neurocirculatory accidents from manipulation. Journal of the Australian Chiropractors' Association 13: 29–33

Terrett A G J 1987a Vascular accidents from cervical spine manipulation: report on 107 cases. Journal of the Australian Chiropractors' Association 17: 15–24

Terrett A G J 1987b Vascular accidents from cervical spine manipulations: the mechanisms. Journal of the Australian Chiropractors' Association 17: 131–144

Thambyrajah K 1972 Fractures of the cervical spine with minimal or no symptoms. Medical Journal of Malaya 26: 244–249

Thierry-Mieg J 1967 Technique des manipulations vertébrales utilisées dans le traitement des cruralgies discales. Indications, contreindications et accidents. Seminar des Hôpitaux de Paris 43: 401–405

Tissington-Tatlow W F, Bammer H G 1957 Syndrome of vertebral artery compression. Neurology 7: 331–340

Tomlinson K M 1955 Purpura following manipulation of the spine. British Medical Journal I: 1260

Toole J F, Tucker S H 1960 Influence of head position upon cerebral circulation. Archives of Neurology 2: 616–623

Turner P G, Green J H, Galasko C S B 1989 Back pain in childhood. Spine 14: 812–814

Urban L M 1986 The straight-leg-raising test: a review. In: Grieve G P 1986 Modern manual therapy. Churchill Livingstone, Edinburgh, ch 53, pp 567–576

Villar R N, Solomon V K, Rangam J 1989 Bonesetters and the Indian child: the enthusiastic amateurs. Journal of Bone and Joint Surgery 71B: 338

Wadia N H 1967 Myelopathy complicating congenital atlanto-axial dislocation. Brain 90: 449–472

Weinstein P R, Ehni G, Wilson C B 1977 Lumbar spondylosis. Year Book Medical Publishers, London, ch 5, pp 115–133

Weinstein J N, McLain R F 1987 Primary tumours of the spine. Spine 12: 843–851

Wilkinson M 1971 Cervical spondylosis. 2nd edn. Heinemann, London. ch 4, p 67

Williams D, Wilson T G 1962 The diagnosis of the major and the minor syndromes of basilar insufficiency. Brain 85: 741–774

Wyke B D 1990 Personal communication

Zimmerman W W, Kumar A J, Gadoth N, Hodges F J 1978 Traumatic vertebrobasilar occlusive disease in childhood. Neurology 28: 185–188

Postscript

Since this chapter was delivered to the Editors, further reports of manipulation accidents have come to the writer's notice, viz:

Cellerier P, Georget A 1984 Dissection des artères vertébrales après manipulation du rachis cervical: apropos d'un cas. Journal de la Radiologie 65: 191–196

Frumkin L R, Baloh R W 1990 Wallenberg's syndrome following neck manipulation. Neurology 40: 611–615

Gallinaro P, Cartesegna M 1983 Three cases of lumbar disc rupture and one of cauda equina syndrome associated with spinal manipulation (chiropractic). Lancet 1: 411

Kornberg E 1988 Lumbar artery aneurysm with acute aortic occlusion resulting from chiropractic manipulation. Surgery 103: 122–124

Lanska D J, Lanska M J, Fenstermaker R, Mapstone T 1987 Thoracic disc herniation associated with chiropractic spinal manipulation. Archives of Neurology 44: 996–997

Malmivaara A, Pohjola R 1982 Cauda equina syndrome caused by chiropraxis on a patient previously free of lumbar spine symptoms. Lancet 2: 986–987

Mas J, Henin D, Bousser M, Chain F, Hauw J 1989 Dissecting aneurysm of the vertebral artery and cervical manipulation: a case report with autopsy. Neurology 39: 512–515

Schmidley J W, Koch T 1984 The non-cerebrovascular complications of chiropractic manipulation. Neurology 34: 684–685

Sherman M, Smialek J, Zane W 1987 Pathogenesis of vertebral artery occlusion following cervical spine manipulation. Archives of Pathology and Laboratory Medicine 111: 851–853

50. Treatment of altered nervous system mechanics

D. S. Butler   M. O. Shacklock   H. Slater

INTRODUCTION

The patient management plan should evolve via clinical reasoning processes that require careful consideration of hypotheses such as sources of symptoms, precautions, prognosis and any further contributing factors. Material to form the hypotheses comes from inquiry and handling skills and previous clinical reasoning experiences that must also include due attention to what is known about patho-anatomy. We propose that with reasoning and handling skills, the nervous system can be effectively and safely mobilized, adding a new dimension to the understanding and treatment of many disorders.

This chapter on treatment of altered nervous system mechanics via mobilization follows chapters on neuroanatomy and neurobiomechanics (Chapter 2), examination and analysis of tension tests (Chapter 44) and clinical reasoning (Chapter 34).

GENERAL POINTS

The ultimate aim of treatment is to restore the patient's range of nervous system movement and stretch capabilities and to normalize the sensitivity of the system. Techniques that alter pathophysiology and pathomechanics will be required. Treatment will invariably be performed while the function of other structures such as joint and muscle is normalized. The idea of mobilizing the nervous system may be new to some readers, but just as muscle, joint and fascial tissue require normal mechanics, so too does the nervous system.

We believe that the best way to determine whether the nervous system is involved in a disorder is to test whether it can conduct normally and can stretch and slide without undue symptom responses during tension tests. These tests are outlined in Chapter 44.

Patients have benefitted in the past with treatment that must mobilize the nervous system, even if inadvertently. For example, 'hamstring' stretches mobilize the neuraxis, meninges and sciatic tract. Stretching of the upper cervical extensor muscles will also mobilize the neuraxis and meninges. We encourage a multistructural approach where an attempt is made to identify the structure(s) requiring mobilization. Making a hypothesis during assessment and treatment about the prime structure(s) at fault is helpful. Treatment can be biased towards a particular structure (the results should support or weaken a hypothesis). For example, a SLR performed in some hip medial rotation rather than in the saggital plane places more emphasis on the nervous system. The accuracy of prognosis is enhanced by utilizing knowledge of the natural history of the injured structure (e.g. the healing rate of muscle is different to that of bone). There are precautionary factors that may be specific to a particular structure.

Familiarity with concepts and techniques of mobilization of the nervous system may take time. It could be argued that it is more difficult than joint mobilization and manipulation. There are no bony levers to push on and it is more difficult to visualize than non-neural structures. Due to the mechanical and physiological continuum, successful treatment requires thinking which encompasses the whole body. Effective treatment invariably requires skilled treatment of surrounding structures. However, what may probably make it more difficult is that, for most physiotherapists, it is a relatively new tissue to contemplate, at least in biomechanical terms, and basic knowledge of the structure is generally less than that of joints and muscles.

Techniques are best considered as mobilization rather than stretch. Thinking 'mobilization', as most physiotherapists know it, creates images of gentle and strong techniques, through range and end-range techniques, movements with regard to symptoms and possible pathologies and most importantly, reassessment.

DISORDERS SUITABLE FOR NEURAL ASSESSMENT AND MOBILIZATION

The management of all disorders involves some consideration of the nervous system. Even if injury is solely non-neural, the nervous system is the pathway for the expression of symptoms and motor output such as muscle spasm and autonomic reactions. Clinical reasoning demands a high level of inquiry skill—it is useful to remember that symptoms are expressed via the nervous system, not just from a particular structure.

There are situations where the nervous system is clearly involved and is the dominant structure in a disorder. Arachnoiditis or acute nerve root compression are examples. There are others where the mechanical shortcomings of the system are just part of the disorder, for example dural sleeve irritation in the presence of gross foraminal stenosis.

It is not only the more overt and obvious neural injuries that require management. Minor meningeal irritation, alterations in the flow of CSF, preneurapraxic cord injuries and intraneural swelling in a dorsal root ganglion are all examples which must be considered. Afferent input to a spinal cord compromized in some way may result in abnormal motor responses, including that of the sympathetic nervous system—especially if that afferent input is abnormal. In some of these patients, the only objective evidence of injury may be the physical findings of the physiotherapist.

Disorders suitable for mobilization can be very broadly separated into those whose origins may result from biomechanical compromise (pathomechanics) or an inflammatory reaction (pathophysiology). The entrapped nerve or abnormally tethered dural ligaments are examples of the former. Intraneural swelling and irritated dura are examples of the latter. These two situations will inevitably co-exist, although one will predominate and consequently determine the emphasis in management. A pathophysiological situation could lead to a pathomechanical sequelae.

TREATMENT GUIDELINES

It is convenient to discuss disorders in the categories of irritable (pathophysiological dominance) and non-irritable (pathomechanical dominance). Assessment and mobilization of the nervous system is applicable for both. The following case study is used to illustrate treatment guidelines for both kinds of disorders.

Case study—irritable disorder

A 40-year-old man fell off the top rung of a step ladder, three days prior to assessment, and landed on top of a steel bucket, causing an apparent lumbar extension and left lateral flexion injury. He could not move after the injury and an ambulance had to convey him to hospital where he stayed for one day under observation and for tests. He is now at home and complains of constant left-sided and central lumbar pain with radiation to the anterior aspect of the knee. He has been unable to sleep since the fall. He said that the whole leg 'does not feel right' and there is paraesthesia in his left foot (see Fig. 50.1). Although the patient had no previous history of lumbar and thoracic symptoms, he has an occasional right-sided neck and arm problem that last required treatment six months ago. There are no general health concerns, no long-term cortisone therapy or indications that the injury has affected the spinal cord or internal organs. X-rays of the lumbar spine show no abnormality or injury. He is under the daily observation of a doctor.

Preliminary thoughts

With this information, the physiotherapist could have a number of thoughts, some of which are hypotheses to guide management:

- Multistructural soft-tissue involvement is likely, including muscle, nerve (symptoms in a dermatome, severe trauma) and joint. There is the likely involvement of multiple joint levels, a number of muscles, and both the central (perhaps meninges) and peripheral nervous system. Fascia, skin and fat could also be affected.
- There are no contraindications at this stage other than to exercise care and pay great respect to the severity and irritability of the disorder.

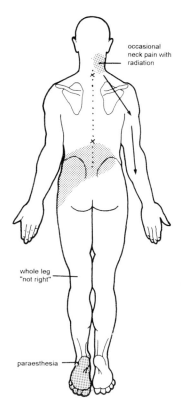

Fig. 50.1 Case study-body chart showing symptom distribution.

● The patient has had a severe injury and the disorder is probably irritable. It may take time for recovery, yet there is only the sudden and severe trauma, the constancy of pain and perhaps the old neck injury that are poor prognostic factors. The nervous system has not been directly stretched. It may have been compressed or, more likely, has been affected by inflammatory exudate or blood from other structures.

● The aims at this stage will be to ease pain and lessen potential for scarring.

Physical findings

The major findings are:

● The patient stands laterally flexed to the left, with his left knee flexed. Neck flexion increases the resting pain as does straightening the left knee. There is widespread left-sided bruising.

● Active spinal movements are markedly restricted and he is unable to laterally flex to the neutral position.

● Reflexes and sensation are normal, Babinski reflex is absent, and muscle power not tested due to the irritable nature of the condition.

● Passive neck flexion (PNF) positive for back pain, left prone knee bend (PKB) positive at 60°, left straight leg raise (SLR) positive at 20°, and left ankle dorsiflexion caused back pain. In addition, right SLR at 45° caused left leg symptoms. All of these movements were performed to a range that was just before an increase in symptoms. The patient was very wary during testing.

TREATMENT OF THE IRRITABLE DISORDER

This is an example of a disorder where the initial considerations in the treatment of the nervous system component must be directed towards pathophysiology. Assessing the contributions of each structure to symptoms and the relative importance of treatment to each structure can be difficult. However, the continuum of the nervous system helps in such a situation. In an irritable disorder, there are advantages in being able to move one structure without interfering too much with the others in the local area. For example, the left ankle dorsiflexion increasing lumbar pain is a useful clue to the sensitivity of the nervous system and the extent of neural involvement. It could be used as a treatment or as a measure of the value of another treatment selected.

Guidelines—starting technique of neural mobilization

In our patient, it may be possible to alter the tension signs by treating relevant interfacing structures some distance away from the injury site. Because the neck and thoracic spine have apparently not been injured these can be treated quite firmly with the aim of affecting the nervous system in the lumbar spine. Treatment of the lumbar spine, not specifically directed at the tension signs will probably improve the tension signs to some extent.

If a nervous system mobilization technique is selected, in such a patient, a technique well removed from the symptom area would be applicable. An example is knee extension in some hip flexion, or even a similar technique on the 'good' leg. In more irritable situations, just dorsiflexion and plantar flexion in some knee flexion may well be a starting treatment. Neural structures can therefore be mobilized in the injured area, and non-neural structures only minimally moved.

The technique should be non-provoking initially, thus remaining short of any increase in symptoms. It is best to undertreat initially until the sensitivity of the neural component of the disorder becomes apparent. There may be some latent responses to treatment that can be determined only on subsequent visits. Suggested grades of technique are large amplitude grade IIs performed slowly and rhythmically through range with maximal respect to symptoms. Grade IV- -techniques, just 'nudging' at resistance, with similar respect for symptoms are also a possibility (for those unfamiliar with grades, consult Maitland 1986). In performing grade IIs, the largest amplitude of movement possible should be done. For example, if it is possible to do 20° of knee extension in hip flexion, why not do more if it can be done without aggravating the disorder?

The symptoms of the disorder must be continually monitored. This requires constant verbal and non-verbal communication with the patient. An increase in the constant ache should be avoided and, if the physiotherapist judges that it is acceptable for some symptoms to be reproduced with the technique, they should be in rhythm with the technique, i.e. on and off rather than a constant ache. It is possible to change symptoms at the time of treatment, or they may change some hours later.

For the optimum movement of the nervous system in relation to interfacing tissues, the patient must be relaxed and comfortable. This may mean spending some time positioning the patient in a pain-relieving position. Use of the idea of 'anti-tension' postures should assist. The most prevalent interfacing tissue to the nervous system is muscle. If these are contracted, it is possible that the sliding of neural structures will be impaired.

If the disorder is deemed to be less irritable, passive movement of the nervous system in a very gentle manner may be applied to, or closer to, the area which is the source of symptoms. For example, hip flexion in knee extension, rather than knee extension in hip flexion. Again, the same guidelines as those listed above are followed.

Rest plays an important part in the treatment. Rest as a

treatment can be biased toward an anti-tension position for the body if required.

Treatment progression

Physiotherapists must carefully explore the therapeutic possibilities. No one patient's signs and symptoms will be the same, and all patients will require different treatments. If an improvement is achieved with a particular technique, the physiotherapist should try to resist the temptation to just repeat that technique. While it may be beneficial, the physiotherapist does not know whether it is the best treatment available. The technique can be used in combination with another technique or it can be performed slightly differently and the responses re-assessed. If signs and symptoms change with treatment, the next technique chosen will require modifications.

There is an infinite number of ways and directions in which techniques can be applied to influence the nervous system:

• The number of repetitions can be increased. In the irritable disorder, we prefer to perform a sequence of gentle oscillations, for example 20 seconds, and then re-assess the effect. The number of these sequences could be increased so the techniques last several minutes.

• The amplitude of the technique can be increased. The technique could be progressed to a point where some symptoms are reproduced or it could be taken to a point where some resistance to the movement is encountered.

• The technique could be repeated with the nervous system in more tension. In the patient example, knee extension in hip flexion could be performed with the cervical spine in some flexion or the lumbar spine in some lateral flexion to the right.

• If a distal technique has been used, such as the knee extension in hip flexion in the patient example, the point of application of technique could be moved closer to the source of symptom area. For instance, the traditional SLR of hip flexion with the knee extended could be employed. Another useful technique in such a situation is hip adduction and hip medial rotation in a few degrees of SLR.

• The effect of treatment on other structures involved in the disorder needs to be re-assessed after a technique of neural mobilization. As discussed, injury to the nervous system cannot exist alone. So, in our patient, after a technique is performed, a re-assessment of related joint (active movements, palpation signs), muscle (length, palpation, spasm) and other structures involved must be performed. This is a basic tenet of manual therapy and one that is crucial to continued learning. In this regard, the patient should be asked how their symptoms are changing. Remember that the nervous system can be responsible for a variety of symptoms and information is required about all symptoms. The patient in severe pain

can easily forget alterations in more minor symptoms (perhaps some abdominal pains or morning stiffness) and this information may be valuable to assist in progression of a technique. There could also be symptoms that at the initial assessment were not originally related to the injury. These may alter with treatment and the only way to find out is to enquire and to encourage the patient to report his symptoms.

• The continuum of the nervous system also allows easy regression of a technique. If the symptoms are being provoked by the technique, then as well as the obvious considerations of performing the technique more gently or abandoning the technique for another, there exists the possibilities of performing it in less tension. A possible example in our patient is performing an SLR in spinal extension or in left lateral flexion.

• Techniques can be modified for self mobilization. Such a prescription should follow the same principles as for physiotherapy mobilization. There are some examples and guidance in this area in Butler (1991).

TREATMENT OF THE NON-IRRITABLE DISORDER

The longer a disorder persists, the greater the likelihood of problems caused by disuse of structures and the products of an inflammatory response causing features of a pathomechanical nature. It follows that the only way to approach a pathomechanical problem is to utilize techniques that address 'mechanics'. Mechanically based treatment is the best way to address a mechanical problem of the nervous system. Treatment such as drugs, bed rest and electrotherapy are unlikely to provide the optimum therapy. Surgery may be an option.

The same patient example can be used:

> This man presents 3 months after the injury following treatment where the physiotherapist utilized only electrotherapy and the patient failed to attend treatment for six weeks. His condition had not improved in the last 5 weeks.
>
> Symptoms were in the same area, though intermittent. The patient was unable to walk more than 200 metres without back symptoms, and if he continued leg symptoms would follow. Since the fall, his neck problem has returned and there was an added symptom of interscapular twinges. There were still problems sleeping at night. Again, there were no precautionary factors to consider.
>
> When asked what he felt he needed to get better, he said 'I just need to be loosened up, both neck and back'.

Major findings on physical examination:

• he still stood with a slight list, towards the left

- lumbar movements were restricted to about half normal range
- L SLR restricted by back pain at 50°
- L PKB restricted by back and leg pain at 90°
- Neck flexion caused interscapular pain which is made worse by the addition of knee extension
- There was general stiffness on palpating the entire lumbar spine and the mid-thoracic spine. The left L3–4 and 4–5 levels were the stiffest and most symptomatic.

Guidelines—starting technique of neural mobilizing

The tension signs may improve with treatment directed at other tissues, such as the stiff lumbar joints. The signs must be monitored and the best treatment may need to be directed at a number of tissues.

If a neural mobilizing technique is selected, the initial technique performed will need to be into some resistance, i.e. through range grade III and/or grade IV. Techniques short of resistance are unlikely to alter mechanics. If there is some concern about irritability, the technique initially performed, should be short of provoking pain. Later techniques are likely to involve some discomfort.

Remember that a grade III mobilization provides considerable nervous system movement in relation to the interfacing structures with a short, low dose of tension at the end of range for a given period. Conversely, a grade IV technique maintains tension at the end of range with very little movement.

The treatment can be directed at the hypothesized site of neural involvement. Some pathologies and clinical findings may make one technique more desirable than another. In terms of pathology, a through-range, large-amplitude movement (grade III) should be employed where abnormalities of mechanics of the nervous system in relation to the interface exist (extraneural). Injury reactions that are intraneural are best managed by placing tension in the nervous system, so small-amplitude movements with the nervous system on some stretch are recommended. In general, grade III techniques will be less symptom-provoking than those at grade IV. Any symptoms provoked during treatment should subside immediately the treatment technique is released. In non-irritable disorders, paraesthesia may occasionally persist for a minute or so after treatment.

The base tests of SLR, PKB and the PNF, so positive in this patient, are probably not the best treatment techniques. Better access to a disorder may be the SLR with some hip adduction and with the lumbar spine in a position of side flexion away (i.e. right lateral flexion). The SLR then makes an excellent re-assessment. The concept of 'hunting out' the best positions to treat using clues from the subjective examination, such as aggravating and easing positions and knowledge of neurobiomechanics,

follows on from the physical examination as discussed by Slater et al in Chapter 44.

Irritability will play a part in the treatment decision. The degree of irritability will differ in the patient group loosely termed 'non-irritable'. It may be desirable to keep a component away from the source of symptoms initially. For example, if the hypothesis was that a source of tension existed in the femoral nerve at the groin, an initial treatment, keeping a component away, might be to flex the knee in some hip flexion. With decreasing irritability and increasing confidence in the treatment, the physiotherapist can move the component treated closer to the hypothesized source of tension, i.e. hip extension performed with the knee in flexion.

After the initial mobilization, all components of the disorder must be re-assessed. This may mean examining the effect on all structures, including other tension tests. The initial treatment selected must be thought of as a hypothesis that has to be proven by re-assessment.

Treatment progression

As with the more irritable disorders, there are a number of ways that treatment of the nervous system may be progressed:

- If required, the starting technique can be performed for a longer period or it can be performed more firmly, i.e. further into resistance and thus expecting some symptoms to be provoked.
- The same starting technique can be performed but with other components in different positions. This will usually involve an increase in overall nervous system tension, e.g. repeat SLR technique with the cervical spine in some flexion.
- The treatment component utilized can be closer to the source of symptoms. From clinical studies (Shacklock 1989) and clinical observation, the technique that best accesses the nervous system will involve taking up the injured component that contains the source of tension and then progressively adding neural tension to it. Then the injured component is treated. For example, if all analysis pointed to the source of symptoms being in the sciatic nerve at the posterior aspect of the hip, the provocative hip position could be taken up first and then tension added above (spine) and below (foot and knee).
- As a progression of treatment of non-neural structures involved in the disorder, these structures can be treated in a tension position. In the example above this may mean, in slump, long-sitting performing a unilateral postero-anterior pressure over a rib or zygapophyseal joint.

Aspects of treatment of the non-irritable disorder

It is difficult to know how vigorously the nervous system

can be treated. If the base tests are exclusively used as the treatment, then more vigour will usually be required to correctly access the nervous system than if the technique involved movements which reproduce signs and symptoms more easily. For example, while an SLR may be affecting a disorder in the lumbar spine, to access that disorder with less force the spine could be placed in a position of lateral flexion and some of the sensitizing movements of the SLR, such as hip adduction and medial rotation, could be used. A corollary for treatment of joints can be given. While strong postero-anterior pressures on the spinous process of a relevant cervical vertebrae may assist restoration of rotation, the same benefit may be achieved with much gentler unilateral pressures or combined physiological movements.

Clinical reasoning skills are required to answer the questions of how many, how much and how long. Treatment can be thought of as a session of slow oscillations, for instance 20–30 seconds in duration, or a number of repetitions. As a broad guide, the greater the concern about the irritability or severity of the disorder, the more likely that oscillatory techniques will be used. It provides the physiotherapist with a greater opportunity to question the patient about symptoms during the technique. In the less irritable disorder, where pathomechanics is the greater concern, the physiotherapist may prefer to perform just one or two firm repetitions of a technique. Here, a further progression is possible by sustaining the technique for a longer time. Some patients report a decrease in symptoms while the position is held. Oscillation may activate the muscles around the nervous system, in which case it seems better to sustain the movement or very slowly oscillate. Our suggestion is that a technique should not have to be sustained for longer than 10 seconds.

There are some patients for whom the technique needs to be performed at speed. The clues will come from the subjective examination. For example, there could be a pain on kicking a ball or a catch of pain that comes on only during a tennis serve. We interpret this as being an inability of the nervous system to respond to the speed of movement of the surrounding structures. The technique can be performed at speed to reproduce and alter the symptoms. Attention to the surrounding structures is also warranted in this kind of presentation.

It is sometimes easy to forget that the nervous system is a continuum. In most adverse tension disorders there will be axial and transverse tension considerations. It should be clear that if a person is to have optimum upper limb tension tests they will require an optimum slump (i.e. longitudinal axial nervous system movement), and vice versa. They will also require an optimum ULTT of the other arm. Similarly, to have the best possible prone knee bend, the SLR will need to be optimal.

Treatment of the non-irritable disorder will probably involve some discomfort. These symptoms provoked are one of the main guides to treatment. With nervous system mobilization in the non-irritable disorder, no matter how strong the treatment, the symptoms reproduced should disappear within seconds of stopping. This is most likely to be due to the replenishment of blood to nerve fibres rendered hypoxic by the stretch or compression. If residual symptoms persist, then non-neural tissues may have been affected or the nervous system treatment is too strong for that particular patient or stage of the disorder. That is, the irritability has been misread.

It is not uncommon for patients to say on re-assessment 'my back is much improved from the treatment but my neck is very sore' when the physiotherapist has not even touched the patient's neck. Unless handled correctly, this situation can result in an instant deterioration of communication. Consideration of biomechanics makes such a presentation feasible. If tension is altered in one area, an altered tension and nervous system relationship with interfacing structures may be set up elsewhere. This may be symptom-provocative and take some time for the patient to adjust to. It can also be a clue that these remote interfaces may need attention.

It is probably therapeutic to give gentle, through-range mobilization of the same or similar movements to help reduce the possibility of treatment pain. Knee extension in hip flexion is a nice technique to perform after vigorous SLRs or slump treatments. Shoulder depressions and elevations appear useful after vigorous ULTTs.

A nerve, where accessible, or the fascia around a nerve can be treated by frictions or mobilized via oscillatory pressures. This is often better performed with the nervous system in tension. For example, the deep friction techniques used by many physiotherapists for 'tennis elbow' are often more effective if performed in the ULTT2 radial nerve bias position. Palpation techniques are discussed by Butler (1991).

It is of no use continuing a technique if it does not produce an improvement. A technique performed should be re-assessed immediately after its cessation. This should incorporate a subjective and a physical re-assessment. As in the irritable disorder, it is worthwhile asking about all symptoms, even if they were symptoms you or the patient did not associate with the disorder. The nervous system is a continuum and the effects of treating part of it could be manifest anywhere in the body. Examples of symptoms often changed early in the treatment are feelings of swelling, night pain and morning stiffness. Often the patient will not volunteer these important alterations unless asked. Another interesting change may be 'nerve crepitus'. This is noted more often in the upper limb, and appears to herald an improvement. The patient will report a creaking along the nerve during mobilization, especially with large through-range movements.

FREQUENTLY ASKED QUESTIONS ABOUT TREATMENT

'Most disorders exhibiting positive tension tests have joint, muscle and fascial components. Is it best to treat these structures first or the nervous system first?'

If the limitation to the tension test appears to be due to extraneural sources, then that extraneural structure (joint, muscle, fascia, other) could be treated first. A trial-and-error approach could be used where one structure is treated first and the result assessed, then subsequent treatment of other structures involved and the result assessed.

Some examples where the nervous system could be treated first are:

- when it is the most comparable structure in the disorder, i.e. its signs outweigh the physical signs of injury to other structures
- when the patient has had adequate treatment of other structures involved in the disorder
- when a familiar pattern of signs and symptoms or pathology known to the physiotherapist implicates the nervous system in the disorder.

A good way to start for those unfamiliar with mobilization of the nervous system and to get a 'feel' for the system is to treat other structures first and then assess the affects of that treatment on the tension test.

'How hard can you stretch the nervous system?'

We usually admonish the person who asks this question and request them to think of mobilization of the nervous system and the structures around it rather than a crude stretch. This would be like asking a joint-based physiotherapist how hard the neck can be tractioned. There is no easy answer. The ultimate aim in treatment is to perform a technique using the minimal force required to achieve a beneficial response.

The answer to this question lies in clinical reasoning skills. The basis is methodical and continual re-assessment. It will take a number of treatments to work up to any vigour, and decisions will be based on results gained from earlier treatments. The clinician with more clinical reasoning experiences and with a greater knowledge base will quickly reach the optimum treatment. Nevertheless, the nervous system is strong, adapted to handling forces, and may require vigorous treatment, especially in the non-irritable disorder. When performing a strong technique, physiotherapists are encouraged to ask themselves continually whether there is an easier, more gentle, or more sensitive way of performing it. For example, rather than performing a strong SLR, better and safer results could be

achieved with the spine in some lateral flexion, and treating hip adduction with the SLR held on the point of symptom reproduction. Perhaps a more skilled treatment of the interfacing structures may be warranted before vigorous mobilization of the nervous system is employed.

'What about causing pins and needles or distal pain during treatment?'

Pins and needles are a neural response, just like pain can be. In the tension tests, especially the median biased tests, pins and needles responses are quite common (Kenneally et al 1988). In most situations, a treatment technique should stop short of reproducing pins and needles. In some other situations it is necessary to cause pins and needles. To get at a disorder of the neural connective tissues such a neural response may need to be provoked. However, the physiotherapist should know before the application of that technique that the pins and needles are a non-irritable symptom and part of a non-progressive disorder, i.e. it is quite 'safe' to perform a strong technique. We would be much less inclined to provoke pins and needles in a patient who had not complained of them previously than one who had pins and needles as part of the disorder. Techniques must not cause a worsening or spread of any numbness. The term 'short of' implies that the movement has provoked that symptom anyway, and treatment including reproduction of the symptom may only be a fraction further into range. Just as in the second question, the process of deciding the vigour and kind of symptoms that may be reproduced is a result of methodical assessment and re-assessment.

'I have improved this patient to a point but progress has plateaued'

Analysing the prognosis is probably the first step in this commonly encountered clinical situation. There may well be a reason why the patient will not get any better and the physiotherapist and the patient are wasting their time. There are a number of answers to this question:

- Have you been fair to yourself and interpreted the prognosis correctly? This important issue is discussed later in this chapter.
- Has the disorder been treated hard enough? (See above: 'How hard can you stretch the nervous system?')
- Are the treatment techniques addressing the disorder adequately or do they need refinement?
- Have you considered other tension-contributing sites along the system and remembered that the nervous system is a continuum? If a movement can alter symptoms, possible sources and contributions to that symptom can be anywhere between the part moved and the symptom. For instance, if a passive neck flexion alters lumbar symptoms,

then, although the lumbar area is the most likely source, contributions to the symptoms can be anywhere between the head and the lumbar spine. In general, physiotherapists need the confidence to examine further than the area of symptoms and known referral sites. Adverse tension in the nervous system gives a valid anatomical reason to examine further.

'What is the difference between active and passive mobilization of the nervous system?'

Both modes of mobilization have a role, but we lean towards passive movement as being the best to influence the nervous system. Most of the tissues interfacing nerve are muscles. To get the best nerve/interface movement, it seems logical to move the nerve with the surrounding structures as lax as possible. On the other hand, an abnormal nerve/muscle movement relationship may be evident only if the muscle is contracted. With a home exercise prescription, part of the exercises will need to be done actively.

'What about hypermobility and the nervous system?'

The nervous system should be thought of as any other system involved in movement. Logically, the hypermobile person requires a more mobile and elastic nervous system than does the hypomobile person. Not only with the nervous system, the mobility must extend to skin, fascia, the circulatory system, joints and muscles. If one of these structures loses its mobility then the others may suffer.

'I seem to aggravate disorders quite easily with nervous system mobilization'

There are a number of suggestions to help this physiotherapist, presuming that the patient has a positive tension test that is relevant to the patient's disorder:

- The irritability of the disorder may not have been interpreted correctly.
- The source of the altered neural mechanics may not reside in the nervous system; it may be in structures around the nervous system, such as ribs, joints, muscles and fascia. The clinician also requires skills in the treatment of non-neural structures.
- Because of the continuum of the nervous system it may be necessary to treat a number of relevant sites along the system to limit aggravation.
- Be aware that an aggravation of symptoms may ultimately be beneficial. With vigorous treatment that results in different tissue mechanics, 'new movement', including different nervous system/mechanical interface relationships, may initially be painful.
- All clinicians need to practice techniques.

'How long will I continue to treat for'?

This question can be answered by considering two distinct group of patients.

The first is the group where it can be decided, after a few treatments, that physiotherapy is not the optimum treatment for that stage in their disorder. The two main issues in that decision are related to the underlying pathology and the response to treatment. These patients may require surgery, drugs, counselling or nothing.

There is also another group who perhaps have had a chronic disorder for many years and begin to slowly improve with mobilization of the nervous system. From the assessment, the physiotherapist should be able to conclude why the patient's disorder is amenable to treatment, for example, there may be no history of severe trauma or disease. In these patients, we believe that treatment over many months can be justified and makes economic sense. With long-term treatment, much will be self mobilization. The major indications however, come from continual re-assessments of treatments. It is no use continuing treatment if the patient does not improve.

'What do you think you are actually doing when you are mobilizing the nervous system and how do you explain your results'?

We cannot answer this question and can only offer hypotheses. The exact mechanisms whereby surgical decompression of an entrapped nerve can ease symptoms at the entrapment site and elsewhere are not known either.

It should be clear that, to mobilize the nervous system effectively, a complete understanding of the pathophysiological and pathomechanical processes behind disorders is not essential, nor is such information complete. If the physiotherapist applies sound clinical reasoning skills (Chapter 34), safe and effective treatment can be delivered. Nevertheless, as well as encouraging physiotherapists at least to attempt to treat the nervous system and trying to prove the clinical hypothesis, they should also attempt to consider or investigate the physiological and/or mechanical alterations their treatment may cause.

Mobilization of the nervous system has a mechanical effect that must affect the vascular dynamics, axonal transport systems and mechanical features of the nerve fibres and connective tissues.

- It is easy to envisage that the 'stuck' peripheral nerve or dura mater surrounded by fresh blood and oedema would benefit from movement.
- Dispersion of an intraneural oedema could be enhanced by alteration of the pressures in the nervous system during movement.
- It is conceivable that dysmyelination could be beneficially altered from mobilizing neural tissue.
- Restoration of normal mechanics of the connective

tissues after injury lessens the possibility of the nerves being entrapped in their surrounding connective tissues. The sinuvertebral nerve could be caught in dural scar. Similar examples are the nervi nervorum caught in the connective tissue sheath or injured or regenerating nerve fibres caught in endoneurial scar.

- It is possible that the nervous system can be trained to lengthen. While some pure stretch is possible, more complex mechanisms probably occur. Bora et al (1980) showed that sutured rat nerve could become more compliant and suggested that this feature allowed repaired nerves to adjust to mobilization. Perhaps the cell body can be signalled from an injury site (presumably by the retrograde axoplasmic flow) and 'requested' to alter the compliance of the nerve. Similar signalling could occur from target tissues. For example, stretch of the hamstring muscle may result in neuronotrophic messages 'requesting' the compliance of the sciatic nerve to be altered. There is an interesting clinical study that would provide support for this hypothesis. Ramamurthi (1980) noted that tension signs in patients with surgically proven disc lesions were significantly more marked in westernized Indian women and men compared to those who followed a more traditional way of life where squatting and bending were more commonly adopted postures. He hypothesized that in these women, the nervous system had stretched over time.

- Where a rapid improvement occurs, at least some of this improvement could be due to improved blood supply to hypoxic nerve fibres. The pressure gradients around the nervous system that allow blood to flow in and out of the system are in a delicate state of balance. Treatment of interfacing tissues and mobilization of the nervous system may normalize the gradients and thus normalize the blood supply. In this regard, the effect of mobilization of the sympathetic trunk, either directly or via the ribs, cannot be underestimated. Distortion and angulation of the sympathetic trunk has not been associated with sympathetic maintained syndromes, although clear pathological evidence of alterations in the sympathetic trunk and ganglia has been provided by Nathan (1986). Marked neuro-ischaemia in rabbit sciatic nerve following stimulation of the lumbar sympathetic chain has been shown (Selander et al 1985).

- The circulation and percolation of cerebrospinal fluid would be assisted by normal movement. At least half of a nerve root's metabolic requirements come from the CSF.

- Normal movement will optimize the axonal transport systems. This may be achieved by altering mechanical restraints on the axoplasm or improving the blood flow and thus increasing the energy available for axonal transport. Normalization of the interface will effect the axoplasmic flow. Korr (1985) suggested that the afferent bombardment from a facilitated segment deprives the nerve fibres related to that segment of some of the energy required

for axonal transport. Manipulation of the segment and improvement of the joint movement eases the energy demand from the facilitated segment.

These hypotheses and thoughts must be taken into account with the fact that the nervous system, especially the peripheral nervous system, has considerable regenerating powers.

COMMUNICATING THROUGHOUT TREATMENT

The value and the skills of communication are well described by Maitland (1986). There are some issues that are particularly related to mobilizing the nervous system.

Patients generally have an awareness and some knowledge of muscles and joints. This may not extend to the nervous system. If they are told that their 'nerves are going to be mobilized', or worse, 'their nerves are going to be stretched', odd impressions may be conjured up. Patients need to be told about the nervous system and how strong and mobile it is. For example, inform them that the sciatic nerve in the buttocks is as thick as their little finger.

A knowledge of pathological processes is extremely useful. The concept of 'double crush' can be utilized. Often a patient may develop symptoms elsewhere during treatment. For example, with our patient disorder, initial treatment to the lumbar spine (joint or nervous system) may help the lumbar area, but cause symptoms elsewhere in the body, most likely in the interscapular area or the neck. This knowledge, all related to, and based on, the fact that the system is a continuum, is of great assistance in explaining increases or decreases in symptoms.

PROGNOSIS MAKING AND ADVERSE TENSION SYNDROMES

Making a prognosis can be difficult. Not only should a prognostic hypothesis be made at the first assessment, this decision must remain flexible during the entire period of physiotherapy management. In many cases, the prognostic decision regarding physiotherapy treatment is made by, rather than in association with, other professionals. Without diminishing the value of interpretation of signs and symptoms and their responses to treatment, in many situations, decisions involving a prognosis for physiotherapy treatment requires some knowledge about the underlying pathology.

Factors that may indicate a poorer prognosis

Severity of the injury

Severe trauma to the nervous system may lead to irreversible fibrosis and alterations in conduction. A fall from a height, or a high-velocity accident—such as a motor vehicle accident—are examples of severe trauma, and they inevitably involve damage to many structures. As well as an injury to the nervous system, products of injury, such as blood and oedema from other structures, could combine to worsen the original nervous system injury. Another consideration is that mobilizing the nervous system may be more difficult because other structures might be too painful or stiff to move.

Site of the injury

If a pathological process has gained access or occurs inside the nervous system, such as intrafascicular or intradural swelling and scarring, then part of this process may be irreversible. If injury occurs at sites of increased vulnerability, such as the T6 vertebral level where the spinal canal is the smallest, the clinical implications may be worse than if the injury were elsewhere.

An unremitting interface

Alterations in the structure next to the nervous system may not allow the improvement that the nervous system is normally capable of. Common examples are spinal stenosis, fixed unphysiological postures such as the 'dowager's hump', bony malalignments secondary to fracture and disc injury.

The patient

For a multitude of reasons, inadvertently or otherwise, the patient may not be allowing the physiotherapist access to the problem. Reasons could range from low pain tolerance, the physiotherapist's poor communication skills, malingering, possible financial gain and the psychological content of the symptoms. There also appears to be a 'nervey' person just as there are 'jointy people' (Maitland 1986). The mechanisms are probably similar. Perhaps lower thresholds for stimuli, interpreted centrally as pain, occurs in the 'nervey person'.

Spread of symptoms

It may be more difficult to achieve an ideal result in a patient who complains of widespread symptoms than someone who complains of localized symptoms. However, the physiotherapist should be optimistic at first. In some situations relief of tension at one site along the nervous system can lead to symptomatic relief at the other site. Clinically, it appears that restoration of normal movement of thoracic spine structures can relieve a widespread variety of symptoms such as abdominal pain, headache and vague limb symptoms.

Spread of signs

A patient who presents with a bilateral limitation of SLR of 30° and limited ULTTs will clearly be more difficult to help than a patient in whom the only tension sign is a unilateral SLR limitation to 60°.

Chronicity

The longer a disorder has been present, the greater are the chances of further anatomical, physiological and psychological involvement. In the absence of severe trauma, it takes time to breach the defences of the nervous system such as the perineurial or the arachnoid diffusion barrier. Although the nervous system may adapt to some injuries (e.g. increased connective tissue to buffer the system), persistent abnormal mechanical and chemical irritants may ultimately lead to a more severe injury.

Occupation

The demands of certain occupations could predispose the worker to further injury, or could have created changes in the nervous system that may contribute to a component of irreversibility. Some examples are occupations involving sustained postures, repeated movements, repeated movements of part of the body with the rest of the body static (keyboard operator), or association with forces such as vibration (jack-hammer operator).

Post-surgery

Occasionally, symptoms persist or may even worsen following surgery. One of the main reasons for this is the scarring that occurs with the trauma of surgery. Failed surgery would further worsen the prognosis.

Congenital abnormalities

Known or unknown congenital abnormalities in the nervous system or the surrounding structures could predispose a person to the development of an adverse tension syndrome and also lessen the potential for successful treatment. Some examples are the nerve root anomalies described by Kadish and Simmons (1984).

Co-existing disease processes may lessen the chances of an optimum result

Common examples are diabetes and herpes zoster. While treatment via mobilization may offer some ease of symptoms, it clearly does not offer any cure. Diseases that may have left neural scarring, such as Guillain-Barré, must also be considered.

Response to early attempts at mobilization

A poor response to early attempts at mobilization could indicate a poor prognosis.

The clinician's impressions of the prognosis may change as treatment progresses, depending on the response to treatment (subjectively and objectively) and also when various features of the disorder are clarified over time. Note that the list above includes features which could contribute to the prognosis although they do not exclude a favourable outcome. A poorer prognosis would exist if a number of these factors occur together.

After a period of treatment, if prognostic goals are not realized, some consideration should be given to the possibility of underlying sinister pathology. Thoughts on prognosis should not be limited to what the physiotherapist can achieve. Mobilization may be in association with treatment from related fields such as surgery, medicine, podiatry and psychology.

PRECAUTIONS IN ASSESSMENT AND TREATMENT

Lists of precautions as outlined by Maitland (1986) should be followed. Remember that the nervous system will never be the only tissue involved; tension tests involve many structures, neural and non-neural, and there may be precautions related to these structures.

There are certain situations where the nervous system is involved in a disorder in a way that requires particular precaution in management:

- Irritable disorders involving the nervous system. The management of an irritable disorder has been discussed earlier in this chapter.
- Mobilization of the nervous system should not be attempted where neurological changes are worsening.
- Great care should be taken in the presence of cord signs.
- Treatment will be limited or contraindicated with inflammatory, systemic and infective disorders that affect the nervous system such as AIDS, diabetes, and multiple sclerosis. While treatment clearly does not offer a cure, some of the symptoms may be eased by treatment.

SUMMARY

If clinical decision-making combines a knowledge of neuropathy and neurobiomechanics in conjunction with handling and inquiry skills, a new assessment and treatment dimension opens for the physiotherapist. The aim of treatment is clear—return the nervous system's normal range and ability to elongate.

REFERENCES

Bora F W, Richardson S, Black J 1980 The biomechanical responses to tension in a peripheral nerve. Journal of Hand Surgery 5: 21–25

Butler D S 1991 Mobilisation of the nervous system. Churchill Livingstone, Melbourne

Kadish L J, Simmons E H 1984 Anomalies of the lumbosacral nerve roots. Journal of Bone and Joint Surgery 66B: 411–416

Kenneally M, Rubenach H, Elvey R 1988 The upper limb tension test: the SLR of the arm. In: Grant R (ed) Physical therapy of the cervical and thoracic spine, Clinics in physical therapy 17. Churchill Livingstone, Edinburgh

Korr I M 1985 Neurochemical and neurotrophic consequences of nerve deformation. In: Glasgow E F et al (eds) Aspects of manipulative therapy, 2nd edn. Churchill Livingstone, Melbourne

Maitland G D 1986 Vertebral manipulation, 5th edn. Butterworths, London

Nathan H 1986 Osteophytes of the spine compressing the sympathetic truck and splanchnic nerves in the thorax. Spine 12: 527–532

Ramamurthi B 1980 Absence of limitation of straight leg raising in proved lumbar disc lesion. Journal of Neurosurgery 52: 852–853

Selander D, Mansson L G, Karlsson L et al 1985 Adrenergetic vasoconstriction in peripheral nerves in the rabbit. Anesthesiology 62: 6–10

Shacklock M 1989 The plantar flexion/inversion straight leg raise. Unpublished thesis. South Australian Institute of Technology, Adelaide

51. Concepts of assessment and rehabilitation for active lumbar stability

C. A. Richardson   G. A. Jull

INTRODUCTION

The lumbar motion segments are quite well designed to carry and resist external forces. Despite the stability provided by the osseous–ligamentous system, the spinal column devoid of musculature is incapable of carrying normal physiological loads (Panjabi et al 1989). Muscle activity is required to stabilize the spine so that it can perform its normal physiological functions. For this reason trunk and lumbar spine muscle insufficiency or weakness can render the spine vulnerable to overload and possible injury. By failing to protect the spinal joints from the high forces associated with functional use, such poor muscular control may also hinder the healing process of injured tissue. The importance of adequate muscle function to stabilize and support the lumbar spine is well recognized by those involved in the prevention and treatment of lumbar spine disorders.

The large movements of the spine especially when under load require the stabilization and protection of many individual joints. This relies on co-ordinated co-contractions of several muscles working in fine balance to provide the background stability while at the same time allowing smooth controlled functional movement.

This chapter is directed towards identifying the key protective stabilizing muscles of the lumbar spine, proposing how the stability function of muscles might be tested, and indicating general guidelines for a suitable rehabilitation programme through which their stabilization role may be enhanced.

IDENTIFICATION OF THE KEY PROTECTIVE STABILIZING MUSCLES OF THE LUMBAR SPINE

While the function of the distal limb musculature is often described in terms of movement or skill activities, a postural antigravity role is usually assigned to the trunk and proximal limb musculature (Edwards et al 1984). This antigravity role is associated with the support and protection of the viscera and the spine especially when the body is subjected to high external loading.

Although all trunk muscles are capable of offering some stability and protection to the lumbar spine, some muscles appear to be more specialized for the task. Identifying these particular muscles would allow therapists to focus more effectively their rehabilitative and preventative exercise programmes. For several reasons it is difficult to establish the muscles ideal for stabilization based on direct research evidence.

The detailed knowledge of how individual muscles work during functional activities involving the lumbar spine is usually gained by monitoring muscle activity in normal pain-free subjects who are often used as the control subjects (Andersson et al 1974, Godfrey et al 1977, Mayhew et al 1983, Hemborg & Moritz 1985, Pope et al 1987, Zetterberg et al 1987). It should be recognized that one of the difficulties in relying on this type of information is that normal pain-free subjects may not demonstrate the 'ideal' pattern in the muscles designed for stabilization. This may be due to the tendency for persons to minimize muscular effort when performing tasks and the basic decline in muscular fitness of the general population concomitant with an increasingly sedentary lifestyle. As evidence of this, Matilla et al (1986) found similar signs of atrophy in the muscle fibres of lumbar multifidus in both normal subjects and patients with back pain.

Despite problems in establishing direct research evidence of the muscles specifically involved in muscular protection of the lumbar spine, it is possible to identify muscles with prime stabilizing roles. Such muscles may be identified by their anatomical features, their fibre type distribution, their ability to support the spine against continuous gravitational load and their relationship with known mechanisms designed to enhance spinal stabilization when the spine is loaded.

Anatomical features

It could be argued that the muscles with a prime stability role for the lumbar spine have some or all of the anatomical features which indicate that they can directly contribute to the support of underlying joints, especially when high forces are involved.

Many are deep muscles overlying the joints which they are controlling (e.g. the short, deep intrinsic muscles of the spine).

They are often muscles which cross over one joint only (e.g. fascicles of lumbar multifidus, gluteus maximus and medius) as opposed to the longer muscles crossing two or more joints.

They are commonly pennate muscles with muscle fibres running more obliquely and terminating in wide fibrous expansions. This type of muscle which is often linked to fascial support systems, is suitable for generating high forces rather than large ranges of movement (Williams et al 1989). Muscles with these features include transversus abdominis and the oblique abdominals.

In contrast, long, fusiform, more superficial muscles which cross over several joints do not provide a structure ideal for protection of individual joints under load. Such muscles are the superficial erector spinae (especially the thoracic components whose tendons traverse the lumbar spine), rectus abdominis and proximal thigh muscles such as rectus femoris and tensor fascia latae.

Fibre type distribution

In animal muscle, the tonic stabilizers consist of high proportions of slow-twitch muscle fibre. It seems however that human muscles which are anatomically designed to enhance stabilization do not necessarily contain higher percentages of tonic fibres. A variable contribution (approximately 50/50) of fast- and slow-twitch fibres exist in most skeletal muscles (Johnson et al 1973, Elder et al 1982). Therefore, most supportive trunk muscles contain both slow-twitch and fast-twitch fibres in order to be able to perform a variety of functional movements at varying load levels.

This variation was confirmed in a specific study on the fibre types of the abdominal muscles (Häggmark & Thorstensson 1979). Large individual variations were found but there were no differences between individual muscles. The exception was the deep, flat transversus abdominis muscle which contained slightly more tonic (slow-twitch fibres) and significantly smaller-diameter fast-twitch fibres than the other more superficial abdominal muscles. This could indicate a specialized tonic supportive role of this muscle.

This may also be true of another important muscle used for stabilization. Multifidus, the more medial of the intrinsic lumbar back muscles, does also appear to contain more tonic fibres (Verbout et al 1989).

Support against continuous gravitational load (in standing posture and gait)

It could be argued that muscles which have been found to be continuously active, even under low spinal loading, may be important in providing background spinal stability.

The antigravity support of the spine during upright stance and gait involves only low economic levels of trunk muscle support (Basmajian & De Luca 1985). Asmussen and Klausen (1962) suggest that gravity is counteracted mainly by continuous activity of the back muscles with contributions from the abdominal musculature in some individuals.

It is not easy to identify the activity in the individual abdominal muscles for the maintenance of upright posture and gait. Transversus abdominis and the internal obliques appear to be active in the standing posture with negligible activity occurring in the rectus abdominis and the external obliques (Machado de Sousa & Furlani 1981). Confirmation of this is difficult as many studies on the abdominal musculature have not included recordings from these deeper muscle layers. Floyd and Silver (1950), in a classical study on relaxed standing, found activity only in the lower portions of the internal oblique muscles. This is probably required to protect the inguinal canal (Basmajian & De Luca 1985).

In a study on gait, Waters and Morris (1972) reported tonic activity of the oblique abdominals (suggestive of a supportive role) compared to slight phasic activity from rectus abdominis. Although abdominal function in gait has not been addressed in many research studies, it is generally recognized that abdominal activity is minimal (Sheffield 1962).

It could be concluded that the tonic supportive role of the abdominal musculature may be confined to the deeper flat musculature. This would be in line with their role in visceral support in upright posture. Rectus abdominis is not included.

It is of interest that Basmajian and De Luca (1985), while recognizing the predominance of rectus abdominis as a head and trunk raiser, do not believe such exercise could be used to promote general tone in the abdominal wall. This is an interesting comment and supports the argument that rectus abdominis does not have a supportive role in posture and gait.

Relationship to the known mechanisms of lumbar stabilization

Additional levels of support from trunk muscles are required when loading to the spine increases. Muscles appear to work in synergistic groups to help stabilize and protect the spine (Pope et al 1987).

The mechanisms studied for their stabilizing and protective role for the lumbar joints have been intra-abdominal pressure (IAP), the thoracolumbar fascia, its connections with the posterior ligamentous system, and the deep extensors of the trunk.

Since the 1960s, IAP has been studied in its role of lessening force on the spine in lifting (Bartelink 1957, Morris et al 1961). The importance and magnitude of the contribution of IAP has been challenged (Bogduk & Twomey 1987). More recently it has been proposed that the role of IAP lies in producing a more general stabilization mechanism for protection of the whole spine (Grew 1980, Tesh et al 1987, Zetterberg et al 1987).

The trunk muscles which are considered to be associated with increasing IAP are the transversus abdominis and oblique abdominals including their attachments to the rectus sheath, the diaphragm and pelvic floor. The rectus abdominis muscle is considered to be only minimally involved (Floyd & Silver 1950, Carmen et al 1972, Rab et al 1977, Jackson & Brown 1983, Basmajian & De Luca 1985).

The thoracolumbar fascia is another mechanism considered to add stability to the lumbar spine (Gracovetsky et al 1985, Macintosh et al 1987). Whereas IAP provides a more general support, the thoracolumbar fascia, through its deep attachments to the spinous processes, is considered to have a more direct effect on the low lumbar levels (Tesh et al 1987). The muscles intimately involved with this mechanism are the transversus abdominis and variably, the internal obliques. Through the tension provided by the contraction of these abdominal muscles, the middle layers of the fascia provide lumbar stability in the coronal plane and the middle and posterior layers together, in the sagittal plane (Bogduk & Twomey 1987, Tesh et al 1987).

The posterior ligamentous system offers restraint in full lumbar flexion (Bogduk & Twomey 1987). In the more intermediate ranges when ligaments are not as taut, the increased bulk of the contracting erector spinae muscles exerts tension on the posterior layer of the thoracolumbar fascia. This mechanism, called the hydraulic amplifier mechanism (Gracovetsky et al 1977), enhances the anti-flexion effect of the fascia.

In addition to these mechanisms, intersegmental lumbar stabilization is enhanced through the contractions of the deep back extensors (Basmajian & Wolf 1990). Within the back muscles, multifidus, with its segmental and multisegmental fascicles, is thought to perform a major stabilizing and protecting role (Valencia & Munro 1985). In an electromyographical study of the segmental levels of multifidus, these researchers concluded that this muscle was often active throughout trunk flexion, during rotation of the trunk in both directions, and was actively stabilizing the lumbar spine and pelvis in extension movements of the lower limb. It is of interest that the muscular control (and hence stabilization) by this muscle during a curl-up exercise was decreased in back pain patients compared to control subjects (Soderberg & Barr 1983). This emphasized its functional and rehabilitative importance.

Although there is still debate about the relative contributions of these mechanisms (Tesh et al 1987), the muscles required to activate dynamic stabilizing mechanisms for the lumbar spine would include most importantly:

- transversus abdominis
- internal and external oblique abdominals
- multifidus and the lumbar erector spinae.

Because of their contribution to IAP, the pelvic floor and diaphragm may also be important. Rectus abdominis is not usually included in the abdominal musculature suggested as having a prime stabilizing role. A study which specifically highlights the prime stabilization role of the oblique abdominals in comparison to rectus abdominis was completed by Zetterberg et al (1987). This electromyographical study of maximal trunk exertions in standing and lifting tasks found that actions of rectus abdominis correlated with biomechanical model predictions for force output but this was not the case with the oblique abdominals. Activity in these muscles was more aligned to a stabilization role.

Clinical and anatomical evidence can be found which supports the importance of the co-contraction of these stability muscles as a synergist group to form a muscular 'corset' to support the spine.

From an anatomical viewpoint, transversus abdominis acting in an isolated fashion could perform the corset action (at the deepest level) due to its line of action and attachments to both the lumbar dorsal fascia and the fascial sheath of rectus abdominis (Lacôte et al 1987).

The obliques, however, due to their diagonal fibre direction, could contribute to the 'corset' action, but due to their ability to produce flexor movements they would require the activation of the lumbar extensors to counteract flexion and shear forces produced in the lumbar vertebral segments. This would explain why, from an anatomical and biomechanical sense, both deep flexors of the antero-lateral abdominal wall and the intervertebral extensor muscles with opposing action would need to contract together for lumbar stabilization (Lefkof 1986).

The need for patterns of co-contraction are advocated by physiotherapists for patients with back pain. The contribution of the 'deep back muscles' and the oblique abdominals was emphasized by Kennedy (1982) when describing the advantages of the active protective technique of abdominal 'bracing'. Sullivan et al (1982) also suggest that the lower abdominals and low back extensors are most important when giving trunk strengthening for low back pain.

Thus, through various complex stabilizing mechanisms, the flat abdominals (transversus and obliques) and the deep low back extensors, through co-contraction in a 'corset' action, are seen as the most important muscles for the enhancement of spinal stability.

In addition to the trunk musculature, the loaded lumbar spine is also dependent on scapular and pelvic stability. The weights and forces of everyday activities are applied to the spine through the limbs. Therefore, for safe and non-injurious function, there needs to be good stability between the shoulder girdles and the trunk and the pelvic girdle and the trunk. Muscles important for these functions include the shoulder girdle retractors and depressors e.g. the middle and lower trapezius, and, at the pelvis, the gluteals and iliopsoas.

TESTING OF STABILIZING FUNCTION OF THE MUSCLES OF THE TRUNK

As the abdominals and low back extensors are often difficult to activate and may weaken in both sedentary individuals (Janda 1964, 1978, Matilla et al 1986) and those with chronic low back pain (Soderberg & Barr 1983), it is necessary to use suitable tests to estimate the level of stabilizing function of these muscles when they work together in a co-contraction pattern to stabilize the spine.

Prior to testing (or attempting to rehabilitate) muscle function, it is essential to first minimize the effects of pain and any reflex inhibition of the muscles concerned. In addition, the effect of any tight opposing structures (joint structures, muscles and fascias, neural tissue) needs to be assessed and treated appropriately.

The use of a static holding test

The aim of objective assessment is to monitor the ability of the patient automatically to hold the lumbar spine steady under increasing levels of load. The level of static holding ability can be ascertained from the limit of load which can be held by the muscles controlling the spine.

This method of assessment for trunk stability differs considerably from other methods of assessing trunk muscle function which rely on measurement of force or torque produced during specific trunk movements (Davies & Gould 1982, Langrana & Lee 1984, Nordin et al 1987, Hoens et al 1990).

A static holding test is advocated because it is similar to the functional stabilizing role required of the muscles. Additionally, there are physiological reasons to support the use of a test to check the ability of the muscles surrounding the spine to hold an isometric contraction for a period of time.

If a muscle has been subjected to decreased use and decreased loading, it develops weakness and atrophy (Goldspink 1980). Besides an increased rate of protein degradation relative to its synthesis (Goldberg 1975), this situation also results in marked reduction in the endurance capabilities of muscle. Studies on the trunk musculature in patients suffering chronic low back pain illustrate that endurance rather than absolute strength is the most obvious deficit in trunk muscular function (Smidt et al 1983, Suzuki & Endo 1983). Thus endurance is an important consideration in the estimation of muscles' contribution to stability.

A further reason for initially testing a static holding contraction considers other changes in muscles as a result of disuse. Results of many research studies have indicated that the contractile characteristics of muscle may change when exposed to disuse or lack of sensory input. Drastic procedures of tenotomy (Henneman & Olson 1965) or spinal cord transection (Lieber et al 1986) performed on animals result in conversion of slow fibre to fast fibre. Chronic disuse and reduction in sensory input has also been linked to similar changes in animal muscle with the tonic (slow) units displaying the more phasic qualities of fast muscle (Fischbach & Robbins 1969, Ianuzzo 1976, Templeton et al 1988).

The results of space research do provide conclusive evidence that changes in muscle fibres can occur in mammals with disuse. In the weightless environment of space the slow muscle fibres gradually change to resemble fast fibres (Oganov et al 1980). The drastic procedures used in animal experiments and in space research, which result in a change from slow-twitch muscle fibres to fast-twitch fibres, do not equate with the common level of disuse or immobilization found in human subjects who are sedentary or suffering some musculoskeletal pathology or dysfunction. For this reason studies on muscle disuse in humans often show changes in contractile characteristics of the motor units which may gradually change without a complete change of fibre type. Two experiments in human muscle which suggest that these changes may occur in disused human muscle are of interest.

Grimby and Hannerz (1976) found that by decreasing proprioceptive input to the tibialis anterior muscle, its tonically firing patterns of motor unit discharge became more phasic. This is compatible to the findings in animals. Richardson (1978a, b) found that when exposed to a fast repetitive knee movement, subjects with a clinically weakened vastus medialis displayed a more phasic pattern of motor unit firing than did normal controls. Thus, it may be changes in the pattern of motor unit firing rather than actual changes in the muscle fibres themselves which could be responsible for these detected changes in human muscles.

It would be reasonable to suggest that, if such changes do occur in human muscle, this should result in disused muscle displaying a decreased ability statically to hold and control a contraction. The muscle would be more likely to display more phasic, erratic patterns of contraction when required to support and hold the body parts. The phasic, inappropriate contractions of the trunk muscles often seen clinically in patients with poor trunk stability would seem to reinforce these research findings (Janda 1978, Watter 1991).

From both clinical observations and research on disused muscle, it seems appropriate to determine whether muscles required for trunk stabilization can control an isometric contraction without phasic irregular movements occurring. Once a muscle can hold and control a contraction it would be important to determine the endurance time for the contraction.

Testing procedure

Active lumbar stabilization is traditionally tested by estimating the ability of the patient or client to hold and control the position of the lumbar spine segments while load is added indirectly to the spine via the upper or lower limbs. Load added via the weight of the lower limbs is an ideal method of performing the test as it requires the action of muscles attached to the lumbar spine and pelvis. If poor muscular control is present, such muscle action could result in movement or lack of active stabilization of the lumbar spine. The measurement of this lumbar movement as a result of poor muscular control can then be used as an indication of the ability of the trunk musculature to stabilize the lumbar spine.

Supine is usually chosen as the starting position for such a test. The lower limbs are taken passively into a loaded position and the patient or client asked to hold the leg(s) and trunk steady. Observation of the changes in position of the lumbar spine and pelvis is used to estimate whether the lumbar segments are stable and controlled during progressive increases in effective weight of the leg(s). The capacity of the muscle to hold the lumbar spine stable over longer periods of time (i.e. endurance) is subsequently tested.

In order to ensure that the test is both reliable and clinically useful there are variables in this testing method which need to be considered. These include the body position in which the test is attempted and the leg position for adding load.

Body position

Functionally, load is transferred to the trunk from the lower limbs predominantly in the upright position. The suggested supine test position, although not as functional, provides a more stable body position which would allow more accurate monitoring of the substitute movements which must be avoided in any objective muscle testing procedure.

Leg positions

Many different leg positions have been used to increase load to the trunk during abdominal muscle testing (Kendall & McCreary 1983, Sahrmann 1988).

An alternative series of positions are suggested here in which hip flexion remains constant as leg load is increased. Figure 51.1 illustrates these positions of increasing loading. By maintaining the thigh at approximately 70° hip flexion, the pelvis and lumbar spine can more easily be maintained in a neutral position. Muscular stabilization would be maximized in such a position when the ligaments and other soft tissues of the lumbar spine and pelvis

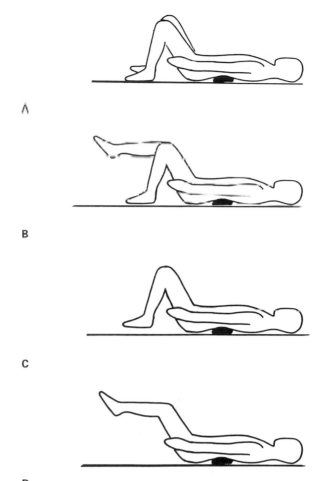

Fig. 51.1 Leg positions for progressive increase in load with constant hip angle. **A.** One heel held 3 cm from supporting surface. **B.** Increased load with the leg straight. **C.** Both heels held 3 cm from supporting surface. **D.** Maximal load with both legs straight.

are not lengthened and therefore unable to contribute significantly to stabilization. It is important in the single leg load positions (a) and (b) to monitor the pressure under the supporting foot to ensure that trunk muscle stabilization was not aided by a 'pushing' action through this foot.

DANGER AND LIMITATIONS IN TRADITIONAL METHODS OF ASSESSING STABILITY

There are inherent dangers to adding load if the associated joint structures are not sufficiently supported. In such situations, the test procedures themselves can be potentially hazardous, especially in the presence of healing tissues or marked pathology. A basic level of muscular control of the lumbar spine must be present before progressive loads are added distally via the lower limbs. Furthermore, the lumbar spine must be monitored at all times during the stability assessments to ensure that the contraction of the appropriate group of muscles has occurred and the spine is constantly maintained in the neutral position.

For these reasons it is necessary to undertake preliminary steps before conducting the traditional tests. The first step is to ensure that the patient or client can activate the appropriate co-contraction pattern for optimizing spinal stability. Secondly, it is necessary to have a method for detecting lumbar spine movement to ensure that the back has been maintained in a constant position throughout the stability test. If these criteria are met, testing should proceed safely and effectively.

Techniques to activate the stability pattern

Stabilization of the spine is optimally achieved through the action of the oblique abdominals, transversus and deep lower back musculature. In order to ensure that these muscles rather than rectus abdominis are predominating in the co-contraction pattern to hold the spine in position during lower limb loading, it is essential that the patient or client consciously activates these muscles prior to adding load.

In instructing the patient in this pretest action, active techniques such as abdominal 'hollowing' or 'bracing' have been shown to activate the appropriate musculature (Richardson et al 1992).

Abdominal 'hollowing'. According to Kendall and McCreary (1983) the use of the obliques for lumbar stabilization with minimal contribution of rectus abdominis requires the effort of pulling upward and inward with the abdominal muscles. (This is referred to as abdominal 'hollowing' in this text.) These authors also suggest descriptive terms such as 'make your lower abdomen cave in' or 'hide your tummy under your chest', as appropriate.

Similar instructions of asking the subject to contemplate their navel and pull it up and against their spine were used by Miller and Medeiros (1987). In an EMG study, these authors found that such a 'visualization cue' increased the level of activity in transversus and internal obliques for their stabilization role during the eccentric phase of a curl up.

The validity of this 'hollowing' procedure for enhancing stabilization (by incorporation of the oblique abdominals as well as the lumbar paraspinal muscles, with lesser activity of rectus abdominis) has recently been verified by Richardson et al (1992). During the performance of this technique, the rib cage should be slightly elevated and breathing checked to make sure that this technique can be achieved during natural relaxed breathing. A depression of the rib cage or a protrusion of the abdominal wall usually indicates that the technique has been performed incorrectly and the rectus abdominis rather than the oblique abdominals are predominating in the co-contraction pattern.

Abdominal 'bracing'. Kennedy (1980) devised and named the technique of active abdominal 'bracing'. This procedure was considered to utilize increased intra-abdominal pressure to stabilize the lumbar spine prior to and during any activity which loads the spine. It was aiming to incorporate a muscle co-contraction of the oblique abdominals and lower back muscles with less emphasis on rectus abdominis activity. This pattern of muscle activity was likewise confirmed in the EMG study by Richardson et al (1992).

Abdominal bracing requires the person to contract the abdominals by actively 'flaring' out laterally in the region of the waist just above the iliac crests. During this technique patients or clients are not permitted to flex their head or trunk forward, elevate their lower ribs, protrude the abdomen or to press through their feet. Breathing in a relaxed manner during the muscle co-contraction pattern is also important.

In summary, to gain a safer and more sensitive stability test by ensuring that the appropriate muscles control the spine, the patient or client is required to preactivate and maintain the co-contraction pattern by either the 'hollowing' or 'bracing' techniques when load is added via the limb(s). Even in the high levels of the stability test, when rectus abdominis will contract strongly, activation and maintenance of the stability co-contraction pattern is still an essential component of the test.

Importantly, clinical experience indicates that many patients (especially those with chronic low back pain) and some symptom-free individuals are unable to perform these active stabilization techniques. In such cases rehabilitation must be commenced at a level to first facilitate the co-contraction pattern (see rehabilitation guidelines — stage 1). IT IS INAPPROPRIATE TO LOAD THE SPINE (EVEN IN TESTING) WHEN A BASIC LEVEL OF ACTIVE PROTECTIVE STABILITY CANNOT BE ACHIEVED.

Measurement of changes of lumbar spine position

In our research and clinical practice we have found that the commonly used methods of observation and manual palpation behind the lumbar spine were often not sufficiently sensitive to detect the sometimes subtle movements of the lumbar spine caused through either weakness, use of inappropriate muscles or muscle fatigue during the suggested testing procedures.

A pressure biofeedback (Fig. 51.2) was devised for the express purpose of detecting flexion, extension and rotation changes in the lumbar spine during testing procedures. An inflatable cushion, with three separate sections, is used to monitor the pressure between the lumbar spine and any supporting surface (Fig. 51.3). Pressure changes in any of the sections of the inflatable pad are detected via a standard pressure gauge calibrated in millimetres of

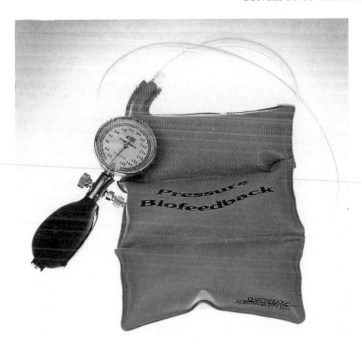

Fig. 51.2 Pressure biofeedback device (Chattanooga Australia Pty Ltd).

mercury (mmHg). Prior to the test, the cushion is inflated to fit into the space between the lumbar curve and exercise surface without forcing the lumbar spine into hyperlordosis. A pressure of approximately 40 mmHg has been found to be suitable for this baseline pressure.

The pressure biofeedback can be used to monitor the effectiveness of the co-contraction pattern as well as monitoring the position of the lumbar spine during testing and exercise to ensure safety during limb loading.

Measurement of co-contraction pattern. The pressure biofeedback is a very helpful device to monitor the lumbar position and ensure correct performance of the 'hollowing' or 'bracing' techniques during testing. Both techniques, when performed correctly, have been found to result in some slight lumbar flattening (flexion). This

raises the baseline pressure of the inflatable bag by approximately 10–15 mmHg (Richardson et al 1992). Inability to perform the technique correctly will result in either a nil increase in pressure (indicating no significant voluntary activation of the pattern) or a marked increase in pressure (e.g. 20–40 mmHg). Such an increase indicates that the patient is moving into posterior pelvic tilt and lumbar flexion through the primary use of rectus abdominis rather than using the desired co-contraction of the flat abdominals.

Measurement of lumbar spine position. The pressure biofeedback operates on the principal that if the spine is actively stabilized and held steady during testing (and exercise), the pressure will remain stable and no increase or decrease will be registered.

When the patient or client can perform the co-contraction pattern, progression to the assessment of stability using limb load still requires very careful and precise monitoring of the lumbar spine position. It is important to ensure that an increase in lumbar extension (as denoted by a decreased 'biofeedback' pressure below that monitored during the co-contraction pattern) or an increase in lumbar flexion (as denoted by an increased biofeedback pressure above that monitored during the co-contraction pattern) does not occur. Such movement out of a neutral position should be avoided as it can result in adverse strain on spinal structures.

It is re-emphasized that our clinical experience has indicated that many back pain patients demonstrate a poor ability to co-contract at a basic level. In such cases, testing stability by adding the load of the limb is undertaken later as progressive assessment following the achievement of the initial stages of the rehabilitation programme. The double leg positions (Fig. 51.1c, d) introduce quite high loads on the lumbar spine. The progression to these tests is not appropriate for all patients, especially those whose pathology or age suggest that such loading may not be warranted or may be detrimental to their condition.

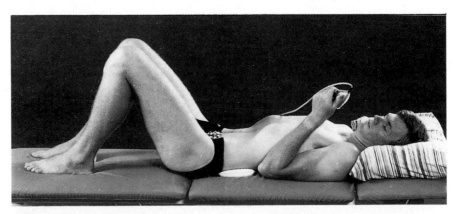

Fig. 51.3 The pressure biofeedback is placed under the lumbar spine to monitor its position.

REHABILITATION GUIDELINES

The general aims of rehabilitation are to promote general tone and holding ability in the appropriate trunk musculature in order to protect the spine during normal everyday activity. It is important to train the trunk musculature so that an appropriate level of spinal stabilization is achieved automatically when higher loads are applied either slowly or rapidly to the spine. To fulfil these aims, the rehabilitation process has four progressive stages. The appropriate stage at which the patient should begin the rehabilitation programme is gained from the assessment of their level of stability.

The effectiveness of the programme and progress of the patient in achieving the progressive levels of trunk stability need to be constantly reassessed. The formal tests described previously can be used initially and can be progressed to more functional tests as appropriate to stages 3 and 4 of the programme.

Stage 1. Development of trunk stabilization mechanisms with the lumbar spine held in neutral

The first stage of rehabilitation is concerned with teaching procedures to the patient or client which will emphasize and train the muscles primarily concerned with stabilization.

Transversus abdominis, internal and external obliques and the deep lumbar paravertebral muscles are the main muscles to be included in specific stabilizing procedures. As discussed previously, high levels of activity in either upper or lower rectus abdominis are not considered appropriate or essential for optimal lumbar spine stabilization. A technique is therefore required which contracts the prime stabilizing muscles in a pattern which fulfils the requirements of support and protection of the lumbar

spine, independent of any trunk, upper or lower limb movement.

As described in the assessment process, two techniques which have been shown to activate appropriate musculature for re-education purposes are abdominal 'hollowing' and abdominal 'bracing'. If, in the initial assessment, it has been found that the patient or client cannot perform these procedures, the first step in stage 1 of the rehabilitation process is to teach the correct 'hollowing' or 'bracing' technique.

The techniques are initially taught to the patient in the supine, crook lying position or in the supported reclined sitting position. If pressure biofeedback is available, it can be used as visual feedback to aid in motor learning to show the therapist that the technique has been performed accurately and safely, and to monitor when fatigue and loss of stability occurs (Fig. 51.3). As a general comment, the lower pressure increases associated with correct 'hollowing' and 'bracing' at this initial stage of rehabilitation are not only appropriate from a muscle activity aspect but also advantageous from a biomechanical viewpoint. They reflect that the lumbar spine is being held in a more 'neutral' position for exercise rather than being subjected to higher stresses which can occur at the extremes of flexion and extension.

In order to achieve and improve the holding capacity of the muscles, additional facilitation techniques may prove useful. These can include:

- conscious activation (including visual/auditory feedback)
- manual guidance
- resistance (note: too much resistance early in rehabilitation may be inhibitory)
- stretch (sweep tapping)

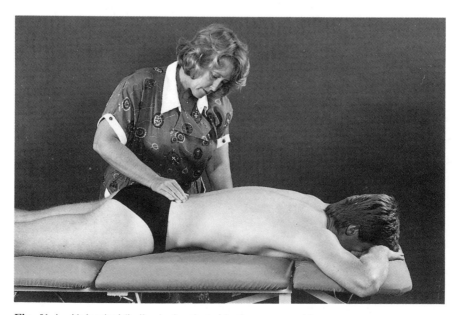

Fig. 51.4 Abdominal 'hollowing' activated in the prone position.

- vibration
- electrical stimulation

Some patients find the muscle co contraction of the 'hollowing' technique difficult to learn in the supine, crook lying or reclined sitting positions. In these instances, the co-contraction pattern can often be more easily facilitated in the prone position (Fig. 51.4). Gentle manual resistance is applied over the multifidus muscle in a downward direction while the client attempts to hollow the abdomen. Furthermore, if it has been determined that multifidus is not activated in the co-contraction pattern, specialized facilitation techniques may be used. Multifidus can be facilitated in its stability role either in the sagittal plane (Fig. 51.5), or during lumbar rotation (Fig. 51.6).

It is important to ensure that these techniques, which require sustained muscle action in order to perform their spinal protection role, are performed at submaximal levels. Furthermore, the co-contraction should not interfere with normal respiration.

Once the correct pattern has been achieved, motor learning will be enhanced by the constant reinforcement through repeated practice. In turn, motor learning can be enhanced by both knowledge of performance and knowledge of results (Carr & Shepherd 1986). Feedback to the patient of level of muscle activity, or position of body parts by visual, auditory or tactile cues are important.

Patients must be encouraged from the outset to incorporate this pattern of muscle co-contraction into their normal postures and daily activities. This immediately provides the spine with some degree of muscle support as well as encouraging the patient to practise continually and reinforce the co-contraction pattern. Clinically it has

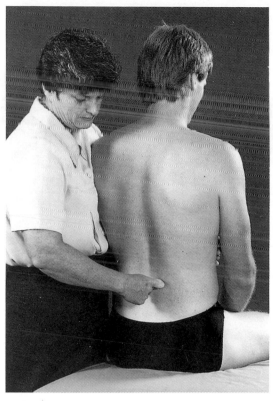

Fig. 51.5 The therapist facilitates multifidus by applying local stretch and requesting the patient to concentrate on 'swelling' the muscle bulk in co-contraction with the other stabilizing muscles. The patient should not achieve this by actively flexing the lumbar spine.

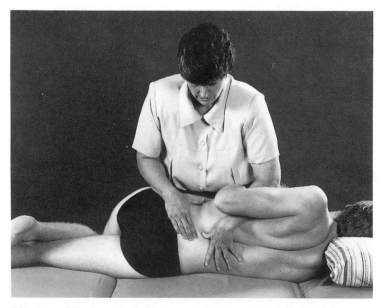

Fig. 51.6 The therapist facilitates multifidus through manual resistance and guidance, via the spinous processes, to the rotary movement at the appropriate level.

been found that patients will often report a lessening of symptoms consistent with this early muscle support.

Stage 2. Enhancing stability through added resistance (lumbar spine in neutral)

Once muscle contractions of the flat abdominals and the lower paravertebral muscles have been activated by a voluntary 'skilled' technique such as 'hollowing', this pattern can be enhanced using additional resistance techniques. This stage allows patterns of stability to develop while still maintaining minimal movement and stress to lumbar spine structures which is especially important in the case of healing tissue.

For all exercise resistance should be applied gradually and smoothly and the patient pre-sets and maintains the 'hollowing' co-contraction throughout all activities. In the first instance load is applied directly to the trunk. This stage can then be progressed by adding more distal load through the upper and lower limbs.

Increased resistance directly to the trunk

In an EMG investigation of eight different types of isometric trunk exercises (Richardson et al 1990), it was shown that those which incorporated resisted trunk rotation activated the most appropriate stabilization patterns for the trunk muscles. That is, these techniques resulted in contractions of the oblique abdominals and lumbar

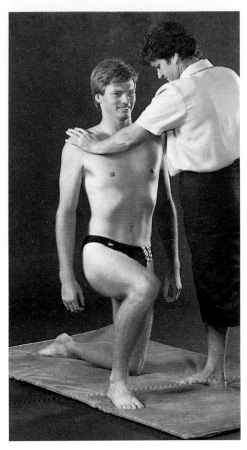

Fig. 51.8 Half kneeling, resisted trunk rotation.

erector spinae with minimal activity of rectus abdominis, especially its upper fibres. Hence the addition of resistance to either the shoulders or pelvis in order to produce an isometric contraction to prevent attempted trunk rotation are suitable techniques for enhancing contractions in the muscles of the trunk primarily concerned with stability. An additional advantage is that the resistance applied to the trunk tends to stretch the muscles directly. This would begin to simulate their role of resisting the force of gravity and functional load on the body.

Positions in which rotatory resistance can be given are bridging, resistance to the pelvis, four foot kneeling, resistance to shoulders or pelvis (Fig. 51.7) kneeling or half kneeling, resistance to the shoulders or pelvis (Fig. 51.8), sitting, resistance to the shoulders.

Manual accommodating resistance is ideal, and this method of applying resistance could be modified and enhanced using the proprioceptive neuromuscular facilitation (PNF) techniques of rhythmic stabilizations (Sullivan & Markos 1987). As mentioned, all exercises should begin and proceed with the patient pre-facilitating their stability muscles with the technique of abdominal 'hollowing'. While the therapist provides the manual exercise in the clinic, exercises should be modified so that they can form part of a home programme (Fig. 51.9).

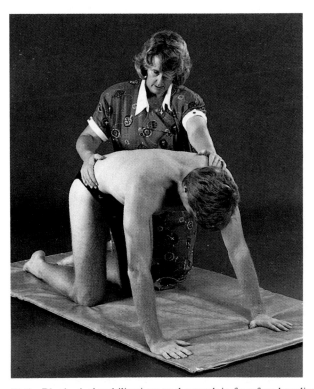

Fig. 51.7 Rhythmical stabilizations to the trunk in four-foot kneeling.

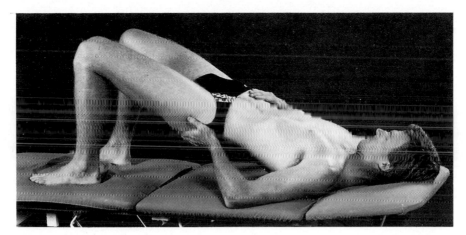

Fig. 51.9 Home programme exercise — resisted trunk rotation in the bridged position (isometric).

Appropriate gym equipment can be used to give resistance to trunk rotation. The level of rotatory resistance of 30–40% maximum voluntary contraction (MVC) suggested by advocates of PNF (Sullivan 1989) would seem an appropriate guide to the amount of resistance necessary to increase the tonic holding, i.e. stabilizing role of these trunk muscles.

Increased resistance/load more distally via the limbs

The aim of this progression is to maintain lumbar stabilization in neutral through the isometric contraction of 'hollowing' while load is gradually added more distally. The addition of load distally would tend to stretch and lengthen the trunk muscles — which would then be required to contract to hold and control the position of the lumbar spine. This begins to simulate their functional eccentric role of trunk stabilization during limb movement.

Where possible it is suggested that the pressure biofeedback is used under the lumbar spine in order to ensure that lumbar stabilization is maintained — and hence to ensure that the exercise will be completed correctly and safely. Alternatively, the clinician or patient can approximately monitor the position of the spine with his or her hand.

Both isometric and slow isotonic (or isokinetic) exercises of the limbs are suitable. Either the load of limb itself or any other appropriate added resistance can be used. Through this method of exercise, both the strength and isometric endurance of the key stabilization muscles of the trunk can be developed while the spine remains in a more safe, neutral position. Some examples of isometric or slow isotonic exercise using the upper or lower limbs are illustrated in Fig. 51.10–51.15. Other exercises — such as increasing lever length via weight of limbs, as used in testing procedures — can be employed.

The formal exercises for increasing the load applied to the stable lumbar spine should be reinforced in functional activities. The patient should be encouraged to maintain abdominal hollowing during loaded functional movement such as carrying, pushing, pulling, lifting as well as during posture and gait.

Stage 3: Development of lumbar stabilization during slow loaded movements of the lumbar spine

When stability mechanisms have been trained through static stabilization procedures, it is necessary to begin loaded movement through range.

The lumbar spine is required to perform co-ordinated efficient movement in order to undertake functional loaded tasks while at the same time ensuring efficient muscular stabilization. Many functional tasks place the lumbar spine at risk. The spine is known to be particularly

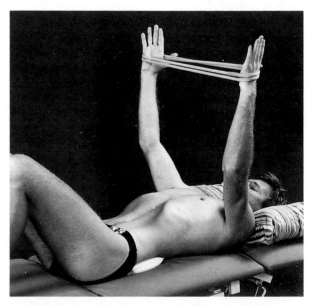

Fig. 51.10 Isometric upper limb exercise with active lumbar stabilization.

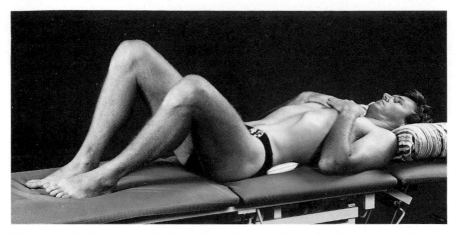

Fig. 51.11 Single leg active hip abduction, adduction while maintaining active lumbar stability.

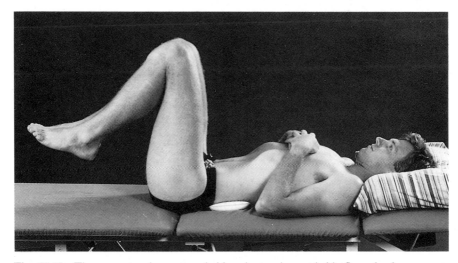

Fig. 51.12 The co-contraction pattern held against an isometric hip flexor load.

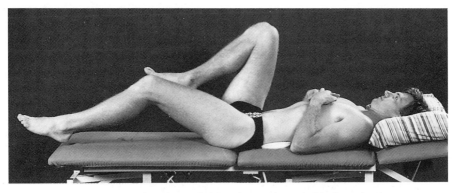

Fig. 51.13 The co-contraction pattern held against an isotonic hip flexor load.

vulnerable during flexion and rotatory movements under load (Farfan et al 1970, Adams & Hutton 1982). Exercises such as 'curl-ups' are also known to produce high intradiscal pressures and high joint loading (Nachemson 1976). While patients can be instructed in many ergonomically sound techniques to minimize stress, there are still many 'high stress' manoeuvres in which the lumbar spine must take part during normal daily functional activities and the muscles must be trained appropriately to a level to cope with the stress demand.

The final level of applied load would depend on the work and leisure requirements of the individual. Manual

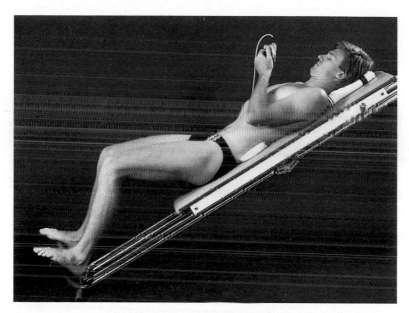

Fig. 51.14 The co-contraction pattern held during leg extension exercise.

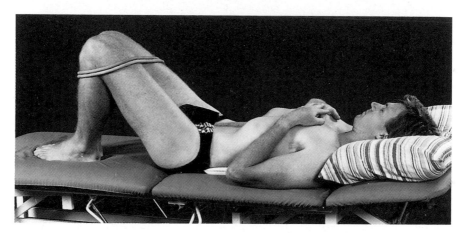

Fig. 51.15 The co-contraction pattern held during resisted hip rotation (using rubber straps).

workers as well as sportsmen may require specialized training as well as the suggested formal exercise programme.

If progressive training has been followed, automatic protective muscle stabilization should now begin to occur during movement. In some cases, it still may be necessary voluntarily to reinforce this muscle activation by the patient performing the abdominal 'hollowing' procedure even during this level of task performance.

Resistance/load can be applied to the lumbar spine using body weight, manual resistance, various types of equipment and through functional training.

Body weight

If undertaken at a slow speed, exercises such as curl-ups and curl-ups with a rotation are appropriate at this later stage. During these movements, the flat abdominals and lumbar paravertebral muscles should be active together with the rectus abdominis. To ensure that this is occurring, the patient should perform the exercises with minimal clothing so that the clinician can observe for a relatively 'flattish' abdominal wall which is indicative of a more balanced activity in the flat abdominals and rectus abdominis (Miller & Medeiros 1987). A markedly convex abdominal wall suggests that rectus abdominis is dominating without the assurance of the protective stability activity of the other abdominal muscles. EMG biofeedback is also useful to monitor muscle performance in these exercises. The clinician also needs to observe for a smoothly rounded spine to ensure an appropriate relationship between the abdominals and hip flexors (Fig. 51.16).

Rotary movement under load could be undertaken using a slow controlled pelvic rotation (Fig. 51.17). This

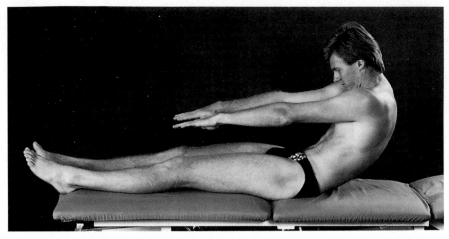

Fig. 51.16   The curl-up exercise — note the flat abdominal wall.

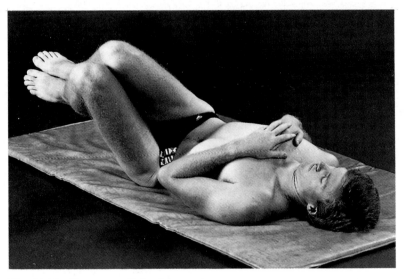

Fig. 51.17   Slow, controlled pelvic rotation.

activity would require maximal control and stabilization of the lumbar spine.

Manual resistance

Trunk PNF patterns may also be used to produce controlled, smooth, loaded movements of the lumbar spine.

Equipment

Load may be increased and progressed safely through the use of trunk exercise machines. The various and more sophisticated types of isokinetic apparatus can provide accommodating resistance to through-range trunk movements in each plane. Programmes can be instituted for concentric and, importantly, eccentric muscle work and movements may be designed with progressive resistance isotonic loading.

Functional movement

Emphasis on quality of movement and active muscle contraction of appropriate muscles is still extremely important as high loaded functional movement is begun.

Lifting, carrying, pushing or other activities as required by the patient's occupation can be gradually progressed to heavier loads. Likewise, sports specific skills or training activities can be progressed to heavier loads and, or speeds.

Stage 4. Development of lumbar stabilization during high-speed movement of the limbs and trunk

It can be observed clinically that maintenance of lumbar and girdle stabilization and control is extremely difficult during rapid limb movements. For example, it is difficult to maintain lumbar–pelvic stability during activities such as running. It is interesting that proximal weakness and instability often occurs in sportsmen spending long periods of time in this type of ballistic activity.

Although difficult to substantiate with objective research measurements, there is some evidence in both animal and human studies that rapid movement could lead to reduced stabilizing capacity of some muscles.

Smith et al (1980) found that during the very rapid movements of 'paw shaking', the gastrocnemius of the cat was extremely active while soleus was inhibited. Similar findings have been reported in a study on humans by Ng and Richardson (1990). After a four-week training session of rapid plantar flexion movements performed in standing, significant increases in jumping height were found but they were accompanied by a significant loss of static function of soleus.

Similar findings have been reported more proximally at the level of the knee. During increasing speeds of ballistic flexion–extension knee movements, Richardson and Bullock (1986) found that increases in muscle activity occurred for rectus femoris and hamstrings but not for the vasti. These muscles appeared inhibited during such a rapid (low load) activity.

There is also some evidence that the repetition of fast trunk movements may be related to reduced trunk stabilization. In a recent study on curl-up exercises performed by army personnel, those who performed the curl-up more rapidly were found to have a significantly reduced level of lumbar stabilization (as estimated by the ability to hold the lumbar spine stable while load was progressively increased via the weight of the legs) as compared to those who performed the exercise at a slower rate. It appeared that exercise at a faster rate was linked with lower levels of lumbar stabilization (Wohlfahrt et al 1993). Once more evidence is produced it could be argued that the training of rapid movement presents the most difficult movement in which to maintain contraction of the muscles designed to protect and control the lumbar spine.

For these reasons rapid movement while maintaining lumbar stabilization is introduced only in the final rehabilitation stage. This may best be trained by increasing speeds at which formal exercise is performed or through functional activities.

CONCLUSIONS

Deep, flat muscles, and those close to the vertebrae themselves, need to be activated in an appropriate pattern to protect and stabilize the lumbar spine. This may be appropriate not only for those suffering back pain or pathology but also for those symptom-free individuals who, due to their particular work or sport, or their sedentary lifestyle, may require activation of these muscles for the prevention of back injury and pain.

Following activation of these muscles, they should ideally be trained isometrically (under progressively increasing loads), then isotonically with a gradual increase in load, and finally — for some individuals to function optimally — during fast repetitive movement.

In this way the muscular system of the lumbar spine can be retrained progressively to support and protect the spine under varying loads and under many functional movement conditions.

REFERENCES

Adams M A, Hutton W C 1982 Prolapsed intervertebral disc. A hyperflexion injury. Spine 7: 184–191

Andersson B J G, Ortengren R, Nachemson A, Elfstrom G 1974 Lumbar disc pressure and myoelectric back activity during sitting. Scandinavian Journal of Rehabilitation Medicine 6: 104–114

Asmussen E, Klausen K 1962 Form and function of the erect human spine. Clinical Orthopaedics 25: 55–63

Bartelink D L 1957 The role of abdominal pressure in relieving pressure on the lumbar intervertebral discs. Journal of Bone and Joint Surgery 39B: 718–725

Basmajian J V, De Luca C J 1985 Muscles alive: their function revealed by electromyography. Williams & Wilkins, Baltimore

Basmajian J V, Wolf S L (eds) 1990 Therapeutic exercise. 5th edn. Williams & Wilkins, Baltimore

Bogduk N, Twomey L T 1987 Clinical anatomy of the lumbar spine. Churchill Livingstone, Melbourne

Carman D J, Blanton P L, Biggs N L 1972 Electromyographic study of the anterolateral abdominal musculature utilizing indwelling electrodes. American Journal of Physical Medicine 51: 113–129

Carr J H, Shepherd R B 1986 Motor training following stroke. In: Banks M A (ed) International perspectives in physical therapy 2: stroke. Churchill Livingstone, London

Davies G, Gould J 1982 Trunk testing using a prototype cybex II isokinetic dynamometer stabilisation system. Journal of Orthopaedic and Sports Physical Therapy 3: 164–170

Edwards R H T, Newham D J, Jones D A et al 1984 Role of mechanical damage in pathogenesis of proximal myopathy in man. Lancet 1(8376): 548–551

Elder G C B, Bradbury K, Roberts R 1982 Variability of fiber type distributions within human muscles. Journal of Applied Physiology 53: 1473–1480

Farfan H F, Cossette J W, Robertson G H et al 1970 The effects of torsion on the lumbar intervertebral joints; the role of torsion in the production of disc degeneration. Journal of Bone and Joint Surgery 52A: 468–497

Fischbach G D, Robbins N 1969 Change in contractile properties of disused soleus muscles. Journal of Physiology 201: 305–320

Floyd W F, Silver P H S 1950 Electromyographic study of patterns of activity of the anterior abdominal wall muscles in man. Journal of Anatomy 84: 132–145

Godfrey K E, Kindig L E, Windell E J 1977 Electromyographic study of duration of muscle activity in sit up variations. Archives of Physical Medicine and Rehabilitation 58: 132–135

Goldberg A L 1975 Mechanisms of growth and atrophy of skeletal muscle. In: Cassens R G & Institute of Muscular Biology (eds) Muscle biology. Marcel Dekker, New York

Goldspink D F 1980 Physiological factors influencing protein and muscle growth in mammals. In: Goldspink D F (ed) Development and specialization of skeletal muscle. Cambridge University Press, Cambridge, pp 65–89

Gracovetsky S, Farfan H F, Lamy C 1977 A mathematical model of the lumbar spine using an optimal system to control muscles and ligaments. Orthopaedic Clinics of North America 8: 135–153

Gracovetsky S, Farfan H, Helleur C 1985 The abdominal mechanism. Spine 10: 317–324

Grew N D 1980 Intraabdominal pressure response to loads applied to the torso in normal subjects. Spine 5: 149–154

Grimby L, Hannerz J 1976 Disturbances in voluntary recruitment order of low and high frequency motor units on blockade of proprioceptive afferent activity. Acta Physiologica Scandinavica 96: 207–216

Häggmark T, Thorstensson A 1979 Fibre types in human abdominal muscles. Acta Physiologica Scandinavica 107: 319–325

Hemborg B, Moritz U 1985 Intra-abdominal pressure and trunk muscle activity during lifting. Scandinavian Journal of Rehabilitation Medicine 17: 5–13

Henneman E, Olson C B 1965 Relations between structure and function in the design of skeletal muscles. Journal of Neurophysiology 29: 581–598

Hoens A, Telfer M, Strauss G 1990 An isokinetic evaluation of trunk strength in elite female field hockey players. Australian Journal of Physiotherapy 36: 163–171

Ianuzzo C D 1976 The cellular composition of human skeletal muscle. In: Knuttgren H G (ed) Neuromuscular mechanisms for therapeutic and conditioning exercise. University Park Press, Baltimore

Jackson C P, Brown M D 1983 Analysis of current approaches and a practical guide to prescription of exercise. Clinical Orthopaedics and Related Research 179: 46–54

Janda V 1964 Movement patterns in the pelvic and hip region with special reference to pathogenesis of vertebrogenic disturbances. Rehabilitation thesis, Charles University, Prague, Czechoslovakia

Janda V 1978 Muscles central nervous motor regulation and back problems. In: Korr I M (ed) Neurobiologic mechanisms in manipulative therapy. Plenum Press, New York

Johnson M A, Polgar J, Weightman D 1973 Data on distribution of fibre types in thirty-six human muscles: an autopsy study. Journal of Neurological Science 18: 111–129

Kendall F P, McCreary E K 1983 Muscles: testing and function. 3rd edn. Williams & Wilkins, Baltimore

Kennedy B 1980 An Australian program for management of back problems. Physiotherapy 66: 108–111

Kennedy B 1982 Dynamic back care through body awareness. Teknidata Services, Sydney

Lacôte M, Chevalier A M, Miranda A et al 1987 Clinical evaluation of muscle function. Churchill Livingstone, London

Langrana N, Lee C 1984 Isokinetic evaluation of trunk muscles. Spine 9: 171–175

Lefkof M B 1986 Trunk flexion in healthy children aged 3 to 7 years. Physical Therapy 66: 39–44

Lieber R L, Johansson C B, Vahlsing H L et al 1986 Long-term effects of spinal cord transection on fast and slow rat skeletal muscle. Experimental Neurology 91: 423–434

Machado de Sousa O, Furlani J 1981 Electromyographic study of some muscles of the anterolateral abdominal wall. Acta Anatomica 111: 231–239

Macintosh J E, Bogduk N, Gracovetsky S 1987 The biomechanics of the thoracolumbar fascia. Clinical Biomechanics 2: 78–83

Matilla M, Hurme M, Alaranta H et al 1986 The multifidus muscle in patients with lumbar disc herniation. Spine 11: 732–738

Mayhew T P, Norton B J, Sahrmann S A 1983 Electromyographic study of the relationship between hamstring and abdominal muscles during a unilateral straight leg raise. Physical Therapy 63: 1769–1175

Miller M I, Medeiros J M 1987 Recruitment of internal oblique and transversus abdominis muscles during the eccentric phase of the curl-up exercise. Physical Therapy 67: 1213–1218

Morris J M, Lucas D B, Bresler B 1961 Role of the trunk in stability of the spine. Journal of Bone and Joint Surgery 43A: 327–351

Nordin M, Kahanovitz N, Verderame R et al 1987 Normal trunk muscle strength in women and the effect of exercises and electrical stimulation: Pt 1. Spine 12: 105–111

Nachemson A L 1976 The lumbar spine, an orthopaedic challenge. Spine 1: 59–71

Ng G, Richardson C A 1990 The effects of training triceps surae using progressive speed loading. Physiotherapy Practice 6: 77–84

Oganov V, Skuratove S, Potapov N et al 1980 Physiological mechanisms of adaption of skeletal muscles of mammals to the weightless state. In: Cuba F, Maredal G, Takacs O (eds) Advances in Physiological Science. Pergamon Press, Hungary

Panjabi M, Abumi K, Duranceau J et al 1989 Spinal stability and intersegmental muscle forces: a biomechanical model. Spine 14: 194–200

Pope M H, Svensson M, Andersson G B J et al 1987 The role of prerotation of the trunk in axial twisting efforts. Spine 12: 1041–1045

Rab G T R, Chao E Y S, Stauffer R N 1977 Muscle force analysis of the lumbar spine. Orthopaedic Clinics of North America 8: 193–199

Richardson C A 1987a Investigations into the optimal approach to exercise for the knee musculature. PhD thesis, University of Queensland

Richardson C A 1987b Atrophy of vastus medialis in patello-femoral pain syndrome. Proceedings of the Tenth International Congress of the World Confederation for Physical Therapy, Sydney, pp 400–403

Richardson C A, Bullock M I 1986 Changes in muscle activity during fast, alternating flexion–extension movements of the knee. Scandinavian Journal of Rehabilitation Medicine 18: 51–58

Richardson C A, Toppenberg R, Jull G 1990 An initial evaluation of eight abdominal exercises for their ability to provide stabilization for the lumbar spine. Australian Journal of Physiotherapy 36: 6–11

Richardson C A, Jull G A, Toppenberg R M K et al 1992 Technique for active lumbar stabilisation for spinal protection: a pilot study. Australian Journal of Physiotherapy 38: 105–112

Sahrmann S A 1988 Sahrmann Techniques. Preconference workshop, Australian Physiotherapy Conference, Canberra

Sheffield F J 1962 Electromyographic study of the abdominal muscles in walking and other movements. American Journal of Physical Medicine 41: 142–147

Smidt G, Herring T, Amundsen L et al 1983 Assessment of abdominal and back extensor function. A quantitative approach and results for chronic low back pain patients. Spine 8: 211–219

Smith J O, Betts B, Ederton V R et al 1980 Rapid ankle extension during paw shakes: selective recruitment of fast ankle extensors. Journal of Neurophysiology 43: 612–620

Soderberg G L, Barr J O 1983 Muscular function in chronic low-back dysfunction. Spine 8: 79–85

Sullivan P E 1989 Therapeutic exercise for patients with low back pain. PNF course, October, Brisbane

Sullivan P E, Markos P D 1987 Clinical procedures in therapeutic exercise. Appleton & Lange, Norwalk, Connecticut

Sullivan P E, Markos P D, Minor M A D 1982 An integrated approach to therapeutic exercise. Reston, Reston, Virginia

Suzuki N, Endo S 1983 A quantitative study of trunk muscle strength and fatiguability in the low-back syndrome. Spine 8: 69–74

Templeton G H, Sweeney H L, Himson B F et al 1988 Changes in fibre composition of soleus muscle during rat hind limb suspension. Journal of Applied Physiology 65: 1191–1195

Tesh K M, Shaw Dunn J, Evans J H 1987 The abdominal muscles and vertebral stability. Spine 12: 501–508

Valencia F P, Munro R R 1985 An electromyographic study on lumbar multifidus in man. Electromyography and Clinical Neurophysiology 25: 205–221

Verbout A J, Wintzen A R, Linthorst P 1989 The distribution of slow and fast twitch fibres in the intrinsic lumbar back muscles. Clinical Anatomy 2: 120–121

Waters R L, Morris J M 1972 Electrical activity of muscles of the trunk during walking. Journal of Anatomy 111: 191–199

Watter P 1991 Director of clinic for the treatment of children with motor coordination difficulties (MCD) University of Queensland: personal communication

Williams P L, Warwick R, Dyson M et al (eds) 1989 Gray's anatomy. 37th edn. Churchill Livingstone, Edinburgh

Wohlfahrt D A, Jull G A, Richardson C A 1993 An initial investigation of the relationship between the static and dynamic function of the abdominal muscles. Australian Journal of Physiotherapy (in press)

Zetterberg C, Andersson G B J, Schultz A B 1987 The activity of individual trunk muscles during heavy physical loading. Spine 12: 1035–1040

52. Principles and practice of muscle energy and functional techniques

D. G. Lee

INTRODUCTION

In the spring of 1987, Rick Hansen realized one of his dreams by successfully completing his 'Man in Motion' tour. With it, he drew attention to a frequently overlooked assumption of life—motion. As physiotherapists, we are presented daily with patients who have either lost the ability to move or to do so without pain. The magnitude and the significance of their loss is variable but none the less pertinent to their function.

Normal motion requires optimal function of the bones, joints, muscles, nerves and circulatory system (Fig. 52.1). The motion of a bone (osteokinematics) is dependent upon the motion of its joints. The motion of a joint (arthrokinematics) is dependent upon contraction of the muscles which cross it. The contractile system (myokinematics) is dependent upon the function of the peripheral and central neurological systems.

Dysfunction in any one of these systems will ultimately effect the motor response, that is, the motion. The resultant altered movement pattern can be very obvious or very subtle. For example, the lateral limp of a patient with an anatomically short leg is easily noticed; however, the shortened stance phase of gait and the excessive compensatory transverse plane rotation of the pelvic girdle which occurs when 10° of hip extension is missing requires closer scrutiny.

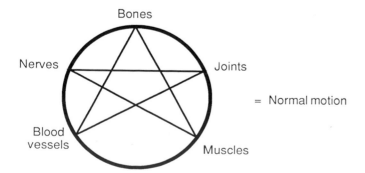

Fig. 52.1 Normal motion requires optimal function of the bones, joints, muscles, nerves and circulatory system.

Restrictions of joint motion are detected by integrating the findings on testing osteokinematic function (movement of the bone) and arthrokinematic function (gliding motion of the joint surfaces). The joint itself is truly restricted when both the bone and the joint demonstrate restricted motion. For example, the occipito-atlantal joint is restricted in flexion when both forward sagittal rotation of the occiput on the atlas *around* a coronal axis and posterior translation of the occiput on the atlas *along* a sagittal axis is reduced. Flexion of the occiput on the atlas may also be limited by the muscular system. In this instance, the osteokinematic function (forward sagittal rotation of the occiput on the atlas) would be restricted while the arthrokinematic function (posterior translation of the occiput on the atlas) would be normal. These findings would suggest that the posterior myofascia was the limiting factor.

In the first instance an articular treatment technique (joint mobilization) would be indicated, whereas in the second instance a myofascial technique (PNF, muscle energy, functional, myofascial release) would be used.

The focus of this chapter is to outline the principles of both muscle energy and functional mobilization techniques and to describe examples of their use in the spinal column. These techniques play a very small, albeit important, role in the restoration of optimal movement patterns. In isolation, their effect is insignificant. By incorporating these techniques into the overall rehabilitation programme (Table 52.1) they can become a powerful tool for the manual therapist.

THEORETICAL CONSIDERATIONS

Muscle energy and functional techniques are used when the limiting factor to motion has been determined to be the neuro/muscular system. 'While usually thinking of muscles as the motors of the body, producing motion by their contraction, it is important to remember that the same contractile forces are also utilized to oppose motion. By the application of controlled counteracting forces,

Table 52.1 Rehabilitation programme for the restoration of optimal movement patterns

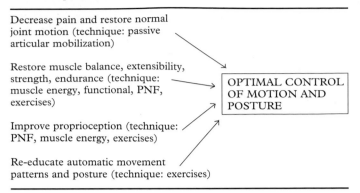

contracting muscle absorbs momentum and regulates, resists, retards, and arrests motion' (Korr 1975).

The extent of the muscular resistance to motion is dependent upon the degree of impulse traffic travelling along the motor axons supplying the muscle. This outflow varies with the level of excitation of the anterior horn cells in the spinal cord which, in turn, varies with the changing afferent input to the cord during motion of the joint.

Muscle tone is a complex neurophysiological state which is controlled by both cortical and spinal reflexes. Resting muscle tone is influenced by the afferent activity from the articular and muscular systems. Afferent input from the type 1 and type 2 mechanoreceptors located in the superficial and deep aspects of the joint capsule is projected polysynaptically (and multisegmentally) to the gamma motoneurons (Wyke 1981). The effect of this afferent discharge on the gamma motoneuron is excitatory (Fig. 52.2).

When the gamma motoneuron discharge to a muscle spindle is facilitated, less external stretch is required to fire the primary annulospiral ending in the muscle spindle. Afferent input from these receptors in the muscle spindle is projected monosynaptically to the alpha motoneuron which controls the extrafusal muscle fibres in the immediate vicinity of the spindle (Korr 1975). The effect of this afferent discharge on the alpha motoneuron is also excitatory (Fig. 52.2). The effect of this excitation on the muscle is an increased resistance to any motion which attempts to lengthen it (hypertonicity) (Korr 1975).

Afferent input from the type 3 mechanoreceptors located in the ligaments of the joint is projected polysynaptically to the alpha motoneurons (Wyke 1981). The effect of this afferent discharge on the alpha motoneuron is inhibitory. Wyke (1981) has noted that the ligaments of the vertebral column do not contain type 3 mechanoreceptors.

The Golgi endings in the tendon of the muscle are stimulated by excessive tension generated within the muscle. This tension is produced by either an active con-traction or a passive stretch of the muscle. Afferent input from these receptors is projected polysynaptically to both the gamma and the alpha motoneurons and the effect is inhibitory.

Dysfunction occurs when abnormal or excessive afferent input maintains a state of constant increased excitation at the spinal cord, a state commonly referred to as a facilitated segment (Patterson 1976). In this state, normally subliminal afferent stimuli evoke an exaggerated efferent output from the facilitated segment causing overactivity in the targeted tissues, one of which is the segmental spinal muscle.

MUSCLE ENERGY TECHNIQUE—PRINCIPLES

Muscle energy technique was developed between 1945 and 1950 by Fred L. Mitchell Sr, an osteopathic physician (Mitchell et al 1979). Muscle energy technique is used in clinical practice to restore mobility of a motion segment, retrain global movement patterns, reduce tissue oedema, stretch fibrotic tissue and retrain the stabilizing function of the intersegmental muscles.

Restoration of mobility

The deep segmental muscles of the spine attach into the posterolateral aspect of the capsule of the zygapophyseal joint (Twomey et al 1989). Muscular hypertonicity secondary to a facilitated segment of the spinal cord can restrict osteokinematic function of the vertebral motion segment (Korr 1975, Hartman 1983). In the restoration of segmental joint mobility, accurate localization of the motion barrier and specific muscle work are key factors to success. The joint is taken to the motion barrier and the patient is instructed to hold against the therapist's gentle resistance. The direction of the resistance applied may be either into or away from the restriction.

According to Sherrington's law of reciprocal innervation (Kabat & Licht 1961), contraction of an agonist muscle reflexly inhibits its antagonist. The gamma motoneuron discharge to the facilitated muscle can be reduced by specific contraction of its antagonist. The stronger the contraction of the antagonist, the greater the relaxation of the agonist. However, too forceful a contraction increases synergistic activity via irradiation, and since the deep spinal muscles are stabilizers of joint motion restoration of mobility is not achieved. Segmental palpation for appropriate muscle relaxation during the application of the technique confirms the magnitude of counterforce necessary.

The principles of autogenic inhibition may also be employed with muscle energy technique. Contraction of the facilitated muscle from a lengthened position generates sufficient tension to activate the Golgi endings in the tendon. This reflexly inhibits both the gamma and the alpha motoneurons (Fig. 52.2). This results in lengthening of the muscle upon relaxation. Accurately localized, low-intensity, isometric contractions of the agonist or antagonist segmental muscle are the most effective for restoring mobility.

Retraining of global movement patterns

Voluntary movement is only as efficient as the individual's neuromuscular co-ordination. Kabat (Kabat & Licht 1961) states that 'Repeated excitation of a pathway in the central nervous system results gradually in easier transmission of nerve impulses through that pathway. This is brought about by a decrease in synaptic resistance and is the basis for the formation of habits and for learning'. Faulty movement patterns become habitual even at a segmental level, and muscle energy techniques can retrain normal movement patterns. Multisegmental motion together with concentric contractions of the agonist and synergist muscles are the most effective.

Reduction of oedema and stretching of myofascial fibrosis

In this instance, high-intensity, eccentric contractions involving multiple segments will achieve the best results. The counterforce applied by the therapist is greater than the patient's force so that the contracting muscle is lengthened and the intramuscular and overlying fascia are stretched.

Restoration of stability

The inability to recruit the segmental musculature is a common finding in spinal instability. The neuromusculature is retrained via highly specific, segmental, eccentric, isometric and concentric muscle work (Pettman 1990).

CLINICAL APPLICATION OF MUSCLE ENERGY TECHNIQUES

The techniques described in this section are used to restore mobility of a motion segment limited by the myofascia. They are classified as low-intensity techniques involving isometric contractions (Hartman 1983). The same techniques can be modified to retrain global movement patterns by allowing multisegmental motion to occur and the muscles to contract concentrically. If the goal is to stretch intramuscular and fascial fibrosis, the same technique can be modified into a high-intensity, multisegmental technique by recruiting the muscles eccentrically. The patient/therapist positioning is identical; the motor recruitment and resistance applied is different.

Since muscle energy techniques follow biomechanical principles, a brief review of the regional osteokinematics and arthrokinematics is necessary. The intention is not to duplicate other chapters in this text but rather to clarify how the motion barrier is reached prior to the application of the muscle energy technique. Selected examples will be described for each region; the reader is referred to Lee (1989) and to Lee and Walsh (1985) for a description of more techniques.

Craniovertebral region

Occipito-atlantal joints—biomechanics

The occiput is capable of two degrees of voluntary motion, flexion/extension and side-flexion/rotation. Flexion/extension of the occiput occurs about a coronal axis through the mastoid processes. Full flexion requires posterior translation of the occipital condyles on the superior facets of the atlas while full extension requires anterior translation. The anterior convergence of the joint surfaces limits the degree of translation possible (Weisl & Rothman 1979) and facilitates a 'rolling' motion at the end of the physiological range. An inextensible rectus capitus posterior minor can limit full flexion; an inextensible rectus capitus anterior minor can limit full extension.

Side-flexion/rotation of the occiput is a unidirectional motion about an oblique anteroposterior axis. Right side-

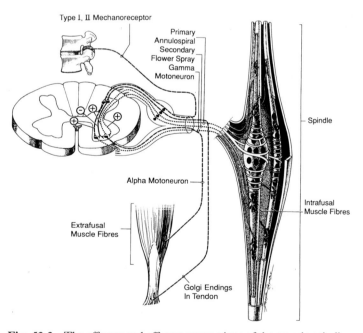

Fig. 52.2 The afferent and efferent connections of the muscle spindle. Segmental facilitation of the spinal cord results in normally subliminal afferent stimuli from the primary annulospiral ending evoking an exaggerated efferent response from the spinal cord causing an increase in the alpha and gamma motoneuron discharge to the extrafusal and intrafusal muscle fibres.

flexion/left rotation requires anterior translation of the right occipito-atlantal joint and posterior translation of the left occipito-atlantal joint. An inextensible left superior oblique and/or right rectus capitus lateralis muscle can limit this motion.

Occipito-atlantal joints—muscle energy techniques

Restricted flexion—occiput/atlas (Fig. 52.3). The aim of the technique is to restore flexion at the occipito-atlantal joints.

Patient: supine lying, head supported on a pillow.

Therapist: standing at the patient's head facing the shoulders.

Palpate: with the lateral aspect of one index finger, palpate transversely the posterior arch of the atlas. With the other hand, cup the occiput.

Localization: the motion barrier is localized by flexing the occiput around a coronal axis through the mastoid processes to the physiological limit, simultaneously allowing the occiput to posteriorly translate on the superior facets of the atlas.

Mobilization: from this position, the patient is instructed to hold the head still while the therapist minimally releases the support of the cranium. This isometric contraction recruits the deep and superficial cervical flexor muscles and reflexly inhibits the deep and superficial cervical extensor muscles. The contraction is held for three to five seconds following which the patient is instructed to relax completely. The new barrier for occipital flexion is localized. The technique is repeated three times.

Restricted right side-flexion/left rotation—occiput/atlas (Fig. 52.4). The aim of the technique is to restore right side-flexion/left rotation at the occipito-atlantal joints.

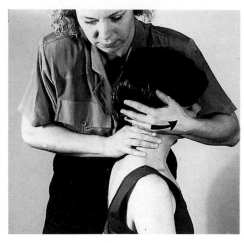

Fig. 52.4 Muscle energy technique to restore right side-flexion/left rotation at the occipito-atlantal joints. The arrow indicates the direction of occipital motion during this technique.

Patient: sitting with the back supported against a chair.

Therapist: standing at the patient's left side.

Palpate: with an open pinch grip, palpate the posterior arch of the atlas with the right hand. The cranium is cradled with the left hand such that the palmar aspect of the fifth digit palpates the temporal/occipital region.

Localization: fix the atlas and localize the motion barrier by side-flexing the occiput around an anteroposterior oblique axis to the physiological limit, simultaneously translating the right occipital condyle anteromedially on the superior facet of the atlas.

Mobilization: from this position, the patient is instructed to hold the head still while the therapist attempts to left side-flex the occiput around the oblique axis. This isometric contraction recruits the right superior oblique and the right rectus lateralis muscles. The contraction is held for three to five seconds following which the patient is instructed to relax completely. The new barrier for occipital right side-flexion/left rotation is localized. The technique is repeated three times.

Atlanto-axial joints—biomechanics

The atlas is capable of two degrees of voluntary motion, flexion/extension and rotation. Flexion/extension of the atlas occurs about a coronal axis through the body of the C2 vertebra. Full flexion requires an anterior roll of the inferior facets of the atlas on the superior facets of the axis together with an inferior translation of the anterior arch of the atlas on the anterior aspect of the dens at the median atlanto-axial joint. Full extension requires a posterior roll of atlas at the lateral joints and a superior translation of the anterior arch of the atlas at the median joint. An inextensible rectus capitus posterior major bilaterally can limit full flexion at the atlanto-axial joint.

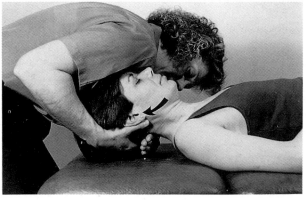

Fig. 52.3 Muscle energy technique to restore flexion at the occipito-atlantal joints. The arrow indicates the direction of occipital motion during this technique.

Rotation of the atlas occurs about a vertical axis through the dens. Left rotation requires an antero-inferior translation of the right lateral atlanto-axial joint, a postero-inferior translation of the left lateral atlanto-axial joint and an inferolateral translation of the atlas at the median joint. An inextensible right inferior oblique muscle can limit this motion. From a rotated position, the atlas is capable of side-flexing both to the left and right (Penning 1978).

Atlanto-axial joints—muscle energy techniques

Restricted left rotation—atlas/axis (Fig. 52.5). The aim of the technique is to restore left rotation at the atlanto-axial joints.

Patient: sitting with the back supported against a chair.
Therapist: standing at the patient's left side.
Palpate: with an open pinch grip, palpate the posterior arch of the axis with the right hand. The cranium is cradled with the left hand and the palmar aspect of the fifth digit palpates the posterior arch of the atlas on the right side.
Localization: fix the axis and localize the motion barrier by rotating the atlas around a vertical axis to the left (Fig. 52.5, black arrow). Simultaneously, side-flex the occiput to the right to release the tension in the right alar ligament (Fig. 52.5, white arrow). The motion barrier for left atlanto-axial rotation will not be achieved unless this side-flexion occurs.
Mobilization: from this position, the patient is instructed to hold the head still while the therapist attempts to increase the left rotation. This isometric contraction recruits the right inferior oblique muscle. The contraction is held for three to five seconds following which the patient is instructed to relax completely. The new barrier

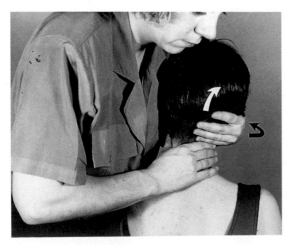

Fig. 52.5 Muscle energy technique to restore left rotation at the atlanto-axial joints. See the text for an explanation of the arrows.

for left rotation of the atlas is localized. The technique is repeated three times.

Midcervical region

Biomechanics

The midcervical motion segment (zygapophyseal joints, uncovertebral joints and interbody joint) is capable of two degrees of voluntary motion, flexion/extension and rotation/side-flexion. Flexion/extension of the superior vertebra occurs about a coronal axis through the body of the inferior vertebra (Penning 1978). At the zygapophyseal joints, full flexion requires an anterosuperior slide of the inferior facets of the superior vertebra on the superior facets of the inferior vertebra. Full extension requires a postero-inferior slide of the inferior facets of the superior vertebra on the superior facets of the inferior vertebra. The degree of anteroposterior translation associated with the sagittal rotation is governed by the level considered and the location of the axis of motion (Penning 1978). There is also a slight 'gapping' of the joint surfaces at the inferior aspect at the limit of flexion and the superior aspect at the limit of extension (Kapandji 1974). Similar arthrokinematics occur at the uncovertebral joints during flexion/extension.

Rotation/side-flexion is a unidirectional motion about an oblique anteroposterior axis (Penning & Wilmink 1987). At the zygapophyseal joints, right rotation/side-flexion requires an anterosuperomedial slide of the inferior facet of the superior vertebra on the left together with a postero-inferomedial slide of the inferior facet of the superior vertebra on the right. The same sliding motion occurs at the uncovertebral joints.

A facilitated segment can result in hypertonicity of the multifidus muscle (Korr 1975, 1976, Patterson 1976), the deep fibres of which attach to the capsule of the zygapophyseal joint. This muscle can then alter the optimal instantaneous axis of motion for rotation. The resultant axis for rotation is displaced posterior to the zygapophyseal joint and runs obliquely lateral from the median plane. Arthrokinematically, this can limit superior, anterior and medial slide of the ipsilateral facet or inferior, posterior and medial slide of the contralateral facet.

Midcervical region—muscle energy techniques

Restricted flexion/right rotation/side-flexion—C4–5 (Fig. 52.6). The aim of the technique is to restore flexion and right rotation/side-flexion at the zygapophyseal and the uncovertebral joints at C4–5.

Patient: supine, head supported on a pillow.
Therapist: standing at the patient's head facing the shoulders.

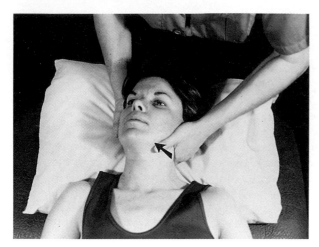

Fig. 52.6 Muscle energy technique to restore flexion and right rotation/side-flexion at C4–5. The arrow indicates the direction of motion of C4–5 during this technique.

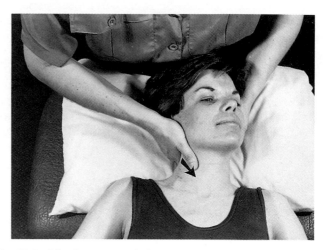

Fig. 52.7 Muscle energy technique to restore extension and right rotation/side-flexion at C4–5. The arrow indicates the direction of motion of C4–5 during this technique.

Palpate: with the lateral aspect of the left index finger, palpate the lamina and spinous process of the C4 vertebra on the left. With the other hand, support the cranium and neck superior to the level being treated on the right.

Localization: the motion barrier of the C4–5 joint is localized using an incongruent lock of the cranial segments. The localization is accomplished by side-flexing C2–3 and C3–4 to the left leaving the craniovertebral region in neutral, and then rotating C2–3 and C3–4 to the right. From this position, the motion barrier for flexion, right rotation/side-flexion at C4–5 is localized by passively rotating C4 about the appropriate oblique axis to the right. This motion induces right rotation of C4–5 or arthrokinematically an anterosuperomedial glide of the left zygapophyseal joint (Fig. 52.6, black arrow).

Mobilization: from this position, the patient is instructed to hold the head still while the therapist attempts to left rotate the head/neck. The contraction is held for three to five seconds following which the patient is instructed to relax completely. The new barrier for flexion, right rotation/side-flexion is localized. The technique is repeated three times.

Restricted extension/right rotation/side-flexion— C4–5 (Fig. 52.7). The aim of the technique is to restore extension and right rotation/side-flexion at the zygapophyseal and uncovertebral joints at C4–5.

Patient: supine, head supported on a pillow.

Therapist: standing at the patient's head facing the shoulders.

Palpate: with the lateral aspect of the left index finger, palpate the lamina and spinous process of the C4 vertebra. With the other hand, support the cranium and neck superior to the level being treated.

Localization: the localization is accomplished by side-flexing the neck to the right to C3–4 leaving the craniovertebral region in neutral, and then rotating the neck to

the left to C3–4. From this position, the motion barrier for extension, right rotation/side-flexion at C4–5 is localized by passively gliding the left inferior articular process of C4 postero-inferomedially on C5 (Fig. 52.7, black arrow).

Mobilization: from this position, the patient is instructed to hold the head still while the therapist attempts to increase the right rotation of the head/neck. The contraction is held for three to five seconds following which the patient is instructed to relax completely. The new barrier for extension, right rotation/side-flexion is localized. The technique is repeated three times.

Thorax region

Biomechanics

The thoracic motion segment is potentially capable of three degrees of voluntary motion, flexion/extension, side-flexion and rotation. Flexion/extension of the superior vertebra occurs about a coronal axis. Flexion requires a superior slide of the inferior facets of the superior vertebra on the superior facets of the inferior vertebra. Full extension requires an inferior slide of the inferior facets of the superior vertebra on the superior facets of the inferior vertebra. There is also a small degree of anteroposterior translation associated with the sagittal rotation (Panjabi et al 1976).

Without the attachment of the ribs at the costotransverse, costochondral and sternocostal joints, the zygapophyseal joints in the thoracic spine would be capable of pure side-flexion and pure rotation (Panjabi et al 1976). However, the intact costal 'ring' influences the resultant motion such that both side-flexion and rotation of the ring are coupled with translation and another rotation. For example, lateral bending of the trunk induces ipsilateral side-flexion and contralateral rotation of the ring below the second thoracic level. Rotation of the trunk, however, induces ipsilateral rotation and ipsilateral side-flexion of the ring. The initial motion appears to guide the direction of the coupled movement.

Thorax region—muscle energy techniques

Restricted flexion/left rotation/left side-flexion—T6–7 (Fig. 52.8). The aim of the technique is to restore flexion and left rotation/side-flexion at T6–7.

Patient: sitting with the arms crossed to opposite shoulders.

Therapist: standing at the patient's left side.

Palpate: with the right hand, palpate the intertransverse space between T6 and T7.

Localization: the motion barrier of the T6–7 joint is localized by flexing and then left rotating the trunk only until the barrier is perceived at the T6–7 level.

Mobilization: from this position, the patient is instructed to hold still while the therapist attempts to right rotate the trunk. The contraction is held for three to five seconds following which the patient is instructed to relax completely. The new barrier for flexion/left rotation/left side-flexion is localized. The technique is repeated three times.

Restricted extension/right rotation/right side-flexion—T6–7 (Fig. 52.9). The aim of the technique is to restore extension and right rotation/side-flexion at T6–7.

Patient: sitting with the arms crossed to opposite shoulders.

Therapist: standing at the patient's left side.

Palpate: with the right hand, palpate the intertransverse space between T6 and T7.

Localization: the motion barrier of the T6–7 joint is localized by extending and then right rotating the trunk only until the barrier is perceived at the T6–7 level.

Mobilization: from this position, the patient is instructed to hold still while the therapist attempts to left rotate the trunk. The contraction is held for three to five seconds following which the patient is instructed to relax completely. The new barrier for extension/right rotation/right side-flexion is localized. The technique is repeated three times.

Lumbar region

Biomechanics

The lumbar motion segment is capable of two degrees of voluntary motion, flexion/extension and side-flexion/rotation. Flexion/extension of the superior vertebra occurs about a coronal axis which moves forward with increasing degrees of flexion (Gracovetsky & Farfan 1986). At the zygapophyseal joints, full flexion requires an antero-

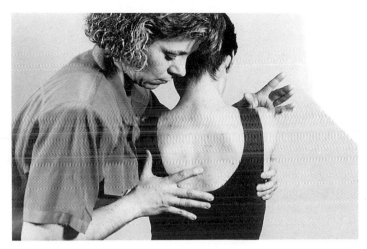

Fig. 52.8 Muscle energy technique to restore flexion and left rotation/side-flexion at T6–7.

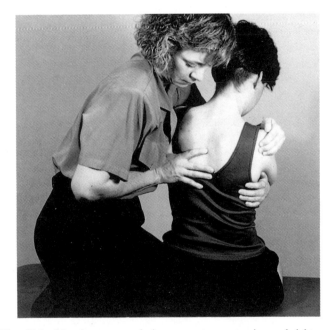

Fig. 52.9 Muscle energy technique to restore extension and right rotation/side-flexion at T6–7.

superior slide of the inferior facets of the superior vertebra on the superior facets of the inferior vertebra. Full extension requires a postero-inferior slide of the inferior facets of the superior vertebra on the superior facets of the inferior vertebra. There is also a slight 'gapping' of the inferior joint surfaces at the limit of flexion and the superior joint surfaces at the limit of extension (Twomey & Taylor 1983).

Side-flexion/rotation (from a neutral position) is a unidirectional motion about an oblique anteroposterior axis (Gracovetsky & Farfan 1986). Rotation to the left induces slight flexion and right side-flexion of the superior vertebra (Fig. 52.10). From a position of hyperextension or hyperflexion, the zygapophyseal joints influence the coupled movement pattern such that ipsilateral side-flexion and rotation occurs (Fig. 52.11).

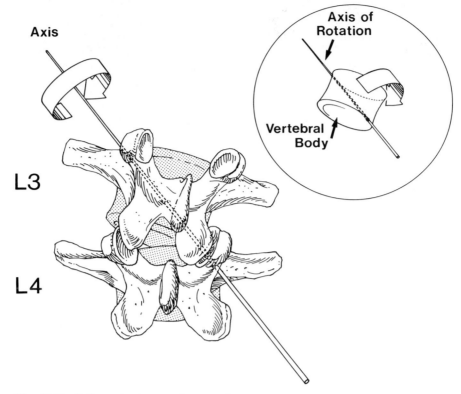

Fig. 52.10 Left rotation in neutral occurs about an anteroposterior oblique axis such that left rotation is coupled with right side-flexion. (Reproduced with permission from Lee 1989 and the publisher, Churchill Livingstone.)

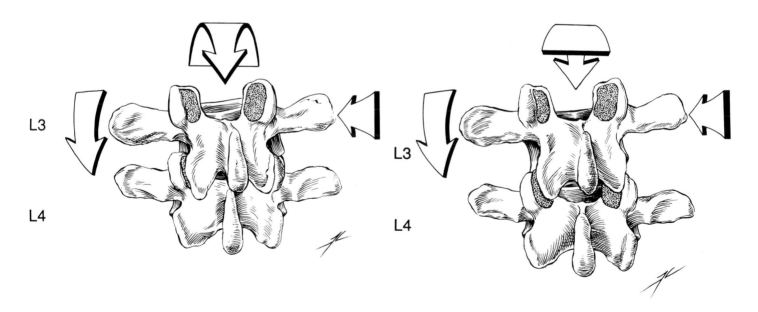

Fig. 52.11 From a position of hyperflexion or hyperextension, the zygapophyseal joints influence the movement pattern such that left rotation is coupled with left side-flexion.

A facilitated segment can result in hypertonicity of the multifidus muscle (Korr 1975, Patterson 1976), the deep fibres of which attach to the capsule of the zygapophyseal joint (Twomey et al 1989, Taylor et al 1990). This muscle can then alter the optimal instantaneous axis of motion for rotation *even in neutral*. The resultant axis for rotation is displaced posterior to the zygapophyseal joint and runs obliquely lateral from the median plane. From all three positions of the trunk, hyperflexion, neutral and hyperextension, the motion segment would side-flex and rotate to the same side (Fig. 52.11). Muscle energy techniques are very effective in restoring the normal muscle balance in these situations.

Lumbar region—muscle energy techniques

Restricted flexion/right side-flexion—L3–4 (Fig. 52.12). The aim of the technique is to restore flexion and right side-flexion at L3–4.

Patient: left side-lying, head supported on a pillow.
Therapist: standing, facing the patient.
Localization: palpate the interspinous space at L2–3. Rotate the thorax to the right (by using the patient's left arm) until full rotation of L2–3 is achieved. Palpate the interspinous space between L4–5. Flex the patient's right hip and knee until full flexion of L4–5 is achieved. Palpate the interspinous space at L3–4. The motion barrier for flexion and right side-flexion is engaged passively through either the pelvic girdle, the thorax or a combination of both. This motion will induce a supero-anterior slide of the left zygapophyseal joint.
Mobilization: from this position, the patient is instructed to hold the pelvis/thorax still while the therapist attempts to increase the right side-flexion (Fig. 52.14, white arrow). The contraction is held for three to five seconds following which the patient is instructed to relax completely. The new barrier for flexion/right side-flexion is localized. The technique is repeated three times.

Restricted extension/left side-flexion—L3–4 (Fig. 52.13). The aim of the technique is to restore extension and left side-flexion at L3–4.

Patient: right side-lying, head supported on a pillow.
Therapist: standing, facing the patient.
Localization: palpate the interspinous space at L2–3. Rotate the thorax to the left (by using the patient's right arm) until full rotation of L2–3 is achieved. Palpate the interspinous space between L4–5. Flex the patient's left hip and knee until full flexion of L4–5 is achieved. Palpate the interspinous space at L3–4. The motion barrier for extension/left side-flexion is engaged passively through either the pelvic girdle, the thorax or a combination of both. This motion will induce an inferoposterior slide of the left zygapophyseal joint.
Mobilization: from this position, the patient is instructed to hold the pelvis/thorax still while the therapist attempts to increase the left side-flexion (Fig. 52.13, white arrow). The contraction is held for three to five seconds following which the patient is instructed to relax completely. The new barrier for extension/left side-flexion is localized. The technique is repeated three times.

Pelvic girdle region

The reader is referred to Fowler (this volume, Ch. 57) for a description of the muscle energy techniques applicable to pelvic girdle disorders. A complete dissertation of the subject is referenced for the interested reader (Lee 1989).

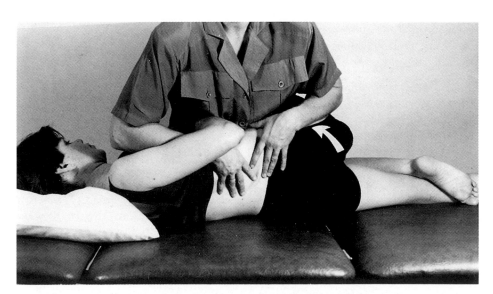

Fig. 52.12 Muscle energy technique to restore flexion and right side-flexion at L3–4. The arrow indicates the direction of resistance applied by the therapist during this technique.

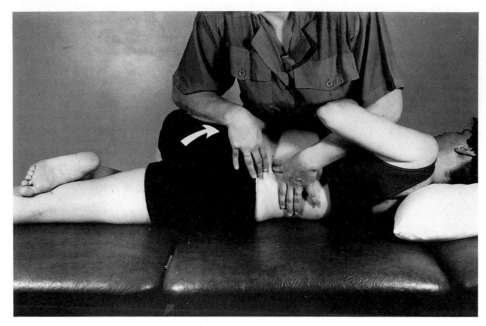

Fig. 52.13 Muscle energy technique to restore extension and left side-flexion at L3–4. The arrow indicates the direction of resistance applied by the therapist during this technique.

Stabilization techniques

Segmental stabilization via muscle energy technique requires specific localization of the unstable joint. The *segmental* musculature is recruited eccentrically, then isometrically, and finally concentrically by very specific resistance applied in a very specific direction following very specific instructions from the therapist (Pettman 1990).

Left rotational instability—L4–5

It is not uncommon to find the motor control of left rotation at L4–5 weak when the joint complex is unstable in the same direction. Rehabilitation of this control is initiated via a stabilization technique (modified muscle energy technique).

Patient: right side-lying, head supported on a pillow.
Therapist: standing, facing the patient.
Localization: the L4–5 segment is localized in the usual manner (see techniques under 'Lumbar region'). The appropriate oblique axis for neutral left rotation (Fig. 52.10) of the segment is found. The patient is instructed to resist gently the attempts of the therapist to right rotate the thorax (Fig. 52.14) (thus recruiting the muscles which left rotate the segment). The patient is then instructed to allow the thorax to right rotate *slowly* such that the left rotary muscles are contracting eccentrically against the therapist's applied resistance. At the limit of the right rotation range, the patient is instructed to hold against an isometric resistance for three to five seconds. This manoeuvre is repeated until eccentric and isometric motor control is efficient. This may take the entire treatment session.

Subsequently, the technique is taken further by instructing the patient to left rotate the thorax (from the limit of right rotation noted above) against the therapist's decreasing resistance, which is now less than the patient's effort, thus inducing a concentric contraction of the left rotary muscles. The goal is to achieve a smooth eccentric contraction of the left rotary muscles followed by an isometric hold followed by a concentric contraction of the muscles which control left rotation of the segment!

These techniques require a motivated patient and a patient therapist. They are difficult to teach but once learned are extremely effective in maintaining segmental control. However, further education and global exercises are necessary if this stability is to be integrated into the patient's activities of daily living.

FUNCTIONAL TECHNIQUE—PRINCIPLES

Functional technique was originated by Harold Hoover, an osteopathic physician. Most of the literature on this subject is found in the yearbooks of the Academy of Applied Osteopathy between 1950 and 1960.

The aim of functional technique is to reduce the exaggerated spindle responses from facilitated segmental muscles to restore normal joint mobility (Fig. 52.2). Contrary to a muscle energy technique, when a functional

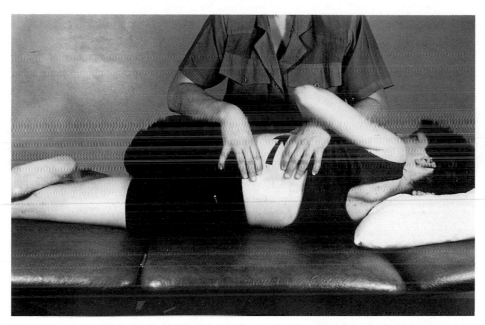

Fig. 52.14   Stabilization therapy. The arrow indicates the direction of the applied resistance.

technique is used the joint is passively taken *away* from the motion barrier and *no muscle effort* from the patient is required. One of the therapist's hands palpates the segmental musculature for an increase and/or decrease in reactivity and hypertonicity. The therapist's other hand (the moving hand) senses the muscular reaction via an increase or decrease in the resistance to motion. This is an indirect technique (Hartman 1983) the aim of which is to find the direction of relative ease of motion and to avoid the direction of resistance to motion. The joint is passively positioned such that the facilitated muscle spindle is shortened. The afferent discharge from the primary annulospiral ending is therefore reduced and the central nervous system decreases the alpha and the gamma motoneuron discharge, thereby allowing the extrafusal muscle fibre to relax (Fig. 52.2). This position of ease is maintained for up to 90 seconds following which the joint is returned to its neutral resting position providing that no increase in resistance to motion occurs during the return route. If the intrafusal/extrafusal muscle fibre length relationship has been restored, the segmental muscles will allow the joint to return to its normal resting position without increasing the resting muscle tone (Korr 1975).

It has been noted that these techniques are difficult to master.

All these techniques are a form of inhibition, in that areas of irritability are quieted, the operator is constantly looking for the state of ease and release, rather than looking for the point of bind and barrier and attempting to fight through it.

Whilst it must be said that anybody can learn to manipulate, the fine details of these subtle types of techniques require constant assiduous practice to ensure their effectiveness. (Hartman 1983)

The key factors in effecting success with a functional technique are accurate palpation of the segmental musculature, low speed of application and sustained duration of the technique. A functional technique can be extremely effective even in acute joint conditions and is contraindicated only when a mechanical dysfunction has not been ascertained.

CLINICAL APPLICATION OF FUNCTIONAL TECHNIQUE

With the patient sitting, the therapist palpates the segment concerned with the dorsal hand while the other supports the head, neck or thorax. The segment is slowly guided into flexion, extension, left and right rotation, left and right side-flexion and combinations thereof (Fig. 52.15) until the exact position which promotes muscular relaxation has been attained. This position is maintained for 90 seconds during which minute ranges of motion are performed in the direction which facilitates relaxation. Any movement which results in increasing resistance is avoided. A sensation of 'release' will often be perceived by the palpating hand following which a dramatic increase in segmental range of motion usually occurs.

CONCLUSION

When the ability to move is lost, optimal function is im-

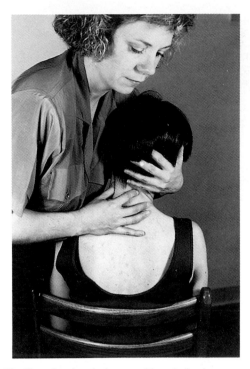

Fig. 52.15 Functional technique—midcervical spine.

paired. The musculoskeletal system will compensate this loss by altering its optimal biomechanics. This can lead to tissue breakdown and pain. The restoration of normal motion requires attention to the bones, joints, muscles, nerves and circulatory system. Muscle energy and functional techniques are but another instrument in the toolbox of the manual therapist. 'No one particular technical approach is the answer to all problems and the wider the spectrum of the operator's armament the more he(she) is liable to be able to help a broader span of patients and a greater number of conditions with greater facility.' (Hartman 1983).

Acknowledgements

The author would like to gratefully acknowledge the assistance of Frank Crymble for preparing the original line drawings, Janet Lowcock for modelling and Thomas Lee for taking the clinical photographs in this chapter.

REFERENCES

Gracovetsky S, Farfan H F 1986 The optimum spine. Spine 11: 543–573

Hartman L S 1983 Handbook of osteopathic technique. NMK Publishers, Herts

Kabat H, Licht S (eds) 1961 Proprioceptive facilitation in therapeutic exercise. Therapeutic exercise, 2nd edn. New Haven Press, New Haven

Kapandji I A 1974 The physiology of joints III: the trunk and vertebral column, 2nd edn. Churchill Livingstone, Edinburgh

Korr I M 1975 Proprioceptors and somatic dysfunction. Journal of the American Osteopathic Association 74: 123–135

Korr I M 1976 The spinal cord as organizer of disease processes: some preliminary perspectives. Journal of the American Osteopathic Association 76: 89–99

Lee D G 1989 The pelvic girdle: an approach to the examination and treatment of the lumbo-pelvic-hip region. Churchill Livingstone, Edinburgh

Lee D G, Walsh M C 1985 A workbook of manual therapy techniques for the vertebral column and pelvic girdle. Nascent, Delta

Mitchell F L, Moran P S, Pruzzo N A 1979 An evaluation and a treatment manual of osteopathic muscle energy procedures. Mitchell Moran and Pruzzo Associates, Valley Park

Panjabi M M, Brand R A, White A A 1976 Mechanical properties of the human thoracic spine. Journal of Bone and Joint Surgery 58A: 642–652

Patterson M M 1976 A model mechanism for spinal segmental facilitation. Journal of the American Osteopathic Association 76: 121–131

Penning L 1978 Normal movements of the cervical spine. American Journal of Roentgenology 130: 317–326

Penning L, Wilmink J T 1987 Rotation of the cervical spine: CT study in normal subjects. Spine 12: 732–738

Pettman E 1990 Personal communication. Upper and Lower Quadrant Courses, Vancouver

Taylor J R, Twomey L T, Corker M 1990 Bone and soft tissue injuries in post-mortem lumbar spines. Paraplegia 28: 119–129

Twomey L T, Taylor J R 1983 Sagittal movements of the human lumbar vertebral column: a quantitative study of the role of the posterior vertebral elements. Archives of Physical Medicine and Rehabilitation 64: 322–326

Twomey L T, Taylor J R, Taylor M M 1989 Unsuspected damage to lumbar zygapophyseal (facet) joints after motor-vehicle accidents. The Medical Journal of Australia 151: 210–217

Weisl S W, Rothman R H 1979 Occipitoatlantal hypermobility. Spine 4: 187–191

Wyke B 1981 The neurology of joints: a review of general principles. Clinics in Rheumatic Diseases 7: 223–239

53. 'SNAGS': mobilizations of the spine with active movement

B. R. Mulligan

INTRODUCTION

This chapter is to acquaint the reader with a new approach to manual therapy which has yet to be scientifically vindicated but which is nevertheless extremely exciting, useful, safe and, when the concept is clearly understood, easy to undertake.

The origin of the term 'SNAGS' is a complex one. Simply stated, it is an acronym for 'sustained natural apophyseal glides'. The term has caught on; it is brief, explicit and therefore useful when writing case notes. With regard to recording, the only added descriptions required are the level and the movement loss being dealt with. Thus, therapist notes may say 'SNAGS left rotation Th 6/7'. If the glide with the active movement was applied, for example, over the left facet and not over the spinous process then this would be indicated, i.e. 'SNAGS left rotation (L) Th 6/7'. This description will be more meaningful when this chapter has been read.

TECHNIQUES

The techniques to be dealt with in this chapter are for the spine. The same principles and techniques can be applied to many extremity joints. The author refers to some of these elsewhere (Mulligan 1989).

There are many texts now available on spinal manual therapy. However, none meet *all* the listed criteria when claiming SNAGS are a new approach. These are:

1. They are weight-bearing.
2. They are carried out at end-of-range.
3. They follow the treatment plane rule that applies to extremity joints.
4. They are sustained.
5. They can be applied to most spinal joints.
6. When indicated they are *painless*. They eliminate any pain associated with the movement taking place.
7. They are mobilizations which are combined with active movement, which is a new concept.
8. Within a couple of minutes you can decide if they are indicated.
9. There is a straightforward procedure for each movement loss.

For clarification, the above list must be discussed in more detail:

1. They are weight-bearing. Many manipulations are done with the patient sitting, and thus weight-bearing, but none for instance for the back with the patient standing. In the case of mobilization, all the texts usually have the patient lying. With SNAGS all procedures are done with the patient sitting or standing. This has many advantages. The improvements, when they occur, take place in a functional posture, making assessment of their efficacy simple. Improvements are real. Before using SNAGS the author had found that, while more conventional manual therapies have shown an immediate improvement in function while the patient is lying, it is often lost when the patient resumes a weight-bearing posture. For all the techniques to be weight-bearing is a new approach.

2. They are carried out at end-of-range. Mobilizations are usually performed with the joints positioned in a resting position. SNAGS are always involved with the end range of movement. They are initiated short of end range and are maintained as the joint is actively moved into this end position. If a joint is restricted, it is expected when applying SNAGS that the restriction will disappear or be dramatically reduced. If the restriction does not alter at the time of delivery then the technique is abandoned as it is obviously not appropriate. These techniques are so good when indicated that, with the very first mobilization with active movement, an improvement in the range will be observed.

3. SNAGS follow the treatment plane rule that applies to extremity joints. Kaltenborn (1980), in his book *Mobilization of the Extremity Joints*, states 'When performing joint mobilization, a bone is moved parallel or at a right angle to the treatment plane'. When examining a mobile joint one facet is usually concave and the other convex. The treatment plane is best described as the plane across the concave articular facet (see Fig. 53.1). Although Kaltenborn's book is dealing with extremity joints the same rule applies when mobilizing spinal joints.

In the laboratory, using spinal dissections where the capsules of the joints have not been disturbed, it is easy to make a superior cervical facet glide on its inferior partner when

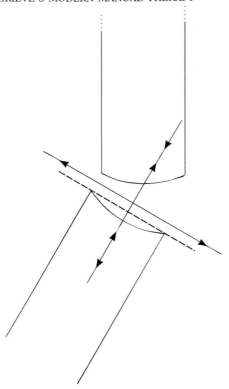

Fig. 53.1 The dotted line shows the treatment plane. Arrows show the direction of glides and traction.

attention is paid to the treatment plane. If a glide was attempted outside the treatment plane this movement was absent (Oliver 1991).

4. They are sustained. Most physiotherapy mobilizations for the spine are oscillatory, i.e. Maitland. SNAGS are mobilizations where the facet glide taking place is sustained while active movement is occurring, and this glide is maintained until the joint returns to its starting position. If a joint in the neck was being SNAGGED for a loss of rotation then the therapist must not stop the procedure until the neck is again in the mid-line. To break this rule might result in a painful response, although no damage would occur.

5. They can be applied to most spinal joints. One is referring here to the mobile facet joints from the occiput to the sacrum and not the mobile articulation between the sacrum and the coccyx.

6. When indicated they are painless and eliminate any pain associated with the movement taking place. The indications for SNAGS hinges around this statement which is, in fact, a rule governing their application. The explanation to the patient, and the patient's cooperation, is absolutely essential for them to be successful. If there is any pain when undertaking a mobilization with movement then *stop*. The therapist will never exacerbate a patient's condition if this rule is followed. The pain of course could be felt because the therapist has chosen the wrong level to mobilize or is not applying the treatment plane rule.

7. They are mobilizations combined with active movements which, of course, is a truly new concept. One should have included in this claim that the active movements are in a weight-bearing mode. When therapists examine patients, active movements are always tested for restrictions and for whether or not they provoke pain. SNAGS are always undertaken in the direction of pain and/or movement loss.

8. Within a couple of minutes you can decide if they are indicated. A patient may present with neck pain. If testing shows a painful loss of extension and right rotation then SNAGS for extension and then rotation can be tried. Provided the therapist is treating the correct level, the pain with movement should disappear and the range of movement increase. If there is any pain, stop, check the level and the technique. If still painful, SNAGS would not be indicated. This whole routine only takes a short time.

9. There is a straightforward procedure for each spinal movement loss. Therapists should in practice be quick to learn these techniques. They have of course had manual therapy backgrounds. The bulk of this chapter will deal in detail with these procedures, and it would help if the reader was familiar with NAGS and REVERSE NAGS which are weight-bearing oscillatory mobilizations for the cervical and upper thoracic spines. These mobilizations preceded and led to the development of SNAGS (Mulligan 1989).

Before continuing, it is necessary to state that SNAGS, just like other forms of manual therapy, are only part of the treatment programme for patients presenting with musculoskeletal disorders. Other therapies are given concurrently together with advice etc. and in this text some of the home SELF SNAGS routines given to patients are described. It is more than worthwhile reading this article just to know of these exercises – especially with regard to restricted neck movements.

DESCRIPTION

As with all therapies before they are initiated, an explanation should be given to the patient. The success of SNAGS is totally dependent on cooperation from the patient. To oblige, they must fully understand what the therapist is doing, and the most important thing to stress is that the technique combined with their active movement *must* be painless. Pain may be experienced for several reasons and these should be checked out. Firstly, the therapist may have chosen the wrong level in the spine. Secondly, the mobilizing direction may not be parallel with the treatment plane. Thirdly, the handling by the therapist rather than the technique may be at fault. If tissues are tender to the touch of the therapist's finger or hand, pressure can be applied through a thin layer of plastic foam. Finally, SNAGS may be inappropriate and should never be applied if they produce pain.

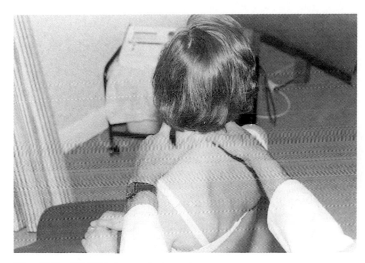

Fig. 53.2 SNAGS for cervical rotation.

It is easier to describe SNAGS as they are used for each movement loss in the spine.

THE CERVICAL AND UPPER THORACIC SPINES

To increase rotation and/or decrease the pain associated with this movement

The patient is seated, with the therapist standing behind. From the history and assessment already done there will be some indication as to which level of the spine is involved. If, for example, restriction is located at cervical 5/6, place the medial border of one thumb on the spinous process of cervical 5. Now glide the spinous process up in the direction of the treatment plane using your other thumb to apply the force (see Fig. 53.2). While this glide is being sustained the patient is asked to turn their head in the painful, restricted direction – provided that it does not hurt. As the head moves around, the therapist's hands must move in the same direction to maintain the glide in the treatment plane. If SNAGS are indicated and the therapist's technique is correct the patient will now be able to rotate their head further and experience no pain. From Figure 53.2 note that the therapist's fingers are resting on each side of the neck pointing in the direction of the facet planes. They tend to guide the neck around. If this technique has the desired effect then repeat it six to ten times and then re-assess the patient's active movement.

Most therapists only see individual patients two or three times a week. Consequently, a very simple way for the patients to SNAG themselves is described for self-administration. Naturally, this routine is called SELF SNAGS. All that is needed is a small hand towel. The selvedge on one side is used to hook under the appropriate spinous process. The ends of the towel are firmly held and an upward pull is applied (along the facet planes) as the head is rotated in the painful direction (see Fig. 53.3).

Provided the direction of pull is right, and the correct level is chosen, patients will improve. Patients are encouraged to repeat the exercise ten times, two-hourly, until their problem is better. It is worthwhile to get patients to start on the incorrect level so that they feel pain with the movement. The patients then stop immediately and try other levels until they get it right.

Various mistakes that patients make are as follows. (i) Patients forget to take their hands around with the movement; this will produce no benefit. (ii) Instead of using the selvedge, patients try to place a gathered towel under a spinous process. This will not work as it is not selective enough, and, when the towel is pulled up, one facet does not specifically glide up on its inferior partner. (iii) Another error is for patients to pull the towel forward instead of up which is useless and, as already mentioned, pulls up on the wrong process. (iv) Finally, patients often let the pressure off before they return to the mid-line – which can result in a sharp pain. Although difficult to explain, it is even better, when pulling up on the towel, to cross one's hands. The right hand grips the left side of the towel and the left hand the right side. If turning to the right the right hand is on top. This assists with the rotation while still maintaining a good facet glide (see Fig. 53.4).

To increase side flexion and/or decrease the pain associated with this movement

The technique is really very much the same as for rotation. The patient is seated, with the therapist standing behind. The therapist places the medial border of the distal phalanx of the thumb on the appropriate spinous process. If cervical 4/5 is the offending joint then the thumb would be on the spine of cervical 4. The other thumb is placed over its partner and provides the upward force as the patient tilts his head in the required direction (see Fig. 53.5). As with rotation, if the correct segment is chosen and SNAGS are indicated, the movement of side-flexion will not only increase but the patient will not experience any pain. Repeat the manoeuvre six to ten times and then re-assess the patient's active movement. Note from Figure 53.5 the position of the fingers which are pointing in the direction of the treatment plane. This ensures that the active movement taking place is that which is required.

As a follow-up to this treatment, the patient is then taught SELF SNAGS. As with rotation, a small towel is used and the selvedge on one side is hooked under the desired spinous process. The patient grips each end of the towel and pulls up along the treatment plane as he side-bends his spine in the restricted direction. When indicated, the movement will increase and be painless. SELF SNAGS should be repeated every two hours in sets of six to ten, or as the therapist feels necessary.

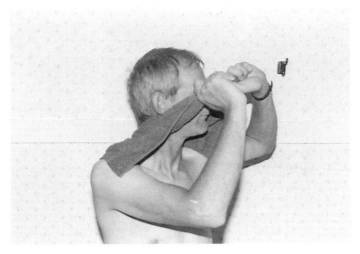

Fig. 53.3   Towel SELF SNAGS for rotation.

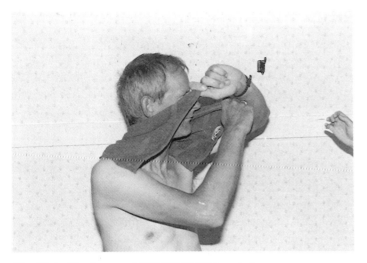

Fig. 53.4   Hands crossed SELF SNAGS for rotation.

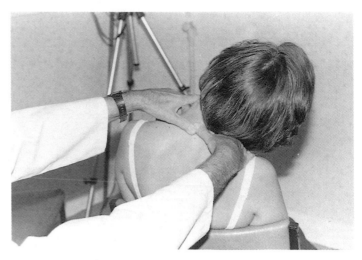

Fig. 53.5   SNAGS for side-flexion.

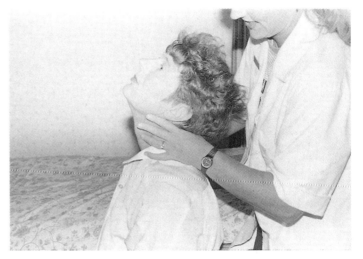

Fig. 53.6   SNAGS for extension.

To increase extension and/or decrease the pain associated with this movement

The patient is seated, and the therapist stands behind. The thumbs are again used under the superior spinous process of the offending segment as with rotation and side-flexion. As the patient extends their neck the therapist pushes up along the facet plane and maintains this pressure until the head is back in the neutral position (see Fig. 53.6). It is emphasized again that SNAGS must not be painful. If they are, they should not be used. The therapist should try two or three levels if the first choice is painful, in the case of starting on the wrong segment. Check also that the gliding direction is accurate.

SELF SNAGS with the towel are often more helpful with extension than SNAGS. This is because when using a thumb on a small spinous process the therapist will often lose the position as the patient extends and the spines approximate. The towel's thin selvedge stays nicely on

target. SELF SNAGS are applied as for side-flexion but a common fault that creeps in when the patients are not being supervised is that they forget to take their hands back with the head as it extends (see Fig. 53.7). This would mean that the glide along the treatment plane is lost and pain will result (see Fig. 53.8).

To increase flexion and/or decrease the pain associated with this movement

There are two techniques that can dramatically improve a patient's painful movement loss. The first to be described is SNAGS, but the second is quite different and is called FIST TRACTION.

SNAGS for flexion

The patient is sitting, and the therapist stands behind. The mobilizations with movement are applied in exactly the same way as those for the other neck restrictions.

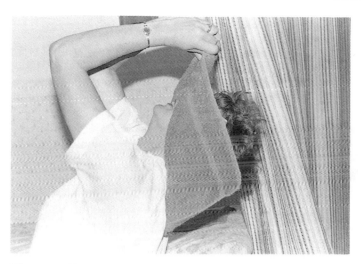

Fig. 53.7 SELF SNAGS for extension.

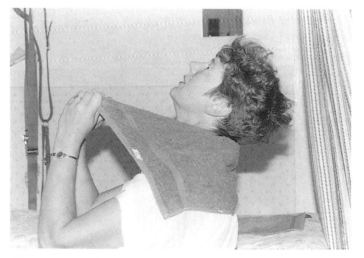

Fig. 53.8 Incorrect SELF SNAGS for extension. The towel is no longer pulling up along the treatment plane.

Place one thumb reinforced by the other under the superior spinous process of the suspected cervical joint and push up along the treatment plane as the patient flexes their neck. When appropriate, flexion is magically restored. As with the other movements, repeat the SNAGS several times and then test to see if the improvement is maintained. As a home programme the patient can be taught to SELF SNAG every two hours if necessary. A towel is again used to slide the superior facet up as flexion is taking place.

FIST TRACTIONS for flexion

This technique is simple to do, and, in over 90% of patients who experience pain with flexion, it is usually successful. It is also easy for a patient to apply; again, this is a bonus as there is an international trend towards self-treatment.

The patient is seated, and the therapist places a clenched fist under the patient's chin so that it lies in the centre of the circle formed by the curled index finger and thumb. The curled little finger lies on top of the sternum. The patient is asked to place a hand around their occiput and pull the head forward and down. The head, of course, cannot flex as the therapist's hand blocks the movement (see Fig. 53.9). The result is that the therapist's fist acts as a fulcrum, allowing the skull to rotate in a small arc around it and causing a traction to take place in the cervical spine. The traction being applied should produce *no* pain (if it does, desist) and should be maintained for at least ten seconds. Repeat three times and then re-assess the range of flexion. If the patient has a long neck, the clenched fist might not be large enough to produce the desired effect; in this case, use a book of sufficient thickness as a wedge instead. A patient can apply SELF FIST TRACTIONS by using his own fist or by placing a book under the chin (See Figs 53.10, 53.11). As with SNAGS, the traction must be painless and can be applied two-hourly by the patient if necessary.

Modifications

All the SNAGS techniques so far described have the therapist placing a thumb over the spinous process and thus applying the gliding force evenly through both facet joints at the offending level. The use of unilateral positioning is more specific. Thus, if the therapist suspects that the facet on the right is the restricted one inhibiting normal segmental movement from taking place, then place one thumb with the other on top on that side. As the active movement takes place, glide the facet up in the desired direction. Remember,

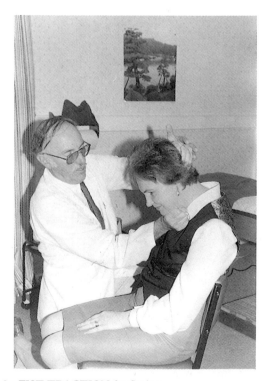

Fig. 53.9 FIST TRACTION for flexion.

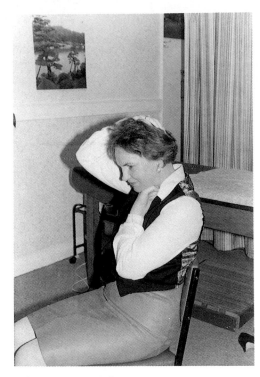

Fig. 53.10   Self traction with fist.

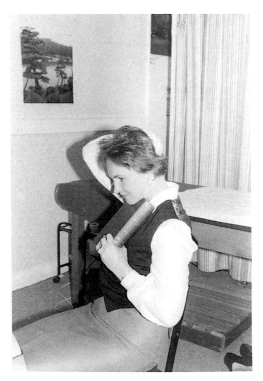

Fig. 53.11   Self traction with book.

as with central pressure, there must be no pain with the procedure. Unilateral SNAGS can be applied for any movement loss in the neck or upper thoracic spine.

THE LUMBAR SPINE

The use of SNAGS in the lumbar spine can be just as effective as in the cervical spine. In the early days of their application to the lumbar spine considerable physical effort was required until a belt was used for patient fixation. SNAGS in the lumbar spine are all undertaken with the patient weight-bearing, that is, sitting or standing.

When assessing the patient's active movements for restrictions and/or pain this should be done in both sitting and standing. If the patient's movement problems are present only when standing, then SNAGS are carried out in standing. If the patient has problems with sitting as well then the initial therapy is carried out in sitting and progresses to standing. The techniques are described as they would be applied for movement losses and/or pain.

To increase flexion and/or decrease the pain associated with this movement

The patient sits on the plinth, with legs over the side. The therapist stands behind the patient and places a fastened 'seat belt' around the patient and themselves, as shown in Figure 53.12. The seat belt is made from car seat belt material; it needs to be 2.5 m long and have a car seat-belt buckle which facilitates easy alteration of the fastened length being used. The seat belt makes the patient stable while mobilization with movement is taking place. The belt should make contact with the patient's lower abdo-

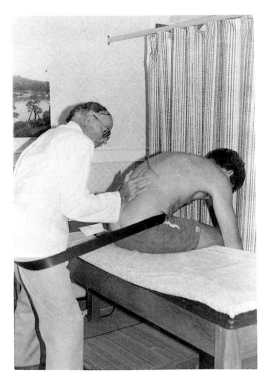

Fig. 53.12   SNAGS for lumbar flexion in sitting.

men so that it lies just below the anterior superior iliac spines. If care is not taken to place it this way, when SNAGS are applied great abdominal discomfort will be experienced. The therapist should have the belt lying over their sacrum. The ulnar border of the right hand is placed under the superior spinous process of the suspected offending segment. The other hand is placed on the bed beside the patient. The patient is now asked to flex forward while the therapist applies a gliding force up along the facet treatment plane provided the patient feels *no* pain. The gliding pressure is sustained until the patient has returned to the starting position. If pain with flexion is experienced choose another level and try again. If alternative levels do not enable the patient to flex without pain then a unilateral SNAGS should be tried. If the patient has a lumbar 4/5 lesion with right-sided symptoms then the therapist can hook the ulnar border of their right hand, just distal to the pisiform, over the superior facet of lumbar 4 on the right. As the patient bends forward the therapist pushes up along the facet plane to see if the patient can move more freely and with no pain. If there is pain then select another level or perhaps try gliding up on the left side. When there is no pain with SNAGS repeat the glide with movement six to ten times and then re-assess the patient. After these painless SNAGS there will now be a definite improvement. At this stage with a very acute lesion it is important that nothing further manually should be done. A minority of patients, as with other forms of manual therapy, can experience either some additional discomfort later on or the next day after treatment. It is of short duration and, when it subsides, they are usually much better – but therapists should be cautious and not over-treat on the first day until the patient's tolerance is known.

The next step would be to apply the technique with the patient standing (see Fig. 53.13). The patient is standing with the belt around both the patient and the therapist as it was for the starting position for the seated technique. The ulnar border of the therapist's right hand is placed under the spinous process at the appropriate level. The patient is asked to bend over while the therapist is gliding the superior facet up, provided there is no pain. It is even better if the patient's knees are slightly flexed while bending over. Remember, the aim is to improve spinal movement, and with the knees slightly flexed the hamstrings are released and there is less tension on the sciatic nerve. It is worth remembering, as with all the other SNAGS that are used, to maintain the spinous pressure until the patient is again standing erect. It may be necessary to use the technique unilaterally, as suggested with sitting, and this is done in the same way. For the lumbosacral segment, when applying unilateral SNAGS it is often necessary to use the thumbs over the superior facet of lumbar 5. This joint is very small, and often the ulnar border of the hand is not selective enough. The thumbs are used in the same

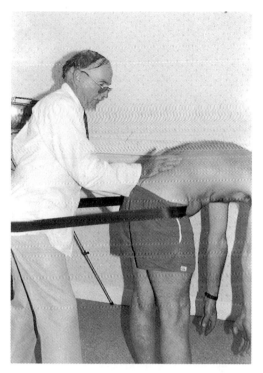

Fig. 53.13 SNAGS for lumbar flexion in standing.

way as described for the cervical spine. The therapist places the medial border of one thumb on the superior facet and uses the other thumb when placed over this to apply the gliding force up as the patient actively bends over (see Fig. 53.14). Remember *no* pain should be experienced. On close examination of the skeleton, the therapist will see that the palpable surfaces of the lumbar 4/5 and lumbosacral facets are indeed very small, and positioning accuracy with the thumbs is very important if the desired effect is to be achieved.

It is worth noting that most people presenting with acute back pain have considerable pain on active flexion and usually a marked loss of this movement. These patients, if SNAGS prove to be of value (i.e. restore flexion) are then taped for 48 h to prevent flexion and help them maintain a good posture (Fig. 53.15). This is to stop the patient from doing anything that might exacerbate the pain. The approach of spinal extension, as taught by therapists using McKenzie's protocols (1981), would be encouraged. However, extension, if it produced any pain, leads conveniently to the next technique.

To increase extension and/or decrease the pain associated with this movement

If extension is limited and/or painful in sitting then start with the patient sitting on the plinth with their legs over the side. Stand behind the patient with the 'seat belt' around both the therapist and the patient as it was for the flexion technique. Place the ulnar border of the therapist's

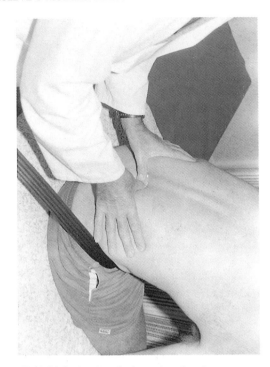

Fig. 53.14 SNAGS for lumbar flexion using thumbs.

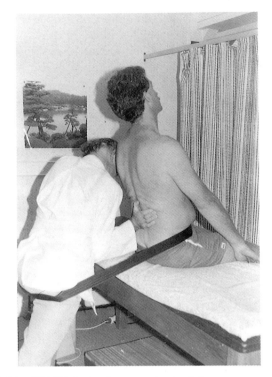

Fig. 53.16 SNAGS for lumbar extension in sitting.

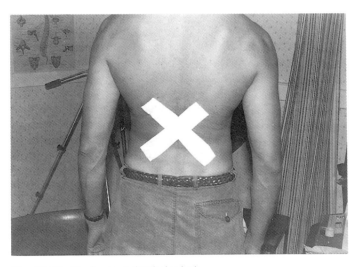

Fig. 53.15 Taping to maintain lordosis.

right hand (or left) under the superior spinous process of the segment involved. The patient is asked to extend while the therapist pushes up, provided that the patient feels no pain (see Fig. 53.16). The patient's co-operation is essential. If painful, stop and try another level. If still painful, try SNAGGING over the left or right articular pillars. Many patients with persistent low-back pain are seen and on examination a common finding is that flexion is unrestricted and pain-free, but not so extension. What is often necessary with these patients, if SNAGS for extension is unsuccessful, is to SNAG them in flexion first. This

would appear to release the facet(s) at the offending level and make a spectacular difference when SNAGS are again repeated for extension. As with the technique for flexion, the therapist would progress to SNAGS for extension in standing. Standing would, of course, be the starting position if extension were faultless in sitting in the first place (see Fig. 53.17).

To increase side-flexion and/or decrease the pain associated with this movement

When side-flexion is painful and limited, these symptoms are usually present in both sitting and standing, so the therapist would start with the patient seated as was the case for flexion and extension. The patient's legs are over the edge and the therapist is standing behind them. The 'seat belt' is around both therapist and patient, as it was for the previous techniques. The therapist now has a choice with, for example, left side-flexion to place the ulnar border of the gliding hand under the superior spinous process or the articular pillar on the right or left of the segment suspected as being involved. While the therapist is gliding the superior facet(s) up along the treatment plane the patient actively side-bends, provided there is no pain (see Fig. 53.18). The same procedure would then be repeated with the patient standing. Remember, when the SNAGS go according to plan, to repeat the routine six to ten times and then re-assess the patient's active movement. Never over-treat the patient on day one. The therapist is

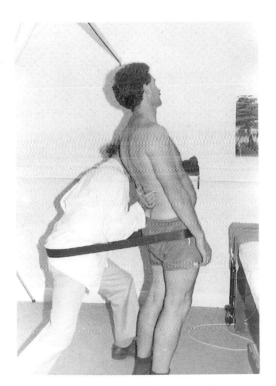

Fig. 53.17 SNAGS for lumbar extension in standing.

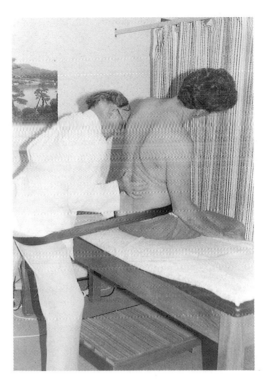

Fig. 53.18 SNAGS for lumbar side-flexion in sitting.

also advised not to be over-zealous with any technique that appears to be working very well. Wait until you re-assess the patient on their next visit as to the efficacy of the treatment given. Some joints can be very irritable.

To increase rotation and/or decrease the pain associated with this movement

The patient sits astride the plinth at one end and the therapist stands behind them. In the case of the patient who has a painful loss of right rotation as a result of a lesion involving the lumbar 3/4 level, the following is done. The patient places their hands behind their neck. The therapist clasps the patient around the waist with the right hand at the desired level and the ulnar border of the left hand is placed under the spinous process of lumbar 3. Provided the patient feels no pain, they are now asked to rotate to the right as the therapist applies a glide up along the treatment plane. The therapist's right hand encourages the active movement to take place at the desired level (see Fig. 53.19). As with the other techniques for the spine, it may be necessary to apply the glide over the appropriate right or left facet, with the active movement, rather than centrally.

SELF SNAGS FOR THE LUMBAR SPINE

Mobilizations with active movements can be performed at home using a belt. McKenzie (1981) refers to the centralization of pain. Repeated extensions in standing, for in-

stance, are encouraged if they centralize a pain that was being experienced in the posterior thigh. When a belt is used successfully by a patient to SELF SNAG they can do repeated extensions standing painlessly, and after several repetitions actively and painlessly extend without the belt. The purpose of any SNAG technique is to bring about an immediate improvement in the patient's movement after its completion. To SNAG a joint successfully only to find that after several repetitions no improvement has been achieved would suggest that the technique was inappropriate. The patient requires a belt (ideally car seat-belt material) long enough to go around their waist and still be gripped at each end at least a forearm's length from their body (see Fig. 53.20). If the lesion is, for example, at lumbar 3/4 and extension is painful, one side of the belt would be hooked under lumbar 3. While the patient actively extends he pulls up through the spinous process with the belt. When indicated and correctly done there should be no pain. Sets of SELF SNAGS would then be repeated two-hourly or at whatever interval the therapist deems necessary. If flexion was limited, and the patient in a great deal of pain, SELF SNAGS for flexion would be inadvisable for a few days. When teaching SELF SNAGS for flexion, have the patient's knees slightly flexed. This greatly enhances the range of movement and patient comfort while still achieving the same end result. After a set of self mobilizations with active flexion the patient would then do a set of extension SELF SNAGS as a precaution. Side-flexion can also be undertaken in the same way with the belt. The common fault

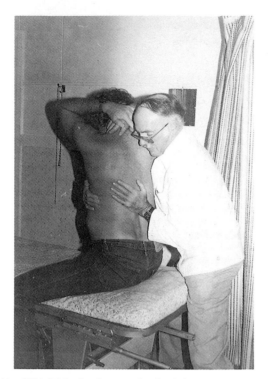

Fig. 53.19   SNAGS for lumbar rotation in sitting.

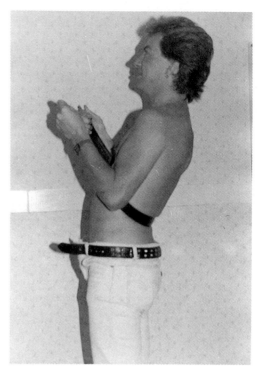

Fig. 53.20   SELF SNAGS standing using belt. Note the upward slope of the belt (compare with cervical spine).

encountered with SELF SNAGS is where the patient does not pull up along the facet planes. Patients tend to pull forwards instead, which will of course not work. SELF SNAGS for the lumbosacral joint will not work if the patient's posterior iliac borders protrude further posteriorly than the spinous process of lumbar 5. The edge of the belt cannot physically make contact with the spinous process.

THE THORACIC SPINE

The reader should now know how to apply SNAGS to the thoracic spine as they are really the same as for the lumbar spine. When dealing with the thoracic spine, rotation is the movement usually requiring attention. The technique of choice for this loss is a unilateral SNAG on the painful side.

WHY DO SNAGS WORK?

The question 'Why are SNAGS successful?' is frequently asked. Another question asked, as it seems paradoxical, why glide the facets up for extension when it has been previously stated to glide them up along the treatment planes for flexion? Why? Why? The explanations given here are conjecture and would not be acceptable to everyone. First, although SNAGS are geared to the mobilization of facet joints, they also involve the intervertebral discs. It is not possible to distort the disc or move either of the facet joints in isolation at an intervertebral segment. The movements that take place between the three articulations at an intervertebral segment are interrelated.

Rather than say that a patient has a disc or facet lesion, simply record the patient as having a segmental lesion. This is convenient as SNAGS really are a segmental technique, remembering that active movement is involved. If the range of movement in a facet joint is reduced, can a disc behave biomechanically as it is designed to – say – with flexion? It can be argued that it cannot. If the patient has a disc problem and a facet joint at the same level is not functioning properly, then unnatural strain would be placed on that disc and hinder its recovery. Restoring function to a restricted facet joint is the main reason that most manipulators would give to justify their treatment. Manipulations have their place, but because the therapist has got a satisfactory 'click' it cannot be assumed that the facet will now move freely enhancing pain-free segmental movement. Many patients do feel instantly better after manipulation, but just as many do not. SNAGS, because they are mobilizations with active movement, influence both the facet and disc in a desirable way and can be justified whether the pain the patient presents with is from the disc or a facet joint.

Secondly, the author has no problem with the fact that, with all the techniques, the gliding force is applied upward. When assessing active movements for pain and restriction the therapist will find that the pain experienced when the facet joints are being compressed as in extension is quite different from that felt with flexion. With the latter movement the joints are being stretched. When a facet joint is restricted and SNAGS work, it can only be presumed that the top facet is jammed caudally in an extension position and with active extension has nowhere to go. It jams further and pain results. Pushing up along the treatment plane repositions the facet so that it can now glide naturally and painlessly down. That is why, when SNAGS for extension do not work, SNAGS for flexion are done first. This helps to release the facet joint so that when SNAGS for extension are again repeated they are more effective. SNAGS for a flexion loss and pain make much more sense as you are gliding the superior facet up in its natural direction. The same hypothesis applies for side-flexion or rotation.

CONCLUSION

If the therapist masters the techniques covered in this chapter they will conclude that the justification for SNAGS in a treatment programme is the fact that when indicated they not only remove pain with active movement but after their application there is an immediate improvement in the patient's signs and symptoms. They are not hard to learn, but care must be taken not to overdo them, especially on the first patient visit. When coupled with other treatment skills that therapists have to offer, patients will be much better off.

It is to be hoped that, in the next decade, research in the manual therapy field will take on a new dimension as magnetic resonance imaging (MRI) becomes more accessible and is capable of imaging active spinal movement. The researcher will then be able to film faulty biomechanical function, film any manual procedure (such as SNAGS) as it is undertaken, and then again observe function to see whether the claimed effects of a technique have in fact taken place. A new breed of manual therapist will then be born — orthodox, effective and scientifically acceptable.

REFERENCES

Kaltenborn F M 1980 Mobilisation of the extremity joints. Dlaf Norlis Bokhandel, Oslo, p 13

McKenzie R A 1981 The lumbar spine. Spinal Publications, Waikanae

Mulligan B R 1989 Manual therapy 'NAGS', 'SNAGS', 'PRPS', etc. Plane View Services, Wellington

Oliver M J 1991 Personal communication

54. Combined movements in the lumbar spine: their use in examination and treatment

B. C. Edwards

INTRODUCTION

Treatment by passive movement has been shown to be a useful therapeutic procedure when compared to other forms of treatment (Glover et al 1974, Rasmussen 1977, Sims-Williams et al 1978, Twomey & Farrell 1982). It is however still empirical in nature. This is because definite movement patterns related to pathology are unclear. A more detailed examination involving the combining of different movements can allow a more accurate choice of technique to be made. It can also help in predicting the result of a technique. The combining of different examining movements can increase or decrease particular signs and symptoms. On some occasions quite unexpected symptoms and signs can be produced. The increase or decrease in signs and symptoms which are produced when combining movements in examination can help to established movement patterns which may assist the therapist in choosing the direction of the passive movement procedures as well as predicting the response.

The movements of the vertebral column are complex and there has been a considerable amount of material published on this subject. Most of the studies seem to have been related to the movements of flexion and extension, presumably as this is the easiest movement to describe, perform and control. Results vary but it would seem that most ranges of movement lie between 60 and 75° (Wiles 1935, Begg & Falconer 1949, Clayson et al 1962, Davis et al 1965, Loebl 1967, Troup et al 1967). Allbrook (1957) found, in his study conducted on individuals not complaining of lumbar pain, that movement between L4 and L5 was greatest and gradually lessened towards the upper lumbar spine. Farfan (1975) showed that the spine elongated as it flexed, revealing that there is about 25% elongation at the level of the facet capsules at 60% of spinal flexion. Not quite as much has been published relating to the movement of lateral flexion. Tanz (1953) concluded that lateral flexion was about 2/3 of the range of flexion and extension for the whole of the lumbar spine, except L5 and SI. Hasner et al (1952) described the spines of each vertebral body combining to form an arcuate line in lateral flexion, and the vertebral bodies angled in

relationship to one another. The results of Moll et al (1972) indicated that there was about 10–45° lateral angular bending and 2.6–7.8 cm of linear movement of the trunk.

There have been relatively few studies of rotation of the lumbar spine. Tanz (1953) reported a range of rotation in the lumbar spine but was not able to measure it. Gregerson and Lucas (1967) compared ranges of rotation during sitting, standing and walking: their results indicated that more rotation occurred in standing, particularly at the lumbosacral joint. Lumsden and Morris (1968) showed that there was an average of 6° of rotation at the lumbosacral joint during maximum rotation of the trunk and that rotation of the joint was always combined with some flexion. Loebl (1973) showed a mean regional rotation of the lumbar spine of 25°.

The combination of movements, namely flexion, lateral flexion and rotation or coupling, as it has been called, has been investigated by a number of authors – Rolander (1966), Troup et al (1967), Loebl (1973) and Farfan (1975). Gregerson and Lucas (1967) found that axial rotation was to the left when the subject bent to the left and to the right when bending to the right. They did find that, in one subject, the reverse was the case. Stoddard (1962) reported the opposite. Schultz et al (1973) showed that counter-clockwise axial rotation towards the concavity of the curve was evident, but was very small. Arkin (1950) showed that, in adults, rotation to the convexity of the curve appeared when the spine was in lateral flexion, whether it was in flexion, extension or neutral. Roaf (1958), using the spines of still-born babies and normal children, showed that lateral flexion and rotation normally occurred independently. Kapandji (1974) stated that contralateral rotation occurs in conjunction with lateral flexion.

Considerable work has been done on the effect of movements on the disc. Rolander (1966) and Farfan et al (1970) discussed the effect of rotation on the disc and pointed out the possibility of damage from forceful rotatory movements. Many authors consider that one of the main functions of the facet joint is to prevent rotation. However, MacConaill (1956) suggested that this is only the case when the spine is not laterally flexed as in this position

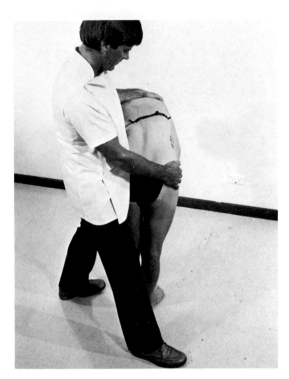

Fig. 54.1 Flexion with left lateral flexion. The therapist stands on the left hand side of the patient so that his left anterior superior iliac spine is in contact with the lateral aspect of the patient's left hip. The therapist's left hand is placed on the posterior aspect of the patient's right shoulder. The therapist's right hand grips the right ilium of the patient, and the patient is then bent forwards and while in the flexed position left lateral flexion is performed.

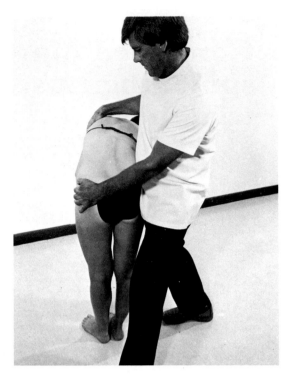

Fig. 54.2 Flexion with right lateral flexion. The same procedure is used as described in Figure 54.1; however, the therapist stands on the right hand side of the patient and the hand positions are reversed.

some conjunct rotation is possible. The biomechanical principles of the lumbar spine are complex. Farfan et al (1970) and Cossette et al (1971) found that the instantaneous centre of axial rotation of the L3–4 disc was anterior to the facet joint in the region of the posterior part of the nucleus, but this centre moved towards the side to which the rotation was forced. Farfan's determination of the centre of rotation (Farfan et al 1970, Farfan 1973) appears to be accurate but where there was obvious asymmetry of facet joints the centre of rotation appeared to be at the intersection of the facet planes.

EXAMINATION OF THE LUMBAR SPINE USING COMBINED MOVEMENTS

The standard orthopaedic examination of lumbar spinal movements are usually done with the patient standing and the therapist standing behind the patient observing the movements. The movements performed are flexion, extension, lateral flexion and rotation. Before any of the examining movements are performed an accurate description of the areas of symptoms must be obtained. It is essential particularly when combining movements that accurate reference is constantly made to the particular symptoms in question.

Following the completion of the standard examination procedures the first movements combined are usually lateral flexion with flexion and extension. (Figs 54.1–54.4). The combining of rotation with flexion or extension is shown in Figures 54.5–54.8.

ESTABLISHMENT OF MOVEMENT PATTERNS

There are certain movements in the lumbar spine which produce similar effects at the intervertebral level, for example, flexion, say, of L1 and L2 causes an upward movement of the inferior articular facets of L1 on the superior articular facets of L2. Extension of L1 on L2 causes a downward movement of the inferior articular facets of L1 on the superior articular facets of L2. Lateral flexion to the left produces a downward movement of the left articular facet of L1 on the left superior facet of L2. The reverse is the case in lateral flexion to the right. As well as the above, there is stretching of the posterior structures of the inter-body joint on flexion and a compression anteriorly. The reverse is the case with extension. On lateral flexion to the left there is a compressing of the left side of the inter-body joint and a stretching of the right; the reverse is the case for right lateral flexion.

From the above it can be seen that there are some aspects of, say, the movement of flexion and left lateral flexion that have similar effects on the right hand side of the vertebral joint. Extension and left lateral flexion have similar effects

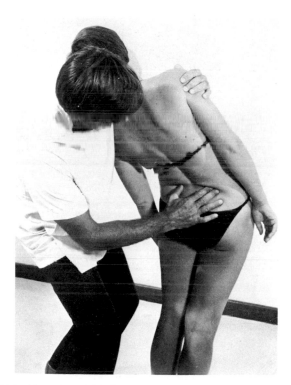

Fig. 54.3   Extension with left lateral flexion. The therapist stands on the left hand side of the patient. His left arm is placed around the chest of the patient so that the left hand grasps the patient's right shoulder. The thumb and index finger of the right hand are placed over the transverse process at the level of the lumbar spine to be examined. The patient is then bent backwards and laterally flexed on the left.

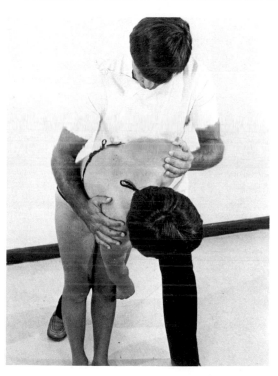

Fig. 54.5   Flexion with left lateral rotation. The therapist stands on the left hand side of the patient and takes hold of the patient's left shoulder by placing his left hand over the anterior aspect of the patient's left shoulder. The therapist takes hold of the patient's right shoulder by placing his right hand over the posterior aspect of the patient's right shoulder. The patient is then asked to bend forward and, in the flexed position, the patient's trunk is rotated to the left.

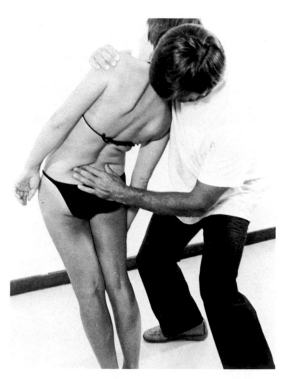

Fig. 54.4   Extension with right lateral flexion. The same procedure is used as described in Figure 54.3; however, the therapist stands on the right hand side of the patient and the hand positions are reversed.

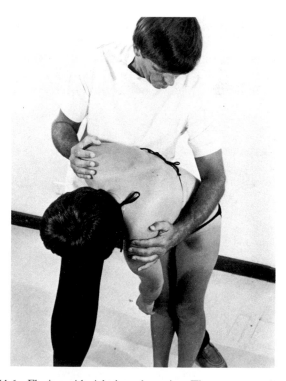

Fig. 54.6   Flexion with right lateral rotation. The same procedure is used as described in Figure 54.5; however, the therapist stands on the right hand side of the patient and the hand positions are reversed.

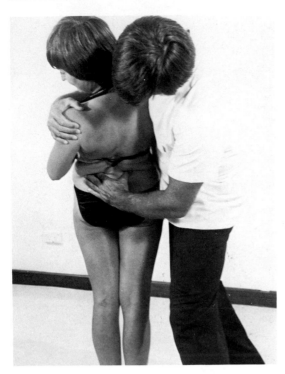

Fig. 54.7 Extension with left lateral rotation. The therapist stands on the right hand side of the patient and takes hold of the patient's left shoulder by placing his right hand around the patient's chest so that the therapist's right hand covers the anterior aspect of the patient's left shoulder. The therapist's left hand is placed so that his thumb and index finger are placed on the transverse process of the level to be examined. The patient is then bent backwards and laterally rotated to the left.

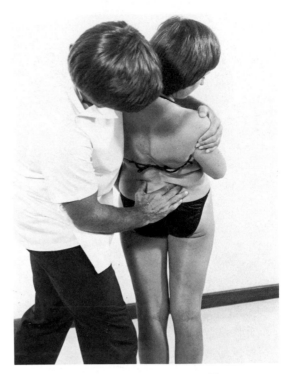

Fig. 54.8 Extension with right lateral rotation. The same procedure is used as described in Figure 54.7; however, the therapist stands on the left hand side of the patient and the hand positions are reversed.

on the left. If the movements are combined, an increase in the stretching or compressing effects can be made. The use of combined movements will help to establish movement patterns. These are classed as either regular or irregular and apply to all regions of the spine.

Regular patterns

These are patterns in which movements produce similar movements at the intervertebral joints while also producing the same symptoms, though these may differ in quality or severity. If the symptoms are on the same side to which the movement is directed, the pattern is a compressing pattern, that is, compressing movements produce the symptoms. The reverse is the case if the symptoms are produced on movement to the opposite side when the pattern would be a stretching pattern.

An example of a compressing regular pattern: right lateral flexion in the lumbar spine produces right buttock pain which is made worse when this movement is done in extension (Fig. 54.4) and eased when done in flexion (Fig. 54.2).

An example of a stretching regular pattern: right lateral flexion of the lumbar spine produces left buttock pain and this pain is accentuated when the movement of right lateral

flexion is performed in flexion (Fig. 54.2) and eased when right lateral flexion is performed in extension (Fig. 54.4).

Irregular patterns of movement

All patterns which are not regular fall into the category of irregular patterns. With irregular patterns there is not the same conformity as described above. Stretching and compressing movements do not follow any recognizable pattern. There appears to be no correlation in the examination findings obtained when combining movements which either compress or stretch. There is a random reproduction of symptoms despite the combining of movements which have similar mechanical effects. Examples of irregular patterns of movements are as follows:

1. Right lateral flexion in the lumbar spine produces right buttock pain, a compressing movement, and this pain is accentuated when the same movement is done in flexion, a stretching not a compressing movement, and eased when done in extension, a compressing movement.

2. Left lateral flexion in the lumbar spine produces right buttock pain, a stretching movement, and this pain is made worse when the same movement is done in extension, a compressing movement, and eased when the movement of lateral flexion is done in flexion, a stretching movement.

There are many examples of irregular patterns, and combinations of movements frequently indicate that there is more than one component to the disorder: for example, zygapophyseal joints, the inter-body joint and the canal and foraminal structures. Generally, traumatic injuries, e.g. whiplash and other traumatic causes of pain, do not have regular patterns of movement. Non-traumatized zygapophyseal and inter-body joint disorders tend to have regular patterns of movement because of the similar effects on the joints which the movements of flexion, extension, lateral flexion and rotation have.

It should be recognized that, within patterns of movements described above, parts of patterns can be present. For example, irregular patterns of movement which may be the result of trauma may have regular patterns or even parts of regular patterns of movement present. This means that, even when irregular patterns of movements are found during examination of a patient's movements, thought must be given to deciding whether they have any regular pattern components which may be forming part of the irregular pattern and thereby indicating a recognizable regular component to part of the patient's disorder.

Recognition of different patterns of movement can assist in:

1. predicting the result of treatment
2. the manner in which the symptoms and movement signs may improve.

Regular patterns of movement tend to respond to treatment in such a way that the least painful movement will improve before the most painful. For example, if right lateral flexion of the lumbar spine in neutral produced the patient's right buttock symptoms and these symptoms are made worse when the movement is done in extension, then right lateral flexion in neutral will improve before right lateral flexion in extension. One can also expect that the treatment of right lateral flexion done in flexion (found on examination to be the painless position) is unlikely to make the symptoms worse. The response in the case of irregular patterns of movement is not as predictable, and the improvement in the symptoms may appear in an apparently random fashion. Care must be taken when choosing the technique, that the correct grade of movement is chosen in relation to the reproduction of pain, spasm or restriction of movement.

Selection of technique

The recognition of regular (or irregular) patterns of movement can help in the selection of technique. The aspects of technique in which combinations of movement assist are:

1. sequence of obtaining the direction
2. the direction.

Sequence of obtaining the direction

It is important to assess accurately which movement of the examining movements is the significant movement in either reducing or increasing the symptoms. This can be considered the primary movement of the examination. For example, if the patient complains of left leg pain extending down the calf, and the calf pain is increased when the patient extends the lumbar spine and other movements of the lumbar spine do not alter the calf symptoms, then extension may be considered to be the primary movement of the examination. When using combined movements one examines the effect of lateral flexion to the right and left performed in extension. If, say, left lateral flexion done in extension increased the left calf pain, it is necessary to assess the effect of doing left lateral flexion first and then to perform extension — comparing this with doing extension and adding in left lateral flexion. The difference in sequence of the movements may be important in terms of the reproduction of the patient's symptoms. The technique of extension may be performed in left lateral flexion or the technique of left lateral flexion may be performed in extension.

For regular patterns

In the case where a patient presents with a regular pattern of movement, the technique chosen is usually the one which is found, on examination, to be the most painful direction of movement, but it is performed in the least painful way. For example, forward flexion of the lumbar spine reproduces right buttock pain and this pain is made worse when left lateral flexion is combined with flexion but eased when left lateral flexion is done in extension. The technique of left lateral flexion is used in the position of extension and progressed to performing left lateral flexion in flexion as the right buttock symptoms improve.

For irregular patterns

The direction of movement chosen for irregular patterns of movement would similarly be the most painful direction of movement done in the least painful way, or if the disorder is one of extreme pain or high irritability, the least painful direction of movement would be used as the technique in the least painful combined position. However, if combining of movements is not part of any obvious pattern, for example, on examination right lateral flexion producing right buttock pain is eased when done in extension and worse in flexion, the chosen direction for treatment technique would be the least painful direction, that is, right lateral flexion done in extension. The response to treatment may not be predictable. Performing the technique in the least painful position may improve the most painful examination movement, right lateral flexion done in flexion. On the other hand the movement of right lateral flexion done in extension may deteriorate. In other words there may be a random response to the technique.

TREATMENT

Although the importance of accurate diagnosis is not to be underestimated, the often ambiguous signs and symptoms in relation to facet and disc leave the practitioner with only physical signs and symptoms by which to ensure the efficacy of treatment.

Determination of the primary movement, primary combination, primary quadrant and accessory movement will assist the practitioner. However, categorization of the patient is also needed. This is based on the examination response.

Three categories are recognized and termed:

acute
subacute
chronic.

Acute category (Fig. 54.9)

(i) Less than 48 h onset.
(ii) Primary movement less than half range.
(iii) Pain score usually greater than 5 on a visual analogue scale (VAS) of 1–10.
(iv) May have irregular or regular patterns.
(v) On a movement diagram, pain resistance and spasm are present and tend to start before half the range. Usually limited by pain.
(vi) Symptoms are usually local; however, they can be referred.

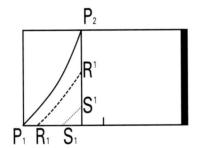

Fig. 54.9   Movement diagram 1.

Subacute category (Fig. 54.10)

(i) Longer than 48 h but less than 6 weeks.
(ii) Primary movement equal to or greater than half range.
(iii) Pain source equal to or less than 5 on VAS.
(iv) A regular pattern may be seen to be dominant, but may have irregular pattern still present.
(v) Movement diagram resistance starting before half-range pain, and spasm usually present but small. Limited by resistance.
(vi) Symptoms may be local or referred.

Chronic category (Fig. 54.11)

(i) Longer than 6 weeks.
(ii) Primary movement greater than half range.

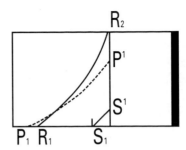

Fig. 54.10   Movement diagram 2.

(iii) Pain sources usually less than 5 on VAS.
(iv) Usually regular patterns dominate.
(v) Movement diagrams show resistance starting early in the range. Pain graph low. Limitations always resistance.
(vi) Symptoms local or referred.

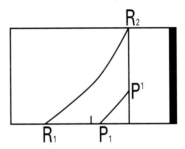

Fig. 54.11   Movement diagram 3.

Once this has been established, the use of the box diagram (Edwards 1992) can also assist in deciding the selection and progression of treatment. The box diagram (Fig. 54.12) is a simple method of deciding patient symptoms.

A, B, C and D quadrants represent anterior and posterior parts of the body. 'A' indicates left anterior, and 'D' right posterior symptoms, and this is indicated by shading the appropriate quadrant.

The primary movement and primary combination can be indicated as shown in Figure 54.13.

In the latter example the primary movement is extension which is limited to half range; the primary combination is left lateral flexion in extension.

In the acute category the sequence of technique would be as follows:

(R) LF in F
(L) LF in E
(L) LF in N
(L) LF in E

or

(R) LF in F
(R) LF in N
(R) LF in E
(L) LF in E

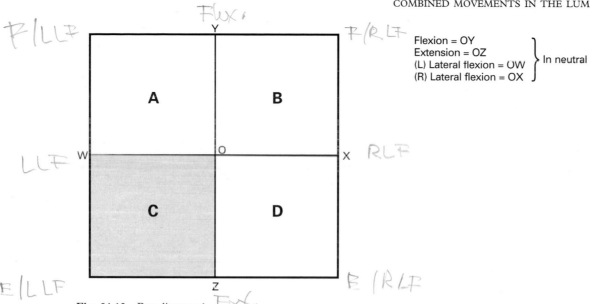

F/LLF   Flux/   F/R LF

LLF   W

E/LLF   Ext.

E/RLF

Flexion = OY
Extension = OZ
(L) Lateral flexion = OW
(R) Lateral flexion = OX
} In neutral

Fig. 54.12   Box diagram 1.

RLF

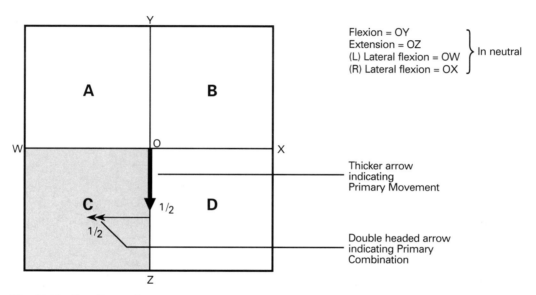

Flexion = OY
Extension = OZ
(L) Lateral flexion = OW
(R) Lateral flexion = OX
} In neutral

Thicker arrow
indicating
Primary Movement

Double headed arrow
indicating Primary
Combination

Fig. 54.13   Box diagram 2.

The sub-acute category with the same primary movement and primary combination:

(R) LF in F
(L) LF in N
(L) LF in E

or

(R) LF in N
(R) LF in E
(L) LF in E

The chronic category with the same primary movement and combination:

(L) LF in N
(L) LF in E

or

(R) LF in E
(L) LF in E

A more detailed account of technique selection has been described by Edwards (1992).

CONCLUSIONS

The combining of various movements may assist in increasing or decreasing the stretch or compression forces on particular joints and therefore highlighting signs which may not be obvious with standard examination procedures. This can lead to the clarification of regular and irregular patterns which assist in the selection of treatment technique. Techniques can then be effectively applied with due regard for the acuteness or chronicity of the patient's condition.

REFERENCES

Allbrook D A 1957 Movements of the lumbar spinal column. Journal of Bone and Joint Surgery 39B: 339–345

Arkin A M 1950 The mechanism of rotation in combination with lateral deviation in the normal spine. Journal of Bone and Joint Surgery 32A: 180–188

Begg A G, Falconer M 1949 Plain radiographs in intraspinal protrusion of lumbar intervertebral discs: a correlation with operative findings. British Journal of Surgery 36: 225–239

Clayson S J, Newman I M, Debevec D F, Anger R W, Skowlund H V, Kottke F J 1962 Evaluation of mobility of hips and lumbar vertebrae of normal young women. Archives of Physical Medicine and Rehabilitation 43: 1–8

Cossette J W, Farfan H F, Robertson G H, Wells R V 1971 The instantaneous centre of rotation of the third lumbar intervertebral joint. Journal of Biomechanics 4: 149–153

Davis P R, Troup J D, Burnard D 1965 Movements of the thoracic and lumbar spine when lifting: a chrono-cyclophotographic study. Journal of Anatomy 99: 13–26

Edwards B C 1992 Manual of combined movements: their use in the examination and treatment of mechanical vertebral column disorders. Churchill Livingstone, Edinburgh

Farfan H F 1973 Mechanical disorders of the low back. Lea & Febiger, Philadelphia, p 50–52

Farfan H F 1975 Muscular mechanism of the lumbar spine and the position of power and efficiency. Orthopaedic Clinics of North America 6: 135–144

Farfan H F, Cossette J W, Robertson G H, Wells R V, Draus H 1970 The effects of torsion on the lumbar intervertebral joints: the role of torsion in the production of disc degeneration. Journal of Bone and Joint Surgery 52A: 468–497

Glover J R, Morris J G, Khosla J 1974 Back pain: a randomised clinical trial of rotational manipulation of the trunk. British Journal of Industrial Medicine 31: 59–64

Gregerson G C, Lucas D B 1967 An in-vivo study of the axial rotation of the human thoraco-lumbar spine. Journal of Bone and Joint Surgery 49A: 247–262

Hasner E, Shalimzek M, Snorrason E 1952 Roentgenological examination of the function of the lumbar spine. Acta Radiologica 37: 141–149

Kapandji I A 1974 Trunk and vertebral column. The physiology of joints, 2nd edn. Churchill Livingstone, Edinburgh, vol 3

Loebl W Y 1967 Measurement of spinal posture and range of spinal movement. Annals of Physical Medicine 9: 103–110

Loebl W Y 1973 Regional rotation of the spine. Rheumatology and Rehabilitation 12: 223

Lumsden R M, Morris J M 1968 An in-vivo study of axial rotation and immobilisation at the lumbo sacral joint. Journal of Bone and Joint Surgery 50A: 1591–1602

MacConaill M A 1956 Mechanical anatomy of motion and posture. In: Licht S (ed) Therapeutic exercise, 2nd edn. Waverley Press, Baltimore

Moll J M H, Liyanage S P, Wright V 1972 An objective clinical method to measure lateral spinal flexion. Rheumatology and Physical Medicine 11: 293–312

Rasmussen G G 1977 Manipulation in the treatment of low back pain: a randomised clinical trial. 5th International Congress, International Federation of Manual Medicine, Copenhagen

Roaf R 1958 Rotation movements of the spine with special reference to scoliosis. Journal of Bone and Joint Surgery 40B: 312–332

Rolander S D 1966 Motion of the lumbar spine with special reference to the stabilising effect of posterior fusion. Acta Orthopaedica Scandinavica supplement no. 90

Schultz A M, Belytschko T B, Andriacchi J P, Galante J L 1973 Analog studies of forces in the human spine: mechanical properties and motion segment behaviour. Journal of Biomechanics 6: 373–383

Sims-Williams H, Jayson M I V, Young S M S, Baddeley H, Collins E 1978 Controlled trial of mobilisation and manipulation for low back pain in general practice. British Medical Journal 2: 1338–1340

Stoddard A 1962 Manual of osteopathic technique, 2nd edn. Hutchinson, London p 157

Tanz S S 1953 Motion of the lumbar spine: a roentgenologic study. American Journal of Roentgenology, Radium Therapy and Nuclear Medicine 69: 399–412

Troup J D G, Hood C A, Chapman A E 1967 Measurements of the sagittal mobility of the lumbar spine and hips. Annals of Physical Medicine 9: 308–321

Twomey L T, Farrell J P 1982 Acute low back pain: a comparison of two conservative treatment approaches. Medical Journal of Australia 1: 160–164

Wiles P 1935 Movements of the lumbar vertebrae during flexion and extension. Proceedings of the Royal Society of Medicine 28: 647–651

55. The McKenzie method of spinal pain management

M. G. Robinson

INTRODUCTION

The management of patients with non-specific mechanical spinal disorders is covered in this chapter and is related to the methods proposed by Robin McKenzie in his two texts (McKenzie 1981, 1990). The McKenzie method of spinal therapy can be said to be a progression of mechanical forces applied by or to the patient in such a way that a minimal amount is utilized to effect a therapeutic change in the presenting mechanical syndrome. In this way the prophylactic concept is engendered in the patient from the beginning of treatment as self-applied therapy is always encouraged. Prophylaxis is a learning process and begins the moment that the patient is able to improve the symptoms, unaided. Indeed, treatment utilizing these principles often begins during the assessment of the patient by the therapist as postural changes and repeated movements are evaluated and found to be providing the desired response (see Ch. 42 on repeated movements).

Therapists are often asked by referring medical colleagues (or at least should be), 'What type of spinal patient are you best able to evaluate and treat?' A comprehensive response to this is to point the questioner in the direction of the Quebec Task Force (QTF) report on activity-related spinal disorders (Spitzer 1987). The similarity between the proposals emerging from the Quebec report for classification of disorders of the spine and McKenzie's three syndromes is referred to in Chapter 28 (diagnosis of syndromes). From this it is possible to state, quite simply, that the categories of patient which are highly likely to respond to mechanical therapy are Quebec groups I–IV. These were labelled the 'non-specific' categories and accounted for 85–90% of patients with mechanical spinal problems. Mechanical evaluation should not necessarily be withheld from patients in groups 7, 8, 9.2 and 10, for useful diagnostic information can be obtained (McKenzie 1990, p 54).

CENTRALIZATION PHENOMENON

During the 1950s it became apparent to Robin McKenzie that there appeared to be a relationship between patients with radiating symptoms who responded rapidly to his newly discovered method of mechanical therapy, and the location of their most distal pain. He noticed that the best responders to lumbar treatment were those whose peripheral pain showed early resolution regardless of the initial effect on central symptoms. In fact a significant proportion of patients undergoing successful therapy complained of increasing pains in or near the mid-line of the body (i.e. centrally) as their distal symptoms were abolished. It became apparent that this process, later to be called the 'centralization phenomenon', occurred only in the derangement syndrome and was equally as relevant to the cervical and thoracic spine. McKenzie now defines centralization as (McKenzie 1990, p 43):

> The phenomenon whereby as a result of the performance of certain repeated movements or the adoption of certain positions, radiating symptoms originating from the spine and referred distally are caused to move proximally towards the midline of the spine. Movements that cause this phenomenon, once identified, can be used to abolish radiating and referred symptoms. Where patients have pain of recent origin this process can be extremely rapid and can, in many cases, occur in a few minutes. The centralisation of pain occurs only in the Derangement Syndrome during the reductive process. As centralisation takes place there may be a significant increase of localised central pain adjacent to or in the spine itself.

The modern mechanical therapist can now confidently utilize this phenomenon as an absolutely reliable predictor of the correct therapeutic motion to be applied by or to the patient with derangement syndrome.

Donelson and co-workers looked at the centralization of pain in a retrospective study (Donelson et al 1990) involving 87 patients evaluated and treated according to McKenzie's principles. They concluded that there was a high statistical correlation between centralization and successful outcome to treatment and, on the opposite score, between lack of centralization and failure to respond. In another study (Williams et al 1991), the effects of sitting with either a kyphotic or lordotic lumbar posture were studied, and it was found that centralization tended to occur with the latter position only. Clinically, patients are very much more likely to have their pain centralize with extension movements of the spine than with flexion (Donelson et al 1991). This has, in no small way, contributed to the widely held misconception that the McKenzie method consists entirely of extension procedures. The direction of therapeutic motion must not be pre-determined but should evolve from the accurate analysis of the moving patient (see Ch. 42 on repeated movements). There can be no doubting the importance of the centralization phenomenon, but is there a rational explanation for its occurrence?

The proposed conceptual model for the derangement syndrome (see Ch. 28) is based upon the known, and speculated, biomechanics of the intervertebral disc. There will be little argument that a full-blown extrusion can be the source of the most severe pain radiating as far as the hand or foot. Relief, in many of these cases, may be gained only by surgical intervention to remove the offending disc material. Patients in this category, and also those with less debilitating distal pain, typically describe their first awareness of the current episode not as pain felt in the limb but as pain felt in or near the spine (i.e. QTF class I). The sitting posture study (Williams et al 1991) showed that only 13% of QTF class III patients had pain which radiated below the knee within one week of onset. In other words, there is a time factor operating during which pain may well peripheralize. The QTF study recognized that the patient whose symptoms are moving to a more distal location is becoming a more complex case and is likely to require more involved and expensive therapy. If the disc is well recognized as the source of the problem in the 'surgical back', it is unlikely that another structure has been the source of trouble in the intermediate stages before extrusion.

The conceptual model proposes that there is an embryonic stage of disc protrusion. The internal displacement is sufficient only to cause distortion of nociceptors in the posterior or posterolateral annulus fibrosus and/or posterior longitudinal ligament. As the derangement progresses the movement of displaced material laterally will irritate more laterally located nociceptors. It has been demonstrated (Smyth & Wright 1958) that the greater the pressure on the nerve root the more distal will the pain be felt. It is not difficult, therefore, to surmise that the movement laterally of an enlarging disc protrusion could explain the time factor noticed in the peripheralization of pain. In a 193-patient study of selective, in vivo, stimulation of lumbar tissues (Kuslich et al 1991) it was found that many of the spinal tissues were insensitive to stimulation. The zygapophyseal joint capsules rarely produced significant low-back pain, and when they did this was never referred below the buttock. Furthermore, it was found that in those cases where a trefoil-shaped central canal produced a narrow lateral recess, the undersurface

of the superior articular facet and its capsule frequently made contact with the posterior surface of the disc. In many cases low-back pain was produced by applying pressure to the disc at this site—which the authors suggest might be interpreted, clinically, as facet syndrome. They also reported that, with the exception of simultaneous stimulation of annulus and nerve root, clinically significant buttock pain could only rarely be produced. They concluded that 'the annulus fibrosus is the tissue of origin in most cases of low-back pain; the facet synovium is never the site of back or leg pain. The facet capsule is sometimes tender, but its true significance in the area of low-back pain and sciatica probably involves its ability to compress or irritate other sensitive local tissues i.e., the nerve root or outer annulus. Sciatica can only be produced by direct pressure or stretch on the inflamed, stretched or compressed nerve root. No other tissues in the spine are capable of producing leg pain.'

This new evidence lends weight to the argument that the disc is active in the production of progressively peripheralizing symptoms.

Centralization can be thought of as a reversal of this process. It will only occur when the annular wall is still competent. Quite clearly, it does not occur when the annulus is completely breached, thereby helping to provide a predictor for the surgical case (Kopp et al 1986, Alexander et al 1990, Donelson et al 1990).

Further weight is given to the centralization and peripheralization phenomena being related to disc pathology by a report from Japan (Fuchioka et al 1988). The investigators were able to show, from an in vivo sample of 69 herniated discs, using CT discography, that in 75.6% of cases perforation had begun in the very centre of the posterior annulus. In 69.6% of these the herniated fragments had then later moved to the left or right. This contradicts the notion that lateral perforation of the annulus is more frequent than at the centre and suggests that the lateral fragment removed at surgery may well have begun its traverse centrally. They also found that primary posterolateral herniation had occurred only in moderate to severely degenerated discs and was not seen in the groups with mild or no degeneration. This leads to speculation that the 'embryonic', central, internal mass displacement or protrusion occurring in well preserved discs may very likely be rapidly reversible using sagittal extension forces. If the displacement has moved laterally and is producing peripheral symptoms, forces in the coronal plane may be required for reduction.

PROGRESSION OF FORCES

The concept of mechanical therapy, now widely known as the 'McKenzie method', can very briefly be defined as: 'a progression of mechanical forces, from patient to therapist generated'. This definition embraces the whole spectrum of mechanical therapy and may come as a surprise to those who believe, erroneously, that the McKenzie method excludes manual procedures. It is true to say that self-treatment plays a major role, but for some patients this is not sufficiently forceful or localized. They are, obviously, not then abandoned for the sake of pursuing some idealistic goal. The following guidance applies to the use of therapist-generated forces: 'Therapist technique should be applied in such a way that the patient is able to self-treat more effectively'. Thus it can be seen that self-treatment and therapist technique are not mutually exhaustive and separate, but are inter-related.

The idea of applying minimal force to maximal effect is perhaps not novel. It is the basis for the McKenzie method for two reasons: (i) to encourage self-treatment (the simplest mechanical force) whenever appropriate and possible, with priority over all other forces, and (ii) for safety reasons, as will become apparent. Robin McKenzie has written (McKenzie 1989): 'It should no longer be necessary to apply Spinal Manipulative Therapy (SMT) to find out retrospectively if the procedure was indicated. SMT should not be dispensed to the entire population with back and neck pain in order to deliver the procedures to the very few who actually require it'. The therapist then needs a means of deciding who those few really are.

To begin with, the therapist will need a logical order in which to lay down a progression of forces, which can be written under the following headings (McKenzie 1990, p 103).

Static patient-generated force

Positioning in mid-range.
Positioning at end-range.

Dynamic patient-generated forces

Patient motion in mid-range.
Patient motion to end-range.
Patient motion to end-range with overpressure.

Therapist-generated forces

Patient motion to end-range with therapist overpressure.
Therapist overpressure—mobilization.
Therapist overpressure—manipulation.
Traction—manual, intermittent or sustained.

'Mobilization' is defined as large-amplitude low-velocity rhythmical passive movement up to the end of the available range. 'Manipulation' is defined as small-amplitude high-velocity single-thrust passive movement at the end of the available range.

The next step for the therapist is to make a decision as to the appropriate mechanical force to be utilized in any given treatment situation. A very simple and effective teaching tool to this end has been proposed by Wayne and Jean Rath of the Spine Center of New Jersey, USA. They call this the 'traffic lights guide to the progression of forces'. This not only applies to the derangement syndrome but can be utilized very effectively in any mechanical syndrome.

Assuming that a mechanical diagnosis has been made (and there is evidence to suggest that failure to diagnose will lead to failure to treat effectively (Roberts 1990)), the simplest mechanical force to apply is that self-generated by the patient. From there on, progressively increasing stresses should be applied in a definite order, and only one new technique should be added per session (Van Wijmen 1986b, p 765).

Providing that the existing pain status is noted it is possible for sustained positioning or repeated, self-applied movements in any given direction to produce one of the following three responses. (It is essential, at this stage, that the reader is familiar with the contents of Table 42.1 in Ch. 42, this volume.)

Red light

In both derangement and dysfunction syndromes pain is *produced* or *increased* and remains *worsened* (but not centralized) as a result.

Inference. (a) In the derangement syndrome the direction of movement is incorrect and has increased the apparent disc displacement. Change the movement or re-check diagnosis. (b) In the derangement syndrome the direction is correct but movement is too rapid to allow reductive movement of fluid nucleus/annulus complex. Use sustained mid-range positions rather than movement. (c) In the dysfunction syndrome overforceful movements are creating microtraumata. Allow 2 or 3 days to settle and re-start programme with less vigour.

Green light

In the derangement syndrome, pain is *decreased* or *abolished* and remains *better* (or centralized) as a result. In the dysfunction syndrome the pain *produced* at end of range disappears when the stretch is released.

Inference. The correct movement and degree of force has been selected to reduce the derangement or stretch the shortened structure. All is well, continue with more of the same until the condition resolves or the 'traffic light' changes colour.

Amber light

In the derangement syndrome, pain that is *produced* or *increased* is *not worsened*, or pain that is *decreased* or *abolished* is *not better* as a result.

Inference. In the derangement syndrome, the applied mechanical forces are not sufficient to produce a lasting change in the patient's symptoms. In effect, nothing has changed and so the careful application of more force is warranted. In the case of the dysfunction syndrome the 'amber light' becomes apparent over a number of days when there is no reported or observable change in the patient's symptoms and signs.

It is only when the 'amber light' response is evident that there is justification for applying more forceful repeated motion to the tissues in question. It is, therefore, possible to predict when greater force is needed. Examples of such indications include:

1. The patient appears to be better with treatment but cannot retain this improvement.
2. The patient is better initially but improvement stops.
3. The patient's pain is failing to centralize fully.

On occasion, some derangements presenting with a temporary deformity require the application of external force before any self-treatment can be contemplated.

The patient who really 'needs' manipulating will be exposed by this system and will already have had several days of treatment. This will have included hundreds of repetitions of self- and therapist-applied end-range movements to the relevant motion segment(s). This approach will, almost certainly, reveal any hidden dangers that might otherwise exclude the use of the high-velocity, low-amplitude technique, by showing the 'red light'. Suspicious pathology, if not already apparent, will be exposed. This is said on the assumption that the therapist has also taken all the usual precautions during the subjective and objective evaluation to exclude pathologies unsuited to mechanical therapy.

Using this method of force progression on acute patient populations, it has been suggested that approximately 75% of patients will require self-treatment alone, leaving about 25–30% who will need some form of additional force, in the form of therapist technique, to gain resolution of their mechanical pathology (McKenzie 1989). The percentage of patients requiring manual therapy is likely to rise in proportion to the chronicity of symptoms. Those actually requiring the high-velocity manipulation will be found to be a very small part of the patient population. Apart from the previously mentioned inbuilt safety aspects of utilizing progressive forces, there are also other justifications to be considered.

THE PROPHYLACTIC CONCEPT

With the rising tide of recurrence rates within the non-specific mechanical spinal pain spectrum it is not possible for any 'school' to claim that it has solved the problem. The only true way to measure effectiveness is to show that the therapies being administered are having a long-term effect for the good on each individual and on the population at large. This has yet to be done. The general picture from the scientific literature supports the proposition that there is no long-term benefit to be gained from SMT (Sims-Williams et al 1978, Hoehler et al 1981, Farrel & Twomey 1982, Brunarski 1984, Hadler et al 1987, MacDonald & Bell 1990). The question remains as to how this issue is to be best tackled. The progression of forces model contains within it the basis of the *prophylactic concept*. This decrees that the emphasis is always placed upon the patient being, or eventually becoming, the main driving force behind any therapeutic application. The use of therapist technique, whenever necessary, does not preclude or override the underlying philosophy that self-treatment is the most important and desirable aspect of any mechanical approach. It was stated earlier in this chapter that therapist technique very much assists and complements self-treatment.

By encouraging the idea within patients that they are able to exert some influence over what is, after all, their pain, it is no giant leap for them to see the pathway to future prevention opening up. If the patient has a particular pain today and is able to apply mechanical force in the shape of a specific exercise which causes the pain to be abolished—then surely the judicious use of the same exercise might well prevent the same pain returning. This may be thought of as the dynamic half of the prophylactic concept. The other half is the static half which involves education of the patient in removing, as far as is practicable, those postural influences which have led to mechanical failure within their spinal system.

A study (Stankovic & Johnell 1990) has compared the McKenzie approach with 'mini back school' and found the former superior in five out of the seven criteria measured (the other two were equal). As well as returning to work more quickly after the initial episode, the McKenzie group showed significantly fewer recurrences in the following year—this may be an indication of prophylaxis working. The Nottingham Back Pain Study (Roberts 1990) has shown, at 1-year follow-up, greater responsibility for personal pain control existing amongst a 'McKenzie treated' group when compared with a group treated with non-steroidal anti-inflammatory medication and advice.

MANAGEMENT OF THE THREE SYNDROMES

The three syndromes of mechanical pain of McKenzie have been described in detail in Chapter 28. Each is a separate entity and can be isolated by the response of body tissues to repeated movements. It follows, therefore, that they will each require a different approach to treatment, certainly initially. The symptoms of postural syndrome will have been felt by everyone at some time in their life, and dysfunction syndrome will probably develop somewhere in all of us at some stage. It is, however, the pain produced by derangement syndrome that mostly drives patients to seek professional help from therapists. The reason for this is found in the nature of the problem. Both postural and dysfunction syndromes are, by definition, 'end-of-range' phenomena, and it is not that difficult for people to learn to adapt their lifestyles accordingly, avoiding end-of-range positions and movements. Failing this, especially with postural pain, the sufferer may well have not been able to convince the referring practitioner that anything is wrong.

In contrast, patients with active derangement syndrome often find that nothing they have tried for themselves will stop the pain, which may be constant, or relieve it more than temporarily. They may have had previous episodes with rapid, spontaneous resolution, but on this occasion symptoms are not resolving.

Rath reported that, of 319 patients classified within QTF groups I–IV, 2.2% were diagnosed as postural, 18.5% dysfunction and 79.3% derangement syndromes (Rath et al 1989). In the light of its frequently complex nature, and potential to worsen if mismanaged, it is wise for the therapist to adopt the attitude that the patient with a non-specific mechanical problem has derangement until proven otherwise. The proof will come out of the dynamic evaluation but, on rare occasions, may not be totally apparent on day one. The value of the repeated movement assessment is that, if necessary, the patient can be sent away for 24 hours, still under evaluation, to apply self-generated forces in a methodical way to clarify the picture. It is not unknown for a patient to be classified as having dysfunction syndrome on day one and then need reclassifying correctly as derangement syndrome on day two. Once again, the 'traffic lights' principle is kept in mind and the patient warned accordingly. Movements should not be prescribed, in this situation, which, logically could be expected to lead to a peripheralization of symptoms on exposing the 'hidden' derangement. The presence of dysfunction syndrome underlying the presenting derangement, however, is not uncommon and should be treated following successful reduction and stabilization of the derangement.

Each of the three syndromes, and the sub-divisions within the derangement category, will take varying lengths of time to treat. This is particularly apparent when comparing derangement syndrome with dysfunction syndrome and the therapist should be fully aware of this. Rapid changes can, and should, be expected when dealing with derangements (especially numbers one to four and seven). The conceptual model of disc mechanics offers an explanation of why this may be so. There is, also, evidence that poor results can be expected if there is no response within six sessions of patient/therapist contact (Kopp et al 1986, Rath et al 1989, Roberts 1990, Stankovic & Johnell 1990). When the shortened structures involved in dys-

function syndrome are considered, however, a much slower response must be anticipated. Many therapists have reported becoming disillusioned with McKenzie's method when rapid results have not been forthcoming. What has often happened is that the vast majority of patients present with derangements and improve rapidly. Becoming used to this, therapists may then expect the same pattern to emerge when treating a pure or underlying dysfunction. It must be clearly understood that the re-modelling of shortened tissues takes time and may require many weeks or even months of regular frequent stretching to regain the desired range of movement.

The management of recurrent mechanical spinal pain does not, by definition, stop once the patient has recovered from the current episode. Prophylaxis is paramount and takes effect from the time the patient first has contact with the therapist. The progression of forces concept encourages this by the utilization of self-treatment, but, before even this can occur, the compliance of the patient is required. Patients who understand what is wrong and what is required of them respond better to therapy (Deyo & Diehl 1986). Therefore, a significant part of patient/therapist contact time on the first and subsequent occasions should involve explanation and encouragement. The 'bent finger syndrome' is a tool which comes in very useful here for posture and dysfunction (McKenzie 1981, pp 10–11). If one finger is bent backwards using over-pressure from its opposite number until the point of 'strain' is reached, this is not really too uncomfortable for short periods. If, however, the pressure were to be maintained, most individuals are astute enough to realize from previous learned experience that the finger will eventually hurt and that this not a desirable thing to do! Postural pain in a nutshell. It is not difficult then to take this a stage further to illustrate dysfunction: if the finger had been previously damaged, leaving shortened scar tissue, the pain would be produced immediately. The difference between these two events lies in the nature of the tissues being stretched (see Ch. 28 on syndromes).

Ready-made diagrams of disc mechanics and flexible models of the spine are probably the best tools for describing the derangement syndrome to the patient.

The verbal explanations should be reinforced by written information for the patient to take away to improve compliance (Moll & Wright 1972, Care et al 1981, Glossop et al 1982). This is particularly important when dealing with the derangement syndrome and needs to consist of general postural instructions and 'dos and don'ts' for when in the acute stage and, later, when recovered (McKenzie 1981, pp 154–157).

It is still a belief held by many referring medical practitioners, and perhaps some therapists, that physical therapy for the spine should take place after the pain has settled, as a sort of rehabilitation and strengthening programme in the vain hope that this will prevent future recurrences. Thousands, maybe millions, of patients around the world have been put through post-pain exercise routines, both individually and in groups, but still the incidence and prevalence of spinal pain has been rising (Cochrane Report 1979, Frymoyer & Mooney 1986, Weber 1986, Kramer 1990 p 12).

The prophylactic concept proposed in this chapter relies upon the patient's compliance from day one of treatment. Patients need to go through the experience of being able to change their own symptoms and, since it is derangement syndrome bearing the recurrent tag, must, preferably be evaluated by the therapist before spontaneous resolution occurs. In an interesting study, patients were assessed, by questionnaire and video, for changes in knowledge and behaviour following attendance at a back school. Although the number of patients was not large ($n = 37$) the results led the author to speculate that back schools may lead to a change in the way people *believe* they use their backs, without necessarily effecting an *observed* behavioural change (Moser 1990). It would seem that education of the patient alone may not be enough. It is proposed here that prophylaxis will work only if, in addition to the passive educational aspect, patients are able to go through the learning experience of influencing their own symptoms. This is irrespective of whether or not any therapist techniques have been used in the treatment programmes. It is also proposed that the use of forces greater than the minimum required will lessen the prophylactic effect by reducing the self-reliance component of treatment. More studies are required to test these hypotheses.

As a treatment tool, the McKenzie method has been compared with a number of other well established systems and found to be superior in every case (Ponte et al 1984, Nwuga & Nwuga 1985, Vanharanta et al 1986, DiMaggio & Mooney 1987, Roberts 1990, Stankovic & Johnell 1990). It is also cost-effective with the average number of patient/therapist contacts required by experienced practitioners being 6.6 (Rath et al 1989). This figure was calculated from an acute through to chronic patient population and included all three syndromes from all areas of the spine.

Full definitions of each of the three syndromes of McKenzie are given in Chapter 28. It is not within the scope of this chapter to describe the full McKenzie treatment approach to each syndrome in detail. To this end the reader is referred to Robin McKenzie's two textbooks (McKenzie 1981, 1990) and the chapters by Paula Van Wijmen in the first edition of this book (Van Wijmen 1986a, b). A brief overview of the treatment rationales will, however, be given to complement the above texts.

POSTURAL SYNDROME

The influence of posture on the pathomechanics of the spine is profound and should never be underestimated. Even though the patient presenting with pure postural

syndrome is a rarity, the understanding of the basic mechanics of postural stresses and their removal is fundamental to the treatment of all three syndromes. Until abnormal postural stresses are removed there will be little or no success in dealing with any spinal patient, using whatever treatment protocol, both in the short term and the long term. Such a simple, underlying fault as poor posture is often neglected by therapists and others looking at the spine as the wonderful, complex structure that it is. They fail to realise that it is still subject to the same physical laws that cause the humble bent finger to hurt (q.v.).

Once poor posture has been identified as the source of the patient's symptoms then treatment, quite obviously, is geared towards postural correction. This cannot be achieved by just telling the patient to sit or stand with better posture. Walter Carrington wrote (Carrington 1970): 'The more we learn of how the organism works, the more we begin to appreciate its vast complexities, the more obvious it becomes that we cannot hope to achieve much by direct cortical intervention (*this is why admonitions are always hopeless*) (MGR's italics). The control that can be consciously exercised is a control of choice, a decision to act or not to act in a certain manner, in a certain direction, at a certain time'.

The re-training of posture requires close co-operation between therapist and patient. The patient must be willing to act and the therapist must have the skill to communicate. Explanation is vital. Patients must understand that by continuing to adopt positions at end-of-range they are exposing their supporting structures to painful stimuli which only they themselves can remove. Tucker (1960) stated: 'Correct upright posture can be defined as an attitude of the mind towards the body promoting both mental and physical equilibrium and poise.' The therapist has to change that state of mind existing within the patient by providing the experience of self-control over pain-producing mechanisms. To this end it is desirable for the patient to be put into the provocative posture (which is most often sitting) until the pain appears. Then, by the simple act of correcting posture (if sitting, forming a lumbar lordosis and retracting the head), the patient is able to feel that the pain can be abolished by volition. Once this 'pain/no pain' pattern emerges the patient is taught, and will quickly realise the value of, the 'slouch/overcorrect' exercise (see Figs 55.1–55.5).

Regular performance of this exercise will enable the most habitual of slouchers to regain their postural awareness, maintain their required position in space and thereby abolish their postural pain. This exercise can also be adapted for the poor standing posture by tilting the pelvis backwards and raising the chest—a very useful teaching tool is for the therapist to place a finger in the patient's sternal notch (see Figs 55.6, 55.7).

Maintenance of the correct sitting posture does also require careful consideration of the seating being used, which is beyond the scope of this chapter. Suffice to say that no one is able to maintain active control over the

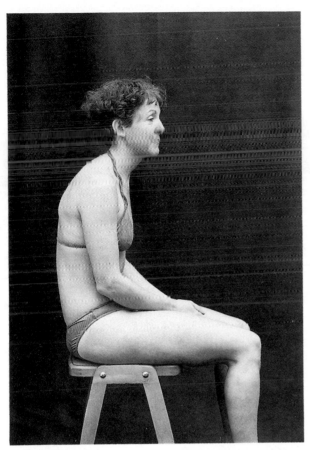

Fig. 55.1 (*see p. 760 for caption*)

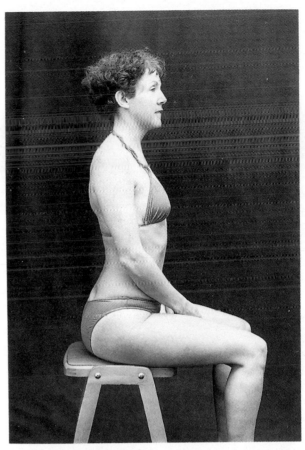

Fig. 55.2 (*see p. 760 for caption*)

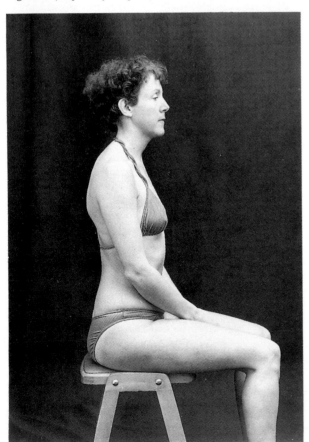

Fig. 55.3 (*see p. 760 for caption*)

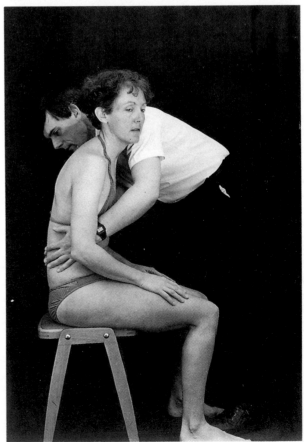

Fig. 55.4 (*see p. 760 for caption*)

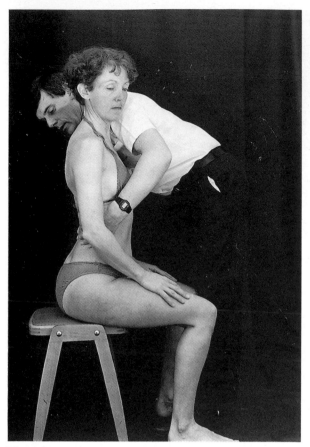

Fig. 55.5

Figs 55.1–55.5 The 'slouch/overcorrect' exercise is used to retrain postural awareness and the ability to maintain good posture whilst sitting. In one variation of this the patient first adopts the fully slouched position, known as '0%' or 'extreme of the bad' (**Fig. 55.1**) and is then instructed to move to '100%' or 'extreme of the good' by rolling the pelvis forwards and raising the chest (**Fig. 55.2**). She repeats this twenty times, moving slowly and smoothly from one end of range to the other, giving her the experience of feeling the difference between the two positions. She then drops back from '100%' to '90%' and attempts, initially, to maintain this for 5 minutes without dropping any further towards a slouched position (**Fig. 55.3**). Manual assistance to the active movement is sometimes required to guide the patient in moving correctly from the slouched to overcorrected position (**Figs 55.4, 55.5**). The therapist gently pulls the patient's waistline forwards and up whilst preventing her torso moving forwards.

sitting posture ad infinitum and so it is most desirable that patients are shown how to use a lumbar support in the correct way to maintain the 90% position as passively as possible. Having said that, a totally stationary sitting or standing position should never be encouraged. Regular, frequent repetitions of the 'slouch/overcorrrect' *movements* should be encouraged in all categories of patients finding themselves in statically loaded situations.

DYSFUNCTION SYNDROME

The Scottish surgeon John Hunter (1728–1793) is quoted as having said 'When all inflammation is gone off and

healing has begun, a little motion frequently repeated is necessary to prevent healing taking place with the parts fixed in one position' (Timbrell Fisher 1948). The lessons from history are sometimes worth exploring.

Once exposed by the repeated movement assessment, the management of the dysfunction syndrome usually follows a fairly straightforward and uncomplicated line. In essence it is a process of remodelling of pathologically shortened structures by stretching manoeuvres. The key words used to describe symptom behaviour are the same when related to the repeated movement assessment and the treatment programme: pain or discomfort should be *produced* at end-of-range only, not during motion, and without increasing with each repetition. It must remain *not worsened* following repetition.

It is this *production* of pain which can sometimes lead to confusion or inadequacy in the treatment of the dysfunction syndrome. For elongation of shortened tissue to occur some pain, or discomfort at least, needs to be experienced by the patient. Clear explanations need to be given to the patient as to the whys and wherefores of the recovery procedure. Clinicians too, as previously indicated, need to be aware of the long-term nature of the treatment plan that is being formulated for the patient.

Despite the fact that pure dysfunction syndrome will be very commonly found in the population at large, especially as age increases, this entity will not make up the largest proportion of the usual spinal case load. A minor loss of movement causes little restriction in many people's daily lives, and by learning to avoid that particular movement or position they can live a relatively pain-free existence. So it is very likely that by the time individuals are driven to seek help, the restriction facing the examining therapist is fairly pronounced and easily exposed.

The postural abuses that are put on our bodies lead to the most common pattern of dysfunction syndrome being loss of spinal extension, except in the upper to mid-cervical spine, where flexion is most likely to be limited. The loss of lower cervical extension correspondingly restricts the lateral movements occurring here since *full* rotation and side-flexion are not possible in the absence of extension which prevents proper posterior glide of the upper on lower facets. This is easily tested by trying to rotate or side-bend from the protracted position—only the upper cervical joints move well. There is, therefore, often an improvement in lateral motion by prescribing sagittal extension stretching alone.

In most cases patient-generated forces are sufficient to complete the therapy programme. As the syndrome will have been exposed by the repeated test movements on examination, these same movements will usually become the initial, and probably the only, treatment tool. It must not be forgotten, however, that some patterns of movement loss may not be straightforward, especially following trauma or, to a lesser extent, derangement, and combined

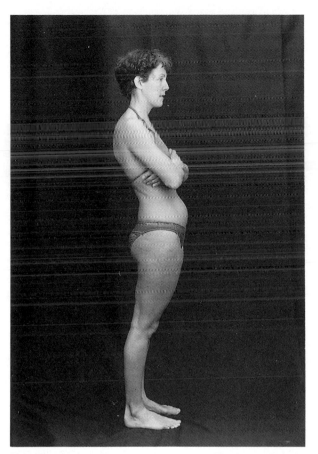 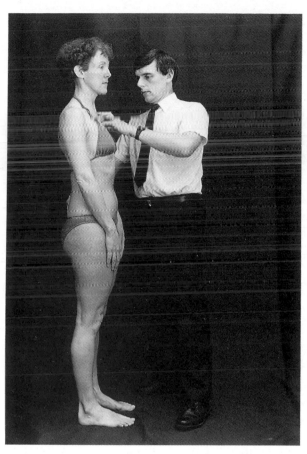

Figs 55.6 & 55.7   Poor standing posture (**Fig. 55.6**). Correction of standing posture (**Fig. 55.7**). One method, as illustrated here, is for the therapist to place a finger into the patient's sternal notch with the instruction 'Lift your chest up into my finger'. The therapist's other hand is placed over the patient's lumbosacral area to provide a stimulus to reduction of lumbosacral extension.

movements may be necessary to expose and treat the shortened structures.

To achieve the tissue response required, stretching procedures to the end of available range are, ideally, performed in a slow repeated movement fashion in sets of 10–15 every 2 hours throughout each day. Not every patient will tolerate this repetition rate, however, particularly when dysfunction accompanies significant degenerative changes or when stretching of neural structures is indicated. Respect must be given to the 'irritability' of the tissues in question so it is wise with such patients to 'test the water' by beginning at a lesser rate and progressing as symptom behaviour dictates. The movement chosen is determined by the spinal region(s) concerned and the loss of movement(s) pattern.

Instructions in postural correction are as necessary to the dysfunction patient as any other. The removal of simple mechanical stresses may play a significant part in symptom reduction. It must be clearly understood by the therapist, however, that the correction of posture alone in no way enhances the lengthening of shortened structures. Cases do occur where patients with flexion dysfunction or neural adherence are prescribed a strict extension principle of treatment and seem to improve dramatically—until,

that is, they apply tension to the shortened tissues again!

It is important to remember, when dealing with extension dysfunction, that the therapist's desire to create a perfectly upright specimen must be tempered with the patient's ability to attain this goal. It is no good forcing too large a lumbar support, for instance, into the back of the patient who cannot achieve the required lordosis. The 90% position applies whatever the available range might be. On the same theme, it is this author's experience that many patients with pronounced lumbar extension and, in many cases, side-gliding dysfunction, make the error of buying a very hard bed in the vain hope of gaining relief. They then find, much to their disappointment, that their night pain has increased in proportion to the drop in their bank balance! Such a bed, the purpose of which is to maintain the lumbar curves, will not help the poor soul whose curves have long deserted them. A similar scenario can be imagined for the thoracic and cervical regions. Sustained end-of-range will not be tolerable. The bed and pillow surfaces must have more 'give' in them without recourse to sagging the mattress—although this may have to be utilized for some thoracic patients. The incentive for the patient in this situation is to restore the lost movements so that the bed becomes useable.

In the treatment of dysfunction syndrome manual procedures are introduced when progress is slow or non-existent and the 'traffic lights' principle is still borne in mind to identify over-stretching which may be causing trauma to the shortened structures. The use of rhythmical end-of-range mobilizations will assist the phenomenon of creep to lengthen soft tissue but *must not replace the exercise programme in any way.* Failure to maintain regular repeated stretches will not produce results. The use of high-velocity end-range manipulations is, basically, illogical since trauma to tissues followed by repair is a source of further shortening. Clinically, however, there will be rare occasions where this approach is necessary to gain the last few degress of movement but it must, once again, be followed up with regular exercises.

Whichever manual technique is chosen, and this is purely at the discretion of the practitioner, the basic treatment principle for the dysfunction syndrome still holds in that the patient's complained-of pain must be *produced* but *not worsened.*

DERANGEMENT SYNDROME

The derangement syndrome confronts therapists with their biggest, and in some ways most rewarding, challenge when dealing with mechanical spinal disorders. With its seven sub-divisions and presence or absence of a number of deformities the variety of clinical presentations may appear to be endless, but there is a common theme running throughout the treatment approach.

Having first established the presence of a non-specific spinal derangement the therapist should carefully consider the following order of events as being very necessary.

Reduction of the derangement

This requires an acceptance of, even if not belief in, the conceptual model of disc pathomechanics proposed earlier. Failure to consider the intervertebral disc as the causative structure may lead to great confusion in the mental processes required of the therapist in analysing the information being gathered in the patient evaluation. No one is able to state categorically that the model is correct but, as McKenzie has written (McKenzie 1990 p xxiii): 'The conceptual models . . . may eventually alter, but the effectiveness of the procedures will not change'.

The reductive process consists essentially of the re-positioning of displaced material that is obstructing spinal curve reversal or even forcing deformity. The diagnosis helps determine the appropriate direction of force required. The therapist should constantly be looking for positions and/or movements that centralize, stop or decrease the pain, with centralization being the most important guide and with the 'traffic lights' principle in action.

A simple posterocentral derangement 1, for instance, in any part of the spine, will be reduced by sagittal extension forces rapidly progressing through to patient overpressure to gain full range (see Figs 55.8–55.11).

A patient with derangement 2, though, may have the same pattern of pain on paper but presents with a very different need in the reductive process. Attempts at rapid reduction, at the rate seen with derangement 1, will show a clear 'red light' and be met with failure. The difference relates, conceptually, to the size of the displacement, although it is still located posterocentrally.

The need for a slower approach here is a clear example of the time factor concept in derangement reduction—we must allow enough time for displacements to be moved (see Figs 55.12–55.19).

Kramer (1990, pp 28–29), quoting the in vitro experiments of Vogel (1977) and Stahl (1977), describes how, by using metal markers, the speed of nucleus pulposus displacement in lumbar and cervical disc was measured. Subjected to prolonged asymmetrical loading, a velocity of 0.6 mm per minute for the first 3 minutes was encountered, followed by continuous displacement for several hours at a lower rate. One can imagine a similar scenario existing in vivo to explain the time factor differences between derangements 1 and 2.

Derangements 2 to 6 are all approached with the aim of being reduced until they resemble derangement 1. Those with a lateral component will require forces directed in the coronal plane to gain centralization of symptoms before sagittal extension is utilized to complete the reduction. The well-known correction of lateral shift technique (McKenzie 1981, pp 76–80) is an example of this when dealing with derangements exhibiting a lateral deformity (numbers 4 and 6).

The odd one out, derangement 7, obviously requires flexion forces to achieve reduction. It also requires confidence from therapists in their diagnostic ability when prescribing forward bending exercises for the acute patient. The same 'traffic light' rules apply, however, and the centralization phenomenon is just as reliable. That it should apply to an apparent anterior displacement does not depart from the conceptual disc model. Cloward's now classic experiments (Cloward 1959) for example, demonstrated that stimulation of the *anterior* annulus fibrosus in the lower cervical discs produced pain in the upper back. Central stimulation produced central inter-scapular pain, and anterolateral stimulation produced medial scapular pain.

Maintenance of the reduction

Just as a skin wound will re-open if pulled on before it has healed sufficiently, so it seems that reduced derangements will recur if stressed too soon. For the posterior derangements this means that the patient must avoid both

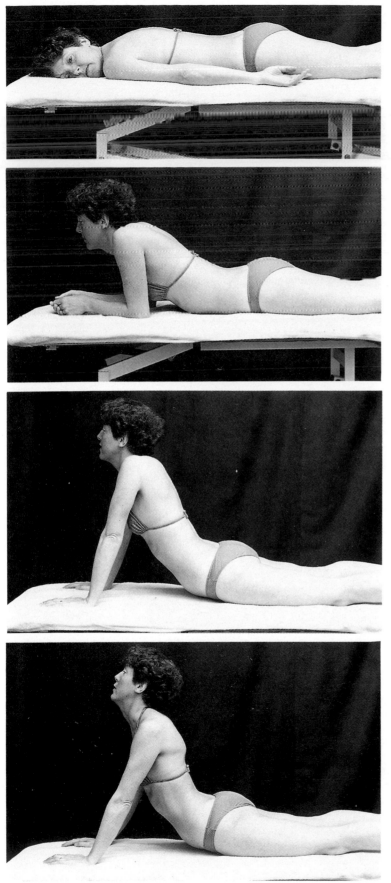

Figs 55.8–55.11   Reduction of the minor posterocentral derangement 1, each stage rapidly progressing to the next. Lying prone (**Fig. 55.8**). This is the first sustained extension procedure; any symptoms are recorded. Lying prone in extension (**Fig. 55.9**). The next progression, sustained to allow for time factor. (May be omitted if pain is not present in lying prone.) Extension in lying (**Fig. 55.10**). Repeated to apply passive reductive pressures. Extension in lying with patient overpressure (**Fig. 55.11**). The patient 'sags' her hips and breathes out fully to gain maximal extension to complete the reductive process.

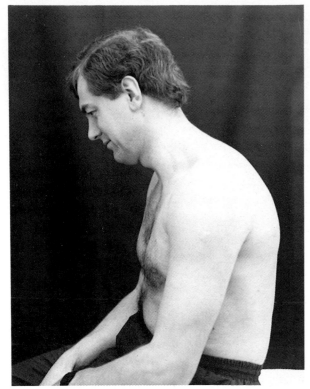

Fig. 55.12 (*see p. 766 for caption*)

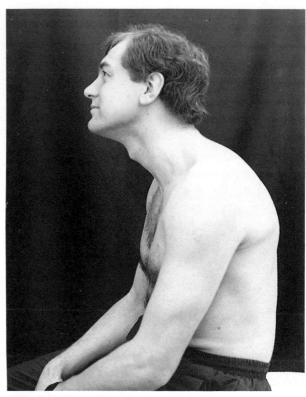

Fig. 55.13 (*see p. 766 for caption*)

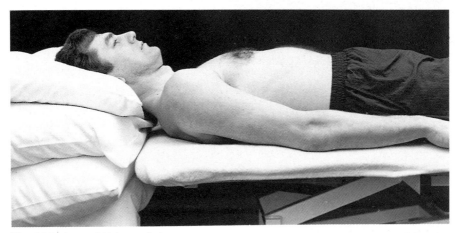

Fig. 55.14 (*see p. 766 for caption*)

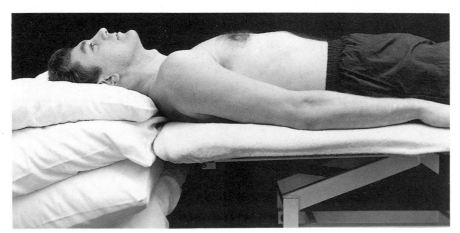

Fig. 55.15 (*see p. 766 for caption*)

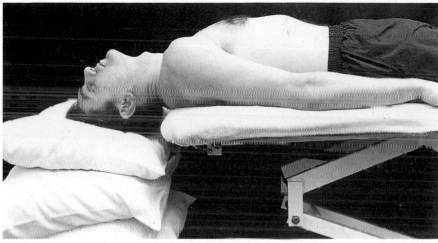

Fig. 55.16 (*see p. 766 for caption*)

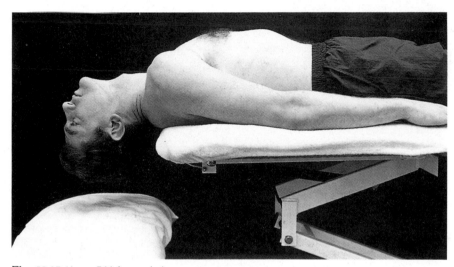

Fig. 55.17 (*see p. 766 for caption*)

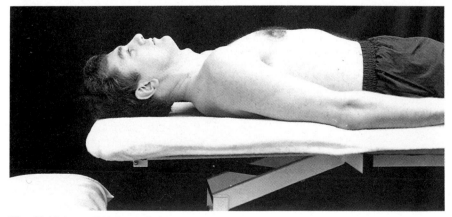

Fig. 55.18 (*see p. 766 for caption*)

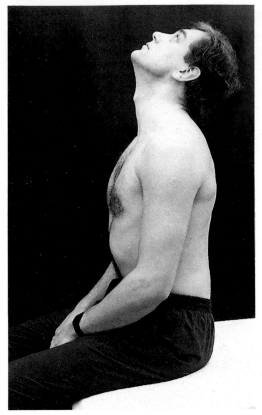

Fig. 55.19

Figs 55.12–55.19 An example of a patient with cervical derangement 2, requiring slow reduction of a major posterocentral displacement. Presenting sitting posture showing lower cervical flexion deformity (**Fig. 55.12**). Initial range of extension, occurring in upper neck only due to obstruction of lower cervical curve reversal (**Fig. 55.13**). The absence of lower cevical extension prevents the patient from being able to lie flat in supine (**Fig. 55.14**). The deformity is accommodated by the use of pillows placed on a stool beyond the end of the plinth to allow for the reductive process which is to follow. Reduction begins (**Fig. 55.15**). The bed is *slowly* raised so that the patient's head and neck move towards extension. Symptom behaviour, as always, is carefully monitored to observe the rules of 'centralization', with 'traffic lights' guidance. Reduction continues (**Fig. 55.16**). Reduction is complete when the patient can lie unsupported over the end of the plinth with little or no discomfort (**Fig. 55.17**). To reach this position may take 10 to 30 minutes from the beginning of reduction. (In some cases it will be impossible to achieve this degree of reduction in the first treatment session.) The patient's head is now slowly lifted by the therapist back to the supine position, which he can now comfortably maintain (**Fig. 55.18**). Great care must be taken to avoid flexing the lower neck during this stage and during rising from the plinth. On resuming the sitting position he is able to extend the lower neck now that the obstruction to curve reversal has been removed (**Fig. 55.19**).

static and dynamic flexion, and for the anterior derangement, extension. Many therapists, from whatever school of thought, having performed a perfectly good reductive procedure, allow their patients to leave the clinic with scant or no regard being payed to the maintenance of correct posture. To omit the removal of provocative forces between treatments results in, at best, a less than perfect result and, at worst, complete failure to respond.

Most patients, for instance, are fully aware of the dangers of lifting a heavy load or the playing of some vigorous sport during the treatment period. Many, however, seem unaware of the slower but just as profound effect that static loading in provocative postures can have. All derangement patients, bar the lumbar anterior type, must be educated in the maintenance of the 90% of full axial extension posture as described above. We must not forget that it is impossible to restore or maintain correct cervical or thoracic posture in sitting without the presence of a lumbar lordosis. On the other hand, correction of lumbar posture does not *automatically* correct cervical posture!

Patients with anterior derangements of the lumbar spine should not be encouraged to remain fully slouched at end-of-range in sitting but rather to maintain some flexion and frequently perform 50–0% movements as a modification of the 'slouch/overcorrect' exercise. As cervical anterior derangements tend to occur in the upper half of the neck, postural instructions are the same as for cervical patients with lower posterior derangements.

A small number of patients, possibly in response to a very enthusiastic therapist, tend to 'overdo' the posture correction and maintain 'extreme of the good' end-of-range positions. They invariably return with significantly increased paraspinal pains which could be confused with centralization but which are in fact due to overstrain. The astute therapist will soon spot the misdemeanour and, once again, alert the patient to the error of sustaining extreme ranges of movement.

During the period of reduction maintenance, the patient's self-treatment programme of appropriate exercises continues unabated with the addition, where necessary, of appropriate manual procedures such as described elsewhere (McKenzie 1981, 1990). The rules to observe in the selection of procedures are according to the 'mechanical diagnosis', 'progression of forces', 'centralization' and 'traffic lights' guides (q.v.). The three-dimensional analysis of symptom behaviour prevails throughout in that the therapist must know the status of the patient's nociceptor activity before, during and after any procedure. Failure to communicate with the patient in this way will lead to unsuccessful mechanical therapy.

Recovery of function

The introduction of gentle natural tension to healing structures (Evans 1980) plays a major role in the prevention of future dysfunction and is one reason for the early introduction of flexion procedures following a posterior derangement. Patients placed on a programme of strict and frequent extension procedures (whether or not preceded by coronal plane forces for any lateral component) cannot continue with this ad infinitum. The continued use of extension leads to the possibility of 'overload' of the posterior joints. The patient who was recovering well starts to complain of renewed spinal pains. The therapist may well think that the patient needs more of the same

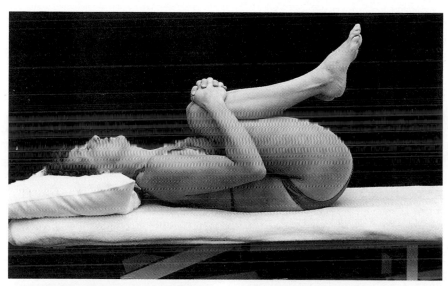

Fig. 55.20

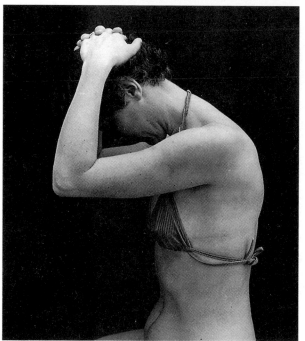

Fig. 55.21

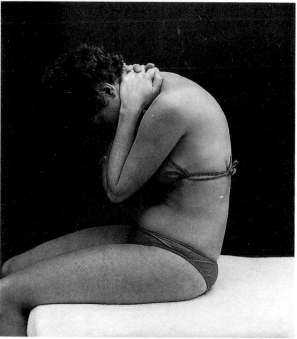

Fig. 55.22

Figs 55.20–55.22   Lumbar flexion in lying (**Fig. 55.20**). The movement is repeated from the crook lying starting position to ascertain the stability of the reduction. Cervical flexion in sitting (**Fig. 55.21**). Overpressure may be added, as illustrated here, *only* when the stability of the derangement has been confirmed. Thoracic flexion in sitting (**Fig. 55.22**). It is important for the patient to bring the shoulders directly down towards the hips to ensure good thoracic movement. Leaning forwards may only flex the hips and lumbar spine. All of the above flexion movements must begin and end in a neutral starting position, with each repetition, to test for 'pain during movement'.

thing to resume the path to recovery, and inadvertently makes matters worse.

When the patient has complained of little or no pain for 2 or 3 days in the thoracolumbar spine and 24 hours in the cervical spine, the time has come to consider the introduction of flexion. This is always done as an exploratory test for the stability of the reduction of the derangement whilst the patient is with the therapist. Testing is carried out in the least forceful manner, which, for the lumbar spine, means flexion in lying (passive), and, for

the cervical and thoracic spine, in sitting (active without overpressure) (see Figs 55.20–55.22).

The three-dimensional symptom evaluation is performed during this repeated movement assessment. The acceptable responses are: no pain produced; pain produced at end-range, not worsened; pain produced at end-range, decreasing and not worsened. If the patient experiences pain during movement, increasing or peripheralizing symptoms, or remains worse following movement, then flexion is not yet safe to introduce as the derangement has not become stable. Those in whom it appears safe to continue with will begin gradually, progressively moving on to weight-bearing or overpressure. Always, following significant posterior derangement, flexion in the first few hours after rising should be avoided due to the increased turgidity of the disc creating a greater risk of recurrence.

Recovery of function is complete when full normal weight-bearing flexion produces no more than the expected 'strain' at end of range. If there is found to be no pain or loss of range on testing flexion then, strictly speaking, there is no need to introduce this procedure to recover function. It is wise, however, to test the integrity of the reduction with some flexion procedures over a few days before allowing the patient to resume full normal activity levels. It is rare for patients to develop extension dysfunction following anterior derangement but this should be explored in the appropriate manner.

Prophylaxis

The conceptual model tells us that a derangement can be prevented if the movement or static force is applied *before* displacement has a chance to recur. Once pain has returned, or obstructions to curve reversals are re-emerging, then treatment—not prevention—is the operative word.

As previously stated, prophylaxis begins on day one with the patient's realization that something good has occurred of their own doing. The educational value of this has to be emphasized. Apart from this essential ingredient the prevention of future recurrences rests very much on the completion of the treatment programme through to full recovery of function. Equally important is the therapist's ability to teach well (and the patient's ability to learn) the general principles of simple body mechanics required to minimize provocative static and dynamic loads on the spine.

Apart from the usual instructions with regard to postures, lifting and other ergonomic advice, patients need to be instructed to introduce extension artificially into their lifestyles, for it rarely occurs naturally in our society. The use of self-applied reductive manoeuvres performed several times a day is essential.

REFERENCES

Alexander A H, Jones A M, Rosenbaum D H Jnr 1990 Nonoperative management of herniated nucleus pulposus: patient selection by the extension sign—long-term follow up. Paper #14, 5th Annual Meeting of the North American Spine Society, Monterey, California, August 8–11
Brunarski D J 1984 Clinical trials of spinal manipulation. Journal of Manipulative Physical Therapy 7: 4
Care G R F, Harfield B, Chamberlain M A 1981 And have you done your exercises? Physiotherapy 67: 180
Carrington W 1970 Balance as a function of intelligence. Systematics 7: 8
Cloward R B 1959 Cervical discography: a contribution to the etiology and mechanism of neck shoulder and arm pain. Annals of Surgery 150: 1052
Cochrane Report 1979 Department of Health and Social Security: report of a working group on back pain. Her Majesty's Stationery Office, London
Deyo R A, Diehl A K 1986 Patient satisfaction with medical care for low back pain. Spine 11: 28–32
DiMaggio A, Mooney V 1987 The McKenzie program: exercise effective against back pain. Journal of Musculoskeletal Medicine 63–74
Donelson R, Murphy K, Silva G 1990 Centralisation phenomenon. Its usefulness in evaluating and treating referred pain. Spine 15: 211–213
Donelson R, Grant W, Kamps C, Medcalf R 1991 Pain response to sagittal end-range spinal motion: a prospective, randomized, multicentered trial. Spine 16: S206–S212
Evans P 1980 The healing process at cellular level. Physiotherapy 66: 256–259
Farrel J P, Twomey L T 1982 Acute low back pain. Comparison of two conservative treatment approaches. Medical Journal of Australia 1: 160–164
Frymoyer J W, Mooney V 1986 Current concepts review: occupational orthopaedics. Journal of Bone and Joint Surgery 68A: 469–474
Fuchioka M, Nakai O, Yamaura I 1988 A topographical study of lumbar disc herniation using CT-discography. International Society for the Study of the Lumbar Spine, Miami, USA, April 13–17

Glossop E S, Goldenberg E, Smith D S, Williams I M 1982 Patient compliance in back and neck pain. Physiotherapy 68: 225–226
Hadler N M, Curtis P, Gillings D B, Stinnett S 1987 A benefit of spinal manipulation as adjunctive therapy for acute low back pain: a stratified controlled trial. Spine 12: 703–706
Hoehler F K, Tobis J S, Buerger A A 1981 Spinal manipulation for low back pain. Journal of the American Medical Association 245: 1835–1838
Kopp J R, Alexander A H, Turocy R H 1986 The use of lumbar extension in the evaluation and treatment of patients with acute herniated nucleus pulposus. A preliminary report. Clinical Orthopaedics and Related Research 202: 211–218
Kramer J 1990 Intervertebral disc diseases, 2nd edn. Thieme Medical Publishers, New York
Kuslich S D, Ulstrom C L, Cami J M 1991 The tissue origin of low back pain and sciatica. A report of pain response to tissue stimulation during operations on the lumbar spine using local anesthesia. Orthopaedic Clinics of North America 22: 181–187
MacDonald R S, Bell C M J 1990 An open controlled assessment of osteopathic manipulation in nonspecific low back pain. Spine 15: 364–370
McKenzie R A 1981 The lumbar spine. Mechanical diagnosis and therapy. Spinal Publications, Waikanae, New Zealand
McKenzie R A 1989 A perspective on manipulative therapy. Physiotherapy 75: 440–444
McKenzie R A 1990 The cervical and thoracic spine. Mechanical diagnosis and therapy. Spinal Publications, Waikanae, New Zealand
Moll V M, Wright V 1972 Evaluation of the Arthritis and Rheumatology Council handbook on gout: an objective study on doctor–patient communication. Annals of the Rheumatic Diseases 31: 405–411
Moser J 1990 An investigation into changes in knowledge and behaviour following attendance at back school. Unpublished thesis in rehabilitation studies housed at Southampton University, UK
Nwuga G, Nwuga V 1985 Relative therapeutic efficacy of the Williams and McKenzie protocols in back pain management. Physiotherapy Practice 1: 99–105
Ponte D J, Jensen G J, Kent B E 1984 A preliminary report on the use of the McKenzie protocol versus Williams protocol in the treatment

of low back pain. Journal of Orthopaedic and Sports Physical Therapy 6: 130–139

Rath W W, Rath J N D, Duffy C G 1989 A comparison of pain location and duration with treatment outcome and frequency. Presented at First International McKenzie Conference, Newport Beach, California, July 20–21

Roberts A P 1990 The conservative treatment of low back pain. Thesis in preparation, Nottingham, UK

Sims-Williams H, Jayson M I V, Young S M S, Baddeley H, Collins E 1978 Controlled trial of mobilisation and manipulation for patients with low back pain in general practice. British Medical Journal 2: 1338–1340

Smyth M J, Wright V 1958 Sciatica and the intervertebral disc. Journal of Bone and Joint Surgery 40A: 1401

Spitzer W Ö 1987 Scientific approach to the assessment and management of activity-related spinal disorders. A monograph for clinicians. Report of the Quebec task force on spinal disorders. Spine 12: 7S

Stahl Ch 1977 Experimentelle Untersuchungen zur Biomechanik der Halswirbelsaule. Diss., Dusseldorf

Stankovic R, Johnell O 1990 Conservative treatment of acute low back pain. A prospective randomized trial: McKenzie method of treatment versus patient education in 'mini back school'. Spine 15: 120–123

Timbrell Fisher A G 1948 Treatment by manipulation, 5th edn. Lewis, London

Tucker W 1960 Active alerted posture. E & S Livingstone, London, pp 1–2

Van Wijmen P M 1986a Lumbar pain syndromes. In: Grieve G P (ed) Modern manual therapy. Churchill Livingstone, Edinburgh

Van Wijmen P M 1986b The management of recurrent low back pain. In: Grieve G P (ed) Modern manual therapy. Churchill Livingstone, Edinburgh

Vanharanta H, Videman T, Mooney V 1986 McKenzie exercise, Back Trac and back school in lumbar syndrome. Annual meeting of International Society for the Study of the Lumbar Spine, Dallas, Texas

Vogel G 1977 Experimentelle Untersuchungen zur Mobilitat des Nucleus Pulposus in lumbalen Bandscheiben. Diss., Dusseldorf

Weber H 1986 Conservative management of back pain: critical evaluation of conservative treatment programmes. Presented at the first European Congress on Back Pain Current Concepts and Recent Advances, Helsinki

Williams M M, Hawley J A, McKenzie R A, Van Wijmen P M, 1991 A comparison of the effects of two sitting postures on back and referred pain. Spine 16: 1185–1191

56. Lumbar zygapophyseal joint syndromes: examination and interpretation of clinical findings

W. Aspinall

INTRODUCTION

Prior to planning a treatment programme and predicting a final outcome the information gathered during the clinical examination is evaluated. Clinical problems may then be developed on which to base the selection and outcome of treatment.

In order that lumbar zygapophyseal joint syndromes may be proposed once the clinical findings are interpreted the analysis should correlate with anatomical, biomechanical and pathological known facts. The clinical problems should address the structure(s) producing the symptoms and the clinical abnormalities which are responsible for the symptoms from that structure. The clinical problems should also address the possible influence of other factors which may predispose these structures to become symptomatic.

PATHOLOGY

The incidence of degenerative joint disease, or osteo-arthrosis increases with age and is the most common pathology of the lumbar zygapophyseal joints (Bogduk 1986). In the younger age groups osteo-arthrosis affects the upper lumbar spinal levels and tends to be localized to one segment. In the later years it is more prevalent at low lumbar spinal levels and may affect more than one spinal segment (Bogduk 1986). Theoretically these joints could be strained by compressive and tensile forces, especially if osteo-arthrosis is established. The joint capsules may become inflamed, causing a chemical irritation of the nociceptive nerve endings, producing pain. The joint capsules may heal in either a lengthened or shortened position, causing zygapophyseal joint hypermobility or hypomobility respectively. Hypomobile joints may predispose other spinal areas to become hypermobile and these could eventually become symptomatic due to repetitive stresses. The hypomobile joints may be the cause of pain from a mechanical irritation of the nociceptive nerve endings in the intra-articular or peri-articular structures.

Once the joint capsules have healed in a lengthened position they are extremely susceptible to further strain following trauma and may produce instability of the zygapophyseal joints.

Subluxations have been alleged to be causes of back pain. In disc narrowing, the zygapophyseal joints may subluxate to such an extent that the inferior articular process may impinge on the laminae below causing erosion of the periosteum, and this could be a cause of pain (Hadley 1935, Vernon-Roberts & Pirie 1977). Subluxations may theoretically occur in hypermobile or unstable joints producing pain from an increased tension on the capsule and increased compression on intra-articular structures due to an aberrant joint movement.

The theory of intra-articular extrapments and entrapments have been discussed in the literature (Bogduk & Jull 1985). These meniscoid structures may be the source of pain or they may produce a traction effect on the joint capsule to elicit the pain.

Fractures of either the inferior or superior articular process may occur from excessive compressive forces and could be a source of back pain. Such fractures may have been underdiagnosed because they are not readily demonstrated by plain radiography (Sims-Williams et al 1978).

CLINICAL FEATURES — SUBJECTIVE EXAMINATION

Area and nature of pain

The local pain distribution of lumbar zygapophyseal joint syndromes is back pain. The back pain may be accompanied by referred pain in the lower limb commonly felt proximal to the knee and into the buttocks and groin (Bogduk & Twomey 1991). Experimental studies have shown that local and referred pain patterns from joints at different levels vary considerably in different individuals, and even in the same individual they may overlap greatly (Bogduk 1986). Consequently, the distribution of referred pain cannot be used to determine the level of the primary source of pain in lumbar zygapophyseal joint syndromes. Complementing these experimental studies are clinical reports of the relief of low-back pain and referred pain in the lower limbs by injections of local anaesthetic into the zygapophyseal joints (Bogduk 1986). The nature of the pain is deep, dull and aching in quality and is difficult to localize (Bogduk & Twomey 1991).

Historical features

Flexion, lateral flexion and torsional injuries have been related to zygapophyseal joint damage (Farfan 1973, Adams & Hutton 1982). The incident may cause sudden acute pain, or the pain may increase over hours or days if inflammatory factors are involved. Apart from injuries from direct trauma a minor incident may cause a major disability which may result from the accumulative effect of postural compensation.

Behaviour of the symptoms

One must equate the activities which provoke and relieve symptoms with known neurophysiological, pathological and mechanical characteristics of zygapophyseal joints. Three case histories of common zygapophyseal joint syndromes are used as illustrations in Figures 56.1–56.3. The definition of 'syndrome' is a set of clinical data which correlate anatomically, pathologically and biomechanically so that a diagnostic hypothesis may be proposed. Tables 56.1–56.3 outline the possible reasons for the behaviour of symptoms in the three case histories.

This hypothesis of zygapophyseal joint syndromes following the subjective examination cannot be made on these clinical features alone, for none of these features are unique to the syndromes. Some form of physical examination is necessary in order to confirm, modify or disprove the diagnostic hypothesis.

Sites of pain and other symptoms

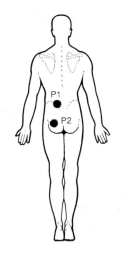

Symptoms
Nature: dull ache

Constant: X; intermittent: ✓

Increasing: ✓; static: X
Decreasing: X

Night pain: X
Sleeping position: no preference
First rising: low back stiff, difficult to bend forward

Eases: repeated flexion in sitting

Aggravates: prolonged standing > 10 min; gardening; prolonged sitting > 0.5 h

Eases: walking several steps

Cough/sneeze: X

Day pain: no pattern; depends on activity level

Fig. 56.1   Case history — patient A.

Name: patient A

Age: 40

Activities: work: teacher, standing and sitting; play: X

Steroids: X

Cord, cauda equina: X

Medication: X

X-ray: mild degenerative disc disease

General health: X

Current history: low-grade gradual onset 1 to 2 years P1; past 6 months P1 more frequent, and onset of P2

Previous history: 3 years ago two episodes of P1, cleared within 2 to 3 weeks; first episode following repetitive carrying and lifting while moving house, and second episode following a day of golf

Treatment and result: X

Table 56.1 Interpretation of functional activities (patient A)

Function	Reaction	Reason
Prolonged standing	↑ Pain	• Fatigue of muscles controlling lordotic curve (Twomey & Taylor 1987) • Gradual creep of tissues ↑ compressive loading (Twomey & Taylor 1987), pain from intra-articular structures ↑ Tensile forces Pain from superior part of the capsule (Hedtmann et al 1989)
Gardening; prolonged sitting (sustained flexion)	↑ Pain	• Gradual creep of tissues (Twomey & Taylor 1987) • ↑ Compressive loads upper and mid zygapophyseal joints (Taylor & Twomey 1987); pain from intra-articular structures • ↑ Tensile forces (Hedtmann et al 1989); pain from dorsal part of capsule
Walking	↓ Pain	• Pain not related to movement through range • Mechanoreceptor influence (Wyke 1976)
First rising (stiffness)		• Altered lubrication of articular cartilage

Sites of pain and other symptoms

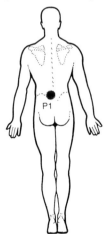

Symptoms

Nature: ache or sharp twinges

Constant: ✓; intermittent: X

Night pain: ↑ P1 with change of position

Aggravates: all movements cause immediate pain

Eases: lying supine, knees over a small pillow; sitting, pain ↓ immediately

Cough/sneeze: P1 ↑

First rising: low back stiffness on flexion

Fig. 56.2 Case history — patient B.

CLINICAL FEATURES — PHYSICAL EXAMINATION — PATIENT A

Postural analysis

There are a number of habitual faulty postures seen on patients with zygapophyseal joint pathology. These postures may give rise to a stretch weakness of the muscles which remain in a lengthened position, however slight, beyond the neutral position. This concept is related to the duration of faulty alignment rather than the severity (Kendall & McCreary 1982). Muscles are made to lengthen by the pull of antagonistic muscles and by the action of gravity. The lengthening of inactive muscle is a passive, not an active process (Kendall & McCreary 1982). Consequently, unless the opposing muscle is able to pull the part back to a neutral position, or some outside force is exerted to lengthen the short muscle, there will be a tendency for the shortened muscle to remain in a somewhat shortened position. Muscle shortness is invariably associated with muscle strength (Gossman et al 1982).

Patient A demonstrated a high lumbar lordotic posture. On observation the lumbar spine was inclined forward from the ideal plumb alignment (Kendall & McCreary 1982) to the level of about the second lumbar vertebra. Above this level there was a sharp deviation backward.

Name: patient B

Age: 28

Activities: work: bank teller (off work); play: ballet and athletics as a teenager

Steroids: X

Cord, cauda equina: X

Medication: anti-inflammatories for 1 day only

X-ray: X

General health: X

Current history: after reaching to adjust curtain and resuming normal posture, immediate low-back pain 48 hours ago

Previous history: one episode, 1 year ago, following a serve at tennis; resolved within 1 week

Treatment and result: X

Table 56.2   Interpretation of functional activities (patient B)

Function	Reaction	Reason
All spinal movements	↑ Pain immediately	• Pain through range intra-articular block
First rising	↑ Stiffness (on flexion)	• ↑ Muscle tone due to pain
Cough/sneeze	↑ Pain	• Mechanical 'jarring' of sudden uncontrolled movement; ↑ compressive loading, pain from intra-articular structures
Sitting; lying with knees bent	↓ Pain immediately	• Zygapophyseal joints in neutral position; ↓ intra-articular compression

This type of posture suggests an increased flexibility of the anterior and lateral fibres of the obliquus externus abdominis muscle.

Muscle function and imbalance

Poor quality and control of a pelvic backward tilt can be either the production or a perpetuation of adverse tensile forces and compressive loads on zygapophyseal joints. Thus the increase flexibility of the obliquus externus abdominis could be the clinical problem to predisposing the zygapophyseal joint dysfunction.

During a curled trunk sit-up, as the hip flexion phase was initiated the anterior superior iliac spines moved inferiorly. The trunk curl was performed with the knees straight and forearms extended forwards. From a supine position hip flexion can be performed only by the hip

Sites of pain and other symptoms

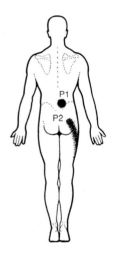

Symptoms
Nature: dull ache

Constant: X; intermittent: ✓

Increasing: ✓; static: X
Decreasing: X

Night pain: P1 occasionally with movement
Sleeping position: side-lying, hips and knees bent
First rising: X

Aggravates: standing > 5 min; walking >10 min; midstance to push off R leg

Eases: sitting in flexion or standing with L foot raised (immediate ↓ pain)

Cough/sneeze: X

Day pain: pattern not time-related

Fig. 56.3   Case history — patient C.

Name: patient C

Age: 52

Activities: work: engineer (desk job); play: golf

Steroids: X

Cord, cauda equina: X

Medication: X

X-ray: ✓

General health: X

Current history: acute episode P1 and P2 2 months ago following a weekend of golf; severity ↓ within 1 week; frequency gradually ↑ over past month

Previous history: low-grade back pain for several years

Previous treatment and results: many chiropractic manipulations in the past

Table 56.3 Interpretation of functional activities (patient C)

Function	Reaction	Reason
Prolonged standing	↑ Pain	• See Table 56.1
Walking 10 minutes; R leg mid-stance to push-off	↑ Pain	• Vertical creep • ↑ Compressive loads (Kirkaldy-Willis & Farfan 1982) • Extension, side flexion/rotation in the lumbar spine • Pain through range of joint movement
Sitting in flexion	↓ Pain immediately	• ↑ Tensile forces on dorsal structures (Hedtmann et al 1989) • Minimal compressive load on lower zygapophyseal joints
Standing, L foot raised	↓ Pain	• L lumbar side flexion • ↓ Tensile and compressive loads on R zygapophyseal joint whilst in the extended position

flexors acting to bring the pelvis in flexion towards the thighs. The external oblique muscles maintain the trunk in flexion by pulling the pelvis in the direction of a posterior tilt. In patient A the abdominals could not overcome the peak tension force of the hip flexors producing an anterior tilt of the pelvis.

Standard active physiological movement

In order to reproduce the patient's symptoms or produce joint signs the physiological movements of trunk extension and of a pelvic forward tilt both increase the lumbar lordosis but often provoke different responses (Magarey 1986). Pelvic forward tilt reproduces the movement most likely to take place during prolonged standing, which was one of the provoking activities for patient A. With prolonged standing, if hyperextension occurs in the lumbar spine it is likely that the axis of movement will shift even further posteriorly to where the tips of the inferior facets articulate with the laminae (Hedtmann et al 1989). During hyperextension the superior part of the zygapophyseal joint capsules may be stretched and cause pain. Osteo-arthritic changes occur at the polar region of the inferior recesses of these joints corresponding to the areas of extension impact and compression and may be the cause of symptoms (Twomey & Taylor 1987). The active physiological movement of pelvic forward tilt causes the sacral base to flex on the fifth lumbar vertebra, and in patient A this movement reproduced P1. Extension from the trunk affects more the upper and mid-lumbar zygapophyseal joints. The sacrum extends with the pelvic girdle, minimizing movement at the lower lumbar

levels, and in this patient extension from the trunk was asymptomatic.

The active physiological movements of trunk flexion and of a pelvic backward tilt both decrease the lumbar lordosis but often produce different responses (Magarey 1986). Pelvic backward tilt reproduces the movement which takes place during squatting whilst gardening and prolonged sitting, two of the provoking activities for patient A. On active pelvic backward tilt the sacral base extends on the fifth lumbar vertebra and may produce tensile forces on the dorsal part of the capsule of the L5/S1 joints. In this patient, pelvic backward tilt in the sitting position was restricted. In sitting, this movement is performed passively, whereas, in standing, active control of the abdominals and hip extensors are required to perform a pelvic backward tilt. Trunk flexion achieves only a neutral position of the lumbar vertebrae (Bogduk & Twomey 1991). This movement would produce less tensile force on the dorsal capsule. The sacrum flexes with the pelvic girdle, hence producing minimal movement at the L5/S1 zygapophyseal joints. In patient A trunk flexion was asymptomatic.

During these functional activities of sustained flexion, anterior sagittal translation is normally performed by gravity (Bogduk & Twomey 1991). Pain may be produced from compression on intra-articular structures in the anteromedial third of the joints. However, in patient A, if the dorsal part of the capsule has healed from trauma in a shortened position this may prevent the anterior sagittal rotation taking place.

Combined physiological movements

Habitually, movements of the spine occur in combination across planes rather than as pure movements in one plane only (Fryette 1954, Gregerson & Lucas 1967, Loebe 1973, Schultz et al 1973, Farfan 1975, Stoddard 1980, Pearcy & Tibrewal 1984). The coupled direction and degree of spinal habitual movements may depend on the control of the joint capsule, shape of the joint surfaces, intra-articular meniscoids and spinal muscle action. The presence of a degenerative process within the zygapophyseal joints may affect the amount and direction of spinal movement. Signs and symptoms produced by active physiological movements may therefore alter when these movements are performed in a combined manner and may be more indicative of the patient's signs and symptoms. Prolonged standing usually involves the transference of weight from one leg to the other — as opposed to even weight continually on both legs. This produces a side flexion/rotation movement of the lumbar spine in the extended position performed from the pelvis rather than the trunk. Pelvic forward tilt provoked only part of the patient's symptoms (P1). The effect of adding lateral flexion to the left by bending the right knee may increase the tensile forces on the superior capsule of the left L5/S1 zygapophyseal joint and increase compressive loads on the intra-articular structures. This combined movement increased P1 and provoked P2. Movements may be combined in different sequences to confirm the dominant component in a movement pattern or to reproduce symptoms more clearly. If one movement is taken to its full range, less movement is available in other directions so that the end position is different with each combination. Consequently the symptoms and signs produced will not necessarily be the same. In patient A a pelvic forward tilt was the dominant component.

The functional movements of gardening and sitting involve transference of weight from one side of the body to the other side. This activity produces a side flexion/rotation movement of the lumbar spine in the flexed position, performed from the trunk rather than the pelvis. The effect of adding lateral flexion to the right from the trunk increased P1. This movement was performed on patient A in the sitting position at the restricted range of a pelvic backward tilt. In this position there may be an increase in tensile forces on the dorsal capsule of the left lumbar zygapophyseal joints which may be the cause of P1 (Behrsin & Briggs 1989).

Spinal accessory movements

The earliest detectable changes in movement that occur with ageing are changes in the quality of the spinal accessory movement (Magarey 1986). These changes are present before any change in physiological movement occurs. Therefore, accessory movements are the most sensitive indicator of abnormality of movement in a joint. Experimental observations have found that manual diagnosis can be as accurate as radiologically controlled blocks for the diagnosis of pain stemming from the cervical spine zygapophyseal joints (Jull & Bogduk 1985). Accessory movements provide more information which may be useful both in confirming the source of symptoms and in directing treatment. Performing these movements when the patient is not bearing weight, as compared to the weight-bearing position, in either the sitting or standing position, will make a difference to the reproduction of symptoms. Accessory movements should be performed as close as possible in the combined physiological movement which produces the patient's signs or symptoms. In patient A the spinal level requires localization and differentiation between tensile and compressive forces producing the symptoms.

Posterior–anterior pressures, angled caudad, were applied to the spinous processes of the lumbar vertebra with patient A standing in the combined habitual position of extension and left-side flexion from the pelvis. These accessory movements increase the compression on the intra-articular structures of the left lumbar zygapophyseal joints (Edwards 1987). In patient A this accessory movement applied to L4 increased P1.

Posterior–anterior pressures on the base of the sacrum, or on L5 spinous process angled cranially with the patient in the same position, may increase tensile forces on the superior part of the capsule of the left zygapophyseal joints of L5/S1 or L4/5 respectively. In this patient, P1 and P2 were increased when the accessory movements was applied to the base of the sacrum.

Posterior–anterior pressures, angled cranially, were applied to the spinous processes of the lumbar vertebra with the patient sitting in flexion and right-side flexion. These accessory movements may increase the tensile forces on the dorsal part of the capsule of the left zygapophyseal joints; a posterior–anterior pressure on L5 increased P1.

Passive physiological intervertebral movement

Where normal joint movement exists there is minimal, if any, gapping of the zygapophyseal joints on physiological intervertebral rotation (McFadden & Taylor 1990). Experimental studies have shown that this gapping exists with zygapophyseal joint hypermobility and instability (McFadden & Taylor 1990).

In this patient it is important to determine whether hypermobility or instability is present at the zygapophyseal joints as this type of joint dysfunction is often the source of pain and should not be subjected to forceful movement. The lumbar vertebral segments are passively moved through a physiological rotation around an axis through the disc as opposed to an axis through the zygapophyseal joints. The amount of movement at each level is compared and the end feel of the joint in an extended position is ascertained. The physiological movement of left rotation at L4/5 and L5/S1 performed in extension may stress the superior part of the left zygapophyseal joint capsules (Behrsin & Briggs 1989). In patient A this test did not seem to demonstrate hypermobility or instability, minimal gapping was detected, and the quality of the end feel was a normal capsular feel. Local discomfort was produced on sustained left physiological intervertebral rotation at L5/S1.

Evaluation — patient A

Before making a prognosis or instituting treatment, information gained during the clinical examination is evaluated. From this information clinical problems can be developed on which to base further management. Clinical problems concern the structure(s) causing symptoms and the specific abnormalities which are responsible for symptoms from that structure. Clinical problems also involve the relationship between different symptoms and the possible influence of other factors on the presenting symptoms. Table 56.4 summarizes the clinical findings

Table 56.4 Clinical findings and clinical problems (patient A)

Physical examination	Clinical findings*
Posture	• High lumbar lordosis
Muscle function	• Trunk curl hip flexion phase, anterior superior iliac spines move inferior bilaterally
Active physiological movement	• Pelvic forward tilt ↑ P1 (standing) • Pelvic backward tilt ↓ range (sitting)
Combined physiological movement	• Pelvic forward tilt ↑ P1 + L side flexion from the pelvis ↑ P1 & P2 (standing) • Pelvic backward tilt ↓ range + R side flexion from trunk ↑ P1 (sitting)
Accessory movement	• Posterior–anterior pressure caudad L4 ↑ P1 in extension and L side flexion • Posterior–anterior pressure cranial base of sacrum ↑ P1 & P2 in extension and L side flexion • Posterior–anterior pressure cranial L5 ↑ P1 in flexion and R side flexion
Passive physiological intervertebral movement	• R rotation L5 in extension local discomfort

Clinical problems
• Intra-articular degenerative changes L L4/5 zygapophyseal joint
• L5/S1 L zygapophyseal joint capsular shortening, maturation stage of healing
• Lengthened obliquus externus abdominis muscle

Clinical syndrome
• L4/5 and L5/S1 zygapophyseal joint arthrosis

* For the location of P1 and P2 see Figure 56.1.

from the physical examination of patient A and outlines the clinical problems and clinical symptoms. A tentative prognosis can also be made of the likely result of treatment and the length of time necessary to achieve that result. Both the clinical problems and prognosis may be changed at any stage during treatment if assessment of the effect of treatment indicates that either were inappropriate or incorrect.

CLINICAL FEATURES — PHYSICAL EXAMINATION — PATIENT B

Postural analysis

This patient demonstrated a flattened low-lumbar spine with a slight shift to the right of the thorax. It was assumed that this was a protective posture.

Combined physiological movements

Lumbar spine extension and left-side flexion from the trunk or pelvis, and in all combinations, increased pain immediately on movement. An intra-articular structure may be blocking the combined physiological movement as pain is demonstrated through the range. Pain through the range may also be produced from an inflammatory condition; this is negated from the analysis of the provoking and easing activities in patient B.

Positional testing

A restrictive fault can be defined as an altered resting position of a vertebral unit which, on subsequent testing, demonstrates a decrease in the total range of movement with the greatest restriction apparent in the opposite direction to which it is held (Lee 1986). In the prone position and slight lumbar spine extension the transverse process of L4 on the right seemed more posterior than on the left. This positional finding suggests a restriction into extension of the left zygapophyseal joint and correlates biomechanically with the combined physiological movement of extension and left-side flexion producing symptoms and the postural finding.

Passive intervertebral movement

Altered gamma input from the symptomatic zygapophyseal joint may change the length/tension of the deep segmental muscles (Patterson 1976). To free an intra-articular block, movement into the opposite direction to the restriction should be available. If the left-sided multifidi have a decrease in flexibility this could restrict right-side flexion and left rotation in the flexed position of the vertebral segment. Patient B demonstrated a passive intervertebral movement restriction of right-side flexion and left rotation in the flexed position at both the L4/5 and L5/S1 segments. This restriction was not obvious on positional testing in a flexed position, probably due to the multifidi not being in a sufficiently lengthened position. One should note that a segmental restriction of a passive intervertebral movement of side flexion and rotation to the same side in a flexed position may suggest a gross shortening of the dorsal capsule of the zygapophyseal joint opposite to the restricted movements.

Evaluation — patient B

Table 56.5 summarizes the clinical findings from the physical examination of patient B and outlines the clinical problems and clinical syndromes. Once these clinical problems have been treated a physical assessment for the underlying cause of the locking would be performed. This would include a postural analysis, passive intervertebral movement testing for hypermobility and instability, and muscle balance testing for the deep segmental muscles and for any other muscles related to the postural findings.

Table 56.5 Clinical findings and clinical problems (patient B)

Physical examination	Clinical findings*
Posture	• Low lumbar flexion with a slight shift R of thorax
Combined physiological movements	• Extension and L side flexion ↑ P1 immediately on movement from trunk and pelvis
Positional testing	• R transverse process L4 posterior in extension
Passive intervertebral movement	• R side flexion and L rotation L4 and L5 restricted in flexion

Clinical problems
• Intra-articular block L4/5 L zygapophyseal joint
• Decrease flexibility L multifidi — low lumbar area

Clinical syndrome
• Locked L zygapophyseal joint L4/5

* For the location of P1 see Figure 56.2.

CLINICAL FEATURES — PHYSICAL EXAMINATION — PATIENT C

Postural analysis

On observing this patient's posture there was a deviation of the pelvis towards the right and a lateral tilt down on the left, the right hip was in postural adduction and the left hip in abduction. The thoracic and lumbar spine had a curve convex towards the left. In this type of posture the right hip abductors, left lateral trunk muscles and left hip adductors are in a somewhat lengthened position. The left hip abductors, right lateral trunk muscles and right hip adductors are in a shortened position.

Walking is one of the functional activities which increased this patient's symptoms during mid-stance to push off on the right leg. Due to the lengthened position of the right hip abductors, the latter may develop a positional weakness and thus be unable to function eccentrically to control hip adduction. To maintain the centre of gravity over the right leg during weight-bearing the thoracolumbar spine compensates by right-side flexion. This postural observation was more apparent on patient C whilst standing on the right leg. This compensation in the thoracolumbar spine may increase the tensile and compressive forces on the right zygapophyseal joints during gait.

Muscle function and imbalance

To assist in confirming this muscle imbalance the patterning of muscle activity during right hip abduction in the left-side lying position was observed. The right quadratus lumborum seemed to initiate hip abduction through a lateral pelvic tilt. If this muscle is truly shortened it will develop positional strength and so tend to come into action quicker than the lengthened muscle. Since abnormal patterning was noticed the length/tension of quadratus lumborum was examined and true shortening was noticed. The left hip abductors and right hip adductors demonstrated only a mild decrease in flexibility. A decreased flexibility of muscle is more common clinically than a true shortening, and, if found, the muscle balance will return if treatment is directed to functionally retraining the lengthened muscles. In this patient's case the truly shortened quadratus lumborum should be addressed first.

During most functional activities a rotation side flexion movement takes place in the lumbar spine. The principal muscles that produce rotation of the thorax are the oblique abdominal muscles, and these muscles impart axial rotation to the lumbar spine (Bogduk & Twomey 1991). The oblique abdominal muscles also simultaneously cause flexion of the trunk and therefore of the lumbar spine (Bogduk & Twomey 1991). To counteract this flexion and maintain pure axial rotation the extensors of the lumbar spine must be recruited to act as stabilizers. In zygapophyseal joint syndromes these muscles, due to their segmental innervation, tend to have altered gamma input from the symptomatic segment (Patterson 1976). This produces either an increase or decrease in flexibility within the muscle belly, and, if this takes place, the muscle balance pattern will be affected. The following test may be used to establish an increase in flexibility within the deep segmental muscles (Aspinall 1988). The patient lies prone, over one pillow to place the lumbar spine in a relatively neutral position. The patient actively raises one leg just off the bed, keeping the knee straight, and the pelvis level, holds it elevated for five seconds and then repeats this manoeuvre on the other leg. It is necessary to repeat this test approximately five times to achieve a true muscular response. On lifting the left leg, extension left-side flexion and right rotation is produced in the lumbar spine. At the same time, in order to keep the lumbar spine and pelvis stable, the right multifidus works as a segmental stabilizer controlling the action of the external oblique which produces flexion and right rotation. If the right multifidus is lengthened and has developed positional weakness one notices an excess of right rotation. In patient C this test was positive on left hip extension.

It should be noted that this test may be misinterpreted if there is an imbalance of muscle activity between the left hip extensors, erector spinae and hamstrings during the action of left hip extension. This imbalance must be corrected prior to testing multifidus.

Combined physiological movements

To reproduce this patient's symptoms or to produce joint signs the combined physiological movements which biomechanically correlated with standing and walking, which are the patient's provoking activities, were assessed. Right-side flexion from the pelvis was the dominant movement producing P1. This was performed by bending the left knee and simulates standing with weight on the right leg. Pelvic forward tilt was added which increased P1, and right-side flexion from the trunk further increased P1. This position produces both tensile forces and compressive loads on the right zygapophyseal joint, which could be the source of pain. If the combination of combined physiological movements was side flexion right from the trunk without side flexion from the pelvis the symptoms were minimal. This could be due to minimal right-side flexion of L5/S1 during trunk side flexion as L5 tends to move with the sacrum. Right-side flexion from the trunk causes the ilium to rotate posteriorly on the left and anteriorly on the right which passively rotates the sacrum to the left, hence a left rotation of L5 (Lee 1989). The coupling action of L5/S1 tends to be rotation and side flexion to the same side regardless of whether the segment is in flexion, neutral or extension (Pearcy & Tibrewal 1984). When the combination of combined movements was pelvic forward tilt followed by right-side flexion from the pelvis less pain and more range was available. The pain may be different but the range should be the same unless there is a subluxation of the right zygapophyseal joint.

Spinal accessory movements

The spinal level reproducing symptoms requires localization and differentiation between compressive and tensile forces as a cause of symptoms. In this patient a posterior–anterior pressure angled cranially on the base of the sacrum with the lumbar spine in right-side flexion and extension increased P1 and P2. This accessory movement may place stress on the superior part of the capsule of L5/S1 right zygapophyseal joint. A posterior–anterior pressure caudad on L5, with the spine in the same position, increases the compressive load on the intra-articular structures of the right L5/S1 zygapophyseal joint; this accessory movement increased P1.

Passive physiological intervertebral movement

On rotating the lumbar vertebral segments to the right, L5/S1 had the most movement and an end feel which seemed 'floppy' compared to the levels above and to the same level on the other side. This finding suggests instability of the L5/S1 right zygapophyseal joint.

Evaluation — patient C

Table 56.6 summarizes the clinical findings from the physical examination of patient C and outlines the clinical problems and clinical syndrome. The tests performed

Table 56.6 Clinical findings and clinical problems (patient C)

Physical examination	Clinical findings*
Posture • standing weight even on both legs • standing with weight on R leg	In both positions: • Deviation pelvis R • R hip postural abduction • L hip postural abduction • Thoracic and lumbar curve convex L
Muscle function • R hip abduction • L hip extension	 • Lateral pelvic tilt • ↑ R rotation lumbar spine
Length tension • quadratus lumborum R	• Sideways push up L in half side lying, lumbar spine straight and increase movement thoracolumbar area
• L hip abductors • R hip adductors	• ↓ Flexibility
Combined physiological movements	• R side flexion from pelvis ↑ P1 + pelvic forward tilt ↑ P1+ and restricted + R side flexion of the trunk ↑ P1++ • Pelvic forward tilt + R side flexion from pelvis greater range than in the above test
Accessory movements	• Posterior–anterior pressure cranial sacrum ↑ P1 & P2 in R side flexion and extension • Posterior–anterior pressure caudad L5 ↑ P1 in R side flexion and extension
Passive physiological intervertebral movement	• R rotation L5/S1 'floppy' end feel

Clinical problems
• L5/S1 superior capsule laxity R zygapophyseal joint
• Intra-articular degenerative changes L5/S1 R zygapophyseal joint
• ↓ Tone R multifidi low lumbar spine
• Short R quadratus lumborum muscle
• Lengthened R hip abductors
• ↓ Flexibility L hip abductors and R hip adductors

Clinical syndrome
• R L5/S1 zygapophyseal joint subluxation

* For the location of P1 and P2 see Figure 56.3.

during the physical examination of these three case histories do not include all the elimination tests for other possible structures involved, e.g. neurological tests, neural tension tests. It is assumed that clinicians would include further testing as appropriate during the physical examination.

SUMMARY

The ability to localize and analyse a patient's problem so that treatment can be directed appropriately is the major concept of the clinical examination. The selection of treatment depends totally on the proposed clinical problems.

Three case histories have been outlined to illustrate common zygapophyseal joint syndromes. However, zygapophyseal joint pathology is often involved with disc pathology at the same or at a different segmental level. Zygapophyseal joints may also influence the nerve root producing both somatic and radicular clinical findings. One must therefore be aware that patients with zygapophyseal joint pathology may have more than one clinical syndrome.

A rationale basis for the interpretation of clinical findings has been outlined. These interpretations need to be explored further with experimental observations so that the hypothesis of zygapophyseal joint syndromes may be substantiated to a greater degree.

REFERENCES

Adams M A, Hutton W C 1982 Prolapsed intervertebral disc: a hyperflexion injury. Spine 7: 184–191

Aspinall W 1988 Clinical testing for degenerative segmental hypermobility in patients with low pain. Proceedings of the Second Annual Orthopaedic Symposium, Orthopaedic Division of the Canadian Physiotherapy Association Montreal, Quebec

Behrsin J F, Briggs C A 1989 Stress in the lumbar zygapophyseal capsule and ligaments during combined movements: a scientific study. Proceedings of the Sixth Biennial Conference of the Manipulative Therapists' Association of Australia

Bogduk N 1986 Lumbar dorsal ramus syndromes. In: Grieve G P (ed) Modern manual therapy of the vertebral column. Churchill Livingstone, Edinburgh, ch 38, pp 396–404

Bogduk N, Jull G 1985 The theoretical pathology of acute locked back: a basis for manipulative therapy. Manual Medicine 1: 78–82

Bogduk N, Twomey L T 1991 Clinical anatomy of the lumbar spine. 2nd edn. Churchill Livingstone, Melbourne

Edwards B C 1987 Clinical assessment: the use of combined movements in assessment and treatment. In: Twomey L T, Taylor J R (eds) Physical therapy of the low back. Clinics in physical therapy. Churchill Livingstone, New York, vol 13, ch 7, pp 175–197

Farfan H F 1973 Mechanical disorders of the low back. Lea & Febiger, Philadelphia

Farfan H F 1975 Muscular mechanism of the lumbar spine and the position of power and efficiency. Orthopaedic Clinics of North America 6: 135–144

Fryette H H 1954 Principles of osteopathic technic. Academy of Applied Osteopathy, California

Gossman M, Sahrmann S A, Rose S J 1982 Review of length associated changes in muscle: experimental evidence and clinical implications. Physical Therapy 62: 1799–1802

Gregerson G C, Lucas D B 1967 An in vivo study of the axial rotation of the human thoraco-lumbar spine. Journal of Bone and Joint Surgery 49A: 247–262

Hadley L A 1935 Subluxation of the apophyseal articulations with bony impingement as a cause of back pain. American Journal of Roentgenology 33: 209–213

Hedtmann A, Steffen R, Methfessel J, Kolditz D, Kramer J, Thols M 1989 Measurement of human lumbar spine ligaments during loaded and unloaded motion. Spine 14: 175–185

Jull G A, Bogduk N 1985 Manual examination: an objective test of cervical joint dysfunction. Proceedings of the Fourth Biennial Conference of the Manipulative Therapists' Association of Australia, Brisbane

Kendall F P, McCreary E K 1982 Muscles testing and function. 3rd edn. Williams & Wilkins, Baltimore

Kirkaldy-Willis W H, Farfan H 1982 Instability of the lumbar spine. Clinical Orthopaedics and Related Research 165: 110–123

Lee D 1986 Principles and practice of muscle energy and functional techniques. In: Grieve G P (ed) Modern manual therapy of the vertebral column. Churchill Livingstone, Edinburgh, ch 59, pp 640–655

Lee D 1989 The pelvic girdle. Churchill Livingstone, London

Loebe W Y 1973 Regional rotation of the spine. Rheumatology and Rehabilitation 12: 223

Magarey M E 1986 Examination and assessment in spinal joint dysfunction. In: Grieve G P (ed) Modern manual therapy of the vertebral column. Churchill Livingstone, Edinburgh, ch 44, pp 481–497

McFadden K D, Taylor F R 1990 Axial rotation in the lumbar spine and gapping of the zygapophyseal joints. Spine 15: 295–299

Patterson M M 1976 A model mechanism for spinal segmental facilitation. Journal of the American Osteopathic Association 76: 62–72

Pearcy M J, Tibrewal S B 1984 Axial rotation and lateral bending in the normal lumbar spine. Measured by three dimensional radiography. Spine 9: 582–587

Schultz A M, Belytschko T B, Andriacchi J P, Galante J L 1973 Analog studies of forces in the human spine: mechanical properties and motion segment behaviour. Journal of Biomechanics 6: 373–383

Sims-Williams H, Jayson M I V, Baddeley H 1978 Small spinal fractures in back patients. Annals of the Rheumatic Diseases 37: 262–265

Stoddard A 1980 Manual of Osteopathic technique. 3rd edn. Hutchison, London

Taylor J R, Twomey L T 1987 The lumbar spine from infancy to old age. In: Twomey L T, Taylor J R (eds) Physical therapy of the low back. Clinics in physical therapy. Churchill Livingstone, New York, vol 13, ch 1, pp 1–49

Twomey L T, Taylor J R 1987 Lumbar posture movement and mechanics. In: Twomey L T, Taylor J R (eds) Physical therapy of the low back. Clinics in physical therapy. Churchill Livingstone, New York, vol 13, ch 2, pp 51–84

Vernon-Roberts B, Pirie C J 1977 Degenerative changes in the vertebral discs of the lumbar spine and their sequelae. Rheumatology and Rehabilitation 16: 13–21

Wyke B 1976 Neurological aspects of low back pain. In: Jayson M (ed) The lumbar spine and back pain. Grune & Stratton, New York, ch 10, pp 189–256

57. Muscle energy techniques for pelvic dysfunction

G. Fowler

INTRODUCTION

Mechanical dysfunction within the pelvic girdle and its contribution to low-back pain has long been recognized and treated by manual therapists.

Some of the common syndromes of pelvic girdle dysfunction together with their clinical findings and the muscle energy treatment technique will be outlined in this chapter. Since pelvic dysfunction rarely occurs in isolation, the chapter will conclude by suggesting an appropriate sequence for treatment.

The following syndromes are seen frequently in clinical practice:

1. pubic symphysis dysfunction
2. sacral torsion syndrome
3. innominate dysfunction
   (a) subluxation
   (b) rotation—anterior, posterior
   (c) flare—in, out.

Dysfunction of the lumbar spine has a dramatic influence on pelvic function and therefore must be thoroughly assessed and, if necessary, treated prior to evaluation of the pelvic girdle.

In the past, asymmetry of pelvic landmarks has been used in isolation to diagnose dysfunction within the pelvic girdle and to direct the subsequent treatment. This has lead to the mobilization of many normal sacro-iliac joints and the false incrimination of the unit as the source of pain. An alteration in the positional relationships of the innominate bones and the sacrum has *not* been found to be indicative of a mobility dysfunction of either the sacro-iliac joint or the pubic symphysis. The positional findings must be correlated with the findings on mobility testing to ascertain a true pelvic girdle dysfunction. The mobility tests used include the kinetic test (vida infra) and the specific intra-articular gliding tests (see Ch. 10). An altered positional relationship within the pelvic girdle is significant only if a mobility restriction of the sacro-iliac joint and/or pubic symphysis is found.

Ipsilateral kinetic test (Fig. 57.1)

The details of this test were investigated by the author and David Lamb during the years 1965 to 1970.

With the patient standing, the clinician places his right thumb on the right posterior superior iliac spine (PSIS) and the left thumb on the median sacral crest of the sacrum directly parallel. The clinician then asks the patient to flex their right hip and knee to 90°. During this movement the right innominate rotates backward on the fixed sacrum; the movement of the right thumb is approximately one-half inch (1.25 cm) caudally. At the same time, left-side flexion of the lumbar spine occurs with right rotation of the lumbar vertebrae (Fryette's Law I—see below).

A positive ipsilateral kinetic test is observed when the

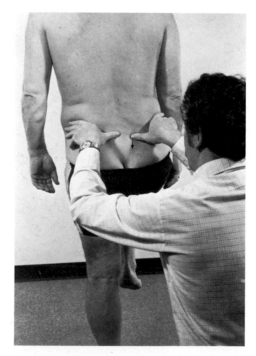

Fig. 57.1 Ipsilateral kinetic test—right.

right thumb moves cranially instead of caudally and the patient hitches the right side of his pelvis. When this occurs a lesion of the right sacro-iliac joint or the lumbar spine is indicated. The potential lesions within the pelvic girdle which render this test positive include:

1. Anteriorly or posteriorly rotated innominate on the right (intra-articular or extra-articular in origin)
2. Pubic symphysis pubic lesion on the right
3. Innominate flare on the right
4. Subluxed innominate on the right (intra-articular in origin).

Contralateral kinetic test (Fig. 57.2)

With the patient standing, place the right thumb on the median sacral crest of the sacrum and the left thumb on the left PSIS and ask the patient to flex their right hip and knee to 90°. During this movement the right thumb travels caudally as a result of the posterior rotation of the right innominate which, at the end of movement, takes the sacrum with it on a fixed left innominate. At the same time the lumbar spine will side-flex to the left, and the vertebral bodies will rotate to the right. When the contralateral kinetic test is positive the right thumb travels either cranially or does not move. The potential sacro-iliac lesions which render this test positive include:

1. left sacral torsions
2. left sacral flexion (which will not be discussed in this chapter).

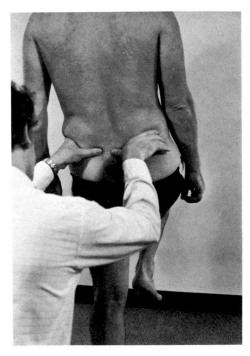

Fig. 57.2   Contralateral kinetic test—right.

The clinician's position relative to the patient must be the same on every test; the level of the operator's eyes should be on the horizontal line of the patient's PSIS. Movement of the PSIS may vary due to the surface and inclination of the sacro-iliac joint being tested. The ipsilateral and contralateral tests have been described on one side only; the clinician would evaluate both sides for comparison.

THE PELVIC SYNDROMES

Pubic symphysis dysfunction

Dysfunction of this cartilaginous articulation may be primary or secondary and, when present, is always treated first. Loss of function or integrity of this joint disrupts the mechanics of the entire pelvic complex. The lesion pattern is determined by palpating the position of the pubic tubercles and correlating the findings with the side of the positive kinetic test. The restricted side indicates the side of the lesion. The position of the affected side can be cranial, caudal, anterior or posterior, or in combinations thereof. The inguinal ligament is usually very tender to palpation on the side of the lesion.

It is common to find the pubic symphysis held in one of the four following positions:

1. anterior/inferior
2. posterior/superior
3. anterior/superior
4. posterior/inferior.

In treatment, only one direction need be chosen for correction since the other occurs as a consequence of the osteokinematic motion. For example, consider the anterior/inferior lesion of the right pubis. To restore the position and mobility using a muscle energy technique, the patient is supine lying with the right hip flexed to 90° and slightly adducted. The therapist places his fist against the right ischial tuberosity while the left hand supports the contralateral anterior superior iliac spine (ASIS) and iliac crest. The patient's right knee rests against the therapist's lateral thorax and axilla. The patient is instructed to resist further hip flexion and adduction while the therapist applies a cranial force through the right ischial tuberosity and a caudal force through the left ASIS and iliac crest. The therapist's right hand may be further supported by bracing elbow against hip. The contraction is held for 3–5 seconds following which the patient is instructed to relax completely. The muscle energy technique is repeated three times following which the positional findings and kinetic test are retested. Improvement of position and decreased pain on palpating the inguinal ligament should be found if the technique has been successful. By restoring the inferior component of the lesion complex, the anterior positional displacement is also corrected.

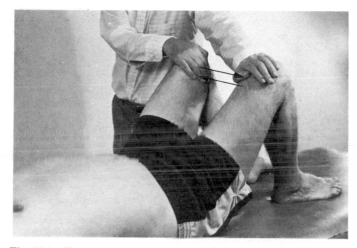

Fig. 57.3 Forced eccentric technique for the pubic symphysis.

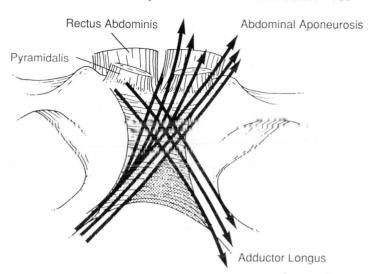

Fig. 57.4 Cruciate arrangement of the short adductors across the anterior aspect of the pubic symphysis (courtesy of Diane Lee).

Consider now the posterior/superior lesion of the right pubis. To restore the position and mobility using a muscle energy technique, the patient is supine lying with the left hip flexed to 90° and the right hip over the side of the table such that the hip joint is extended and slightly abducted. The therapist places his left hand over the left ASIS and the right hand over the medial aspect of the distal right thigh. The patient is instructed to resist further extension/abduction while the therapist applies a counterforce. The contraction is held for 3–5 seconds following which the patient is instructed to relax completely. The muscle energy technique is repeated three times following which the positional findings and kinetic test are retested. Improvement of position and decreased pain on palpating the inguinal ligament should be found if the technique has been successful. By restoring the posterior component of the lesion complex, the superior positional displacement is also corrected.

Alternatively, a forced eccentric technique applied to the adductors can be used for lesions which do not respond to the above techniques (Fig. 57.3). The short adductors cross the inferior aspect of the pubic articulation in a cruciate manner (Fig. 57.4), and, when recruited, bring the joint into a level position. Since a slight 'popping' noise is often elicited, which can be of concern and surprise to the patient as the operator overcomes the muscle resistance by a short high velocity movement in the opposite direction, a preliminary word of warning is necessary.

Following treatment, the kinetic test and positional findings are re-evaluated. If no change has occurred a sacro-iliac dysfunction is the probable cause.

Sacral torsion syndrome

To understand clearly the changes that occur in the sacral torsion syndrome, a review of the physiological movements of the pelvic girdle and lumbar spine is necessary.

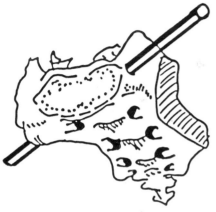

Fig. 57.5 The oblique axis of sacral torsion (courtesy of Alun Morgan).

Torsion of the sacrum occurs through an oblique axis (Fig. 57.5) which runs from the superior articular surface on one side of the sacrum to the inferior articular surface on the other side of the sacrum. This axis has never been proven but is used clinically in treating torsion syndromes.

Due to the shape of the articular surface, minute motion can occur in either a forward or backward direction. The definition of forward motion would be as follows: an inferior movement of the sacrum along the upper limb of each articular surface together with a posterior movement along the lower limb of each articular surface (Fig. 57.6). Backward motion of the sacrum would be the reverse; an anterior movement of the sacrum along the lower limb of each articular surface together with a superior movement along the upper limb of each articular surface (Fig. 57.7).

A left torsion of the sacrum is defined as an unphysiological occurrence when osteokinematically the sacrum rotates to the left and side-flexes to the left. Arthrokinematically, the sacrum glides antero-inferiorly along the short arm on the right and postero-inferiorly along the

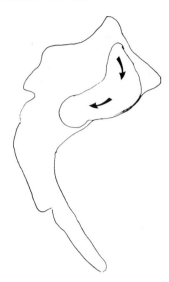

Fig. 57.6   Forward sacral motion.

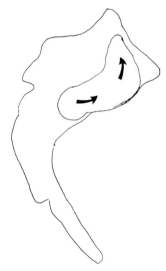

Fig. 57.7   Backward sacral motion.

long arm on the left. When the sacrum is held in this unphysiological torsion, the effect on the lumbar spine varies according to Fryette's laws of physiological spinal motion.

Fryette's laws of physiological motion

Law I

Whenever the spine moves from easy normal, lateral flexion occurs before rotation except during pure flexion or extension. The lateral flexion produces a bending movement about which the rotation occurs. This combined motion is referred to as *latexion*, and the lateral flexion and rotation occur to opposite sides; the vertebral body rotates into the convexity of the curve. Spinal dysfunctions presenting as latexion are referred to as type I lesions.

Law II

From a position of full flexion or full extension, rotation precedes lateral flexion when movement occurs other than return to easy normal. Capsular and ligamentous tension restricts lateral flexion from occurring initially and must therefore be preceded by rotation to relieve the restrictive forces. This combined motion is referred to as *rotexion*, and the rotation and lateral flexion occur to the same side; the vertebral body rotates into the concavity of the curve. Spinal dysfunctions presenting as rotexion are referred to as type II lesions.

With this knowledge it is now relatively easy to describe the clinical findings of the sacral torsion syndrome.

Clinical findings of the sacral torsion syndrome

With the left sacral torsion the sacrum will have moved inferiorly and posteriorly on the left articular surface and inferiorly and anteriorly on the right. Relative to the sacrum, the left innominate will have moved superiorly and the right innominate will have moved posteriorly. The lumbar spine will follow the first or second law of Fryette. This depends on the lumbosacral angle. If the lumbosacral angle is increased—and the iliolumbar ligaments therefore become taut—the pull of the right iliolumbar ligament will cause the 5th and sometimes the 4th lumbar vertebrae to move with the left innominate superiorly and anteriorly on the left, which, considering the second law of Fryette, would find the vertebrae in a right-rotated and right-side flexed position. The lumbar vertebrae above L5 and L4 would gradually counter-rotate, giving the clinical appearance of a left convexity (Fig. 57.8).

If the lumbosacral angle is within easy normal with no tension on the iliolumbar ligaments, the 5th lumbar vertebrae will be free to follow Fryette's first law of physiological spinal motion and side-flex to the right and rotate to the left. The remainder of the lumbar spine will follow L5, giving a convexity to the left (Fig. 57.9).

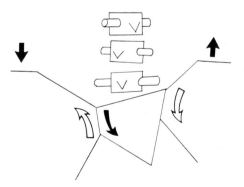

Fig. 57.8   Left sacral torsion in the presence of an increased lumbosacral angle.

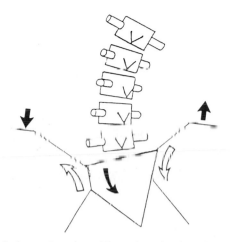

Fig. 57.9 Left sacral torsion with resultant lumbar adaptation.

The left sacral torsion syndrome, type I

The type I left sacral torsion syndrome exists when the anterior sacrum is held in a left-rotated position and the lumbar vertebrae adapt by following the first law of physiological spinal motion and side-flex to the right and rotate to the left (Fig. 57.9). The contralateral kinetic test is positive on the left, and the positional findings of the pelvic girdle include:

1. Standing position:
   a. the right iliac crest will be cephalad due to depression of the sacral base on the left and elevation of the sacral base on the right
   b. the left ASIS will be slightly ventral due to the forward and upward position of the left innominate bone
   c. the spine will have a left convex curve.
2. Sitting position:
   a. the right iliac crest will be cephalad due to depression of the sacral base on the left and elevation of the sacral base on the right
   b. the left ASIS will be ventral due to the upward and forward rotation of the left innominate
   c. a point of tenderness will be found on the crest of the left ilium at the origin of the lateral margin of the iliocostalis lumborum muscle.
3. Supine:
   a. left iliac crest will be cephalad. This reversal in position of the crests from sitting and standing to lying is due to the release of tension from iliopsoas and quadratus lumborum muscles which, in standing, were counteracting the effects of gravity. Relaxation of these muscles in the supine position allows the true position of the left iliac crest relative to the sacrum to be seen
   b. the left leg will appear shorter than the right
   c. the left iliotibial band will be tender on palpation and feel tense.

4. Prone:
   a. fullness will be found posterior to the left transverse process of the 5th lumbar vertebrae due to the left rotation of L5 and the sacrum in the transverse (body) plane
   b. the lumbar lordosis will be increased
   c. sacral sulcus will be deeper on the right than on the left
   d. sacral lateral angle (ILA) will be posterior on the left
   e. sacral ILA will be inferior on the left.

The left torsion syndrome, type II

The type II sacral torsion syndrome exists when the anterior surface of the sacrum is held in a left rotated position and the lower lumbar vertebrae follow the second law of physiological motion; L5 and L4 rotate and side-flex to the right (Fig. 57.8). Both the ipsilateral and contralateral kinetic test is positive on the left, and the positional findings of the pelvic girdle include:

1. Standing position:
   a. the right iliac crest will be cephalad due to the depression of the sacral base on the left
   b. the left ASIS will be considerably more ventral because of the upward and forward motion of the left innominate bone and the right rotation of the lower lumbar vertebrae
   c. the spine will have a left convex curve and be held in a fixed position.
2. Sitting position:
   a. the left iliac crest will be cephalad because of the right side-bending of the 4th and 5th lumbar vertebrae
   b. the left ASIS will be considerably more ventral because of the upward and forward movement of the left innominate bone and the right side bending and rotation of the 4th and 5th lumbar vertebrae
   c. a point of tenderness will be found at the origin of the left iliocostalis on the left iliac crest.
3. Supine:
   a. the right iliac crest will be cephalad because of the relative fixation of the type II right rotation lesions of the L4 and L5 vertebrae which do not allow the relaxation of the psoas and quadratus lumborum muscles
   b. the left leg will appear shorter than the right
   c. the left iliotibial band will appear tender on palpation and feel tense.
4. Prone:
   a. fullness will be found posterior to the right transverse process of the 5th lumbar vertebrae because of its right rotation

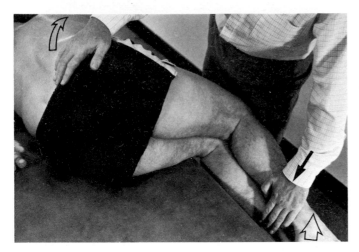

Fig. 57.10 Treatment of the type I left sacral torsion lesion.

b. the lumbar lordosis will be decreased
c. sacral sulcus will be deeper on the right than on the left
d. sacral ILA will be posterior on the left
e. sacral ILA will be inferior on the left.

Treatment of the left sacral torsion syndrome, type I (Fig. 57.10)

The patient lies on his left side with his left arm placed behind him. His right arm reaches to the floor, which produces left rotation of the trunk on the pelvis. The clinician monitors this rotation at the L5–S1 articulation. The clinician subsequently flexes the patient's hips and knees until motion is perceived at the L5–S1 joint. The patient's feet are then directed towards the floor, thereby externally rotating the right hip joint and internally rotating the left to the point of muscular resistance (muscular barrier). The clinician then directs the patient to raise the lower legs to the ceiling. This effort is resisted isometrically. Simultaneously, the patient is asked to reach further towards the floor with his right arm. This contraction is held for 5 seconds and upon relaxation the clinician engages the new muscular barrier by depressing the feet further towards the floor. This sequence of contraction and relaxation is repeated three times following which the kinetic test and pelvic landmarks are re-evaluated.

Treatment of the left sacral torsion syndrome, type II

The standing patient lies prone across the treatment table with his anterior superior iliac spine level with the surface and his hands beneath the shoulders in a push-up position. The clinician stands to the left of the patient and with his right pisiform applies an anterior pressure over the left ILA (Fig. 57.11). From this position, the patient is asked to extend slowly the thoracolumbar spine by bringing al-

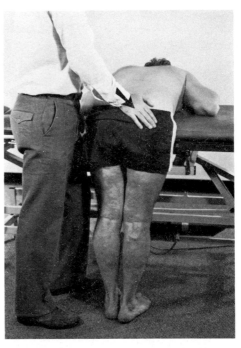

Fig. 57.11 Treatment of the type II left sacral torsion lesion—starting position of patient and the operator's sacral pressure.

ternately the left and then the right hand towards the operator. (This motion could be equated to watching a duck walk backwards!) Simultaneously, the clinician maintains the anterior pressure over the left ILA (Fig. 57.12) until the patient assumes an erect position. This procedure may be repeated two to three times fol-

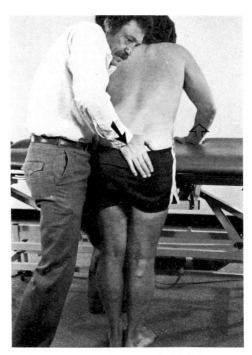

Fig. 57.12 Treatment of the type II left sacral torsion lesion midway through the treatment technique.

lowing which the kinetic test and positional findings are re-evaluated.

The clinical appearance of the type II sacral torsion is very similar to the acute lumbar disc prolapse, and caution is advised when making this diagnosis. The subjective examination is often helpful in differentiating the two, i.e. type II sacral torsions are *not* aggravated by sitting whereas the patient with an acute lumbar disc prolapse finds this position intolerable.

Innominate dysfunctions

Subluxation

The 'upslip', as it is known in osteopathic terminology, can be defined as a superior subluxation of the innominate upon the sacrum at the sacro-iliac joint. The dysfunction is primarily articular with secondary muscular imbalances as opposed to anterior and posterior innominate rotations which are primarily the result of muscular imbalances which secondarily restrict sacro-iliac joint motion. There are two kinds of upslip: those which render the joint hypomobile and those which result in hypermobility. Figure 57.13 illustrates the articular surface of the sacro-iliac joint. The potential for subluxation of the innominate of 1 mm is possible in a multitude of directions. The character of the lesion depends on the resting posture of the pelvis at the time the force was applied to it, as well as the direction of the force. If the force is applied posterior to the instantaneous centre of innominate rotation, the superior subluxation will occur combined with an element of anterior rotation. If, however, the force is applied anterior to the instantaneous centre of innominate rotation, the superior subluxation will occur with an element of posterior rotation. As long as the joint capsule and ligamentous system remains intact, the articular mechanics dictate that a conjunct rotation will occur with any translation or slide of the innominate along either of

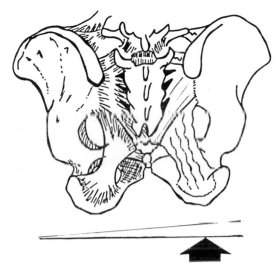

Fig. 57.14 Anterior rotated upslip on the right (courtesy of Alun Morgan).

the 'arms' of the sacro-iliac joint. If the joint integrity is compromised, a pure superior subluxation without an element of rotation can occur; however, the joint is now hypermobile.

The simple superior subluxation of the innominate, with or without rotation, can also be complicated by dysfunctions of the sacrum on the opposite innominate and/ or L5–S1 articular or discogenic dysfunction, none of which will be covered here.

The aetiology of this dysfunction is commonly a fall on the ischial tuberosities; however, any cranial force through the lower extremity may be sufficient to sublux the joint. The traumatic incident may be recent or remote, and the site of pain is not necessarily local to the side of the dysfunction. The pain behaviour is totally dependent upon the patient's occupation, leisure activities and habitual postures.

The superior innominate subluxation (the upslip) in anterior rotation (right) (Fig. 57.14): ***clinical signs.*** The kinetic test will be ipsilateral positive on the right. The positional findings include:

1. Standing:
   (a) right iliac crest superior to the left
   (b) right PSIS superior to the left
   (c) right ASIS inferior to the left
   (d) spine has a left scoliosis (could be marginal).
2. Sitting:
   (a) right iliac crest superior to the left
   (b) right PSIS superior to the left
   (c) scoliosis to the left
   (d) paravertebral muscle bulk remains the same in the standing or the sitting position on forward flexion of the spine.
3. Supine:
   (a) right leg shorter than the left

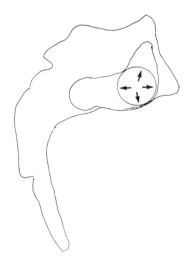

Fig. 57.13 Direction of potential subluxation of the innominate.

(b) right pubic symphysis anterior/inferior compared to the left.

(c) Fabere test (hip flexion, abduction, external rotation, extension) may be restricted slightly in the last 5° of motion.

4. Prone:

(a) right ischial tuberosity more cranial than the left

(b) right sacrotuberous ligament slack compared to the left and may be tender to palpation.

Treatment of the superior innominate subluxation in anterior rotation on the right. The preferred technique is a high-velocity, low-amplitude manipulation of the innominate on the sacrum through the lower extremity. The innominate is manipulated caudally in its rotated position to minimize torque forces through the joint. Therefore, the patient with an anteriorly rotated upslip is positioned in a prone position so that the hip joint can be extended and thus the caudal force through the lower extremity can be directed parallel to the line of the subluxation (Fig. 57.15). A gentle, caudal traction force is initially applied through the lower leg with the knee joint extended until the exact degree of hip abduction, flexion or extension necessary to localize the force to the sacro-iliac joint is attained. From this position, a high-velocity, low-amplitude tug is applied through the lower extremity following which mobility and positional findings are re-evaluated. Mobility should be restored within the first treatment session.

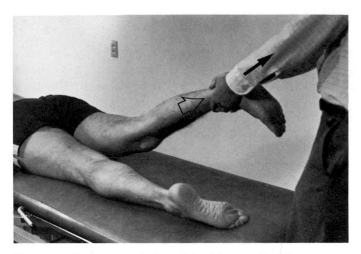

Fig. 57.15 Treatment technique of the right rotated upslip.

The superior innominate subluxation in posterior rotation (left) (Fig. 57.16): ***clinical signs.*** The kinetic test will be ipsilateral positive on the left. The positional findings include:

1. Standing:

(a) iliac crest superior to the left

(b) scoliosis to the left

(c) left PSIS inferior to the right

(d) left ASIS superior to the right.

2. Sitting:

(a) left iliac crest superior to the right

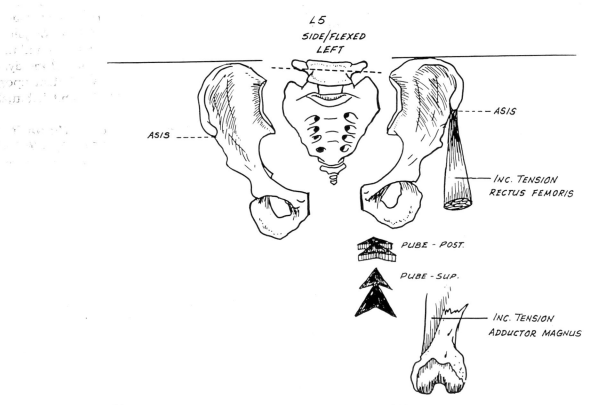

Fig. 57.16 Posterior rotated upslip on the left (courtesy of Alun Morgan).

(b) left PSIS inferior to the right

(c) scoliosis to the left.

3. Supine:

(a) left leg may be shorter or equal to the right

(b) left symphysis pubic posterior/superior to the right

(c) left inguinal ligament tender to palpation

(d) hypertonicity of adductor magnus and rectus femoris on the left.

4. Prone:

(a) left ischial tuberosity is level or slightly cranial to the right

(b) left sacrotuberous ligament tension is normal due to the posterior innominate rotation

(c) left interosseous sacro-iliac ligament is tender to palpation.

Treatment of the superior innominate subluxation in posterior rotation on the left. The patient with a posteriorly rotated unslip is treated in the supine position so that the hip joint can be flexed and abducted and thus the caudal force through the lower extremity can be directed parallel to the line of the subluxation (Fig. 57.17).

The above examples are the syndromes most commonly seen. However, a left upslip may also be found in anterior rotation, and a right upslip in posterior rotation.

Rotation

Innominate rotation lesions can occur as the result of muscular imbalance between the axial and appendicular musculature. This occurs when the lumbopelvic mechanism has exceeded its adaptive potential.

Clinical signs of the right anteriorly rotated innominate. The kinetic test will be ipsilateral positive on the right. Articular movements of the lumbar spine may show restriction of backward bending of the lumbar spine. The positional findings include:

1. Standing:

(a) right PSIS superior to the left

(b) right ASIS inferior to the left

(c) pelvis as a unit rotated to the left

(d) increased lumbosacral angle.

2. Supine:

(a) right leg longer than the left

(b) pelvis as a unit rotated to the left.

3. Prone:

(a) right sacrotuberous ligament is firm

(b) right interosseous sacro-iliac ligament is tender to palpation.

Treatment of the right anteriorly rotated innominate (Fig. 57.18). The patient lies on his left side. The clinician faces the patient and with his right hand flexes the patient's right hip and knee simultaneously, monitoring the right iliosacral joint with his left hand until the barrier is reached. From this position the patient is given an isometric resistance to right hip flexion. The iliopsoas muscle is recruited which reciprocally inhibits the ipsilateral hamstring. Upon relaxation, the new barrier is engaged, which may be assisted by passive innominate rotation via the left hand. This procedure is repeated three times followed by evaluation of innominate mobility.

Clinical signs of the left posteriorly rotated innominate. The kinetic test will be ipsilateral positive on the left. Articular movements of the lumbar spine may show restriction of forward bending and left side flexion associated with the subjective complaint of a 'pulling sensation' over the right lower lumbar area. The positional findings include:

1. Standing:

(a) left PSIS inferior to the right

(b) left ASIS superior to the right

(c) right foot tends to be pronated.

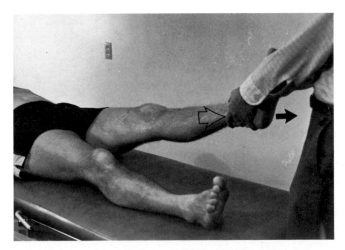

Fig. 57.17 Treatment technique of the posterior rotated upslip.

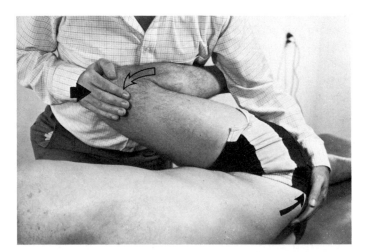

Fig. 57.18 Treatment technique of the right anterior rotated innominate.

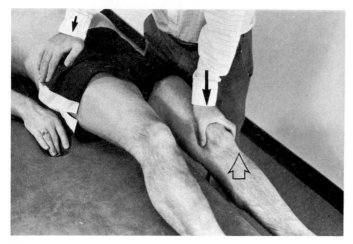

Fig. 57.19   Treatment technique of posterior rotated innominate.

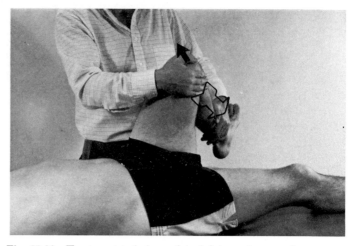

Fig. 57.20   Treatment technique of the left innominate outflare.

2. Supine:
  (a) left leg shorter than the right
  (b) pelvis as a unit rotates to the left
  (c) hamstrings are tight on the left.
3. Prone:
  (a) left sacrotuberous ligament is taut as opposed to firm
  (b) left interosseous sacro-iliac ligament is tender to palpation.

Treatment of the left posteriorly rotated innominate (Fig. 57.19). A tight left hamstring muscle may mimic this lesion and therefore must be stretched initially prior to treatment of the innominate dysfunction.

The patient lies supine close to the left side of the table such that the left leg may be extended below its surface. The clinician stands to the left of the patient and fixes the right innominate with his right hand. The patient's left leg is extended until the barrier of left anterior innominate rotation is reached. From this position, the patient is given an isometric resistance to straight leg raising. The rectus femoris muscle is recruited with a reverse origin and insertion which subsequently pulls the innominate into anterior rotation. Upon relaxation, the new barrier is engaged by extending the lower extremity towards the floor. This procedure is repeated three times followed by evaluation of innominate mobility.

Flare

This innominate dysfunction is probably a consequence of articular asymmetry when the plane of the joint is excessively anteromedial or posterolateral. This is a clinical opinion as opposed to proven anatomical fact. This lesion tends to occur in those with very wide, short innominate bones.

Clinical signs of the left innominate outflare. The kinetic test will be ipsilateral positive on the left. Weight-

bearing through the left lower extremity dramatically increases the symptoms. The patient walks with a 'toeing out' of the left leg. A positional fault of the left hip joint is present with an apparent restriction of medial rotation, which is also painful. The positional findings include:

1. Standing:
  left PSIS is medial to the midline (median sacral crest) in comparison with the right.
2. Supine:
  (a) left ASIS is lateral to the mid-line (line between the xyphoid process and symphysis pubis) in comparison with the right
  (b) left leg is shorter than the right
  (c) left inguinal ligament is tender to palpation.
3. Prone:
  (a) left PSIS is medial to the mid-line (median sacral crest) in comparison with the right
  (b) left PSIS is tender to palpation.

Treatment of the left innominate outflare (Fig. 57.20). The patient lies supine. The clinician stands to the left of the patient and flexes the left hip joint to 90°, adducts and medially rotates the left hip joint until the innominate barrier is reached. From this position, the patient is given an isometric resistance to left hip adduction via the operator's right hand which is held for 5 seconds. Upon relaxation the new barrier is engaged by further adduction and medial rotation of the left hip joint. This procedure is repeated three times followed by evaluation of innominate mobility.

Clinical signs of the left innominate inflare. The kinetic test will be ipsilateral positive on the left. Weight-bearing through the left lower extremity is painful. The patient walks with a 'toeing in' of the left leg. A positional fault of the left hip joint is present with an apparent restriction of lateral rotation which is also painful. The positional findings include:

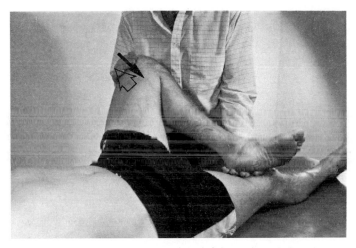

Fig. 57.21 Treatment technique of the left innominate inflare.

1. Standing:
   left PSIS is lateral to the mid-line in comparison with the right.
2. Supine:
   (a) left ASIS is medial to the mid-line in comparison with the right
   (b) left leg is slightly longer than the right.
3. Prone:
   (a) left PSIS is lateral to the mid-line in comparison with the right
   (b) left PSIS is exquisitely tender to palpation with swelling over the left sacral sulcus.

Treatment of the left innominate inflare (Fig. 57.21). The patient lies supine. The clinician stands to the left of the patient and flexes, abducts and externally rotates the left hip joint until the innominate barrier is reached. From this position, the patient is given an isometric resistance to left hip abduction via the operator's right hand which is held for 5 seconds. Upon relaxation, the new barrier is engaged by further abduction and lateral rotation of the left hip joint. This procedure is repeated three times followed by evaluation of innominate mobility.

CONCLUSION

The preceding pelvic dysfunctions have been presented as isolated entities when, in fact, clinically, they tend to occur in combination. Therefore, a sequence of treatment progression is necessary. The pelvic dysfunctions should be treated in the following order:

1. segmental restrictive faults of the lumbar spine
2. pubic symphysis dysfunction
3. sacral torsion syndrome
4. innominate subluxation
5. innominate rotation
6. innominate flare
7. any dysfunction of the lower limb and foot.

The author also recognizes the existence of hypermobile sacro-iliac joint dysfunction with its attendant ligamentous insufficiency; however, aside from pelvic stabilization via strapping, treatment of this disorder is the physician's prerogative.

Contrary to orthodox beliefs, sacro-iliac or iliosacral joint dysfunction is not rare. Evaluation of the pelvic complex can be most challenging, and its successful diagnosis and treatment most rewarding. To quote Harrison H. Fryette, D.O.: 'Dare to be different, so many would rather be orthodox than right'.

REFERENCES

Fowler C 1984 Proceedings of the International Federation of Orthopaedic Manipulative Therapists Congress, Vancouver

Fryette H H 1954 Principles of osteopathic technique. Academy of Applied Osteopathy, Carmel, California

Lee D 1989 The pelvic girdle. An approach to the examination and treatment of the lumbo-pelvic-hip region. Churchill Livingstone, Edinburgh

Mitchell F L, Moran P S, Pruzzo N A 1979 An evaluation and treatment manual of osteopathic muscle energy procedures. ICEOP, Valley Park, Missouri

Pratt W A 1952 The lumbopelvic torsion syndrome. Journal of the American Osteopathic Association 51: 97–103

Vleeming A 1990 The sacroiliac joint. A clinical–anatomical, biomechanical and radiological study. Proefschrift

Walheim G G, Olerud S, Ribbe T 1984 Mobility of the pubic symphysis. Acta Orthopaedica Scandinavica 55: 319–324

58. A flexible approach to traction

J. Sherriff

INTRODUCTION

In the realm of passive handling it is probable that traction has lagged behind during recent advances, and over the last 10 years there have been few English-language articles that have substantially influenced the current use of traction (Saunders 1981, Petulla 1986). New ideas are constantly appearing for 'hands on' techniques, but with few exceptions traction continues to be approached in a traditional and rather standardized style. This chapter attempts to expand the use of positioning to increase the flexibility with which traction may be approached.

Traction is not a unique and separate form of treatment, but simply one form of passive mobilization and it should be considered in this context. Almost any form of passive handling may be used either with some form of oscillation or as a static hold: a longitudinal movement may be performed as an oscillatory mobilization, as a slow rhythmic stretch, or as a static traction. In any passive mobilization the starting position is important; in traction it can be vital, and it can make the difference between the success and failure of the technique. Traction can be varied in many ways; it may be manual or mechanical, static or rhythmic, fast or slow; the force applied may be strong or gentle, and, in the lumbar spine, it may be applied symmetrically or asymmetrically. The effects of traction are not localized, but may be made more specific by careful positioning: there will also be maximization of the effect at any damaged or degenerate levels (Colachis & Strohm 1966) regardless of whether or not these levels contribute to the patient's current problem. When using any type of passive mobilization it is usually more effective to be guided by the signs and symptoms rather than be restricted by the diagnosis. A diagnosis of 'acute cervical nerve root compression' will indicate the need for careful handling, but only the behaviour of the pain and of the signs of power and/or sensory loss will indicate the precise positioning necessary to relieve the compression.

PRINCIPLES OF POSITIONING

Positioning aims to maximize the effect of the treatment on the structures which are responsible for the patient's signs and symptoms, and may be designed to affect a region of the spine or one particular level. Positioning is usually governed by the response of the signs and symptoms, if possible at the time of application, and, in the case of nerve root involvement, may need to be extremely precise. There are several ways of discovering the optimum position: by the behaviour of local or referred symptoms, by the behaviour of any affected peripheral joint movements, or by the behaviour of nerve root signs. In default of any of these, mid-positioning of the joint may suffice. Clues to positioning may exist in a change of the patient's sleeping position necessitated by pain, in the response of signs and symptoms to movement, or in a change in posture. Postural changes may be either the cause or the effect of pain; the former should be changed, the latter should not. Any antalgic (pain relieving) position should be maintained during treatment or the symptoms and signs may become worse; as the condition improves the posture will usually normalize.

CERVICAL SPINE POSITIONING

It is usual to apply traction to the cervical spine either in some variant of the sitting position or in supine lying. The probability is that unless there is a good reason for the patient to sit up, e.g. the presence of a hiatus hernia etc., it is most effective to position the spine in lying. This also reduces the effect of gravity on the spine and is more conducive to relaxation. Alternative positioning is possible; the patient may be placed in side-lying or even prone, but this is rarely necessary.

The actual positioning of the spine differs depending on which particular structures are deemed to be the culprits in producing the symptoms. If, for example, the patient presents with a long-term protracted posture of the cervical spine, which is producing both upper cervical and cervicothoracic symptoms, the probability is that both muscular and ligamentous tissue has become adaptively shortened around these two areas. It may then be helpful, in conjunction with other techniques, to position the patient towards the end of the available range of retraction and apply a gentle traction to the neck, aiming for a regional effect. If the symptoms arise from one specific level and are local, or referred only a short distance and are symmetrical, the appropriate spinal level may be positioned simply in mid flexion/extension as is often the current standard practice, and this may be effective. For symptoms which refer to a greater extent down a limb, or which are unilateral, the spinal segment may additionally be placed in some degree of rotation and/or side-flexion.

If a patient presents with referred pain this may be due to involvement of a nerve root, or may be produced by other structures around the spine; it is important to differentiate between the two different types of referred pain as the approach to each must be different (Grieve 1981a). If the patient's referred pain is of the non-nerve root type, the presentation may also involve limitation of movement of a peripheral joint due to pain or to stiffness. This loss of movement can be used as a guide to positioning the spine for traction. For instance, if a cervical spine problem involves referred pain to the arm and reduced elevation of the arm, changing the position of the neck may change the range of elevation of the arm. The movement of the shoulder should be tested in supine lying before positioning, as a change from a weight-bearing neck to a non-weight-bearing neck may, in itself, influence the shoulder movement. If the shoulder responds to changes in the neck position, that position which gives maximum movement or least pain will be the one in which traction, or any other suitable passive mobilization, will have the greatest effect.

Elbow pain or restriction may also be used to guide positioning for traction, but it may be found that elbow symptoms of the 'tennis elbow' type originate in the thoracic spine at a level which necessitates a thoracic rather than a cervical approach.

The most logical way to position seems to be to test the effect of changes in flexion/extension first, to enable the correct number of pillows to be used, and then to test the effect of rotation and side-flexion, or a combination of both directions.

Positioning for a problem which involves a nerve root needs to be approached differently, as frequently a nerve root will respond adversely to mid-positioning of the joint. If the nerve root involvement does not include disturbances of conduction pain alone is the only guide to positioning. If, however, there are signs of loss or diminution of power and/or sensation, then these may be used to position the spinal segment correctly. The use of reflexes for positioning is rarely helpful, as reflex changes are much

less likely to recover quickly. Positioning for nerve roots must be extremely accurate; frequently an extremely small change in position will make the difference between success and failure. A weight-bearing posture can have an adverse effect on a nerve root problem, and it is essential to test any power or sensation loss in both the standing or sitting and lying positions. It may be noted that positioning the spine may reduce nerve-root-type pain without altering the signs, and these may not change until traction is added. Usually, nerve roots respond to either rotation or side-flexion away from the painful side, and if it is found that the pain is reduced by movement towards the painful side very careful testing should exclude the possibility of increased compression of the root with decreased conduction being responsible for the reduced pain.

Having correctly positioned the neck it is obvious that the angle of pull which is then applied, either manually or mechanically, must maintain the neck in the chosen position. This can sometimes be difficult to achieve mechanically, and in these circumstances manual traction may be the approach of choice, although it is more difficult to maintain an accurate amount of force manually.

If a side-flexed position is found to be necessary, manual traction is to be recommended for the cervical spine as the position is most easily maintained in this way. It is possible to traction the cervical spine in side-lying, with the neck appropriately supported, and for some patients this can be an easy way of self-traction, using the weight of the head to effect the traction. As with any self-treatment, the method needs to be carefully taught and monitored. When using mechanical traction for side-flexion in supine it may be necessary to angle the plinth, or use mesh on a side-wall to maintain the correct position.

When using static traction it is undoubtedly easier to use a simple cord and pulley system with a spring balance and a hook as this is more versatile than a 'traction unit', unless intermittent traction is considered necessary. A mechanical 'neck guide' must be used with care as these devices may only position the one area of the spine and perhaps not allow correct positioning of any other areas. Care must always be taken of the position of the upper cervical spine when an area lower down is positioned, to avoid undue extension and rotation which might compromise the vertebral artery or produce upper cervical symptoms. Having carefully positioned the spine an accurate record must then be made of the exact position to allow repetition of the treatment.

LUMBAR SPINE POSITIONING

The principles of positioning the lumbar spine are the same as for the cervical spine: identify the spinal position in which the signs and symptoms are least and maintain this during traction; in the lumbar spine, however, there is the added possibility of using a variety of starting positions, and of using symmetrical or asymmetrical traction (Sherriff 1988).

The starting position may be chosen with one of several objectives: to ensure maintenance of the patient's antalgic position, to use a position in which the patient can relax most easily, or simply to use the position in which the selected form of traction is most easily applied. In any starting position, supine, prone, or side-lying, the spine may be positioned in some degree of flexion or extension, in side-flexion or in rotation; or in a combination position. The exact position to choose may be indicated by an antalgic position that the patient adopts, by a change in sleeping position necessitated by pain, or by a careful study of the effects of movement on the signs and symptom. When studying flexion in the lumbar spine it is often useful to look at flexion in sitting as this reduces tension on neuromeningeal structures as compared to the standing position. If the chosen position does not involve side-flexion symmetrical traction is appropriate; if the position does include side-flexion then asymmetric traction is necessary to maintain the side-flexion.

In order to use symmetrical traction the harness must be applied to the patient so that the pull comes centrally over the spine, either anteriorly or posteriorly; in either form of traction it is most accurate to use the type of harness with one central 'tail' rather than two straps. With the 'tail' central the patient may be positioned in supine, if some degree of flexion is needed (Fig. 58.1), in prone, if extension is suitable, or in side-lying. If the side-lying position is chosen, care should be taken to ensure that the spine is not side-flexed, supporting as necessary with a small pad, and that the pull is applied in a direction parallel to the traction plinth (Fig. 58.2). A flexion or extension component may be added by moving the patient closer to one side or other of the plinth, and it is therefore helpful to have as wide a top to the traction plinth as possible. Any amount of rotation necessary may be readily added in side-lying (Fig. 58.3); it is possible in prone or supine but much less easy to achieve, necessitating padding under one hip and knee and the opposite shoulder, and rarely being comfortable. With symmetrical traction the 'friction free' mechanism can be used.

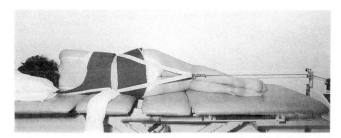

Fig. 58.2 Symmetrical traction—similar position to that in Fig. 58.1 but here in side-lying—with 'free float' in use.

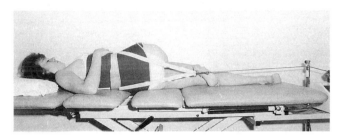

Fig. 58.3 Symmetrical traction with rotation in side-lying, with 'free float' in use.

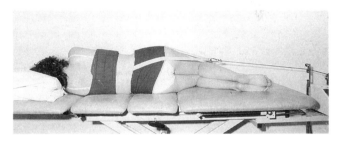

Fig. 58.4 Asymmetrical traction in side-lying with 'free float' closed.

Asymmetrical traction may be achieved by placing the 'tail' of the harness laterally anywhere between the sacro-iliac joint and the anterior superior iliac spine. The easiest body position in which to apply asymmetric traction is side-lying (Fig. 58.4), and the position of the belt allows control of flexion, with the 'tail' posterolateral, or extension with the 'tail' anterolateral. Rotation may also be added. With asymmetric traction a certain amount of lateral stretching occurs, and the probability is that the pull should be applied from a point as close to the top of the traction table as possible in order to emphasize this tendency. The 'free float' mechanism should not be used as this negates the tendency to stretch laterally. To emphasize the side-flexion a firm support such as a rolled-up towel or two may be used under the patient's waist, and the upper leg may stretched down to reinforce the position (Fig. 58.5). If asymmetric traction must be used in supine or prone the side-flexion may be maintained by moving the hips across to the side of the plinth.

If for any reason it is undesirable to use a pelvic belt for traction it is sometimes successful to use either an ankle

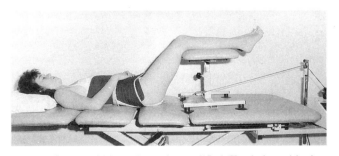

Fig. 58.1 Symmetrical traction—the modified 'Fowler's position'—with 'free float' in use.

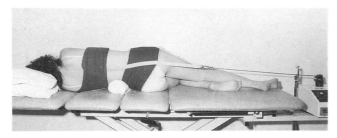

Fig. 58.5 Asymmetrical traction in increased side-flexion.

cuff, unilaterally for asymmetric traction and bilaterally for symmetric, or, with the lower legs on a stool, a wide band over the thigh. Either is clipped onto the traction cord as a belt would be.

THORACIC SPINE POSITIONING

Upper thoracic traction is most easily effected via the cervical spine; middle and lower thoracic traction may be set up as for lumbar traction, with the placement of the harness around the affected level. It may not always be possible to place the affected level at or near the gap in the plinth and therefore some other friction-reducing mechanism may be necessary; the use of a flat plastic sheet may be suitable but it should be inserted after positioning, if possible, to avoid slippage. If a roll is used with asymmetric traction this should be placed directly under the affected level, rather than the waist, as this is usually the most comfortable position for a lumbar roll.

APPLICATION OF FORCE

Having positioned the patient, the next step is to consider the force to be applied. Generally speaking, there appear to be two distinctly different approaches to the question of the force, or weight, to be applied for traction. One school of thought advocates the approach in which a large amount of force is applied in an attempt to 'separate the vertebral levels'. The other approach advocates the use of the minimum effective force necessary to achieve relief of signs and symptoms. Given the fact that any symptomatic vertebral level may be damaged or degenerate, the probability is that using the minimum effective force is the most appropriate, and, allied to careful positioning, very low poundage may relieve even severe nerve root signs and symptoms. When handling nerve root problems, signs and symptoms may be made worse by using too great a force—it is safest to start with a poundage that may appear to be too low, and to increase this slowly if signs and symptoms do not change. Generally speaking, if nerve root signs do not improve with traction it is more effective to alter the position rather than increase the force applied.

When a low force is effective the hypothesis that traction may have an effect due to the separation of vertebral bodies becomes somewhat debatable. The question then is: if this is not the mode of action of traction, then how does it have an effect? (Grieve 1981b).

SPEED OF RESPONSE TO TRACTION

It is sometimes assumed that traction takes time to have an effect, and that improvement should not be looked for in one treatment, but this may depend on the culprit structures. If, for instance, the traction is aimed at tight collagen structures the probability is that there will be a slow response. If a 'joint' problem is being treated the response should be as immediate as it would be with any other passive handling technique. Nerve root problems which will respond to traction may do so, to some extent, during the treatment, and it is vital to re-test continually for changes in signs and symptoms. Initially, re-testing should take place at every step, first with the spine in a weight-bearing position if possible; then, non-weight bearing; then with every change in positioning; then after traction is applied; then at the end of the treatment time while the traction is still on; then after the rest period, and finally on weight-bearing again. In this way a clear and detailed picture may be built up of the exact response of the signs and symptoms to each change. It may be found that reduction in signs and symptoms may occur with simply positioning the spine, before any traction is applied, and often in this circumstance a very slight amount of traction is all that is necessary to improve the condition further. The position may then be used by the patient as home treatment to maintain and increase the reduction of symptoms. If a drastic change is found between weight-bearing signs and symptoms and non-weight-bearing signs and symptoms, it may be more helpful for the patient to have a period of bed-rest rather than traction.

Even with good positioning there will be some nerve root problems that will still respond slowly, and some that will not respond at all. Symptoms due to the presence of inflammation around the root are unlikely to respond just to traction, and conditions in which the signs and symptoms are not influenced by changes in posture or by movement may respond slowly, or not at all.

SUMMARY

Traction can be a very powerful tool when used with precision. To achieve maximum success in the minimum time, position the patient accurately, use the minimum effective force, re-test signs and symptoms frequently, and base each patient's treatment on the signs and symptoms rather than the diagnosis.

REFERENCES

Colachis S C, Strohm B R 1966 Effect of duration of intermittent cervical traction on vertebral separation. Archives of Physical Medicine Rehabilitation 46: 820

Grieve G P 1981a Common vertebral joint problems. Churchill Livingstone, Edinburgh, pp 170–176

Grieve G P 1981b Common vertebral joint problems. Churchill Livingstone, Edinburgh, p 397

Petullo L R 1986 Clinical observations with respect to progressive/regressive traction. Journal of Orthopaedic and Sports Physical Therapy 7: 261–263

Saunders H D 1981 Unilateral lumbar traction. Physical Therapy 61(2): 221–225

Sherriff J 1988 A flexible approach to traction. International Federation of Orthopaedic Manipulative Therapists Papers and Poster Abstracts, Cambridge

Walker G L 1986 Goodley polyaxial cervical traction. Physical Therapy 66(9): 1255–1259

59. Back pain in the childbearing year

J. Mantle

The phrase 'the childbearing year' has been coined to encapsulate the totality of the physiological sequence through which a woman's body passes in order to grow, deliver and suckle a child. Usually more than a year, it consists of the pregnancy (normally about 40 weeks), labour, which, with modern obstetrics, is now rarely more than 24 hours, the puerperium, a period of about 8 weeks following delivery during which the mother's body substantially returns in most respects both anatomically and physiologically to its pre-pregnancy state, and finally—and particularly where lactation is established and continued for some months—a further open-ended period to allow for the gradual completion of the whole process.

This chapter will seek to review the problem of pain associated with the back and pelvic joints occurring during the childbearing year and to suggest ways in which the physiotherapist may contribute to prevention and relief. From the very outset it must be clearly understood that research has shown that many women in their fertile years, i.e. commonly 15–42 years, experience back pain from time to time regardless of whether or not they are pregnant or have had a child recently. General population surveys, such as those conducted by the Consumers Association (1986) and Cats (1986), suggest that, at any point in time, about 20% of this age group have back pain, and obviously a larger percentage will be able to recall having suffered it at some time in the previous year. The findings of researchers such as Biering-Sørensen (1984) and Scholey and Hair (1989) lead one to consider that this latter figure may be as high as 40%; these facts have been frequently ignored when appraising the issue of back pain in pregnant or recently delivered women. The natural inclination of mainstream medical carers has often been to accept the patient's logic and seek to attribute the causation solely to the childbearing process. However, this cannot be the case, for, although childbearing undoubtedly brings additional possible causal factors and heightens others, there is at this moment no reason to suppose that—with the exception of menstruation—it protects a woman from the factors, both known and as yet unknown, which contribute to the multifactorial causation of back pain in that whole peer group.

PREGNANCY

Pain associated with spine and/or pelvic joints is a common complaint in pregnancy. The number, severity and duration of pain episodes vary greatly between individuals and from pregnancy to pregnancy in the same individual. For some there are very minor transient discomforts; for a few there is totally disabling agony. This fact must be remembered when appraising the literature on the incidence of backache in pregnancy. Nwuga (1982) found an incidence of 90% but included any degree of pain, while Mantle et al (1977) found 48% had troublesome or severe pain. In fact there seems to be general agreement that about 50% of all pregnant women experience at some stage back pain of sufficient intensity and duration to affect lifestyle in some way, and that one-third of these women will experience severe pain (Mantle et al 1977, 1981, Nwuga 1982, Fast et al 1987, Bullock et al 1987, Berg et al 1988). The majority suffer low-back pain; in the study conducted by Mantle et al (1981) about 50% of women felt the pain chiefly in the lumbar region, and for most of the remainder it was sacral spreading into buttocks and thighs. Pain radiating down one or both legs has also been reported (Mantle et al 1977, Fast et al 1987). Berg et al (1988) found that for 50% of women pain was experienced for short periods, and only a few (6%) suffered backache for more than six months.

A tendency for backache in pregnancy to be felt at a lower anatomical level than in the non-pregnant state was reported (Mantle et al 1981). Pain may also be experienced over the symphysis pubis, in the cervical, thoracic and/or coccygeal regions, either in addition to low-back pain or separately.

For a majority of sufferers the first back pain of a pregnancy occurs between the fifth and seventh months of pregnancy (Mantle et al 1977, 1981, Fast et al 1987, Berg et al 1988). Fast et al (1987) shrewdly suggested that the aetiology of the pain may vary with each trimester. For some women it will be their first experience of back pain (Mantle et al 1981, Svensson et al 1990) and such people inevitably attribute it to the pregnancy. There is evidence to suggest that back pain in second and subsequent pregnancies is both more common and more severe than in the first (Mantle et al 1977, Fast et al 1987, Berg et al 1988). There are a few women for whom the return of 'the pain' is a reliable predictor of a new pregnancy. There is no evidence that back pain prior to pregnancy results in inevitable backache in childbearing (Mantle et al 1977), but a study of 804 women of mixed parity (Ostgaard & Andersson 1991) showed that it was more likely where there was a pre-pregnancy history, and where it did occur it lasted longer. So it is unquestionably wise to seek to cure or control back pain in advance of a pregnancy. However, there are some women whose back problem clearly improves during pregnancy only to return again after delivery. It has been suggested that this could be due to the strut effect of the rising uterus with resulting reduction in trunk mobility, to a general reduction in activity and taking more rest, to slight joint laxity, and/or to small but evidently beneficial changes in posture or loading. Backache in pregnancy is typically aggravated by fatigue, sitting, standing, walking, forward bending and lifting—particularly when combined with twisting, e.g. ironing (Mantle et al 1977, 1981, Fast et al 1987, Berg 1988). Work by Nicholls (1989) and Nicholls & Grieve (1992) reported that women found the performance of many everyday tasks becoming more difficult with advancing pregnancy and that back pain in particular limited the performance of ironing, washing up, carrying a food tray, vacuuming, mopping, and sitting in an upright chair for one hour. The consequences of the increasingly protuberant abdomen on workspace usage, and particularly on forward arm reach in standing and sitting, were explored. A further small preliminary study of a group of secretaries (Nicholls & Grieve 1992) showed an increase in back pain from the second to third trimester of pregnancy both before and after completing a typing task in sitting. The implications for work-station design need speedy evaluation and implementaion by employers.

Additional causal factors of back pain in pregnancy

It is considered that the following may act as additional factors to heighten a woman's susceptibility to, or actually cause, back pain in pregnancy: fatigue, weight gain, fluid retention, change in centre of gravity, effects of hormones on connective tissue, anxiety.

Fatigue

Women commonly complain of quite severe tiredness, a sapping of strength and some emotional lability, particu-

larly in the first and third trimesters of pregnancy. This will naturally predispose toward poor posture, carelessness and clumsiness in performing activities, strains and accidents. In the first trimester this is attributed to hormonal changes; in the early weeks some experience nausea—thought to be caused by the chorionic gonadotrophic hormone—and a few feel thoroughly unwell. There is also a gradual increase in blood plasma volume without a complementary increase in erythrocytes with resulting lowering in haemoglobin level—dilution anaemia. In the third trimester increased effort is required to carry around the additional body volume and weight; these can also make it difficult 'to get comfortable' and cause restlessness and disturbed sleep.

Weight gain

The average weight gain is said to be 10–12 kg (Table 59.1), but some women increase their weight by as much as 20–25 kg. The increase in breast size and weight occurs quite early, but in general the weight gain is predominantly in the latter half of pregnancy. This has obvious implications for compression and torsional strains on all the spinal and pelvic joints in all positions, even lying, e.g. turning over in bed with an enlarged heavy tense abdomen. The rising uterus eventually pushes up on the diaphragm and the lower rib margin causing the latter to lift and flare—thoracic girth increases.

Fluid retention

An increased blood volume of about 40%, and raised oestrogen levels tending to favour fluid retention, may result in oedema which directly presses on nerves causing paraesthesia and muscle weakness—e.g. carpal tunnel syndrome (Voitk et al 1983), meralgia paraesthetic—and is affected by warm weather and gravity. In addition, or alternatively, increased fluid retention means increased weight and, for example, this results in increased gravitational drag on the shoulder girdle and brachial plexus—like permanently carrying a small suitcase.

Change in centre of gravity

Because the weight gain is predominantly anteriorly placed and thereby affects the body's centre of gravity, it is

Table 59.1 The distribution of average weight gain in pregnancy

Breasts	0.5 kg
Increased blood volume	1.2 kg
Fetus	3.3 kg
Placenta	0.6 kg
Amniotic fluid	0.8 kg
Enlarged uterus	0.9 kg
Fat deposits, e.g. hips, thighs	4.0 kg
Extracellular fluid	1.2 kg

necessary for most women to adapt their posture. A large study of 855 pregnant women of mixed parity (Ostgaard et al 1993) found three factors correlating with back pain in pregnancy—a large sagittal abdominal diameter, large transverse abdominal diameter, and deep lumbar lordosis. Others have suggested that the increasing abdominal girth and the need to sustain adequate arm reach results in an increase in trunk inclination in the performance of some tasks (Nicholls & Grieve 1991, 1992). Bullock (1987) and Bullock et al (1987) showed an increase in both lumbar and thoracic curves; interestingly, the development of these did not seem to correlate with the onset of back pain. It is also noteworthy that, contrary to apocryphal wisdom, increased pelvic inclination (downward and forward) was not found. However, such postural changes must further alter spinal loading and torsional strains. Overriding of the facet joints in the lumbar region can cause irritability.

Effects of hormones on connective tissue

Before the hazards of X-rays were appreciated an increase in the average width of the symphysis pubis from 4 inches to 9 inches (10 cm to 23 cm) through pregnancy was documented, and Abramson et al (1934) noted that relaxation of the symphysis pubis began in the early months of pregnancy, reached a peak just before labour, and took about five months to return to normal. It is said that mobility at the symphysis increases by two and a half times; extremely rarely it separates completely in pregnancy or labour. The mobility of the sacro-iliac joints may also increase but not necessarily equally; sclerosis—osteitis condensans ilii—is sometimes seen on X-ray after childbirth and indicates transient stress. Both anterior and posterior dysfunction (rotation of the ilium on the sacrum) have been described (Fraser 1976, Berg et al 1988) but there is disagreement as to which is the most common in pregnancy (Golightly 1982, DonTigny 1985, Lee 1989). Any hypermobility of one or more of the pelvic joints obviously affects the others, and strains all. A hypermobile joint can also lock, throwing greater strain on the others.

Animal work (Hisaw 1926, Chihal & Epsey 1973, Mercado-Simmen et al 1980, MacLennan 1981, MacLennan et al 1986a) suggests that a combination of raised levels of oestrogens, progesterone, endogenous cortisols and especially relaxin—early and late in pregnancy—are responsible for this. There seems to be a gradual breakdown in collagen in the target tissues, e.g. ligaments, and replacement with a modified form which is more pliable and extensible, which has a higher water content and a greater volume. Increased volume could result in pressure on pain-sensitive structures. MacLennan et al (1986b) found higher levels of serum relaxin in women experiencing severe pelvic pain and pelvic joint instability late in pregnancy compared to those with little

or no pain. Could there also be a connection between these changes and the occasional new lumbar disc lesion with neurological deficit seen in early pregnancy, as the increased pliability is the last straw for a beleaguered annulus?

Nor are these changes limited to pelvic joints. Calguneri et al (1982) reported an increase in range of the metacarpo-phalangeal joints, with greater laxity in the second and subsequent pregnancies compared to the first, while the obvious dramatic increase in pliability and extensibility of other collagenous structures, such as the linear alba, is rarely mentioned.

Anxiety

Some have tried to correlate back pain with certain personality characteristics (Wolkind 1976). Mantle et al (1981) found no connection between previous depression and back pain in pregnancy, although there can be little doubt that a new unfamiliar pain increases the constant and universal anxiety about the welfare of the fetus which transcends any fear about self. Back pain also adds to the other stresses which commonly beset pregnant women, e.g. the need to continue employment, finance, housing with a baby, relationships, impending labour. Anxiety tends to increase tension, pain and fatigue—the topic with which this section commenced.

Prevention

Prevention of back pain in pregnancy starts from the mother's own birth or, some would even say, from her parentage. Congenital spinal and pelvic anomalies and asymmetries are commonplace and cannot be changed. However, it is vital that parents and teachers are sufficiently well informed to be guardians, role models and trainers through the critical growing years. What is wanted is for each young person to develop a strong healthy body, with an understanding of its limitations and of what are realistic and safe loadings and activities. School days should provide a wonderfully controlled environment for this. Such a preparation is then ideally reinforced and developed in the ergonomically friendly work place as a result of initiatives by a management who has realized the cost-effective benefits of promoting and maintaining the health of the work force. Women who passed through such a utopian system would be fit and have heightened kinaesthetic sense, and they would need little additional help to adapt to the very real strains and stresses—physical and mental—of childbearing and rearing.

In reality, most women have had little or no instruction in wise back usage (Mantle et al 1981) but have heard that fitness may be advantageous in procreation (Hall & Kaufman 1987). This can lead to disastrous results where courses and/or unsuitable activities are undertaken with inappropriate supervision. Well Women Clinics would do well to provide assessment, advice, and instruction, including backcare, by a physiotherapist to avoid this iatrogenic damage. Such a positive programme would integrate with a comprehensive parentcraft programme. It is so difficult for the first-time mother to anticipate without help the effects of changing physiology, weight and shape. Yet anticipation and prophylactic action is essential to prevention; waiting for a problem to arise and then trying to deal with it is second best.

It will take a thoroughly competent physiotherapist at least one hour with a small group of women to go through and give opportunity to test out the chief issues in relation to wise back usage and pain prevention or limitation in pregnancy. How this might be done has already been described in detail (Mantle et al 1981, Mantle 1988, Polden & Mantle 1990); the following are the priority areas to be considered:

- comfortable supported sleeping positions related to changing weight and shape, and avoiding trunk rotation
- getting in and out of bed, avoiding back strain related to restlessness, and increased need to micturate at night
- turning over in bed keeping knees crooked and pressed together related to lax pelvic joints and drag of abdomen
- sitting positions, chairs that fit, and the importance of firmly supporting the lumbar curve (Mantle et al 1977, 1981)
- work environment at work and at home related to a pregnant woman's changing ergonomic workspace envelope
- best posture: sitting, standing and walking 'TALL'
- avoiding, reducing or coping with excessive stress and fatigue both mental and physical
- wise lifting and handling; avoiding heavy weights
- general lifestyle in relation to present and future as parent; travel and sport
- avoiding doing any activity for too long.

ASSESSMENT

It is an interesting fact that pregnant women with back pain are rarely fully assessed or treated. This positive discrimination against pregnant women seems to be due in part to obstetricians considering back pain in pregnancy inevitable or unimportant and/or not referring women for assessment. Perhaps they are unaware that therapy is available. However, on the other hand, physiotherapists are often strangely reluctant to treat a woman once they know she is pregnant, a reluctance not shared by osteopaths, except in the earliest weeks of pregnancy (up to 16 weeks). It has been suggested that the current physiotherapy training pays insufficient attention to the childbearing process as compared to osteopathy training.

The assessment of a pregnant woman with back pain follows the classic pattern with only minor adaptations according to the gestational stage. However, a basic understanding of the process of pregnancy is essential to the interpretation of findings as the following comments seek to illustrate.

Subjective examination

Details of present pain and other symptoms

Flaring of the ribs may cause costochondral margin pain (or even disruption of a junction), pain may emanate from the costovertebral joints and there may be intercostal neuralgia. Fluid retention may be responsible for para-aesthesia and/or muscle weakness. Sharp stabs of stitch-like lower abdominal or groin pain may be attributable to tension on and/or stretch of the uterine suspensory ligaments or to abdominal adhesions. There is also the rare possibility of osteoporosis of pregnancy (Smith et al 1985); vertebral collapse and even hip fractures have been reported.

Any reported recent onset of malaise, headaches or oedema require immediate referral to exclude pre-eclamptic toxaemia or urinary tract infections; the latter are common in pregnancy and can also cause low-back pain.

Mandatory questions concerning the perineum and micturition

Pregnant women commonly experience changes in continence, e.g. frequency, urgency, and latterly there is a tendency to stress incontinence. There is also a predisposition to constipation, and pain, hyperalgia or numbness of the perineum may accompany piles, haemorrhoids or varicosities of the vulva.

Onset and history of this and any previous episodes

The stage of pregnancy at onset is relevant in interpreting findings. Hormone-mediated changes in collagen commence quite early, enlargement of the abdomen and serious weight gain occurs later, back pain toward the end of pregnancy can herald labour. The possibility of a greater degree of joint laxity in second pregnancies, compared with the first, has already been mentioned (Calguneri et al 1982) and several authors have noted and tried to explain the increase in incidence and severity of back pain with increased parity (Mantle et al 1977, 1981, Nwuga 1982, Fast et al 1987, Berg et al 1988, Ostgaard & Andersson 1991).

General physical health, occupation and lifestyle

The present social philosophy toward women, and the employment climate, are leading some women, their partners and employers to underestimate the demand—both physical and mental—that pregnancy places on a body. Every body has its limits, and the physiotherapist is an ideal impartial assessor. Berg et al (1988) and Cherry (1987) found a strong association between type of work—especially lifting and twisting—and back pain and sacro-iliac dysfunction.

Objective examination

The balance of a heavily pregnant woman is unreliable, so it is wise to carry out the examination in standing adjacent to a plinth which can safely be used for support. Supine-lying for any length or time can lead to faintness due to pressure of the gravid uterus on the inferior vena cava and aorta—pregnancy hypotensive syndrome. The infallible remedy for this is to turn the patient into side-lying. Prone-lying with the innovative use of pillows is an examination position option further into pregnancy than might be imagined. Side-lying may be preferred with a small firm pillow at the waist and a pillow between the legs.

From quite early in pregnancy in some women, increases in joint laxity may be discernible but may not be so bilaterally; less pressure is needed in testing, and the 'end feel' is spongier. Later in pregnancy the strut effect of the rising uterus limits all spinal movements; thoracic and lumbar curves can be expected to increase (Bullock 1987, Bullock et al 1987), and oedema may also reduce joint range, especially at the periphery. Shoulder levels, abdominal and waist contours may be changed temporarily according to the lie of the mobile fetus.

Recording

This clinical speciality area is prone to litigation, so record-keeping must be meticulous. It is wise to record patients' comments and complaints verbatim. The physiotherapist should keep abreast of the obstetric notes and enter a synopsis of physiotherapy findings and treatment regularly in order that the whole obstetric team has all the relevant data at all times.

TREATMENT

Once the initial assessment is complete and the problems analysed, the patient should be fully informed and encouraged to participate as an equal in considering the treatment options for solving the problems. The obstetrician should also be involved in the decision-making process in order that no obstetric consideration is overlooked.

The sooner treatment is instituted the better (Sims-Williams et al 1978), and rest and relaxation, instruction and advice on posture and backcare, support, mobilization and/or manipulation, and exercise on land or in the water are the chief modalities used. Heat, massage, traction and TENS also have a place, while short-wave diathermy, interferential therapy and ultrasound are considered, certainly by the machine manufacturers, to be contraindicated. However, it is an interesting fact that improvement often follows informed reassurance that all is well with the fetus and an explanation of what is causing the back pain.

Rest and relaxation

As intimated earlier, pregnant women frequently expect and are expected to do too much; often the total daily work load is too great or unsuitable. There are also financial pressures to work right up to the end of pregnancy. Where there is acute pain and/or neurological deficit bed rest is the treatment of choice but dramatic improvements are achieved by two or three days modified bed rest and/or discontinuing paid employment. First it must be established whether rest at home is a realistic possibility. Then women need very clear and specific instructions as to what they should and should not do, and help to find several really comfortable pain-free positions in which to rest. Teaching a woman a relaxation technique, e.g. the Mitchel Method (Mitchel 1987) can both encourage resting and counter stress, but it also heightens body awareness as to activities most aggravating to stress and fatigue. Daytime resting positions for simple postural backache include sitting astride an upright chair leaning forward onto the chair back, the psoas position (early pregnancy), and crook prone kneeling resting head on forearms.

Instruction and advice on posture and backcare

Because of the changing centre of gravity in pregnancy, posture usually has to adapt. Considerable professional wisdom is needed to evaluate the current result with respect to the patient presenting with back pain symptoms and to judge whether it is the best possible compromise.

A common adaptation in the third trimester is like that of a yacht with the spinnaker out: the abdomen is thrust forward with an accentuated lumbar cure, the mid-thoracic region is thrust back to counter balance, the lower cervical spine is straightened, the head is extended and the chin juts forward. A simple but effective approach is, using a long mirror, to show the woman her position and then ask her to stand as TALL as possible and observe the difference. The same concept can be used in sitting and walking.

For any advice to be effective it must be inherently good and appropriate, clearly communicated and acceptable, and then be implemented by the recipient. Much time is wasted by physiotherapists, on backcare advice because insufficient time is devoted to it and one or more of these criteria are not met. For example, it is useless to recommend using hips and knees for bending and lifting if the pregnant body weight is too great for the quadriceps to raise the body to standing again. Broadly, the instruction and advice is similar to that of the prophylactic approach discussed earlier, but time spent with each patient allows active testing and adapting of the principles to a tailor-made realistic and individual solution. Anything less than this can be a total waste of time.

Support

When pain in the thoracic region is associated with increased size and weight of the breasts it is important to ensure that the patient has a well-fitting and supportive brassière.

As is discussed elsewhere in some detail (Mantle 1988), physiotherapists in different parts of the world have found that many women, particularly those with back pain emanating from the sacro-iliac joints, derive benefit from firm supra trochanteric support. This has taken a variety of forms in composition and width. In the UK, the Fembrace—a wide band of elastic material drawn posteriorly across the sacro-iliac joints and crossing over to fix beneath the abdomen—and similar derivatives have been popular. It should be applied in crook lying and following manipulative reduction of any abnormal pelvic torsion. It can also be useful to support a lax pendulant abdomen which is considered to be dragging adversely on the sacro-iliac or lumbar region. A narrow supra-trochanteric belt has also been produced to support lax symphysis pubis joints.

Mobilization and manipulation

Generally quite gentle mobilizations are successful, and resourceful innovation, as advocated by Maitland (1986a), enables the pregnant patient to be treated whatever the size and shape of the abdomen. The following sections are by no means an exhaustive list but are designed to show examples of what is possible.

Thoracic region

Posterior–anterior central, unilateral or transverse vertebral pressures are mercifully most usually needed in the first half of pregnancy—associated with the early increase in size and weight of breasts—so that the patient is often able to lie prone for treatment. However, if the breasts are too tender, or pressure on the abdomen is considered uncomfortable, transverse vertebral pressures can be done with the patient in crook side-lying on the least painful side. This position is also very suitable for soft-tissue massage either side of the spine in the painful area.

Later in pregnancy where a combination of increasing thoracic curve and a rising uterus are causing rib flare and thoracic pain, a gentle stretch of the anterior thoracic soft tissue may be achieved with the patient sitting on a stool with hands interlocked behind the neck. The physiotherapist stands behind and applies pressure with hip or thigh to the patient's back, while grasping the patient's upper arms close to the axillae. By rhythmically leaning back and forth the therapist can produce gentle extensions of the thorax. Maitland (1986b) described a similar movement with sharp upward traction, the therapist having threaded her arms under the patient's axillae to grasp the wrists. It is also possible to perform thoracic rotation in a similar position or in crook supine lying with the patient's arms crossed, as described by Maitland (1986c). Costovertebral and costotransverse joint mobilizations can be performed in a similar way in crook supine lying if the patient is toward the end of pregnancy; the physiotherapist must just be alert for signs of pregnancy hypotensive syndrome as already described.

A patient can often ease costal margin pain or rib ache by resting forward sitting the wrong way around astride and well back on an upright chair, with forearms supported on the chair back or resting back, sitting in a high backed easy chair with arms raised above the head or with arm raised and trunk side flexed away from the pain where there is unilateral pain.

Lumbar region

Posterior–anterior central, unilateral or transverse vertebral pressures can be applied in prone up to about the sixth month in many cases. However, transverse vertebral pressure may be done in crook side-lying with a small pillow or towel at waist level. Grade I and II rotations can also be achieved in side-lying by simply moving the pelvis. Pain symptoms from below L4 may respond to a double leg longitudinal movement with the legs grasped at 25–30° from horizontal (Maitland 1986). A single leg technique is used for unilateral pain. Alternatively, gentle small-range flexion, extension and rotation mobilizations can be performed in crook lying with the physiotherapist grasping the pelvis.

Sacro-iliac region

Posterior–anterior pressures may be performed in prone-lying in early pregnancy. To correct torsions in the later months, gentle mobilizations can be performed very effectively in either direction in crook lying with the physiotherapist cradling the ischial tuberosity in one hand and applying complimentary pressure over either the anterior or posterior aspect of the appropriate ilium with the other hand.

Fraser (1976) and Golightly (1982) favoured the Cyriax technique for gapping the sacro-iliac to correct iliac torsion, and this is entirely possible with a pregnant woman. The patient lies supine with the knee of the affected side flexed and the toes hooked under the straight knee. The therapist takes the flexed knee across the body while holding the shoulder of the affected side against the plinth. Thus tension is applied to the affected sacro-iliac joint and any slack is taken up. At the end of range the therapist applies a single gentle thrust. In pregnancy it is surely wise to consider the state of the soft tissues and manipulate as infrequently as possible. A Fembrace-type support may be applied after treatment. The woman may be recommended to repeat the same movement (without the thrust) at home or to cross the affected leg over the other and, combining this with sufficient trunk rotation, to dangle the lower leg over the side of the bed to gain traction. Alternatively, DonTigny (1985) suggests a movement performed by the patient in a sitting or standing position with the affected hip and knee flexed and the foot on the chair or stool. The patient rocks forward to the knee and back.

Both Fraser and Golightly assume that the ilial torsion will be forward and downward and recommend that the patient perform a maintenance movement once or twice a day, both sides, affected side first. For the left sacro-iliac joint, the patient lies supine and grasps the left flexed knee at the level of the tibial tubercle with the left hand. The left hip is then rotated laterally to allow the left calcaneum to be cupped in the right hand. With the trunk fully supported and the right leg relaxed and straight, the left knee is gently pulled towards a point just lateral to the left shoulder and the heel eased toward the right groin. The pressure is then released and re-applied once or twice before repeating the procedure with the opposite leg.

Golightly (1982) reported good success with sacro-iliac torsion by using a sharp longitudinal leg pull, first to the leg on the affected side and then to the other with the patient supine. Patients sometimes report relief from slow hyperextension in standing with hands firmly applied either side in the small of the back. DonTigny's (1985) explanation for this was that 'the posterior shift of the line of gravity behind the centre of the acetabula creates a powerful strain in posterior rotation that would help correct an anterior dysfunction (rotation) to the sacroiliac joints'.

Sciatica is best treated by a reduction in activity or even bed rest (Bell & Rothman 1984). Coccydynia is usually associated with previous injury but sometimes benefits from gentle posterior–anterior mobilizations—grasping the coccyx using a gloved lubricated index finger in the anus and the thumb posteriorly. A rubber ring to relieve pressure in sitting is essential.

Other techniques

Many women use heat in the form of a hot water bottle for their back pain, and massage, already mentioned, is a greatly undervalued, underused, non-invasive modality appreciated by women. Many physiotherapists shrink from using traction in pregnancy but with lowered poundage it may be useful. TENS has no known adverse side-effects but should be used cautiously in selected cases (Mantle 1988).

LABOUR

Intermittent backache correlated with labour uterine contractions is a common and excepted feature in addition to low abdominal, perineal and thigh pain; the pain zones with each stage of labour have been described (Bonica 1984). Generations of sufferers and carers have collaborated in finding the most comfortable position and using massage—stroking, kneading and simple firm hand pressure—over the most painful site which is usually the lower lumbar and sacral region. There is still some mystery as to why the normal physiological process of labour should cause so much pain (Polden & Mantle 1990); uterine muscle ischaemia, stretching of the cervix and other soft tissue, and pressure from the firm fetal head are common suggestions. It is recognized that certain presenting positions of the fetus (e.g. the occipitoposterior position) cause more back pain than others. MacLennan et al (1986) found an increase in the serum level of the hormone relaxin during labour; and pelvic joint laxity is traditionally accepted as occurring and gives plasticity to the boney pelvic ring which favours the passage through it of the irregularly shaped fetus. It is suggested, for example, that such flexibility allows all sorts of unusual outward movements to increase diameters of the pelvic outlet, and delivery positions (like squatting), which encourage full backward movement freedom for the apex of the sacrum and permit lateral movement of the ischial tuberosities, have become popular. Few have questioned whether back pain in labour or in the puerperium is caused by these torsional stresses and strains or injudicious positioning, particularly when pain perception is dulled or removed pharmaceutically (MacArthur et al 1990).

The relevance of the process and management of labour to the physiotherapist is in two contexts. Firstly, when treating a patient for back pain in pregnancy, there should be prospective consideration of and planning for the management of labour as a damage-limitation exercise. In modern obstetrics, providing the labour is progressing satisfactorily, the labouring woman is usually free to walk, stand, sit and lie as she feels is most comforting, moving around and using a wide range of positions. While the physiotherapist regrettably is rarely with her labouring patient she has an unrivalled understanding of the nature of a particular patient's back pain in the pregnancy and is well equipped to recommend how exacerbating the trauma might best be avoided. Knowledge of a particular maternity unit's policies and practices, direct communication with and, in some cases, instruction of, the midwives is essential. Midwives are not trained to deal with such special needs.

The second context concerns patients presenting with back pain in the puerperium and beyond, where the precise events of labour are a very relevant area of enquiry. However, unless the physiotherapist has a considerable all-round knowledge, appropriate questions will not be asked and valuable insight will be lost. For example, in the second stage, prolonged strong bearing down in lying with hips and knees flexed—rather than half-lying—and fixing the shoulders by gripping behind the thighs, often strains the upper thoracic area. If in addition the partner seeks to help the woman flex her head, neck and thorax, but in a rather forceful manner, then a stiff neck may result. The lithotomy position in stirrups is used for forceps delivery and sometimes for perineal stitching after delivery. If both legs are not raised and lowered simultaneously sacro-iliac torsion can result. The implication of epidural anaesthesia in persistent backache following childbirth will be discussed in the next section (MacArthur et al 1990).

PUERPERIUM

Postnatally, back pain may be a continuation of that experience antenatally, or there may be new pain. The whole process of labouring and delivering, and caring for the infant brings in new causative factors. Tiredness and lack of sleep, stretched and slack abdominal muscles, sore perineum making sitting awkward, heavy engorged breasts, poor or unsupported positions, particularly when feeding perhaps every two hours, mild depression, the cot and nappy-changing surface too low, carrying a carrycot, a baby increasing in weight, other children and partner demanding extra reassurance and attention are just some of the commonest early adverse factors postpartum as far as back health are concerned. Bullock et al (1987) found that the increased thoracic and lumbar curves of pregnancy were substantially still present at 12 weeks postpartum. They point out that, although there is no longer the weight of the fetus, and there is reduction in abdominal size, the adaptive lengthening and shortening of ligaments and muscles associated with the increased kyphosis and lordosis could result in perpetuation of the pregnancy posture and muscle imbalances. It seems generally agreed that relaxin levels remain slightly raised for some months (MacLennan et al 1986a) and the joint laxity can take as much as 6 months to fully stabilize. Hagan (1974) noted that, out of 23 postpartum women with severe symptoms including pain and tenderness over the pelvic joints, snapping sounds occurred on vertical symphysial movement, and Berg et al (1988) found that 65% of those with sacro-iliac joint disfunction in pregnancy were continuing to suffer from 0.5–12 months after delivery. Fraser (1976) reported on 115 women examined postpartum. He claimed to find 96% with sacro-iliac tor-

sions (apparently forward and downward rotation of the ilium) predominately on the right and, though not all were complaining of significant back pain, he recommended manipulation using the Cyriax gapping technique followed by regular practice by the patient of the self-help manoeuvre already described. Finally, pain is often experienced for a day or two round the catheter insertion site following epidural anesthetic, and MacArthur et al (1990) reported a relationship between persistent backache and epidural anaesthesia which is probably causal and seems to result from a combination of effective analgesia and stressed postures during labour. Physiotherapists should be aware of this possibility, which should increase their interest in ensuring that their obstetrician and midwife colleagues are fully aware of and competent in all the non-invasive pain-relieving and pain-coping strategies relevant to labour, and of how to protect the spine and pelvic joints from stress.

Prevention can never be total, but an understanding of the principles, and good backcare habits must be established wherever possible antenatally. Postpartum, the woman's interest in herself is small, and her concentration span is short, yet she is at considerable risk; and this is compounded if there are other children to care for and little supportive help. Never is it more essential for the physiotherapist to assess the whole situation in a holistic way than when called to treat a recently delivered woman with back pain. The challenge for the physiotherapist is that it is not possible for a mother with a new baby to keep regular appointments, to travel long distances, to be kept waiting or to devote time to lengthy treatment sessions. Care in the first three months postpartum has to be supremely time-efficient, it has to give maximum immediate relief, and it must allow the woman first and foremost to continue mothering; cure may have to wait. Ideally the community physiotherapist treats the woman at home and, with the midwife and health visitor, mobilizes the appropriate agencies to provide the practical help deemed necessary.

There are anecdotal reports of women with continuing postpartum joint laxity with back pain being advised to discontinue breast feeding on the basis that this will speed the return of hormonal levels to normal. Certainly, continuation of lactation is governed by the necessary neurohormonal stimulation provided by the sight, sound, and the touching of the baby combined with suckling and removal of the milk. Certainly too, hormonal effects are demonstrated by the fact that continuation of full breast feeding usually delays resumption of ovulation and menstruation for several months. However, stopping breast feeding early is of unproven benefit for back pain, and it would seem to be in the best interest of the infant to try every other reasonable alternative first. Most particularly, a postpartum woman must not expect—or be expected—to do too much.

TREATMENT

The commonest pain postpartum is pain in the thoracolumbar region. It is almost always a direct result of slumped or unsupported positions when breast- or bottle-feeding. It is imperative that the mother's back is well supported and, whether she sits on a chair or in bed, a firm pillow in the small of the back is needed. The baby should rest on one or more pillows on the lap to raise him to breast height. When sitting on a chair some women find a footstool gives additional comfort, and shoulder-circling exercises after feeding relieves residual tension. It is entirely possible to breast-feed in side-lying; this has many advantages for the weary mother whatever the site of the back pain. Relaxation can be practised at the same time. Occasionally thoracic pain persists because one or more ribs have locked in a rib flare position; mobilizations soon release this.

Poor posture and lumbar pain are often associated with lax stretched abdominal muscles; in some cases there is also a degree of diastasis recti, and these rob the lumbar spine of the supportive corset it needs. Temporary help can be given to the more pendulant abdomens with double-thickness Tubigrip (size K or L) but there is no substitute for gentle repetitive abdominal exercises. It may take three or four months for abdominal muscle strength to return to normal. Tubigrip or a firm pantigirdle is also useful to give some support to pelvic joints still showing signs of instability, and where sacro-iliac torsion was a problem antenatally, careful monitoring is critical. There are a few anecdotal reports from physiotherapist mothers who claim that their sacro-iliac joint tightened up in the 'wrong' position postpartum, only to be corrected at the next pregnancy!

A detailed appraisal of baby care activities is essential whether or not a mother has back pain, e.g. heights for nappy changing, baby bathing, pram handle, and lifting and handing should be revised. Otherwise, providing the physiotherapist includes the childbearing aspect in her interpretation of findings, it is likely that she will reach appropriate conclusions.

REFERENCES

Abramson D, Roberts S M, Wilson P D 1934 Relaxation of the pelvic joints. Surgical Gynaecology and Obstetrics 58: 595

Bell G R, Rothman R H 1984 The conservative treatment of sciatica. Spine 9: 54–56

Berg G, Hammar M, Moller-Nielsen J et al 1988 Low back pain during pregnancy. Obstetrics and Gynecology 71: 71–75

Biering-Sörensen F 1984 A one-year prospective study of low back trouble in a general population. Danish Medical Bulletin 30: 362–375

Bonica J J 1984 In: Wall P, Melzack R (eds) Texbook of pain. Churchill Livingstone, Edinburgh, p 380

Bullock J E 1987 A study of postural changes associated with pregnancy. Proceedings of 10th International Congress of World Confederation for Physical Therapy, Book 1, pp 177–181

Bullock J E, Jull G A, Bullock M I 1987 The relationship of low back pain to postural changes during pregnancy. Australian Journal of Physiotherapy 33: 10–17

Calguneri M, Bird H A, Wright V 1982 Changes in joint laxity occurring during pregnancy. Annals of Rheumatic Disease 41: 126–128

Cats A 1986 Inflammatory disease and the spine. International Back Pain, Society Seminar, London

Cherry N 1987 Physical demands of work and health complaints among women working late in pregnancy. Ergonomics 30: 689–701

Chihal H J, Espey L L 1973 Utilization of the relaxed symphysis pubis of guinea pigs for clues to the mechanism of ovulation. Endocrinology 93: 1441–1445

Consumers Association 1986 Backpain and how to keep it at bay. Which? February: 58–63

DonTigny R L 1985 Function and pathomechanics of the sacro-iliac joint. Physical Therapy 65: 35–44

Fast A, Shapiro D, Ducommun E J et al 1987 Low back pain in pregnancy. Spine 12: 368–371

Fraser D 1976 Postpartum backache: a preventable condition? Canadian Family Practitioner 22: 1434–1436

Golightly R 1982 Pelvic arthropathy in pregnancy and the puerperium. Physiotherapy 68: 216–220

Hagan R 1974 Pelvic girdle relaxation from an orthopaedic point of view. Acta Orthopaedica Scandinavica 45: 550

Hall D C, Kaufman D A 1987 Effects of aerobic and strength conditioning on pregnancy outcomes. American Journal of Obstetrics and Gynecology 11: 1199–1203

Lee D 1989 The pelvic girdle. Churchill Livingstone, Edinburgh

MacArthur C, Lewis M, Knox E G, Crawford S J 1990 Epidural anaesthesia and long term backache after childbirth. British Medical Journal 301: 9–12

MacLennan A H 1981 Relaxin—a review. Australian and New Zealand Journal of Obstetrics and Gynaecology 21: 195–202

MacLennan A H, Nicolson R, Green R C 1986a Serum relaxin in pregnancy. Lancet 2(8501): 241–243

MacLennan A H, Nicolson R, Green R C et al 1986b Serum relaxin and pelvic pain in pregnancy. Lancet 2(8501): 243–245

Maitland G D 1986a Vertebral manipulation. Butterworths, London pp 4–5

Maitland G D 1986b Vertebral manipulation. Butterworths, London p 225

Maitland G D 1986c Vertebral manipulation. Butterworths, London p 25

Mantle J 1988 Back pain in pregnancy. In: McKenna J (ed) Obstetrics and gynaecology, no. 3 International perspectives in physical therapy. Churchill Livingstone, Edinburgh, ch 5

Mantle M J, Greenwood R M, Currey H L F 1977 Backache in pregnancy. Rheumatology and Rehabilitation 16: 95–101

Mantle M L, Holmes J, Currey H L F 1981 Backache in pregnancy II: prophylactic influence of back care classes. Rheumatology and Rehabilitation 20: 227–232

Mercado-Simmen R C, Bryant Greenwood G D, Greenwood F C 1980 Characterization of the binding of 1251- relaxin to rat uterus. Journal of Biological Chemistry 255: 3617–3623

Mitchel L 1987 Simple relaxation. John Murray

Nicholls J 1989 Ergonomic aspects of pregnancy. MSc thesis, University College, London

Nicholls J A, Grieve D W 1992 Performance of physical tasks in pregnancy. Ergonomics 35: 301–311

Nicholls J A, Grieve D W 1992 Posture, performance and discomfort in pregnancy. Applied Ergonomics 23: 128–132

Nwuga V 1982 Pregnancy and back pain among upper class Nigerian women. Australian Journal of Physiotherapy 28: 8–11

Ostgaard H C, Andersson G B 1991 Previous back pain and risk of developing back pain in a future pregnancy. Spine 16: 432–436

Ostgaard H C, Andersson G B, Schultz A B, Miller J A 1993 Influence of some biomechanical factors on low-back pain in pregnancy. Spine 18: 61–65

Polden M, Mantle J 1990 Physiotherapy in obstetrics and gynaecology. Butterworth Heinemann, London

Scholey M, Hair M 1989 Back pain in physiotherapists involved in back care education. Ergonomics 32: 179–190

Sims-Williams H, Jayson M V, Young S M S et al 1978 Controlled trial of mobilisation and manipulation for patients with low back pain in general practice. British Medical Journal 2: 1338

Smith R, Winearls C G, Stevenson J C et al 1985 Osteoporosis of pregnancy. Lancet 1: 1178–1180

Svensson H, Andersson G, Hagstad A et al 1990 The relationship of low back pain to pregnancy and gynecologic factors. Spine 15: 371–375

Voitk A J, Mueller J C, Farlinger D E, Johnston R U 1983 Carpal tunnel syndrome in pregnancy. Canadian Medical Journal 128: 227–282

Wolkind S N 1976 Psychogenic low back pain. British Journal of Hospital Medicine 22: 17–24

FURTHER READING

Bennet V R, Brown L K (eds) 1993 Myles textbook for midwives, 12th edn. Churchill Livingstone, Edinburgh

Lee D 1989 The pelvic girdle. Butterworths,

Polden M, Mantle J 1990 Physiotherapy in obstetrics and gynaecology. Butterworth Heinemann

60. Soft-tissue manipulative techniques

N. Palastanga

SOFT-TISSUE MANIPULATIVE TECHNIQUES

The use of the hands in the treatment of fellow human beings is one of the earliest recorded forms of medical intervention. Many cultures have used types of massage to treat a variety of musculoskeletal conditions with techniques first used by the Chinese around 2700 BC followed later by the Greeks and Romans. Hippocrates described how massage should be applied as a medical treatment in 400 BC. The French are accredited with the modern introduction of massage into Europe, and this accounts for many of the massage techniques still bearing the French names (Licht 1960).

The very formation of the physiotherapy profession in the United Kingdom was the direct result of massage becoming a specialized branch of nursing. As the practice of this new treatment of patients became widespread an unpleasant series of scandals arose in 1894. The basis of these was that some unfortunate nurses trained in massage were enticed to work in 'houses of ill-repute' on false pretences. So strong was the outcry that in July 1894, the British Medical Journal published a warning to its readers urging them not to send patients for massage treatments because of the number of unscrupulous people practising it (Wickstead 1948).

These trained nurses, who, by now, had enough clinical practice to establish their firm belief in the therapeutic value of massage, were concerned by the effect of the scandals. Their response was to form a professional body which, as the Society of Trained Masseuses, in 1895 established training courses and examinations in order to make massage 'a safe, clean and honourable profession for women'. This professional body was to be the forerunner of the Chartered Society of Physiotherapy which was formed in 1942.

The start of the physiotherapy profession in the United States of America can be traced back to the First World War when the American Surgeon General assigned an American trained in massage in the United Kingdom, Mary McMillan, to set up a rehabilitation service for wounded soldiers in 1917 (Granger 1923). The British model of massage, which had been heavily influenced by Ling from Sweden, was gradually exported to the then extensive British Empire and Commonwealth. In the early days of the British physiotherapy profession, massage was the only form of treatment offered, but this soon expanded to include exercise in 1903 and medical electricity in 1915 (Wickstead 1948).

This brief history of the development of the physiotherapy profession is offered to serve as a reminder of just where physiotherapy came from. Massage was the core skill and as such was an examined subject on courses operated by the Chartered Society of Physiotherapy until 1977. As part of the necessary development of any profession there has to be a continuing assessment of the basis upon which it is founded. This has been taking place in physiotherapy, and while manual skills are still a central part of the repertoire of treatment skills there has been rapid development in the fields of electrotherapy and cryotherapy (Forster & Palastanga 1985, Low & Reed 1990). The range of manual skills offered by physiotherapists has also expanded to include mobilization and manipulation of joints (Grieve 1986, Maitland 1986, 1991, Blackman 1986, 1988), mobilization of neural tissue (Butler 1991), and facilitation techniques to strengthen and mobilize (Knott & Voss 1967, Guymer 1986).

In this short chapter an attempt will be made to put together some of the techniques applied to the soft tissue by the therapist's hands, and to explain the rationale behind their use and effects.

TRADITIONAL MASSAGE TECHNIQUES

The term 'traditional massage' is applied to the techniques which were those used at the origin of the physiotherapy profession. Massage means 'to knead' and is the term applied to manipulations of the soft tissues of the body using hands to produce effects on the nervous, musculoskeletal and circulatory systems (Beard & Wood 1964). Although there have been some minor variations made to techniques over the years they are still basically the same as those of the 1890s. Some of the individual techniques will be described in outline along with their effects.

Stroking techniques

Stroking techniques are long massage strokes applied over the whole length of a limb or the trunk. The depth of the stroke can be very superficial or deeper.

Effleurage

Effleurage is a stroking, superficial type of manipulation where the pressure from the hands is applied in a centripetal direction (from distal to proximal) at a depth which is both comfortable yet effective (Hollis 1987). The therapist makes a firm but comfortable contact with the part using the whole surface of their hand, and the pressure will encourage drainage in veins and lymphatics in a proximal direction. At the end of the stroke the hands are lifted from the patient's skin and are replaced at the starting position. This could well have a useful effect in reducing swelling as the pressure at the venous end of the capillary could be reduced sufficiently to allow reabsorbtion of excess tissue fluid (Beard & Wood 1964). The technique is modified depending upon the size of the part to be treated and, where possible, other factors such as gravity are used to assist drainage.

Stroking

Stroking is a very superficial massage technique where the strokes are applied along the whole length of a surface. The superficial nature of the contact will not have any direct mechanical effect, but the skin contact will have an effect on cutaneous nerve endings. The effect usually required by the therapist is to prepare the patient for the deeper techniques which are to follow, in other words, the patient gets used to being touched and will therefore relax. In some instances this relaxing effect could in fact be the primary aim of treatment, and the technique could be applied with the object of reducing muscle spasm (Mennell 1945).

Petrissage

Petrissage is the term used to describe a group of techniques where the tissues, usually muscles, are compressed against other structures (Hollis 1987).

Kneading

This technique involves the application of circular manipulations to the tissues. The pressure is applied in a circular manner such that the circles overlap and the pressure is maximal for half the circle and minimal for the other half. The pressure used will vary with the area being treated and could be maximal over the gluteals or back, where a reinforced double-handed technique is used—or minimal, as over the face, where only the pads of the fingers are used. The technique of kneading can be very effectively applied using the pads of the thumbs.

Picking-up

Picking-up is a complex technique where the therapist first compresses the muscle against the underlying bone and then picks it up in a scooping manner in their hand, squeezes it, and puts it down again. The squeezing effect is achieved by a counter pressure between the thumb and thenar eminence on one side of the hand, and the little and ring finger and hypothenar eminence on the other.

Wringing

Wringing is another complex technique where the tissues are 'wrung' between the two hands of the therapist. This is achieved by an interaction of the hands which turn in opposite directions to put tension on the patient's tissues.

Wringing, kneading and picking-up are all useful techniques to reduce swelling as they will encourage venous and lymphatic return. They will also mobilize tissues against one another.

Rolling

Rolling can be applied in a superficial manner to the skin. To achieve skin rolling the therapist moves a roll of the patient's tissues across the surface of the body by applying a forward pressure with both thumbs while the fingers pull the roll in a backwards direction without stopping the movement. This technique has the effect of assisting the superficial circulation, but more importantly, of mobilizing the skin against the deeper structures.

Percussive techniques or tapotement

Clapping

When using this technique a cup-like shape is produced with the hand and this is used to strike the body part. An attempt is made to trap air in the hand between it and the patient's skin in order to cushion the impact and make it more comfortable. This technique has traditionally been used to assist drainage of the respiratory passages of secretions when the patient is placed in a postural drainage position.

Hacking

Hacking is a complex technique where the ulnar borders

of the therapist's little and ring finger are used to strike the patient's tissues. The therapist achieves this by producing an alternate pronation and supination of their forearm with the wrist in extension. This technique may be modified in well developed muscular areas into pounding or beating, where a clenched fist is used to make the impact (Hollis 1987).

These vigorous percussive impacts are thought to be very stimulating and to produce reflex responses in the skin in terms of increased circulation which can be clearly seen as an erythema following even a brief treatment. This reaction is the same as would be produced by any vigorous scratching or slapping and has traditionally been described as part of the 'triple response'. They will also have a stimulating effect on voluntary muscle as the impact could well invoke a reflex type of contraction which will increase tone.

Effects of traditional massage

Much of the older literature describes massage as having circulatory, muscular and psychological effects (Beard & Wood 1964, Wood 1974), whereas in more recent texts the effects are divided into mechanical, physiological and psychological (Hollis 1987). A simpler method of considering the effects will follow below.

Circulatory effects

As described earlier, these effects are partly produced by mechanical and partly physiological factors. The mechanical effects are related to the changes of pressure the massage techniques impart on the tissues. If these pressures are centripetal (effleurage), or alternately compressing and relaxing (picking-up, wringing, kneading), then venous and lymphatic return is encouraged. If the problem being managed is swelling then this removal of blood and lymph from the vessels will effectively reduce the hydrostatic pressure at the venous end of the capillary. This reduction of pressure will have an effect on the pressure gradient such that tissue fluid can be drawn from the tissues into the capillaries and lymphatics, thus removing it from the area and thereby reducing swelling (Beard & Wood 1964, Wood 1974).

More vigorous massage techniques can be used where an increase in circulation is considered to be necessary in muscles. It is claimed that when muscles are at rest there is very little circulation of lymph and that massage can be usefully applied to athletes to remove the products of fatigue and injury which could cause post-activity muscle soreness (Briggs 1991).

Effect on pain

Massage has a tradition of being used to reduce pain, and the age old remedy of 'rubbing it better' (Bowsher 1988) still operates in most cultures. The physiological basis for the reduction of pain can be considered from a number of stand points. Firstly, the gentle soothing techniques where slow smooth strokes are applied to the tissues in a rhythmical way, will cause stimulation of cutaneous mechanoreceptors. This sensory information will enter the central nervous system via the posterior root and could well have an inhibitory effect on the transmission of pain at the substantia gelatinosa or 'pain gate' of Melzack and Wall (Wall 1970, 1989).

The physical removal of extracellular fluid could well reduce pressure on nociceptive endings in the tissues to a level where they are no longer stimulated and so would reduce pain. Similarly, the physical removal of pain-stimulating chemicals in the vicinity of nociceptive endings could also reduce pain. Lastly, the more vigorous techniques such as hacking or pounding could in themselves cause stimuli of a painful type to be transmitted to the central nervous system. As this traffic passes through the brainstem it will stimulate areas of the mid-brain and other centres to then release the body's endogenous opiate-like substances at a spinal level, thus inhibiting the transmission of further pain.

A more detailed account of the mechanisms by which pain is mediated can be found in Chapter 18.

Effects on adhesions

Massage by its very nature will mobilize one tissue against adjacent tissues. In normal tissues this will serve to maintain their relative mobility. In tissues which have been immobile or damaged, massage may be used to attempt to restore mobility by stretching the structures or by stretching or breaking down adhesions between them (Beard & Wood 1964, Wood 1974).

Psychological effects

The physical contact of massage performed by a professionally educated physiotherapist is bound to have strong psychological effects. These may simply be perceived as the placebo effect which is recognized as having a very strong effect on the reduction of pain (Weisenberg 1989). Massage is, however, a pleasant experience and many people will pay large sums of money just to be massaged. Patients with pain and stiffness or people who wish only to enjoy the experience and to relax and reduce tension seek the service of a good masseur (Wells 1988). The vacuum left by physiotherapists who no longer wish to practise traditional massage has already been filled in the United Kingdom by new professions who now base their whole approach on massage. These new professions are able to exist because of the desire of the general public to employ the skills of these non-medical masseuses (Wells 1988).

Traditional massage is still taught to pre-registration physiotherapy students on all of the physiotherapy degree courses in the United Kingdom. This is partly because it is required by the Core Curriculum of the Chartered Society of Physiotherapy (Chartered Society of Physiotherapy 1991), but probably more importantly because it allows students to develop a sensitivity of touch. This sensitivity of touch is a skill which has to be developed in all therapists who handle human tissues. The feel of normal and abnormal tension and movement can be achieved only by extensive practice. As with any manual skill, practice is the essential component which has to be brought into the student's programme; one cannot learn the feel of normal and abnormal structures by reading about it in a book. Many pre- and post-registration teachers of physiotherapists would agree that the development of sensitive handling skills takes place more easily in therapists as a result of the basic massage techniques which they have been required to master in the past. This applies equally to manipulative skills and to sensitive neurological, respiratory and manual resistance techniques.

Traditional massage has in the past been an important form of treatment for patients. While this could still be true today, therapists tend to shy away from the image of being a 'masseur', possibly because of its more seedy connotations, and traditional massage is seldom used as a treatment in its own right. However, traditional massage will continue to be a skill taught to students in order to prepare them for their role in handling patients' tissues. This skill will be lying dormant ready to be reactivated should the opportunity or necessity arise.

DEEPER SOFT-TISSUE TECHNIQUES APPLIED TO CONNECTIVE TISSUES

While there has been a decline in the application of the more traditional massage techniques described earlier, other techniques have to some extent taken their place. These techniques will now be described separately, although there is a degree of overlap between some of them.

Deep transverse frictions

The very title 'deep transverse frictions' suggests that they will be applied at a greater depth than traditional massage techniques. Transverse frictions were first described by Dr J. Cyriax, and a whole generation of therapists is indebted to him for his detailed description of the techniques (Cyriax 1984).

For the application of transverse frictions the therapist must have an accurate knowledge of the anatomy of the soft tissues, not just their position and attachments, but also the direction of their fibres. Without this background it is impossible for the technique to be applied properly. Application of transverse frictions must be accurate in terms of the position of the therapist's finger, the direction in which the finger is moved, and the tension in the structure which is being treated.

Mode of action

Following injury of sufficient magnitude to fibrous tissue or muscle, repair will take place by the formation of a fibrin mesh which becomes infiltrated with fibroblasts to form a scar. Often this scar will involve adjacent unaffected structures, severely affecting their mobility and function (Johnson & Saliba 1991). This scar may also prove to be a source of pain for some considerable time after its formation as a result of local nociceptive stimulation. The basic aim of applying transverse frictions to this area of scar tissue is to make it as small as possible (while still allowing repair) and to allow pain-free normal mobility by preventing the scar becoming tethered to adjacent structures by adhesions. Adhesions tend to form between the mobile structure and adjacent tissues as the result of the organization of excess inflammatory exudate (Johnson & Saliba 1991). Mechanical movement of the tissues is in itself a most effective method of either preventing or breaking down these adhesions and reducing pain (Cyriax 1984). Movement of the therapist's digit should be across the fibres of the ligament, tendon or muscle being treated because movement applied transverse to their long axis will mobilize the structure relative to bone, sheath or fascia. This will free it for movement.

After injury a joint is often too painful to move and this reduces the amount of movement between normally mobile structures. Transverse frictions can produce some of this movement passively, thus inhibiting pain and allowing a more normal active/passive range to be carried out on the affected joints.

The chronic stress seen in tissues surrounding osteoarthritic joints may eventually be the cause of considerable pain. In these chronic cases transverse frictions can also be a very useful, if less spectacular, form of treatment.

Physiological effects

Transverse frictions involve the application of friction and pressure at depth to the offending lesion which is considered to be the cause of pain or reduced function (Cyriax 1978). This pressure and movement is in itself of sufficient insult to normal tissues as to cause minor damage, resulting in the release of inflammatory chemicals such as histamine and bradykinin. These chemicals will have an effect upon the local circulation and on nociceptors (Williams et al 1989, Campbell et al 1989).

First, the inflammatory chemicals will cause a local vasodilatation seen as traumatic hyperaemia. This lasts for some considerable time and may in itself have beneficial effects in terms of accelerating repair. The increased circulation could also help to reduce the oedema around a chronically inflamed ligament or tendon, reducing pressure and therefore nociceptive stimulation, thereby reducing pain.

Secondly, the local inflammatory chemicals will stimulate local nociceptive endings directly and cause pain. This may seem to be a contradiction in terms, the application of a pain-producing technique to an already painful structure, but advances in the understanding of pain modulation mechanisms help to explain the anomaly. Deep pain from the lesion itself tends to be of a dull aching nature, transmitted to the CNS along slow conducting, small-diameter fibres (Bowsher 1988). The function of this deep pain seems to be to indicate centrally that there has been tissue damage. These impulses are transmitted across the substantia gelatinosa (the 'gate') at the spinal cord and pain is eventually perceived at a conscious level (Bowsher 1988).

Deep transverse frictions cause the stimulation of nociceptive endings connected to Aδ fibres and mechanoreceptors found in soft tissues which are connected to larger diameter Aβ fibres (Wyke 1967, 1972). These endings are stimulated by traumatic or mechanical events, the information being conducted to the posterior root of the cord by fast-conducting, large-diameter fibres. This traffic will initially be allowed to pass to consciousness, and a sharp pain or pressure may be perceived. However, these large-diameter fibres have an effect on cells in the posterior horn of the cord, tending to inhibit forward transmission of the small-diameter nociceptive information, i.e the 'pain gate' is closed. Hence it is suggested that presynaptic inhibition at cord level will modulate peripheral pain and reduce its perception (Watson 1986, Bowsher 1988).

There may also be inhibition of neurotransmission exerted from higher centres, as the arrival of nociceptive stimuli at certain central inhibitory nuclei in the CNS (Raphé nuclei and periaqueductal area of grey matter in the mid-brain) causes release of chemicals from neurones at cord level which block the action of nociceptive neurotransmitters. These chemicals include encephalin, beta-endorphin and dynorphin (Bowsher 1988). Consequently, in terms of modulation of pain, transverse frictions can be justified on both counts as they will cause presynaptic inhibition at cord level and inhibit pain by the central production of encephalins. In the past this phenomenon was called 'massage analgesia' (Cyriax 1980) and was in fact one of the aims of treatment prior to more vigorous manipulative procedures. However, this chapter is concerned with the techniques used, and for a more detailed description of the mechanisms of pain modulation the reader is referred to Chapter 18 in this book.

Examination of the patient prior to treatment with transverse frictions

The most important point which cannot be overstressed

is that the technique MUST be applied specifically to the lesion itself. An accurate knowledge of anatomy is essential in order that assessment, which includes a detailed history, palpation and movement can localize the lesion to an exact point in a specific tissue. Often this is made more difficult by the problem of referred pain and tenderness. The lesion itself may refer pain for some considerable distance; conversely, the therapist may be misled by pain referred from a spinal joint which mimics a more peripheral problem. In fact, a vertebral joint problem which refers pain into the region of a limb girdle joint or even further into a limb, may eventually lead to actual changes in these more distal soft tissues (Grieve 1988). For example, C5–C6 joint problems may produce changes in the supraspinatus tendon which itself requires treatment and could respond to transverse frictions. The same is true for many other lesions in the upper limb and thorax. However, the origin is, and was, a spinal structure and as such warrants attention too. Hence, examination of the spinal joints should be undertaken whenever lesions of the soft tissues around a peripheral joint are to be treated.

Lesions may occur in the fibrous capsule of a synovial joint, in a ligament which blends with this capsule, or in an accessory ligament some distance from it. Careful palpation and passive stretching of these structures helps the therapist to determine whether a lesion is present. If the lesion is in muscle tissue, palpation is still important but resisted static contraction of the muscle helps to localize the exact point within the muscle belly. Lesions in the attachment tissues of the muscle will produce pain on contraction of the muscle, but palpation will allow exact localization. Lesions in the synovial sheath of a tendon or in the tendon itself (either with or without a sheath) usually produce most pain on active resisted movement.

Accurate examination techniques are vital as the exact location of the lesion is the point at which the technique of transverse frictions has to be applied. This in itself justifies the time spent teaching detailed anatomy and examination procedures. It is essential that the therapist knows exactly where the structure is, what direction its fibres run in and when they are put under tension.

Technique for transverse frictions

Transverse frictions can be usefully applied to muscles, tendons, ligaments and joint capsules with slight modifications being needed for each of these.

Position of the patient. The patient must be properly supported in a comfortable position, with the tissue containing the lesion placed in an appropriate position of accessibility and tension. For example, the supraspinatus tendon is made accessible by extending and medially rotating the shoulder joint, thus bringing the tendon from below the acromion process of the scapula.

If frictions are to be applied to a tendon with a synovial

sheath, then the tendon is placed at maximum stretch in order that the transverse friction technique can develop maximum frictional force between these two elements.

Transverse frictions applied to a lesion within the substance of a muscle are directed transversely across the muscle which is in a relaxed and shortened position. The aim of this is to broaden fully the muscle and break down adhesions between muscle fibres (Cyriax 1984).

The position adopted for the treatment of a ligament or joint capsule requires that it be accessible, and also that it can be moved relative to adjacent tissue by the transverse frictions.

Position and technique of the therapist. The position of the therapist is important as he or she could well be applying the technique for up to 20 minutes. The therapist should be comfortable and should be able to apply the right amount of pressure in the correct direction.

The therapist's finger and the patient's skin must move together as one. This allows the friction to be developed between the subcutaneous tissues and the offending lesion in muscle, tendon or ligament. Friction between the finger and skin will result if there is any movement between them, and this may cause blisters or even erosions of the skin. Consequently, the technique involves carrying the patient's skin and the therapist's digits as one over the offending lesion. To ensure that this is the case, the patient's skin must be dry and grease-free in order to avoid any slipping between the two. If the technique is carried out correctly the patient's skin will tolerate transverse frictions very well, but may show some redness (traumatic hyperaemia) and even bruising after treatment. The natural laxity of the skin allows the bruise to be drawn to one side before application of pressure at the next treatment, so giving the bruised area some time to recover.

Transverse frictions must be applied with sufficient pressure to penetrate to the depth of the lesion. This requirement is one of the major limitations of the technique as certain structures are too deep or inaccessible to the therapist's digits. This pressure should not replace the frictional element of the technique, which is developed by movement.

The amplitude of movement of the patient's skin and the therapist's digit, which is traditionally called the 'sweep' (Cyriax 1984), should be great enough to produce sufficient friction between the subcutaneous fascia and the lesion, and to move the offending tissue relative to its neighbours.

Direction of the transverse friction technique. The technique is applied at right angles to the fibres comprising the tissue containing the lesion—hence the term 'transverse frictions' (Cyriax 1984). Frictions applied across the fibres of a ligament will mobilize the whole ligament relative to the bone below, and individual fibres within the ligament relative to one another.

Tendons are placed under tension and the frictions are applied across them in order to mobilize tendons enclosed in a synovial sheath against this sheath (to smooth off elevations or break down adhesions), or tendons without sheaths against adjacent structures.

Muscles are first shortened and the transverse frictions are applied across the muscle fibres in an attempt to break down adhesions between muscle fibres or between adjacent muscles. This gives the appearance of flattening out and then broadening the muscle.

Method of application

There are a number of ways in which the friction can be applied, all of which incorporate the use of the therapist's digits. Where possible the large muscle groups in the arm should be used to produce the transverse movement as the small intrinsic muscles in the hand fatigue rapidly.

One finger reinforcing another. A single finger tip is applied above the lesion and reinforcing pressure is given by another finger, e.g. index over middle, or middle over index. This is a very suitable technique for a small localized lesion (see Figs 60.1, 60.3, 60.4, 60.5, 60.6).

One thumb. One thumb can be used, but often it is difficult to sustain sufficient pressure or amplitude for a whole treatment session. There is also a temptation to make small circular movements which are not as effective as transverse movements. However, in certain situations it can be a useful alternative technique (see Fig. 60.2).

Two or three fingers side-by-side. If a long structure is to be treated, e.g. a tendon or long fascial attachment to bone, then two or three finger tips side-by-side can be used to apply the frictions.

Opposed fingers and thumb. If the structure to be treated is of a rounded nature, e.g. the achilles tendon, then a pinching technique between the thumb and fingers can be used to apply the friction.

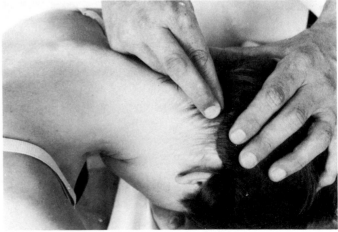

Fig. 60.1 Transverse frictions to the occipital attachment of the trapezius or splenius capitis muscles, using a reinforced finger technique.

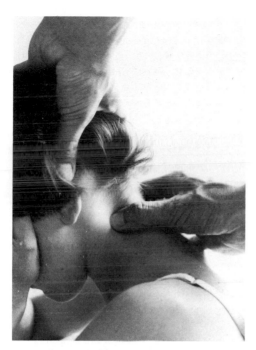

Fig. 60.2 Transverse frictions to a cervical apophyseal joint capsule using the thumb with the patient in sitting.

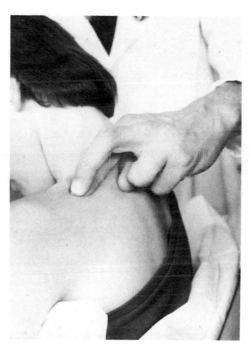

Fig. 60.4 Transverse frictions to the musculotendinous junction of supraspinatus, achieved by a pronation/supination movement of the therapists forearm.

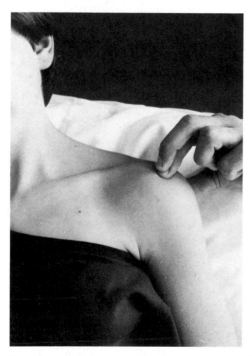

Fig. 60.3 Transverse frictions to the left acromioclavicular joint.

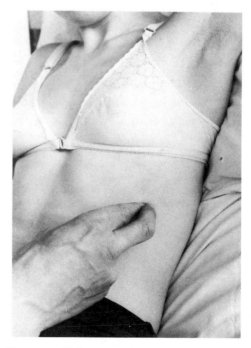

Fig. 60.5 Transverse frictions to an intercostal muscle.

Contraindications to frictions

Rheumatoid arthritis. Transverse frictions should not be applied to tissues involved in rheumatoid disease as the active inflammation in and around joints could well be made worse by these techniques. The same is true for infective arthritis.

Calcification of soft tissues. Calcification in liga- ments or tendons, e.g. supraspinatus, can be shown on X-ray, and transverse frictions applied in these cases will make the condition more painful.

Peripheral and spinal nerves. Peripheral and spinal nerves could be damaged by the pressure and frictional elements of transverse frictions to such an extent as to cause neurapraxia or even axonotmesis. Consequently, peripheral nerves and their branches are avoided.

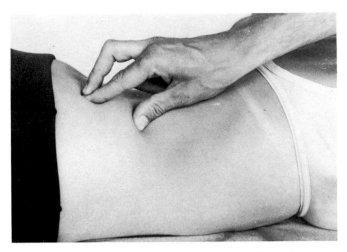

Fig. 60.6 Transverse friction to the posterior sacro-iliac region.

Duration and frequency of treatment

The duration of treatment is initially governed by the lesion being treated. In the acute stage pain may make prolonged treatment at depth difficult. The therapist starts the transverse friction technique with reduced pressure (depth) but as the session progresses the pain from the lesion normally decreases and the pressure of the frictions can be gradually increased until normal depth is reached. Following the frictions, full-range active or passive movements are carried out to produce physiological movement of the tissues involved.

In more chronic conditions a gradual build up of pressure can still be applied, but the eventual deep frictional pressure is arrived at fairly quickly. From this point the transverse frictions are applied in an appropriate direction (across the fibres), with sufficient amplitude (sweep), at the correct pressure (depth), moving the therapist's digit and the patient's skin as one.

Treatment should continue for at least 10 minutes but can be for as long as 20 minutes in some conditions. The long duration of treatment has been one of the major drawbacks to the application of this technique as therapists are sometimes reluctant to commit such long periods of time to an individual patient. These long treatment times are however necessary if good results are to be achieved. Short sessions of frictions are of little or no use to the patient.

In both the acute and chronic case it is difficult to treat the patient more often than every other day, as treatment soreness precludes daily treatment. Treatment soreness may delay treatment for even longer, but when the next session is given the therapist must gradually increase the pressure of technique until the original depth is reached. This can be moderately uncomfortable to the patient for the first few minutes of treatment.

Examples of treatment techniques

In the earlier section it was difficult to give an in-depth description of the techniques as they necessarily involve long strokes or movements repeated over the whole surface of a limb. This is not the case with transverse frictions as they are applied to a specific tissue which is often very small and localized.

In an attempt to introduce the reader who is not familiar with these techniques, or to remind those who do not regularly use them, some techniques of application will now be described. The inclusion or omission of any technique does not imply a judgement as to its usefulness, but a range have been selected in order to illustrate general principles. For more detailed descriptions and further techniques the reader is referred to more specific texts on the subject (Cyriax 1984).

Insertion of trapezius and splenius capitis muscles onto occipital bone. Lesions at this site produce pain on local palpation and on isometric contraction of these muscles just below the nuchal line. The genesis of this lesion may be traumatic or referred from high cervical vertebral joint problems. The patient should be positioned prone with the neck slightly flexed to place the muscles under tension. The therapist, sitting or standing level with the patient's neck, steadies the occiput with one hand and applies a reinforced finger technique across the fibres of insertion at their attachment. Frictions are produced by using the whole of the therapist's arm, and upward pressure against the occiput is maintained at the same time as inward frictional pressure (Fig. 60.1).

Cervical facet joint capsule. The cervical facet joint capsule can be palpated in the mid-cervical region but tends to be painful on palpation even in a normal neck. It is suggested that treatment is applicable in osteoarthritis of the cervical spine (Cyriax 1980) but could be useful in conditions of a non-degenerative origin. The patient is positioned in the sitting position supporting head in hands, with the cervical spine in slight flexion. The therapist stands behind the patient and applies the frictional pressure with the pad of one thumb, the fingers giving counter-pressure on the other side of the neck. Once the lateral aspect of the facet joint has been palpated, the thumb is moved along the joint line (i.e. at right angles to the fibres of the capsule) by moving it backwards and downwards (Fig. 60.2). The angle of the movement will vary according to the level of the cervical spine being treated.

This is an extremely uncomfortable technique and requires considerable tolerance from the patient and determination from the therapist. For once, the sessions tend to be necessarily short, but this technique may prove a useful alternative when those suggested by other practitioners have been unsuccessful.

Acromioclavicular joint capsule. Pain in the acromioclavicular joint is usually the result of direct trauma and is provoked when the joint is forced to move at the extreme of elevation of the shoulder girdle, or when horizontally flexing the arm across the chest. The patient sits with the therapist standing behind. A reinforced finger technique is used with the line of the joint being used as the direction of movement (at right angles to the fibres of the joint capsule and superior acromioclavicular ligament) (Fig. 60.3).

Supraspinatus tendon. Lesions in the tendon of supraspinatus are common as the result of trauma or overuse, but they may accompany vertebral joint problems originating from the C5–C6 region of the cervical spine (Grieve 1988). Swelling within the tendon means that it will be compressed below the acromion process as it moves and thus produce a painful arc of movement on active abduction. The patient is positioned in long sitting, with the arm extended, adducted and medially rotated (placing the hand in the small of the back achieves this but the arm can be allowed to hang straight if the former position is uncomfortable). This position moves the tendon from below cover of the acromion process of scapula and also places the tendon under tension.

The therapist is positioned on the side of the lesion facing the shoulder and palpates the tendon with reinforced finger technique. The direction of movement of the finger is across the tendon. The deep, sweeping friction is applied across the tendon just proximal to its attachment to the bone. Many variations of technique can be employed when treating supraspinatus tendon but as long as the basic principles are followed any of them can be effective.

Results of the treatment of supraspinatus tendon are very good, and it is one lesion that most therapists will have treated with frictions. Poor results can usually be attributed to insufficient depth or sweep, or to too short a treatment application.

Supraspinatus musculotendinous junction. Lesions in the musculotendinous junction of supraspinatus may be caused by trauma or overuse. There is usually pain on contraction of the muscle but as the lesion is more medial than the tendon the painful arc of movement is not present. As treatment is to be applied to the musculotendinous junction the muscle is placed off tension by abducting the arm. This also makes the lesion more accessible to the friction technique. The therapist stands on the side opposite to the lesion and reaches across the patient's back. A reinforced finger technique is used but the anatomy of the supraspinatus fossa is such that the transverse friction technique across the muscle fibres is achieved by a pronation/supination of the therapists forearm (Fig. 60.4).

The tendon of the long head of biceps brachii. Lesions can occur in the tendon of the long head of biceps brachii as it passes through the intertubercular sulcus of humerus. In this sulcus it is covered by the transverse ligament (Palastanga et al 1989) and so considerable pressure has to be applied by the therapist to achieve sufficient depth. The patient is positioned with their affected arm adducted and laterally rotated to make the tendon more accessible. The friction technique is applied by the therapist's thumb which is moved medially and laterally across the tendon with the fingers providing counter-pressure posteriorly.

Intercostal muscle. Lesions in the intercostal muscles often occur following trauma to the thorax, and tenderness is elicited in the muscle on palpation. A reinforced finger technique is used with the finger tip being moved in a horizontal direction between the ribs at right angles to the muscle fibres (Fig 60.5).

Posterior sacro-iliac ligament. A painful sacro-iliac joint often presents acute tenderness on palpation of the soft tissues in the sulcus on the medial side of the posterior superior iliac spine. In this situation the lesion could be either in the fascial origin of the erector spinae muscle or in the posterior sacro-iliac ligament. The patient is positioned prone with the therapist on the same side as the lesion, facing the patient's feet. Frictions are applied along the line of the joint sulcus (across the fibres) using a reinforced finger technique (Fig. 60.6). This technique can often be successful when other techniques have failed.

Many lesions in muscles, tendons and ligaments can be successfully treated using transverse frictions (Cyriax 1984). Consequently, they can be a useful form of treatment as far as relief of patients' signs and symptoms are concerned, and also for therapists regarding results. Literature pertaining to the use of frictions appears from time to time (Chamberlain 1982), suggesting that more clinical research is needed, but there is currently a resurgence of interest in the teaching and learning of these techniques if the number of validated courses currently available in the United Kingdom can be used as a guide.

Connective tissue massage

Connective tissue massage (CTM) is a specific manipulative technique applied to the connective tissues close to the body surface. It was first described by a German physical therapist named Dicke (Bischof & Elminger 1963) who called the technique *Bindegewebsmassage*. Historically, the technique developed more quickly in the Germanic countries and was slow to spread to English-speaking regions until the development of books on the subject in the English language (Ebner 1975).

The development of CTM coincided with the rapid rise in the use of other manipulative techniques, the production of more effective anti-inflammatory drugs and the application of electrotherapy techniques more scientifically to achieve specific therapeutic effects. All of these, plus the time taken to first learn the CTM technique and the long treatment times required to apply it, has meant that only relatively few therapists have developed the skill. Research into the effects of CTM is somewhat limited, with most of it being conducted in Germany and

Switzerland, but some accounts have been produced in English (Ebner 1975, Frazer 1975, Gifford & Gifford 1988).

The technique of CTM is applied via the therapist's middle and ring fingers to the patient's skin, with the tensile force of the application being transmitted from the epidermis to the deeper connective tissues.

Connective tissues

Connective tissues are derived from the embryonic mesoderm and are either specialized as bone, cartilage, etc., or of an ordinary type. Ordinary connective tissue (CT) has two components, cells and an extracellular matrix which contains fibres.

Cells. Six types of cell are associated with ordinary CT (Williams et al 1989), of which fibroblasts and mast cells are of the greatest significance to CTM. Fibroblasts are usually the most numerous, being flat and irregular in shape, and are responsible for the production of the matrix and fibres. Mast cells occur particularly in loose CT, being oval with many vesicles which contain histamine and serotonin, agents important in inflammatory processes. Mast cells also contain the anticoagulant heparin.

Matrix. The matrix consists of fibres and ground substance. The important fibres are of collagen and elastin. Collagen fibres are the most numerous in ordinary CT and are often collected in bundles. Although soft and flexible they have a high tensile strength and are relatively inelastic. These collagen fibres are a tri-helix chain formed from nine amino acids which, at rest, is coiled, but the fibre can elongate by uncoiling (Cailliet 1988). Elastin fibres are more yellow and branching, and are extensible with good recoil due to their elastin content. The ground substance is a viscous gel in which the cells and fibres are supported. It contains carbohydrate and protein molecules in the form of proteoglycans which have the ability to hold water molecules. The water content of the matrix is vital as it allows the diffusion of metabolites, gases and electrolytes between the capillaries and the cells. This water content affects the 'tension' of the CT as a whole, and thus its sensitivity to stretch. This is an important palpable sign in the assessment prior to CTM.

Ordinary CT can further be sub-divided into:

1. Loose CT, which has the function of binding structures together, but, by virtue of considerable extensibility, allows mobility. The term 'functional joints' has been used to describe the spaces maintained by fascia and built for motion which exists between adjoining structures (Johnson & Saliba 1991). In man, loose CT provides for space and lubrication between all bodily structures and thus facilitates ease of movement. If these 'functional joints' were to become restricted they would limit normal biomechanical function of the tissues.

2. Dense CT, where a large proportion of collagen fibres forms dense strong sheets to ensheath organs; more important to CTM, it forms the deep fascia. Many nerve endings have been demonstrated in this dense CT.

The skin

In the skin the deep fascia lies immediately below the superficial fascia, and in most areas of the body there is considerable mobility between the two layers. In some places however, the skin may be anchored to the periosteum of superficial bone, or to the deep fascia—as in the flexural lines in the palm. These factors are of significance in the application of CTM as in some areas considerable slack has to be taken up in the skin before tension is applied to the deep fascia, whereas in others there is little or none.

Innervation of the skin is very complex and extensive via many afferent and efferent fibres. Sensory endings of a free type permeate the whole of the skin as far as the deep layers of the epidermis, while encapsulated endings are found in the dermis and fascia only. The complexity and variety of sensory endings situated in the skin allow performance of its vital sensory role via thermal, chemical and mechanical stimulation which is transmitted to the CNS for interpretation and analysis. Efferent nerve fibres give autonomic supply to blood vessels, sweat glands and the arrectores pylorum muscles of the skin.

Rationale of CTM

There are a number of philosophies upon which CTM is based. First, the term 'reflex zone', referred to by some authorities (Bischof & Elminger 1963, Ebner 1975), where it has been observed that disease affecting internal organs could produce reflex changes in the skin of specific and constant areas. Similarly, Mackenzie's zones relate to areas of increased muscle tone as a result of internal disease, the most common example being the spasm of abdominal muscles in the lower right quadrant in appendicitis. Secondly, connective tissue zones were first described by Dicke and explained further by Ebner (1975) where the principle was that all connective tissue in the body is continuous, and that changes in normal tension or mobility in one area of CT will be reflected in CT elsewhere. Lastly, the concept of functional joints described earlier implies that the spaces between connective tissues are essential in order to allow the normal biomechanical movement of one tissue upon adjacent tissues (Johnson & Saliba 1991).

The technique of CTM may have both a reflex and a physical effect, the reflex affecting circulation and pain, the physical by stretching and mobilizing the CT. One of the interesting uses of CTM has been in the diagnosis and treatment of disorders of internal organs by the application of CTM strokes to specific areas of skin (an application of Head's principle). The effect is termed a 'cutaneovisceral' reflex by which the treatment of CT produces a beneficial effect in terms of pain reduction or increased circulation in a deeply placed organ or distant area (Ebner 1975).

Assessment technique prior to CTM

Assessment is carried out in order to detect changes in the tension of the CT, caused either by physical shortening and/or alteration in its fluid content.

Observation. The patient is usually seated with thighs supported, hips and knees at 90°, feet supported, hands resting on thighs. The therapist looks for changes in symmetry (Gifford & Gifford 1988).

Palpation. General palpation is undertaken when the skin is moved against the deep fascia by small symmetrical pushes using the middle three fingertips of slightly flexed fingers. The movement produced should be the same on both sides, differences indicating increased tension in one side. These small movements are initially started at the sacrum and symmetrically moved up the back (Gifford & Gifford 1988). A second technique of investigation is to use a vertical 'diagnostic stroke' (see Fig 60.7) performed by the therapist's middle and ring finger, positioned at an angle of 40–60° to the skin. Starting alongside L5, the fingers are 'pulled' up along the back to finish the stroke alongside C7. The movement and resulting pressure should cause a bulge of tissue to appear in front of the ascending fingers as shown in Figure 60.7. Alteration of the tension in the CT will cause a reduction in the size of the bulge and a change in the sensation produced. Tension varies from patient to patient depending upon age, build and the area being investigated; however, the sensation produced from normal CT (assuming a proper technique of application) should be a tolerable pulling, scratching or cutting sensation. If tension in the CT is increased, then the stroke produces a stronger intolerable sensation. One of the aims of CTM should be to return this sensation to normal, and once areas of increased tension have been identified CTM can be used as a treatment. The techniques of CTM can be applied to any body segment.

Technique of application

With any manual skill demonstration, practice and correction are the essential components of developing the ability to apply it and to evaluate its effectiveness. Tissue tension can be interpreted only by the perceptive sensation of the therapist's fingers. The essential feature of CTM is that a tensile strain is applied to the CT in order to produce physical and reflex effects. To achieve this the finger position or grip described by Ebner (1975) is advocated. In this position the middle finger is supported by the ring and they make an angle of 40–60° with the skin; the stroke is always a pull, with the wrist leading the movement. Tension has to be developed between the fingers and the skin, so sufficient pressure is required for adherence, and lubricants are not used. The depth of application can be altered by varying the angle of the fingers or speed of the pull; decreasing the angle or reducing the speed makes the effect more superficial.

Types of stroke

Two types of stroke may be used, either short or long.

Short strokes. Depending upon the patients size, area under treatment and tension of the CT, these strokes are up to 3 cm long. The sequence of events should be:

1. Achieve adequate adherence of the pads of the third and fourth fingers with the skin.
2. With the wrist leading the movement, the slack is taken up in the superficial skin tissues and the tension then applied to the deeper CT. This should be achieved without a sliding movement between the skin and finger pads (see Fig. 60.8). The sensation experienced by the patient should be of a cutting or scratching nature, but should not be unduly uncomfortable. These short strokes are usually applied in a set sequence depending upon the body segment under treatment (see Fig. 60.10).

Long strokes. The major difference between long and short strokes is that movement is allowed between the finger pads and the skin. Once again, appropriate pressure is applied and the slack of the skin is taken up. The fingers

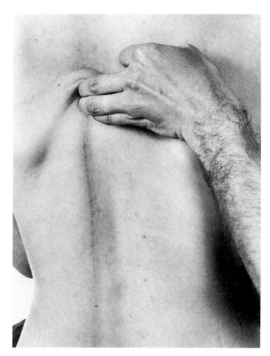

Fig. 60.7   The long diagnostic stroke.

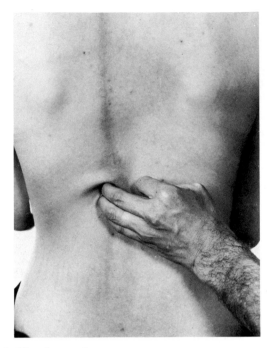

Fig. 60.8   The short stroke.

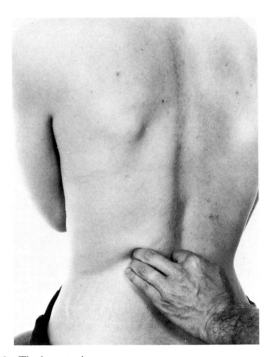

Fig. 60.9   The long stroke.

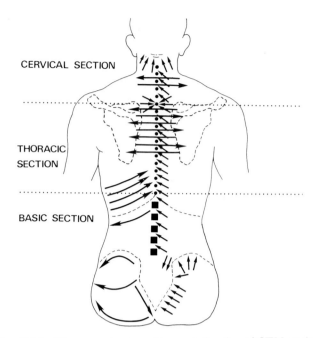

Fig. 60.10   The approximate position and direction of CTM strokes applied to basic, thoracic and cervical sections.

sacrum and work up along the trunk and neck. Treatment may then progress out along the limbs as necessary. Figure 60.10 gives an illustration of the pattern by which the strokes are applied to the lumbosacral region (called the 'basic section' as all CTM starts here), thoracic section and cervical section of the trunk. For a fuller description of application of the technique to other body section the reader is referred to more detailed texts (Ebner 1975).

Effect of connective tissue massage

Circulatory. The effects of CTM on the circulation are both local and general. Local effects are produced as a result of the tensile strength placed on CT by the stroke applied. The stroke is sufficiently traumatic to cause mast cells to release histamine-like substances and these will produce a local vasodilatation which leads to a triple response. A local axon reflex may also occur whereby local sensory stimulation produced in the skin by CTM causes local arteriolar dilatation in the area. The subsequent rise in capillary pressure may cause transudation of fluid into the tissues which is seen as a wheal in some patients. The benefits of this local increase in circulation could be to affect the fluid level within the matrix of the CT and help to restore normal tension and, thus, its sensitivity. In the presence of local inflammation the circulatory increase could help resolution and remove pain-producing chemicals (Watson 1986).

General circulatory effects are produced by stimulation of the autonomic nervous system by the CTM strokes. This can produce reflex effects on the circulation in

are drawn along the surface with constant pressure and speed in a direction which will apply appropriate tension to the CT. A fold of skin should precede the stroking finger (see Fig. 60.9)

The portions of the body to which CTM is applied are called sections (Ebner 1975), and a specific set of CTM strokes is applied to each section. The premise that all CT is connected requires that all treatment strokes start at the specific areas. These areas may be superficial or deep, and the technique of CTM has been used to affect the circulation of both (Bischof & Elminger 1963, Ebner 1975). However, the general circulatory effect can have detrimental effects and may cause certain sensitive individuals to faint because of a drop in blood pressure.

Reduction of pain. As stated in the preceding sections, the modulation of pain is a complex subject, and for an in-depth review of the mechanisms the reader is referred to Chapter 18 in this text. Only a brief description of the probable mechanisms of pain modulation caused by the application of CTM will be offered here.

CTM is a sufficiently strong physical stimulus to produce trauma and release appropriate chemicals which can stimulate nociceptive endings. CTM can also stimulate mechanoreceptors within the CT. Both of these effects could be useful in the treatment of painful areas. Briefly, it is proposed that there are three methods by which CTM can help to modulate pain:

1. The increased circulation already described could remove chemicals stimulating nociceptors or remove excess fluid which is causing pressure on them.

2. The mechanical stimulation of mechanoreceptors in the CT will be conducted to the spinal cord along large-diameter afferent nerves. This large-diameter traffic could well inhibit the forward transmission of small-diameter pain traffic at the substantia gelatinosa and nucleus proprius at the posterior horn of the spinal cord. The 'pain gate' of Melzack and Wall is closed (Wall 1978, 1989, Watson 1986, Bowsher 1988).

3. The CTM stroke itself can be considered a painful episode which will be transmitted to a conscious level in the CNS. As this newly created painful stimulus passes through certain areas of the brain-stem it will cause the release of the body's own opiate-like substances (e.g. encephalin) into areas of the CNS which will block the forward transmission of other pain stimuli (Watson 1980, Bowsher 1988).

Physical effects of CTM. The CTM strokes, whether short or long, will affect the mobility of CT. In the presence of reduced mobility the short strokes of a hook-on nature attempt to stretch and release the CT. Once this has been achieved, long strokes are applied to make the CT move in a more physiological way. Restoration of normal mobility of CT will mean that tissues will be allowed to move through a more normal excursion without encroaching on the function of other adjacent tissues, or producing painful stress. Exercises of a stretching nature may be appropriate when this stage is reached.

CTM is a manual technique which places the therapist in direct contact with the patient's tissues. The sensitivity of touch and skill of technique required for its successful application make it a manual skill of the most complex nature. However, in skilled hands it is a very useful technique and as such deserves to be placed on a par with other techniques applied by manipulative therapists.

Neuromuscular technique

Neuromuscular technique (NMT) has many similarities with CTM and has been applied to patients since the 1800s (Chaitow 1980). The technique is applied to CT where it is at its densest, predominantly close to its attachments to ribs, vertebrae and iliac crests. The basic philosophy in NMT, as in CTM, is that shortened connective tissue is stretched and mobilized relative to adjacent structures.

The patient is examined in the same position as for CTM, sitting over the side of a plinth, and the tissues are examined in a similar way for tenderness and tension. Some of the techniques of NMT are also very similar to CTM, especially the finger technique where the index or middle finger is drawn towards the operator. Other techniques involve the use of the thumb where it is drawn towards the fingers which act as a fulcrum to produce a 2–3 inch (5–7.5 cm) stroke. A skin-rolling technique involves the gathering of tissues into a roll between the fingers and thumb and moving this roll across the area in a similar manner to traditional massage techniques. The depth and tension developed when using the technique should be such as to produce an uncomfortable feeling.

The concept of 'trigger points' is also important in NMT and relates to an area in skeletal muscle which is identified by deep local tenderness in a firm band of muscle. At the point of maximum deep hyperalgesia the palpating fingers can detect a tight band in the muscle (Travell 1960, Travell & Simons 1983). To treat a trigger point, a 'pressure technique' is used in which the trigger point is squeezed between the thumb and underlying tissues with sufficient pressure to produce vascular and neurological changes. Alternatively, the trigger point can be pinched between the fingers and thumb. There would also appear to be similarities between this and the deep friction techniques applied by Cyriax (1980) to broaden muscle. Tissue release techniques are described (Chaitow 1980) where a flat hand is placed over the tissues and a direct downward and rotational stretch is applied with the aim of breaking down adhesions between layers of CT.

Effects of NMT

The effects claimed for NMT are related to the mobilization of CT which it produces. These are very similar to those previously described for CTM but in addition an effect on muscle is also described where the muscle fibre damage is literally 'ironed out', and healing facilitated by a reduction in swelling and inflammation. The benefits claimed include a more rapid rate of recovery, treatment of the cause and not just the symptoms, and encouragement to the body to normalize itself (Chaitow 1980).

NMT has been applied by its advocates in North America for many years but has not made great inroads into treatment regimes applied in Europe. The reverse situation is true for CTM.

Summary

Many forms of soft-tissue manipulative technique exist, and an attempt has been made to describe some of the most commonly applied. The inclusion or exclusion of any particular technique should not be seen as an indication of its value. There are obvious overlaps in the way some techniques are applied and even more obvious overlaps in the effects achieved. The normal mobility and tone of the soft tissues is an essential requirement for the normal functioning and movement of the body parts (Johnson & Saliba 1991). The absence of this normal tone and mobility is an indication for the application of soft-tissue manipulative techniques applied by a skilled therapist. The value of these techniques in the repertoire available to the manual therapist should not be underestimated.

REFERENCES

Beard G, Wood C 1964 Massage, principles and techniques. W B Saunders, Philadelphia

Bischof I, Elminger G 1963 Connective tissue massage. In: Licht S (ed) Massage, manipulation and traction. Waverley press, Baltimore

Blackman J 1986 Manipulation: a personal view. In: Grieve G (ed) Modern manual therapy. Churchill Livingstone, Edinburgh

Blackman J 1988 Mobilisation techniques, 2nd edn. Churchill Livingstone, Edinburgh

Bowsher D 1988 Modulation of nociceptive input. In: Wells P, Frampton V, Bowsher D (eds) Pain management and control in physiotherapy. Heinemann, London

Briggs J 1991 Are sports people getting the massage? Sports therapy 2: 11–13

Butler D S 1991 Mobilisation of the nervous system. Churchill Livingstone, Edinburgh

Cailliet R 1988 Soft tissue pain and disability. F A Davis, Philadelphia

Campbell J, Rata S, Cohen R, Manning D, Khan A, Meyer R 1989 Peripheral neural mechanisms of nociception. In: Wall P, Melzack R (eds) Textbook of pain, 2nd edn. Churchill Livingstone, Edinburgh

Chaitow L 1988 Soft tissue manipulation. Thorsons, Northamptonshire

Chamberlain G J 1982 Cyriax's friction massage: a review. Journal of Orthopaedic and Sports Physical Therapy 4: 16–22

Chartered Society of Physiotherapy 1991 Curriculum of study. Chartered Society of Physiotherapy, London

Cyriax J 1978 Textbook of orthopaedic medicine, 7th edn. Bailliere Tindall, London, vol 1

Cyriax J 1980 Textbook of orthopaedic medicine, 10th edn. Bailliere Tindall, London, vol 2

Cyriax J 1984 Textbook of orthopaedic medicine, 11th edn. Bailliere Tindall, London, vol 2

Ebner M 1975 Connective tissue massage, theory and practice. Churchill Livingstone, Edinburgh

Forster A, Palastanga N 1985 Claytons electrotherapy, 9th edn. Bailliere Tindall, Eastbourne

Frazer F 1978 Persistent post herpetic pain treated by connective tissue massage. Physiotherapy 64: 211–212

Gifford L, Gifford J 1988 Connective tissue massage. In: Wells P, Frampton V, Bowsher D (eds) Pain management and control in physiotherapy. Heinemann, London

Granger F B 1923 The development of physiotherapy. Reprinted in: Physical Therapy 1976 56: 13–21

Grieve G P (ed) 1986 Modern manual therapy. Churchill Livingstone, Edinburgh

Grieve G P 1988 Common vertebral joint problems, 2nd edn. Churchill Livingstone, Edinburgh

Guymer G 1986 Proprioceptive neuromuscular facilitation for vertebral joint conditions. In: Grieve G (ed) Modern manual therapy. Churchill Livingstone, Edinburgh

Hollis M 1987 Massage for therapists. Blackwell, Oxford

Johnson G, Saliba V 1991 Soft tissue mobilisation. In: White A, Anderson A (eds) Conservative care of low back pain. Williams & Wilkins, Baltimore

Knott M, Voss D 1967 Proprioceptive neuromuscular facilitation, 2nd edn. Moeber, New York

Licht S 1960 Massage, manipulation and traction. E Licht, Connecticut

Low J, Reed A 1990 Electrotherapy explained. Heinemann, Oxford

Maitland G D 1986 Vertebral manipulation, 5th edn. Butterworth, London

Maitland G D 1991 Peripheral manipulation, 3rd edn. Butterworth Heinemann, Oxford

Mennell J B 1945 Physical treatment, 5th edn. Blakinstow, Philadelphia

Pastalanga N, Field D, Soames R 1989 Anatomy and human movement. Heinemann Medical, Oxford

Travell J 1960 Temperomandibular joint pain referred from the Muscles of head and neck. Journal of prosth. dent. 10: 745–763

Travell J, Simons D 1983 Myofascial pain and dysfunction: the Trigger point manual. Williams & Wilkins, Baltimore

Wall P D 1978 The gate control theory of pain mechanisms—a re-examination and restatement. Brain 101: 1-18

Wall P D 1989 The dorsal horn. In: Wall P D, Melzack R (eds) Textbook of pain. Churchill Livingstone, Edinburgh

Watson J 1986 Pain and nociception—mechanisms and modulation. In: Grieve G (ed) Modern manual therapy. Churchill Livingstone, Edinburgh

Weisenberg M 1989 Cognitive aspects of pain. In: Wall P D, Melzack R (eds) Textbook of pain. Churchill Livingstone, Edinburgh

Wells P 1988 Manipulative procedures. In: Wells P, Frampton V, Bowsher D (eds) Pain management and control in physiotherapy. Heinemann, London

Wickstead J H 1948 The growth of a profession. Arnold, London

Williams P, Warwick R, Dyson M, Bannister L 1989 Gray's anatomy, 37th edn. Churchill Livingstone, Edinburgh

Wood E 1974 Beards massage. Principles and techniques, 2nd edn. W B Saunders, Philadelphia

Wyke B 1967 The neurology of joints. Annals of the Royal College of Surgeons of England 41: 25–50

Wyke B 1972 Articular neurology—a review. Physiotherapy 58: 94–99

61. Hydrotherapy for spinal problems

A. T. Skinner   A. M. Thomson

INTRODUCTION

Hydrotherapy is the therapeutic use of water, and the main form of hydrotherapy used in the treatment of spinal conditions is pool therapy; this can be enhanced by the use of underwater douches. Pool therapy is of special value when the physiotherapist considers that the patient will benefit from movement and relaxation in a medium of weight relief and warmth. Freedom of movement and water sport recreation are aspects not obtainable on dry land.

APPLICATION OF THE PROPERTIES OF WATER

Buoyancy

Buoyancy is the force experienced as an upthrust on a body in water. It may be used for support, weight relief and grading resisted exercises.

Support

The whole body may be supported in supine with or without floats, or one limb may be supported. The effect of gravity is counteracted. It enables a greater freedom of movement than on land, facilitates relaxation, and contributes to pain relief.

Weight relief

Buoyancy reduces the weight taken through the feet in standing. This effect increases with water depth and enables a patient to exercise is a position which is nearly non-weight-bearing. Progression is made by moving the patient to shallower water. In sitting, there is also reduced weight through the ischial tuberosities and vertebrae. Patients are able to perform exercises which are limited by pain on land so that scar tissue may be stretched, muscle spasm relaxed, gait re-educated and mobility and nutrition restored to injured tissues.

Grading of exercises

Strengthening of muscles starts with buoyancy assisting the movement, and progresses to buoyancy counterbalanced (the moving part is supported by buoyancy with or without floats and the movement is in a horizontal plane). Then, the movement is performed against buoyancy (in a downward direction and vertical plane) and may be progressed by the addition of floats which are available in different densities and offer increasing resistance with decreasing density (Harrison 1980).

Turbulence

This refers to irregular movement of water molecules. In the therapeutic pool it is created by movement of the body through the water. It acts as a resistance (or 'drag') to movement. The greater the speed at which a movement is performed the greater is the effect of turbulence. It is also related to the shape of the body. Less turbulence is created by a smooth streamlined shape and more is created by a broad unstreamlined shape. Turbulence may therefore be used to progress strengthening exercises. It may also be created near to a stationary patient by a physiotherapist moving hands or bats through the water, in which case the patient tends to be drawn towards the turbulence. This effect is useful for retraining balance and for propelling a patient through the water.

Hydrostatic pressure

This is the thrust exerted by a fluid on the surfaces of any body immersed within it. A patient standing or sitting in the pool is subjected to this pressure which helps to stabilize the body, resists thoracic expansion and (because it decreases from deep to shallow) assists venous and lymphatic return from the legs and lower trunk.

STARTING POSITIONS

Commonly used positions are shown in Figures 61.1 to 61.8 and are listed below:

float-lying (Fig. 61.1)
head-support float-lying (Fig. 61.2)

lying half-plinth (Fig. 61.3)
prone-lying half-plinth (Fig. 61.4)
sitting (Fig. 61.5)
side-lying half-plinth (Fig. 61.6)
side-lying with floats (Fig. 61.7)
lying across the corner of the pool (Fig. 61.8).

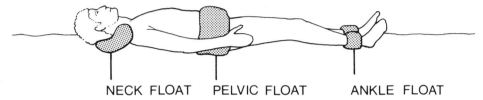

NECK FLOAT   PELVIC FLOAT   ANKLE FLOAT

Fig. 61.1   Float-lying.

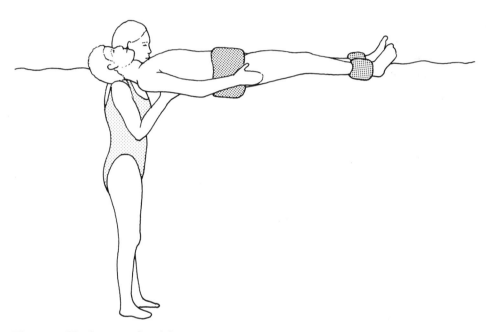

Fig. 61.2   Head-support float-lying.

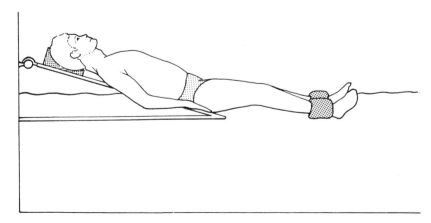

Fig. 61.3   Lying half-plinth.

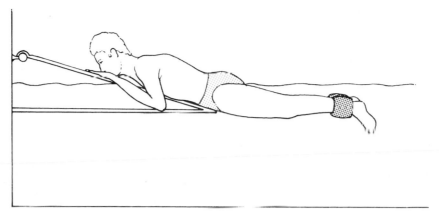

Fig. 61.4 Prone-lying half-plinth.

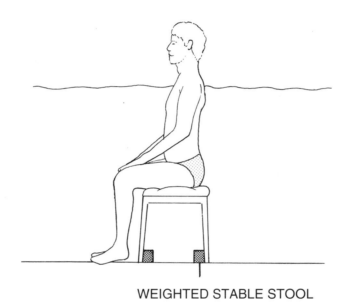

WEIGHTED STABLE STOOL

Fig. 61.5 Sitting.

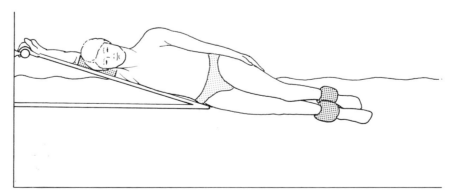

Fig. 61.6 Side-lying half-plinth.

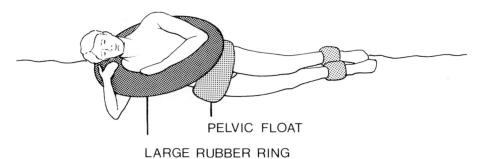

PELVIC FLOAT

LARGE RUBBER RING

Fig. 61.7　Side-lying with floats.

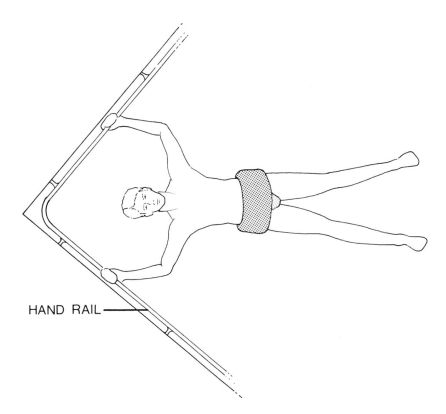

HAND RAIL

Fig. 61.8　Lying across the corner of the pool.

INDICATIONS AND CONTRAINDICATIONS TO POOL THERAPY FOR SPINAL PROBLEMS

Physiotherapists should consider pool therapy for patients with spinal problems arising from the conditions listed in Table 61.1. Absolute contraindications are listed in Table 61.2. Physiotherapists need to exercise care in the situations listed in Table 61.3.

Table 61.1　Spinal problems indicated for pool therapy

Ankylosing spondylitis
Spondylosis
Osteo-arthritis of the facet joints
Mechanical spinal disorders
Intervertebral disc lesions
Ante- and post-natal spinal problems
Spinal pain associated with postural abnormalities
Weakness of the paraspinal muscles – symmetrical or asymmetrical
Postoperative rehabilitation for spinal surgery
Rehabilitation following spinal injury with and without neurological deficit

Table 61.2 Absolute contraindications to pool therapy

Wound infections
Skin infections
Severe gastrointestinal infections
Recent CVA (particularly following haemorrhage)
Recent pulmonary embolus
Deep venous thrombosis with positive signs
Systemic illness or pyrexia
Severe or unstable cardiac disease
Incontinence of faeces unless on a controlled regime

Table 61.3 Situations requiring care to be taken

Open wounds – cover with plastic adhesive dressing, e.g. Opsite
Hypo/hypertension.
Vertigo
Epilepsy
Low vital capacity – below 1000 ml
Kidney disease
Tracheostomies and lines insitu
Recent radiotherapy
Uncontrolled diabetes
Tinea pedis and verrucae – special tight rubber socks should be worn
AIDS – patients with this syndrome should not be allowed into the
    pool if there are abrasions of the skin
Contact lenses and hearing aids should be removed
Severe learning difficulties
Haemophilia – avoid forceful movements to prevent bleeding into the
    joints
Incontinence of urine – prior to pool treatment the bladder must be
    manually or reflexly expressed or, if the patient is catheterized, the
    bag must be emptied
Hydrophobia – a patient who is hydrophobic may benefit from
    exercises in water provided he/she is standing in water to chest level
    or supported in an upright position; progression to the lying position
    is possible when the patient is more water-confident
Spinal extensor spasm – it is important that a patient with spasm of the
    spinal extensor muscles is not put straight into float-lying because if
    he/she holds the head up there can be an increase in the spinal
    extensor spasm and consequent exacerbation of pain
People with cervical or cervicothoracic problems often find that
    swimming increases the pain; this is usually due to the fact that these
    people hold the head out of the water all the time they are swimming
    – which exaggerates extension in the upper and flexion in the lower
    cervical spine; lying positions cannot be used for patients who refuse
    to get their hair wet, and this may preclude the value of pool
    treatment

EXAMINATION OF PATIENTS FOR POOL TREATMENTS

This should be undertaken both on land and in the water at the beginning of treatment and at regular intervals throughout the programme. The particular points which apply to examination of patients with spinal pain for whom hydrotherapy is suitable (in addition to the dry-land examination) (see Ch. 35) are given below.

Subjective

Questions

Is the patient at ease in a swimming pool?

Can the patient swim?
What is the level of swimming ability/regularity, e.g. recreational, daily, weekly, holiday, competitive?
Has back pain stopped the swimming – does swimming exacerbate the pain?
Has the patient attended recreational exercises in water, if so, what activities were undertaken and how do these relate to the back pain?
Are bladder and bowel control normal?

Objective

Tests for joint range, muscle power, and balance are measured on land and in water. The range of movement is often greater in the pool than on land because the warmth and support of the water reduces pain and muscle spasm. The patient is observed before any tests are undertaken.

Observation

Skin – feet are examined to rule out tinea pedis.
    – open wounds, (which may be covered with a plastic adhesive dressing, e.g. Opsite.)
    – eczema, dermatitis, infections.

Body shape/type

It is important to note any asymmetry which will have rotational effects on the patient in water; for example, if, when the patient is in supine lying, one leg is in flexion with the knee out of the water, there is a tendency for the body to turn towards the flexed knee. People with excess fat tissue will float more readily than thin people. Muscles in spasm tend to increase the density of the patient, so extra floats are required to avoid sinking.

Tests

Blood pressure should be measured before and after pool treatment. Vital capacity should be measured if it may be below 1500 ml so that the pace of the treatment is appropriate.

Joint range

Lateral flexion is examined with the patient in float-lying or supine lying on a half-plinth. If the therapist supports the patient's head on her shoulder (head-support float-lying) her hands can be placed at different levels to palpate intersegmental movement and associated soft-tissue reaction. Flexion and extension are examined with the patient in side-lying; again, the therapist palpates the different spinal levels. Rotation is examined with the patient in sitting. Intersegmental movement must be palpated because refraction distorts the view of the part of the trunk below water level.

Muscle power

This is recorded and assessed using the modified Oxford Scale in water (Skinner & Thomson 1983). This scale is as follows:

1. Contraction with buoyancy assisting
2. Contraction with buoyancy conterbalanced (supporting)
2+. Contraction against buoyancy
3. Contraction against buoyancy at speed
4. Contraction against buoyancy plus light (low density) float
5. Contraction against buoyancy plus heavy (high density) float.

Grade 5 is not normal as on land because normal function cannot be assessed in the medium of water. This scale is used to determine strength of muscles as prime movers and is not appropriate for patients with central nervous system disorders because of altered synergic and fixator control or lack of smooth, controlled lengthening of antagonists.

Balance

Balance in sitting and standing is assisted by the hydrostatic pressure of the water. If balance is to be tested, turbulence is created by the therapist moving her hands backwards and forwards near the patient. The patient tends to be drawn towards the area of turbulence, and trunk muscle work is required to counteract this effect.

Gait

In standing, buoyancy reduces the weight going through the feet by 20–30% when the water is at xiphisternum level (Harrison & Bulstrode 1987). A patient's gait pattern may therefore be observed in the pool when there is too much pain for walking or the patient is non-weight bearing on dry land. The muscle work of walking in water is different from that on land because buoyancy acts in the opposite direction to gravity, e.g. during the swing phase buoyancy assists the push off and swing components then resists the heel strike component. The patient has to lean forwards from the hips to retain balance when walking forwards because as the leg in swing phase is carried forwards buoyancy tends to displace it upwards and the patient tends to fall backwards.

TREATMENT

The treatment programme devised for each patient is designed for individual requirements from the main categories of:

relaxation methods
mobilizing methods
strengthening methods
confidence building and fitness
prevention of recurrence.

Relaxation methods

Relaxation is aided by the warmth of the water, the support provided by buoyancy and freedom of movement.

Contrast relaxation

Float-lying: the patient lifts the pelvis out of the pelvic float (contraction of spinal extensors), holds and rests back into the float (relaxation of extensors).

Float-lying (large float round feet): the patient pushes the head and feet against the floats (contraction of spinal extensors), holds and rests (relaxation of extensors).

Assisted relaxation

1. Float-lying. The therapist holds the patient's feet with one hand. The patient's feet are moved: (a) from side to side, (b) up and down, (c) in an arc up to the right down to the centre and, up to the left, (d) in a figure-of-eight. Movements are at first slow, rhythmical and small-range. Progression is made by increasing the range of movement, increasing the speed, and moving the patient through the water from end to end of the pool.

2. Float-lying. The therapist holds the pelvis. The patient is moved slowly from side to side.

3. Head-support float-lying. The therapist places her hands at different levels of the trunk on either side of the spine and establishes a movement which is in resonance with the patient's natural rhythm.

4. Float-lying. The therapist stands sideways to the patient at the level of the spinal problem, and places the forearms parallel to each other under the patient's trunk. One forearm and hand remains fixed, and the other moves the patient from side to side with the focus of movement at the problem level (Fig. 61.9).

Mobilizing methods

These may be active or passive, general or local.

Active exercises

1. Sitting – knees and hips bending with pelvis tilting backwards (buoyancy assisting to gain lumbar flexion). The therapist encourages small movements at end of range.

2. Side-lying (half-plinth), thoracic strap round plinth and thorax – buoyancy supporting legs – hips, knees and pelvis; bend – add small movements to end of range.

3. Standing, grasp rail with one hand, knees slightly flexed, pelvis tilting backwards and relaxing.

4. Hold relax technique to gain lumbar flexion, (Fig. 61.10). With the patient sitting, the therapist stands on the patient's right, places the right forearm under patient's thighs and the left forearm across the anterior aspect of the patient's thorax. The therapist instructs the patient to hold the thighs steady, to relax, and to allow the knees and hips to flex (buoyancy assisting), repeat encouraging backward pelvic tilt.

5. Repeated contractions for lumbar flexion (Fig. 61.11) with the patient in float side-lying, the therapist holds the thorax. The patient is instructed to flex hips, knees and lumbar spine and to hold; while the therapist moves the thorax backwards and then instructs the patient to bend a little further. The sequence is repeated. (Turbulence is resisting the hold of the flexors as the body moves through the water.)

6. Prone lying on half-plinth, legs lifting to gain lumbar spine extension (buoyancy assisting).

7. Standing holding bar at arm's length, keep hands and feet steady, arch forwards to extend lumbar spine and back to stretch lumbar spine (Fig. 61.12).

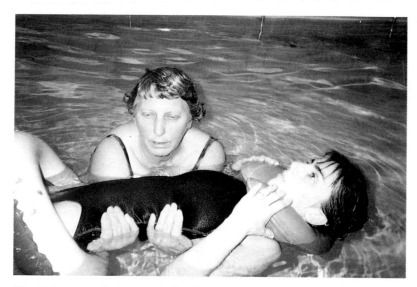

Fig. 61.9 Assisted relaxation in float-lying.

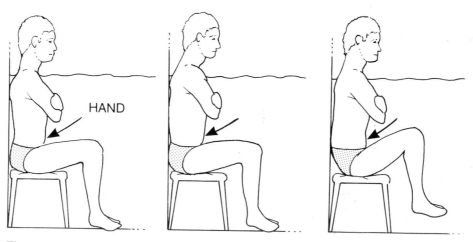

Fig. 61.10 Hold-relax to gain lumbar flexion.

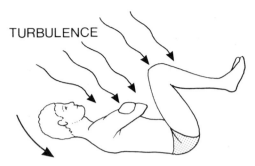

Fig. 61.11 Repeated contractions for lumbar spine flexors.

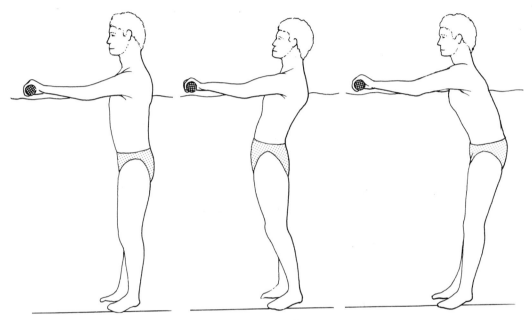

Fig. 61.12 Standing, trunk arching forwards and backwards.

8. Side-lying on half-plinth, stretch legs back, hold; arch a little further to gain lumbar extension.

9. Hold–relax technique may be applied to number 8 above.

10. Repeated contractions for extension are performed in the direction opposite to flexion (number 5).

11. Standing, hip hitching buoyancy assisting side-flexion of the lumbar spine.

12. Float-lying, trunk bending sideways to slide hand down side of thigh, hold; add small movements to end of range.

13. Lying on half-plinth, swing legs to one side, hold; swing a little further, repeat to opposite side to gain side flexion.

14. Head-support float-lying. The therapist places the hands on either side of the thoracic spine and moves the patient's thorax from side to side to obtain reciprocal movement of the legs and gain side flexion; the patient gradually joins in the movement until the therapist is fixing the thorax and the patient is performing the movement entirely.

15. Patient stands with forearms crossed on the bar, legs swinging from side to side (floats added to the ankles increase the effect).

Oscillatory passive movements (mobilizations)

Mobilizations can be applied very effectively to patients in the pool. Examples are as follows:

1. Longitudinal to lumbar spine. With the patient lying, fixed to the half-plinth, the longitudinal technique is applied to both legs. The therapist may hold the patient's feet to apply the force or may stand between the patient's legs and hold the thighs.

2. Side flexion of the lumbar spine, e.g. to the right (Fig. 61.13). With the patient lying on the half-plinth, the therapist stands on the patient's right, fixes the thorax with the left hand, places the right hand on the patient's left thigh, and the patient's legs and pelvis are moved to the right.

3. Postero-anterior central technique. Lumbar and thoracic spine. With the patient in float-lying or head-support float-lying, the therapist cups her hands so that the finger tips can apply central vertebral pressure in the direction of buoyancy.

4. Rotation technique for the lumbar spine. The patient may lie on a half-plinth or hold the bar across the corner of the pool. The patient's knees are flexed and then carried over to one side with the top knee going over a little further. This technique may be purely passive, or the patient may join in the movement, thrusting the top knee a little further down into the water.

5. Side flexion mid-thoracic spine. With the patient in head-support float-lying, the therapist places her hands over the scapulae with the fingers resting on the vertebral spines. The therapist performs side-flexion to one side with the fingers palpating the level of movement.

6. Cervical spine rotation (rotating head to right) (Fig. 61.14). With the patient in float-lying, and with the head on the therapist's right shoulder, the therapist's right hand and forearm holds the patient's head turned slightly to the right. The patient crosses her arms and places her hands on her shoulders. The therapist places the left hand and forearm over the patient's arms and moves the patient's left shoulder down into the water.

7. Cervical spine side flexion (to the right) (Fig. 61.15). With the patient in head-support float-lying with the head on the therapist's right shoulder, the therapist's right hand holds the patient's head and the left hand is placed on the patient's left shoulder. The technique is performed by the patient's left shoulder being pushed down towards the patient's feet. A sustained stretch to the cervical spine left side flexors may be applied in the same position.

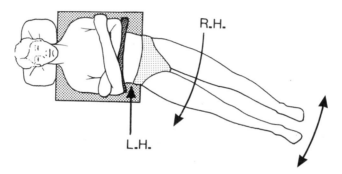

Fig. 61.13 Oscillatory lateral flexion.

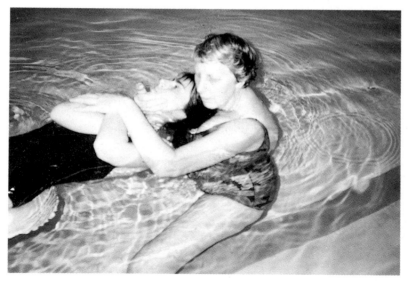

Fig. 61.14 Cervical spine rotation mobilization.

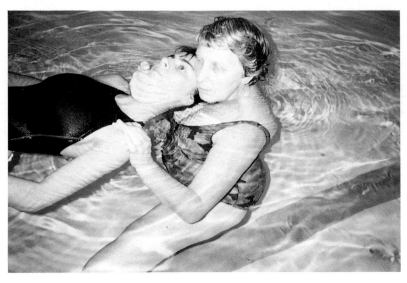

Fig. 61.15   Cervical spine lateral flexion mobilization.

Stretching

Stretching of soft tissues is a very important part of mobilizing and maintaining mobility. Examples of stretching which may be used are as follows:

1. Stride standing, side to bar, grasping bar with hand. Stretch head and trunk back to touch the water with back of head and shoulders; hold and rest. Stretches neck and trunk flexors.

2. Lying, grasp bar. Push legs and trunk down to floor, hold and rest. Stretches trunk and hip flexors.

3. Standing facing wall, grasping bar. 'Walk' feet up the wall, bending the hips and knees to stretch the lumbar spine extensors; hold and rest.

4. Standing facing wall, grasping bar with spine straight and hips flexed to about 120°. Push the thorax into the water, stretch the thoracic spine and retract the shoulders; hold, and rest. Stretches pectorals.

5. Lying across corner of pool, grasping bar. Turn the pelvis and legs to the right, push left leg further, hold, push a little further, and rest. Stretches trunk rotators.

6. Standing facing wall, grasping bar. Keep feet flat and press forward to arch the spine, holding the head in extension; hold and rest. Stretches trunk flexors.

7. Side-lying on half-plinth, with edge of plinth at mid-lumbar level. Push both legs down to touch floor or pool; hold and rest. Stretches side flexors.

8. Standing facing wall, grasping bar, feet hip-width apart; bend forward at the hips to bring the trunk level with the water surface. Carry the left leg forward, keeping the knee straight and allow buoyancy to produce hamstring stretch. (The effect may be enhanced by adding a float to the ankle.)

Under water douche

This is a single jet of water applied to localized areas of the body at a distance of approximately 10 cm from the skin surface. The jet is moved in circles or straight lines over the skin for up to 5 minutes. There is a massaging effect in the tissues with relief of pain, a local increase in circulation, and restoration of mobility to the tissues. It is useful for treating local areas of muscle spasm, chronic pain, fascial/muscle thickenings. It should be applied prior to exercise.

Strengthening methods

The properties of water utilized for strengthening are buoyancy and turbulence. Unstreamlining of a body's shape creates turbulence. The effects of buoyancy are increased by floats, and increasing speed creates more turbulence.

Examples of exercises for the lumbar and thoracic spine extensor muscles:

1. Prone-lying on half-plinth; legs raising to horizontal (buoyancy assisting).
2. Side-lying on half-plinth; legs swinging back in extension (buoyancy supporting); increase speed; add flippers to progress.
3. Lying on half-plinth, legs pushing down (buoyancy resisted); progress as above.
4. Float-lying (floats on feet), legs pushing down (progression on number 3 because the starting position is less fixed).
5. Right side-lying with ring under left arm and supporting head (Fig. 61.7). The therapist supports the patient's thighs and pelvis from in front and flexes the patient's trunk. Patient extends head and spine while the therapist returns patient to starting position and repeats movement (Fig. 61.16).

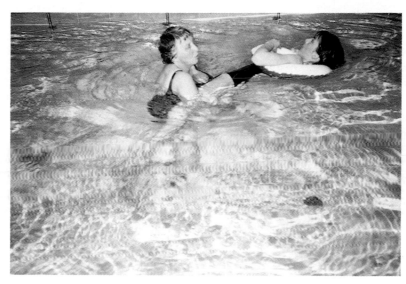

Fig. 61.16 Lumbar and thoracic spine strengthening exercises.

Examples of exercises for lumbar and thoracic spine flexors muscles:

1. Sitting; knees and hips bending (buoyancy assisting inner range).
2. Side-lying on half-plinth; hips and knees bending (buoyancy supporting); increase speed and add flippers to progress.
3. Prone-lying on half-plinth, legs pushing down (buoyancy resisting outer range).
4. Patient lying across corner of pool, grasping bar. The therapist holds the patient's feet. The patient is instructed to push her buttocks down into the water with the knees moving along the surface of the water towards the chest (buoyancy resisting middle to inner range).
5. Right side-lying with ring under left arm and supporting the head (Fig. 61.7). The therapist stands behind the patient and supports the patient's thighs. Patient flexes trunk as therapist moves back then relaxes as therapist extends the patient to return to starting position. The movement is then repeated.

Examples of exercises for lumbar and thoracic spine side flexor muscles:

1. Standing, holding bar; alternate hip updrawing (buoyancy assisting).
2. Lying on half-plinth, feet supported by one float, legs swinging from side to side (buoyancy supporting).
3. Float-lying, with therapist fixing patient's feet or pelvis or thighs. Patient bends slowly from side to side (buoyancy supporting). Progression is made by having the patient's arms by the side, to hands on hips, to hands on shoulders, to arms stretched sideways, to arms stretched above the head.
4. Side-lying on half-plinth. Push both legs down into

the water (buoyancy resisting). Progress by adding floats to the ankles.
5. Float-lying, hands clasped behind head (Fig 61.17). The therapist holds the patient's elbows, left hand on cephalad aspect of left elbow and right hand on caudad aspect of right elbow. Patient swings legs and trunk to right, therapist changes hands and patient swings to left. Progression is made by increasing the speed.

Examples of exercises for lumbar and thoracic spine rotators muscles:

1. Sitting, arms crossed hands on shoulders, head and shoulders turning from side to side (buoyancy supporting). Progress by holding arms stretched forwards, then out to the side. Progress by holding bats horizontal, then vertical.
2. Lying on half-plinth. Push the left leg down and carry the right leg over – repeat to opposite side.
3. Grasp bar with back to wall, hold knees and hips in flexion. Carry knees from side to side.

Confidence building and fitness

This consists of helping the patient to believe that the structure and musculature of the spine have recovered from injury and can be relied upon to perform to full function during the everyday activities comprising the patient's lifestyle. Some of the above exercises will help to achieve this, especially the strengthening ones performed at speed. Combined movements in patterns are important at this stage. Examples of activities:

1. Stride standing, hands clasped arms stretched forwards. Swing arms and trunk from side to side. Progress by holding a bat vertically.

2. Prone-lying, holding bar. Swing legs shown, bend hips and knees to touch wall with feet; return to starting position by thrusting legs back.

3. Standing. Bend right knee and left elbow, touch together and repeat with opposite arm and leg.

4. Sitting position, with feet and knees held firmly together, hands beside hips. Paddle with hands to move forwards, backwards and turning.

5. Walking quickly forwards, backwards and sideways. Take bigger strides.

6. Standing with broad elastic band round waist and fixed to bar. 'Walk' or 'run' against resistance of band.

7. Stride standing, holding floats. Push left arm forwards and bend right arm back; change arm position quickly.

8. Float-lying, hands clasped behind head (Fig. 61.17). The therapist holds the patient's elbows, left hand on cephalad aspect of left elbow and right hand on caudad aspect of right elbow. Patient swings legs and trunk to the right while rotating the right hip up (trunk extensors and side flexors) or while rotating the left hip up (trunk flexors and side flexors). The therapist changes hands and the patient swings to the left.

9. Right side-lying with ring under the left arm and supporting the head. The therapist supports the patient's thighs and pelvis from behind. The patient brings right shoulder to left hip, moving along the surface of the water, while the therapist moves backwards. Repeat to opposite side.

10. Prone-lying, grasping bar. Leg action of breast-stroke or crawl.

11. Lying grasping bar. Leg action of back crawl.

12. Grasping bar, feet on wall. Swing hips up to right then down and up to left.

13. Prone-lying, grasping bar at arms length with right hand. Carry left arm straight under right and carry back out to left. Progress by adding a float to the hand.

14. Patient supported upright with ring under both arms. Bicycling action with legs.

15. Group work (see below).

Once a patient is water-confident, and knows various activities well, it may be of benefit to encourage group work. This may take different forms, as follows. A formal group of six to nine patients can perform the same exercises at the same time under the therapist's instructions. The therapist has the opportunity to observe and correct individuals, and this method is therefore suitable for early progression from individual treatment — and for patients who are not particularly athletic. A big advantage of this type of group is that the exercises may be performed to music, which adds rhythm and enjoyment to the treatment.

Informal groups can be organized where patients are 'doing their own thing'. This method allows patients to have an individual programme progressed at their own pace. Numbers need to be limited to four so that the physiotherapist can give enough attention to each patient.

Circuit training is useful for final rehabilitation to restore musculoskeletal fitness — which is an important factor in preventing further injury. The programme of exercises can be very vigorous, or gentle, according to the age, body type and disabilities of the group. The programme is designed to work all muscle groups and to improve cardiovascular fitness.

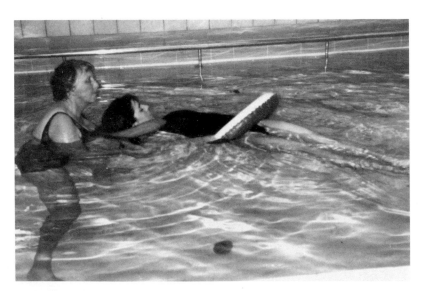

Fig. 61.17 Lumbar and thoracic spine exercise for confidence and fitness.

Prevention of recurrence

The therapist in the course of examining and treating the patient will have identified aggravating and causative factors of the patient's problems. Both therapist and patient will have developed plans for avoiding recurrence. Prior to discharge it may be necessary to advise the patient to continue with some form of exercise. The classical example is the patient who has a style of life dominated by flexion who rarely moves into extension and who must be educated to stretch into extension. There is also the patient who has hyperextension at lumbar 3–5 level and tightness of the associated soft tissues who must be taught how to keep these tissues stretched.

It may be appropriate to help the patient to identify a local exercise group which will suit. This is important because, with the best will in the world, most people whose pain has disappeared forget to continue with exercise. In relation to hydrotherapy, there may be a class of exercises in water suitable for the patient to attend. There is a difference between this and swimming. A class taken by a recognized teacher (e.g. approved by the Sports Council in the UK or a similar body) may be better for a person than unsupervised swimming. Before recommending swimming it is important that the therapist remembers that this activity emphasizes extension and is good for the patient who requires this – but is disastrous for the patient who is already hyperextended.

HYDROTHERAPY AND MANIPULATIVE THERAPY

The importance of hydrotherapy in the management of spinal problems is particularly related to the freedom of movement, pain reduction due to weight relief and warmth, and the enjoyment factor of exercises in water. Mobilizations can be carried out very successfully, as indicated, although high-velocity thrusts are inappropriate because of the difficulty of fixation. Water is a comfortable medium for most people, and the feeling of well-being which follows exercises in water is particularly important for patients with long-standing problems and chronic spinal pain. Often it is of great benefit for a patient to have individual manipulative therapy on land and then to have pool therapy afterwards.

REFERENCES

Harrison R A 1980 A quantitative approach to strengthening exerciss in the hydrotherapy pool. Physiotherapy 66: 2
Harrison R A, Bulstrode S 1987 Percentage weight bearing during part immersion in the pool. Physiotherapy Practice 3: 60–63
Skinner A T, Thomson A M 1983 Duffield's exercises in water, 3rd edn. Bailliere Tindall, London, p 126

FURTHER READING

Barefoot J 1981 Intensive treatment for ankylosing spondylitis. Therapy Weekly 7: 32
Baum G 1991 Aquarobics. Arrow Books, London
Davis B C, Harrison R A 1988 Hydrotherapy in practice. Churchill Livingstone, Edinburgh
Reid Campion M 1990 Adult hydrotherapy. Butterworth-Heinemann, London

62. Ergonomics: spinal stress reduction

J. D. Boyling

INTRODUCTION

This book has covered issues such as the structure and function of the spine, spinal pain, common clinical problems, examination and assessment as well as clinical procedures. Manipulative physiotherapists need to be aware of these issues so that they can effectively treat those patients presenting with spinal pain. However, thought needs to be given as to why patients present with spinal pain. Some cases are due to trauma, e.g. motor vehicle accidents, while others are due to congenital disorders. However, many are due to degenerative changes and work-related problems, be they factory- or office-based. Yet, with the work-related group, how much thought is given to prevention? A quick review of seating or how to pick up a box may be given in the confines of the treatment cubicle, but what resemblance does this bear to the tasks undertaken in the workplace over a prolonged period of time? If manipulative therapists are going to provide a full service to the patient, greater emphasis has to be given to prevention of spinal stress. Ergonomics has a part to play.

ERGONOMICS

Ergonomics is a relatively new word since it was coined only in the early 1950s. Numerous definitions have been applied since then. Murrell (1965) defined ergonomics as 'the scientific study of the relationship between man and the working environment'. 'Fitting the task to the man' was the title of the book by Grandjean (1982), and this definition has been widely used. More recently, Pheasant (1991) has stated that 'ergonomics is the scientific study of human work'. With this definition, work needs to be considered in the broad sense of any human activity and it need not necessarily be for financial gain.

Singleton (1972) stated that ergonomics was based on the disciplines of anatomy, physiology and psychology. These particular groupings can be expanded to cover anthropometry, biomechanics, work physiology, environmental physiology, skill psychology and occupational psychology. What then is the relationship of ergonomics to the spine? This requires a deeper examination of some of the components of ergonomics and the spine.

Anthropometry

Anthropometry deals with the dimensions of the human body. Humans vary in shape and size, and this can lead to spinal stress, particularly when they have to share workplaces.

Pheasant (1986) has combined a variety of data sources to provide dimensions for the human spine. Table 62.1 gives a summary, and it is clear that human variation does occur. The table indicates a variation of 190 mm for occipital height down to 70 mm for sacral height. In the context of a person sitting on a chair, or using a screen, adequate support may not be possible in the former if it is designed with a fixed dimension. Lack of adjustability for a VDU screen may lead to spinal stress in an operator. Ascertaining the resulting musculoskeletal discomfort requires a questionnaire – but what type?

Questionnaire methods

Ascertaining the extent of any musculoskeletal problem in the workplace requires a survey of the work force. This is not a task lightly undertaken. The first problem arises in designing a questionnaire to elicit the required information. Dickinson et al (1992) have constructed a flow chart to guide the individual undertaking this process. The Nordic Musculoskeletal Questionnaire (NMQ) has been used frequently but it was considered improvements could be made. The purpose of the study by Dickinson et al (1992) was to achieve an improved format. Studying a range of workers (data entry clerks, technical staff, administrative, and 481 subjects employed in 10 supermarkets) led to improvements being made in the layout and wording. The improved version will allow a databank of responses to be accumulated and, in particular, the prevalence of reported symptoms in many types of occupational groups. There still remains the problem of how to resolve existing problems. Once again, ergonomics can help in reducing neck and spinal pain.

Neck pain

It is not uncommon to see an increased thoracic kyphosis

Table 62.1 Variation in UK human spinal size for specified percentiles (%le)

Dimension	Female				Male			
	5th (%le)	50th (%le)	95th (%le)	SD	5th (%le)	50th (%le)	95th (%le)	SD
Occipital height	710	770	825	35	765	830	900	38
C7 height	565	615	665	31	605	660	710	33
Lumbar height	195	230	265	22	195	240	285	26
Sacral height	130	165	200	21	125	165	200	23

in an individual whose working life has been spent dealing with paperwork on a flat surface. At the same time it is generally accepted that a correctly adjusted chair and table improve the sitting posture.

Reading and writing at a desk are common and daily tasks for many people and, as such, can lead to musculoskeletal symptoms if the posture is constrained and sustained. Most of this work is carried out on a work surface which is horizontal. Slanting the work surface is presumed to reduce the neck tension and complaints, and to increase work efficiency.

Bendix and Hagberg (1984) studied sitting posture in relation to three different desk slopes of 45, 22 and 0°. The study utilized ten subjects who were given a task of reading, and EMG recordings were taken from the descending part of the trapezius muscle during both reading and writing tasks. The results indicated that acceptability for reading increased from 0° to 22° to 45°. However, acceptability for writing decreased from 0° to 22° to 45°. The authors concluded that a sloping desk on a horizontal table seemed preferable to slanting of the total table. Slanting more than 10° usually resulted in papers and pencils sliding off the work surface. However, lower inclinations are expected to have only minor effects on the posture.

Further research has been undertaken by De Wall et al (1991) who studied the effect of a desk with a 10° inclination on the sitting posture of ten subjects while reading and writing. Recordings of trunk postures were taken during the activity which lasted 1.5 h on different days. The result of using a slope of 10° inclination was that the head was more erect by 6°, and the position of the trunk was 7° more erect. This equated to a maximal decrease in load observed on the cervical spine of 35% and on the thoracic spine of 95%. The head–trunk angle did not change significantly when using the inclined desk. Although the study was not tied to a clinical examination of those taking part, the authors expected that neck complaints should be reduced.

Freudenthal et al (1991) have also studied the change in neck posture when a tilted work surface was used. The work surface had a tilt of 10°. This research reported that the posture assumed by a person who is doing mixed reading and writing work at a table with the Erasmus office-desk is more upright than the posture of the same person doing the same work without the desk. This applies for both the head and the trunk. The moment of force caused by gravity is proportional to the sine of the angle. The average change in the position of the head was from 38.5° to 29.6°, resulting in an average decrease of the moment of force at C7–T1 of 21%. The largest individual decrease was 51%.

Of course, the provision of equipment designed to reduce spinal stress – especially that on the neck – does not necessarily mean that it will be used. Verbeek (1991) investigated this. The findings, although significant, were discounted due to the low practical value. The reasons for this were assumed to be the arbitrary concept of an ideal sitting posture, the social acceptability of the advice given, and practical impediments that can occur while adopting an ideal sitting posture.

The problem of neck pain is not confined to the office environment. Neck and shoulder complaints among sewing-machine operators were investigated by Blader et al (1991). Some 224 sewing-machine operators from four textile factories were studied, and it was found that the one-year prevalence rate for neck–shoulder complaints was 75%. This dropped to 51% for the last seven days of the study period. The daily prevalence rate was 26%. The extent of these complaints led to a restraint in work time in 27% of cases and 37% in leisure time. The application of ergonomic principles could have been investigated and the prevalence rates monitored for improvement.

Spinal pain

Spinal pain affects the majority of the population at some stage of their life. The extent of this has been shown in a study which looked at a large cross-section of a Danish town. In this study Biering-Sorensen (1982) reported a point prevalence of 14%, a one-year prevalence of 45% and a lifetime prevalence of 62% for low-back pain. Pheasant (1991, p. 68) has concluded after reviewing the literature that low-back pain is predominantly work-related. One occupation studied has been that of nurses.

Pheasant and Stubbs (1992) studied back pain in nurses and, in particular, epidemiology and risk assessment.

They found a point prevalence of 17% while the one-year prevalence was 43.1%. This compared with the work of Magora (1972) who reported a 16.8% point prevalence. It is widely believed that nurses suffer back injuries because they are under-trained. Pheasant and Stubbs (1992) believe that the truth is probably much more that they are overworked (i.e. physically overloaded). To deal with this type of problem it is necessary to identify those features of the working system which are responsible for the overload. Some of these are under the individual nurse's control and can, at least in principle, be corrected by training. However, many are not and require an engineering solution, design solutions or changes in the accepted working practice. Frequently, the individual nurse is not in a position to make these changes but senior nurse managers are. The authors concluded that training is necessary but should be seen as an adjunct and not an alternative to safer systems of work.

In the office environment various studies have been made. The work of Cantoni et al (1984) showed that work place modifications can have a positive effect on the postural loading of the spine. The major difference noted in this study of operators on a telephone switchboard was that, in the old work station, the supported back was only adopted for a small percentage of the working day whereas in the new work station it was by far the most common posture adopted. The average load on the intervertebral disc was calculated and a marked decrease was noted.

The study of Occhipinti et al (1985) clearly shows that supporting the upper limbs has a definite effect on the discal load. Freudenthal et al (1991) studied the change in trunk posture when a tilted work surface was used by a person who was doing mixed reading and writing work. The work surface had a tilt of 10°. The average position of the trunk was changed from 26° to 18.2° when working with the desk placed on the table. The moment of force caused by gravity is proportional to the sine of the angle. Therefore the change of angle results in a decrease of the average moment of force on the back at L5–S1 of 29%. The largest individual decrease found was 86%. Lateral flexion of the back was less often assumed when the subjects were using the desk.

In the factory, Andersson and Ortengren (1984) have analysed myo-electric signals in the lumbar region in the back when the back is loaded. Doing this they have found that the myo-electric signals correlate well to the compression force in the spine measured by means of disc pressure. These authors studied assembly line work, and 13 male workers participated in a study of three strenuous work stations on the assembly line of the car factory. The strenuous work stations were mounting of a side panel and a sound insulator in the front compartment, mounting of floor mats and mounting of the left front seat. The

study showed that the use of a lifting aid at one work station gave a significant decrease in high-amplitude levels.

Electromyography is not the only technique available for studying spinal loading. Shrinkage has been used to measure the effect of load on the spine. Eklund et al (1984) developed a system to measure the shrinkage as a measure of the effect of the load on the spine. Since this initial work was done, the actual technique has been put to good effect to see changes in spinal stature as a result of work and leisure activities.

With regard to leisure activities, Boocock et al (1988) have studied the effect of gravity inversion on exercise-induced spinal loading. In this particular study eight males were subjected to periods of standing and gravity inversion as well as exercise. Standing pre-exercise caused little change in the stature whereas gravity inversion caused a mean increase in stature of 2.7 mm. The exercise regime consisted of ten sets of five standing broad jumps with 15 seconds recovery between each set. This series of exercises caused a mean shrinkage of 1.7 mm when it was performed immediately after standing. However, a shrinkage of 3.5 mm occurred when exercise followed gravity inversion. The authors concluded that the benefits gained by unloading the spine were short-lived in this particular experiment.

Ergonomics and manual handling

The rise in manual handling injuries in the United Kingdom and elsewhere has resulted in codes of practice and legislation being introduced. There has been an associated increase in the advertising of aids to assist those involved in manual handling tasks. In particular, there has been an increase in emphasis given to the use of spinal belts. Are they a valuable adjunct?

Spinal belts

With greater attention being applied to the reduction of manual handling injuries there has been an associated rise in the number of aids available. These range from mechanical devices to reduce the load, to spinal belts. The advertising of these belts is rarely if ever accompanied by research data to validate the claims made by the supplier of the equipment. Two studies throw doubt on the efficiency of these devices. In the first, McGill et al (1990) studied six subjects lifting loads with and without a weight-lifting belt. EMG recordings of abdominal, intercostal and low-back muscles were recorded, along with intra-abdominal pressure. No significant differences were reported and the authors concluded that prescribing the belt could not be justified.

A more recent study by Reddell et al (1992) examined the role of a weight-lifting belt in airline baggage handlers. The study was conducted over an eight-month period and involved 642 handlers. The purpose of the study was to ascertain the effect on lumbar injury rates and severity. The study design used four groups. One group was issued with the belt; another group received the belt plus training; a third group received training and no belt; the fourth group was a control. The authors reported no significant difference in injury rate for the groups. It was noted that 58% of participants discontinued use of the belt before the eight-month trial was concluded. Reasons for this included the belt being hot, it rubbed etc. Wearers who then fail to use the equipment may be at risk of injury. In summary, belts seem to be treating the symptom and not the cause. The application of ergonomics to the problem of manual handling may be a more effective option.

CONCLUSION

Many occupations have a high prevalence of spinal pain. Some occupations appear to be affected more than others. However, irrespective of occupation, ergonomics can have a role in reducing spinal load. The examples quoted here support this.

REFERENCES

Aaras A, Westgaard R H, Stranden E 1988 Postural angles as an indicator of postural load and muscular injury in occupational work situations. Ergonomics 31: 915–933

Andersson G B J, Ortengren R 1984 Assessment of back load in assembly-line work using electromyography. Ergonomics 27: 1157–1168

Bendix T, Hagberg M 1984 Trunk posture and load on the trapezius muscle whilst sitting at sloping desks. Ergonomics 27: 873–882

Biering-Sorensen F 1982 Low back trouble in a population of 30-, 40-, 50- and 60-year-old men and women. Danish Medical Bulletin 29: 289–298

Blader S, Barck-Holst U, Danielsson S, Ferhm E, Kalpamaa M, Leijon M, Lindh M, Markhede G 1991 Neck and shoulder complaints among sewing-machine operators. Applied Ergonomics 22: 251–257

Boocock M G, Garbutt G, Reilly T, Linge K, Troup J D G 1988 The effects of gravity inversion on exercise-induced spinal loading. Ergonomics 31: 1631–1636

Cantoni S, Colombini D, Occhipinti E, Grieco A, Frigo C, Pedotti A 1984 Postural analysis and evaluation at the old and new workplace in a telephone company. In: Grandjean E (ed) Ergonomics and health in modern offices. Taylor & Francis, London

De Wall M, Van Riel M P J M, Snijders C J 1991 The effect on sitting posture of a desk with a ten degree inclination for reading and writing. Ergonomics 34: 575–584

Dickinson C E, Campion K, Foster A F, Newman S J, O'Rourke A M T, Thomas P G 1992 Questionnaire development: an examination of the Nordic Musculoskeletal Questionnaire. Applied Ergonomics 23: 197–201

Eklund J A E, Corlett E N, Johnson F 1984 A method for measuring the load imposed on the back of a sitting person. Ergonomics 26: 1063–1076

Freudenthal A, van Riel M P J M, Molenbroek J F M, Snijders C J 1991 The effect on sitting posture of a desk and with a ten-degree inclination using an adjustable chair and table. Applied Ergonomics 22: 329–336

Grandjean E 1982 Fitting the task to the man. Taylor & Francis, London

McGill S M, Norman R W, Sharratt M T 1990 The effect of an abdominal belt on trunk muscle activity and intra-abdominal pressure during squat lifts. Ergonomics 33: 147–160

Magora A 1972 Investigation of the relation between low back pain and occupation. Industrial Medicine and Surgery 39: 28–34

Murrell K F H 1965 Ergonomics: man in his working environment. Chapman Hall, London, p xiii

Occhipinti E, Colombini D, Frigo C, Pedotti A, Grieco A 1985 Sitting posture: analysis of lumbar stresses with upper limbs supported. Ergonomics 28: 1333–1346

Pheasant S T 1986 Bodyspace: anthropometry, ergonomics and design. Taylor & Francis, London

Pheasant S T 1991 Ergonomics, work and health. Macmillan Press, Basingstoke

Pheasant S, Stubbs D 1992 Back pain in nurses: epidemiology and risk assessment. Applied Ergonomics 23: 226–232

Reddell C R, Congleton J J, Huchingson R D, Montgomery J F 1992 An evaluation of a weightlifting belt and back injury prevention training class for airline baggage handlers. Applied Ergonomics 23: 319–329

Singleton W T 1972 Introduction to ergonomics. World Health Organization, Geneva

Verbeek J 1991 The use of adjustable furniture: evaluation of an instruction programme for office workers. Applied Ergonomics 22: 179–184

Westgaarn R H, Aaras A 1984 Postural muscle strain as a causal factor in the development of musculo skeletal illnesses. Applied Ergonomics 15: 162–174

63. The masqueraders

G. P. Grieve

INTRODUCTION

Since physiotherapists are now 'first contact' clinicians, and we decide the manual or other physiotherapy treatment, where indicated, we have assumed greater responsibilities. While those interested in manipulation and allied treatments energetically improve their expertise in the various techniques and applications, perhaps we should spend more time considering what we are doing all this *to*. If we take patients off the street, we need more than ever to be awake for those conditions which may be other than musculoskeletal; this is not 'diagnosis', only an enlightened awareness of when manual or other physical therapy may be more than merely unsuitable and perhaps foolish. There is also the factor of possibly delaying more appropriate treatment. It is not in patients' best interest to foster the notion that 'first contact clinician' also means 'diagnostician' (Grieve 1988). Our concern is to recognize when the non-musculoskeletal condition should promptly be directed elsewhere for the best chance of skilled detection and proper help.

Provocation and relief

A common view is that benign musculoskeletal conditions are recognisable because the clinical features are provoked by certain posture(s) and activities, and lessened by others — this pattern of provocation/relief being the confirming factor. In contrast, the features of systemic, neoplastic or other (non-musculoskeletal) conditions are said, in broad terms, to be identifiable in being less influenced by postures or activity.

This rule of thumb is too simplistic; many conditions, in either category, do *not* behave in this way. The writer recalls two patients: one who, with a clear history of recent trauma to the left upper thorax, developed the classical features of a simple rib joint lesion, and another who presented with a watertight history of episodic bouts of low-back pain, closely related to periods of prolonged sitting or stooping. In each case the physical signs confirmed the opinion that these were musculoskeletal problems. Both were neoplasms, in fact, and both patients soon succumbed. Fortunately, manual treatment was not aggressive or enthusiastic, and quickly stopped.

Visceral conditions

These conditions, particularly, can easily mislead, unless one maintains a lively awareness of how they commonly present. Some examples follow:

- Angina can affect face, jaw and neck only and true anginal pain can, on occasion, be posterior thoracic as well as precordial, although simple thoracic joint lesions often simulate anginal pain, of course (see Ch. 29).
- Hiatus hernia may present with widespread chest and bilateral shoulder pain, as may oesophageal spasm with, in this case, added radiation to the back.
- Virtually anything in the abdomen can present with back pain; examples are peptic ulcer, cancer of the colon or rectum, retroperitoneal disease (e.g. cancer of pancreas) or abdominal arterial disease. Some suggest that a peptic ulcer must be a gross lesion to refer pain to the back, yet individuals with an ulcer shallow enough to escape detection on barium meal examination may have back pain from the ulcer. Even when the ulcer is healing, a glass of milk will ease the backache which follows gardening.

Benign gynaecological problems rarely refer pain to the back (see Ch. 19, p. 288), although pelvic neoplastic disease may do so.

Summation of pain-producing factors should be borne in mind. The severity of pain, and the pattern of pain projection or reference from a visceral condition, occurring in the presence of a mild and covert spinal musculoskeletal problem, may be potentiated by premenstrual changes, for example Brewerton (1990). True anginal pain is more likely to be referred to the neck if there is an existing mild and covert cervical joint condition, and more especially into the arm if there exists a concurrent neck and shoulder problem. The factor of summation is an important component of the neural mechanisms being considered.

Because serious conditions may masquerade as musculoskeletal problems, it may be useful to categorize examples of those which confusingly present as the tip of a very different kind of iceberg.

The conditions which may misrepresent themselves are marshalled under:

1. misleading presentation; idiosyncrasies of pain and other clinical features
2. patterns of provocation/relief by certain postures and activities in non-musculoskeletal conditions
3. Low-back pain with listing (scoliosis) — variety of causes
4. Neoplasms.

Perhaps successors might take up this important theme, broadening the material and incorporating it as a larger part of formal training in manual therapy — particularly now that the word 'diagnosis' is often appearing, not always justifiably, in paramedical writing. Some of the conditions will be mentioned several times in different contexts. A few of them may never be seen, but most therapists will encounter a high proportion of these conditions during a professional career — increased awareness reduces time-wasting and inappropriate treatment.

1. Misleading presentation — some examples

—Gall bladder conditions may refer pain only to the thoracic region of the back, on one or both sides, in the territory of T6–T11 dermatomes (Doran 1967) (see Ch. 29, p. 412).

—Perforation of the ileum, in Crohn's disease (regional ileitis), can present just like a sacro-iliac problem with right buttock pain (Aitken 1986).

—Urolithiasis or stone in the ureter — 'renal colic' closely simulates an acute episode of severe spinal thoracolumbar junction pain (Blandy 1982, Grieve 1988).

—Aneurysm of the abdominal aorta may present with severe low-back pain; the addition of testicular pain is ominous and often precedes fatal rupture (Richardson 1960, Sokoloff & Bland 1975, Appenzeller 1978, Adams 1981).

—The onset of dissection of an aneurysm in the ascending aorta or aortic arch is characterized by a sudden, tearing chest pain; this often radiates into the neck, dorsal trunk, abdomen and legs (Macleod 1981). The suddenness, severity and spread of pain should be sufficient evidence of serious visceral disease, as opposed to an acute thoracic musculoskeletal problem.

—Varicosis of vertebral veins may underlie chronic, indeterminate back ache, secondary to heart disease, pul-

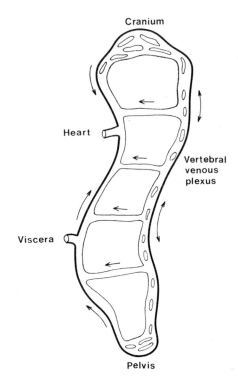

Fig. 63.1   A scheme of the vertebral veins and their valveless connections with other major venous systems of the thoracic and abdominal cavities.

monary or bronchial neoplasms, for example (Hanraets 1959). The venous drainage of the vertebral column is especially rich, and by its direct connection with other major venous systems (Fig. 63.1), the vertebral venous system acts as a 'pressure-absorber' when the trunk cavity pressure rises. As elsewhere in the body, the adventitia of vertebral veins and venules, as well as arteries and arterioles, are supplied with a dense plexiform arrangement of unmyelinated nerve fibres (Wyke 1987) which constitute an important part of the nociceptor system of the vertebral column, and which may be irritated in a variety of ways to give rise to pain.

—Paget's disease (osteitis deformans) is often symptomless but some patients may present with virtuously continuous, deep, aching pain (Fig. 63.2). It is never a generalized bone disease, and frequently only a single vertebra will be affected (Murray et al 1989).

—Ankylosing spondylitis, although commonly manifest in young men, may occur in young women, for the most part in a mild, covert and atypical form (Fig. 63.3). Radiographically, there may be sacro-iliac and cervical changes, sometimes with normal lumbar and thoracic spines, and, on occasion, severe osteitis pubis. There is a higher incidence of peripheral joint involvement (Braunstein et al 1982, Marks et al 1983). Many young women may not be fully investigated, as it is common to blame the pelvic organs, and X-ray of the pelvis is understandably avoided.

—Tight filum terminale is a tethering lesion of meninges;

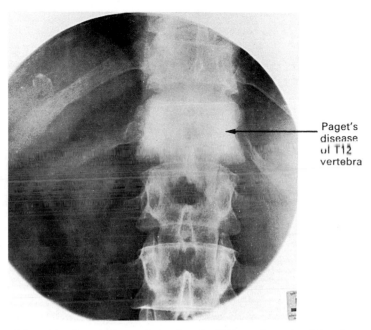

Paget's disease of T12 vertebra

Fig. 63.2 Paget's disease isolated to the T12 vertebra only, although the left iliac crest was also involved. Closed needle biopsy confirmed Paget's disease at both areas.

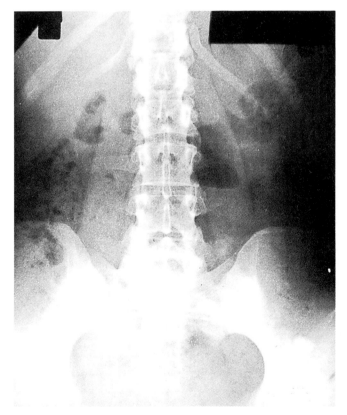

Fig. 63.3 The a–p view reveals the changes of ankylosing spondylitis in this young lady. Observe the characteristic changes at the lower border of the T12 vertebral body. A proportion of young women, with the same condition, may present with normal thoracic and lumbar X-ray appearances.

young people afflicted may complain of back pain and other spinal problems during the adolescent growth spurt (girls 12–14 years, boys 14–16 years). The presence of mild bilateral pes cavus, shortening of the tendocalcaneus and a history of childhood enuresis, without a clear history of any neurological disease, might indicate a meningeal anomaly as the cause (James & Lassman 1972, Govendos & Charles 1988).

— Concurrent musculoskeletal and visceral lesions are not uncommon, e.g. heart disease and chest wall pain (Edwards 1955, Prinzmetal & Massumi 1955) or gallstones and T7 segment problems, especially in women (Kellgren 1940) (see Ch. 29). Many writers, for example Lewit (1985), have discussed this phenomenon and it is of interest to chiropractors, of course, but the preponderance of enthusiastic folklore over proven fact in much of their writing discounts its validity.

Some conditions initially simulating non-inflammatory musculoskeletal conditions

— Brucellosis (undulant fever, abortus fever, Malta fever) occurs uncommonly in agricultural communities, nowadays in mild and obscure forms. A farm worker, for example, may present with migraine and vague muscle pains, and clinicians in country districts should be aware of the possibility (Glasgow 1976, Dixon 1980, Golding 1982).
— Systemic lupus erythematosus, a generalized multi-system connective tissue disorder, tends to occur in young females. Milder forms are common, and in some 25% the typical skin lesions may not occur. Joint pain, of apparently cervical origin, may be reported. There may be migraine with tiredness and lassitude, with a previous history of migraine (Jacobs et al 1979, Macleod 1981, Golding 1982).
— Acute infective polyneuritis (Guillain–Barré syndrome) can initially present like an acute back pain episode, with leg weakness like acute mechanical derangement (Porter 1986).
— Polymyalgia rheumatica, with 'central' joint pain and severe morning stiffness of limb girdles, occurs in mature individuals and in the early stages can easily mislead. It is important to institute quickly skilled diagnosis and correct management, because of the possibility of temporal arteritis and consequent loss of vision (O'Duffy et al 1980, Golding 1982).
— Maxillary or mandibular abscesses may cause neck, suboccipital and head pain, in the presence of palpable changes in cervical joints which are then inculpated as the cause. Wheeler et al (1985) describe a mandibular abscess of some severity, and the writer himself harboured a grumbling maxillary abscess for some years. His recurrent ipsilateral head pains were relieved to a degree by periodic unilateral mobilisation of C1–C2,

but never completely cleared until the abscess was surgically drained — the head pains have not recurred. It is known that teeth commonly refer pain to the suboccipital area, too.

Idiosyncrasies of pain and other clinical features

N.B. 'Idiosyncrasy' is perhaps the wrong word. For example, the 'classical' history and findings occur in less than 50% of appendicitis cases (Macleod 1981) and 'classical' migraine occurs in only about 10% of headache (Friedman 1975) (see also Ch. 19). Hence, clinical features which do not match classical descriptions can scarcely be thought of as idiosyncratic. *In truth, it is the classical descriptions themselves which merit the description 'idiosyncratic', so wide of the mark are so many of the hoary clinical assertions faithfully copied from text to text.* In the writer's opinion, much orthodox nonsense is believed, written and taught regarding the qualities and behaviour of so-called root pain (Grieve 1991). There is a pressing need to learn to live with a little confusion and doubt. Newcomers frequently 'solve' clinical problems in terms of the authoritarian black-and-white statements of dogmatic teachers. Weed (1968) suggested that students must be encouraged to acquire a capacity for 'sustained muddleheadedness' and a tolerance for ambiguity when difficult, unexplained findings are being dealt with. It is wise to remember that the musculoskeletal and nervous systems cannot read the textbook.

Many examples of the vagaries of so-called 'root' signs and symptoms have already been given in Chapter 19; for example, thoracic root pain (Kikta et al 1982) and lumbosacral radiculopathy (Johnson & Fletcher 1981).

Further examples are (i) in 50 disc herniations at the lumbosacral segment, knee-jerk reflex changes (L3–L4) were observed in six cases (Epstein 1976); (ii) in 18 patients with reduced or absent reflex changes, only 10 were confirmed as abnormal on electrical testing of ankle reflex latency (Leyshon et al 1981); (iii) Ross and Jameson (1971) mentioned a series of 470 surgically proven lumbar disc lesions, in which 39% had no neurological signs; (iv) Phillips (1975) regarded clinical neurological findings to be of extremely limited use in assessing the segmental levels involved — they may actively mislead; (v) Brodsky (1985), and several others (see Ch. 19) have indicated that so-called root pain of C7 origin, for example, is not only referred to the scapular area and the post-axial border of the upper limb, but into the precordium, too; (vi) discogenic compression of the cauda equina may cause shooting pains into genitalia and perineum, with severe disturbance of micturition, yet there is no sciatica (O'Ladire et al 1981).

Shifting patterns of spinal cord facilitation may be a factor in the day to day shifting patterns of distal responses, such as pain and paraesthesiae, to central verte-

Salient Palpation Findings

○	Locally tender	‖‖	Deep thickening
●	Locally sore ++	⊛	Prominent segment
Ƨ	Elicited spasm	⊙	Depressed segment
x	Stiff Segment	p	Provokes peripheral pain
͡ᴎᴎ	Hypermobile segment	ps	Provokes peripheral paraesthesiae

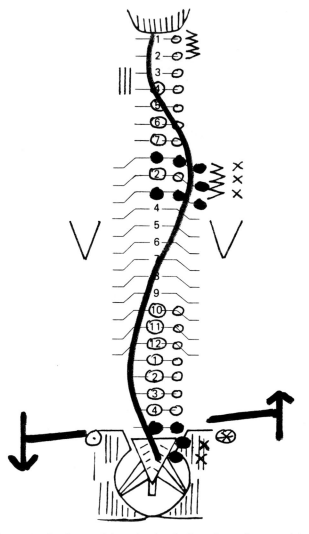

Fig. 63.4 A scheme of the palpation findings (posterior aspect) in a young woman with a lateral pelvic tilt upwards on the right side, and right unilateral dorsal pain from pelvis to occiput. Virtually all her chronic symptoms were relieved within 12 days by a simple unilateral heel raise. The degree of scoliosis has been exaggerated.

bral testing pressures. This is an unresearched clinical impression, yet observation over the years has convinced the writer of its validity.

Lesions of the symphysis pubis may refer pain felt only over the sacro-iliac joint. Chamberlain (1932) described three cases. Coccydynia is often referred from L5, even after local trauma to the coccyx, e.g. sitting heavily or falling onto the behind. After the local effects have been dealt with, there will be persistent coccydynia until L5, too, is mobilized (Grieve 1988).

— Unilateral pain, continuously from buttock to occiput, may be secondary to a lateral pelvic tilt, of less than 2 cm, in healthy young women (Grieve 1988). A simple unilateral heel raise frequently relieves all symptoms without further attention, other than periodic assessment (Fig. 63.4).

— Episacro-iliac lipoma (Grieve 1990), a benign aggregation of fat in the sacro-iliac sulcus, may present just like an intractable sacro iliac joint problem (Fig. 63.5). Physical treatment of the spine itself is generally unavailing.

— During the enthusiastic performance of slump tests, in pursuit of possible lesions of intracanal structures believed to be underlying this or that provocation of symptoms, it is easy to overlook the factor of stress simultaneously being applied to the long extrasegmental muscles of the thoracic region, as has been mentioned elsewhere (Grieve 1988).

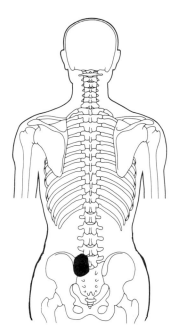

Fig. 63.5 A common site for aggregations of fat in the soft tissues overlying the sacroiliac sulcus. The size of the fatty mass will vary between a few millimetres to two or more centimetres across.

2. Patterns of provocation/relief by certain postures and activities in non-musculoskeletal conditions, some of them serious

— Episacro-iliac lipoma presents just like an intractable sacro-iliac joint problem. The unilateral sacro-iliac region pain is aggravated by certain postures and by coughing. Some patients have an antalgic gait and prefer antalgic sitting positions (Faille 1978).

— Renal colic (urolithiasis) is provoked by jolting and jarring, but not by spinal movements (Adams 1981).

— Upper urinary tract inflammation in women is provoked by activity and relieved by rest. Generally there is dysuria too, of course, but patients may not mention this (Fox & Saunders 1978).

— In elderly men with bladder stone and prostatic outflow obstruction, pain in the genital area is made worse by walking and exercise, and relieved by lying down (Blandy 1982).

— Hiatus hernia; discomfort is provoked by bending to dress, and other stooping postures, as well as lying down (Grieve 1988).

— Bornholm disease, epidemic cervical myalgia — a virus inflammation of muscle; there is pain in upper abdomen and costal margins provoked by coughing, deep breathing, yawning, laughing and thoracic movement. Neck pain is also aggravated on movement (Grieve 1988).

— Dry pleurisy; there is severe pain over scapula, axilla or nipple provoked by respiration and thoracic movement (Macleod 1981).

— Perinephric abscess and retrocaecal appendicitis; pain is provoked by movement, and subdued by rest (Kellgren 1940).

— Spinal Paget's disease is worst at night in some, and aggravated by weightbearing in some (Grieve 1989).

— Bone tumours of the spine; pain is provoked when supine, less so when up and about (Sim et al 1977).

— Headache due to brain tumour is sometimes provoked more by being upright than lying down (Dalessio 1990).

— Intradural tumour; the pain can be walked off, yet provoked by sneezing and lying down.

— Thoracic neurofibroma; the pain can be provoked by coughing, bending, sneezing, but relieved by rest in some and exercise in others (Black 1944).

— Spinal cord vascular malformations (angiomas) in middle-aged men can be provoked by stooping and exercise, and relieved by rest (lying) (Aminoff & Logue 1974).

— Backache of testicular malignancy in young men is aggravated by coughing and sneezing (Cole 1987).

3. Low-back pain with listing (scoliosis) — variety of causes

Uncommon bony lesions of neural arch structures which can cause painful scoliosis are osteoid osteoma, eosinophilic granuloma, aneurysmal bone cyst, pyogenic osteomyelitis and Ewing's sarcoma (Kornberg 1986). Although Ewing's sarcoma is relatively rare, comprising less than 10% of all primary malignant bone neoplasms in a Mayo Clinic series (Dahlin et al 1961), it is surpassed in incidence of this category of tumour only by plasma cell myeloma and osteosarcoma. Primary Ewing's sarcoma is often misdiagnosed as a disc herniation.

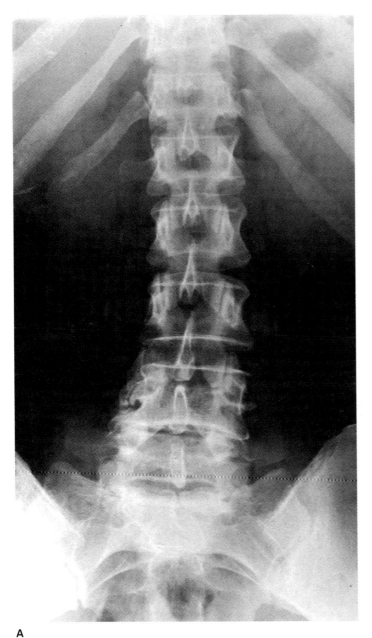

A

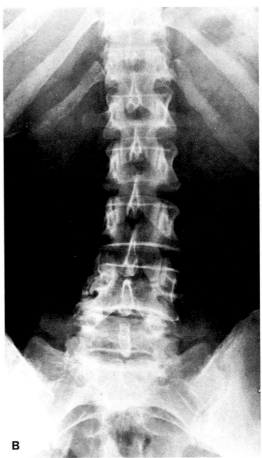

B

Fig. 63.6 This young lady has group II (**A**) spondylolisthesis at L4–5. Her right upper sacral surface is higher than the left and she is consequently listing to the left, despite having a slight lateral pelvic tilt upwards on the left. The 12th ribs are asymmetrical, suggesting the rule of thumb 'When one anomaly is found, be on the lookout for others'.

Osteoid osteoma/osteoblastoma is the most common of these bony lesions. It can occur at various levels — Jones (1987) described an osteoid osteoma of atlas, and Murray et al (1989) illustrated lesions at L2 and L4. Occasionally the lesion is of a rib (Lynch & Dorgan 1986). The main presenting symptoms are severe spinal pain, stiffness and scoliosis concave to the affected side (Schulman & Dorfman 1970, Sim et al 1977, Dixon 1980, Kirwan et al 1984).

Group II (isthmic) spondylolisthesis in young people may present with lateral deviation as a spastic or functional scoliosis (Macnab & McCullough 1990), a listing scoliosis similar to that encountered in acute lumbar pain episodes and secondary to muscle spasm (Fig. 63.6) (Turner & Bianco 1971).

Neurofibromatosis — scoliosis is the most frequent clinical and skeletal manifestations of this disease, and the most common reason for clinical presentation. It has usually been picked up already, but the therapist may be the first contact. One patient with a single neurofibroma remained undiagnosed for 3½ years (Black 1944). Anomalies of lumbosacral facet formation (Onimus et al 1986), a tilted upper sacral surface, a wedge-shaped or trapezoidal L5 vertebra (Fig 63.7) and unequal leg lengths (Grieve 1988) may also underlie lateral spinal listing.

The coexistence of severe backache and scoliosis may indicate a benign tumour. Idiopathic scoliosis is rarely painful (Macnab & McCullough 1990).

Unequal leg lengths

We usually discuss lateral lumbar deviation on the basis

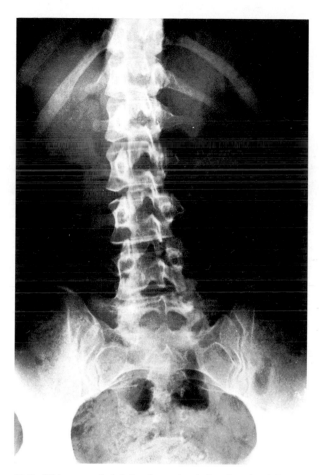

Fig. 63.7 This young lady's lumbar spine is listed to the right, on a level pelvis, because of a trapezoidal and partially sacralized L5 vertebra. The 11th and 12th ribs are asymmetrically positioned.

that the pelvis is level, yet true equality of leg lengths is uncommon (Giles & Taylor 1981).

There are two factors, perhaps not unconnected:

1. Most unilateral low-back pain in adults, associated with a frank lateral tilt of the pelvis, occurs on the side of the longer leg.

2. In most lateral listing or deviation, associated with a low-back pain episode, the spine is deviated away from the painful side.

We know that if the patient deviates towards the side of pain (perhaps some 10%) we will savagely provoke their discomfort by trying to straighten them up and extend them. If there is proximal limb pain we may provoke this and send it more distally.

It may well be that some transient lumbar deviations are merely an *exaggeration of the patient's normal tendency*. There is also the perennial factor that neither patient nor therapist had any knowledge of whether the patient was previously a little deviated anyway — whether in pain or not.

Stoddard (1987) mentioned that nearly two-thirds of all patients with low-back pain have a one-quarter inch (6 mm) discrepancy between leg lengths. This statistic, as such, has only limited significance until an equal number of individuals without leg length discrepancy is studied — and the incidence of low-back pain compared.

Besides leg length inequality, there are so many factors which may underlie the laterally deviated lumbar spine — a few examples are old unilateral slipped femoral epiphysis,

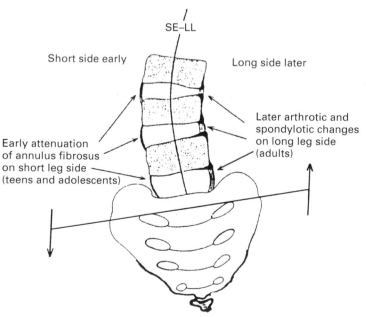

Fig. 63.8 A scheme (anterior aspect) of a laterally tilted pelvis due to leg-length inequality. If symptoms *are* caused by the asymmetry they are more likely to be on the short-leg side during the teenage years and on the long-leg side in adulthood. A proportion of patients with leg-length inequality are asymptomatic, of course.

congenital intra-pelvic asymmetry, acquired sacroiliac/symphysis pubis joint asymmetry, tilted upper sacral surface, trapezoidal L5, unilateral muscle spasm (psoas, quadratus lumborum) or any combination of these.

Besides correction of deviation and lumbar extension posturing, (when indicated), it is wise to suggest a suitable raise (Grieve 1988) on the short leg side if such be present — it often is (Fig. 63.8).

4. Spinal neoplasms

Since the writer does not have the competence to dissertate at length on vertebral neoplastic disease, neoplasms might briefly be considered under the headings of Incidence, Aggression and Clinical Features, followed by notes on examples of benign and malignant tumours of bone and soft tissue. No more is intended than to provide short illustrative examples of the way in which neoplastic conditions may, for some considerable time, simulate the clinical features of innocuous lesions. Neoplasms are sly, surreptitious things, often masquerading as quite ordinary musculoskeletal syndromes.

Incidence

(a) Most primary neoplasms occur in the first half of life. Primary bone tumours, benign or malignant, are uncommon; they have a tendency to affect the ilium and sacrum (Fig. 63.9).

Of 1000+ patients presenting with surgically proven benign or malignant primary bone tumours of the spine, pelvis and lower limb (Table 63.1), 38 were pre-

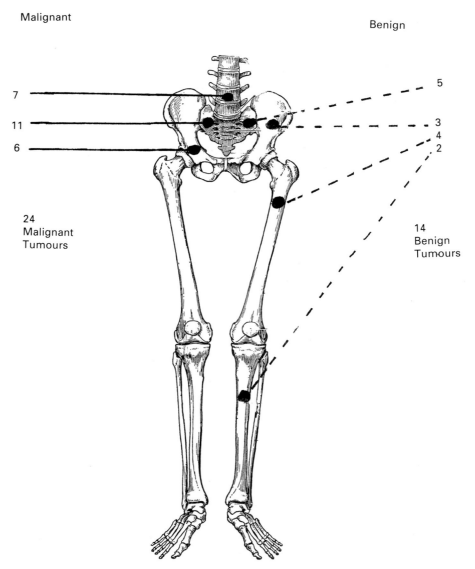

Malignant

Benign

7

11

6

5

3

4

2

24
Malignant
Tumours

14
Benign
Tumours

Fig. 63.9 The *general* localities of primary benign and malignant bone tumours which simulated the clinical features of lumbar disc syndrome. Left and right are of no significance in this representative scheme of the localities. (After Sim et al 1977.)

Table 63.1 Primary bone tumours simulating lumbar disc syndrome (after Sim et al 1977)

Type	Patients
Benign	
Osteoid osteoma	7
Benign giant-cell tumour	5
Chondromyxoid fibroma	2
Total	14
Malignant	
Multiple myeloma	6
Lymphoma	4
Osteogenic sarcoma	5
Chondrosarcoma	4
Chordoma	2
Ewing's sarcoma	2
Fibrosarcoma	1
Total	24
Total (combined)	38

Table 63.2 Categories and distribution of 557 spinal cord tumours (after Black 1944)

Classification	Numbers	(%)
Neurofibromas	163	29
Meningiomas	140	25
Intramedullary tumours	64	11.5
Sarcomas	55	10
Extramedullary haemangio-endotheliomas	47	8.5
Extramedullary ependymomas	32	6
Chordomas	23	4
Miscellaneous extramedullary tumours	33	6
Total	557	100
Region of spinal cord		
Cervical	100	18
Thoracic	304	54
Lumbar	117	21
Sacral	35	7
Multiple levels	1	—
Total	557	100

operatively diagnosed as lumbar disc lesions (Sim et al 1977). Of these, 18 had a myelogram and operation for a supposed 'disc'.

(b) Metastases (secondaries) account for the great majority of spinal neoplasms (Murray et al 1989). In 4000 autopsies, only 35 cases of primary bone tumours were found, and more than 500 cases of secondary tumours (Sim 1983).

Secondaries also represent the most common malignant bone tumours. The greater majority of secondaries occur in the latter half of life (usually 50+) hence age is important, and the primary tumours most often responsible for skeletal metastases are those of breast, bronchus and prostate — less frequent are those of thyroid and kidney. The spine is one of the most frequent sites for metastases, the lumbar spine rather more commonly than other districts, although the thoracic region shows a striking predilection as the site of *spinal cord compression* by a variety of tumours (Black 1944, Table 63.2; Simeone & Lawner 1982).

Over 25% of patients with spinal metastases present with neurological dysfunction, and over 80% of the tumours producing neurological deficit occur at *thoracic* cord level (Macnab & McCullough 1990).

In 57 patients (undergoing 60 operations for secondaries) the sites of metastases were 11 cervical, 39 thoracic and 10 lumbar (Onimus et al 1986, Tables 63.3, 63.4).

In another series, of 179 patients with spinal metastases, the lumbar spine was the most frequently involved (Schaberg & Gainor 1985) (Fig. 63.10).

(c) Soft-tissue tumours. Nerve-sheath tumours and meningiomas are more common than tumours of the spinal cord itself (Sissons 1959).

Aggression

The prognosis is poorer the more cranially the lesion,

Table 63.3 Sites of metastases (after Onimus et al 1986)

District	Numbers
Cervical (C1–T1)	11
Thoracic (T2–L1)	39
Lumbar (L2–L5)	10
Total	60

Table 63.4 Origins of metastases (after Onimus et al 1986)

Origins	Number
Breast	21
Bronchus	12
Myeloma*	6
Uterus	3
Kidney	3
Prostate	2
Bladder	1
Oesophagus	1
Unknown	11

* The six patients who presented with a spinal localization of myeloma were classified in this category because the disease behaves similarly to a metastasis from the mechanical viewpoint.

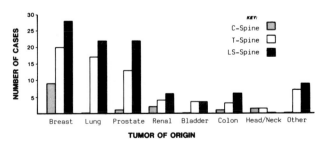

Segmental distribution of bony metastases from primary carcinomata

Fig. 63.10 The segmental distribution of bony metastases from primary carcinomata. (Reproduced from Schaberg & Gainor 1985 with permission.)

the more rapid the onset, the longer the signs have been present and the more manifest is sphincter involvement.

The relatively younger the patient, the more aggressive is the spread of secondaries (Murray et al 1989). Metastases from the bronchus initiate more aggressive secondaries than do those from breast or prostate. Hence secondary lesions from prostate, kidney and thyroid tumours are relatively indolent and grow slowly, even without treatment. When the bronchus is the primary site, in patients who come to surgery for the secondary, the patient is usually dead within a year (Onimus et al 1986), but if the primary is in the breast, some 63% of patients are still alive a year later. Upper thoracic secondaries have a poorer prognosis after surgery than do lower thoracic secondaries.

Clinical features

Some 19 features which may provide warning of the possibility of spinal neoplastic disease have been summarized elsewhere (Grieve 1991). The recognition of neoplasms, earlier rather than later, depends more on awareness, vigilance and suspicion rather than a set of rules. Grimer and Sneath (1990) discussed the diagnosis of malignant bone tumours. While their remarks apply largely to limb tumours the authors make points which are sufficiently general to merit attention here. While aches and pains are of course very common in clinical practice, the duration and progressive nature of symptoms should alert clinicians to the possible underlying pathology. A survey revealed how long patients had endured their symptoms before going to see a doctor: averages of 6 weeks for those with osteosarcoma, 16 weeks for patients with Ewing's sarcoma, and 21 weeks for those with chondrosarcomas. Even more concerning was the time taken, after the initial consultation, for the diagnosis to be made and the treatment started — a further 7 weeks for osteosarcoma, 31 weeks for Ewing's sarcoma and 30 weeks for chondro-sarcoma. *The usual cause of this delay was a low level of suspicion.*

The initial radiograph was passed as normal by clinician and radiologist, in 13 out of 70 cases, although the evidence was present on retrospective review.

When the diagnosis was not suspected a variety of treatments were employed; these were of no benefit and simply delayed the making of a correct diagnosis. Tumours of the pelvis were especially difficult to diagnose, taking an average of 61 weeks from start of symptoms to start of treatment. This long delay probably arose because the symptoms can masquerade as spinal and/or abdominal disorders.

All of the clinical features associated with disc changes, including abnormal movement patterns (Table 63.5), may occur in tumours of vertebral bone (Sim et al 1977).

Although parosteal osteosarcoma is rare, it is of interest

Table 63.5 Clinical features of primary bone tumours (after Sim et al 1977)

Feature	Benign (14 patients)	Malignant (24 patients)
Back pain	10	23
Sciatic pain	14	23
Night accentuation	11	12
Cough–sneeze accentuation	2	11
Limited lumbar motion	4	14
Tenderness to percussion	6	16
Positive Lasègue test	5	13
Reflex changes	6	15
Sensory changes	1	6
Motor weakness	1	6
Sphincter disturbance	1	4
Muscle atrophy	5	6

to physical therapists in that, of 20 cases reviewed, 16 involved the proximal half of the lower limb (Kavanagh et al 1990). This primary malignant bone tumour tends to occur in the first half of life; a local swelling is the predominant early feature, yet simulation of lumbar disc disease may occur in the early stages.

It is of interest that, of 38 cases of primary bone tumour (Table 63.5), 20 had no restriction of straight-leg-raising, i.e. absence of a positive SLR test does not preclude a neoplasm. Extensive bony metastases can exist without symptoms referable to the vertebra involved. In multiple metastases, bone may be riddled with metastases and yet not cause symptoms.

(i) Pain. Neoplastic pain is not necessarily continuous and progressive. It can be intermittent for lengthy periods, mimicking the features of benign conditions. When cervical pain of some duration is due to malignant deposits or infection of *cervical* structures, the neck may be held virtually rigid (Yates 1969), but the early clinical presentation may simulate cervical spondylosis. A Pancoast tumour in the early stages, for example, may amount to no more than aching over the upper trapezius on that side, and some vague but persistent discomfort on cervical movements away from the affected side. Slowly expanding lymphomas in the epidural space can for some time mimic the clinical presentation of disc disease.

Lange et al (1986) reported the simultaneous occurrence, in two separate low-thoracic segments of a 19-year-old male, of an osteoblastoma and a haemangioendothelioma. The intermittent pain, for six months, was not aggravated by activity and was worse at night. Spinal motion was full and straight-leg-raising was normal, as were the responses to neurological tests. Biopsy revealed the lesions. Ker and Jones (1985) reported on 32 patients with primary tumours of the cauda equina who were initially diagnosed as having prolapsed discs and treated accordingly. Considerable delay, in correctly diagnosing their condition, was frequent. Several were labelled neurotic and discharged from clinics. The correct diagnosis was eventually made, in all cases, by myelography. Features suggesting malignancy are pain, warmth, tenderness — easier to note in the limbs than in the spine. In very general terms progressive pain, accentuated by the supine position, favours a diagnosis of bone tumour (Sim et al 1977). Some authorities suggest that back pain is the first symptom in most cases and disquieting when it occurs at night (Onimus et al 1986). Others report that back pain was absent in one-third (36%) of patients with spinal secondaries, and that more than 50% of the patients with thoracic secondaries were asymptomatic (Schoberg & Gainor 1985). Again, of 17 patients (5 cervical, 7 thoracic, 5 lumbar), all had spinal pain (De Wald et al 1985).

The pain is characteristically worse on rest, and particularly at night; early in the history it will awaken the patient from sound sleep, but later the patient is awake for more time than asleep. Discogenic pain may be bad at night, but is more commonly provoked by *movement* in bed, and its intensity is generally less than when the patient is trying to move about during the day and suffering the effects of gravitational compression (Bianco 1968).

Turning over and changing limb positions often relieves the pain of degenerative joint disease, but gives no relief from the pain of malignancy, and frequently the patient must get up and walk about in an attempt to distract himself.

It should be remembered that disc space infection has a different characteristic in that it may be so severe at night that movement in bed is not even possible, and the patient is *unable* to sit up, or get out of bed (Bianco 1968).

Once the pain begins, the symptoms eventually become virtually constant, tending to remain so regardless of position or movement. This does not mean to say that active movements, asked of the patient during clinical examination, will not provoke pain. Contrary to what seems to be believed, an active movement may provoke a very severe jab of pain; rotation of the thoracic spine, for example, may make a patient gasp with the viciousness of provoked fulgurant pain which settles to the previous level as quickly as it arose. The usual analgesics provide no relief. In myelomatosis, the disease may be declared by the sudden onset of severely painful backache because of a pathological fracture.

(ii) X-ray appearance — in general terms. Large metastases can exist without visible changes in bone contours or density. An area of bone destruction of 1 cm diameter, in the middle of a vertebral body, may be present without any radiographic sign of it (see Fig. 49.1, p. 680).

Benign tumours. These remain local, and usually have a well-defined edge on X-ray. Most occur in young people and their growth usually ceases when bone growth is complete (Apley & Solomon 1982). Benign osteogenic tumours usually involve the vertebral apophyses rather than the vertebral body (Macnab & McCullough 1990). They present with pain which is not especially severe,

and it may have been present for some time before X-ray reveals the bone lesion.

Malignant tumours. These have the potential to metastasize. Edges look ill-defined on X-ray. Other factors suggesting malignancy are cortical destruction, calcification extending into the soft tissues and 'hot spots' on bone scans. Asymmetrical loss of pedicle shadow in a–p films makes a neoplasm virtually certain (Fig. 63.11, a and b). Malignant secondaries in the lumbar spine usually involve the vertebral body rather than the apophyses. Backache is commonly the presenting symptom, and it is wise not to rely on X-ray appearances; in autopsy specimens with neoplastic changes, quite gross disease may not be visible on post mortem radiographs in 85% of the specimens (Macnab & McCullough 1990).

Occasionally, excessive vertebral involvement may be manifest only as an apparent diffuse osteoporosis, and this may be the X-ray appearance of multiple myeloma.

Secondaries may be osteolytic, osteoblastic or mixed, i.e. a metastasis of any origin may give rise to new bone as part of the pathological process (Murray et al 1989).

Perkins (1961) mentioned that osteolytic secondary deposits in bone give a speckled appearance, and osteoblastic secondaries a mottled appearance. He remarked that, in multiple metastases, the bone may be riddled with secondary deposits (carcinomatosis) yet there are no symptoms; a woman with a primary carcinoma of breast and a skull swarming with secondary deposits did not complain of her head.

Examples may be grouped as shown in Table 63.6.

Table 63.6

Benign	Malignant
Bone	
(a) Osteoid osteoma/osteoblastoma complex	(e) Ca secondaries
	(f) Multiple myeloma (myelomatosis)
Soft tissue	
(b) Spinal vascular malformations (angioma)	(g) Pancoast tumour
(c) Neurofibromatosis	(h) Testicular malignancy
(d) Episacro-iliac lipoma	
(i) Clinical features of headache due to brain tumour	

(a) Osteoid osteoma. In young people with actual bony lesions of the posterior elements, the most common cause of painful scoliosis is the *osteoid osteoma/osteoblastoma complex* (Kirwan et al 1984). There is severe pain, not always in the locality of the lesion. The pain is worse at night, usually, and is dramatically relieved by aspirin. It is a small, painful bone lesion, occurring mostly in children, adolescents and young adults. It is rarely seen after 30 years. The patient is often misdiagnosed as 'neurotic' or 'a chronic malingerer'. The poorly localized pain is out of all

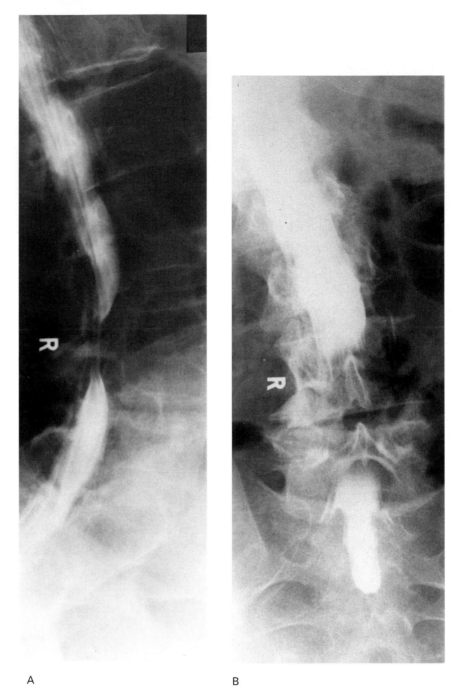

A   B

Fig. 63.11 The myelographic appearances of a suspected myeloma in a mature woman.
A. A space-occupying mass is evident at the L4 level in this lateral view. **B**. Besides the
evidence of trespass at the L4–L5 segments, the loss of the left L4 pedicle shadow in this
a–p view is strongly suggestive of a neoplasm.

proportion to the small size of the lesion (1 cm or less),
which is the archetypal diagnostic trap! (Dixon 1980).
The bone lesion (in sacrum, pelvis or vertebral pedicles)
may easily be missed on X-ray. The pain is often referred
elsewhere — rather than occurring in the vicinity of the
lesion itself — and the wrong part is X-rayed.

When identified on X-ray, there is an area of bone

sclerosis, often with a central translucency, in which osteoid material is proliferating — the nidus (Schulman &
Dorfman 1970). There is severe and unremitting pain, yet
no indication of disease in the usual routine screening
tests. In spinal lesions, a scoliosis concave to the side of
the lesion is characteristic, i.e. the scoliosis is such as to
shut down the affected side because of muscle spasm

(Murray et al 1989). As we have seen, it can occur at various levels, including a rib. Of 18 cases (Kirwan et al 1984):

— Eleven were lumbar, four thoracic and three cervical, and plain X-rays revealed the lesion in only six of them (one-third).
— The average delay in diagnosis was 19 months.
— Three-quarters of the patients had consulted three or more specialists before being correctly diagnosed.
— The most reliable investigation procedures were bone scan and CAT.

Sim et al (1977) observed that of all the bone tumours which simulate the intervertebral disc syndrome, the osteoid osteoma is probably the most confusing. Laminal osteoid osteoma can simulate nerve root involvement and concomitant symptoms, physical findings and cerebrospinal fluid changes. Numerous reports in the literature mention the long delay in diagnosis, and the fact that many patients are treated unsuccessfully as having intervertebral disc lesions.

(b) Spinal cord vascular malformations (angiomas) in middle-aged males. Haemangiomas in vertebral bodies are fairly common (10.7% in 3829 autopsies) (Schmorl & Junghanns 1951) but seldom cause symptoms. Spinal cord angiomas are less common but their clinical features are distressing. The majority of these angiomas occur at the thoracolumbar junction region and the diagnosis is established radiographically (Aminoff & Logue 1974).

The most frequent initial symptom is pain, which may be 'radicular' in distribution. Back pain is often lower lumbar. In several of a group of 60 patients, PID was diagnosed initially. Severe disturbance of micturition develops early.

Weakness of legs leads to severe restriction of exercise tolerance, but *pain may be the only early symptom*. Symptoms are clearly provoked by exercise and relieved by rest, often similar to intermittent claudication. Little wonder that PID was diagnosed in some.

(c) Neurofibromatosis. This is an autosomal dominant disorder characterized by cranial and peripheral nerve tumours, and pigmented areas on the skin (Black 1944, Macleod 1981, Cummine & Kirwan 1989, Murray et al 1989). Because the tumours may involve any nerve the clinical features may be numerous and bizarre. Swellings enlarge slowly and are rarely malignant. These benign tumours affect the thoracic spine mainly (Table 63.7), hence the prevalence of scoliosis.

A 'dumb-bell' tumour may occupy both IVF and neural canal, involving both the spinal cord and the somatic root.

Although a sacral neurofibroma is unusual, Figure 63.12 depicts one such in a female dancer, whose main complaint was that the discomfort interfered with her dancing!

Table 63.7 Distribution of 163 neurofibromas (after Black 1944)

Situation	Tumours	(%)
Cervical	35	22
Thoracic	70	43
Lumbar	55	33.5
Sacral	2	1
Multiple levels	1	0.5
Total	163	100

(d) Episacro-iliac lipoma. This is an acutely painful and localized fatty tumour over one sacro-iliac joint (Grieve 1990). Until the therapist has seen one, and noted all symptoms relieved by a single anaesthetic injection, it is unbelievable that the lesion is not a straightforward sacro-iliac joint lesion. It is superficial, very localized and very painful to pressure, which declares the condition at once. Relief by injection of local anaesthetic or excision of the nodule confirms the diagnosis. The nodule is more an aggregation or herniation of fat than a tumour.

(e) Ca secondaries (Murray et al 1989). Since space has already been devoted to metastases and their behaviour, it may be sufficient to illustrate an osteolytic secondary of the C6 vertebral body (Fig. 63.13). The patient said his neck was sore and cervical movements were limited. There was no clinical feature to suggest a secondary neoplasm, and the prescribed physiotherapy was wisely withheld until the X-ray was seen. After a sudden worsening of his condition, he died three weeks later despite a decompression operation for paraplegia.

(f) Multiple myeloma (myelomatosis). This is a neoplastic disorder of plasma cells — whether the growths are polyfocal or metastases is not known (Macleod 1981).

The X-ray appearance is often that of an apparent dif-

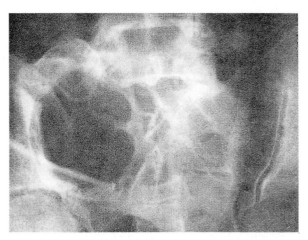

Fig. 63.12 An anteroposterior view of a massive neurofibroma of the sacrum and adjacent right ilium of a dancer. She complained that the discomfort interfered with her performance. (Reproduced from Stripp 1979 with permission.)

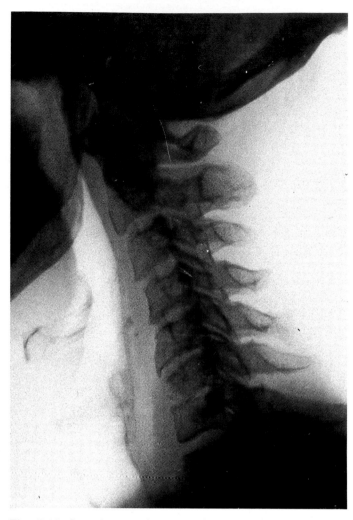

Fig. 63.13 Lateral aspect of an osteolytic secondary carcinoma of the 6th cervical body in a mature adult.

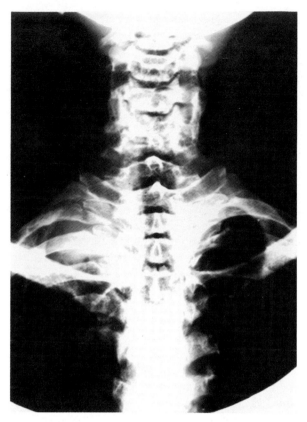

Fig. 63.14 Anteroposterior aspect of a right bronchogenic (Pancoast) carcinoma in the apex of the lung of a middle-aged man. The opacity was initially shown on a chest film. A penetrated view of the apex revealed extensive erosion by the tumour of the right 1st and 2nd ribs. The diagnosis was confirmed at biopsy. (Radiograph kindly provided by Dr D. J. Stoker, Dean of the Institute of Orthopaedics, London.)

fuse osteoporosis. A good rule of thumb is 'over 45, high ESR plus X-ray evidence of osteoporosis = myelomatosis until proved otherwise' (Apley & Solomon 1982). Peak incidence is 60–70 years. There is a preclinical phase of up to 25 years. The diffuse osteoporosis plus local erosion cause stress pain and eventually pathological fracture — which may be the first intimation of trouble.

Symptoms arise mainly in weight-bearing bones (spine, pelvis, femur), and stress pain may be wandering and difficult to pin down. Whatever the cause, the pain is often severe, prolonged and exhausting.

(g) Pancoast tumour. This bronchogenic carcinoma of upper lobe, with direct invasion of first and second ribs, frequently produces Horner's syndrome, plus wasting of C8–T1 distribution muscles and distal paraesthesiae (Murray et al 1989). Pain in the upper chest and shoulder is an almost constant symptom, and as mentioned earlier this may amount to no more than persistent discomfort in the early stages (Fig. 63.14).

(h) Testicular malignancy. Of 42 young men with malignant neoplasms of the testicle, 9 presented with back pain as the major symptom. The incidence is 1% of cancers in male patients, but this is the commonest solid tumour in young men aged 20–34 and its incidence is increasing. Watch for low-back pain without a history of stress in young men (Cole 1987, Cantwell et al 1987).

(i) Headache due to brain tumour. Because therapists deal with many cases of headache of musculoskeletal origin, it may be useful to mention the features of head pain due to brain tumour (Dalessio 1990). It will be seen that there are some significant distinctions between the presentation of an intracranial neoplasm and head pain referred from an upper cervical musculoskeletal problem.

Commonly, a brain tumour declares itself as follows:

— deep, dull, steady ache — not rhythmic or throbbing
— severe only sometimes — not intense like meningitis or so-called migraine
— usually relieved by aspirin or cold packs
— usually does not disturb sleep
— provoked by coughing, straining and being upright (recumbency is less provocative)
— nausea is not a common feature
— may be associated with stiffness or aching of neck muscles.

CONCLUSION

This chapter has been devoted to a variety of clinical misrepresentations, the features of which are counterfeit and should not be taken at their face value. Hence it can be summarized by a short apothegm:

THINGS ARE NOT ALWAYS WHAT THEY SEEM INITIALLY — BE INFORMED AND AWAKE.

REFERENCES

Adams G J 1981 Outline of orthopaedics. 9th edn. Churchill Livingstone, Edinburgh, p 225

Aitken G S 1986 Syndromes of lumbopelvic dysfunction. In: Grieve G P (ed) Modern manual therapy of the vertebral column. Churchill Livingstone, Edinburgh, pp 473–478

Aminoff M J, Logue V 1974 Clinical features of spinal vascular malformations. Brain 97: 197–210

Apley A G, Solomon L 1982 Apley's system of orthopaedics and fractures 6th edn. Butterworth, London, ch 9

Appenzeller O 1978 Somatoautonomic reflexology — normal and abnormal. In: Korr I M (ed) The neurobiologic mechanisms of manipulation therapy. Plenum Press, London, pp 179–217

Bianco A J 1968 Low back pain and sciatica: diagnosis and treatment. Journal of Bone and Joint Surgery 50A: 170–186

Black W A 1944 Pain produced by intraspinal tumour simulating pain caused by gall-bladder disease. Surgical Clinics of North America 24: 893–902

Blandy J 1982 Lectures in urology. 3rd edn. Blackwell Scientific, Oxford

Braunstein E M, Martel W, Moidel R 1982 Ankylosing spondylitis in men and women. Radiology 144: 91–103

Brewerton D A 1990 Personal communication

Brodsky A E 1985 Cervical angina. Spine 10: 699–709

Cantwell B M J, Mannix K A, Harris A L 1987 Back pain — a presentation of metastatic testicular germ cell tumours. Lancet 1: 262–265

Chamberlain W E 1932 The X-ray examination of the sacroiliac joint. Delaware State Medical Journal 4: 195–204

Cole R P 1987 Low back pain and testicular cancer. British Medical Journal 295: 840–841

Cummine J L, Kirwan D 1989 The management of intraspinal neurofibromata. Journal of Bone and Joint Surgery 71B: 165

Dahlin D C, Coventry M B, Scanlon P W 1961 Ewing's sarcoma. Journal of Bone and Joint Surgery 43A: 185–192

Dalessio D J 1990 Headache. In: Wall P D, Melzack R (eds) Textbook of pain. 2nd edn. Churchill Livingstone, Edinburgh, p 386

De Wald E L, Bridwell K H, Prodromas C, Rodts N F 1985 Reconstructive spinal surgery as palliation for metastatic malignancies of the spine. Spine 10: 21–26

Dixon A S J 1980 Diagnosis of low back pain. In: Jayson M I V (ed) The lumbar spine and back pain. 2nd edn. Pitman Medical, Tunbridge Wells p 135

Doran F S A 1967 The sites to which pain is referred from the common bile duct in man, and its implications for the theory of referred pain. British Journal of Surgery 54: 599–606

Edwards W L J 1955 Musculoskeletal chest pain following myocardial infarction. American Heart Journal 49: 713–719

Epstein B S 1976 The spine: a radiological text and atlas, 4th edn. Lee & Febiger, Philadelphia, ch 7

Faille R J 1978 Low back pain and lumbar fat herniation. American Surgeon 44: 359–361

Fox M, Saunders E R 1978 Significance of loin pain in women. Lancet 1: 115–116

Friedman A P 1975 Migraine. Psychiatric Annals 5: 29–36

Giles L G F, Taylor J R 1981 Low back pain associated with leg length inequality. Spine 6: 510–521

Glasgow M M S 1976 Brucellosis of the spine. British Journal of Surgery 63: 283–288

Golding D N 1982 A synopsis of rheumatic disease. 4th edn. Wright, Bristol, p 111

Govendos S, Charles R W 1988 Level of termination of the spinal cord during foetal development. Journal of Bone and Joint Surgery 70B: 504

Grieve G P 1988 Common vertebral joint problems. 2nd edn. Churchill Livingstone, Edinburgh, pp 1, 38–9, 62, 66, 160, 243, 288, 296–8, 300, 356, 453, 457, 465

Grieve G P 1989 Contraindications to manipulation and allied treatments. Physiotherapy 75: 445–453

Grieve G P 1990 Episacroiliac lipoma. Physiotherapy 76: 308–310

Grieve G P 1991 Mobilisation of the spine: a primary handbook of clinical method. 5th edn. Churchill Livingstone, Edinburgh

Grimer R J, Sneath R S 1990 Editorial: diagnosing malignant bone tumours. Journal of Bone and Joint Surgery 72B: 754–756

Hanraets P R M J 1959 The degenerative back. Elsevier, Amsterdam, pp 176, 183, 197

Jacobs J R, Walters R C, Toomey J M 1979 Head and neck manifestations of systemic lupus erythematosus. American Family Physician 20: 97–99

James C C M, Lassman L P 1972 Spinal dysraphism. Butterworth, London, p 84

Johnson E W, Fletcher F R 1981 Lumbosacral radiculopathy: review of 100 consecutive cases. Archives of Physical Medicine and Rehabilitation 62: 321–323

Jones D A 1987 Osteoid osteoma of the atlas. Journal of Bone and Joint Surgery 69B: 149

Kavanagh T G, Cannon S R, Pringle J, Stoker D J, Kemp H B S 1990 Parosteal osteosarcoma. Journal of Bone and Joint Surgery 72B: 959–965

Kellgren J H 1940 Somatic simulating visceral pain. Clinical Science 4: 303–309

Ker N B, Jones C B 1985 Tumours of the cauda equina: the problem of differential diagnosis. Journal of Bone and Joint Surgery 67B: 358–362

Kikta D G, Brever A C, Wilburn A J 1982 Thoracic root pain in diabetes: the spectrum of clinical and electromyographic findings. Annals of Neurology 11: 80–85

Kirwan E O'G, Hutton P, Pozo J, Ransford A 1984 The osteoid osteoma/osteoblastoma complex of the spine. Proceedings of the International Society for the study of the Lumbar Spine, Montreal (abstr)

Kornberg M 1986 Primary Ewing's sarcoma of the spine (T11). Spine 11: 54–57

Lange T A, Zoltan D, Hafez G R 1986 Simultaneous occurrence in the spine of osteoblastoma and haemangioendothelioma. Spine 11: 92–95

Lewit K 1985 Manipulative therapy in rehabilitation of the motor system. Butterworth, London

Leyshon A, Kirwan E O'G, Wynn-Parry L 1981 Electrical studies in the diagnosis of compression of the lumbar root. Journal of Bone and Joint Surgery 63B: 71–75

Lynch M C, Dorgan J C 1986 Osteoid osteoma of rib as a cause of scoliosis. Spine 11: 480–482

McLeod J (ed)1981 Davidson's principles and practice of medicine. 13th edn. Churchill Livingstone, Edinburgh, pp 213, 298, 627, 642

Macnab I, McCullough J A 1990 Backache. 2nd edn. Williams & Wilkins, Baltimore

Marks S H, Barnett M, Calin A 1983 Ankylosing spondylitis in men and women: a case-control study. Journal of Rheumatology 10: 624–633

Murray R O, Jacobson H G, Stoker D J 1989 The radiology of skeletal disease. 3rd edn. Churchill Livingstone, Edinburgh

O'Duffy J D, Hunder G G, Wahner H W 1980 A follow-up study of polymyalgia rheumatica: evidence of chronic axial synovitis. Journal of Rheumatology 7: 685–693

O'Ladire S A, Crockard H A, Thomas D G 1981 Prognosis for sphincter recovery after operation for cauda equina compression owing to lumbar disc prolapse. British Medical Journal 282: 1852–1854

Onimus M, Schraub S, Bartin D, Bosset J P, Guidet M 1986 Surgical treatment of vertebral metastases. Spine 11: 883–891

Perkins G 1961 Orthopaedics. Athlone Press, London, p 162

Phillips D G 1975 Upper limb involvement in cervical spondylosis. Journal of Neurology, Neurosurgery and Psychiatry 38: 386–390

Porter R W 1986 Management of back pain. Churchill Livingstone, Edinburgh, pp 7, 9

Prinzmetal M, Massumi R A 1955 The anterior chest wall syndrome — chest pain resembling pain of cardiac origin. Journal of the American Medical Association 169: 177–182

Richardson J 1960 The practice of medicine. Churchill, London, pp 233, 508

Ross J C, Jameson R M 1971 Vesical dysfunction due to prolapsed disc. British Medical Journal 3: 752–754

Schaberg J, Gainor B J 1985 A profile of metatastic carcinoma of the spine. Spine 10: 19–20

Schmorl G, Junghanns H 1951 Die Gerunde und Kranke Wirbelsäule in Röntgenbild und Klinik. 2nd edn. Georg Thieme, Stuttgart

Schulman L, Dorfman H D 1970 Nerve fibres in osteoid osteoma. Journal of Bone and Joint Surgery 52A: 1351–1356

Sim F H 1983 Metastatic bone disease and myeloma. In: Evarts C M (ed) Surgery of the musculoskeletal system. Churchill Livingstone, Edinburgh, vol 4 p11: 393

Sim F H, Dahlin D C, Stauffer R N, Lewis E R 1977 Primary bone tumours simulating lumbar spine disc syndrome. Spine 2: 65–74

Simeone F A, Lawner P M 1982 Intraspinal neoplasms. In: Rothman R H, Simeone F A (eds) The Spine. 2nd edn. W B Saunders, Philadelphia, p 1041

Sissons H A 1959 Tumours of the vertebral column. In: Nassim R, Burrows H J (eds) Modern trends in diseases of the vertebral column. Butterworths, London, ch 10

Sokoloff L, Bland J E 1975 The musculoskeletal system. Williams & Wilkins, Baltimore p 151

Stoddard A 1987 Short leg syndrome. British Association of Manipulative Medicine Newsletter April: 5

Stripp J 1979 Special techniques in orthopaedic radiography. Churchill Livingstone, Edinburgh

Turner R H, Bianco A J 1971 Spondylolysis and spondylolisthesis in children and teenagers. Journal of Bone and Joint Surgery 53A: 1298–1306

Weed L L 1968 Medical records that guide and teach I and II. New England Journal of Medicine 278: 593–657

Wheeler D C, Calvey H D, Wicks A C B 1985 A difficult pain in the neck. British Medical Journal 291: 804

Wyke B D 1987 The neurology of low back pain. In: Jayson M I V (ed) The lumbar spine and back pain. 3rd edn. Churchill Livingstone, Edinburgh, p 56

Yates D A H 1969 Cervical spine. British Medical Journal 2: 807–811

Index